PEDIATRIC SECRETS

PEDIATRIC SECRETS

SIXTH EDITION

RICHARD A. POLIN, MD
William T. Speck Professor of Pediatrics, College of Physicians and Surgeons, Columbia University; Director of Neonatology, New York-Presbyterian/Morgan Stanley Children's Hospital, New York, New York

MARK F. DITMAR, MD
Medical Officer, Health Resources and Services Administration, U.S. Department of Health and Human Services, Rockville, Maryland; Clinical Associate Professor of Pediatrics, Jefferson Medical College, Philadelphia, Pennsylvania

ELSEVIER

ELSEVIER

1600 John F. Kennedy Blvd.
Ste 1800
Philadelphia, PA 19103-2899

PEDIATRIC SECRETS, SIXTH EDITION

ISBN: 978-0-323-31030-7

Notices

Knowledge and best practice in this field are constantly changing. As new research and experience broaden our understanding, changes in research methods, professional practices, or medical treatment may become necessary.

Practitioners and researchers must always rely on their own experience and knowledge in evaluating and using any information, methods, compounds, or experiments described herein. In using such information or methods they should be mindful of their own safety and the safety of others, including parties for whom they have a professional responsibility.

With respect to any drug or pharmaceutical products identified, readers are advised to check the most current information provided (i) on procedures featured or (ii) by the manufacturer of each product to be administered, to verify the recommended dose or formula, the method and duration of administration, and contraindications. It is the responsibility of practitioners, relying on their own experience and knowledge of their patients, to make diagnoses, to determine dosages and the best treatment for each individual patient, and to take all appropriate safety precautions.

To the fullest extent of the law, neither the Publisher nor the authors, contributors, or editors, assume any liability for any injury and/or damage to persons or property as a matter of products liability, negligence or otherwise, or from any use or operation of any methods, products, instructions, or ideas contained in the material herein.

Library of Congress Cataloging-in-Publication Data

Pediatric secrets / [edited by] Richard A. Polin, MD, Professor of Pediatrics, Columbia University College of Physicians and Surgeons, Vice Chairman for Clinical and Academic Affairs, Director, Division of Neonatology, Morgan Stanley Children Hospital of New York, New York City, NY, Mark F. Ditmar, MD, Medical Officer, Health Resources and Services Administration, U.S. Department of Health and Human Services, Rockville, Maryland, Clinical Associate Professor of Pediatrics, Jefferson Medical College, Philadelphia, Pennsylvania. – Sixth edition.
    pages cm
Includes bibliographical references and index.
ISBN 978-0-323-31030-7 (pbk. : alk. paper) 1. Pediatrics–Examinations, questions, etc. 2. Pediatrics. I. Polin, Richard A. (Richard Alan), 1945- II. Ditmar, Mark F.
RJ48.2.P65 2016
618.9200076–dc23

    2015008063

Senior Content Strategist: James Merritt
Content Development Specialist: Lisa Barnes
Publishing Services Manager: Hemamalini Rajendrababu
Senior Project Manager: Beula Christopher
Design Direction: Ryan Cook

Printed in United States
Last digit is the print number: 9 8 7 6 5 4 3 2 1

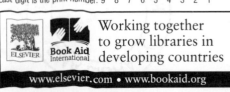

Working together
to grow libraries in
developing countries

www.elsevier.com • www.bookaid.org

PREFACE

It has been 26 years since the publication of the first edition of *Pediatric Secrets*. During this time, diagnostic and therapeutic advances along with social, economic, and political changes have very much reshaped the landscape of pediatric medicine.

While the content of this edition reflects many of those changes, the format remains the same. Someone once remarked that a question mark is shaped like a hook in an effort to pull a reader more deeply into a topic. While chapters do include questions about well-documented and more straightforward aspects of pediatric pathophysiology, differential diagnoses, and treatments, we have continued to include topics of clinical controversy and uncertainty so that the reader might feel compelled to explore these subjects in greater detail.

Sadly, we have lost two gifted authors since the publication of the first edition, Drs. Ed Charney and Steve Miller, as well as two mentors from the Children's Hospital of Philadelphia, Drs. David Cornfeld and Jean Cortner, who provided valuable suggestions in the early years of the book. All were revered as clinicians, colleagues, and friends. They remain very much missed.

We are grateful to the chapter authors of the sixth edition for their diligence and flexibility during busy clinical and research lives; to Lisa Barnes and the editorial staff of Elsevier for their assistance in guiding this edition through the shoals of deadlines and bibliomegaly; and to our families—children and grandchildren—and especially our wives, Helene Polin and Nina Ditmar, for their patience, support, and inspiration. Given our often convoluted schedules over the past 26+ years, we are grateful to them for always leaving the light on for us.

Richard A. Polin, MD

Mark F. Ditmar, MD

CONTRIBUTORS

Kwame Anyane-Yeboa, MD
Professor of Pediatrics
Department of Pediatrics
Columbia University Medical Center
New York, New York

Bradley A. Becker, MD
Professor
Department of Pediatrics
Saint Louis University School of Medicine
St. Louis, Missouri

Joan S. Bregstein, MD
Associate Professor of Pediatrics
Department of Pediatrics
Columbia University Medical Center;
Director of Community Outreach
Pediatric Emergency Medicine
New York-Presbyterian/Morgan Stanley Children's
    Hospital
New York, New York

Kathleen G. Brennan, MD
Neonatology Fellow
Department of Pediatrics
Columbia University College of Physicians and
    Surgeons;
Fellow
Division of Neonatology, Department of Pediatrics
New York-Presbyterian/Morgan Stanley Children's
    Hospital
New York, New York

Elizabeth Candell Chalom, MD
Clinical Associate Professor of Pediatrics
Department of Pediatrics
Rutgers University
Newark, New Jersey;
Director, Pediatric Rheumatology
Pediatrics
Saint Barnabas Health
Livingston, New Jersey

Marisa Censani, MD
Assistant Professor of Pediatrics
Department of Pediatrics
Division of Pediatric Endocrinology
Weill Cornell Medical College;
Assistant Attending Physician

Department of Pediatrics
New York Presbyterian Hospital/Weill Cornell Medical
    Center
New York, New York

Maire Conrad, MD, MS
Fellow
Department of Pediatric Gastroenterology
The Children's Hospital of Philadelphia
Philadelphia, Pennsylvania

Mark F. Ditmar, MD
Medical Officer
Health Resources and Services Administration
U.S. Department of Health and Human
    Services
Rockville, Maryland;
Clinical Associate Professor of Pediatrics
Jefferson Medical College
Philadelphia, Pennsylvania

Jennifer Duchon, MDCM, MPH
Clinical Fellow
Division of Pediatric Infectious Disease
Columbia -Presbyterian Medical Center
New York, New York

Andrew H. Eichenfield, MD
Assistant Professor of Pediatrics at Columbia
    University Medical Center
Division of Pediatric Allergy, Immunology, and
    Rheumatology
Columbia University Medical Center;
Attending Physician
Division of Allergy, Immunology, and
    Rheumatology
New York-Presbyterian/Morgan Stanley Children's
    Hospital
New York, New York

Marc D. Foca, MD
Associate Professor of Pediatrics at Columbia
    University Medical Center
Department of Pediatrics, Division of Infectious
    Diseases
Columbia University;
Associate Attending
Department of Pediatrics
New York-Presbyterian/Morgan Stanley Children's
    Hospital
New York, New York

Mary Patricia Gallagher, MD
Assistant Professor at Columbia University Medical Center
Department of Pediatrics
Division of Pediatric Endocrinology
Columbia University;
Co-Director, Pediatric Diabetes Program
Naoml Berrie Diabetes Center
Columbia University
New York, New York

Maria C. Garzon, MD
Professor of Dermatology and Pediatrics at CUMC
Columbia University;
Director, Pediatric Dermatology
New York-Presbyterian/Morgan Stanley Children's Hospital
New York, New York

Constance J. Hayes, MD
Pediatric Cardiologist
New York-Presbyterian/Morgan Stanley Children's Hospital
New York, New York

Noah J.F. Hoffman, MD
Fellow
Division of Gastroenterology, Hepatology, and Nutrition
The Children's Hospital of Philadelphia
Philadelphia, Pennsylvania

Allan J. Hordof, MD
Pediatric Cardiologist
Department of Pediatrics
Division of Pediatric Cardiology
New York-Presbyterian/Morgan Stanley Children's Hospital
New York, New York

Alejandro Iglesias, MD
Assistant Professor
Department of Pediatrics
Division of Medical Genetics
Columbia University Medical Center
New York, New York

Candi Jump, MD
Fellow
Department of Pediatric Gastroenterology, Hepatology and Nutrition
Children's Hospital of Philadelphia
Philadelphia, Pennsylvania

Bernard S. Kaplan, MB BCh
Nephrologist
Department of Pediatrics
The Children's Hospita of Philadelphia;
Professor
Department of Pediatrics

The Perelman School of Medicine at the University of Pennsylvania
Philadelphia, Pennsylvania

Christine T. Lauren, MD
Assistant Professor of Dermatology and Pediatrics and CUMC
Department of Dermatology
Columbia University Medical Center
New York, New York

Alice Lee, MD
Assistant Professor of Pediatrics
Department of Pediatrics
Columbia University
New York, New York

Tina A. Leone, MD
Assistant Professor of Pediatrics at CUMC
Department of Pediatrics
Columbia University College of Physicians and Surgeons
New York, New York

Chris A. Liacouras, MD
Professor of Pediatrics
Division of Gastroenterology, Hepatology and Nutrition
Perelman School of Medicine
Philadelphia, Pennsylvania

Elizabeth C. Maxwell, MD
Fellow
Department of Pediatric Gastroenterology Hepatology and Nutrition
Children's Hospital of Philadelphia
Philadelphia, Pennsylvania

Tiffani L. McDonough, MD
Assistant Professor
Division of Child Neurology
Department of Neurology
Columbia University Medical Center
New York-Presbyterian/Morgan Stanley Children's Hospital
New York, New York

Steven E. McKenzie, MD, PhD
Professor
Department of Medicine and Pediatrics
Thomas Jefferson University
Thomas Jefferson University Hospitals;
Attending Physician
Department of Hematology
Philadelphia, Pennsylvania

Kevin E.C. Meyers, MB BCh
Professor of Pediatrics
Department of Nephrology/Pediatrics
The Children's Hospital of Philadelphia
University of Pennsylvania,
Philadelphia, Pennsylvania

Kimberly D. Morel, MD
Associate Professor of Dermatology and Pediatrics
   at CUMC
Department of Dermatology
Columbia University
New York, New York

Amanda Muir, MD
Instructor of Pediatrics
Department of Gastroenterology, Hepatology, and
   Nutrition
The Children's Hospital of Philadelphia
Philadelphia, Pennsylvania

Sharon E. Oberfield, MD
Professor of Pediatrics and Director of Pediatric
   Endocrinology
Department of Pediatrics
Columbia University Medical Center
New York, New York

Kerice Pinkney, MBBS
Chief Fellow
Division of Pediatric Hematology/Oncology/Stem Cell
   Transplant
Columbia University
New York, New York

Julia Potter, MD
Adolescent Medicine Fellow
Department of Child and Adolescent Health
Columbia University Medical Center
New York, New York

James J. Riviello, Jr., MD
Sergievsky Family Professor of Neurology and
   Pediatrics
Chief, Division of Child Neurology
Department of Neurology
Columbia University Medical Center;
Chief of Child Neurology
New York-Presbyterian/Morgan Stanley Children's
   Hospital
New York, New York

Dina L. Romo, MD
Columbia University
Department of Adolescent Medicine
New York, New York

Carlos D. Rosé, MD, CIP
Professor of Pediatrics
Department of Pediatrics
Thomas Jefferson University
Philadelphia, Pennsylvania;
Chief of Rheumatology
Department of Pediatrics
duPont Children's Hospital
Wilmington, Delaware

Cindy Ganis Roskind, MD
Assistant Professor
Department of Pediatrics
Columbia University Medical Center
New York, New York

Benjamin D. Roye, MD, MPH
Assistant Professor
Department of Orthopedic Surgery
Columbia University
New York, New York

Lisa Saiman, MD, MPH
Professor of Clinical Pediatrics
Department of Pediatrics
Columbia University
New York, New York

F. Meridith Sonnett, MD
Associate Professor of Pediatrics
Department of Pediatrics
Columbia College of Physicians and
   Surgeons/Columbia University Medical
   Center;
Chief, Division of Pediatric Emergency
   Medicine
Department of Pediatrics
New York-Presbyterian/Morgan Stanley Children's
   Hospital
New York, New York

Karen Soren, MD
Associate Professor
Department of Pediatrics
Columbia University Medical Center;
Director, Adolescent Medicine
New York-Presbyterian/Morgan Stanley Children's
   Hospital
New York, New York

Thomas J. Starc, MD, MPH
Professor
Department of Pediatrics
Columbia University
New York, New York

Randi Teplow-Phipps, MD
Clinical Fellow in Adolescent Medicine
Department of Pediatrics
Columbia University Medical Center
New York, New York

Orith Waisbourd-Zinman, MD
Fellow Physician
Division of Gastroenterology, Hepatology and
   Nutrition
Children's Hospital of Philadelphia
Philadelphia, Pennsylvania

Jennifer L. Webb, MD
Assistant Professor
Department of Pediatrics
George Washington School of Medicine;
Pediatric Hematologist
Department of Pediatrics
Children's National Medical Center
Washington, DC

Danielle Wendel, MD
Pediatric Gastroenterology Fellow
Department of Gastroenterology, Hepatology, and
    Nutrition
Children's Hospital of Philadelphia
Philadelphia, Pennsylvania

Robert W. Wilmott, MD
IMMUNO Professor and Chair
Department of Pediatrics
Saint Louis University;
Pediatrician-in-Chief
SSM Cardinal Glennon Children's Medical Center
St. Louis, Missouri

CONTENTS

TOP 100 SECRETS

These secrets are 100 of the top board alerts. They summarize the concepts, principles, and most salient details of clinical practice.

1. Acne vulgaris that begins before age 7 years warrants further investigation for endocrine abnormalities such as androgen excess or precocious puberty.

2. After iron supplementation for iron deficiency anemia, the reticulocyte count should double in 1 to 2 weeks, and hemoglobin should increase by 1 g/dL in 2 to 4 weeks. The most common reason for persistence of iron deficiency anemia is poor compliance with supplementation.

3. It is rare for an infant to develop congestive heart failure (CHF) from supraventricular tachycardia (SVT) in <24 hours. When SVT is present for 24 to 36 hours, about 20% develop CHF. At 48 hours, the number increases to 50%.

4. After age 7 years, nocturnal enuresis (which affects 10% of children at that age) resolves spontaneously at a rate of approximately 15% per year, so that by age 15 years about 1% to 2% of teenagers are still affected.

5. The "atopic march" is the phenomenon in which about half of infants with atopic dermatitis eventually develop asthma, and two-thirds develop allergic rhinitis.

6. While leukemias constitute the most common group of pediatric cancer diagnoses overall, neuroblastomas are the most commonly occurring cancer in children <1 year of age.

7. Coughing and choking (witnessed or by history) occur in 80% to 90% of children with suspected foreign body aspiration, which highlights the importance of questioning about choking in a child who is evaluated for cough.

8. Idiopathic scoliosis (with a Cobb angle of 10 degrees or more) occurs in about 3% of children, but only 0.3% to 0.5% will have progression of curves that require treatment.

9. IgA nephropathy is the most common type of primary glomerular disease worldwide. Compared with adults, pediatric patients are more likely to have minimal histologic lesions and less likely to have advanced chronic lesions.

10. The most common worldwide cause of chronic gastrointestinal (GI) blood loss is hookworm infection, which is often associated with iron deficiency anemia.

11. Neonates with midline lumbosacral lesions (e.g., sacral pits, hypertrichosis, lipomas) above the gluteal crease should have screening imaging of the spine performed to search for occult spinal dysraphism.

12. A falling serum sodium concentration during diabetic ketoacidosis (DKA) treatment is worrisome because it indicates either inappropriate fluid management or the onset of syndrome of inappropriate antidiuretic hormone (SIADH) and can herald impending cerebral edema.

13. The most identifiable cause of microscopic hematuria is hypercalciuria, defined as elevated urinary calcium excretion without concomitant hypercalcemia.

14. The median time for the rash of Lyme disease to appear after a tick bite is 7 to 10 days, but the range can be 1 to 36 days.

15. 2011 AAP guidelines no longer recommend routine voiding cystourethrogram (VCUG) for a first urinary tract infection (UTI) unless an ultrasound reveals hydronephrosis, scarring,

or other findings that would suggest either high-grade vesicoureteral reflux or obstructive uropathy.

16. Always consider ovarian torsion in the differential diagnosis of abdominal pain in girls, particularly during the ages of 9 to 14 years, when ovarian cysts as potential lead points are more common because of the maturing reproductive hormonal axis.

17. Left shoulder pain after abdominal trauma is a worrisome sign that could represent blood accumulating under the diaphragm, which results in pain referred to the left shoulder (Kehr sign) due to splenic injury.

18. Because irreversible histologic changes can develop in 4 to 8 hours after the onset of testicular torsion, timely diagnosis is critical. Testicular salvage rates are <10% if symptom duration is ≥24 hours.

19. Carbon monoxide poisoning is often misdiagnosed because the presenting symptoms can be flu-like.

20. Most umbilical hernias <0.5 cm spontaneously close before a patient is 2 years old. A hernia >2 cm may still close spontaneously, but it may take up to 6 years.

21. Although precocious puberty occurs much more frequently in girls (80% of cases are girls), boys are more likely to have identifiable pathology.

22. Consider the use of prostaglandin E_1 to maintain the patency of the ductus arteriosus in a newborn <1 month who presents in shock with evidence of CHF and cyanosis because of the possibility of a ductal-dependent cardiac lesion, such as hypoplastic left heart syndrome.

23. A hemoglobin A_1C level ≥6.5% on two occasions is sufficient for the diagnosis of diabetes. Levels between 5.7% and 6.4% place a person at increased risk for diabetes.

24. Isolated primary nocturnal enuresis rarely has identifiable organic pathology.

25. Only 20% of patients with intussusception present with the classic triad of colicky pain, vomiting, and passage of bloody stool.

26. In patients with suspected rheumatic disease, clinical features that are concerning for malignancy include nonarticular bone pain, back pain as the primary presenting symptom, bone tenderness, and severe constitutional symptoms.

27. Three or more minor malformations should raise concern about the presence of a major malformation.

28. Patients with atypical Kawasaki disease are usually younger (<1 year old) and most commonly lack cervical adenopathy and extremity changes.

29. Older children with unexplained unilateral deformities of an extremity (e.g., pes cavus) should have screening magnetic resonance imaging to evaluate for intraspinal disease.

30. In patients with sickle cell disease, use of transcranial Doppler ultrasound to measure intracranial blood flow and regular transfusions to reduce the hemoglobin S content for those with abnormal values can significantly lower the likelihood of stroke.

31. Methanol, present in antifreeze and windshield washer fluid, is considered the most lethal alcohol and can cause severe, refractory metabolic acidosis and permanent retinal damage leading to blindness.

32. Hyperbilirubinemia generally is not an indication for the cessation of breastfeeding but rather for increasing its frequency.

33. Fractures that have been shown to have a high specificity for child abuse are rib fractures (particularly posteromedial) in infants, classic metaphyseal lesions of long bones, and fractures of the scapula, spinous process, and sternum.

34. About 6% of children are streptococcal carriers and will have positive throat cultures between episodes of pharyngitis.

35. The two most consistent prognostic factors for outcome for childhood acute lymphoblastic leukemia (ALL) are age at presentation (<1 year or >10 years have a worse prognosis) and extent of elevation of initial white blood cell (WBC) count ($\geq$50,000/mm^3 have a worse prognosis).

36. Infants with unexplained failure to thrive, weakness, hypotonia, and metabolic acidosis (particularly lactic acidosis) should be evaluated for a possible mitochondrial disorder.

37. Polycystic ovarian syndrome, which affects up to 10% of reproductive age women, should be suspected in overweight or obese teenagers with amenorrhea/oligomenorrhea and signs of hyperandrogenism (hirsutism, acne).

38. Women with primary genital herpes simplex virus (HSV) infections who are shedding HSV at delivery are 10 to 30 times more likely to transmit the virus than women with recurrent infection.

39. The two essential features of autism are (1) impaired social interaction and social communication and (2) restricted and repetitive patterns of behavior.

40. The daily spiking fevers of systemic juvenile idiopathic arthritis can precede the development of arthritis by weeks to months.

41. Syncope is more likely to be of a cardiac nature if there is sudden onset without prior dizziness or awareness, occurrence during exercise, history of palpitations before fainting, syncope results in an injury from a fall, and/or a positive family history of sudden death.

42. About 10% to 20% of patients with Rocky Mountain spotted fever do not develop a rash, so a high index of suspicion is needed for any patient in an endemic area who presents with fever, myalgia, severe headaches, and vomiting.

43. An overweight 5-year-old is $4\times$ as likely to be an overweight teenager, which highlights the importance of addressing obesity at an early age.

44. The earliest evidence of nephropathy in patients with type 1 diabetes mellitus is microalbuminuria, which is the presence of small quantities of albumin in the urine, preferably measured in a first morning sample.

45. The best measure of cognitive function in a younger child is receptive language, which should be assessed in a fashion that is free of motor requirements.

46. In a toddler with suspected idiopathic thrombocytopenic purpura (ITP), the presence of splenomegaly warrants more aggressive evaluation for an associated problem (e.g., collagen-vascular disease, hypersplenism, leukemia, glycogen storage disease).

47. The most common cause of overdose deaths in children and adolescents in the United States is acetaminophen, owing to its widespread availability and frequency of use in accidental and suicidal intoxications.

48. The most reliable physical exam finding for a developmentally dysplastic hip in an older infant is limited hip abduction, which occurs as a result of shortening of the adductor muscles.

49. The most common cause of persistent seizures is an inadequate serum antiepileptic level.

50. Midline neck masses usually involve the thyroid gland or thyroid remnants, such as a thyroglossal duct cyst.

51. Most amblyopia is unilateral; vision testing solely with both eyes open is inadequate.

52. Emergency contraception should be discussed with all sexually active adolescents; 90% of teenage pregnancies are unintended.

53. An infant with vomiting, lethargy, hypoglycemia and no ketones on urinalysis should be evaluated for a fatty-acid oxidation defect.

54. Without a booster after age 5 years, pertussis protection against infection is about 80% during the first 3 years after immunization, dropping to 50% after 4 to 7 years, and to near 0% after 11 years.

55. Asthma rarely causes clubbing in children. Consider other diseases, particularly cystic fibrosis.

56. Only 5% of obese adolescents have an identifiable pathologic cause, such as an endocrine problem (e.g., hypothyroidism) or an uncommon syndrome (e.g., Prader-Willi) for their obesity.

57. Bilingual children develop speech milestones normally; two-language households should not be presumed as a cause of speech delay.

58. Sulfonamides and antiepileptic medications (especially phenobarbital, carbamazepine and lamotrigine) are the medications most commonly associated with Stevens-Johnson syndrome and toxic epidermal necrolysis.

59. The most common specific etiology diagnosed in pediatric patients with a systemic febrile illness after international travel is malaria. More than half of the world's population lives in areas where malaria is endemic.

60. The most common condition presenting as a food impaction in an adolescent is eosinophilic esophagitis.

61. The optimal time for surgical repair of an undescended testicle is 12 months of age or shortly thereafter as spontaneous descent after 9 months is unlikely and ultrastructural changes in the seminiferous tubules can occur in the second year of life unless orchidopexy is performed.

62. The classic picture of appendicitis is anorexia followed by pain, then by nausea and vomiting, with subsequent localization of findings to the right lower quadrant. However, there is a large degree of variability, particularly in younger patients.

63. An infant with nonsyndromic sensorineural hearing loss should be tested for mutations in the connexin 26 gene. Mutations in that gene contribute to at least 50% of autosomal recessive hearing loss and about 10% to 20% of all prelingual hearing loss.

64. The Gorlin sign is the ability to touch the tip of the nose with the tongue, which can be seen in conditions associated with hypermobility syndromes, such as Ehlers-Danlos syndrome.

65. A pelvic examination is not required before prescribing oral contraceptives for teenagers without risk factors. Appropriate screening for sexually transmitted infections and possible cervical dysplasia can be scheduled, but delaying oral contraception unnecessarily increases the risk for pregnancy.

66. A skin scale that bleeds easily on removal (Auspitz sign) is characteristic of psoriasis and is related to the rupture of capillaries high in the papillary dermis.

67. The most frequent cause of chronically elevated aminotransferases among children and adolescents in the United States is nonalcoholic fatty liver disease (NAFLD), which is commonly seen in obese patients with the metabolic syndrome.

68. Seizures with fever in patients >6 years should not be considered febrile seizures.

69. A pop or snap sensation in the setting of acute knee injury is usually associated with an anterior cruciate ligament injury, a meniscal injury, and/or patellar subluxation.

70. Hypercapnia (elevated P_{CO_2}) in a patient with an acute asthma attack is a serious sign that the child may be tiring or becoming severely obstructed.

71. Signs and symptoms of acute poststreptococcal glomerulonephritis (e.g., gross hematuria, hypertension, oliguria) begin about 7 to 14 days after pharyngitis and as long as 6 weeks after a pyoderma.

72. Premature babies should be immunized in accordance with postnatal chronologic age.

73. During the first year of life, hypotonia is more common than hypertonia in patients who are ultimately diagnosed with cerebral palsy.

74. A male child with a liver abscess should be considered to have chronic granulomatous disease until proven otherwise.

75. Items in the preparticipation sports physical exam that identify a patient at risk for sudden death include Marfanoid features, pathologic murmurs, weak or delayed femoral pulses, and evidence of an arrhythmia (rapid or irregular heartbeat).

76. Up to 10% of normal, healthy children may have low-level (1:10) positive antinuclear antibody testing that will remain positive. Without clinical or laboratory features of disease, it is of no significance.

77. The most common cause of chronic pelvic pain in adolescents without a history of pelvic inflammatory disease is endometriosis.

78. Headaches that awaken children from sleep, are associated with vomiting without nausea, are made worse by straining or coughing, and have intensity changes with changes in body position are concerning for pathology that is causing increased intracranial pressure.

79. Pulse oximetry screening for complex congenital heart disease in asymptomatic infants in the nursery is abnormal if oxygen levels are <90% in either limb or if oxygen saturation is ≥90% and <95% in both limbs or >3% difference between limbs on initial and repeat testing.

80. Significant proteinuria, in addition to hematuria, is much more likely to be caused by an underlying renal pathology compared with hematuria alone.

81. In the evaluation of children with constipation, the most important physical exam component is the rectal exam because large amounts of stool in the rectal vault almost always indicate functional constipation.

82. In children with simple obesity (e.g., familial), linear growth is typically enhanced; in children with endocrinopathies (e.g., Cushing syndrome, hypothyroidism), linear growth is usually impaired.

83. Telogen effluvium, the most common cause of diffuse hair loss in children, develops 2 to 5 months after a stressful event (e.g., surgery, birth, large weight loss) and resolves gradually without therapy.

84. The most important variable that influences mortality in necrotizing fasciitis is the time to surgical debridement.

85. Crawling is one of the least valuable markers of development because there is enormous variability in the timing of crawling and a significant percentage of normal infants never crawl before walking.

86. Newborns diagnosed with chlamydial conjunctivitis should not be treated with topical therapy alone because this will not eradicate the organism from the upper respiratory tract and may fail to prevent the development of chlamydial pneumonia. Oral macrolide therapy is required.

87. Psychogenic cough should be considered in a child with persistent dry, honking, explosive daytime cough that disappears with sleep or during the weekend.

88. Up to 20% of adolescents with menorrhagia may have a bleeding disorder, most commonly von Willebrand disease.

89. Intelligibility increases by about 25% per year from 25% at age 1 year to 100% at age 4 years. Significantly delayed intelligibility should prompt hearing and language evaluation.

90. Infants infected in the perinatal period with hepatitis B have a >90% chance of developing chronic hepatitis B infection, and of these, 25% go on to develop hepatocellular carcinoma.

91. Following an episode of acute otitis media, about 70% of patients will continue to have a middle ear effusion at 2 weeks, 40% at 1 month, 20% at 2 months and 10% at 3 months.

92. Acute kidney injury (AKI) has replaced the term acute renal failure (ARF) to reflect the more appropriate concept that smaller reductions in kidney function (short of complete organ failure) have significant clinical repercussions in terms of morbidity and mortality.

93. Since the introduction of pneumococcal conjugate vaccines, bacteremia rates for *Streptococcus pneumoniae* have fallen dramatically to <1% in febrile, nontoxic-appearing children from ages 3 to 36 months.

94. Most pediatric deaths in the United States associated with influenza tend to result from either (1) an exacerbation of an underlying medical condition or an invasive procedure, or (2) coinfection from another pathogen, most commonly *Staphylococcus aureus*.

95. The most common genetic lethal disease, defined as a disease that interferes with a person's ability to reproduce as a result of early death or impaired sexual function, is cystic fibrosis.

96. Measles, after an incubation period of 4 to 12 days, typically presents with cough, coryza, and conjunctivitis followed by the characteristic morbilliform rash with macular and papular features.

97. Cytomegalovirus is the most common congenital infection, up to 1.3% in some studies, but 80% to 90% of infected neonates are asymptomatic at birth or in early infancy.

98. A ciliary flush, which is circumcorneal hyperemia in which conjunctival redness is concentrated in the area adjacent to the cornea (limbus), is worrisome as a possible sign of significant ocular pathology (e.g., keratitis, anterior uveitis, acute angle-closure glaucoma). Urgent referral to an ophthalmologist is required.

99. Recommendations to decrease the risk of sudden infant death syndrome (SIDS) include placing infants in a nonprone position for sleep; use of a firm sleep surface; breastfeeding; room-sharing without bed-sharing; routine immunizations; consideration of a pacifier; and avoidance of soft bedding, overheating and exposure to tobacco smoke, alcohol and illicit drugs.

100. Occasional strabismus is common in young infants because the macula and fovea are poorly developed at birth, but intervention should be considered for symptoms that persist beyond 2 to 3 months of age.

ADOLESCENT MEDICINE

Karen Soren, MD, Randi Teplow-Phipps, MD, Julia Potter, MD and Dina L. Romo, MD

CHAPTER 1

CLINICAL ISSUES

1. What are the three leading causes of mortality in adolescents?

1. **Unintentional injury** is the leading cause of death with the majority of injuries caused by car crashes. The fatal crash rate per mile driven for 16- to 17-year-olds is about 3 times greater than the rate for drivers 20 and older.
2. **Violence**, specifically homicide, is the *second* leading cause of death among 15- to 24-year-olds and the leading cause for black males in this age range. In 2013, about 28% of males compared with 8% of females reported having carried a weapon (gun, knife, or club) on at least 1 day in the previous month.
3. **Suicide** is the third leading cause of death in adolescents aged 10 to 19 years.

Highway Loss Data Institute, 2014: www.iihs.org. Accessed Oct. 29, 2014.
Heron M: Deaths: leading causes for 2010. National vital statistics reports: from the Centers for Disease Control and Prevention, National Center for Health Statistics, *Natl Vital Stat System*, 62:1–97, 2013.
Kann L, Kinchen S, Shanklin SL, et al: Youth risk behavior surveillance—United States, 2013, *MMWR*, 63:4,2014.

2. How common is dating violence among adolescents?

Dating violence, also referred to as intimate partner violence (IPV), can be defined as being hit, slapped, or intentionally physically hurt by a boyfriend or girlfriend. Almost 10% of high school students have reported IPV and 7% report having ever been forced to have sexual intercourse.

Kann L, Kinchen S, Shanklin SL, et al: Youth risk behavior surveillance—United States, 2013, *MMWR* 63:4,2014.

3. Which sports cause the greatest number of concussions in teenagers?

Among individuals 15 to 24 years of age, sports are second only to motor vehicle crashes as the leading cause of concussions. In 2012, the majority of concussions resulted from participation in *football*, followed by girls' *soccer*. The most common mechanism of injury was player-player contact. In gender-comparable sports, girls had a higher concussion rate (OR = 1.7) than boys.

Marar M, McIlvain NM, Fields SK, et al:. Epidemiology of concussions among United States high school athletes in 20 sports, *Am J Sports Med* 40:747–755, 2012.

4. Which diagnoses require mandatory disclosure regardless of confidentiality?

Most states require:

- Notification of child welfare authorities under state **child-abuse** (physical and sexual) reporting laws
- Notification of law enforcement officials of **gunshot** and **stab wounds**
- Warning from a psychotherapist to a reasonably identifiable victim of a patient's **threat of violence**
- Notification to parents or other authorities if a patient represents a reasonable threat to himself or herself (i.e., **suicidal ideation**)

5. How does the "HEADS" mnemonic assist in adolescent interviewing?

This mnemonic allows for a systematic approach to the evaluation of multiple health issues and risk factors that affect teenagers:

H–Home (living arrangement, family relationships, support)
E–Education (school issues, study habits, achievement, expectations)
A–Activities (recreation, friends, exercise, employment)

D–Drugs (alcohol, tobacco, marijuana, cocaine, pills, etc.)
    Depression
S–Sexuality (sexual activity, sexual orientation)
    Self-esteem (body image)
    Safety (abuse, intimate partner violence, risk of self-harm)
    Suicidality

6. **When does sexual orientation usually emerge?**
   Sexual orientation emerges before or in early adolescence. Sexual minority youth are often referred to as *LGBTQ* or Lesbian, Gay, Bisexual, Transgender, and Questioning youth. Sexual experimentation is common in adolescence and may not predict future sexual orientation.

7. **What characterizes gender identity, gender expression, and gender dysphoria?**
   - *Gender identity* is how one identifies one's own gender.
   - *Gender expression* is the outward display of gender characteristics. This usually conforms to anatomic sex for both heterosexual and homosexual teenagers.
   - *Gender dysphoria* refers to the emotional stress of having a gender identity that is different from natal or anatomic sex.

Levine DA: Office-based care for lesbian, gay, bisexual, transgender, and questioning youth, *Pediatrics* 132: e297–313, 2013.

8. **What health disparities are particular to LGBTQ youth?**
   LGBTQ youth have higher rates of being bullied, stigmatization, and/or parental rejection. This may result in issues with self-esteem, depression, and suicidality. LGBTQ youth have also been found to have higher rates of drug and alcohol use, STIs (particularly human immunodeficiency virus [HIV]), and homelessness. Protective factors include family connectedness, caring adults, and school safety.

9. **How may social media impact adolescent behavior?**
   Social media (e.g., Facebook, Instagram, Snapchat, YouTube) can strongly influence adolescents' attitudes and behavior. It has become an integral part of many adolescents' lives. Many teens use the Internet daily to communicate with friends and maintain and form new social relationships. Teens often post on social media venues pictures of risky behaviors that reflect their actual behavior. They may display postings of risky sexual behaviors, substance use, or violence. Their peers may perceive these public displays as acceptable, and this false perception may entice others to engage in such high-risk behaviors as well.

Moreno MA, Parks MR, Zimmerman FJ, et al: Display of health risk behaviors on MySpace by adolescents: prevalence and associations, *Arch Pediatr Adolesc Med* 163:27–34, 2009.

10. **What is cyberbullying?**
    Cyberbullying is using the Internet, cell phones, or social media venues to communicate false, embarrassing, or hostile information about someone else. This can range from insults to peer exclusion to sexual harassment. Cyber victims can develop emotional, behavioral, and school-related problems.

Suzuki K, Asaga R, Sourander A, et al: Cyberbullying and adolescent mental health. *Int J Adolesc Med Health* 24:27–35, 2012.

11. **Which teenagers <18 years can give consent for their medical care?**
    Those who are <18 years old must be considered "emancipated" or "mature" minors in order to give consent. However, the definition varies from state to state. Emancipated minors include those who are married, are parents themselves, are members of the armed forces, are living apart from their parents, and/or those who have evidence of independence (financial or otherwise).

Berlan ED, Bravender T: Confidentiality, consent and caring for the adolescent patient, *Curr Opin Pediatr* 21:450–456, 2009.
Bruce CR, Berg SL, McGuire AL: Please don't call my mom: pediatric consent and confidentiality, *Clin Pediatr* 48:243–246, 2009.

EATING DISORDERS

12. How is the diagnosis of anorexia nervosa made?

Anorexia nervosa consists of a spectrum of psychological, behavioral, and medical abnormalities. The 2013 *Diagnostic and Statistical Manual of Mental Disorders*, 5th Edition (DSM-5) lists three components needed for the diagnosis:

1. *Restriction of energy intake relative to requirements, leading to a significantly low body weight*—a weight that is less than minimally expected. (This replaces the older criterion of refusal to maintain a weight that is >85% of expected weight for height.)
2. Intense *fear of gaining weight* or of becoming fat *or persistent behavior that interferes with weight gain,* even though the affected individual is at a significantly low weight. Often, adolescents insist that they are trying to gain weight but are unable to do so.
3. *Disturbances of perception* of body shape and size, undue influence of body weight or shape on self-evaluation, *or persistent lack of recognition of the seriousness of the current low body weight.*
   The presence of amenorrhea is no longer necessary for the diagnosis of anorexia nervosa in postmenarchal girls.

American Psychiatric Association: *Diagnostic and Statistical Manual of Mental Disorders, ed 5.* Washington, DC, 2013, American Psychiatric Association.

13. What are signs of anorexia nervosa on physical examination?
    - Sinus bradycardia (or other dysrhythmias)
    - Hypothermia
    - Orthostatic changes in blood pressure and heart rate
    - Dull, thinning hair
    - Dry skin, lanugo (downy hair on body)
    - Cachexia (especially facial wasting)
    - Acrocyanosis (cold, bluish hands and feet)
    - Extremity edema
    - Heart murmur (mitral valve prolapse)
    - Growth retardation
    - Pubertal delay or arrest

14. What are the differential diagnoses that one must consider when evaluating a patient with anorexia nervosa?

    One should consider gastrointestinal disorders (inflammatory bowel, celiac, or peptic ulcer disease), occult malignancies, endocrine disorders (hyperthyroidism, diabetes), and infection (tuberculosis, HIV). Depression, anxiety, obsessive–compulsive disorder, and substance abuse can also present with weight loss. Superior mesenteric artery (SMA) syndrome is a consequence of severe weight loss but can present like anorexia.

15. What are good and bad prognosticators for recovery from anorexia?

    Good: Early age at onset (<14 years), supportive family, shorter duration of illness
    Bad: Late age at onset, purging behavior, more significant weight loss, family dysfunction, comorbid mental illness, longer duration of illness

16. Why are adolescent girls with anorexia nervosa at risk for low bone mineral density?

    Decreased FSH and LH levels result in anovulation and subsequent low levels of serum estrogen. Because estrogen is necessary to incorporate calcium into bone, osteopenia may be a consequence.

17. What are the clinical differences between males and females with anorexia nervosa?

    It is estimated that less than 5% of anorexia nervosa involves boys. Males are more likely to:
    - Have been obese before the onset of symptoms
    - Be ambivalent regarding the desire to gain or lose weight

- Have more issues about gender and sexual identity
- Involve dieting with sports participation
- Engage in "defensive dieting" (avoiding weight gain after an athletic injury)

Domine F, Berchtold A, Akre C, et al: Disordered eating behaviors: what about boys? *J Adolesc Health* 44:111–117, 2009.

18. **What electrolyte disturbances occur in patients with severe anorexia nervosa and what are the potential clinical effects?**
   Hypocalcemia: Muscle spasm and tetany, stridor, seizures
   Hyponatremia: Seizures, coma, death
   Hypokalemia: Dysrhythmias, poor gut motility, skeletal muscle myopathy, nephropathy
   Hypomagnesemia: Muscle cramps, weakness, irritability, psychosis, seizures, dysrhythmias
   Hypophosphatemia: Muscle weakness, paresthesia, central nervous system (CNS) disturbances (e.g., irritability, delirium, seizures)

Norrington A, Stanley R, Tremlett M, Birrell G: Medical management of acute severe anorexia nervosa, *Arch Dis Child Educ Pract Ed* 97:48–54, 2012.

19. **What causes sudden death in patients with anorexia nervosa?**
   The main cause of sudden death is related to *cardiac* complications. Chronic malnutrition, prolonged hypokalemia, low serum albumin, and prolonged QT intervals on electrocardiogram are related to sudden cardiovascular death in eating disorder patients. Cardiovascular complications include bradycardia, orthostatic hypotension, dysrhythmias (often related to prolonged QT interval), and decreased left ventricular mass and myocardial contractility.

Jauergui-Garrido B, Jauregui-Lobera I: Sudden death in eating disorders, *Vasc Health Risk Manag* 8: 91–98, 2012.

20. **What are indications for hospital admission for a patient with anorexia nervosa?**
   - Refusal to eat with ongoing weight loss despite intensive management
   - Dehydration and orthostatic changes in pulse (>20 beats per minute) or blood pressure (>10 mm Hg)
   - Electrolyte abnormalities (e.g., hypokalemia, hyponatremia, hypophosphatemia)
   - Heart rate less than 50 beats per minute during the day, less than 45 beats per minute overnight
   - Systolic blood pressure < 80 mm Hg
   - Temperature < 96° F
   - Cardiac dysrhythmia
   - Acute medical complication of malnutrition (syncope, seizure, congestive heart failure, pancreatitis)
   - Severe coexisting psychiatric disease (e.g., suicidality, psychosis)

Rosen DS: American Academy of Pediatrics Committee on Adolescence: Identification and management of eating disorders in children and adolescents, *Pediatrics* 126:1240–1253, 2010.

21. **What are the medical complications of bulimia nervosa?**
   Electrolyte abnormalities: Hypokalemia, hypochloremia, and metabolic alkalosis may occur. The hypokalemia can cause a prolonged QT interval and T-wave abnormalities.
   Esophageal: Acid reflux with esophagitis and (rarely) Mallory-Weiss tear may be found.
   Central nervous system: Neurotransmitters can be affected, thereby causing changes in the patient's perceptions of satiety.

Miscellaneous: Enamel erosion, salivary gland enlargement, cheilosis, and knuckle calluses are signs of recurrent vomiting.

Mehler PS: Bulimia nervosa, *N Engl J Med* 349:875–881, 2003.

22. An 11-year-old with weight loss due to avoidance of food because of its sensory characteristics has what condition?

    Avoidant/Restrictive Food Intake Disorder (ARFID). This is a new DSM-5 diagnostic category of eating disorder not explained by a concurrent medical condition or a mental disorder. The condition is distinct from anorexia nervosa or bulimia nervosa. Children and younger teens in this category may avoid foods because of problems with digestion, they may have an aversion to colors or textures, or they may eat in very small portions because of previous frightening episodes of choking or vomiting. The food restriction leads to weight loss, nutritional deficiencies, or interference with psychosocial functioning.

23. What is the primary biochemical feature of the refeeding syndrome?

    Hypophosphatemia. The *refeeding syndrome* is a potentially fatal process that results from fluid shifts and electrolyte abnormalities, which occurs when someone who has been chronically malnourished is refed, either orally or parenterally. In starvation, total body phosphorus is depleted although the serum phosphorus level usually remains normal because of adjustments in renal excretion. When carbohydrates are added through feeding, insulin is secreted, which stimulates anabolic protein synthesis and enhances the intracellular uptake of glucose, phosphate, and water. This can lead to significant extracellular hypophosphatemia. Because phosphate is needed for metabolic processes, potentially fatal cardiac, respiratory, and neurologic complications can ensue.

Mehanna HM, Moledina J, Travis J: Refeeding syndrome: what it is, and how to prevent and treat it, *BMJ* 336:1495–1498, 2008.

24. Name the three features that constitute the "female athlete triad."

    Low energy availability (with or without disordered eating), menstrual dysfunction, and low bone mineral density. This triad can present in active girls and young women, particularly in those who engage in sports that emphasize leanness such as gymnastics, ballet, or diving. Diagnosis is based on history, physical examination, and laboratory evaluation. The basic laboratory workup should include a urine pregnancy test, thyroid-stimulating hormone, prolactin, FSH, LH, and estradiol. Evaluation for bone mineral density and vitamin D levels may be helpful. Ongoing counseling regarding eating behaviors and need for adequate weight gain is important. The use of oral contraceptives may give patients a false sense of security by inducing menses, but it has not been shown to increase bone mineral density.

DeSouza MJ, Nattiv A, Joy E: 2014 Female athlete triad coalition consensus statement on treatment and return to play of the female athlete triad, *Br J Sports Med* 48:289, 2014.

KEY POINTS: EATING DISORDERS

1. Eating disorders can affect both females and males and young people of all ethnicities and from all socioeconomic backgrounds.
2. Eating disorders put young people at risk for serious electrolyte disturbances, as well as for other physiological, metabolic, and hormonal disturbances.
3. Anorexia nervosa has the highest mortality of any psychiatric disorder.
4. When treating a patient with anorexia nervosa on an inpatient unit, be on the lookout for fluid overload, and monitor electrolytes in order to avoid refeeding syndrome.
5. Treatment for a patient with an eating disorder is best done using a collaborative approach and involving a mental health professional and a nutritionist.

MENSTRUAL DISORDERS

25. **What is the median age of menarche in the United States?**
12.4 years. Non-Hispanic black females experience menarche slightly earlier than non-Hispanic white and Mexican-American females. Menstruation typically begins 2 to 2.5 years after breast development begins and occurs at sexual maturity rating (SMR) 3 to 4.

Gray SH: Menstrual disorders, *Pediatr Rev* 34:6–17, 2013.

26. **How do you define a normal menstrual cycle?**
    - *Interval:* count from the first day of one period to the first day of the next period; range is from 21 to 45 days in adolescents
    - *Duration:* 3 to 7 days; more than 8 days is considered prolonged
    - *Quantity:* average is about 30 mL per cycle; >80 mL of blood loss is considered excessive (but can be hard to quantify). Changing a blood-soaked pad or tampon every 1 to 2 hours, bleeding through clothing, and using secondary protection are all signs of excessive bleeding.

ACOG Committee on Adolescent Health Care: ACOG Committee Opinion No. 349, November 2006: Menstruation in girls and adolescents: using the menstrual cycle as a vital sign, *Obstet Gynecol* 108:1323–1328, 2006.

27. **What is the physiology of a normal menstrual cycle?**
Three phases: follicular (proliferative), ovulation, and luteal (secretory phase)
See Figure 1-1.

28. **What is the difference between primary and secondary amenorrhea?**
Primary amenorrhea is the failure to achieve menarche by 15 years or no menses by 3 years after the development of secondary sex characteristics.
Secondary amenorrhea is ≥3 months of amenorrhea after achievement of menarche.

29. **What is the value of a progesterone challenge test in a patient with amenorrhea?**
If bleeding ensues within 2 weeks after the administration of oral medroxyprogesterone (5 to 10 mg daily for 5 to 10 days), the test is positive. This indicates that the endometrium has been primed by estrogen and that the outflow tract is functioning. No response indicates hypothalamic-pituitary dysfunction, anatomic obstruction, or ovarian failure.

30. **What are some of the causes of amenorrhea in adolescents?**
Causes of amenorrhea in adolescents include pregnancy, contraceptive use, stress, chronic illness, iatrogenic (i.e., medications, chemotherapy), disordered eating (e.g., anorexia nervosa), female athlete triad, anatomic anomalies (e.g., imperforate hymen, vaginal septum, uterine or vaginal agenesis), and endocrinologic causes. Endocrine disorders that can result in amenorrhea include hypothalamic/pituitary dysfunction, ovarian pathology, thyroid abnormalities, adrenal abnormalities, androgen insensitivity syndrome, and polycystic ovarian syndrome (PCOS).

Talib HJ, Coupey SM: Excessive uterine bleeding, *Adolesc Med State Art Rev* 23:53–72, 2012.

31. **How do you define the different types of "rrhagias"?**
    - **Menorrhagia**: large quantity of bleeding
    - **Metrorrhagia**: irregular interval bleeding
    - **Menometrorrhagia**: heavy and irregular bleeding

32. **What is the differential diagnosis of heavy menstrual bleeding?**
Heavy menstrual bleeding, also sometimes referred to as abnormal uterine or vaginal bleeding, was formerly called dysfunctional uterine bleeding (DUB). This is usually caused by anovulation secondary to an immature hypothalalmic-pituitary-ovarian axis. However, the differential diagnosis also includes *pregnancy* (ectopic, miscarriage), *bleeding disorders* (such as von Willebrand disease, often with onset of first menstrual cycle and affecting about 1% of the population), *pelvic infection* (gonorrhea, chlamydia), *foreign body/trauma*, and *endocrinopathies* (PCOS, thyroid disease).

The Menstrual Cycle

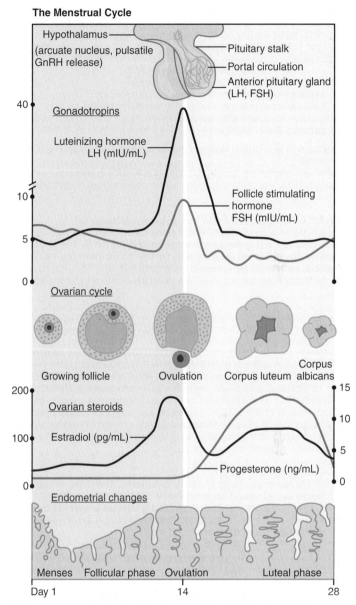

Figure 1-1. The normal menstrual cycle, with relationship among levels of gonadotropins, physiologic activity in the ovary, levels of ovarian steroids, and changes in the endometrium. *(From Braverman PK, Sondheimer SJ: Menstrual disorders, Pediatr Rev 18(1):18, 1997.)*

33. You see an 18-year-old female who comes to your office complaining of 10 days of heavy menstrual bleeding, including soaking through a pad every 2 hours and passing clots. What are key points in the assessment of this patient?
    - *Vital signs*: look for orthostatic hypotension, tachycardia
    - *Physical exam*:
        - Skin for acne, hirsutism, striae consistent with PCOS
        - Petechiae/bruising suggestive of a bleeding disorder
        - Palpation of abdomen to evaluate for undetected pregnancy
        - If sexually active: pelvic/bimanual exam to examine for infection and PID
    - *Labs*: complete blood count (CBC) (assessing for anemia and platelet count), reticulocyte count, TSH, pregnancy test

34. What are the two key clinical features that determine the management of abnormal uterine bleeding?
    Hemoglobin concentration (i.e., anemia) and **signs of orthostatic hypotension**. The more severe the clinical feature, the more urgent and aggressive the management must be, particularly in the setting of acute hemorrhage.

35. How would you treat a patient with heavy menstrual bleeding?
    Treatment is based on extent of bleeding. First, it is important to stabilize the endometrium by giving estrogen (hemostasis) and progestin (for endometrial stability). This can be done by using a combined birth control pill. Iron replacement should be given. Consider a blood transfusion if the patient is hemodynamically unstable. An alternative is to use an antifibrinolytic agent such as tranexamic acid to prevent breakdown of blood clots, especially if the patient has a contraindication to estrogen-containing medication.

36. You see a 16-year-old overweight female who reports having irregular periods, acne, and having to remove hair on her upper lip and chin. What is her most likely diagnosis?
    Polycystic ovary syndrome (PCOS), which can affect up to 10% of reproductive age women, is the most likely diagnosis. Symptoms include amenorrhea/oligomenorrhea, hyperandrogenism (hirsutism, acne), overweight/obesity, and polycystic ovaries on ultrasound. Not all patients with PCOS will have all of these symptoms. Endocrinologic abnormalities may include insulin resistance (with elevated blood insulin levels), elevated LH/FSH ratios, and elevated free and total testosterone. It is important to rule out other causes of symptoms by obtaining DHEA-S (marked elevation suggests a possible adrenal tumor), TSH, prolactin (elevation suggests a possible pituitary tumor), and a morning 17-hydroxyprogesterone (to rule-out late-onset congenital adrenal hyperplasia). Long-term risks and sequelae of PCOS include infertility, endometrial cancer, metabolic syndrome, and diabetes.

37. How common is dysmenorrhea?
    Up to 90% of adolescents are affected by primary dysmenorrhea (pain during menses). The condition remains the single greatest cause of lost school hours in females. However, fewer than 15% of teenage females with dysmenorrhea will seek medical care, so it is important to screen for the problem. Most cases are primary, but about 10% of patients with severe dysmenorrhea symptoms will have uterine or pelvic abnormalities, such as endometriosis.

Harel Z: Dysmenorrhea in adolescents and young adults: an update on pharmacological treatments and management strategies, *Expert Opin Pharmacother* 13:2157–2170, 2012.

38. Does dysmenorrhea occur more commonly in early or late adolescence?
    Dysmenorrhea occurs almost entirely with ovulatory cycles due to prostaglandin release. Menstrual periods shortly after the onset of menarche are usually anovulatory. With the establishment of more regular ovulatory cycles after 2 to 3 years, primary dysmenorrhea becomes more likely.

39. What is the difference between primary and secondary dysmenorrhea?
    Primary dysmenorrhea, also called functional dysmenorrhea, is pain in the absence of pelvic disease. This usually presents in the second to third year after menarche; occurs with ovulatory cycles due to prostaglandin release and uterine hyperactivity; and may be associated with nausea, vomiting, and/or diarrhea. Pain is usually in the lower abdomen, back, or upper thighs.

Secondary dysmenorrhea is dysmenorrhea due to a pathologic process. Some of these processes include endometriosis (endometrial tissue outside the uterus), pelvic infections, intrauterine device (IUD)-related pain (specifically from the nonhormonal copper IUD), pregnancy (either pregnancy-related bleeding or complication such as miscarriage), and genital tract anomalies (especially if dysmenorrhea has been present since menarche).

Gray SH: Menstrual disorders, *Pediatr Rev* 34:6–17, 2013.

40. What two classes of medications are most commonly used for dysmenorrhea?

- **Nonsteroidal anti-inflammatory drugs (NSAIDs):** These limit local prostaglandin production. Naproxen or ibuprofen may be effective in up to 80% of patients.
- **Hormonal therapies:** Oral contraceptives act by reducing endometrial growth, which limits the total production of endometrial prostaglandin. Ovulation is suppressed, which also minimizes pain. A combined estrogen-progestin pill is preferred. Improvement may not be seen for up to 3 months.

41. What is a common cause of chronic pelvic pain in adolescents without a history of pelvic inflammatory disease (PID)?

Endometriosis. This condition results from the implantation of endometrial tissue in areas of the peritoneum outside the uterine cavity. It is reported in 25% to 38% of adolescents with chronic pelvic pain. The pain can be noncyclic (may occur with intercourse or defecation) or cyclic (often most severe just before menses, and dysmenorrhea is common). Studies show that endometriosis can be diagnosed in 50% to 70% of patients with dysmenorrhea who do not respond to NSAIDs. Definitive diagnosis is made by laparoscopy and biopsy. Therapy can be surgical (e.g., excision, coagulation, laser vaporization) and/or medical (e.g., gonadotropin-releasing hormone analogues [GnRHa], combination oral contraceptives, medroxyprogesterone acetate).

Hickey M, Ballard K, Farquhar C: Endometriosis, *BMJ* 348:1752, 2014.

42. What is the peak age for ovarian torsion?

National data reveal that almost 90% of those with ovarian torsion are >11 years old, with a mean age of 14.5 years and an estimated incidence of approximately 5 per 100,000 females aged 1 to 20 years old. A pubertal peak of ovarian torsion is thought to be due to the increasing likelihood of the development of ovarian cysts by the maturing reproductive hormonal axis. These cysts then act as lead points for torsion. Ovarian torsion should be considered in the evaluation of abdominal pain in an adolescent.

Guthrie BD, Adler MD, Powell EC: Incidence and trends of pediatric ovarian torsion hospitalizations in the United States, 2000-2006, *Pediatrics* 125:532–538, 2010.

43. In what setting should ectopic pregnancy be suspected?

Amenorrhea with **unilateral abdominal** or **pelvic pain, irregular vaginal bleeding, and a positive pregnancy test** is indicative of ectopic pregnancy until proven otherwise. A teenager with a ruptured ectopic pregnancy can present with features of shock (hypotension, tachycardia) and rebound tenderness. Sequential hCG levels can help with differentiating an ectopic from an intrauterine pregnancy. For a viable intrauterine pregnancy, the doubling time of hCG levels is about 48 hours; in ectopic pregnancy, there is usually a significant lag. Other causes of lag include missed abortion and spontaneous abortion. Ultrasound is the first-line imaging modality for diagnosis. Laparoscopy may be necessary if the diagnosis remains unclear.

Barnhart KT: Ectopic pregnancy, *N Engl J Med* 361:379–387, 2009.

KEY POINTS: MENSTRUAL DISORDERS

1. Consider von Willebrand disease for abnormally heavy bleeding at menarche or unusually long menstrual periods.
2. Irregular menstrual bleeding patterns are common in early adolescence because regular ovulatory menstrual cycles typically do not develop for 2 to 3 years after the onset of menarche. If irregularity continues >2 years after menarche, consider a workup for PCOS or other causes.

Continued on following page

KEY POINTS: MENSTRUAL DISORDERS *(Continued)*

3. Always consider pregnancy in a patient with secondary amenorrhea.
4. Signs of androgen excess (hirsutism and/or acne) in the setting of menstrual irregularities suggest polycystic ovarian syndrome.
5. Ask about dysmenorrhea; it affects >50% of teenage girls and causes considerable school absence.
   PCOS, Polycystic ovarian syndrome.

OBESITY

44. **What is the body mass index (BMI)?**
    BMI = (weight [kg]/height [m²]). BMI is an indicator of body fat, is age and sex-specific, and is recommended by the Centers for Disease Control and Prevention (CDC) as the main screening tool for obesity. When plotted on standard charts for age and gender, a BMI from the 85th to 95th percentile indicates "overweight" and a BMI > 95th percentile indicates "obese." Data from 2011 to 2012 show that among 12- to 19-year-olds, 35% are overweight, and 21% are obese. BMI growth charts for age and gender are available at http://www.cdc.gov/growthcharts/.

Centers for Disease Control: http://www.cdc.gov/growthcharts/. Growth charts accessed on Dec. 3, 2014.
Ogden CL, Carroll MD, Kit BK, et al: Prevalence of childhood and adult obesity in the United States, 2011-2012, *JAMA* 311:806–814, 2014.
Endocrine Society: http://obesityinamerica.org. Accessed on Mar 19, 2015.

45. **How predictive is early childhood obesity of later adolescent obesity?**
    An overweight 5-year-old is 4 times as likely to be an overweight teenager, which highlights the importance of addressing obesity at an early age.

Cunningham SA, Kramer MR, Narayan KMV: Incidence of childhood obesity in the United States, *N Engl J Med* 370:403–411, 2014.

46. **What are some of the health risk factors related to obesity?**
    A variety of physical, social, and emotional potential problems are involved (Fig. 1-2).

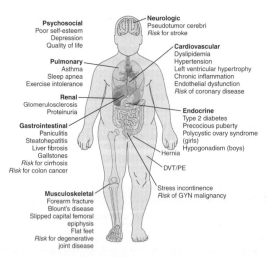

Figure 1-2. Complications of adolescent obesity. *DVT/PE,* Deep vein thrombosis/pulmonary embolism; *GYN,* gynecologic; (*From Slap GB:* Adolescent Medicine: The Requisites in Pediatrics. *Philadelphia, 2011, Elsevier Mosby, p 67.).*

47. **What variety of factors may contribute to obesity?**

Both *genetic* and *environmental* factors are associated with obesity in most cases. *Endocrine* disorders and genetic syndromes leading to obesity are uncommon. An emerging area of interest is *epigenetics*, which is defined as the study of heritable changes in gene expression that occur without a change in the deoxyribonucleic acid (DNA) sequence. Epigenetic mechanisms would include alterations in DNA methylation, histone modifications, or other epigenetically related processes that might increase susceptibility to weight gain.

- *Genetic* factors may explain the variance of fat distribution and metabolism rate.
- *Genetic syndromes* include Prader-Willi, Cohen, and Bardet-Biedl syndromes and are rare.
- *Environmental* factors include increased caloric intake and decreased physical activity.
- *Psychological* disordered eating may result in obesity.
- *Endocrine* causes such as hypothyroidism, Cushing's syndrome, and growth hormone deficiency are rare.

Marinez JA, Milagro FI, Claycombe KJ, et al: Epigenetics in adipose tissue, obesity, weight loss and diabetes, *Adv Nutr* 5:71–81, 2014.

Martos-Moreno GA, Vincente Barrios, Munoz-Calvo, et al: Principles and pitfalls in the differential diagnosis and management of childhood obesity, *Adv Nutr* 5:2995–3055, 2014.

48. **What features on physical examination are particularly important in the evaluation of the obese patient?**

- Blood pressure (hypertension)
- Acanthosis nigricans (type 2 diabetes)
- Hirsutism (polycystic ovarian syndrome)
- Thyroid (goiter, possible hypothyroidism)
- Right upper quadrant (RUQ) tenderness (gallbladder disease)
- Striae (Cushing syndrome)
- Tonsils (hypertrophy; potential for obstructive sleep apnea)
- Facial dysmorphic features (evidence of genetic syndrome)
- Limited hip range of motion (slipped capital femoral epiphysis)
- Small hands and feet, cryptorchidism (Prader-Willi syndrome)
- Lower-leg bowing (Blount disease)

49. **How does sleep affect weight?**

Lack of sleep increases the risk of obesity, and with each hour of sleep lost, the odds of becoming obese increase. People who sleep fewer hours also seem to prefer eating foods that are higher in calories and carbohydrates, which can lead to overeating, weight gain, and obesity. Sleep helps maintain a healthy balance of the hormones that regulate hunger (ghrelin) or satiety (leptin). Insufficient sleep causes levels of ghrelin to increase and levels of leptin to decrease. Sleep also affects the body's response to insulin and lack of sleep results in a higher than normal blood glucose level, increasing the risk for diabetes.

National Institutes of Health: "What causes overweight and obesity?" Accessed at http://www.nhlbi.nih.gov/health/health-topics/topics/obe/causes.html on Oct. 1, 2014.

50. **What are the diagnostic criteria for the metabolic syndrome?**

For children age 10 or older, metabolic syndrome can be diagnosed by abdominal obesity (using waist circumference percentiles >90%) *and* the presence of two or more other clinical features: triglycerides >150 mg/dL, HDL <40 mg/dL, BP systolic ≥130/diastolic ≥85 mm Hg, and known type 2 diabetes or elevated glucose.

Zimmer P, Alberti KG, Kaufman F, et al: The metabolic syndrome in children and adolescents—an IDF consensus report, *Pediatr Diabetes* 8:299–306, 2007.

51. **Why is a short obese 11-year-old of more clinical concern than a tall obese 11-year-old?**

Being overweight is associated with an advanced skeletal age in preadolescents and younger adolescents, and thus, increased height compared with nonobese peers. Therefore, you expect them to be taller. Short stature in an obese 11-year-old could be a sign of possible endocrine disease.

52. **What are some key points when discussing weight reduction counseling and management with a teenager?**

It is important to assess current diet history, encourage healthy dietary practices, and identify problem areas and behaviors. Providers should:

- Help the adolescent set small attainable goals
- Discourage the use of food as reward/comfort and avoid emotional eating
- Encourage physical activity
- Encourage family mealtimes; involve the family to help modify behaviors and lifestyle
- Limit screen-time, including TV, videogames, Internet, and cell phone use when not related to school work, and discourage a TV in the teen's bedroom

Centers for Disease Control and Prevention: "How much physical activity do children need? Accessed at http://www.cdc.gov/physicalactivity/everyone/guidelines/children.html on October 1, 2014.

53. **What are the indications for bariatric surgery in adolescents?**

Surgery can be considered when adolescents have a BMI $\geq$ 35 kg/m^2 with a severe comorbid condition (i.e., type 2 diabetes mellitus, severe obstructive sleep apnea (OSA), pseudotumor cerebri, or severe steatohepatitis) **or** a BMI >40 kg/m^2 with mild comorbidities (mild OSA, hypertension, insulin resistance, dyslipidemia, impaired quality of life). The patient must be Tanner stage IV or V; have completed at least 95% of skeletal maturity; be able to understand diet and lifestyle changes after surgery; and have evidence of mature decision making, social support, and motivation to comply with preoperative and postoperative treatments. Many experts also recommend that before surgery a patient should have failed sustained organized efforts through lifestyle intervention to lose weight. Assent from the adolescent should always be obtained separately from the parents to avoid coercion.

Black JA, White B, Viner RM, et al: Bariatric surgery for obese children and adolescents: a systematic review and meta-analysis, *Obes Rev* 14: 634–644, 2013.
Apovian CM, Baker C, Ludwig DS, et al: Best practice guidelines in pediatric/adolescent weight loss surgery, *Obes Research* 13: 274–282, 2005.

KEY POINTS: OBESITY

1. Obesity is the most common chronic condition in children.
2. With obesity and short stature, think thyroid abnormalities and evaluate thyroid-stimulating hormone and T$_4$ levels.
3. Only 5% of obese children have an identifiable underlying pathologic cause.
4. If a child is at risk as a result of family history, the earlier the modifications (e.g., limiting television time, encouraging exercise, and healthy diet), the better.
5. Keep weight reduction or stabilization goals reasonable; if too unrealistic, discouragement and weight cycling are more likely.

SEXUAL DEVELOPMENT

54. **What is Tanner staging for boys?**

In 1969 and 1970, Dr. James Tanner categorized the progression of stages of puberty, (Table 1-1). It is now commonly referred to as sexual maturity rating (SMR) staging of sexual development. Separate

Table 1-1. Tanner Staging for Boys

STAGE	DESCRIPTION
Pubic Hair	
I	None
II	Countable; straight; increased pigmentation and length; primarily at base of penis
III	Darker; begins to curl; increased quantity
IV	Increased quantity; coarser texture; covers most of pubic area
V	Adult distribution; spread to medial thighs and lower abdomen

Table 1-1. Tanner Staging for Boys (*Continued*)

STAGE	DESCRIPTION
Genital Development	
I	Prepubertal
II	Testicular enlargement (>4 mL volume); slight rugation of scrotum
III	Further testicular enlargement; penile lengthening begins
IV	Testicular enlargement continues; increased rugation of scrotum; increased penile breadth
V	Adult

scales define staging for males based on pubic hair and genital appearance. Of note, the limitation of this rating system is that it relies only on visual inspection. Accurate staging requires palpation for assessment of testicular volume.

55. **What is the normal progression of sexual development and growth for boys during puberty?**
Nearly all boys begin puberty with testicular enlargement. This is followed in about 1 to 1.5 years by pubic hair and then about 12 months later by phallic enlargement. For boys, puberty lasts an average of 3.5 years and begins an average of 2 years later than it does in girls (Fig. 1-3).

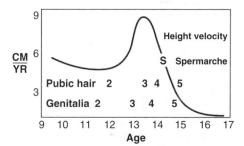

Figure 1-3. Summary of pubertal development in boys. *(From Rosen DS: Physiologic growth and development during adolescence,* Pediatr Rev *25:194–200, 2004.)*

56. **What are the ranges of normal in the stages of pubertal development in girls?**
Tanner divided pubertal development in girls according to pubic hair and breast development (Table 1-2).

Table 1-2. Tanner Stages for Girls

STAGE	DESCRIPTION
Pubic Hair	
I	None
II	Countable; straight; increased pigmentation and length; primarily on medial border of labia
III	Darker; begins to curl; increased quantity on mons pubis
IV	Increased quantity; coarser texture; labia and mons well covered
V	Adult distribution; with feminine triangle and spread to medial thighs
Breast Development	
I	Prepubertal
II	Breast bud present; increased areolar size
III	Further enlargement of breast; no secondary contour
IV	Areolar area forms secondary mound on breast contour
V	Mature; areolar area is part of breast contour; nipple projects

57. **What is the normal progression of sexual development and growth for girls during puberty?**
The majority of girls typically begin puberty with thelarche, or breast development. The appearance of breast buds may initially be asymmetric. Pubic hair usually starts to appear 1 to 1.5 years later, although this may occur first or simultaneously in some girls. In about 15% of girls, axillary hair may appear first. Menarche usually occurs about 18 to 24 months after the onset of breast development. For girls, the duration of puberty is about 4.5 years, which is longer than that for boys (Fig. 1-4).

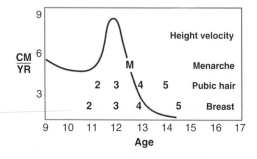

Figure 1-4. Summary of pubertal development in girls. *(From Rosen DS: Physiologic growth and development during adolescence, Pediatr Rev 25:198, 2004.)*

58. **Has the age of menarche declined in the United States during the century?**
Survey data of women over the last several decades indicate a general decline in age over this time period for the initiation of puberty by about 15 months for black girls, 12 months for Mexican-American girls, and 10 months for white girls. A variety of factors may be contributing, including environmental (dietary changes and increasing obesity), socioeconomic, and genetic. Currently the average age of menarche is 12.6 years in white girls and 12.1 years in black girls of normal weight, and Mexican-American girls falling intermediate to this range.

McDowell MA, Brody DJ, Hughes JP: Has age at menarche changed? Results from the National Health and Nutrition Examination Survey (NHANES), *J Adolesc Health* 40:227–231, 2007.

59. **When do boys develop the ability to reproduce?**
The average age of **spermarche** (as demonstrated by the presence of spermatozoa in the first morning urine) is 13.3 years or at Tanner stage (SMR) 3. Unlike what occurs in girls (in whom menarche follows the peak height velocity), in boys, spermarche occurs before the growth spurt. Ejaculation usually occurs by Tanner stage (SMR) 4.

60. **How is delayed puberty defined?**
Delayed puberty is defined as the **absence of testicular enlargement (>4 cm) in boys** and **absence of breast development in girls** at an age that is 2 to 2.5 standard deviations later than the population mean. This has traditionally been defined as age 14 years in boys and age 13 in girls, but given downward trends in pubertal timing in the United States and racial and ethnic disparities, some experts have advocated for younger age cutoffs.

Palmert MR, Dunkel L: Delayed puberty, *N Engl J Med* 366:443, 2012.

61. **Why should the sense of smell be tested in a teenager with delayed puberty?**
Kallmann syndrome is characterized by a defect in gonadotropin-releasing hormone [GnRH] with resultant gonadotropin deficiency and hypogonadism. Maldevelopment of the olfactory lobes also occurs, with resultant anosmia or hyposmia. Less commonly, cleft palate, congenital deafness, kidney malformation, pes cavus, and color blindness can co-occur. Boys who have GnRH deficiency often have a small phallus and testes, but physical exam may be significant only for sexual immaturity. Delayed bone age is the only consistent lab finding. These patients require hormonal therapy to achieve puberty and fertility.

62. **What is the most common cause of delayed puberty?**
Constitutional delay of growth and puberty (CDGP) is the cause of delayed puberty in 70% to 90% of cases, boys more commonly than girls. This is a form of hypogonadotropic hypogonadism in

which there is delayed secretion of GnRH and activation of the gonadal axis. Fifty percent to 75% of children with CDGP have a family history of late-onset puberty, which indicates a strong genetic component. Children often are small for their age (5%) but have grown steadily. Bone age is delayed. Once puberty does begin, its progression is normal. Although it is considered a normal variant of growth, there are some consequences to adult height. Once the pubertal growth spurt occurs, its duration and peak height velocity achieved are both reduced, resulting in a reduction in total pubertal height gain.

Frank Graeme. Growth Disorders. In Martin M, Alderman E, Kreipe R, Rosenfeld W, editors: *Textbook of Adolescent Health Care*. Elk Grove Village, IL, 2011, American Academy of Pediatrics, pp 656–666.

63. What features suggest constitutional delay of puberty?
- Family history of delayed puberty
- Short stature (boys are usually below the 10th percentile for height)
- Slowed growth velocity (4 to 5 cm/year in preadolescent girls and 3.5 to 4.5 cm/year in preadolescent boys) compared with same-age, same-sex peers (8 to 11 cm/year)
- Delayed bone age (from 1.5 to 4 years) compared with chronologic age; bone age is typically 12 to 13.5 years before the onset of puberty
- Normal prepubertal anatomy, sense of smell, and prepubertal LH, FSH levels

64. Which laboratory tests should you consider in a boy or girl with delayed puberty?
If history or physical examination does not suggest an underlying cause (e.g., anorexia nervosa, chronic disease), tests should include **LH, FSH**, **testosterone** (male), and **bone age.** These tests help categorize the condition as *hypergonadotropic* with increased GnRH, FSH, and LH (implying possible gonadal defects, androgen insensitivity, or enzyme defects) or *hypogonadotropic* with decreased GnRH and low to normal FSH and LH (implying constitutional delay or primary hypothalamic-pituitary problems). Most cases involve decreased GnRH.

65. What is the most common cause of primary gonadal failure in boys?
Klinefelter syndrome. The frequency of this condition is 1:1000 males. It is characterized in adolescence by gynecomastia and small, firm testes with seminiferous tubule dysgenesis. It is found in more than 80% of XXY males (i.e., males with 47 chromosomes). Onset of puberty is usually not delayed, and testosterone levels are usually adequate to initiate pubertal development. Levels of FSH and LH are elevated in these patients after the onset of puberty.

66. Can puberty be safely accelerated?
In some teenagers—more commonly boys—the constitutional delay in puberty has significant psychological effects. Studies have shown that, in *boys*, puberty can be accelerated without any compromise in expected adult height. In boys older than 14 years with plasma testosterone levels of less than 10 ng/dL, intramuscular testosterone can be given every 2 to 4 weeks for 4 to 6 months. Treatment for *girls* who are constitutionally delayed is less well studied. Conjugated estrogen or estradiol for 4 to 6 months has been used in girls older than 13 years without breast buds.

Palmert MR, Dunkel L: Delayed puberty, *N Engl J Med* 366:443–453, 2012.

67. How do you evaluate a breast lump noted by a teenage girl on self-examination?
Although the incidence of cancerous lesions is extremely low in adolescents, breast lumps do require careful evaluation. *Fibrocystic changes* (i.e., the proliferation of stromal and epithelial elements, ductal dilation, cyst formation) are common in later adolescence and are characterized by variations in size and tenderness with menstrual periods. Cystic changes will often resolve over 1 to 2 menstrual cycles. Reassurance and observation should be provided. The most common tumor (70% to 95%) is a fibroadenoma, which is a firm, discrete, rubbery, smooth mass that is usually found laterally. This is the most surgically treated or biopsied mass in adolescents. Other causes of masses include lipomas; hematomas; abscesses; simple cysts; and rarely, adenocarcinomas (especially if a bloody nipple discharge is present).

The size, location, and other characteristics of a mass should be documented and reevaluated over the next one to three menstrual periods. A persistent or slowly growing mass should be evaluated with *fine-needle aspiration*. *Ultrasound* can be helpful for distinguishing cystic from solid masses.

Mammography is a very poor tool for identifying distinct pathologic lesions in teenagers because the breast density of adolescents makes interpretation difficult.

Huppert JS, Zidenberg N: Breast disorders in females. In Slap GB, editor: *Adolescent Medicine: The Requisites in Pediatrics*. Philadelphia, 2008, Mosby Elsevier, pp 146–151.

68. **Should breast self-examination be taught and emphasized for all teenage girls?**
Because the incidence of malignancy is very low in this age group, no data support benefits for breast self-examination, and it may cause unnecessary anxiety and testing. Exceptions would be all adolescents with a history of malignancy, those who have had radiation therapy to the chest more than 10 years ago, and adolescents 18 to 21 years old whose mothers carry the *BRCA1* or *BRCA2* gene.

Huppert JS, Zidenberg N: Breast disorders in females. In Slap GB, editor: *Adolescent Medicine: The Requisites in Pediatrics*. Philadelphia, 2008, Mosby Elsevier, p 150.

KEY POINTS: SEXUAL DEVELOPMENT

1. If there are no signs of puberty by age 13 in girls and age 14 in boys, evaluate for an underlying medical cause.
2. Most cases of late puberty are constitutional delay.
3. Nearly all boys begin puberty with testicular enlargement; 85% of girls begin puberty with breast enlargement.
4. Following onset, puberty lasts about 4.5 years for girls and 3.5 years for boys.
5. Mean time between the onset of breast development and menarche is slightly more than 2 years.

SEXUALLY TRANSMITTED INFECTIONS

69. **How does the prevalence of sexually transmitted infections (STIs) in adolescents compare with that of adults?**
Among sexually active people, adolescents have a **higher likelihood** than adults of being infected with an STI. About 25% of adolescents contract at least one STI by the time of high school graduation. Reinfection is also more common in adolescents. About 40% of the annual incidence of chlamydia or gonorrhea infections occurs in teens previously infected with the causative organism. Many adolescents are reinfected within a few months of the index infection. Reasons for the increased susceptibility in teens include the following:

  - Cervical ectropion: *Neisseria gonorrhoeae* and *Chlamydia trachomatis* more readily infect columnar epithelium, and the adolescent ectocervix has more of this type of epithelium than does that of an adult.
  - Cervical metaplasia in the transformation zone (from columnar to squamous epithelium) is more susceptible to human papillomavirus (HPV) infection.
  - There is less frequent use of barrier methods of contraception among this population.
  - Adolescents and young adults account for approximately one fourth of new human immunodeficiency virus (HIV) infections in the United States. In general, the number of cases of HIV is increasing among youth ages 13 to 24 years.

70. **What is the best way to screen for STIs?**
Nucleic acid amplification tests (NAATs), such as polymerase chain reaction or transcription-mediated amplification, are highly sensitive and specific, primarily for chlamydial and gonococcal infections. Advantages of NAATs include more rapid results and less invasiveness. Disadvantages include higher costs and lack of antibiotic sensitivity testing.
The gold standard for STI diagnosis in cases of possible sexual abuse has traditionally been culture. However, as fewer laboratories perform culture tests and more use NAATs for diagnosis, the recommendations are evolving. The American Academy of Pediatrics now recommends the use of NAATs for such evaluations.

Crawford-Jakubiak JC, Committee on Child Abuse and Neglect of the American Academy of Pediatrics: The evaluation of children in the primary care setting when sexual abuse is suspected, *Pediatrics* 132:e558–e567, 2013.

71. **What is the most common STI in sexually active adolescent females?**
    Among females, the most common STI is **HPV infection** followed by chlamydial infection.

72. **How should we screen for STIs in adolescent females?**
    For all sexually active females younger than 25 years, the CDC recommends screening *annually* for chlamydia. High risk adolescent females should also be screened yearly for gonorrhea. Universal screening for HIV is recommended. Screening for syphilis and hepatitis B is on a case-by-case basis. Routine screening for other STIs such as trichomoniasis, herpes simplex virus (HSV), and HPV is not recommended. Risky sexual behaviors should determine screening frequency. Other populations, such as pregnant or HIV-infected adolescent females, may require more thorough evaluation.

CDC: Sexually Transmitted Diseases Treatment Guidelines, 2010, *MMWR* 59 (No. RR-12), 2010.
Screening for HIV: Clinical Summary of U.S. Preventive Services Task Force, 2013.
AHRQ Publication No. 12-05173-EF-4: Accessed at http://www.uspreventiveservicestaskforce.org/uspstf13/hiv/hivfinalrs.htmon Dec. 3, 2014.

73. **How should we screen for STIs in adolescent males?**
    National recommendations for STI screening among sexually active heterosexual males have not yet been officially determined. Annual gonorrhea and chlamydia screening should be considered in sexually active adolescent males. Universal screening for HIV is now also recommended. For males who have had sex with males, the CDC recommendations include annual HIV and syphilis serologies, with more frequent screening based on specific sexual practices.

74. **Are pelvic examinations with specula always required to obtain specimens for STI diagnosis in teenagers?**
    Trends in screening for STIs in teenage girls have shifted from endocervical sampling to urine-based and vaginal swab collection. Optimal specimen type for NAATs in females is a vaginal swab.
    - The chlamydia load in females has been found to be greater in vaginal fluid than in urine.
    - Vaginal specimens obtained without the use of a speculum have a high screening validity for trichomonas, bacterial vaginosis, and yeast infections.
    - Self-collection by teenagers of vaginal specimens has yielded comparable results compared with physician-obtained cervical specimens when nucleic acid amplification testing was used.
    - Urine testing for chlamydia and gonorrhea is also useful if a vaginal specimen is not obtainable or if the adolescent resists obtaining a vaginal swab sample. Urine-based screening tests (NAATS) also have good sensitivity and specificity similar to that of specimens obtained using a speculum.

Fang J, Husman C, DeSilva L, et al: Evaluation of self-collected vaginal swab, first void urine, and endocervical swab specimens for the detection of *Chlamydia trachomatis* and *Neisseria gonorrhoeae* in adolescent females, *J Pediatr Adolesc Gynecol* 21:355–360, 2008.
Michel CE, Sonnex C, Carne CA, et al: *Chlamydia trachomatis* load at matched anatomic sites: implications for screening strategies, *J Clin Microbiol* 45:1395, 2007.

75. **Which STI is most closely linked to cervical cancer?**
    Human papillomavirus. HPV affects 20% to 40% of sexually active adolescent females. More than 100 HPV types have been identified, of which about 30% are known to infect the genital tract. They differ in their clinical presentation. Types 6 and 11 classically cause 90% of genital warts. Types 16 and 18 cause the majority of cervical cancers. Because of this association, HPV vaccination is recommended by the Advisory Committee on Immunization Practices for boys and girls beginning at the 11- to 12-year visit. Catch-up vaccination is also recommended for unvaccinated adolescents.

http://www.cdc.gov/hpv/ (Accessed Mar 23, 2015).

76. **What are the manifestations of HPV infection?**
    HPV infection is typically **subclinical,** but infection can present with **anogenital condyloma acuminata (genital warts). Cervical HPV infection** may lead to cervical dysplasia and cervical cancer. Other complications may include vulvar and vaginal cancers. HPV is also a cause of nonsexually transmitted disease, including **deep plantar warts, palmar warts,** and **common warts.**

Cervical infection with both the low-risk and the high-risk types of HPV in adolescent girls often clears spontaneously over a 6- to 8-month period. In males, HPV infection has been associated with anal cancers, particularly among men who have sex with men (MSM) and patients who are HIV infected. Oropharyngeal and penile cancers have also been associated with HPV infection.

77. **When are Pap smears indicated in teenagers?**
The American College of Obstetricians and Gynecologists recommends that routine cervical cytology screening (Pap smear) for healthy women begins at age 21. Only in certain circumstances (HIV infection, immunocompromised state) are pap smears indicated in younger women. This is because most HPV infections in healthy adolescents self-resolve.

Whitlock EP, Vesco KK, Eder M, et al: Liquid based cytology and human papillomavirus testing to screen for cervical cancer: a systematic review for the U.S. Preventive Services Task Force, *Ann Intern Med* 155:687–697, 2011.

78. **Describe the appearance of condylomata acuminata**
Condyloma acuminata (anogenital warts) are soft, fleshy, polypoid or pedunculated papules that appear in the genital and perianal area (Fig. 1-5). They may coalesce and take on a cauliflower-like appearance. Visualization of anogenital warts can be enhanced by wetting the area with 3% to 5% acetic acid (vinegar), which whitens the lesions. They may be located in the urethra or on the penis, scrotum, or perianal area of men and on the vulva, perineum, vagina, cervix, periurethral, or perianal area in women. They may also be found periorally.

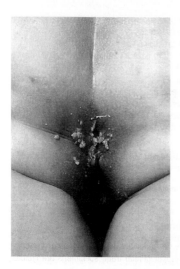

Figure 1-5. Perianal condylomata acuminata. *(From Gates RH: Infectious Disease Secrets, ed 2. Philadelphia, 2003, Hanley & Belfus, p 221.)*

79. **What is the natural history of genital warts?**
Left untreated, 40% of genital warts may spontaneously resolve, but the timing is unpredictable (months to years). The lesions are not oncogenic and will not progress to malignancy. Treatment, often done for cosmetic purposes or symptoms of itching or burning, consists of topical products, cryotherapy, or surgical removal. Recurrence can occur in as many as one third of cases and usually manifests within the first 3 months after therapy.

80. **What is the typical presentation of chlamydial genital infections in both female and male teenagers?**
Most are **asymptomatic** (up to 80% in females and 75% in males) and infection can persist for several months. Those with asymptomatic infection contribute to the high rates of transmission, which is the

reason for screening asymptomatic adolescents. In females with symptoms, chlamydia should be suspected if vaginal discharge and bleeding are noted, especially after intercourse. This may be due to endocervical friability. In males, the most typical symptoms are dysuria and a penile discharge, which is usually scant and watery or mucoid. Occasionally penile itching or tingling may occur without discharge. Less frequently, urinary frequency, dysuria, hematuria, or hematospermia may occur.

Siqueira LM: Chlamydia infections in children and adolescents, *Pediatr Rev* 35;145–154. 2014.

81. What is the typical appearance of *N. gonorrhoeae* on Gram stain?
    Intracellular gram-negative diplococci (Fig. 1-6) are found on Gram stain.

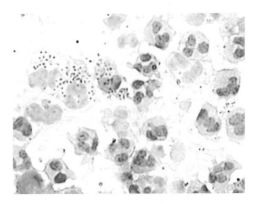

Figure 1-6. Gram stain of Neisseria gonorrhoeae. *(From Gates RH:* Infectious Disease Secrets, *ed 2. Philadelphia, 2003, Hanley & Belfus, p 207.)*

82. What are the minimal criteria for the diagnosis of PID?
    Pelvic or lower abdominal pain with no other cause likely other than PID and one or more of the following must be present:
    - Uterine tenderness
    - Cervical motion tenderness
    - Adnexal tenderness

83. What additional criteria support the diagnosis of PID?
    - Oral temperature > 38.3°C (101 ° F)
    - Abnormal cervical or vaginal discharge (with leukocytes > epithelial cells)
    - Elevated erythrocyte sedimentation rate (usually >15 mm/hr)
    - Elevated C-reactive protein
    - Cervical infection with *N. gonorrhoeae* or *C. trachomatis*
      Because no single clinical aspect or laboratory test is definitive for PID, a constellation of findings is used to support the diagnosis. Of note, tests for gonorrhea and chlamydia are often negative in PID because, although the disease is in the upper genital tract, specimens are typically obtained from the lower tract.

CDC: Sexually transmitted diseases treatment guidelines, 2010, *MMWR Recomm Rep* 59 (RR-12), 1–110, 2010.

84. Which adolescents with PID should be hospitalized for intravenous antibiotics?
    Those with any of the following conditions:
    - Surgical emergency (e.g., appendicitis or ectopic pregnancy [or if such a diagnosis cannot be excluded])
    - Severe illness (e.g., overt peritonitis, vomiting, high fever)
    - Tubo-ovarian abscess
    - Pregnancy
    - Immunodeficiency

- High suspicion for unreliable compliance or timely follow-up within 72 hours
- Failure of outpatient therapy
  These are the same criteria that are used for older women when considering hospitalization for PID. No evidence is available that supports adolescents have better outcomes from hospitalizations for treatment for PID as compared with adults if none of these conditions are present.

American Academy of Pediatrics: Pelvic inflammatory disease. In Pickering LK, editor: *2012 Red Book*, ed 28. Elk Grove Village, IL, 2012, American Academy of Pediatrics, p 550.

85. **What are the common causative pathogens for PID?**
    PID is typically a polymicrobial ascending infection causing endometritis, salpingitis, and oophoritis. It is most commonly caused by gonococcal or chlamydial infections. Other pathogens include *Gardnerella* species, *Haemophilus influenza*, gram negative rods, mycoplasma, *Ureaplasma urealyticum*, and cytomegalovirus.

86. **A sexually active 17-year-old girl with adnexal and RUQ tenderness probably has what condition?**
    Fitz-Hugh–Curtis syndrome. This is an infectious perihepatitis that is caused by gonococci or by chlamydia. It should be suspected in any patient with PID who has RUQ tenderness. It may be mistaken for acute hepatitis or cholecystitis. The pathophysiology is thought to be the direct spread from a pelvic infection along the paracolic gutters to the liver, where inflammation develops and capsular adhesions form (the so-called violin-string adhesions seen on surgical exploration). If RUQ pain persists despite treatment for PID, ultrasonography should be done to rule out a perihepatic abscess.

87. **What are the sequelae of PID?**
    Twenty-five percent of patients with a history of PID will have one or more major sequelae of the disease, including the following:
    - Tubo-ovarian abscess
    - Recurrent PID (about 1 in 5 patients)
    - Chronic abdominal pain: May include exacerbated dysmenorrhea and dyspareunia related to pelvic adhesions in about 20% of patients with PID
    - Ectopic pregnancy: Risk is increased 6- to 10-fold
    - Infertility: Up to 21% after 1 episode of PID, 30% after 2 episodes, and 55% after 3 or more episodes

Trent M, Haggerty CM, Jennings JJ, et al: Adverse adolescent reproductive health outcomes after pelvic inflammatory disease, *Arch Pediatr Adolesc Med* 165:49–54, 2011.
Bortot AT, Risser WL, Cromwell, PF: Coping with pelvic inflammatory disease in the adolescent, *Contemp Pediatr* 21:33–48, 2004.

88. **How are the genital ulcer syndromes differentiated?**
    Genital ulcers may be seen in herpes simplex, syphilis, chancroid, lymphogranuloma venereum, and granuloma inguinale (donovanosis). Herpes and syphilis are the most common, and granuloma inguinale is very rare. Although there is overlap, clinical distinction is summarized in Table 1-3.

Table 1-3. Differentiation of Genital Ulcer Syndromes

	HERPES SIMPLEX	SYPHILIS (PRIMARY, SECONDARY)	CHANCROID	LYMPHO-GRANULOMA VENEREUM
Agent	Herpes simplex virus	*Treponema pallidum*	*Haemophilus ducreyi*	*Chlamydia trachomatis*
Primary lesions	Vesicle	Papule	Papule-pustule	Papule-vesicle
Size (mm)	1-2	5-15	2-20	2-10

Table 1-3. Differentiation of Genital Ulcer Syndromes (*Continued*)

	HERPES SIMPLEX	SYPHILIS (PRIMARY, SECONDARY)	CHANCROID	LYMPHO-GRANULOMA VENEREUM
Number	Multiple, clusters (coalesce ±)	Single	Multiple (coalesce ±)	Single
Depth	Superficial	Superficial or deep	Deep	Superficial or deep
Base	Erythematous, nonpurulent	Sharp, indurated, nonpurulent	Ragged border, purulent, friable	Varies
Pain	Yes	No	Yes	No
Lymphadenopathy	Tender, bilateral	Nontender, bilateral	Tender, unilateral, may suppurate, unilocular fluctuance	Tender, unilateral, may suppurate, multilocular fluctuance

From Shafer MA: Sexually transmitted disease syndromes. In McAnarney ER, Kreipe RE, Orr DP, et al, editors: Textbook of Adolescent Medicine. *Philadelphia, 1992, WB Saunders, p 708.*

89. What are risk factors for the acquisition of genital ulcer disease?
    - Lack of circumcision in males
    - High-risk sexual behaviors (unprotected sex, MSM have a 6-fold increased risk)
    - Unprotected skin-skin contact with ulcers
    - Infection with HIV

Braverman PK: Genital ulcer disease: herpes simplex virus, syphilis, and chancroid. In Slap GB, editor: *Adolescent Medicine: The Requisites in Pediatrics.* Philadelphia, 2008, Mosby Elsevier, p 211.
Roett MA, Mayor MT, Uduhiri KA: Diagnosis and management of genital ulcers, *Am Fam Physician* 85:254–262, 2012.

90. What are the main differences between HSV-1 and HSV-2?
    HSV-1 is typically associated with gingivostomatitis. It is usually transmitted nonsexually through contact with oral secretions (i.e., kissing) during childhood, whereas HSV-2 is associated with genital infection acquired via genital-genital contact. HSV-1 is being increasingly recognized as a cause of genital herpes in industrialized countries in adolescents and college students, which may result from oral sex in the setting of a declining prevalence of early childhood acquisition of HSV-1. This means more young people are susceptible to genital HSV-1 infection.

Bradley H, Marowitz LE, Gibson T, et al: Seroprevalence of herpes simplex virus types 1 and 2—United States, 1999-2010, *J Infect Dis* 209:325–333, 2014.

91. How do recurrent episodes of genital herpes simplex infections compare with the primary episode?
    - Usually less severe, with faster resolution
    - Less likely to have prodromal symptoms (buttock, leg, or hip pain or tingling)
    - Less likely to have neurologic complications (e.g., aseptic meningitis)
    - More likely to have asymptomatic infections
    - Duration of viral shedding is shorter (4 versus 11 days)

Chayavichitsilp J, Buckwalter JV, Krakowski AC, et al: Herpes simplex, *Pediatr Rev* 30:119–129, 2009.
Kimberlin DW, Rouse DJ: Genital herpes, *N Engl J Med* 350:1970–1977, 2004.

92. **How are the three most common causes of postpubertal vaginitis clinically distinguished?**
   Candidal vaginitis: Vulvar itching, erythema and excoriations, vaginal discharge (thick, white, curdlike, lack of odor)
   Trichomonal vaginitis: Vulvar itching and soreness and erythema, vaginal discharge (gray, yellow-green, frothy; rarely malodorous)
   Bacterial vaginosis: Minimal erythema, vaginal discharge (malodorous fishy smell; thin white discharge clings to vaginal walls)

93. **How does the vaginal pH help determine the cause of a vaginal discharge?**
   Ordinarily, the vaginal pH in a pubertal girl is less than 4.5 (compared with 7.0 in prepubertal girls). If the pH is greater than 4.5, infection with trichomonas or bacterial vaginosis should be suspected.

94. **How does evaluation of the vaginal discharge help identify the etiology?**
   See Table 1-4.

Table 1-4. Evaluation of Vaginal Discharge

	CANDIDAL VAGINITIS	TRICHOMONAL VAGINITIS	BACTERIAL VAGINOSIS
pH	≤4.5	>4.5	>4.5
KOH prep	Mycelia pseudohyphae	Normal	Fishy odor (positive "whiff" test)
NaCl prep	Few WBCs	Many WBCs; motile trichomonads	Clue cells

KOH = Potassium hydroxide; NaCl = sodium chloride (salt); WBCs = white blood cells.

95. **How is trichomoniasis diagnosed?**
   Wet mount microscopy has been the most common method of diagnosis. For a wet mount, a sample of vaginal fluid is rolled onto a glass slide, and normal saline is added; look for the lashing flagella and jerky motility of the trichomonads (Fig. 1-7). Wet mounts, however, can be falsely negative in up to one third of cases. *Nucleic acid amplification tests* are now available for detection of *Trichomonas vaginalis*, with higher sensitivities than the wet mount.

Gallion HR, Dupree LJ, Scott TA, et al: Diagnosis of *Trichomonas vaginalis* in female children and adolescents evaluated for possible sexual abuse: a comparison of the InPouch *Trichomonas vaginalis* culture method and wet mount microscopy, *J Pediatr Adolesc Gynecol* 32:300–305, 2009.

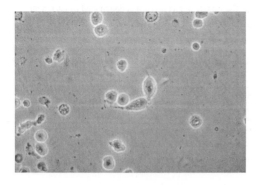

Figure 1-7. Wet mount of vaginal secretions with leukocytes and flagellated trichomonads. *(From Mandell GL, Bennett JE, Dolin R, editors: Principles and Practice of Infectious Diseases, ed 6. Philadelphia, 2004, Churchill Livingstone, p 1361.)*

96. If a patient is receiving a standard treatment for a trichomonal infection, why should alcohol be avoided?

The recommended treatment is single dose administration of metronidazole or tinidazole. Both medications interfere with the processing of ingested alcohol and may cause a disulfiram-like reaction in patients who drink alcohol within 24 hours of dosing. Symptoms may include abdominal pain, cramps, nausea/vomiting, facial flushing, and headaches.

97. What are "clue cells"?

Clue cells are vaginal squamous epithelial cells to which many bacteria are attached. This gives the cell a stippled appearance when viewed in a normal saline preparation (Fig. 1-8). Clue cells are characteristic—but not diagnostic—of bacterial vaginosis.

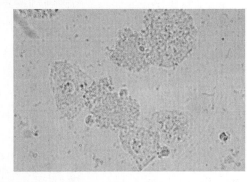

Figure 1-8. "Clue cells" are squamous cells with folded cytoplasm and numerous bacteria (typically *Gardnerella vaginalis*) attached to their surface. *(From Mandell GL, Bennett JE, Dolin R, editors:* Principles and Practice of Infectious Diseases, *ed 6. Philadelphia, 2004, Churchill Livingstone, p 1366.)*

98. What is the etiology of bacterial vaginosis?

Formerly called nonspecific, *Gardnerella*, or *Haemophilus* vaginitis, bacterial vaginosis is the replacement of normal vaginal lactobacilli with a variety of bacteria, including *Gardnerella vaginalis*, genital mycoplasmas, and an overgrowth of anaerobic species.

99. What are the criteria for the diagnosis of bacterial vaginosis?

Clinical diagnosis requires three of the four following criteria (Amsel criteria):
- Homogeneous thin white or gray homogeneous vaginal discharge
- Discharge pH greater than 4.5
- On wet mount, more than 20% of cells are clue cells
- Positive "whiff" test: addition of 10% KOH to discharge results in fishy odor

---

Hwang LY, Shafer M-A: Vaginitis and vaginosis. In Neinstein LS, editor: *Adolescent Health Care*, ed 5. Philadelphia, 2008, Wolters Kluwer, pp 728–729.

100. What is expedited partner therapy?

Expedited partner therapy is treating the patient's sexual partner(s) for presumed infection of gonorrhea or chlamydia without examining the partner(s) before dispensing treatment. The CDC has recommended this option to facilitate partner treatment. The legality of this practice is determined by each state.

101. What are CDC treatment recommendations for common STIs?

See Table 1-5.

Table 1-5. CDC STI treatment guidelines

COMMON INFECTION	RECOMMENDED TREATMENT
Gonorrhea urethritis/cervicitis	Ceftriaxone 250 mg intramuscular (IM), single dose PLUS Azithromycin 1 g orally, single dose
Chlamydia urethritis/cervicitis	Azithromycin 1 g orally, single dose

Continued on following page

Table 1-5. CDC STI treatment guidelines (*Continued*)

COMMON INFECTION	RECOMMENDED TREATMENT
PID	Ceftriaxone 250 mg IM, single dose 　PLUS Doxycycline 100 mg orally twice daily for 14 days **WITH or WITHOUT** Metronidazole 500 mg orally twice daily for 14 days PARENTERAL REGIMEN: Cefotetan 2 g IV every 12 hrs OR Cefoxitin 2 g IV every 6 hrs 　PLUS Doxycycline 100 mg oral or IV every 12 hours **OR** Clindamycin 900 mg IV every 8 hrs 　PLUS Gentamycin (loading) 2 mg/kg IV once, followed by 1.5 mg/kg IV every 8 hrs
Genital HSV	PRIMARY LESION: Acyclovir 400 mg orally three times a day for 7-10 days **OR** Valacyclovir 1 g orally twice a day for 7-10 days EPISODIC THERAPY FOR RECURRENT GENITAL HERPES: Acyclovir 800 mg orally twice a day for 5 days **OR** Valacyclovir 1 g orally once a day for 5 days SUPPRESSION: Acyclovir 400 mg orally twice a day **OR** Valcyclovir 1 g orally once a day (decrease to 500 mg once a day if <10 outbreaks/year)
Primary Syphilis	Benzathine Penicillin G 2.4 million units IM in a single dose

HSV = Herpes simplex virus; IM = intramuscular; IV = intravenous; PID = pelvic inflammatory disease; STI = sexually transmitted infection.
http://www.cdc.gov/std/treatment/update.htm (Accessed Mar 23, 2015).

KEY POINTS: SEXUALLY TRANSMITTED INFECTIONS

1. Regardless of the pathogen, most sexually transmitted infections (STIs) can be asymptomatic.
2. Nucleic acid amplification tests for chlamydia and gonorrhea are particularly useful when screening for STIs in males and females.
3. STI screening in girls is best done via vaginal swab or urine collection rather than through endocervical sampling. Vaginal samples are the most sensitive.
4. No single symptom, exam finding, or laboratory test is definitive for PID.
5. Cultures are often negative in PID because the disease is in the upper genital tract and specimens are obtained from the lower tract.
6. Despite high rates of STIs in adolescents, clinicians frequently do not inquire about sexual activity, risk factors, or means of reducing risks.

SUBSTANCE ABUSE

102. What are the categories of abused drugs?
    - **Sedative-hypnotics:** Alcohol, barbiturates, benzodiazepines, γ-hydroxybutyrate, flunitrazepam (Rohypnol), other sedatives
    - **Stimulants:** Caffeine, cocaine, amphetamines, decongestants

- **Tobacco**
- **Cannabinoids:** Marijuana, hashish, synthetic cannabinoids
- **Opioids:** Heroin, opium, pharmaceutical opioid painkillers including methadone and oxycodone/ oxycodone derivatives
- **Hallucinogens:** Lysergic acid diethylamide (LSD), phencyclidine, mescaline, psilocybin, hallucinogenic mushrooms, methylenedioxy-methamphetamine (MDMA, ecstasy, Molly)
- **Inhalants:** Aliphatic, halogenated, and aromatic hydrocarbons; nitrous oxide; ketones; esters
- **Steroids**

Liepman MR, Calles JL, Kizilbash L, et al: Genetic and nongenetic factors influencing substance abuse by adolescents, *Adolesc Med* 13:375–401, 2002.

103. What is the CRAFFT screen?

This is a six-item screening test for adolescent substance abuse. Two or more "yes" answers indicate with more than 90% sensitivity and more than 80% specificity potential significant substance abuse. A number of screening instruments are available for interviewing adolescents, and the search for alcohol or drug use should be part of routine medical care.

- **C**ar: Have you driven a car (or ridden with a driver) under the influence of drugs or alcohol?
- **R**elax: Do you use drugs or alcohol to relax, feel better, or fit in?
- **A**lone: Do you use drugs or alcohol while you are alone?
- **F**orget: Do you sometimes forget what you did while using drugs or alcohol?
- **F**amily/Friends: Do they ever tell you to cut down on drug or alcohol use?
- **T**rouble: Have you gotten into trouble when using drugs or alcohol?

American Academy of Pediatrics, Committee on Substance Abuse: policy statement—alcohol use by youth and adolescents: a pediatric concern, *Pediatrics* 125: 1078–1087, 2010.

104. What are characteristic physical signs of illicit drug use?

See Table 1-6.

Kaul P, Coupey SM: Clinical evaluation of substance abuse, *Pediatr Rev* 23:85–94, 2002.

Table 1-6. Physical Signs of Illicit Drug Use

PHYSICAL SIGN	DRUG OF ABUSE
Hypothermia	Phencyclidine, ketamine
Hyperthermia	Mescaline, LSD
Increased heart rate	Amphetamine, cocaine, marijuana, MDMA, LSD
Increased blood pressure	Amphetamine, cocaine, phencyclidine, MDMA, LSD
Decreased gag reflex	Heroin, morphine, oxycodone, other opiates, benzodiazepines
Conjunctival redness	Marijuana
Pinpoint pupils	Heroin, morphine, oxycodone, other opiates
Sluggish pupillary response	Barbiturates
Irritation/ulceration of nasal mucosa	Intranasal cocaine, heroin, inhalants
Oral sores/burns, perioral pyodermas	Inhalants
Cutaneous scars ("tracks")	Intravenous use
Gynecomastia, small testes	Marijuana
Subcutaneous fat necrosis	Intravenous and intradermal use

Continued on following page

Table 1-6. Physical Signs of Illicit Drug Use (*Continued*)	
PHYSICAL SIGN	**DRUG OF ABUSE**
Tattoos in antecubital fossa	Intravenous use
Skin abscesses and cellulitis	Intravenous and intradermal use

LSD = Lysergic acid diethylamide; MDMA = methylenedioxy-methamphetamine.

105. Should an adolescent be screened for drug abuse without his or her consent?

The American Academy of Pediatrics (AAP) advises against involuntarily drug testing of adolescents. The AAP recommends that pediatricians discuss who will receive results with adolescents and their parents before ordering a drug test. Others have argued that a teenager's right to privacy and confidentiality does not supersede potential risks for serious damage from drug abuse, particularly if there is strong clinical suspicion or parental concern. Drug screening may be obtained without consent in cases of emergency where the minor is unable to give consent and/or the course of management may be dependent on the drug screen results. The legal ramifications are evolving and vary from state to state. In 1995, the U.S. Supreme Court ruled that random drug testing of high-school athletes and participants in extracurricular activities is legal.

Levy S, Siqueira LM and Committee on Substance Abuse: Testing for drugs of abuse in children and adolescents, *Pediatrics* 133:e1798–e1807, 2014.

106. How long do illicit drugs remain detectable in urine specimens?

There is variability depending on a patient's hydration status and method of intake, but, as a rule, metabolites can be detected after ingestion, as shown in Table 1-7. Most urine screens are very sensitive and may detect drugs up to 99% of the time in concentrations established as analytic cutoff points. However, the screens can be much less specific, sometimes with false-positive rates of up to 35%. Therefore, second tests using the analytic methodology most specific for the suspected drug should be used. Furthermore, the use of urine drug screening is of limited value because many drugs are not included in screening panels.

Levy S, Siqueira LM, and Committee on Substance Abuse: Testing for drugs of abuse in children and adolescents, *Pediatrics* 133:e1803, 2014.

Table 1-7. Detection of Illicit Drug Metabolites	
Alcohol	7-12 hours
Amphetamines	1-3 days
Barbiturates (short acting)	4-6 days
Benzodiazepines (short acting)	1 day
Cocaine	1-3 days
Heroin	<24 hours up to 1-2 days
Marijuana	1-3 days for single use; 3-5 weeks after last use for chronic smoker
Methadone	1-7 days
Morphine	1-2 days
Oxycodone	2-4 days
Phencyclidine	2-8 days for casual use; several weeks for chronic use

107. **What is the genetic predisposition for alcoholism?**
A male child of an alcoholic father is five times more likely to become an alcoholic than a child with a nonalcoholic father. Twin studies have demonstrated heritability patterns to be between 50% to 75%.

108. **What are other individual risk factors for alcohol abuse?**
Risk factors include poor school performance, conduct disorder, and untreated attention-deficit/hyperactivity disorder (ADHD). Mood disorders and psychiatric conditions such as anxiety, depression, schizophrenia and bulimia tend to co-occur with alcohol abuse.

109. **Which type of substance abuse is more common in younger adolescents than older adolescents?**
Inhalant abuse. These substances are used at a higher rate among 12- to 13-year-olds as compared with older adolescents. Household products are typically abused, including aliphatic hydrocarbons (e.g., gasoline, butane in cigarette lighters), aromatic hydrocarbons (e.g., benzene and toluene in glues and acrylic paints), alkyl halides (e.g., methylene chloride and trichloroethylene in paint thinners and spot removers), and ketones (e.g., acetone in nail polish remover). Inhalants are the first illicit drugs used in about 6% of adolescents. Marijuana and pain relievers are the next most common drug types to be used for the first time by adolescents. Inhalants have short durations of action and usually cannot be detected by toxicology screen.

110. **What is the leading cause of fatality related to inhalant abuse?**
Fatal arrhythmias. The volatile hydrocarbons sensitize the myocardium to the effect of epinephrine and also affect depolarization of the myocardial cell membranes. Abnormal propagation of impulses can occur, sometimes associated with adrenaline surge (as when hallucinating or running from an authority figure), resulting in fatal arrhythmias. In adolescents who die from this entity, about 1 in 5 is using inhalants for the first time. This phenomenon may be referred to as Sudden Sniffing Death Syndrome.

Crocetti M. Inhalants, *Pediatr Rev* 29; 33–34. 2008.
Williams JF, Storck M: Inhalant abuse, *Pediatrics* 119:1009–1017, 2007.

111. **What are the toxicities of chronic marijuana use?**
Pulmonary: Decreased pulmonary function. Compared with cigarette smoke, marijuana smoke contains more carcinogens and respiratory irritants and produces higher carboxyhemoglobin levels and greater tar deposition. Studies have demonstrated premalignant changes in those who smoke marijuana but not tobacco. The long-term significance of this has not yet been determined. Chronic use is associated with symptoms of chronic bronchitis.
Endocrine: Decreased sperm count and motility in boys. Marijuana use may interfere with hypothalamic-pituitary function and increase the likelihood of anovulation in girls. Chronic use also antagonizes insulin, which may affect diabetic management. Marijuana use may also impair cortisol and growth hormone secretion but the clinical implications are not yet known.
Neurologic/behavioral: Diminished short-term memory, concentration, and ability for complex decision making. Reaction time and motor coordination may be affected as well. There may also be interference with learning, possible "amotivational syndrome." Use early in adolescence may alter brain development and result in cognitive impairment. Regular use is associated with an increased risk of anxiety and depression (although causality has not been established).

112. **Is marijuana a "gateway" drug?**
A *gateway drug* is one with apparent less deleterious side effects, which is believed to lead to future risks of the use of more dangerous drugs. Epidemiologic and preclinical data indicate that marijuana use by adolescents could influence multiple addictive behaviors in adulthood. Additionally, long-term marijuana use itself can lead to addiction. One in 6 who starts using marijuana as a teenager and 25% to 50% among those who smoke marijuana daily will become addicted.

Volkow ND, Baler RD, Compton WM, Weiss SRB: Adverse health effects of marijuana use, *N Engl J Med* 370:1724–1731, 2014.

113. **What performance-enhancing drugs are used by teenagers?**
The different classes of these drugs include *anabolic steroids* (e.g., androstenedione), *nutritional supplements* (e.g., creatine, protein shakes), *stimulants* (e.g., ephedrine, caffeine, or guarana), and *others*,

including human growth hormone and blood-enhancing products. Many adolescents using these products do not participate in sports, but take these products in an effort to improve their appearance.

Dandoy C, Gereige RS: Performance-enhancing drugs. *Pediatr Rev* 33;265–271, 2012.

114. What are the potential side effects of anabolic steroids?
    See Table 1-8.

Table 1-8. Potential Side Effects of Anabolic Steroids

Endocrine	In males—testicular atrophy, oligospermia, gynecomastia
	In females—amenorrhea, breast atrophy, clitoromegaly
Musculoskeletal	Premature epiphyseal closure
Dermatologic	Acne, hirsutism, striae, male pattern baldness
Hepatic	Impaired excretory function with cholestatic jaundice, elevated liver function test results, peliosis hepatis (a form of hepatitis in which hepatic lobules have microscopic pools of blood), benign and malignant tumors
Cardiovascular	Hypertension, decreased high-density lipoprotein, thrombosis
Psychological	Aggressive behavior, mood swings, depression

Smith DV, McCambridge TM: Performance-enhancing substances in teens, *Contemp Pediatr* 26:41, 2009.

115. When does cigarette smoking begin?
    In the United States, about three fourths of daily adult smokers started smoking when they were *between the ages of 13 and 17 years*. Nearly 9 out of 10 smokers begin by age 18 years; worldwide, the average age is lower. Cigarette smoking remains the major preventable cause of premature death in the world. In the United States, rates for teenagers younger than 18 years have been declining since the late 1990s. In 2014, 14% of 8th graders and 34% of high school seniors reported any lifetime use of cigarettes.

http://monitoringthefuture.org//pressreleases/14drugpr_complete.pdf (Accessed Mar 23, 2015).

116. What are the main reasons that cigarette smoking begins?
    • Peer pressure (the strongest influence)
    • Curiosity or wanting to experiment
    • Family member smoking
    • As a method of weight control by girls
    • As a way of risk-taking by boys
    • Low self-esteem and depression
    • LGBTQ youth smoke over 50% more than their straight counterparts and are more likely to use smokeless tobacco products as well.

117. What are the risks of chewing tobacco?
    As a result of the decreased gingival blood flow caused by nicotine, chronic ischemia and necrosis can occur. Chronic use results in **gingival recession** and **inflammation, periodontal disease,** and **oral leukoplakia** (a premalignant change). The risk for oral and pharyngeal cancer is increased. Although more commonly used by males, smokeless tobacco used by pregnant females may be associated with low-birth-weight infants and premature birth. Chewing tobacco, like cigarettes, is addictive.

Lenney W, Enderby B: "Blowing in the wind": a review of teenage smoking, *Arch Dis Child* 93:72–75, 2008.

118. What are the risks of E-cigarette use among adolescents?
    E-cigarettes electronically aerosolize nicotine and therefore have a similar side effect profile to that of cigarettes. Little is known about their long-term health effects; however, because e-cigarettes contain

concentrated nicotine, there is a greater risk of nicotine overdose. The Food and Drug Administration (FDA) has not approved their sale to teenagers, given these safety concerns.

119. **What are the 5 "A's" of smoking cessation counseling?**
- Ask about tobacco use
- Advise to quit
- Assess willingness to attempt quitting
- Assist in attempt to quit (e.g., pharmacotherapy such as nicotine gum or patch)
- Arrange follow-up

Klein JD, Camenga DR: Tobacco prevention and cessation in pediatric patients, *Pediatr Rev* 25:17–26, 2004.
www.smokefree.gov: This is the national site with information for individuals interested in quitting, including smoking quitlines. Accessed May 2, 2014.

120. **Are tattoos a tip-off to high-risk behaviors?**
Yes. Permanent tattoos are obtained by 10% to 16% of adolescents between the ages of 12 and 18 years in the United States. The more tattoos an adolescent has, the stronger is the association with high-risk behaviors, including substance abuse, early initiation of sexual intercourse, interpersonal violence, and school failure.

Owen DC, Armstrong ML, Koch JR, Roberts AE. College students with body art: well-being or high risk behavior? *J Psychosoc Nurs Ment Health Serv* 51(10):20–28, 2013.
Desai NA, Smith ML: Body art in adolescents: paint, piercings, and perils. *Adolesc Med State Art Rev* 22:97–118, 2011.
Roberts TA, Ryan SA: Tattooing and high-risk behavior in adolescents, *Pediatrics* 110:1058–1063, 2002.

TEENAGE MALE DISORDERS

121. **How common is gynecomastia in teenage boys?**
As many as 60% to 70% of adolescent boys have some breast development. In most, it spontaneously resolves in 1 to 2 years; 25% have persistence ≥ 2 years. It occurs most commonly during Tanner stages II and III, and it usually consists of subareolar enlargement (breast bud). It may be unilateral or bilateral. The breast bud may be tender, which indicates the recent rapid growth of tissue. Obese boys often have breast enlargement due to the deposition of adipose tissue, and differentiation from gynecomastia (true breast budding) is sometimes difficult.

Bell DL, Breland DJ, Ott MA: Adolescent and young adult male health: a review, *Pediatrics* 132:540, 2013.
Cakan N, Kamat D: Gynecomastia: evaluation and treatment recommendations for primary care providers, *Clin Pediatr* 46:487–490, 2007.

122. **Why does gynecomastia occur so commonly in young teenage boys?**
Early during puberty, the production of estrogen (a stimulator of ductal proliferation) increases relatively faster than does that of testosterone (an inhibitor of breast development). This slight imbalance causes the breast enlargement. In obese teenagers, the enzyme aromatase (found in higher concentrations in adipose tissue) converts testosterone to estrogen.

123. **Which boys with gynecomastia warrant further evaluation?**
- Prepubertal or postpubertal boys
- Pubertal-age boys with little or no virilization and small testes
- Boys with hepatomegaly or abdominal mass palpated
- Boys with CNS complaints

Evaluation may include testing for hypothalamic or pituitary disease, feminizing tumors of the adrenal or testes, and genetic abnormalities (e.g., Klinefelter syndrome). Although breast cancer is extremely rare in men (0.2%), the rate increases to 3% to 6% in patients with Klinefelter syndrome. Benign cases of gynecomastia should be managed with reassurance. Plastic surgery is a last resort option if the gynecomastia does not resolve and is causing significant distress.

124. What are the clinical manifestations of testicular torsion?

Testicular torsion in adolescents usually presents with acute-onset hemiscrotal pain that may radiate to the groin and lower abdomen. Nausea and vomiting are also common. The testis is acutely tender and may be elevated, indicating a twisted and foreshortened spermatic cord. The cremasteric reflex (the testicle retracts after light stroking of the ipsilateral thigh) is typically absent. Many patients report previous episodes of severe acute scrotal pain.

125. When is testicular torsion likely to occur?

Testicular torsion has a peak incidence at ages 15 to 16, with two thirds of cases occurring between ages 12 to 18. The most common underlying factor leading to testicular torsion is a congenital malformation called the "bell-clapper" deformity. The bell-clapper deformity refers to an abnormal fixation of the tunica vaginalis to the testicle, resulting in a horizontal lie of the testis and increased mobility of the testis. Of note, the other peak of testicular torsion occurs in the neonatal period.

Sharp VJ, Kieran K, Arlen AM: Testicular torsion: diagnosis, evaluation, and management, *Am Fam Physician* 88:835-840, 2013.

126. How is testicular torsion diagnosed?

Because salvage of the testis depends on the timely restoration of blood flow, imaging studies should not delay surgical exploration if symptoms and physical exam findings strongly suggest torsion. **Ultrasound with color Doppler** is sensitive and specific, fast to perform, and often readily available, making it the modality of choice for imaging if the presentation warrants further investigation. Low or absent blood flow to the testis seen on Doppler is suggestive of torsion.

127. How is testicular torsion treated?

Manual detorsion of the spermatic cord may be attempted if prompt surgical intervention is not available. However, surgical exploration is still required for fixation to prevent recurrence. Bilateral orchiopexy should be performed because the bell-clapper deformity is bilateral in up to 80% of cases.

Gatti JM, Murphy JP: Acute testicular disorders, *Pediatr Rev* 29:235–240, 2008.

128. If complete testicular torsion has occurred, how long is it before irreversible changes develop?

Irreversible changes develop in **4 to 8 hours.** Reported testicular salvage rates are 90% to 100% if surgical exploration occurs within 6 hours of symptoms, 50% if symptoms are present for more than 12 hours, and less than 10% if symptom duration is 24 hours or longer.

129. How is testicular torsion clinically differentiated from other causes of the acute painful scrotum?

- **Epididymitis:** An inflammatory process that is usually slower in onset; pain is initially localized to epididymis, but as inflammation spreads, whole testis may become painful; may be associated with nausea, fever, abdominal or flank pain, dysuria, and/or urethral discharge; pain does not usually radiate to the groin; often caused by *C. trachomatis* and *N. gonorrhoeae*; history of STIs is suggestive; unusual in non–sexually active teenagers
- **Orchitis:** Usually slower in onset; often systemic symptoms (nausea, vomiting, fever, chills) as a result of diffuse viral infection; in patients with mumps, occurs about 4 to 8 days after parotitis; bilateral involvement more common, most commonly affects 7- to 12-year-olds
- **Torsion of appendix testis:** Sudden onset of pain; localized, isolate tenderness at the superior aspect of the testicle (occasionally with bluish discoloration, the so-called blue-dot sign); nausea and vomiting uncommon; more common in prepubertal boys; cremasteric reflex is usually present
- **Incarcerated hernia:** Acute onset; pain not localized to hemiscrotum; usually palpable inguinal mass; testes not painful; symptoms and signs of bowel obstruction (vomiting, abdominal distention, guarding, rebound tenderness)

Yin S, Trainor JL: Diagnosis and management of testicular torsion, torsion of the appendix testis, and epididymitis, *Clin Pediatr Emerg Med* 10:38–44, 2009.

130. How does the Prehn sign help distinguish between epididymitis and testicular torsion?

Relief of pain with elevation of the testis (*positive Prehn sign*) is associated with epididymitis, whereas persistent pain (*negative Prehn sign*) is more indicative of testicular torsion. However, this relatively nonspecific sign should be interpreted in the context of other signs and symptoms.

131. What is the most frequent solid cancer in older adolescent males?

Testicular cancer. Testicular cancer is most common in males 15 to 35 years of age. Those with a history of cryptorchidism (undescended testicle) are at increased risk, as are males with a history of hypospadias. The most common type is a seminoma, which, if detected when confined to the testicle (stage I), has a cure rate of up to 97% with orchiectomy and radiation. There is currently no evidence that testicular self-exam is associated with improved outcomes in testicular cancer and is therefore controversial.

Bell DL, Breland DJ, Ott MA: Adolescent and young adult male health: a review, *Pediatrics* 132:535–546, 2013.

132. What is the significance of a varicocele in a teenager?

A *varicocele* is an enlargement of either the pampiniform or cremasteric venous plexus of the spermatic cord, which results in a boggy enlargement ("bag of worms") of the upper scrotum. These are rare before puberty. About 15% of boys between the ages of 12 to 18 have a varicocele, and about 10% of those are symptomatic (pain, discomfort). Longitudinal studies of adolescents show that large varicoceles may interfere with normal testicular growth and result in decreased spermatogenesis.

133. Which varicoceles warrant surgical intervention?

It is controversial whether surgery can prevent the potential fertility consequences. Referral for possible intervention is warranted in the following situations:

- Varicocele with testicular atrophy (>20% volume difference)
- Large varicocele
- Bilateral varicoceles (higher potential for infertility)
- Scrotal pain

Fine RG, Poppas DP: Varicocele: standard and alternative indications for repair, *Curr Opin Urol* 22:513–516, 2012.
Hayes JH: Inguinal and scrotal disorders, *Surg Clin North Am* 86:371–381, 2006.

134. On which side do varicoceles more commonly occur?

The left side: The left spermatic vein drains into the left renal vein at a right angle, and the right spermatic vein drains into the inferior vena cava at an obtuse angle. These hemodynamics favor higher left-sided pressures, which predispose patients to left-sided varicoceles. Unilateral left-sided varicoceles are the most common type, occurring in 90% of patients; the remainder are bilateral. A unilateral right-sided lesion is rare, and many experts consider its presence a reason to search for other causes of venous obstruction, such as a renal or retroperitoneal tumor.

135. What is the difference between phimosis and paraphimosis?

Phimosis is constriction of the prepuce orifice that prevents the foreskin from being withdrawn to reveal the glans penis. It can be secondary to minor inflammation from normal erections and from poor hygiene. Treatment is initially conservative with topical steroid creams, but circumcision may be considered in resistant cases.

Paraphimosis, on the other hand, is retraction of the foreskin behind the glans with inability to reposition it back. This is a medical emergency and requires surgical intervention. If untreated, paraphimosis can lead to penile ischemia.

136. What are pearly penile papules and should a teen worry about them?

Pearly penile papules (*hirsuties coronae glandis*) are 1- to 3-mm papules of the same size and shape distributed symmetrically along the corona of the glans penis. These papules are an anatomic variation and not infectious. They occur in about 15% to 20% of adolescent boys. There is a higher incidence in uncircumcised males. No treatment is indicated. Providers should reassure the teen that this is a normal finding.

Leung AK, Barankin B: Pearly penile papules, *J Pediatr* 165:409, 2014.

TEENAGE PREGNANCY AND CONTRACEPTION

137. **What are trends in teenage pregnancy in the United States?**

Teenage pregnancy rates have fallen steadily from 1990 to 2009, except for a brief increase between 2006 and 2007. Pregnancy rates fell 51% for non-Hispanic white and non-Hispanic black teenagers and 40% for Hispanic teenagers between 1990 and 2009. However, U.S. teen pregnancy rates are among the highest in the developed world. Teen pregnancy rates for black and Hispanic teens remain consistently at least twice that of white teenagers. About 80% of teen pregnancies are unintended and about one-third end in abortion. The teenage abortion rate in 2008 was the lowest since abortion was legalized (in 1973). About half of U.S. teen pregnancies progress to delivery.

Curtain SC, Abma JC, Ventura SJ, et al: Pregnancy Rates for U.S. Women Continue to Drop. *NCHS Data Brief* 136:1–8, 2013.

138. **What factors make it more likely that a teenager will become pregnant?**

- **Early initiation of sexual intercourse:** Risk factors for early initiation include low socioeconomic status, low future-achievement orientation, and academic difficulties.
- **Influence from peers and sisters:** If surrounded by sexually active friends and siblings, a teenager is more likely to engage in sexual behavior. For many teens, pregnancy is not viewed as a negative experience.
- **History of physical or sexual abuse**
- **Family history of adolescent pregnancy**
- **Lack of family support and structure**
- **Barriers to contraception:** Inaccurate information, lack of accessibility, improper use
- **History of pregnancy**
- **History of negative pregnancy tests**
- **Race:** Blacks and Hispanics have higher rates of pregnancy than whites, although rates significantly vary by race according to socioeconomic status.

Cox JE: Teenage pregnancy. In Neinstein LS, editor: *Adolescent Health Care*, ed 5. Philadelphia, 2008, Wolters Kluwer, pp 565–569.

139. **If a teenager has been pregnant once, how likely is she to become pregnant again during her teenage years?**

Repeat adolescent pregnancy is common. Studies show that 28% to 63% of teen mothers will have a repeat pregnancy within 18 months and about 40% will have a repeat pregnancy within 2 years. Factors associated with a repeat teen pregnancy include young age at first conception, intended first pregnancy, lack of contraceptive use, poor outcome of first birth, low school achievement, regular use of alcohol or drugs, poor family involvement, low level of parental education, and being the product of a teen pregnancy.

Crittenden CP, Boris NW, Rice JC, et al: The role of mental health factors, behavioral factors, and past experiences in the prediction of rapid repeat pregnancy in adolescence, *J Adolesc Health* 44:25–32, 2009.

140. **What are the risks for infants of teenage mothers?**

Babies born to young teenage mothers are more likely to be preterm, have low birth weight, or be small for gestational age. In addition, infant mortality is greater for the infants of teenage mothers. It is unclear whether these risks are due to physiologic effects of adolescent pregnancy or to sociodemographic factors associated with teenage pregnancy (e.g., poverty, inadequate prenatal care).

Ganchimeg T, Ota E, Morisaki N, et al: Pregnancy and childbirth outcomes among adolescent mothers: a World Health Organization multicountry study, *BJOG* 121:40–48, 2014.

141. **How soon after conception will a urine pregnancy test become positive?**

Human chorionic gonadotropin (hCG) is a glycoprotein that is produced by trophoblastic tissue. Urine pregnancy tests can detect pregnancy by measuring total hCG, hyperglycosolated hCG, or the free β subunit of hCG. Urine levels of 25 mIU/mL hCG are detectable by the most sensitive tests by about 7 days after fertilization. Although many home pregnancy tests can detect these low levels, some are less sensitive and can only accurately diagnose pregnancy by about 3 days after the missed menstrual period.

Cole LA: The utility of 6 over-the-counter (home) pregnancy tests, *Clin Chem Lab Med* 49:1317–1322, 2011.

142. **Which contraceptive methods are appropriate for adolescents?**
     All available reversible methods of contraception are appropriate for use in adolescents, barring specific medical contraindications.
     - **Long-acting reversible contraception (LARC):** Long-acting reversible contraceptive methods available include IUDs and subdermal implants. In the past, myths about the safety of IUD use in adolescents and in nulliparous women discouraged providers from taking advantage of these highly effective methods. However, it is now known that methodologic flaws in prior studies exaggerated the risks in the adolescent population and that these methods are safe for use in teens. IUDs do not significantly increase the risk of PID, outside of the 3 weeks after insertion, and do not cause infertility.
     - **Progestin-only injectable contraception:** The injectable progestin-only contraception available in the United States (Depo-Provera®) is a common type of hormonal contraception used by adolescents. It is dosed every 3 months. Weight gain and intermenstrual bleeding are side effects associated with this method. While bone mineral loss may be associated with this method, users do not appear to have an increased risk of fractures.
     - **Combined hormonal contraception:** Combined estrogen and progestin contraception methods include the combined oral contraceptive pill (COC), patch, and vaginal ring. These methods have the same mechanism of action, but vary in their delivery systems and dosing intervals, from daily dosing (COCs) to monthly dosing (vaginal ring). Despite excellent efficacy with perfect use, failure rates for typical use are about 9 pregnancies per 100 women and may be higher for adolescents because missed doses are common.
     - **Barrier methods:** The male and female condoms are the only contraceptive methods that also provide protection against STIs. However, condoms have relatively high typical use failure rates for pregnancy prevention and therefore dual contraceptive method use (i.e., hormonal contraception together with a barrier method) should be encouraged.

Upadhya KK: Contraception for adolescents, *Pediatr Rev* 34:384–394, 2013.

143. **What are contraindications to the use of estrogen-containing contraceptive methods?**
     Estrogen is the hormonal component of contraception with the greatest number of medical contraindications. Absolute contraindications that should be screened for before starting an estrogen-containing method include:
     - Migraine headaches with aura
     - Personal history of deep venous thrombosis
     - Known thromboembolic disorder, including lupus with antiphospholipid antibody syndrome and familial factor V Leiden deficiency
     - Untreated hypertension (>160/100)
     - Major surgery with prolonged immobilization
     - Complicated valvular heart disease
     - Coronary artery disease
     - Stroke
     - Acute or chronic liver disease with abnormal liver function
     - Breast, endometrial, or other estrogen-sensitive cancer

Straw F, Porter C: Sexual health and contraception, *Arch Dis Child Educ Pract Ed* 97:177–184, 2012.

144. **How likely are teenagers to use contraception?**
     About 25% of teenagers use no contraception at the time of first intercourse and about two-thirds report using condoms, with or without another contraceptive method. Among sexually experienced adolescent females ages 15 to 19, the majority report having used a contraceptive method, with the condom being the most popular method used (96%), followed by withdrawal (57%), and then the

contraceptive pill (56%). The approximate time between first sex and seeking family planning services for adolescent females is just over 1 year.

145. **Is a pelvic examination mandatory before starting a patient on contraception?**
No. Numerous professional organizations, including the American College of Obstetricians and Gynecologists, concur that a pelvic examination is not required for safe initiation of contraception. A large percentage of teenagers will delay seeking contraceptive care if they believe a pelvic examination is required. Routine pelvic examination and pap smears should begin at age 21, regardless of sexual activity or contraceptive use.

ACOG Committee Opinion No. 463: Cervical cancer in adolescents: screening, evaluation, and management, *Obstet Gynecol* 116:469–472, 2010.

146. **What oral treatment is most commonly used for emergency postcoital contraception?**
Levonorgestrel (Plan B® and generics) is a U.S. FDA-approved progestin-only method, now available in a one-pill formulation (1.5 mg of levonorgestrel) taken as soon as possible after intercourse. This method has been approved for over-the-counter sale (without a prescription) in the United States to all women, regardless of age. Progestin-only emergency contraception acts by inhibiting or delaying ovulation, disrupting follicular development, thickening cervical mucus to impede sperm penetration, and affecting the maturation of the corpus luteum. Levonorgestrel can reduce the risk for pregnancy by at least 75% when given within 72 hours of unprotected intercourse, and studies show that it maintains good efficacy when taken up to 120 hours later. Ulipristal acetate (Ella®) is another FDA-approved emergency contraceptive method available by prescription only in the United States. This method maintains stable efficacy up to 5 days following intercourse. The copper IUD can also be used as emergency contraception when inserted within 5 days of unprotected intercourse and is the most effective method of emergency contraception.

Upadhya KK: Contraception for adolescents, *Pediatr Rev* 34:384–394, 2013.

TEENAGE SUICIDE

147. **What is the main predictor of suicidal ideation in teenagers?**
Depression. Up to 85% of adolescents with major depressive disorder (MDD) or dysthymia (less severe chronic depression) will report suicidal ideation. About one-third will make a suicide attempt sometime during adolescence or young adulthood. This is one of the reasons the AAP has advised screening for depression, including the use of various screening tools, at ages 11 through 21 at all well-visits.

Committee on Practice and Ambulatory Medicine: 2014 Recommendations for Pediatric Preventive Health Care, *Pediatrics* 133:568–570, 2014.
Cash SJ, Bridge JA: Epidemiology of youth suicide and suicidal behavior, *Curr Opin Pediatr* 21:615, 2009.

148. **How often do adolescents attempt suicide in the United States?**
Suicide is the third leading cause of death in youth ages 15 to 24 in the United States, killing about 4600 youth each year. About 12% to 16% of adolescents report ever having contemplated suicide, and 4% to 8% report ever having made a suicide attempt. Among high school students in the United States, the prevalence of suicide attempt remained fairly stable between 1991 through 2011, although suicidal ideation has decreased over the same time period. About 15% to 30% of teens who attempt suicide will re-attempt within 1 year. Suicide attempt is a significant risk factor for completed suicide.

Nock MK, Green JG, Hwang I, et al: Prevalence, correlates, and treatment of lifetime suicidal behavior among adolescents: results from the National Comorbidity Survey Replication Adolescent Supplement, *JAMA Psychiatry* 70:300–310, 2013.

149. **Who are more likely to attempt suicide, males or females?**
Females have greater odds of both suicidal ideation and suicide attempt compared with males. However, males (particularly white males) are much more likely to succeed, due in large part to the choice

of more lethal methods (especially firearms). In younger patients (10 to 14 years), suffocation (such as hanging) is the most common method used.

150. **Which adolescents are at increased risk for suicide?**

Those with any of the following characteristics:

- History of previous attempts, especially those involving very lethal methods and those within the past 2 years
- Psychiatric disorder, especially MDD, bipolar disorder, conduct disorder
- Easy access to firearms (most common location for teenage suicide involving firearms is in the home)
- Substance abuse (both illicit drugs and alcohol)
- Family history of suicide and depression
- Family discord
- Loss of a parent to death or divorce
- History of impulsive aggression (tendency to react to frustration with hostility or aggression)
- Sexual minority (LGBTQ) adolescents, especially if unsupportive family or hostile school environment
- History of physical and/or sexual abuse

Cash SJ, Bridge JA: Epidemiology of youth suicide and suicidal behavior, *Curr Opin Pediatr* 21:613–619, 2009.

CHAPTER 2

BEHAVIOR AND DEVELOPMENT

Mark F. Ditmar, MD

ATTENTION-DEFICIT/HYPERACTIVITY DISORDER

1. **What are the characteristics of attention-deficit/hyperactivity disorder (ADHD)?**
   ADHD is a chronic neurodevelopmental and behavioral disorder, considered to have neurobiologic origins, that is diagnosed on the basis of the number, severity, and duration of three clusters of behavioral problems: *inattention*, *hyperactivity*, and *impulsivity*. It is the most commonly diagnosed behavior disorder in children. According to the *Diagnostic and Statistical Manual of Mental Disorders, 5th edition* (DSM-5), symptoms of inattention, hyperactivity, and impulsivity must have lasted for more than 6 months and be inconsistent with the child's developmental level. These symptoms have to involve more than one setting and result in significant functional impairment at home, school, or in social settings. Some symptoms must have begun before the age of 13 years.

   American Psychiatric Association: Diagnostic and Statistical Manual of Mental Disorders, ed 5, Arlington, VA, 2013, American Psychiatric Association.
   National Resource Center on ADHD: http://www.help4adhd.org. Accessed on Nov. 17, 2014.

2. **How common is ADHD?**
   Community prevalence studies indicate that 4% to 12% of school-age children are affected by ADHD.

3. **Are boys or girls more likely to be diagnosed with ADHD?**
   Males are three to four times more frequently diagnosed with ADHD. Their symptoms tend to be more disruptive, particularly with hyperactivity, whereas girls present more commonly with problems of attention.

4. **Is there a genetic predisposition to ADHD?**
   ADHD has a **high rate of heritability.** In studies of identical twins raised apart, if one twin has ADHD, the other has up to a 75% likelihood of being diagnosed with ADHD. In nonidentical twin studies, the concordance rate is as high as 33%. Studies of siblings of patients with ADHD indicate a 20% to 30% likelihood. About 25% of children with ADHD have at least one parent with symptoms or diagnosis of ADHD. Genome-wide linkage and fine mapping studies support the linkage between ADHD and various chromosomal bands and candidate genes. Genes that regulate dopaminergic pathways are suspected to be involved in the ADHD's pathogenesis.

   Zhang L, Chang S, Li Z, et al: ADHD gene: a genetic database for attention deficit hyperactivity disorder, *Nucleic Acids Res* 40:D1003–D1009, 2012.
   Thapar A, Cooper M, Jefferies R, et al: What causes attention deficit hyperactivity disorder? *Arch Dis Child* 97:260–265, 2012.

5. **What conditions can mimic ADHD?**
   Medical: Lead toxicity, iron deficiency, thyroid dysfunction, visual or hearing impairment, sleep disorders, mass lesions (e.g., hydrocephalus), seizures, complex migraines, fetal alcohol syndrome, fragile X syndrome, Williams syndrome, neurofibromatosis, tuberous sclerosis, medication side effects (e.g., cold preparations, steroids), and substance abuse
   Developmental or learning disorders: Intellectual disability (mental retardation), autistic spectrum disorders, and specific learning disabilities. Central auditory processing difficulties have also been investigated, although it is still unclear as to whether such difficulties are a different disorder or whether they represent the cognitive deficits seen with ADHD.
   Behavioral or emotional disorders: Affective disorders (e.g., dysthymia, bipolar disorder), anxiety disorders, stress reactions (e.g., post-traumatic stress disorder, adjustment disorder), other disruptive behavior disorders (e.g., oppositional defiant disorder), and personality disorders
   Psychosocial factors: Family dysfunction, parenting dysfunction, and abuse

6. **Is there a definitive diagnostic test for ADHD?**
   No. Diagnosis requires evidence of characteristic symptoms occurring in high frequency over an extended period of time. This information, which is ideally obtained from at least two settings or sources (e.g., school and home), can be garnered from observation, narrative histories, and the use of various standardized rating scales.

   American Academy of Pediatrics: ADHD clinical practice guideline for the diagnosis, evaluation, and treatment of attention-deficit/hyperactivity disorder in children and adolescents, *Pediatrics* 128:1007–1022, 2011.

7. **How should ADHD be treated?**
   A multimodal approach is recommended, which may include psychotropic medication, behavioral therapies, family education and counseling, and educational interventions.

   Feldman HM, Reiff MI: Attention deficit-hyperactivity disorder in children and adolescents, *N Engl J Med* 370:838–846, 2014.

8. **What are the best medications for treating ADHD?**
   Stimulant medications (methylphenidate, mixed amphetamine salts, and dextroamphetamine). Randomized, controlled trials support their benefits, usually by demonstrating the improvement of core ADHD symptoms in 70% to 80% of children. Of the 20% to 30% of nonresponders to one medication, about half will respond to the other stimulant. Other medications used to treat ADHD include atomoxetine (a norepinephrine-reuptake inhibitor), α-adrenergic agonists (e.g., clonidine), tricyclic antidepressants, and atypical antidepressants (e.g., bupropion). There is concern about the possible overuse of stimulants in children of all ages.

   Feldman HM, Reiff MI: Attention deficit-hyperactivity disorder in children and adolescents, *N Engl J Med* 370:838–846, 2014.
   Rappley MD: Attention-deficit/hyperactivity disorder, *N Engl J Med* 352:165–173, 2005.

9. **Is a positive response to stimulant medication diagnostic of ADHD?**
   A positive response is not diagnostic because (1) children without symptoms of ADHD given stimulants demonstrate positive responses in sustained and focused attention, and (2) observer bias (i.e., parent or teacher) can be considerable. Thus, many experts recommend a placebo-controlled trial when stimulant medication is used.

   Nahlilk J: Issues in diagnosis of attention-deficit/hyperactivity disorder in adolescents, *Clin Pediatr* 43:1–10, 2004.

10. **Is an electrocardiogram (ECG) required before beginning patients on stimulant medication for ADHD?**
    This is controversial. Case reports of sudden death among pediatric patients treated with ADHD medications prompted the U.S. Food and Drug Administration (FDA) in 2005 to 2006 to issue warnings on stimulant medication use in ADHD patients. The American Heart Association listed the indication for an ECG in this setting as class II, indicating uncertainty as to its need or lack of need. Large studies subsequently did not demonstrate an increased risk compared with the background rate of sudden death.
    Many pediatric cardiologists do not recommend an ECG because, in a population with a very low risk, the ECG as a screening test has low predictive values, both positive and negative.

    Shahani SA, Evans WN, Mayman GA, et al: Attention deficit hyperactivity disorder screening electrocardiograms: a community-based perspective, *Pediatr Cardiol* 35:485–489, 2014.
    Cooper WO, Habel LA, et al: ADHD drugs and serious cardiovascular events in children and young adults, *N Engl J Med* 365:1896–1904, 2011.
    Vetter VL, Elia J, Erickson C, et al: Cardiovascular monitoring of children and adolescents with heart disease receiving stimulant drugs, *Circulation* 117:2407–2423, 2008.

11. **How young is "too young" to diagnose ADHD and prescribe stimulant medications?**
    The American Academy of Pediatrics (AAP) recommends an initial evaluation for ADHD for any child **as young as age 4 years** with academic or behavioral problems and symptoms of inattention, hyperactivity, or impulsivity. Behavior therapy is advised as the first line of treatment, but methylphenidate may be

prescribed if behavior therapy results in no significant improvement and moderate-to-severe disturbance is occurring in the child's function. Treatment of preschool children, however, is controversial.

American Academy of Pediatrics: ADHD clinical practice guideline for the diagnosis, evaluation, and treatment of attention-deficit/hyperactivity disorder in children and adolescents, *Pediatrics* 128(5):1007-1022, 2011.

12. What are the risks for adolescents with ADHD?

Risks for adolescents involve **increased high-risk behaviors,** including higher rates of sexually transmitted infections and pregnancies, and **increased school problems,** including higher rates of grade failure, dropping out, and expulsion. Untreated ADHD has also been found to be a significant risk factor for future substance abuse.

Wolraich ML, Wibbelsman CJ, Brown TE, et al: Attention-deficit/hyperactivity disorder among adolescents: a review of the diagnosis, treatment, and clinical implications, *Pediatrics* 115:1734–1746, 2005.

KEY POINTS: THE "I"SSENTIALS OF ADHD

Inattention
Increased activity
Impulsiveness
Impairment in multiple settings
Inappropriate (for developmental stage)
Incessant (persists for >6 months)

---

13. Does sugar or food additives make children hyperactive?

Although it would be gratifying if complex behavioral problems could be attributable solely or in large measure to dietary causes, the majority of controlled studies have failed to demonstrate any significant exacerbations of symptoms from the intake of sucrose or aspartame.

Millichap JG, Yee MM: The diet factor in attention-deficit/hyperactivity disorder, *Pediatrics* 129:330–337, 2012.

14. Are complementary or alternative medicine (CAM) therapies beneficial for ADHD?

Many are tried by frustrated parents (often unbeknownst to the primary care provider), such as megadose vitamin therapy, herbals, antifungal therapy, and others. However, randomized controlled trials are few and, when done, typically demonstrate no benefit. Although the AAP recommends no specific CAM therapy for ADHD, essential fatty acid (omega-3 and omega-6) supplementation is well tolerated and may be modestly effective in some patients.

Bader A, Adesman A: Complementary and alternative therapies for children and adolescents with ADHD, *Curr Opin Pediatr* 24:760–769, 2012.
Chalon S: The role of fatty acids in the treatment of ADHD, *Neuropharmacology* 57:636–639, 2009.

15. Do children with ADHD become teenagers and adults with ADHD?

Ongoing observations of children initially diagnosed with ADHD note that 70% to 80% will continue to have symptoms present during adolescence and up to 60% will show symptoms as adults. Of the features of ADHD, hyperactivity is the symptom most likely to be outgrown. Inattention, distractibility, and failure to finish things are more likely to persist. Adolescents and adults also have continued problems with anxiety and depression, as well as with tobacco and substance abuse. Motor vehicle infractions, employment difficulties, and intimate relationships have also been described as problematic for adults. Children and adolescents with symptoms of conduct disorder and ADHD are at the highest risk for severe problems as adults.

Harpin VA: The effect of ADHD on the life of an individual, their family, and community from preschool to adult life, *Arch Dis Child* 90:12–17, 2005.
Attention Deficit Disorder Association: http://www.add.org. Accessed on Mar. 23, 2015.

AUTISM

16. **What is the DSM-5?**

The DSM is the *Diagnostic and Statistical Manual of Mental Disorders*, which is published by the American Psychiatric Association on a periodic basis to diagnose and classify mental and behavioral disorders. Criteria for diagnoses are commonly changed to improve diagnostic accuracy based on new research and ongoing psychiatric practice, but classifications can be controversial. The latest version, DSM-5, was released in May 2013. It replaced the DSM-4, which had been introduced in 1994 and had undergone a number of revisions.

Baker JP: Autism at 70—redrawing the boundaries, *N Engl J Med* 369:1089–1091, 2013.

17. **How did classifications change for disorders of autism in the DSM-5?**

Previously, autism spectrum disorders were classified into groups including Asperger syndrome, pervasive developmental disorder, not otherwise specified (PDD-NOS), childhood disintegrative disorder (with developmental deterioration after 24 months of age), and autistic disorder. DSM-5 eliminated these separate subcategories and folded all individual groups into the broader term of autism spectrum disorder (ASD) with two essential features (see question 18). Clinicians rate the severity of autistic features to classify patients.

American Psychiatric Association: *Diagnosis and Statistical Manual of Mental Disorders, ed 5*, Washington, DC, 2013, American Psychiatric Association.
Autism Society of America: http://www.autism-society.org. Accessed on Nov. 17, 2014.
Autism Speaks: http://www.autismspeaks.org. Accessed on Mar. 20, 2015.

18. **What are the two essential features of autism?**

1. *Impaired social interaction and social communication* (e.g., extreme aloneness, failure to make eye contact, deficit in nonverbal communicative behaviors for social interaction, deficits in maintaining and understanding relationships)
2. *Restricted and repetitive patterns of behavior* (e.g., insistence on sameness or inflexible adherence to routines, stereotyped or repetitive responses to objects, narrow range of interests, hyperreactivity to sensory input, unusual interest in sensory aspects of the environment)

KEY POINTS: TWO ESSENTIAL FEATURES OF AUTISM

1. Impaired social interaction and social communication
2. Restricted and repetitive patterns of behavior

19. **Which behaviors of children should arouse suspicion of possible autism?**

- Avoidance of eye contact during infancy ("gaze aversion)"
- Relating to only part of a person's body (e.g., the lap) rather than to the whole person
- Failure to acquire speech or speech acquisition in an unusual manner (e.g., echolalia [repeating another person's speech])
- Failure to respond to name when called
- Spending long periods of time in repetitive activities and fascination with movement (e.g., spinning records, dripping water)
- Failure to look in the same direction when directed by an adult ("gaze monitoring")
- Absence of pointing to show or request something ("protodeclarative pointing")
- Excessively lining up toys or other objects
- Limited pretend or symbolic play

Johnson CP, Myers SM: Identification and evaluation of children with autism spectrum disorders, *Pediatrics* 120:1183–1215, 2007.

20. **When should screening be done for autism?**

The AAP recommends that all children receive autism-specific screening at 18 and 24 months and whenever there is a concern for autism. Younger siblings of patients with autism have a 10- to 20-fold increased risk. Problems with preverbal gestural language and deficits in social skills are present in most children by 18 months of age. Early recognition of autism can lead to earlier intervention, which can improve outcomes markedly. A 20-question M-CHAT-R/F (Modified Checklist for Autism in Toddlers, Revised with Follow-up) will likely become the most commonly used screening questionnaire for children ages 18 to 30 months. Other screening tools are available for children younger and older than this age range.

Robins DL, Casagrande K, Barton M, et al: Validation of the modified checklist for autism in toddlers, revised with follow-up (M-CHAT-R/F), *Pediatrics* 133:37–45, 2014.
Harrington JW, Allen K: The clinician's guide to autism, *Pediatr Rev* 35:62–77, 2014.

21. What studies should be considered in the evaluation of a child with suspected autism?
    - Hearing screening
    - Metabolic screening: Urine for organic acids, serum for lactate, amino acids, ammonia, and very long-chain fatty acids (if developmental regression, intellectual disability, dysmorphic features, hypotonia, vomiting or dehydration, feeding intolerance, early-onset seizures, episodic vomiting)
    - Karyotype, chromosomal microarray analysis, other genetic testing (if dysmorphic features or intellectual disability; more than two dozen genetic syndromes are associated with autism)
    - DNA fragile X analysis (if intellectual disability or phenotype of long, thin face and prominent ears)
    - Electroencephalogram (especially if history of seizures, staring spells, or regression of milestones)
    - Neuroimaging with magnetic resonance imaging (especially if abnormal head shape or circumference, focal neurologic abnormalities, or seizures)
    - Lead level (if history of pica)

Pickler L, Elias E: Genetic evaluation of the child with an autism spectrum disorder, *Pediatr Ann* 38:26–29, 2009.

22. What accounts for the apparent increase in autism in the United States?
    Centers for Disease Control and Prevention (CDC) data published in 2014 indicated a prevalence rate of autism spectrum disorders (ASD) of 1 in 68, which was a 30% increase from 2012 estimates of 1 in 88. While some experts believe the condition *per se* is truly increasing in prevalence, other reasons may include diagnostic substitution (which assumes children were previously characterized as developmentally-delayed rather than having ASD), broadening of the definition of ASD, and better screening and ascertainment. The largest increase in diagnosed cases has occurred among the higher-functioning patients with less severe disease and in black and Hispanic populations.

CDC. Prevalence of autism spectrum disorder among children aged 8 years—autism and developmental disabilities monitoring network, 11 sites, United States, 2010, *MMWR* 63(SS02):1–21, March 28, 2014.
Harrington JW, Allen K: The clinician's guide to autism, *Pediatr Rev* 35:62–77, 2014.

23. Do vaccines cause autism?
    Many claims have been made regarding possible environmental triggers for autism, especially vaccines, particularly measles-mumps-rubella (MMR), and vaccine components, particularly thimerosal (a mercury-containing compound used as a preservative in some vaccines). The Institute of Medicine has found no link between the use of thimerosal or MMR as a cause of autism.

IOM (Institute of Medicine). 2012. *Adverse Effects of Vaccines: Evidence of Causality*. Washington, DC: The National Academies Press, pp 145–153.

24. Does early intervention and/or therapy improve the outcome in children with autism?
    In general, earlier diagnosis and involvement of therapies for children with autism does appear to improve outcomes such as a decreased need for special education in later years and an increase in the chance for independence as an adult. Certain subsets of children with autism, such as those with no coexisting cognitive deficits, will fare better. Additionally, earlier recognition and intervention may assist families in understanding and coping with potentially challenging medical comorbidities and social and behavioral issues.

Zwaigenbaum L, Bryson S, Lord C, et al: Clinical assessment and management of toddlers with suspected autism spectrum disorder: insights from studies of high-risk infants, *Pediatrics* 123:1383–1391, 2009.

BEHAVIOR PROBLEMS

25. What are the most common types of behavior problems in children?
    - **Problems of daily routine** (e.g., food refusal, sleep abnormalities, toilet difficulties)
    - **Aggressive-resistant behavior** (e.g., temper tantrums, aggressiveness with peers)
    - **Overdependent-withdrawing behavior** (e.g., separation upset, fears, shyness)
    - **Hyperactivity**
    - **Undesirable habits** (e.g., thumb-sucking, head banging, nail biting, playing with genitals)
    - **School problems**

Chamberlin RW: Prevention of behavioral problems in young children, *Pediatr Clin North Am* 29:239–247, 1982.

26. How much do babies normally cry each day?
    In Brazelton's oft-quoted 1962 study of 80 infants, it was found that, at 2 weeks of age, the average crying time was nearly 2 hours per day. This increased to nearly 3 hours per day at 6 weeks and then declined to about 1 hour per day at 12 weeks.

Brazelton TB: Crying in infancy, *Pediatrics* 29:579–588, 1962.

27. What is infantile colic?
    Colic is excessive crying or fussiness, which occurs in 5% to 20% of infants depending on the criteria used. For study purposes, it is defined as paroxysms of crying in an otherwise healthy infant for more than 3 hours per day on more than 3 days per week for more than 3 weeks. The typical clinical picture is that of an otherwise healthy and well-fed baby (usually between the ages of 2 weeks and 3 months) who cries intensely and inconsolably for several hours at a time, usually during the late afternoon or evening. Often the infant appears to be in pain and has a slightly distended abdomen, with the legs drawn up; occasional temporary relief occurs if gas is passed.

    The symptoms nearly always resolve by the time the infant is 3 to 4 months old, but the problem can have repercussions, including early discontinuation of breastfeeding, multiple formula changes, heightened maternal anxiety and distress, diminished maternal-infant interaction, and increased risk for child abuse.

28. What causes colic?
    No precise cause has been identified, and the etiology is likely multifactorial. Theories have involved gastrointestinal dysfunction (e.g., intolerance or allergy to cow milk or soy protein, gastroesophageal reflux, lactose intolerance, immaturity of the gastrointestinal tract), neurologic problems (immaturity of the central nervous system [CNS], neurotransmitter imbalance), hormonal processes (e.g., increased serotonin), difficult infant temperament, and interaction problems between the infant and the caregiver (e.g., misinterpreted infant cues, transfer of parental anxiety).

29. Are there any treatments that are useful for colic?
    As is the case for most self-resolving conditions without a known cause, **counseling** is the most effective treatment. However, multiple interventions with minimal effectiveness are often tried, and these often involve the gastrointestinal tract: elimination of cow milk from the breastfeeding mother's diet, formula changes (to soy or to protein hydrolysates), or a trial of herbal tea or simethicone to decrease intestinal gas. Probiotics have been studied as possible remedies, but clinical results are mixed. Medications such as antispasmodics are not recommended because of the risk for side effects. Other sensory modifiers (e.g., car rides, massage, swaddling) are also attempted to provide some course of action until the expected 3- to 4-month resolution.

Chumpitazi BP, Shulman RJ: Five probiotic drops a day to keep infantile colic away? *JAMA Pediatr* 168:204–205, 2014.
Drug and Therapeutics Bulletin: Management of infantile colic, *BMJ* 347:f4102, 2013.

30. What evaluations should be done for the excessively crying infant?
    The infant with acute excessive crying (interpreted by caretakers as differing in quality and persisting beyond a reasonable time, generally 1 to 2 hours, without adequate explanation) can be a taxing problem for pediatricians and emergency room physicians. The differential diagnosis is broad, but infantile colic remains the most common diagnosis (but a diagnosis of exclusion). History and physical examination

make the diagnosis in most infants. However, other tests to consider include stool for occult blood (possible intussusception), fluorescein testing of both eyes (possible corneal abrasion), urinalysis and urine culture (possible urinary tract infection), pulse oximetry (hypoxia from cardiac causes may manifest as increased irritability), and electrolytes and blood glucose (possible endocrine or metabolic disturbance).

Ditmar MF: Crying. In Schwartz MW, editor: *The 5-Minute Pediatric Consult*, ed 6. Philadelphia, 2012, Wolters Kluwer, pp 236–237.
Douglas PS, Hill PS: The crying baby: what approach? *Curr Opin Pediatr* 23:523–529, 2011.

31. How should children be punished?

The goal of punishment should be to teach children that a specific behavior was wrong and to discourage the behavior in the future. To meet this goal, punishment should be consistent and relatively brief. It should be carried out in a calm manner as soon as possible after the infraction. Time-out from ongoing activity and removal of privileges are two punishment techniques that can be used. The use of corporal punishment is controversial. Although spanking and other physical forms of punishment are widely practiced, most developmental authorities argue against their use because they do not foster the internalization of rules of behavior and may legitimize violence.

Larsen MA, Tentis E: The art and science of disciplining children, *Pediatr Clin North Am* 50:817–840, 2003.

32. How valid is the proverb "spare the rod and spoil the child" as a defense for corporal punishment?

The actual biblical proverb (Proverbs 13:24) reads, "He who spares the rod hates his son, but he who loves him is careful to discipline him." Although the proverb has often been used as a justification for spanking, in actuality it does not refer to specific discipline strategies but rather to the need for love and discipline. In addition, the rod may refer to the shepherd's staff, which was used to guide—rather than hit—sheep.

Carey TA: Spare the rod and spoil the child: is this a sensible justification for the use of punishment in child rearing? *Child Abuse Negl* 18:1005–1010, 1994.

33. Is physical injury a concern in children with head banging?

Head banging, which is a common problem that occurs in 5% to 15% of normal children, rarely results in physical injury. When injury does occur, it is usually in children with autism or other developmental disabilities. Normal children often show signs of bliss as they bang away, and the activity usually resolves by the time the child is 4 years old. (It may resume spontaneously during pediatric board examinations.)

34. What is the difference between a "blue" breath-holding spell and a "white" breath-holding spell?

Both are syncopal attacks with involuntary cessation of breathing that occur in up to 4% of children between the ages of 6 months and 4 years.

"Blue" or cyanotic spell: More common. Vigorous crying provoked by physical or emotional upset leads to apnea at end of expiration. This is followed by cyanosis, opisthotonus, rigidity, and loss of tone. Brief convulsive jerking may occur. The episode lasts from 10 to 60 seconds. A short period of sleepiness may ensue.

"White" or pallid spell: More commonly precipitated by an unexpected event that frightens the child. Crying is limited or absent. Breath holding and loss of consciousness occur simultaneously. On testing, children prone to these spells demonstrate increased responsiveness to vagal maneuvers. This parasympathetic hypersensitivity may cause cardiac slowing, diminished cardiac output, and diminished arterial pressure, which result in a pale appearance.

35. When should a diagnosis of seizure disorder be considered rather than a breath-holding spell?

- Precipitating event is minor or nonexistent
- History of no or minimal crying or breath holding
- Episode lasts >1 minute
- Period of post-episode sleepiness lasts >10 minutes

- Convulsive component of episode is prominent and occurs before cyanosis
- Occurs in child <6 months or >4 years old
- Associated with incontinence

36. **Does treatment with iron decrease the frequency of breath-holding spells?**
    In the 1960s, it was observed that children with breath-holding spells had lower hemoglobin levels than controls. Treatment with iron has decreased the frequency of breath-holding spells in some children, most notably those with iron deficiency anemia. Interestingly, some of the children whose breath-holding spells respond to iron are not anemic, and the mechanism by which iron decreases breath-holding spells is not known.

Zehetner AA, Orr N, et al: Iron supplementation for breath-holding attacks in children, *Cochrane Database of Systematic Reviews* (5):CD008132,2010.

37. **When does prolonged thumb-sucking warrant intervention?**
    If frequent thumb-sucking persists in a child who is older than 4 to 5 years or in whom permanent teeth have begun to erupt, treatment is usually indicated. Persistent thumb-sucking after the eruption of permanent teeth can lead to malocclusion.

38. **What treatments are used for thumb-sucking?**
    Treatment commonly has two components: (1) physical modifications such as an application of a substance with an unpleasant taste at frequent intervals (such products are commercially available) and/or use of a thumb splint or glove for nighttime sucking, and (2) behavior modification with positive reinforcement (small rewards) given when a child is observed not sucking his or her thumb. Occlusive dental appliances are generally not needed.

39. **When should "toilet training" be started?**
    When a child has language readiness (use of two-word phrases and two-step commands), understands the cause and effect of toileting, seems to desire independence without worsening oppositional behaviors, and has sufficient motor skills and body awareness, training can be begun. The physical prerequisite of the neurologic maturation of bladder and bowel control usually occurs between 18 and 30 months of age. The child's emotional readiness is often influenced by his or her temperament, parental attitudes, and parent-child interactions. The "potty chair" is typically introduced when the child is between 2 and 3 years old. In the United States, about one-fourth of children achieve daytime continence by 2 years and 98% by 3 years. There are distinct racial disparities regarding parental beliefs. Black parents believe training should be initiated around 18 months compared with 25 months for white parents.

Kaerts N, Van Hal G, et al: Readiness signs used to define the proper moment to start toilet training: a review of the literature, *Neurourol Urodyn* 31:437–440, 2012.
Horn IB, Brenner R, Rao M, et al: Beliefs about the appropriate age for initiating toilet training: are there racial and socioeconomic differences? *J Pediatr* 149:165–168, 2006.

40. **Are girls or boys toilet trained earlier?**
    On average, **girls** are toilet trained earlier than boys. With regard to most other developmental milestones during the first years of life, however, there do not appear to be significant sex differences (i.e., in walking or running, sleep patterns, or verbal ability). Girls do show more rapid bone development.

CRANIAL DISORDERS

41. **How many fontanels are present at birth?**
    Although there are six fontanels present at birth (two anterior lateral, two posterior lateral, one anterior, and one posterior), only two (the anterior and posterior fontanels) are usually palpable on physical examination (Fig. 2-1).

42. **When does the anterior fontanel close?**
    On the basis of studies using physical exam, classic teaching indicated between 10 and 14 months. However, computed tomography (CT) scans indicate that closure is quite variable and occurs later than previously thought. Only 16% of anterior fontanels are closed at 10 months, 50% at 16 months and 88%

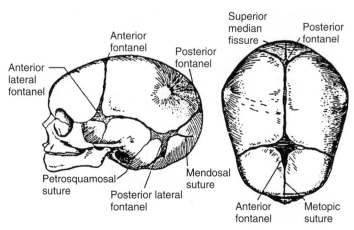

Figure 2-1. The cranium at birth, showing major sutures and fontanels. No attempt is made to show molding or overlapping of bones, which sometimes occurs at birth. *(From Silverman FN, Kuhn JP, editors:* Caffey's Pediatric X-ray Diagnosis, *ed 9. St. Louis, 1993, Mosby, p 5.)*

at 20 months. Thus, about 10% of normal infants may not have complete closure until 20 to 24 months of age. Of note, 3% to 5% of normal infants have closure at 5 to 6 months.

Pindrik F, Ye X, Ji BG, et al: Anterior fontanelle closure and size in full-term children based on head computed tomography, *Clin Pediatr* 53:1149–1157, 2014.

43. Which conditions are most commonly associated with premature or delayed closure of the fontanel?
Premature closure: Microcephaly, high calcium-to-vitamin D ratio in pregnancy, craniosynostosis, hyperthyroidism, or variation of normal
Delayed closure: Achondroplasia, Down syndrome, increased intracranial pressure, familial macrocephaly, rickets, or variation of normal

44. When is an anterior fontanel too big?
The size of the fontanel can be calculated using the formula: (length + width)/2, where length equals anterior-posterior dimension and width equals transverse dimension. However, there is wide variability in the normal size range of the anterior fontanel. Mean fontanel size on day 1 of life is 2.1 cm, with an upper limit of normal of 3.6 cm in white infants and 4.7 cm in black infants. These upper limits may be helpful for identifying disorders in which a large fontanel may be a feature (e.g., hypothyroidism, hypophosphatasia, skeletal dysplasias, increased intracranial pressure). Of note is that the posterior fontanel is normally about the size of a fingertip or smaller in 97% of full-term newborns.

Kiesler J, Ricer R: The anterior fontanel, *Am Fam Physician* 67:2547–2552, 2003.

45. What are the types of primary craniosynostosis?
Craniosynostosis is the premature fusion of various cranial suture lines that results in the ridging of the sutures, asymmetric growth, and deformity of the skull. Suture lines (with resultant disorders listed in parentheses) include sagittal (scaphocephaly or dolichocephaly); coronal (brachycephaly); unilateral, coronal, or lambdoidal (plagiocephaly); and metopic (trigonocephaly). Multiple fused sutures can result in a high and pointed skull (oxycephaly or acrocephaly) (Fig. 2-2).

46. What is the most common type of primary craniosynostosis?
Sagittal (60%); coronal synostosis accounts for 20% of cases.

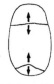

Normocephaly   Dolichocephaly   Trigonocephaly   Plagiocephaly

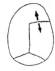

Plagiocephaly   Brachycephaly

Figure 2-2. Types of primary craniosynostosis.

47. What causes craniosynostosis?

Most cases of isolated craniosynostosis have no known etiology. *Primary* craniosynostosis may be observed as part of craniofacial syndromes, including Apert, Crouzon, and Carpenter syndromes. *Secondary* causes can include abnormalities of calcium and phosphorus metabolism (e.g., hypophosphatasia, rickets); hematologic disorders (e.g., thalassemia), mucopolysaccharidoses, and hyperthyroidism. Inadequate brain growth (e.g., microcephaly) can lead to craniosynostosis.

Williams H: Lumps, bumps and funny shaped heads, *Arch Dis Child Educ Pract Ed* 93:120–128, 2008.

48. What is positional or deformational plagiocephaly?

Since the implementation of the "back-to-sleep" program by the AAP in 1992 to reduce the risk for sudden infant death syndrome (SIDS), an estimated 13% to 20% of infants develop occipital flattening (posterior or lambdoidal plagiocephaly) due to transient calvarial deformation from prolonged supine sleeping positions. The condition can be prevented by varying the infant's head position during sleep and feeding and by observing prone positioning ("tummy time)" for at least 5 minutes daily during the first 6 weeks of life. Therapy for severe cases consists of repositioning; physiotherapy; and rarely, surgery. Helmet therapy, while widely used, has not been shown to be effective in one randomized study.

van Wijk RM, van Vlimmeren LA, Groothuis-Oudshoorn CGM, et al: Helmet therapy in infants with positional skull deformation: randomised controlled trial, *BMJ* 348:2741, 2014.
American Academy of Pediatrics Committee on Practice and Ambulatory Medicine: Prevention and management of positional skull deformities in infants, *Pediatrics* 128:1236–1241, 2011.

49. How is positional plagiocephaly differentiated from plagiocephaly caused by craniosynostosis?

Synostotic lambdoidal plagiocephaly is much more rare. It is usually associated with ridging of the involved suture lines, and it causes a different pattern of frontal bossing and ear displacement when the infant's head is viewed from above (Fig. 2-3).

50. What conditions are associated with skull softening?

- Cleidocranial dysostosis
- Craniotabes
- Lacunar skull (associated with spina bifida and major CNS anomalies)
- Osteogenesis imperfecta
- Multiple wormian bones (associated with hypothyroidism, hypophosphatasia, and chronic hydrocephalus)
- Rickets

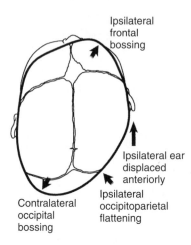
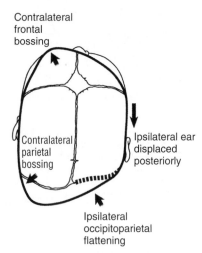

Figure 2-3. Factors distinguishing *(left)* positional plagiocephaly from *(right)* lambdoidal craniosynostosis. *(From Kabbani H, Raghuveer TS: Craniosynostosis, Am Fam Physician 69:2866, 2004.)*

51. What is the significance of craniotabes?

In this condition, abnormally soft, thin skull bones buckle under pressure and recoil like a ping-pong ball. It is best elicited on the parietal or frontal bones and is often associated with rickets in infancy. It may also be seen in hypervitaminosis A, syphilis, and hydrocephalus. Craniotabes may be a normal finding during the first 3 months of life.

52. What evaluations should be done in a child with microcephaly?

The extent of evaluation depends on various factors: prenatal versus postnatal acquisition, presence of minor or major anomalies, developmental problems, and neurologic abnormalities. The diagnosis can be as straightforward as a simple familial variant (autosomal dominant) in a child with normal intelligence, or it can range to a variety of conditions associated with abnormal brain growth (e.g., intrauterine infections, heritable syndromes, chromosomal abnormalities). Evaluation may include the following:

- Parental head-size measurements
- Ophthalmologic evaluation (abnormal optic nerve or retinal findings may be found in various syndromes)
- Genetic testing (e.g., karyotype, chromosomal microarray analysis)
- Neuroimaging (cranial magnetic resonance imaging (MRI) or CT to evaluate for structural abnormalities or intracranial calcifications)
- Metabolic screening
- Cultures and serology if suspected intrauterine infection (e.g., cytomegalovirus)

Von der Hagen M, Pivarcsi M, et al: Diagnostic approach to microcephaly in childhood: a two-center study and review of the literature, *Dev Med Child Neuro* 56: 732–741, 2014.

53. What are the three main general causes of macrocephaly?

- **Increased intracranial pressure:** Caused by dilated ventricles (e.g., progressive hydrocephalus of various causes), subdural fluid collections, intracranial tumors, or idiopathic intracranial hypertension (i.e., pseudotumor cerebri)
- **Thickened skull:** Caused by cranioskeletal dysplasias (e.g., osteopetrosis) and various anemias
- **Megalencephaly** (enlarged brain): May be familial or syndromic (e.g., Sotos syndrome) or caused by storage diseases, leukodystrophies, or neurocutaneous disorders (e.g., neurofibromatosis)

DENTAL DEVELOPMENT AND DISORDERS

54. When do primary and permanent teeth erupt?

Mandibular teeth usually erupt first. The central incisors appear by the age of 5 to 7 months, with about 1 new tooth per month thereafter until 23 to 30 months, at which time the second molars (and thus all 20 primary or deciduous teeth) are in place. Of the 32 permanent teeth, the central incisors erupt first between 5 and 7 years, and the third molars are in place by 17 to 22 years.

American Academy of Pediatric Dentistry: http://www.aapd.org. Accessed on Nov. 17, 2014.

55. What is the significance of natal teeth?

Occasionally, teeth are present at birth (natal teeth) or erupt within 30 days after birth (neonatal teeth). When x-rays are taken, 95% of natal teeth are primary incisors, and 5% are supernumerary teeth or extra teeth. Very sharp teeth that can cause tongue lacerations and very loose teeth that can be aspirated should be removed. Females are affected more commonly than males, and the prevalence is 1 in 2000 to 3500. Most cases are familial and without consequence, but natal teeth can be associated with genetic syndromes, including the Ellis-van Creveld and Hallermann-Streiff syndromes.

56. How common is the congenital absence of teeth?

The congenital absence of primary teeth is very rare, but up to 25% of individuals may have an absence of one or more third molars, and up to 5% may have an absence of another secondary or permanent tooth (most commonly the maxillary lateral incisors and mandibular second premolar).

57. What are mesiodentes?

These are **peg-shaped supernumerary teeth** that occur in up to 5% of individuals, and they are most commonly situated in the maxillary midline. They should be considered for removal because they interfere with the eruption of permanent incisors.

58. What is the significance of an infant presenting with a single central upper tooth?

A solitary median maxillary central incisor (Fig. 2-4) may be associated with developmental defects, short stature (due to growth hormone deficiency), mild craniofacial dysmorphology and intellectual disability. It is another example of a midline defect having potential significance regarding accompanying CNS abnormalities.

Viana ES, Kramer PF, Closs LQ, Scalco G: Solitary median maxillary central incisor syndrome and holoprosencephaly: a case report, *Pediatr Dent* 32:424–427, 2010.

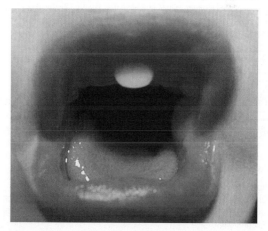

Figure 2-4. Central maxillary incisor. *(From Zitelli BJ, Davis HW: Atlas of Pediatric Physical Diagnosis, ed 5, Philadelphia, 2011, Mosby Elsevier, p 353.)*

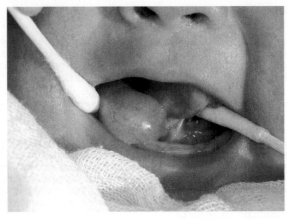

Figure 2-5. Sublingual ranula of right floor mouth in 1-month infant. *(From Zhi K, Wen Y, Ren W, Zhang Y: Management of infant ranula,* Int J Pediatr Otolaryngol *72:823–826, 2008.)*

59. **What is a ranula?**
    A large **mucocele,** usually bluish, painless, soft, and unilateral, that occurs under the tongue. (Fig. 2-5) Most of these self-resolve. If a patient has a large one, surgical marsupialization can be done. If the ranula is recurrent, excision may be needed.

60. **Where are Epstein pearls located?**
    These white, superficial, mobile nodules are usually midline and often paired on the hard palate in many newborns. They are keratin-containing cysts that are asymptomatic, do not increase in size, and usually exfoliate spontaneously within a few weeks.

61. **What is the most common chronic disease of childhood?**
    Early childhood dental caries affect nearly half of children ages 2 to 11 years, which is 2½ times the rate of obesity, 4 times the rate of asthma, and 7 times the rate of allergic rhinitis. By 17 years of age, only 15% to 20% of individuals are free from dental caries, and the average child has 8 decayed, missing, or filled tooth surfaces. Prevention of dental caries involves a decrease in the frequency of tooth exposure to carbohydrates (frequency is more important than total amount), the use of fluoride supplements at age 6 months for children whose water supply is deficient in fluoride, application of fluoride varnish to all infants and children beginning at the age of primary tooth eruption, increased brushing of the teeth, and the use of dental sealants.

    Moyer V: Prevention of dental caries in children from birth through age 5 years: US Preventive Services Task Force recommendation statement, *Pediatrics* 133:1102–1111, 2014.

62. **What are milk-bottle caries?**
    Frequent contact of cariogenic liquids (e.g., milk, formula, breast milk, juice) with teeth, as occurs in infants who fall asleep with a bottle or who are breastfed frequently at night after the age of 1 year ("nursing caries"), has been associated with a significant increase in the development of caries (Fig. 2-6). The AAP recommends that infants not be put to sleep with a bottle (unless it is filled with water), that nocturnal ad lib breastfeeding be limited as dental development progresses, and that cup feedings be introduced when the child is 1 year old.

63. **How does fluoride minimize the development of dental caries?**
    - Topical fluoride from toothbrushing is thought to increase the remineralization of enamel.
    - Bacterial fermentation of sugar into acid plays a major role in the development of caries, and fluoride inhibits this process.
    - As teeth are developing, fluoride incorporates into the hydroxyapatite crystal of enamel, thereby making it less soluble and less susceptible to erosion.

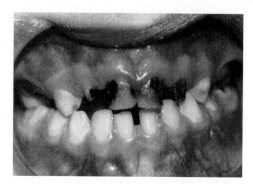

Figure 2-6. Classic nursing bottle decay involving the maxillary anterior teeth. Mandibular incisors are protected by the tongue during feeding and are usually caries free. *(From Gessner IH, Victorica BE:* Pediatric Cardiology: A Problem-Oriented Approach, *Philadelphia, 1993, WB Saunders, p 232.)*

64. **What is fluorosis?**

Exposure to excessive levels of fluoride during tooth development, primarily in a patient younger than 8 years, can damage enamel, causing changes that range from mild (lacy white markings) to severe (pitting, mottling, striations).

65. **How long should fluoride supplementation be continued?**

Fluoride supplementation should continue until a child is 14 to 16 years old, when the third molar crowns are completely calcified.

KEY POINTS: DENTAL PROBLEMS

1. Prolonged pacifier use beyond the age of 18 months can result in oral and dental distortions.
2. Dental caries is the most common chronic disease of childhood.
3. Appropriate use of fluoride and dental sealants could prevent caries in most children.
4. Use of formula or breastfeeding at bedtime after dental eruption leads to higher incidences of caries.
5. Excessive fluoride is associated initially with a white, speckled, or lacy appearance of the enamel.

66. **How effective are dental sealants for preventing cavities?**

Dental sealants may reduce the development of caries by up to 80% compared with rates in untreated teeth. Although fluoride acts primarily by protecting smooth surfaces, dental sealants (commonly bisphenol A and glycidyl methacrylate) act by protecting the pits and fissures of the surface, especially in posterior teeth. Reapplication may be needed every 2 years. As a preventive dental procedure, it is relatively underused.

67. **How common is gingivitis in children?**

Gingivitis is **extremely common,** affecting nearly 50% of children. The disorder is usually painless and is manifested by the bluish-red discoloration of gums, which are swollen and bleed easily. The cause is bacteria in plaque deposits between teeth; the cure is improved dental hygiene and daily flossing.

68. **What is the largest health-related expense before adulthood for normally developing children?**

Dental braces. More than 50% of children have dental malocclusions that could be improved with treatment, but only 10% to 20% have severe malocclusions that require treatment. For others, the costs and benefits of braces need to be weighed individually. Besides the financial expense, the costs of braces include physical discomfort and some increases in the risk for tooth decay and periodontal disease.

69. **What causes halitosis is children?**

Halitosis (bad breath) is usually the result of oral factors, including microbial activity on the dorsal tongue and between the teeth. Conditions associated with postnasal drip, including chronic sinusitis, upper and lower respiratory tract infections, and various systemic diseases, are also causes.

Amir E, Shimonov R, Rosenberg M: Halitosis in children, *J Pediatr* 134:338–343, 1999.

70. Pacifiers: friend or foe?

Pros: Appear to reduce the risk for SIDS (for this reason, use in infancy is now encouraged by the AAP after breastfeeding is well established or shortly after birth in formula-fed infants); role as soother

Cons: May (or may not) promote early discontinuation of breastfeeding; may modestly increase the risk for otitis media; if improperly cleaned, may serve as bacterial reservoir; with two-piece design, potential for aspiration; potential for compulsive use (pacifier addiction); persistent use (years) can interfere with normal teeth positioning.

Home RSC, Hauck FR, Moon RY, et al: Dummy (pacifier) use and sudden infant death syndrome: Potential advantages and disadvantages, *J Paediatr Child Health* 50:170–174, 2014.

O'Connor NR, Tanabe KO, et al: Pacifiers and breastfeeding: a systematic review, *Arch Pediatr Adolesc Med* 163:378–382, 2009.

DEVELOPMENTAL ASSESSMENT

71. What aspects of development are typically monitored?
    - Motor skills (gross and fine motor)
    - Speech and language
    - Activities of daily living (social and personal)
    - Cognition

Bellman M, Byrne O, Sege R: Developmental assessment of children, *BMJ* 346:8687, 2013.

72. What are primitive reflexes?

Primitive reflexes are *automatisms* that are usually triggered by an external stimulus. They are thought to emanate from primitive regions of the CNS: the spine, the inner ear labyrinths, and the brainstem. Examples are rooting, which is triggered by touching the corner of the mouth, and the asymmetric tonic neck reflex (ATNR), which is triggered by rotating the head. Some reflexes (e.g., rooting, sucking, and grasp) have survival value. Others, such as the ATNR or the tonic labyrinthine reflex, have no obvious purpose. Placing and stepping reflexes usually disappear by 2 months. Moro and grasp reflexes and the ATNR usually disappear by 5 months.

73. What three primitive reflexes, if persistent beyond 4 to 6 months, can interfere with the development of the ability to roll, sit, and use both hands together?
    - **Moro reflex:** Sudden neck extension results in extension, abduction, and then adduction of the upper extremities with flexion of fingers, wrists, and elbows.
    - **ATNR:** In a calm supine infant, turning of the head laterally results in relative extension of the arm and leg on the side of the turn and flexion of both on the side away from the turn (the "fencer" position).
    - **Tonic labyrinthine reflex:** In an infant who is being held suspended in the prone position, flexion of the neck results in shoulder protraction and hip flexion, whereas neck extension causes shoulder retraction and hip extension.

Zafeiriou DI: Primitive reflexes and postural reactions in the neurodevelopmental examination, *Pediatr Neurol* 31:1–8, 2004.

74. At what age do children develop handedness?

Usually by **18 to 24 months.** Hand preference is usually fixed by the time a child is 5 years old. Handedness before 1 year may be indicative of a problem with the nonpreferred side (e.g., hemiparesis, brachial plexus injury).

75. What percentage of children are left-handed?

Various studies put the prevalence at **between 7% and 10%.** However, in former premature infants without cerebral palsy, the rate increases to 20% to 25%. Although antecedent brain injury has been hypothesized to account for this increase in prevalence of left-handedness, studies of unilateral intraventricular hemorrhage and handedness have not demonstrated a relationship. Of note is that animals such as mice, dogs, and cats show paw preferences, but, in these groups, 50% prefer the left paw and 50% prefer the right paw.

Marlow N, Roberts BL, Cooke RW: Laterality and prematurity, *Arch Dis Child* 64:1713–1716, 1989.

76. **Are there ethnic differences in development in the first year of life?**
Yes. Even after correcting for potential variables such as social, economic, environmental, and household characteristics, ethnic differences in the attainment of developmental milestones occur. A large-scale population-based study in the United Kingdom found that Indian, black Caribbean, and black African children were much less likely to show delays in gross motor milestones compared with white children.

Kelly Y, Sacker A, et al: Ethnic differences in achievement of developmental milestones by 9 months of age: The Millennium Cohort Study, *Dev Med Child Neurol* 48:825–830, 2006.

77. **What are the major developmental landmarks for motor skills during the first 2 years of life?**
See Table 2-1.

Table 2-1 Major Developmental Landmarks for Motor Skills

DEVELOPMENTAL LANDMARK	AGE RANGE (MO)
Major Gross Motor	
Steadiness of head when placed in supported position	1-4
Sits without support for >30 seconds	5-8
Cruises or walks holding on to things	7-13
Stands alone	9-16
Walks alone	9-17
Walks up stairs with help	12-23
Major Fine Motor	
Grasp	2-4
Reach	3-5
Transfers objects from hand to hand	5-7
Fine pincer grasp with index finger and thumb apposition	9-14
Spontaneous scribbling	12-24

78. **How valuable is the timing of crawling as a marker of development?**
Crawling is one of the least valuable milestones because there is enormous variability in the timing of crawling. A significant percentage of normal infants never crawl before walking.

Wong K: Crawling may be unnecessary for normal child development, *Scientific American* 301: 11, 2009.

79. **What are the most common causes of gross motor delay?**
Normal variation is the most common, followed by **mental retardation. Cerebral palsy** is a distant third, and all other conditions combined (e.g., spinal muscular atrophy, myopathies) run a distant fourth. The most common pathologic cause of gross motor delay is mental retardation (MR), although most children with this condition have normal gross motor milestones.

80. **What are major red flags that a child's development is abnormal?**
Presence of:
* loss of developmental skills at any age
* parental concerns about a child's vision or ability to follow objects

- persistently low muscle tone or floppiness
- no speech (or other efforts to communicate) by 18 months
- asymmetry of movements
- persistent toe walking
- evidence of microcephaly or macrocephaly, particularly if discordant with parental head circumference percentiles

Inability to:
- sit unsupported by 12 months
- walk by 18 months (boys) or 2 years (girls)
- walk other than on tiptoes
- run by 2½ years
- reach for objects by 6 months (corrected for prematurity, if applicable)
- point at objects to demonstrate to others by 2 years

Bellman M, Byrne O, Sege R: Developmental assessment of children, *BMJ* 346:8692, 2013.

81. **What features suggest a possible metabolic cause for disordered development?**
    - Parental consanguinity
    - Family history of unexplained death in childhood
    - Progressive or intermittent symptoms (such as vomiting), which are unexplained
    - Symptom-free intervals
    - Slowing of developmental skill acquisition
    - Loss of skills
    - Evidence of encephalopathy (e.g., personality changes, periods of lethargy)
    - Specific phenotype
    - Coarse facial features
    - Organomegaly

Horridge KA: Assessment and investigation of the child with disordered development, *Arch Dis Child Educ Pract Ed* 96:9–20, 2011.

82. **Do infant walkers promote physical strength or development of the lower extremities?**
    No. On the contrary, published data confirm that infants in walkers actually manifest mild but statistically significant gross motor delays. Infants with walkers were found to sit and crawl later than those without walkers. However, most walk unaided within a normal time frame. Safety hazards can include head trauma, fractures, burns, finger entrapments, and dental injuries. Most of the serious injuries involve falls down stairs.

Pin TP, Eldridge B, Galea MP: A review of the effects of sleep position, play position and equipment use on motor development in infants, *Dev Med Child Neuro* 49:858–867, 2007.

83. **Do twins develop at a rate that is comparable to infants of single birth?**
    Twins exhibit **significant verbal and motor delay** during the first year of life. The difficulty lies not in the lack of potential but in the relative lack of individual stimulation. In general, children who are more closely spaced in a family have slower acquisition of verbal skills. Twins with significant language delay or with excessive use of "twin language" (language understood only by the twins themselves) may be candidates for interventional therapy.

84. **Do premature infants develop at the same rate as term infants?**
    For the most part, premature infants do develop at the same rate as term infants. In ongoing developmental assessments, they eventually "catch up" to their chronologic peers, not by accelerated development, but rather through the arithmetic of time. As they age, their degree of prematurity (in months) becomes less of a percentage of their chronologic age. Early in life, the extent of prematurity is key and must be taken into account during assessments. Such "correction factors" are generally unnecessary after the age of 2 to 3 years, depending on the degree of prematurity.

85. **When can an infant smell?**

The sense of smell is present **at birth.** Newborn infants show preferential head turning toward gauze pads soaked with their mother's milk as opposed to the milk of another woman. The same holds for axillary odor. In one study, infants exposed to familiar odors before heel-stick procedures had lower pain responses.

Marin MM, Rapisardi G, Tani F: Two-day-old newborn infants recognise their mother by her axillary odour, *Acta Paediatr* 104:237–240, 2015.

Goubet N, Strasbaugh K, Chesney J: Familiarity breeds content? Soothing effect of a familiar odor on full-term newborns, *J Dev Behav Pediatr* 28:189–194, 2007.

86. **What are the best measures of cognitive development?**

Ideally, cognitive development should be assessed in a fashion that is free of motor requirements. **Receptive language** is the best measure of cognitive function. Even an eye blink or a voluntary eye gaze can be used to assess cognition independently of motor disability. Adaptive skills such as tool use (e.g., spoon, crayon) are also useful, although they may be delayed because of purely motoric reasons. Gross motor milestones such as walking raise concerns about MR if they are delayed, but normal gross motor milestones cannot be used to infer normal cognitive development.

87. **What do the stages of play tell us about a child's development?**

A well-taken history of a child's play is a valuable adjunct to more traditional milestones such as language and adaptive skills (Table 2-2).

Table 2-2 Play Activity and Child Development

AGE RANGE (MO)	PLAY ACTIVITY	UNDERLYING SKILLS
3	Midline hand play	Sensorimotor; self-discovery
4-5	Bats at objects	Ability to affect environment
6-7	Directed reaching; transfers	
7-9	Banging and mouthing objects	
12	Casting ("I throw it down, and you pick it up for me"); explores objects by visual inspection and handling rather than orally	Object permanence; social reciprocity; use of pointing, joint attention (eye gaze), and simple language to effect response in caregiver
16-18+	Stacking and dumping; exploring; lids; light switches; simple mechanical toys (jack-in-the-box; shape ball)	Means-ends behavior: experimenting with causality
24	Imitative play ("helping" with the dishes; doll play with a physical doll)	Language and socialization; development of "inner language"
36	Make-believe play (e.g., doll play with a pillow to represent the doll)	Distinguish between "real" and "not real"
48	Simple board games, rule-based playground games (e.g., "tag")	Concrete operations (Piaget)

Data from http://www.parentcenter.com. Accessed on Nov. 17, 2014.

88. **What can one learn about a child's developmental level with regard to the use of a crayon?**

A lot. At less than 9 months, the infant will use the crayon as a teething object. Between 10 and 14 months, the infant will make marks on a piece of paper, almost as a by-product of holding the crayon and "banging" it against the paper. By 14 to 16 months, the infant will make marks spontaneously, and by 18 to 20 months, he or she will make marks with vigorous scribbling. By 20 to 22 months, an infant will begin copying specific geometric patterns as presented by the examiner (Table 2-3). The ability to execute these figures requires visual-perceptual, fine-motor, and cognitive abilities. Delay in the ability to complete these tasks suggests difficulty with one or more of these underlying streams of development.

Table 2-3 Crayon Use and Development Level

AGE	TASK
20-22 mo	Alternates from scribble to stroke on imitation of examiner
27-30 mo	Alternates from horizontal to vertical on imitation of examiner
36 mo	Copies circle from illustration
3 yr	Copies cross
4 yr	Copies square
5 yr	Copies triangle
6 yr	Copies "Union Jack"

89. What is the value of the Goodenough-Harris drawing test?
This "draw a person" test is a screening tool used to evaluate a child's cognition and intellect, visual perception, and visual-motor integration. The child is asked to draw a person, and a point is given for each body part drawn with pairs (e.g., legs) that is considered as one part. An average child that is 4 years and 9 months will draw a person with three parts; most children by the age of 5 years and 3 months will draw a person with six parts.

90. What are key physical exam features in the evaluation of a child with possible developmental delay?
- *Head circumference:* possible microcephaly or macrocephaly
- *Dysmorphic features:* possible genetic, metabolic, or syndromic conditions
- *Skin abnormalities* (e.g., café au lait spots, neurofibromas): possible neurocutaneous syndrome
- *Observations of movements* (e.g., unsteadiness, weakness, spasticity): possible underlying neurologic disorder
- *Assessment of tone, strength, and reflexes:* possible underlying neurologic disorder
- *Eye examination* (e.g., nystagmus, cataract): possible disorder of vision due to neurologic disorder
- *Liver size* (e.g., hepatomegaly): possible metabolic disorder

Bellman M, Byrne O, Sege R: Developmental assessment of children, *BMJ* 346:8687, 2013.

91. In infants with global developmental delay, what are the likely causes?
The majority of patients have an antenatal or perinatal insult (e.g., intrauterine infection), but 1% with global delay may have an inborn error of metabolism and 3.5% to 10% have a chromosomal disorder.

Shevell M, Ashwal S, Donley D, et al: Practice parameter: evaluation of the child with global developmental delay. Report of the Quality Standards Committee of the American Academy of Neurology and the Practice Committee of the Child Neurology Society, *Neurology* 60:367–380, 2003.

92. What factors increase the likelihood of finding a potentially progressive disease in patients with global delay?
- Affected family member
- Parental consanguinity
- Organomegaly
- Absent tendon reflexes

Fenichel GM: *Clinical Pediatric Neurology,* ed 6. Elsevier, 2009, Philadelphia, p 121.

LANGUAGE DEVELOPMENT AND DISORDERS

93. What are average times for the development of expressive, receptive, and visual language milestones?
See Table 2-4.

Table 2-4 Development of Expressive, Receptive, and Visual Language

AGE (MO)	EXPRESSIVE	RECEPTIVE	VISUAL
0-3	Coo	Alerts to voice	Recognizes parents; visual tracking
4-6	Monosyllabic babbling, laugh, "raspberry"	Turns to voice and sounds	Responds to facial expressions
7-9	Polysyllabic babbling; mama/dada, nonspecific	Recognizes own name; inhibits to command "No"	Imitates games (patty cake; peek-a-boo)
10-12	Mama/dada specific; first word other than mama/dada or names of other family members or pets	Follows at least 1 one-step command without a gestural cue (e.g., "Come here," "Give me")	Points to desired objects
16-18	Uses words to indicate wants	Follows many one-step commands; points to body parts on command	
22-24	Two-word phrases	Follows two-step commands	
30	Telegraphic speech	Follows prepositional commands	
36	Simple sentences		

94. **What are signs of significantly delayed receptive and expressive speech warranting evaluation?**
See Table 2-5.

American Speech-Language-Hearing Association: http://www.asha.org. Accessed on Mar. 24, 2015.

95. **Do deaf infants babble?**
Yes. Babbling begins at about the same time in both deaf and hearing infants, but deaf infants stop babbling without the normal progression to meaningful communicative speech.

Locke JL: Babbling and early speech: continuity and individual differences, *First Language* 9:191–205, 1989.
Laurent Clerc National Deaf Education Center: http://clerccenter.gallaudet.edu. Accessed on Nov. 17, 2014.

96. **At what age does a child's speech become intelligible?**
Intelligibility increases by about 25% per year. A 1-year-old child has about 25% intelligibility, a 2-year-old has 50%, a 3-year-old has 75%, and a 4-year-old has 100%. Significantly delayed intelligibility should prompt a hearing and language evaluation.

97. **What are the most common causes of so-called delayed speech?**
The most common causes of speech or language delay include the following: developmental language disorders (i.e., normal cognition, impaired intelligibility, and delayed emergence of phrases, sentences, and grammatical markers), intellectual disability, hearing loss, and autistic spectrum disorder.

Feldman HM: Evaluation and management of language and speech disorders in preschool children, *Pediatr Rev* 26:131–142, 2005.

98. **What risk factors make hearing loss more likely in a newborn or young infant?**
- Craniofacial anomaly
- Family history of permanent childhood hearing loss

Table 2-5 Signs of Speech-Language Problems Absolutely Needing Further Evaluation

AT AGE (MO)	RECEPTIVE	EXPRESSIVE
15	Does not look/point at 5 to 10 objects/people named by parent	Not using 3 words
18	Does not follow simple commands ("roll the ball")	No use of single words (including mama, dada)
24	Does not point to pictures or body parts when they are named	Single-word vocabulary of ≤10 words
30	Does not verbally respond or nod/shake head to questions	Not using unique 2-word phrases, including noun-verb combinations; unintelligible speech
36	Does not understand prepositions or action words; does not follow 2-step directions	Vocabulary <200 words; does not ask for things by name; echolalia to questions; regression of language after acquiring 2-word phrases

Data from Harlor ADB Jr, Bower C, et al: Clinical report—hearing assessment in infants and children: recommendations beyond neonatal screening, Pediatrics 124:1252–1263, 2009; and Schum RL: Language screening in the pediatric office setting, Pediatr Clin North Am 54:432, 2007.

- Head trauma requiring hospitalization
- *In utero* infections (such as cytomegalovirus [CMV], herpes, rubella, syphilis, toxoplasmosis)
- Neonatal intensive care unit (NICU) care for >5 days
- Need for extracorporeal membrane oxygenation (ECMO) therapy
- Exposure to ototoxic medications (gentamicin, tobramycin, furosemide)
- Hyperbilirubinemia that required exchange transfusion
- Stigmata of a syndrome associated with hearing loss

Yelverton JC, Dominguez LM, Chapman DA, et al: Risk factors associated with unilateral hearing loss, *JAMA Otolaryngol Head Neck Surg* 139:59–63, 2013.

99. **What causes flat tympanograms?**

Tympanometry is an objective measurement of the compliance of the tympanic membrane and the middle ear compartment that involves varying the air pressure in the external ear canal from about −200 to +400 mm H_2O while measuring the reflected energy of a simultaneous acoustic tone. A normal tracing looks like an inverted "V" with the peak occurring at an air pressure of 0 mm H_2O; this indicates a functionally normal external canal, an intact tympanic membrane, and a lack of excess of middle ear fluid. Flat tympanograms occur with perforation of the tympanic membrane, occlusion of the tympanometry probe against the wall of the canal, obstruction of the canal by a foreign body or impaction by cerumen, or large middle ear effusion. Flat tympanograms due to middle ear effusion are usually associated with a 20- to 30-dB conductive hearing loss, although in occasional instances, the loss may be as great as 50 dB.

100. **A toddler with a bifid uvula and hypernasal speech most likely has what condition?**

Velopharyngeal insufficiency with a possible submucosal cleft palate. The velum (soft palate) moves posteriorly during swallowing and speech, thereby separating the oropharynx from the nasopharynx. Velopharyngeal insufficiency exists when this separation is incomplete, which may occur after cleft palate repair or adenoidectomy (usually transient). In severe cases, nasopharyngeal regurgitation of food may occur. In milder cases, the only manifestation may be hypernasal speech as a result of the nasal emission of air during phonation. If a bifid uvula is present, one should palpate the palate carefully for the presence of a submucous cleft.

KEY POINTS: LANGUAGE DEVELOPMENT

1. Very red flags include no meaningful words by 18 months or no meaningful phrases by 2 years.
2. Intelligibility should increase yearly by 25%, from 25% at 1 year of age up to 100% at 4 years of age.
3. Stuttering is common in younger children, but beyond the age of 5 to 6 years, it warrants speech evaluation.
4. Autism, intellectual disability, and cerebral palsy can present with speech delay.
5. Evaluation of hearing is mandatory in any setting of significant speech delay.

101. **When is stuttering abnormal?**

Stuttering is a common characteristic of the speech of preschool children. However, most children do not persist with stuttering beyond 5 or 6 years of age. Preschoolers at increased risk for persistence of stuttering include those with a positive family history of stuttering and those with anxiety-provoking stress related to talking. A child older than 5 or 6 years who stutters should be referred to a speech-language pathologist for assessment and treatment.

National Stuttering Association: www.westutter.org. Accessed on Mar. 23, 2015.

102. **What advice should be given to parents of a child who stutters?**

- Do not give the child directives about how to deal with his or her speech (e.g., "Slow down," or "Take a breath.").
- Provide a relaxed, easy speech model in your own manner of speaking to the child.
- Reduce the need and expectations for the child to speak to strangers, adults, or authority figures or to compete with others (such as siblings) to be heard.
- Listen attentively to the child with patience and without showing concern.
- Seek professional guidance if speech is not noticeably more fluent in 2 to 3 months.

103. **Which infants with "tongue tie" should have surgical correction?**

"Tongue tie," complete or partial ankyloglossia, is the restriction of mobility of the tongue due to a short or thickened lingual frenulum (Fig. 2-7). Complete ankyloglossia, with the tongue unable to protrude past the alveolar ridge or to move laterally, is uncommon but, when present, requires frenuloplasty. Partial ankyloglossia with variability in lingual range of motion occurs in up to 5% of newborns. There is a wide range of opinion regarding the need for "clipping." Partial ankyloglossia can interfere with breastfeeding when there is limited lingual extension or inability to touch the hard palate with the mouth wide open. Ankyloglossia is less commonly associated with speech problems. A video of a frenuloplasty is available at http://www.youtube.com/watch?v=XN-vVYd1m-o.

Bowley DM, Arul GS: Fifteen minute consultation: the infant with a tongue tie, *Arch Dis Child Educ Pract Ed* 99:127–129, 2014.
Webb AN, Hao W, Hong P: The effect of tongue-tie division on breastfeeding and speech articulation: a systematic review, *Int J Pediatr Otorhinolaryngol* 77:635 – 646, 2013.

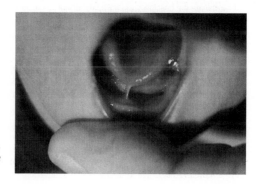

Figure 2-7. Newborn with ankyloglossia. *(From Clark DA:* Atlas of Neonatology. *Philadelphia, WB Saunders, 2000, p 146.)*

MENTAL RETARDATION/INTELLECTUAL DISABILITY

104. Why is the term *mental retardation* being changed?
There is controversy that the term is stigmatizing and pejorative. Indeed, the term is being phased out. DSM-5 replaces "mental retardation" with the term *intellectual disability*. However, because of numerous statutes and programs that use the term *mental retardation* and thus carry legal ramifications, the change will likely be a gradual process.

Harns JC: New terminology for mental retardation in DSM-5 and ICD-11, *Curr Opin Psychiatry* 26:260–262, 2013.

105. How is intellectual disability defined?
The American Association on Intellectual and Developmental Disabilities defines intellectual disability (formerly mental retardation) as "a disability characterized by significant limitations both in intellectual functioning and in adaptive behavior as expressed in conceptual, social, and practical adaptive skills. This disability originates before the age of 18."

American Association on Intellectual and Developmental Disabilities: www.aaidd.org. Accessed on Nov. 17, 2014.

106. How is intelligence classified with IQ scores?
Most IQ tests are constructed to yield a mean IQ of 100 and a standard deviation of 15 points (Table 2-6).

Table 2-6 Construction of Intelligence Quotient Scores

INTELLIGENCE QUOTIENT	STANDARD DEVIATION	CATEGORY
>130	>+2	Very superior
116-130	+1 to +2	High average to superior
115-85	Mean ± 1	Average
84-70	−1 to −2	Low average to borderline ID
69-55	−2 to −3	Mild ID
54-40	−3 to −4	Moderate ID
39-25	−4 to −5	Severe ID
<25	<-5	Profound ID

ID = intellectual disability.

107. What features can indicate cognitive problems in infants and young children?
In younger infants and toddlers, fine motor skill development and especially language development are the usual best correlates of cognitive achievement. As the child ages, the various milestones can be evaluated. Significant sequential delay should warrant referral for formal developmental testing to evaluate the possibility of intellectual disability (Table 2-7).

First LR, Palfrey JS: The infant or young child with developmental delay, *N Engl J Med* 330:478–483, 1994.

Table 2-7 Signs of Sequential Delay in Cognitive Achievement

2-3 mo	Not alerting to mother with special interest
6-7 mo	Not searching for dropped object
8-9 mo	No interest in peek-a-boo
12 mo	Does not search for hidden object
15-18 mo	No interest in cause-and-effect games

Table 2-7 Signs of Sequential Delay in Cognitive Achievement (*Continued*)	
2 yr	Does not categorize similarities (e.g., animals versus vehicles)
3 yr	Does not know own full name
4 yr	Cannot pick shorter or longer of two lines
4½ yr	Cannot count sequentially
5 yr	Does not know colors or any letters
5½ yr	Does not know own birthday or address

108. **Worldwide, what is the most common preventable cause of intellectual disability?**
     Iodine deficiency leads to maternal and fetal hypothyroxinemia during gestation, which causes brain developmental injury. Severe endemic iodine deficiency can cause cretinism (characterized by deaf-mutism, severe intellectual deficiency, and often hypothyroidism) and may occur in 2% to 10% of isolated world communities. Moderate iodine deficiency, which is even more common, leads to milder degrees of cognitive impairment.

Zimmermann MB, Jooste PL, Pandav CS: Iodine-deficiency disorders, *Lancet* 372:1251–1262, 2008.
Cao XY, Jiang XM, Dou ZH, et al: Timing of vulnerability of the brain to iodine deficiency in endemic cretinism, *N Engl J Med* 331:1739–1744, 1994.

PSYCHIATRIC DISORDERS

109. **What is the prevalence of childhood psychiatric disorders?**
     Overall, 15% to 20% of children 4 to 20 years old in community samples are diagnosed with a specific psychiatric disorder. The most common disorders are as follows:
     - ADHD (4% to 12%)
     - Anxiety disorder (5% to 15%)
     - Oppositional disorder (5% to 10%)
     - Overanxious disorder (2% to 5%)
     - Conduct disorder (1% to 5%)
     - Depression (2% to 12%)

National Institute of Mental Health: http://www.nimh.nih.gov. Accessed on Nov. 17, 2014.
American Academy of Child and Adolescent Psychiatry: http://www.aacap.org. Accessed on Nov. 17, 2014.

110. **What items constitute the "11 Action Signs"?**
     Developed as a screening tool by a number of national experts in pediatric mental health, these are a list of 11 items designed to identify early issues in children and adolescents. If any one of these signs is present, significant impairment is highly possible and expert evaluation is warranted (Table 2-8).

Table 2-8 11 Action Signs Suggestive of Significant Mental Health Problems	
POTENTIAL DISORDER	**SIGN**
Severe depression	Feeling very sad or withdrawn for more than 2 weeks
Suicidal ideation	Seriously trying to harm or kill yourself or making plans to do so
Panic attack	Sudden overwhelming fear for no reason, sometimes with a racing heart or fast breathing
Severe aggression	Involved in multiple fights, using a weapon, or wanting badly to hurt others

Continued on following page

Table 2-8 11 Action Signs Suggestive of Significant Mental Health Problems (*Continued*)

POTENTIAL DISORDER	SIGN
Poor impulse control	Severe out-of-control behavior that can hurt yourself or others
Eating disorder	Not eating, throwing up, or using laxatives to make yourself lose weight
Anxiety	Intense worries or fears that get in the way of your daily activity
Severe inattention/ hyperactivity	Extreme difficulty in concentrating or staying still that puts you in physical danger or causes school failure
Substance abuse	Repeated use of drugs or alcohol
Mood swings	Severe mood swings that cause problems in relationships
Personality changes	Drastic changes in your behavior or personality

Adapted from Jensen PS, Goldman E, Offord E, et al: Overlooked and underserved: "action signs" for identifying children with unmet mental health needs, Pediatrics 128:970–979, 2011.

111. **If a parent has an affective disorder, what is the likelihood that an offspring will have similar problems?**
Approximately 20% to 25% of these children will develop a major affective disorder, and as many as 40% to 45% will have a psychiatric problem.

112. **How does mania differ in children and adolescents?**
Mania occurs in about 0.5% to 1% of adolescents and occurs less frequently in prepubertal children. *Younger children* may present with extreme irritability, emotional lability, and aggression. Dysphoria, hypomania, and agitation may be intermixed. Hyperactivity, distractibility, and pressured speech often occur in all age groups. Symptoms in *adolescents* more closely resemble those seen in adults. They include elated mood, flight of ideas, sleeplessness, bizarre behavior, delusions of grandeur, paranoia, and euphoria.

113. **What ritualistic behaviors are common in children with obsessive-compulsive disorder?**
The most common rituals involve **excessive cleaning, repeating gross motor rituals** (e.g., going up and down stairs), and **repetitive checking behaviors** (e.g., checking that doors are locked or that homework is correct). Obsessions most commonly deal with fear of contamination. Symptoms tend to wax and wane in severity, and the specific obsessions or compulsions change over time. Most children attempt to disguise their rituals. Anxiety and distress that interfere with school or family life can occur when children fail in their efforts to resist the thoughts or activities. Cognitive behavioral therapy and selective serotonin reuptake inhibitor (SSRI) medications (e.g., sertraline), particularly in combination, can be beneficial.

Gilbert AR, Maalouf FT: Pediatric obsessive-compulsive disorder: management in primary care, *Curr Opin Pediatr* 20:544–550, 2008.

114. **What are the differences between child-onset OCD and adult-onset OCD?**
Compared with adult-onset OCD, a patient with child-onset OCD is more likely to:
- have an associated tic disorder
- have an associated disruptive behavior disorder (e.g., ADHD)
- have a first-degree relative with OCD (i.e., increased inheritability in child-onset)
- be male (adult-onset OCD has female:male predominance)
- have a better prognosis (nearly half of patients with childhood-onset OCD have subclinical levels of symptom severity, which are signs of remission, by early adulthood; only 20% of untreated adults have remission)

Grant JE: Obsessive-compulsive disorder, *N Engl J Med* 371: 1324–1331, 2014
Sarvet B: Childhood obsessive-compulsive disorder, *Pediatr Rev* 34:20, 2013

115. **What distinguishes a conduct disorder from an oppositional defiant disorder?**
Both are disruptive behavior disorders of childhood and early adolescence. **Conduct disorder** is the more serious disorder in that it is diagnosed when the child's behaviors violate the rights of others (e.g., assault) or are in conflict with major societal norms (e.g., stealing, truancy, setting fires). Children with conduct disorder are at risk for developing the antisocial personality disorder seen in adults.
Oppositional defiant disorder is characterized by recurrent negative and defiant behaviors toward authority figures.

116. **What are common symptoms of depression in children and adolescents?**
    - Sadness
    - School problems
    - Tearfulness
    - Somatic complaints
    - Irritability
    - Suicidal ideation
    - Negative self-imagery
    - Changes in appetite
    - Lack of concentration
    - Unintended weight changes
    - Decreased interest in usual activities
    - Sleep problems, including hypersomnia
    - Fatigue
    - Delusions

117. **How is major depressive disorder in children diagnosed?**
The DSM-5 criteria require the presence of 5 or more symptoms (out of 9 possible) from the categories of sleep, interest, guilt, concentration, appetite, psychomotor, and suicide during the same 2-week period. A variety of ratings scales (e.g., the Hamilton Depression Rating Scale, the Childhood Depression Inventory, the Child Behavioral Checklist, the Beck Depression Inventory) are available to assist with evaluation.

118. **What are treatments for major depressive disorder in children and adolescents?**
Psychotherapy: Various types of therapy may be used, including cognitive-behavioral therapy, interpersonal therapy, and family therapy.
Pharmacotherapy: SSRIs have been recommended by the American Academy of Child and Adolescent Psychiatry as the treatment of choice for children who warrant pharmacotherapy. There have been controversial warnings by regulatory agencies in Britain and the United States that antidepressant medications may be associated with an increased risk for suicide.

Clark MS, Jansen KL, Cloy JA: Treatment of childhood and adolescent depression, *Am Fam Physician* 86:442–448, 2012.

119. **How likely is it that a depressed teenager will be a depressed adult?**
Despite being a treatable condition, depression is chronic and recurrent, and up to 60% of teenagers will have recurrence as an adult.

Weissman MM, Wolk S, Goldstein RB, et al: Depressed adolescents grow up, *JAMA* 281:1707–1713, 1999.

120. **What are types of anxiety disorders in children?**
Separation anxiety disorder: Developmentally inappropriate, unrealistic, persistent fears of separation from caregivers that interfere with daily activities
Panic disorder: Recurrent, discrete periods of intense fear or discomfort; rare in prepubertal children; may occur with or without agoraphobia (fear or distress in or about places that may limit egress, such as a restaurant)
Social anxiety disorder: Extreme anxiety about social interactions with peers and adults; may manifest as generalized or specific (e.g., public speaking)

121. Which is preferable for children with anxiety disorders, cognitive behavioral therapy (CBT) or medication?

Actually, a **combination of both.** In a study of 488 children using CBT alone, medication (sertraline) alone, combination therapy, or placebo, the combination therapy resulted in 80% very much or much improved as measured by ratings scales compared with either therapy alone or placebo.

Walkup JT, Albano AM, Piacentini J, et al: Cognitive behavioral therapy, sertraline, or a combination in childhood anxiety, *N Engl J Med* 359:2753–2766, 2008.

122. What characterizes bipolar disorder?

This is a *mood disorder* with fluctuations of *mania* followed by *depression* and interludes of relatively normal behavior. In children, there are often out-of-control mood swings with dramatic behavior changes including marked irritability and rage.

- **Manic episode:** Inflated self-esteem, decreased need for sleep, flight of ideas or racing thoughts, distractibility, increase in goal-directed activity, excessive involvement in dangerous activities that have a high potential for dangerous consequences
- **Major depressive episode:** Depressed mood, markedly diminished interest or pleasure in activities, significant changes in weight and appetite, insomnia or hypersomnia, fatigue or loss of energy, diminished ability to concentrate, indecisiveness, recurrent thoughts of death or suicide

Cummings CM, Fristad MA: Pediatric bipolar disorder: recognition in primary care, *Curr Opin Pediatr* 20:560–565, 2008.

PSYCHOSOCIAL FAMILY ISSUES

123. How likely is it that children in the United States will experience the separation or divorce of their parents?

About half of first marriages end in divorce. In the United States, about 1.5 million children experience parental divorce each year. It is estimated that nearly 75% of black children and 40% of white children born to married parents will experience their parents' divorce before they are 18 years old. An addition to this stressor is that 50% of individuals who divorce will remarry within 4 years, thus creating another major family transition for a child. Of stepfamilies, nearly 90% consist of a biologic mother and a stepfather.

Tanner JL: Separation, divorce and remarriage. In: Carey WB, Crocker AC, Coleman WL, et al, editors: *Developmental-Behavioral Pediatrics*, ed 4, Philadelphia, 2009, Saunders Elsevier, p 126.

124. How do children of different ages vary in their response to parental divorce?

Preschool age (2 to 5 years): Most likely to show regression in developmental milestones (e.g., toilet training); irritability; sleep disturbances; preoccupation with fear of abandonment; demanding with remaining parent

Early school age (6 to 8 years): Most likely to demonstrate open grieving; preoccupied with fear of rejection and of being replaced; half may have a decrease in school performance

Later school age (9 to 12 years): More likely to demonstrate profound anger at one or both parents; more likely to distinguish one parent as the culprit causing the divorce; deterioration in school performance and peer relationships; sense of loneliness and powerlessness

Adolescence: Significant potential for acute depression and even suicidal ideation; acting-out behavior (substance abuse, truancy, sexual activity); self-doubts about own potential for marital success

Hetherington EM: Divorce and the adjustment of children, *Pediatr Rev* 26:163–169, 2005.
Kelly JB: Children's adjustment in conflicted marriage and divorce: a decade review of research, *J Am Acad Child Adolesc Psychiatry* 39:963–973, 2000.

125. What factors are central to a good outcome after a divorce?

- Ability of parents to set aside or resolve conflicts without involving children
- Emotional and physical availability of custodial parent to the child
- Parenting skills of custodial parent

- Extent to which child does not feel rejected by noncustodial parent
- Child's temperament
- Presence of supportive family network
- Absence of continuing anger or depression in the child

Cohen GJ: Helping children deal with divorce and separation, *Pediatrics* 110:1019–1023, 2002.

126. What is the "vulnerable child syndrome"?

The *vulnerable child syndrome* is characterized by excessive parental concern about the health and development of their child. It usually occurs after a medical illness in which the parents are understandably upset or worried about the child's health (e.g., prematurity, congenital heart disease). However, this concern persists despite the child's recovery. Problems of the syndrome can include pathologic separation difficulties for parent and child, sleep problems, overprotectiveness, and overindulgence. Children are at risk for behavioral, school, and peer-relationship problems.

Pearson SR, Boyce WT: The vulnerable child syndrome, *Pediatr Rev* 25:345–348, 2004.

127. How does the cognitive understanding of death evolve?

Toddler (<2 years): Death as separation, abandonment, or change; may become irritable or withdrawn

Preschool (2 to 6 years): Prelogical thought with magical and egocentric beliefs that the child may be responsible for the death; death as temporary and reversible

School age (6 to 10 years): Concrete logical thinking; death as permanent and universal but due to a specific illness or injury rather than as a biologic process; death is something that occurs to others; may develop a morbid interest in death

Adolescence (>10 years): Abstract logical thinking; more complete comprehension of death; death as a possibility for self

Linebarger JS, Sahler OJZ, Egan KA: Coping with death, *Pediatr Rev* 30:350–355, 2009.

128. Should adopted children be informed of their adoption?

Yes. It should not occur as a one-time event, but rather increasing amounts of information can be given over time. Most preschool children will not understand the process or meaning of adoption, and for them, disclosure should be guided by what the child wants to know. School-age children should be aware of their adoption and feel comfortable discussing it with their parents.

Borchers D, for the American Academy of Pediatrics Committee on Early Childhood, Adoption, and Dependent Care: Families and adoption: The pediatrician's role in supporting communication, *Pediatrics* 112:1437–1441, 2003.

129. How common is domestic violence?

Statistics indicate that about 1 in 4 women are physically assaulted by a spouse or cohabitant during their lifetime. The term *domestic violence* is now more commonly referred to as "intimate partner violence." The potential impact on children in these families is enormous, including behavioral and mental health problems, developmental delay, and potential for child abuse. Children who witness intimate partner violence are at greater risk for developing psychiatric disorders, school failure, and initiating violence against others, including future partners. The AAP has recommended since 1998 that all pediatricians incorporate screening for domestic violence as part of anticipatory guidance.

Gilbert AL, Bauer NS, Carroll AE, et al: Child exposure to parental violence and psychological distress associated with delayed milestones, *Pediatrics* 132:e1577–e1583, 2013.
Tjaden P, Thoennes N: *Extent, nature, and consequences of intimate partner violence, National Violence Against Women Survey.* Washington, 2000, National Institute of Justice and the Centers for Disease Control and Prevention, p iii.

130. Who are "latchkey" children?

The term refers to the millions of children <18 years of age who are in unsupervised care after school because they are members of families in which 1 or 2 parents work. Because of the enormous variability of circumstances, the consequences may be positive (e.g., increased maturity, self-reliance) or negative (e.g., isolation, feelings of neglect). Increased after-school programs may minimize negative consequences.

131. **What are the effects of heavy television watching in young children?**
It is hard not to overestimate the television exposure of children. Thirty percent of preschoolers have a television in their bedroom. Young children in some studies spend up to one-third of their waking hours watching television. By the time of an individual's high school graduation, more hours will have been spent watching television than in the classroom. Although the AAP discourages television viewing in the first 2 years of life, most children begin watching television at 5 months of age. Studies have documented the effects of heavy television viewing in the following areas: increased aggressive behavior (if exposed to more violent programming), increase in general level of arousal, increased risk for attentional problems, increased obesity, and decreased school performance. The long-term implications of this excessive early exposure to television are unclear, but negative effects on development, obesity, sleep, cognition, and attention have been demonstrated.

SCHOOL PROBLEMS

132. **How is "learning disability" defined?**
Currently, as defined by federal legislation, *learning disability* (LD) "means a disorder in one or more of the basic psychological processes involved in understanding or in using language, spoken or written, which may manifest itself in an imperfect ability to listen, think, speak, read, write, spell, or to do mathematical calculations." Such difficulties are not due to visual, hearing, or motor handicaps; emotional problems; MR; or environmental, social, cultural, or economic issues. This implies a discrepancy between academic achievement and that expected for age, schooling, and intelligence.

Dworkin PH: School failure. In Augustyn M, Zuckerman B, Caronna EB, editors: *The Zuckerman Parker Handbook of Developmental and Behavioral Pediatrics for Primary Care*, ed 3, Philadelphia, 2011, Lippincott Williams & Wilkins, p 317.

133. **What distinguishes dyslexia, dyscalculia, and dysgraphia?**
Dyslexia is a reading LD. It is the most common LD, affecting 3% to 15% of school-age children. About 80% of children identified as learning disabled have dyslexia (or a specific reading difficulty) as their primary diagnosis. Characterized by problems decoding single words (i.e., reading single words in isolation), dyslexia is usually the result of deficits in phonological processing.
Dyscalculia, or specific mathematics disability, affects 1% to 6% of children. Mathematics disabilities involve difficulties in computation, math concepts, and/or the application of those concepts to everyday situations.
Dysgraphia, or disorder of written expression, affects up to 10% of children. Difficulties with writing have several possible etiologies, including problems with fine motor control, linguistic abilities, visual-spatial skills, motor planning, proprioception, attention, memory, and sequencing.

Feder KP, Majnemer A: Handwriting development, competency, and intervention, *Dev Med Child Neurol* 49:312–317, 2007.
Shaywitz SE, Shaywitz BA: Dyslexia, *Pediatr Rev* 24:147–152, 2003.

134. **What are clues that a school-age child may have dyslexia?**
Problems in speaking: Mispronunciation of multisyllable words; hesitant, choppy speech; imprecise language
Problems in reading: Trouble reading and sounding out unfamiliar words; reading aloud is hesitant and choppy; handwriting is very messy; extremely poor speller; great difficulties in learning a foreign language; often a family history of reading or spelling difficulties

Shaywitz SE, Gruen JR, Shaywitz BA: Management of dyslexia, its rationale, and underlying neurobiology, *Pediatr Clin North Am* 54:609–623, 2007.

135. How are the two types of school avoidance behaviors distinguished?
    - **Anxiety-related avoidance:** Excessive fears (about peers, potential for teasing, grades); often an overprotective parent; typically excellent students with no classroom behavioral issues; girls affected more often than boys; symptoms are often physiologic manifestations of anxiety (e.g., headache, abdominal pain)
    - **Secondary-gain avoidance:** No anxiety about school; absence often follows lingering illness; "rewarded" at home for absence (e.g., sympathy, television); often are poor students; boys affected more often than girls; symptoms are fabricated or exaggerated (e.g., sore throat, extremity pain)

Schmitt BD: School avoidance. In Augustyn M, Zuckerman B, Caronna EB, editors: *The Zuckerman Parker Handbook of Developmental and Behavioral Pediatrics for Primary Care*, ed 3, Philadelphia, 2011, Lippincott Williams & Wilkins, pp 309–314.

136. How much of a problem are bullies?
    Bullying has been defined as "intentional, unprovoked abuse of power by one or more children to inflict pain or cause distress to another child on repeated occasions." It is a universal problem in schools worldwide. The victims frequently experience a range of psychological, psychosomatic, and behavioral problems that include anxiety, insecurity, low self-esteem, sleeping difficulties, bedwetting, sadness, and frequent bouts of headache and abdominal pain. In this age of social media and social networking, electronic bullying (or cyberbullying) is a rapidly growing problem.

Juvonen J, Graham S: Bullying in schools: The power of bullies and the plight of victims, *Ann Rev Psychol* 65:159–185, 2014.

SLEEP PROBLEMS

137. What is the average daily sleep requirement by age?
    - Newborns: 16 to 20 hours
    - 6 months: 13 to 14 hours
    - Toddlers (1 to 3 years): 12 hours
    - Preschoolers (3 to 6 years): 11 to 12 hours
    - Middle childhood (6 to 12 years): 10 to 11 hours
    - Adolescents (>12 years): 9 hours

Chamness JA: Taking a pediatric sleep history, *Pediatr Ann* 37:503, 2008.

138. Why is the supine sleeping position recommended for infants?
    In countries that have advocated the supine sleeping position as a preventive measure for SIDS, there have been dramatic decreases in the incidence of the syndrome. Hypotheses on why the prone position is more dangerous for infants have included the potential for airway obstruction and the possibility of rebreathing carbon dioxide, particularly when soft bedding is used.

139. When do infants begin to sleep through the night?
    By the time they are about 3 months old, about 70% of infants (slightly more for bottle-fed babies and slightly less for breast-fed babies) will not cry or awaken their parents between midnight and 6 AM. By 6 months, 90% of infants fit into this category, but between 6 and 9 months, the percentage of infants with night awakenings increases.

140. What advice to parents may minimize the problem of night waking?
    - After a parent-child bedtime routine, place the infant in the sleep setting while he or she is still awake (i.e., do not rock an infant to sleep).
    - The parent should not be present as the child falls asleep.
    - Gradually eliminate night feedings (infants by 6 months receive sufficient daytime nutrition to allow this).
    - Transitional objects (e.g., blanket, teddy bear) may minimize separation issues.

- Create a consistent sleep schedule and a bedtime routine of 20 to 30 minutes.
- Avoid giving a child items in late afternoon or evening that contain caffeine (e.g., chocolate, soda).

Meltzer LJ, Mindell JA: Nonpharmacologic treatments for pediatric sleeplessness, *Pediatr Clin North Am* 51:135–151, 2004.

141. How common are sleep problems in elementary school-age children?
About 40% of children between 7 and 12 years old experience sleep-onset delay, 10% experience night awakening, and 10% have significant daytime sleepiness. Some studies have shown that the extent of sleep is also inversely related to teacher-reported psychiatric symptoms.

Chamness JA: Taking a pediatric sleep history, *Pediatr Ann* 37:503, 2008.

142. What are parasomnias?
Parasomnias are undesirable physical phenomena that occur during sleep. Examples include night terrors, nightmares, sleepwalking, sleeptalking, nocturnal enuresis, sleep bruxism, somniloquy, and body rocking. Between the ages of 3 and 13 years, nearly 80% of all children will have had at least one parasomnia.

143. At what age do sleepwalking and sleeptalking occur?
Sleepwalking occurs most commonly between the ages of 5 and 10 years. As many as 15% of children between the ages of 5 and 12 years may have somnambulated once, and as many as 10% of 3- to 10-year-old children may sleepwalk regularly. The sleepwalking child is clumsy, restless, and walking without purpose, and the episode is not remembered. Injury is common during this outing. **Sleeptalking** is monosyllabic and often incomprehensible. Both conditions usually end before the age of 15 years. Severe cases may benefit from diazepam or imipramine therapy.

144. What is the difference between nightmares and night terrors?
Nightmares are frightening dreams that occur during rapid eye movement (REM) sleep (usually during the last half of the night) and that may be readily recalled on awakening. The child is aroused without difficulty and is usually easily consolable, but returning to sleep after a nightmare may be problematic.

Night terrors are brief episodes that occur during non-REM stage IV sleep. They usually last 30 seconds to 5 minutes, during which a child sits up, screams, and appears aroused, often staring and sweating profusely. The child cannot be consoled, rapidly goes back to sleep, and does not recall the episode in the morning. The onset of night terrors in an older child or persistent multiple attacks may indicate more serious psychopathology.

145. What recommendation should be given to a parent whose child is having night terrors?
An explanation of the phenomenon to the parent, with emphasis on the fact that the child is still asleep during the episode and should not be awakened, is all that is needed. If stress or sleep deprivation coincides with the night terrors, these factors should be addressed. If this is not successful, other approaches may be considered.
- When night terrors occur at the same time each night, the parent may awaken the child 15 minutes before the anticipated event over a 7-day period and keep him or her awake for at least 5 minutes. This often disrupts the sleep cycle and results in resolution of the problem.
- Rarely, for severe night terrors, a short course of diazepam will suppress REM sleep, reset the sleep cycles, and result in cessation of the problem.

VISUAL DEVELOPMENT AND DISORDERS

146. How well does a newborn see?
Because of the short diameter of the eye as well as retinal immaturity, a newborn's visual acuity is roughly 20/200 to 20/400. The human face is the most preferred object of fixation during early infancy. The light sense is one of the most primitive of all visual functions and is present by the seventh fetal month.

147. Do babies make tears?
Alacrima, or the absence of tear secretion, is not uncommon during the newborn period, although some infants may produce reflexive tearing at birth. In most others, tearing is delayed and typically not seen until the infant is 2 to 4 months old. Persistent lack of tearing is seen in Riley-Day syndrome (familial

dysautonomia). This is a rare genetic syndrome seen in the Ashkenazi Jewish population, affecting 1 in 10,000 newborns. Other symptoms include diaphoresis, skin blotching or marbling, hyporeflexia, and indifference to pain.

148. **At what age does an infant's eye color assume its permanent color?**
A neonate's eyes will never be lighter than they are at birth. The pigmentation of the iris in all races increases over the first 6 to 12 months. The eye color is usually defined by 6 months and always by 1 year.

149. **A 2-week-old infant with intermittent eye discharge and clear conjunctiva has what likely diagnosis?**
Nasolacrimal duct obstruction, seen in roughly 5% of newborns, is typically due to an intermittent blockage at the lower end of the duct. Massaging the area and watchful waiting are generally all that is needed. Almost all cases (95%) resolve by 6 months, and a few resolve thereafter. Occasionally, *acute dacryocystitis* can develop with pain, erythema, and edema in the lacrimal sac region, which, depending on the severity and age of the patient, may warrant IV antibiotics (Fig. 2-8). Ophthalmologic referral during the first 6 months is usually unnecessary, unless there are multiple episodes of dacryocystitis or a large congenital mucocele. Most ophthalmologists advise referral between 6 and 13 months because during this period, simple probing of the duct is curative in 95% of patients. After 13 months, the cure rate by probing alone falls to 75%, and silicone intubation of the duct is often necessary.

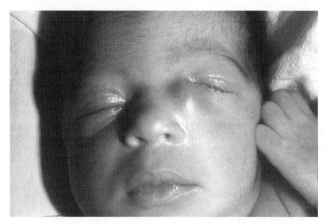

Figure 2-8. Congenital nasolacrimal duct obstruction with infected dacryocele (dacryocystitis) with swelling and erythema along the left side of the nose. *(From Bergelson JM, Shah SS, Zaoutis TE: Pediatric Infectious Diseases: The Requisites in Pediatrics, Philadelphia, Elsevier Mosby, 2008, p 76.)*

150. **What are the valves of Rosenmüller and Hasner?**
These are narrowings of the nasolacrimal drainage system where blockage can commonly occur in infancy, particularly at the Hasner valve due to persistence of an embryonic membrane (Fig. 2-9).

151. **What is normal visual acuity for children?**
- **Birth to 6 months:** Gradually improves from 20/400 to 20/80
- **6 months to 3 years:** Improves from 20/80 to 20/50
- **2 to 5 years:** Improves to 20/40 or better, with a less than 2-line difference between left and right eyes on visual charts
- **>5 years:** 20/30 or better, with a less than 2-line difference between eyes on visual charts
 It should be noted that almost 20% of children require eyeglasses for correction of refractive errors before adulthood.

152. **When do binocular fixation and depth perception develop in children?**
Binocularity of vision depends primarily on the adequate coordination of the extraocular muscles and is normally established by 3 to 6 months of age. At about 6 to 8 months, early evidence of depth perception

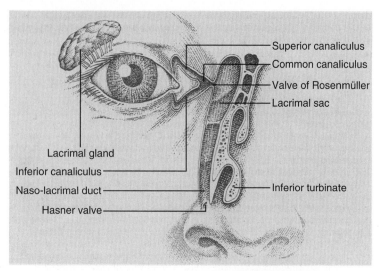

Figure 2-9. The nasolacrimal drainage system. *(From Ogawa GSH, Gonnering RS:* Congenital nasolacrimal duct obstruction, *J Pediatr 119:13, 1991.)*

is seen, but it is still poorly developed. Depth perception becomes very accurate at 6 or 7 years and continues to improve through the early teenage years.

153. **How does refractive capacity vary with age?**
The newborn infant is typically slightly hyperopic (farsighted). The mild hyperopia actually increases slowly for about the first 8 years. It then decreases gradually until adolescence, when vision is emmetropic (no refractive error). After 20 years, there is a tendency for myopia (nearsightedness).

154. **How are the degrees of blindness classified?**
The World Health Organization defines blindness as follows:
- **Visual impairment:** Snellen visual acuity of ≤20/60 (best eye corrected)
- **Social blindness:** Snellen visual acuity of ≤20/200 or a visual field of ≤20
- **Virtual blindness:** Snellen visual acuity of <20/1200 or a visual field of ≤10
- **Total blindness:** No light perception

American Foundation for the Blind: www.afb.org. Accessed on Mar. 20, 2015.
Prevent Blindness America: www.preventblindness.org. Accessed on Mar. 20, 2015.

155. **What is strabismus?**
Strabismus is the misalignment of the eyes with either an in-turning (esotropia), out-turning (exotropia), or up-turning (hypertropia) of one eye.

156. **A 2-month-old baby is noted to have eyes that appear to turn outward rather than looking forward. Is this strabismus?**
Yes, but intervention is not needed unless the symptom persists beyond 2 to 3 months of age. Strabismus is defined as any deviation from perfect ocular alignment. However, most newborns (up to 70%) will be found to have an exodeviated alignment (i.e., looking somewhat out) rather than an orthotropic (i.e., straight) alignment. Most infants will become orthotropic by the time they are 4 months old.

Infants do not focus well because the macula and fovea are poorly developed at birth. Therefore, it is not uncommon for infants to occasionally have an inward crossing of the eyes or for their eyes to be turned slightly outward to 10 or 15 degrees. Persistent in-turning of the eyes for more than a few seconds or outward deviation of more than 10 to 15 degrees requires ophthalmologic referral.

157. Name the types of childhood strabismus
    - **Strabismus of visual deprivation** occurs when normal vision in one or both eyes is disrupted by any cause. The most serious varieties occur with tumors (e.g., retinoblastoma). In children with ocular tumors, strabismus may be the presenting sign.
    - **Infantile** or **congenital esotropia** occurs within the first few months of life, usually as an isolated condition and often with large-angle strabismus. Corrective surgery is usually required.
    - **Accommodative esotropia** commonly occurs between the ages of 3 months and 5 years in very farsighted (hyperopic) children. These children use extra lens accommodation because of their visual problems, which leads to persistent convergence. Eyeglasses to correct the hyperopia often correct the esotropia.
    - **Intermittent exotropia** appears between the ages of 2 and 8 years as misalignment that is often brought on by fatigue, visual inattention, or bright sunlight. There is a strong hereditary component. Surgery is often necessary after the correction of refractive errors and the elimination of any pathology that might have caused visual deprivation.
    - **Incomitant strabismus** is caused by limited eye movement due to restriction (e.g., periocular scarring) or muscle paresis, most commonly from neurologic (e.g., cranial nerve palsies) or muscle pathology. The size of the deviation changes depending on the gaze because of the restrictions of eye movement.

Wright KW. *Pediatric Ophthalmology for Primary Care*, ed 3, Elk Grove Village, IL, 2008, American Academy of Pediatrics, pp 49–70.

158. What separates pseudostrabismus from true strabismus?
    Often a cause of unnecessary ophthalmologic referrals, **pseudostrabismus** is the appearance of ocular misalignment (usually esotropia) that occurs in children with a broad and flat nasal bridge and prominent epicanthal folds. The iris appears to be shifted to the midline, with differing amounts of white sclera on each side (Fig. 2-10). This is a common condition that may occur in up to 30% of newborns and is more common in Asian children. No treatment is required. It may be distinguished from true esotropia (or strabismus) by the observation of full extraocular movements, by symmetric reflections of a flashlight on the cornea from a distance of about 12 inches (although this test as a measure of strabismus is more accurate in infants ≥6 months old), and by normal visualization of red reflexes by direct ophthalmoscopy.

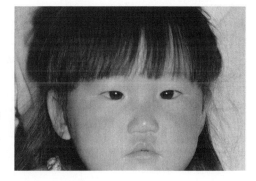

Figure 2-10. Pseudoesotropia. Note that the wide nasal bridge and prominent epicanthal folds create the illusion of an esotropia. The corneal light reflexes are centered in each eye; therefore, the eyes are straight. (*From Gault JA:* Ophthalmology Pearls. *Philadelphia, Hanley & Belfus, 2003, p 45.*)

159. **What is amblyopia?**

Amblyopia refers to decreased visual acuity in one eye that is not correctable by glasses and is a result of decreased visual stimulation of that eye. The visual cortex adheres to the concept of "use it or lose it." Amblyopia is the most common cause of vision loss in children younger than 6 years, and it occurs in 1% to 2% of this age group and in 2% to 2.5% of the general population.

160. **What are the causes of amblyopia?**
- **Strabismus:** Input from one eye is suppressed to avoid double vision.
- **Anisometropic amblyopia:** Significant refraction differences cause the suppression of images from the weaker eye.
- **Deprivation:** Images received are unclear (e.g., from congenital cataracts or ptosis).
- **Occlusion amblyopia:** This is typically iatrogenic. Prolonged covering of the preferred eye as a treatment for amblyopia can cause changes in visual acuity in the preferred eye.

Mittelman D: Amblyopia, *Pediatr Clin North Am* 50:189–196, 2003.

161. **Which treatments are effective for amblyopia?**

The first step involves providing a clear retinal image with use of eyeglasses or contact lenses for refractive errors and with removal of any obstructing opacities such as cataracts. Occlusion of the good eye allows stimulation of the visual cortex correlating to the amblyopic eye. Traditionally, prolonged patching has been the therapeutic mainstay. By causing papillary dilation and paralysis of accommodation, 1% atropine drops in the better eye cause blurring, particularly for patients who are hyperopic, and reliance on the amblyopic eye. Recent studies have shown that both atropine and patching are effective treatments for patients from 3 to 12 years and that shorter durations of patching are as effective as longer periods.

Repka MX, Kraker RT, Holmes JM, et al: Atropine vs patching for treatment of moderate amblyopia, *JAMA Ophthalmol* 132:799–805, 2014.

162. **What is the red reflex test?**

An essential component of any eye examination in an infant or child, the red reflex test is an evaluation of reflected light off the ocular fundus. A direct ophthalmoscope, set to a lens power of "0," is projected onto both eyes from a distance of 18 inches. A red image, symmetric from both eyes, should be visible. Abnormal color (particularly white), incomplete coloring (dark spots present), or asymmetric coloring warrant ophthalmologic consultation because these can represent cataracts, glaucoma, retinoblastoma, strabismus, or high refractive errors.

American Academy of Pediatrics, Section on Ophthalmology: Red reflex examination in neonates, infants, and children, *Pediatrics* 112:1401–1404, 2008.

163. **Why are early diagnosis and treatment critical for patients with congenital cataracts?**

Delay in treatment can lead to irreversible vision loss as a result of deprivation amblyopia. Cataracts undiagnosed for as little as 4 to 8 weeks after birth can result in permanent deficits. In general, the younger the child, the more urgent the need for evaluation if cataracts are suspected.

164. **What is ectopia lentis?**

Ectopia lentis refers to the displacement or dislocation of the lens. It may be due to trauma, but it has also been associated with systemic diseases such as Marfan syndrome, homocystinuria, and congenital syphilis.

165. **What diseases may present with a white pupil?**

Leukocoria, or white pupil, may be a result of any intraocular abnormality behind the pupillary space whereby light is obstructed (Fig. 2-11). This includes infants with cataracts, retinoblastoma, or retinopathy of prematurity who develop retinal detachment.

Varughese R: Fifteen minute consultation: A structured approach to the child with a white red reflex, *Arch Dis Child Educ Pract Ed* 99:162–165, 2014.

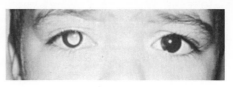

Figure 2-11. Leukocoria. White papillary reflex in a child with retinoblastoma. (*From Kleigman RM, Stanton BF, Schor NF, et al:* Nelson Textbook of Pediatrics, *ed 19, Philadelphia, Elsevier Saunders, 2011, p 2157.*)

166. **How common are unequally sized pupils?**

Up to 20% of the normal population can have physiologic **anisocoria** (inequality of pupil size) of up to 0.5 mm. The percentage of difference remains the same in bright or dim lighting.

167. **Is heterochromia normal?**

Yes, if it is an *isolated* finding. Heterochromia irides, or difference in iris colors, can be a familial autosomal dominant trait. It is also seen in some syndromes (e.g., Waardenburg, Horner). However, changes in color can occur from trauma, hemorrhage, inflammation (uveitis, iridocyclitis), malignancy (retinoblastoma, neuroblastoma), or glaucoma, or after intraocular surgery.

KEY POINTS: VISION

1. Red reflex testing should be done routinely for all infants.
2. Suspected cataracts require urgent evaluation, particularly in newborns and younger infants.
3. Uncorrected visual acuity errors in children <8 years old can cause irreversible, lifelong problems.
4. Amblyopia accompanies strabismus in 30% to 60% of cases.
5. Pseudoesotropia, a normal variant, mimics strabismus as a result of widened epicanthal folds. Unlike strabismus, corneal light reflections are equal.
6. Nasolacrimal duct obstruction is common in infants and resolves spontaneously in >95% of cases by 6 months of age.

168. **When are children aware of color differences?**

By 6 months of age, infants have perceptual awareness of colors. By age 2½ years, 50% of children can match cubes or cards by color. By 3½ to 4 years, 50% can name 4 colors correctly.

Sharma A: Developmental examination: birth to 5 years, *Arch Dis Child Educ Pract Ed* 96:162–175, 2011.

169. **How is color blindness inherited?**

Color blindness typically involves the variable loss of the ability to distinguish colors, especially red, green, and blue. The defects can be partial (anomaly) or complete (anopia). Defects in appreciating red or green color are transmitted in an X-linked recessive manner and affect up to 1% and 6%, respectively, of the male population. Blue color blindness is an autosomal dominant phenomenon and occurs in 0.1% of the population.

Acknowledgment

The editors gratefully acknowledge contributions by Drs. Nathan J. Blum, Mark Clayton, and James Coplan that were retained from the first three editions of *Pediatric Secrets*.

CHAPTER 3

CARDIOLOGY

Thomas J. Starc, MD, MPH, Constance J. Hayes, MD and Allan J. Hordof, MD

CLINICAL ISSUES

1. **Is cardiac pathology the most common cause of chest pain in children?**
   A cardiac cause of chest pain is **very uncommon and represents** less than 1% of cases in a published series. The most common identifiable causes involve *musculoskeletal* pain (e.g., strained intercostal muscles, costochondritis, Tietze syndrome, precordial catch syndrome), which occurs in one-quarter to one-half of cases. Other causes are *pulmonary* disease (e.g., asthma, cough illness, pneumonia, pleurisy), *gastrointestinal* disease (e.g., reflux, esophagitis, gastroenteritis), and miscellaneous diseases (e.g., sickle cell crisis, herpes zoster). Other possibilities include *psychogenic* (e.g., anxiety, hyperventilation/disordered breathing) and the always present *idiopathic* diseases (which may represent the largest category).

Collins SA, Griksaitis MJ, Legg JP: 15-minute consultation: a structured approach to the assessment of chest pain in a child, *Arch Dis Child Educ Pract Ed* 99:122–126, 2014.

2. **What is the clinical distinction between costochondritis and Tietze syndrome?**
   Costochondritis involves sharp, anterior chest wall pain that emanates from *multiple* costochondral and costosternal junctions. Causes can be inflammatory; post-traumatic; or, less commonly, infectious (including bacterial or fungal). Because the costal cartilage is avascular, it is susceptible to infection following surgery or trauma. This can be delayed and insidious in presentation. Palpation and percussion over the affected areas typically reproduce the pain. Swelling is not a prominent feature.
   Tietze syndrome is a localized form of costochondritis, usually involving just one costochondral junction (typically the second or third costochondral junction). A tender, swollen (but not hot) 1- to 4-cm mass is frequently palpable at the site. Onset is more commonly related to trauma.

3. **What are potential red flags that increase the likelihood of a cardiac cause for chest pain?**
   - Personal history of acquired or congenital cardiac disease
   - Exertional syncope
   - Exertional cardiac-type chest pain (e.g., centrally located with radiation to left arm/jaw, crushing pain or heaviness)
   - Hypercoagulable or hypercholesterolemic state
   - Family history of sudden death <35 years, young-onset ischemic heart disease, inherited arrhythmias (such as long QT syndrome)
   - Connective tissue disorders
   - History of cocaine/amphetamine use

Collins SA, Griksaitis MJ, Legg JP: 15-minute consultation: a structured approach to the assessment of chest pain in a child, *Arch Dis Child Educ Pract Ed* 99:123, 2014.

4. **A child with sharp, stabbing, very localized chest pain that occurs at rest and resolves completely without associated symptoms after 1 minute likely has what condition?**
   Precordial catch syndrome, also called *Texidor twinge* after the original 1955 describer, may be an underappreciated phenomenon in children with characteristic features that often prompt extensive and unproductive diagnostic workups. It manifests as a sudden-onset chest pain in children, very localized (patient points to area with one or two fingers), which occurs most commonly over the left sternal border, right anterior chest, or flanks with variation of site from episode to episode. The pain occurs typically at rest without provocation, is exacerbated by deep breaths (so the patient breathes very

shallowly), and usually lasts 30 seconds to 3 minutes. Unlike cardiac, pulmonary, gastrointestinal, or chest wall causes, there is a paucity of associated symptoms (e.g., no palpitations, pallor, flushing, fever, tenderness, or near-syncope). Physical examination, when done during the episode, is normal. The cause is unknown. Pain may originate from the parietal pleura or chest wall (e.g., rib or cartilage), but is not cardiac or pericardial in origin. Ancillary testing, when done, is normal. Management is expectant with reassurance.

Gumbiner CH: Precordial catch syndrome, *South Med J* 96:38–41, 2003.

5. What is the significance of mitral valve prolapse (MVP)?

MVP occurs when one or both mitral valve leaflets billow excessively into the left atrium near the end of systole. Some studies show that up to 13% of normal children have some degree of posterior leaflet prolapse on echocardiography. There is a spectrum of anatomic abnormalities, the most minor of which are variations of normal. Children with clinical features of mitral valve insufficiency constitute the pathologic category. Whenever auscultation reveals the classic findings of MVP, referral to a pediatric cardiologist is recommended. This allows for evaluation of the child for possible accompanying cardiac abnormalities (e.g., mitral insufficiency, secundum atrial septal defects) and confirmation of the diagnosis.

6. What connective tissue diseases may be associated with MVP?

Marfan syndrome, Ehlers-Danlos syndrome, pseudoxanthoma elasticum, osteogenesis imperfecta, and Hurler syndrome may be associated with MVP.

7. What are the common types of vascular rings and slings?

Vascular rings occur when the trachea and/or the esophagus is encircled by aberrant vascular structures. *Vascular slings* are compressions (typically anterior) that are caused by nonencircling aberrant vessels (Table 3-1).

Table 3-1. Vascular Rings and Slings

	FREQUENCY (%)	SYMPTOMS	TREATMENT
"Complete" Rings			
Double aortic arch	50	Respiratory difficulty, worsened by feeding or exertion (onset <3 mo)	Surgical division of a smaller arch (usually the left)
Right aortic arch with left ligamentum arteriosum	45	Mild respiratory difficulty (onset later in infancy); swallowing dysfunction	Surgical division of ligamentum arteriosum
"Incomplete" Rings			
Anomalous innominate artery	<5	Stridor and/or cough in infancy	Conservative management or surgical suturing of artery to the sternum
Aberrant right subclavian artery	<5	Occasional swallowing dysfunction	Usually no treatment necessary
Vascular sling or anomalous left pulmonary artery	Rare	Wheezing and cyanotic episodes during first weeks of life	Surgical division of anomalous left pulmonary artery and anastomosis to the main pulmonary artery; may also need tracheal reconstruction

Adapted from Park MK: Pediatric Cardiology for Practitioners, ed 5. St. Louis, 2008, Mosby Elsevier, p 578.

8. What evaluations are commonly done if a vascular ring is suspected?
   - **Chest radiograph:** For detection of possible right-sided aortic arch
   - **Barium esophagram:** Previously considered the gold standard for diagnosis (before magnetic resonance imaging); confirms external indentation of esophagus in up to 95% of cases (Fig. 3-1)
   - **Magnetic resonance imaging (MRI):** Noninvasive and now used as the primary diagnostic modality
   - **Arteriogram:** Precise delineation of vascular anatomy; rarely needed because of MRI
   - **Echocardiogram:** Should not be relied on for identifying the ring itself, but important when evaluating for other congenital heart lesions that can occur in patients with vascular rings

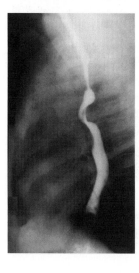

Figure 3-1. Barium swallow in a toddler with posterior compression of the esophagus and trachea from a vascular ring. *(From Zitelli BJ, Davis HW: Atlas of Pediatric Physical Diagnosis, ed 4. St. Louis, Mosby, 2002, p 540.)*

9. Describe four categories of cardiomyopathy in children
   - **Dilated cardiomyopathy** is the most common. Etiology is usually unknown. Anatomically, the heart is normal, but both ventricles are dilated. Older children exhibit symptoms of congestive heart failure (CHF). Infants demonstrate poor weight gain, feeding difficulty, and respiratory distress. In all pediatric age groups, a more acute presenting symptom can be shock.
   - **Hypertrophic cardiomyopathy with left ventricular (LV) outflow obstruction** is also known as idiopathic hypertrophic subaortic stenosis and asymmetric septal hypertrophy. Of patients with this condition, most have some degree of LV outflow tract obstruction as a result of abnormal hypertrophy of the subaortic region of the intraventricular septum. Most of these defects are inherited in an autosomal dominant fashion.
   - **Hypertrophic cardiomyopathy without LV outflow obstruction** is also usually of unknown etiology. It may be associated with systemic metabolic disease, particularly a storage disease. Cardiomegaly is a constant feature.
   - **Restrictive cardiomyopathy** is associated with abnormal diastolic function of the ventricles. The ventricles may be of normal size, or they may be hypertrophied with normal systolic function. The atria are typically enlarged. The etiology is usually unknown but restrictive cardiomyopathy may be seen with storage diseases.

Pettersen MD: Cardiomyopathies encountered commonly in the teenage years and their presentation, *Pediatr Clin North Am* 61:173–186, 2014.
Watkins H, Ashrafian H, Redwood C: Inherited cardiomyopathies, *N Engl J Med* 364:1643–1656, 2011.

10. **What mineral is added to hyperalimentation fluids to prevent a potential cardiomyopathy?**

    Selenium is routinely added to hyperalimentation fluids to prevent selenium deficiency, which can be a cause of both skeletal weakness and cardiomyopathy. This "acquired" heart disease has been described in patients on long-term hyperalimentation (before modern hyperalimentation); patients with acquired immunodeficiency syndrome (AIDS), chronic diarrhea, and wasting disease. It has also been described in children living in the Keshan province of China, where the soil is naturally low in selenium. It is typically reversible with the addition of selenium to the diet or intravenous fluids.

11. **What are the cardiac causes of sudden cardiac death in children and adolescents?**

    Sudden death occurs because of ventricular fibrillation in the setting of myocardial or coronary abnormalities or underlying primary rhythm disorders. The main structural causes are hypertrophic cardiomyopathy (particularly with extreme LV hypertrophy), anomalies of the coronary artery (congenital or acquired), Marfan syndrome, and arrhythmogenic right ventricular (RV) dysplasia. Children with CHD (e.g., severe aortic stenosis, Ebstein anomaly) are at higher risk for sudden death. ECG abnormalities which can lead to sudden death include Wolff Parkinson White (WPW) syndrome, prolonged QT syndrome, AV block and Brugada syndrome.

Rowland T: Sudden unexpected death in young athletes: reconsidering "hypertrophic cardiomyopathy," *Pediatrics* 123:1217–1222, 2009.

12. **What historical features may identify the patient who is at risk for sudden death?**
    - Sudden death may be associated with previous symptoms of exertional chest discomfort; dizziness; or prolonged dyspnea with exercise, syncope, and palpitations.
    - A family history of premature cardiovascular disease (<50 years), hypertrophic or dilated cardiomyopathy, Marfan syndrome, long QT syndrome, other clinically significant arrhythmias or sudden death may be elicited.
    - Previous recognition of a heart murmur or elevated systemic blood pressure are significant findings.

Mahmood S, Lim L, Akram Y, et al: Screening for sudden cardiac death before participation in high school and collegiate sports, *Am J Prev Med* 45:130–133, 2013.

13. **What features in the preparticipation sports physical examination identify patients at risk for sudden death?**
    - **Marfanoid features**: Tall and thin habitus, hyperextensible joints, pectus excavatum, click and murmur suggestive of MVP
    - **Pathologic murmurs** (any systolic murmur grade 3/6 or greater, any diastolic murmur)
    - **Weak or delayed femoral pulses**
    - **Arrhythmia:** Rapid or irregular heartbeat

Singh A, Silberbach M: Cardiovascular preparticipation sports screening, *Pediatr Rev* 27:418–423, 2006.

14. **Should an electrocardiogram (ECG) be included in the preparticipation screening of young athletes?**

    This remains a hotly debated topic. The potential value is that an ECG could identify at-risk athletes with hypertrophic cardiomyopathy, severe cardiac hypertrophy, arrhythmogenic RV cardiomyopathy, WPW, AV block and long QT syndrome. Proponents argue that the use of history and physical examination alone is not decreasing the rate of sudden cardiac death. Some even call for universal screening of all children. Opponents argue that sudden cardiac death is a rare event and that the ECG is an inexact screening tool because of the overlap between normal and abnormal tracings. The European Society of Cardiology recommends ECG screening, but the American Heart Association, as of 2014, has not endorsed ECG use as part of the preparticipation process.

Friedman RA: Electrocardiographic screening should not be implemented for children and adolescents between ages 1 and 19 in the United States, *Circulation* 130:698–702, 2014.
Vetter VL: Electrocardiographic screening of all infants, children and teenagers should be performed, *Circulation* 130: 688–697, 2014.

15. Name five disorders in which a screening ECG might identify a subject at risk for sudden death
    - **Wolf-Parkinson-White syndrome:** short PR, delta wave, T wave abnormalities leading to supraventricular tachycardia and ventricular fibrillation
    - **Prolonged QT syndrome:** Secondary to congenital channelopathy, electrolyte or drug-induced abnormality leading to ventricular tachycardia and torsades de pointes
    - **Brugada syndrome:** Right ventricular conduction delay with profound ST elevation in V_1-V_3 leading to ventricular fibrillation
    - **Hypertrophic cardiomyopathy**
    - **AV block**

16. What is the likely diagnosis in a 10-year-old little leaguer who develops sudden cardiac arrest after being struck in the chest by a batted baseball?
    Commotio cordis. This is a life-threatening arrhythmia that occurs as a result of a blunt, nonpenetrating direct blow to the chest. The precordial force is often only low or moderate and typically not associated with structural injury. Ventricular fibrillation is thought to occur when impact is applied during the vulnerable phase of repolarization, which occurs 30 to 15 milliseconds before the peak of the T wave. Prompt cardiopulmonary resuscitation followed by defibrillation improves the chance of survival.

Maron BJ, Estes NAM III: Commotio cordis, *N Engl J Med* 362:917–927, 2010.

17. In which patients is syncope more likely to be of a cardiac nature?
    - Sudden onset without any prodromal period of dizziness or imminent awareness
    - Syncope during exercise or exertion
    - History of palpitations or abnormal heartbeat before fainting
    - Syncope leading to a fall which results in an injury
    - Family history of sudden death

18. What arrhythmias may be associated with syncope?
    See Table 3-2.

Table 3-2. Syncope

DIAGNOSIS	HISTORY AND PHYSICAL EXAMINATION	ELECTROCARDIOGRAPHIC FINDINGS
WPW	Family history of WPW, known hypertrophic cardiomyopathy, or Ebstein anomaly	Short PR interval, presence of delta waves
Prolonged QT syndrome	Family history of prolonged QT, sudden death, and/or deafness	Borderline QTc = 440–460 msec Prolonged QTc = > 460 msec
Atrioventricular block	Myocarditis, Lyme disease, acute rheumatic fever, maternal history of lupus	First-, second-, or third-degree heart block
Arrhythmogenic right ventricular dysplasia	Syncope, palpitations, positive family history	PVCs, ventricular tachycardia, left bundle branch block
Ventricular tachycardia	Most ventricular tachycardia occurs in abnormal hearts; requires extensive evaluation	Ventricular tachycardia

PVCs = Premature ventricular contractions; QTc = corrected QT interval; WPW = Wolff-Parkinson-White syndrome.
From Feinberg AN, Lane-Davies A: Syncope in the adolescent, Adolesc Med *13:553–567, 2002.*

KEY POINTS: SYNCOPE MORE LIKELY TO BE OF A CARDIAC NATURE

1. Occurring during exercise
2. Sudden onset without prodromal symptoms or awareness
3. Complete loss of tone or awareness leading to injury
4. Palpitations or abnormal heartbeat noted before event
5. Abnormal heart rate (fast or slow) after event
6. Family history of sudden death

19. **What are the most common clinical signs of coarctation of the aorta (Fig. 3-2) in *older* children?**
    - Differential blood pressure: arms > legs (100%)
    - Systolic murmur or bruit in the back (96%)
    - Systolic hypertension in the upper extremities (96%)
    - Diminished or absent femoral or lower-extremity pulses (92%)

Ing FF, Starc TJ, Griffiths SP, Gersony WM: Early diagnosis of coarctation of the aorta in children: a continuing dilemma, *Pediatrics* 98:378–382, 1996.

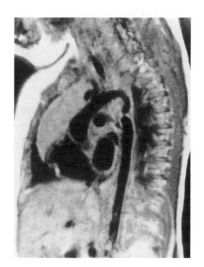

Figure 3-2. Magnetic resonance imaging of coarctation of the aorta. *(From Clark DA:* Atlas of Neonatology. *Philadelphia, 2000, WB Saunders, p 119.)*

20. **How much does peak exercise affect cardiac output?**
    Cardiac output is calculated by the formula: *Cardiac output = Heart rate x Stroke volume.* Cardiac output at peak exercise will increase up to approximately 5 times the baseline value. In upright exercise, stroke volume increases early in exercise by 1½ to 2 times baseline values, but then plateaus at that level. Heart rate will also increase early in exercise, but will continue to rise up to the maximum predicted value of about 200 beats/minute at peak exercise.

21. **What cardiac lesions can lead to thrombosis and stroke?**
    - **Arrhythmias:** chronic atrial fibrillation, atrial flutter
    - **Cardiomyopathies:** decreased cardiac function is associated with increased risk for thrombus formation; therefore, many of these patients are on aspirin or warfarin.
    - **Mechanical valves**: These patients require lifelong anticoagulation.
    - Patients with **Fontan circulation** are at increased risk for thrombosis.
    - Patients with **systemic-to-pulmonary shunts,** such as Blalock-Taussig shunts, are at risk for shunt thrombosis.
    - Patients with **Kawasaki disease** with coronary aneurysms are at risk for thrombosis in the coronary arteries.

22. What are two of the more common neuromuscular diseases in which a cardiac consultation is routinely recommended?
    - **Duchenne muscular dystrophy** is an X-recessive disease with an abnormality in the dystrophin gene, which leads to muscle necrosis and fibrosis. Although the majority of deaths are due to respiratory insufficiency, death from cardiomyopathy can occur in up to 25% of patients. Symptoms of heart disease are typically hidden by the skeletal myopathy that masks any exercise-induced complaints such as shortness of breath with exertion. Therefore, screening echocardiograms and ECGs are recommended for long-term follow-up.
    - **Friedrich ataxia** is an autosomal recessive disorder involving a gene encoding frataxin, a mitochondrial protein. Symptoms include ataxia and muscle weakness, typically manifesting by 9 years of age. Cardiac abnormalities include both dilated and concentric cardiomyopathies. Atrial fibrillation and atrial flutter are commonly reported arrhythmias. Because muscle weakness and ataxia will prevent prolonged exertion, periodic echocardiograms and ECGs are recommended.

23. Why are chemotherapeutic agents that use arsenic of cardiac concern?
    Arsenic may cause prolonged QT and lead to torsades de pointes and ventricular fibrillation. Periodic ECG monitoring is recommended in these patients.

CONGENITAL HEART DISEASE

24. What prenatal maternal factors may be associated with cardiac disease in the neonate?
    See Table 3-3.

Table 3-3. Prenatal Maternal Factors Associated With Cardiac Disease in Neonates

PRENATAL HISTORICAL FACTOR	ASSOCIATED CARDIAC DEFECT
Diabetes mellitus	Left ventricular outflow obstruction (asymmetric septal hypertrophy, aortic stenosis), D-transposition of great arteries, ventricular septal defect
Lupus erythematosus	Heart block, pericarditis, endomyocardial fibrosis
Rubella	Patent ductus arteriosus, pulmonic stenosis (peripheral)
Alcohol use	Pulmonic stenosis, ventricular septal defect
Aspirin use	Persistent pulmonary hypertension syndrome
Lithium	Ebstein anomaly
Diphenylhydantoin	Aortic stenosis, pulmonary stenosis
Coxsackie B infection	Myocarditis

From Gewitz MH: Cardiac disease in the newborn infant. In Polin RA, Yoder MC, Burg FD, editors: Workbook in Practical Neonatology, *ed 3. Philadelphia, 2001, WB Saunders, p 269.*

25. In a cyanotic newborn, what test can help distinguish pulmonary disease from cyanotic congenital heart disease (CHD)?
    Hyperoxia test. The infant is placed on 100% oxygen, and an arterial blood gas level is obtained. A Pao_2 of greater than 100 mm Hg is usually achieved in infants with primary lung disease, whereas a Pao_2 of less than 100 mm Hg is characteristic of heart disease. Typically, children with cyanotic heart disease also have a low or normal Pco_2, whereas children with lung disease have an elevated Pco_2. However, the hyperoxia test does not usually distinguish children with cyanotic heart disease from those with persistent pulmonary hypertension.

26. Which congenital heart lesions commonly appear with cyanosis during the newborn period?

Independent pulmonary and systemic circulations (severe cyanosis)
- Transposition of great arteries with an intact ventricular septum

Inadequate pulmonary blood flow (severe cyanosis)
- Tricuspid valve atresia
- Pulmonary valve atresia with intact ventricular septum
- Tetralogy of Fallot
- Severe Ebstein anomaly of the tricuspid valve

Admixture lesions (moderate cyanosis)
- Total anomalous pulmonary venous return
- Hypoplastic left heart syndrome (HLHS)
- Truncus arteriosus

Victoria BE: Cyanotic newborns. In Gessner IH, Victoria BE, editors: Pediatric Cardiology: A Problem Oriented Approach. *Philadelphia, 1993, WB Saunders, p 101.*

KEY POINTS: CARDIAC CAUSES OF CYANOSIS IN THE NEWBORN

1. Transposition of the great arteries
2. Tetralogy of Fallot
3. Truncus arteriosus
4. Pulmonary atresia
5. Total anomalous pulmonary venous return
6. Tricuspid atresia
7. Hypoplastic left heart

---

27. In the patient with suspected heart disease, what bony abnormalities seen on a chest radiograph increase the likelihood of CHD?
- **Hemivertebrae, rib anomalies:** Associated with tetralogy of Fallot, truncus arteriosus, and VACTERL syndrome (**v**ertebral abnormalities, **a**nal atresia, **c**ardiac abnormalities, **t**racheoesophageal fistula and/or **e**sophageal atresia, **r**enal agenesis and dysplasia, and **l**imb defects)
- **11 pairs of ribs:** Seen in patients with Down syndrome
- **Skeletal chest deformities** (e.g., scoliosis, pectus excavatum, narrow anterior-posterior diameter): Associated with Marfan syndrome and mitral valve prolapse
- **Bilateral rib notching:** Coarctation of the aorta (seen in older children)

28. How do pulmonary vascular markings on a chest radiograph help in the differential diagnosis of a cyanotic newborn with suspected cardiac disease?

The chest radiograph may help differentiate the types of congenital heart defects. An increase or decrease in pulmonary vascular markings is indicative of the amount of pulmonary blood flow:

Decreased pulmonary markings (diminished pulmonary blood flow)
- Pulmonary atresia or severe stenosis
- Tetralogy of Fallot
- Tricuspid atresia
- Ebstein anomaly

Increased pulmonary markings (increased pulmonary blood flow)
- Transposition of great arteries
- Total anomalous pulmonary venous return
- Truncus arteriosus

29. What ECG findings suggest specific congenital heart conditions?
- **Left axis deviation:** Endocardial cushion defects (both complete atrioventricular [AV] canal and ostium primum atrial septal defects), tricuspid atresia
- **WPW syndrome:** Ebstein anomaly, L-transposition of the great arteries (L-TGA)
- **Complete heart block:** L-TGA, polysplenia syndrome, maternal lupus

30. What chest radiograph findings (Fig. 3-3) are considered characteristic for various CHDs?
    - **Boot-shaped heart:** Tetralogy of Fallot
    - **Egg-shaped heart:** Transposition of great arteries
    - **Snowman silhouette:** Total anomalous pulmonary venous return (supracardiac)
    - **Rib notching:** Coarctation of the aorta (older children)

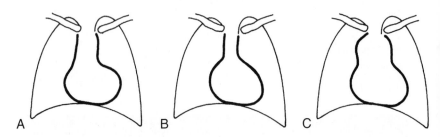

Figure 3-3. Abnormal cardiac silhouettes. **A,** "Boot-shaped" heart seen in cyanotic tetralogy of Fallot or tricuspid atresia. **B,** "Egg-shaped" heart seen in transposition of the great arteries. **C,** "Snowman" silhouette seen in total anomalous pulmonary artery venous return (supracardiac type). *(From Park MK: Pediatric Cardiology for Practitioners, ed 5. Philadelphia, Mosby Elsevier, 2008, p 68.)*

31. What are the common ductal-dependent cardiac lesions?
    Ductal-dependent pulmonary blood flow
    - Critical pulmonary valve stenosis
    - Pulmonary atresia
    - Tetralogy of Fallot with severe pulmonary stenosis
    - Tricuspid atresia with pulmonary stenosis or pulmonary atresia
    Ductal-dependent systemic blood flow
    - Coarctation of the aorta
    - HLHS
    - Interrupted aortic arch

32. What types of CHDs are associated with the right aortic arch?
    - Tetralogy of Fallot with pulmonary atresia (50%)
    - Truncus arteriosus (35%)
    - Classic tetralogy of Fallot (25%)
    - Double-outlet right ventricle (25%)
    - Single ventricle (12.5%)

Crowley JJ, Oh KS, Newman B, et al: Telltale signs of congenital heart disease, *Radiol Clin North Am* 31:573–582, 1993.

33. Name 5 different types of left ventricular outflow tract stenosis
    - Aortic valve stenosis (more common in males)
    - Supravalvular aortic stenosis (Williams syndrome)
    - Subvalvular aortic stenosis due to a subaortic membrane
    - Subvalvular aortic stenosis due to hypertrophic obstructive cardiomyopathy
    - Subvalvular aortic stenosis due to fibromuscular tunnel

34. Which genetic syndromes are most commonly associated with CHD?
    See Table 3-4.

Table 3-4. Genetic Syndromes Associated with Congenital Heart Disease

SYNDROME	PERCENTAGE OF PATIENTS WITH CHD	PREDOMINANT HEART DEFECTS
Down	50	ECD, VSD, TOF
Turner	20	COA
Noonan	65	PS, ASD, ASH
Marfan	60	MVP, AoAn, AR
Trisomy 18	90	VSD, PDA
Trisomy 13	80	VSD, PDA
DiGeorge	80	IAA-B, TA
Williams	75	SVAS, peripheral PS

AoAn = Aortic aneurysm; AR = aortic regurgitation; ASD = atrial sepal defect; ASH = asymmetric septal hypertrophy; CHD = congenital heart disease; COA = coarctation of the aorta; ECD = endocardial cushion defect; IAA-B = interrupted aortic arch type B; MVP = mitral valve prolapse; PDA = patent ductus arteriosus; PS = pulmonary stenosis; SVAS = supravalvular aortic stenosis; TA = truncus arteriosus; TOF = tetralogy of Fallot; VSD = ventricular septal defect.
From Frias JL: Genetic issues of congenital heart defects. In Gessner IH, Victoria BE, editors: Pediatric Cardiology: A Problem Oriented Approach. *Philadelphia, 1993, WB Saunders, p 238.*

35. Which infants with CHD should be evaluated for other anomalies?
In the evaluation of the newborn with heart disease, several known associations between CHD and other anomalies should be considered, especially for the patient with more complex disease. Syndromes such as CHARGE (**c**oloboma, **h**eart disease, choanal **a**tresia, **r**etarded growth and development or central nervous system anomalies, **g**enital hypoplasia, **e**ar anomalies and/or deafness) or VACTERL may first be identified by the presence of heart disease. An association between conotruncal defects (tetralogy of Fallot, truncus arteriosus, and interrupted aortic arch) and deletions on chromosome 22 is often seen. Some of these patients may have DiGeorge syndrome or velocardiofacial syndrome, but others may have only minimal palatal dysfunction. For this reason, patients with conotruncal cardiac defects should undergo screening for deletions on chromosome 22; if these are found, these patients should be referred to a geneticist for special testing and evaluation.

36. Describe the clinical manifestations of a large patent ductus arteriosus (PDA)
   • Tachypnea and tachycardia
   • Bounding pulses
   • Hyperdynamic precordium
   • Wide pulse pressure
   • Continuous murmur (older child)
   • Systolic murmur (premature infant)
   • Labile oxygenation (premature infant)
   • Apnea (premature infant)

37. How commonly do PDAs occur in premature infants?
They are evident in 40% to 60% of infants with birth weights of 501 to 1500 g.

38. Is a "to-and-fro" murmur a good description for the heart murmur of a PDA?
No. The heart murmur of a typical PDA is usually *continuous* or at least "spills from systole into diastole." In a small preterm infant, the diastolic portion may be difficult to discern. The direction of blood flow is from the aorta to the pulmonary artery in systole and continues from the aorta to the pulmonary artery during diastole. A to-and-fro murmur describes blood flow in semilunar valvular lesions such as the combination of aortic stenosis with aortic insufficiency or pulmonary stenosis with pulmonary insufficiency. The blood flow in these examples goes "antegrade" during systole and "retrograde" during diastole. This back and forth flow is aptly described as to-and-fro.

39. **How can you explain a PaO$_2$ of more than 400 mm Hg in a blood sample from an umbilical catheter in a newborn with transposition of the great arteries?**
A very elevated PaO$_2$ can be observed if the umbilical vein catheter has passed from the inferior vena cava to the right atrium and into the left atrium. The PO$_2$ in the left atrium represents the pulmonary venous oxygenation and not the arterial oxygen level. In cyanotic heart disease, the alveolar and pulmonary vein PO$_2$ values are usually normal. It is the arterial oxygenation concentration that is severely diminished in children with cyanotic heart disease.

40. **How do the presenting symptoms of ventricular septal defect (VSD) and atrial septal defect (ASD) differ?**
VSD: In an infant with a large VSD, signs of CHF generally appear at 4 to 8 weeks of age, when the pulmonary vascular resistance drops and pulmonary blood flow increases. CHF is due to a large left-to-right shunt and increased pulmonary blood flow and may be associated with failure to thrive or recurrent respiratory infections. The child with a small VSD may have a systolic murmur during the first few weeks of life. These infants do not develop CHF, and spontaneous closure often occurs.

　　ASD: Most children with an isolated ASD are not clinically diagnosed until they are 3 to 5 years old. Most are asymptomatic at the time of diagnosis. Rarely, infants with an ASD demonstrate signs of CHF during the first year of life.

41. **What is the primary concern of the pediatric cardiologist if a child with a large VSD is lost to follow-up and comes back after 2 years of age?**
Although even large VSDs may close spontaneously in childhood, the child with a large VSD can develop **irreversible pulmonary vascular disease** as a sequela of the long-term increased pulmonary blood flow and **pulmonary hypertension** (Eisenmenger syndrome). This complication is usually preventable if the VSD is closed before 18 to 24 months of age.

42. **What are some of the common presenting symptoms in older children with primary pulmonary hypertension?**
In the early stages of the disease, children are asymptomatic at rest. Children with primary pulmonary hypertension may present with symptoms such as fatigue, dyspnea, chronic cough and shortness of breath with exercise. They may also present with chest pain, syncope, and atypical seizures. These symptoms are easily confused with other chronic diseases such as asthma, recurrent pneumonia, or a seizure disorder.

Nicolarsen J, Ivy D: Progress in the diagnosis and management of pulmonary hypertension in children, *Curr Opin Pediatr* 26:527–535, 2014.

43. **What examination features are suggestive of pulmonary hypertension?**
Physical examination may reveal a RV heave or lift suggestive of RV hypertrophy. The pulmonary component of the second heart sound is usually loud. There may be a 1-2/6 diastolic decrescendo murmur of pulmonary insufficiency at the left upper sternal border and a 1-2/6 holosystolic murmur of tricuspid insufficiency at the left lower sternal border. Eventually, signs of right heart failure with peripheral edema, neck vein distention, ascites, and hepatomegaly may develop.

44. **What is the anomaly in Ebstein anomaly?**
The septal and posterior leaflets of the tricuspid valve are thickened and displaced inferiorly into the right ventricle. In its most severe form, the tricuspid valve is severely incompetent, profound right atrial enlargement results, and signs of CHF predominate.

45. **What are the four structural abnormalities of tetralogy of Fallot?**
- Pulmonary stenosis with RV outflow tract obstruction
- VSD
- Aorta overriding the VSD
- RV hypertrophy

46. **What occurs during a "Tet spell"?**
Tet spells are hyper cyanotic episodes that occur in patients with tetralogy of Fallot. The pathophysiology is thought to be related to a change in the balance of systemic-to-pulmonary vascular resistance. Spells

may be initiated by events that cause a decrease in systemic vascular resistance (e.g., fever, crying, hypotension) or by events that cause an increase in pulmonary outflow tract obstruction. Both types of events lead to more right-to-left shunting and increased cyanosis. Hypoxia and cyanosis can result in metabolic acidosis and systemic vasodilation, which cause a further increase in cyanosis. Anemia may be a predisposing factor. Although most episodes are self-limited, a prolonged Tet spell can lead to stroke or death; therefore, a spell is an indication for surgery.

47. **Name two conditions in which the murmur has disappeared or diminished in intensity and yet the patient is actually worse**
    Tetralogy of Fallot. The systolic heart murmur represents blood flow across the narrow RV outflow tract. With worsening RV outflow tract obstruction or during a cyanotic spell, less blood crosses the valve, and the heart murmur consequently diminishes and may actually disappear completely.
    VSD with Eisenmenger syndrome. The left-to-right shunt across the VSD diminishes because of the increase in pulmonary vascular resistance. The heart murmur lessens and may disappear. A "honeymoon period" with no shunting is then followed by the progression of increased right-to-left shunting and cyanosis. The pulmonary component of the second heart sound begins to increase in intensity, and visible cyanosis and clubbing of the nail beds are often seen.

48. **After what age does a presumed peripheral pulmonic branch stenosis murmur deserve more detailed study?**
    The murmur of peripheral pulmonic branch stenosis—a low-intensity systolic ejection murmur heard frequently in newborns—is the result of the relative hypoplasia of the pulmonary arteries as well as the acute angle of the branching of pulmonary arteries in the early newborn period. A murmur which persists **beyond 6 months of age** should be investigated.

49. **What is the role of pulse oximetry in screening for complex congenital heart disease (CCHD) in asymptomatic infants in the newborn nursery?**
    Of the approximate 1 in 100 children born with congenital heart disease, 25% will have CCHD, defined as a condition that requires surgical or catheter intervention in the first year of life. When the diagnosis is delayed, there can be a significant impact on morbidity and mortality. These delays can occur because of limitations in the value of the physical exam (particularly in those lesions without distinct murmurs), difficulty in identifying cyanosis in anemic or dark-pigmented neonates, and early hospital discharge for ductal-dependent lesions when the ductus arteriosus has not yet closed. Discharged infants may later present *in extremis* with sudden and profound clinical worsening, including shock, due to changes in pulmonary vascular resistance and ductal closure. Universal pulse oximetry screening of newborns, ideally done after 24 hours, is now recommended by the AAP as a means of identifying infants with CCHD before leaving the nursery. The rationale is based on the fact that hypoxemia is present to some degree in the majority of cases of CCHD. The screen is felt to have a sensitivity of 60% to 70% for CCHD, so a normal screen does not rule out heart disease.

Thangaratinam S, Brown K, Zamora J, et al: Pulse oximetry screening for critical congenital heart defects in asymptomatic newborn babies: a systemic review and meta-analysis, *Lancet* 379:2459–2464, 2012.

50. **What is the AAP screening protocol for CCHD using pulse oximetry?**
    Oxygen saturation is measured in the right hand and either foot. The screen is failed if oxygen level is <90% in either limb. If oxygen saturation is ≥90% and <95% in both limbs or there is >3% difference between the hand and foot, repeat testing should be done in 1 hour. If persistent, the screen is failed. For a failed screen, cardiology consultation is recommended and an echocardiography is generally indicated.

Mahle WT, Martin GR, Beekman RH III, et al: Endorsement of Health and Human Services recommendation for pulse oximetry screening for critical congenital heart disease, *Pediatrics* 129:190–192, 2012.
Kemper AR, Mahle WT, Martin GR, et al: Strategies for implementing screening for critical congenital heart disease, *Pediatrics* 128:e1259–e1267, 2011.

51. Which ductal-dependent lesions are the AAP's primary targets for screening with the use of pulse oximetry?
HLHS, pulmonary atresia, tetralogy of Fallot, total anomalous pulmonary venous return, transposition of the great arteries, and truncus arteriosus are the primary targets for screening with pulse oximetry.

52. What should parents be told about the risk for recurrence of common heart defects?
The risk for CHD in pregnancies after the birth of one affected child is about 1% to 4%. With two affected first-degree relatives, the risk is about 10%. With three affected children, the family may be considered at even higher risk.

Congenital Heart Information Network: www.tchin.org. Accessed on Jan. 6, 2015.

53. Can you think of a "handy" way to remember the congenital cyanotic heart diseases?
See Figure 3-4.

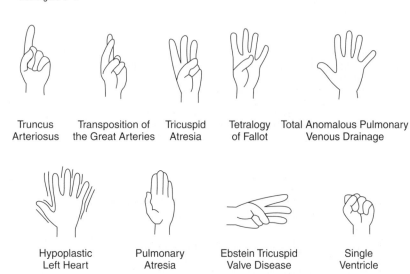

| Truncus Arteriosus | Transposition of the Great Arteries | Tricuspid Atresia | Tetralogy of Fallot | Total Anomalous Pulmonary Venous Drainage |

| Hypoplastic Left Heart | Pulmonary Atresia | Ebstein Tricuspid Valve Disease | Single Ventricle |

Figure 3-4. Congenital cyanotic heart disease hand signatures.

CONGESTIVE HEART FAILURE

54. Identify the clinical signs and symptoms associated with CHF in children.
These may be grouped into three categories:
- **Signs or symptoms of impaired myocardial performance:** cardiomegaly, tachycardia, gallop rhythm, cold extremities or mottling, growth failure, sweating with feeding, pallor
- **Signs or symptoms of pulmonary congestion:** tachypnea, wheezing, rales, cyanosis, dyspnea, cough
- **Signs or symptoms of systemic venous congestion:** hepatomegaly, neck vein distention, peripheral edema (seen in the older patient)

55. How is heart size assessed in older children?
Cardiothoracic (CT) ratio: This is derived by comparing the largest transverse diameter of the heart to the widest internal diameter of the chest: CT ratio = (A + B)/C, as shown in Figure 3-5. A CT ratio of >0.5 indicates cardiomegaly.

56. In infancy, how does the likely cause of CHF vary by age?
See Table 3-5.

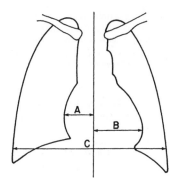

Figure 3-5. The cardiothoracic ratio is obtained by dividing the largest horizontal diameter of the heart *(A + B)* by the longest internal diameter of the chest *(C)*. *(From Park MK:* Pediatric Cardiology for Practitioners, *ed 5. Philadelphia, 2008, Mosby Elsevier, p 66.)*

Table 3-5. Causes of Congestive Heart Failure

AGE OF ONSET	CAUSE
At birth	HLHS with restrictive foramen ovale Volume overload lesions: Severe tricuspid or pulmonary insufficiency (i.e., severe Ebstein, tetralogy of Fallot with absent pulmonary valve) Large systemic arteriovenous fistula Arrhythmia
0-7 days	TGA and VSD PDA in small premature infants HLHS TAPVR, particularly those with pulmonary venous obstruction Systemic arteriovenous fistula Critical AS or PS
1-6 wk	COA isolated or with associated anomalies Critical AS Large left-to-right shunt lesions (VSD, PDA, AVC) All other lesions previously listed
6 wk-4 mo	Large VSD Large PDA Others such as anomalous left coronary artery from the PA

AS = aortic stenosis; AVC = atrioventricular canal; COA = coarctation of the aorta; HLHS = hypoplastic left heart syndrome; PA = pulmonary artery; PDA = patent ductus arteriosus; PS = pulmonary stenosis; TAPVR = total anomalous pulmonary venous return; TGA = transposition of the great arteries; VSD = ventricular septal defect.
Adapted from Park, Myung K: Pediatric Cardiology for Practitioners, *ed 5. St. Louis, 2008, Mosby, p 462.*

KEY POINTS: COMMON CARDIAC CAUSES OF CONGESTIVE HEART FAILURE IN A 6-WEEK-OLD INFANT

1. Ventricular septal defect
2. Atrioventricular canal
3. Patent ductus arteriosus
4. Coarctation of the aorta

57. **What are the typical ages for the presentation of CHF with CHD?**
As a general rule, large-volume overload lesions (e.g., Ebstein anomaly or arteriovenous (AV) malformations) present soon after birth, ductal-dependent lesions present in the first week when the ductus closes, and lesions with significant left-to-right shunting present over the first 1 to 2 months as the normal pulmonary vascular resistance falls (with increased systemic-to-pulmonary shunting).

58. **If a patient develops CHF and cardiomegaly during the newborn period, but no heart murmur is heard, what is the differential diagnosis?**
   - Myocarditis
   - Cardiomyopathy as a result of asphyxia or sepsis
   - Glycogen storage disease (Pompe disease)
   - Cardiac arrhythmia: paroxysmal supraventricular tachycardia, congenital heart block, atrial flutter
   - Arteriovenous malformations (e.g., liver, vein of Galen)

59. **If a patient develops CHF and cardiomegaly after the newborn period, but no murmur is heard, what is the differential diagnosis?**
   Myocardial diseases
   - Myocarditis (viral or idiopathic)
   - Glycogen storage disease (Pompe disease)
   - Endocardial fibroelastosis

   Coronary artery diseases resulting in myocardial insufficiency
   - Anomalous origin of left coronary artery from pulmonary artery
   - Kawasaki syndrome (acute vasculitis of infancy and early childhood)
   - Calcification of the coronary arteries

   CHD with severe heart failure
   - Coarctation of the aorta in infants
   - Ebstein anomaly (may have gallop rhythm)

ELECTROCARDIOGRAMS AND ARRHYTHMIAS

60. **How does the ECG of a term infant differ from that of the older child?**
   - **Birth:** At birth, the ECG reflects RV dominance. The QRS complex consists of a tall R wave in the right precordial leads (V_1 and V_2) and an S wave in the left precordial leads (V_5 and V_6). The axis is also rightward (90 to 150 degrees). T waves are initially variable with relatively low voltage. They are upright in anterior precordial leads (V_1 to V_{3-4}), invert beyond 7 days of age and can remain inverted until about 12 to 13 years.
   - **Toddler age (2 to 4 years):** There is an axis shift from the right to the normal quadrant, and the R wave diminishes over the right precordial leads. The S wave disappears from the left precordium.
   - **School age:** At this age, the ECG has a nearly adult pattern, with a small R and a dominant S in the right precordial leads and an axis in the normal quadrant.

Price A, Kaski J: How to use the paediatric ECG, *Arch Dis Child Educ Pract Ed* 99:53–60, 2014.

61. **What are the characteristic features of the ECG of a premature infant?**
In the premature infant, there is less RV dominance. The R wave may be small in the right precordial leads, and there may be no significant S wave over the left precordium. The electrical axis is often in the normal quadrant (0 to 90 degrees).

62. **Describe the ECG abnormalities associated with potassium and calcium imbalances**
See Figure 3-6.

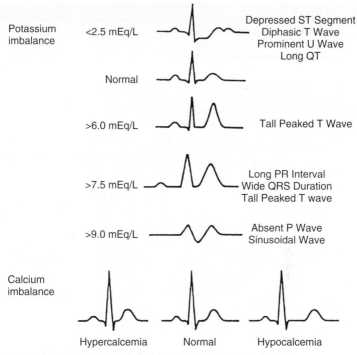

Figure 3-6. Electrocardiogram abnormalities associated with potassium and calcium imbalances. *(From Park MK, Guntheroth WG: How to Read Pediatric ECGs, ed 3. St. Louis, 1992, Mosby, pp 106–107.)*

63. **What is the difference between a QT interval and a corrected QT interval (QTc)?**
The QT interval represents the time required for ventricular depolarization and repolarization. It begins at the onset of the QRS complex and continues through the end of the T wave. This interval varies with the heart rate. The QTc adjusts for heart rate differences. As a rule, a prolonged QTc interval is diagnosed when the QTc exceeds 0.44 second using the following formula, known as the *Bazett formula*, with RR representing the interval from the onset of the preceeding QRS complex to the onset of the next QRS complex:

$$QT_c = QT \text{ (in seconds)} / \sqrt{RR} \text{ interval (in seconds)}$$

Al-Khatib SM, LaPointe NM, Kramer JM, Califf RM: What clinicians should know about the QT interval, *JAMA* 289:2120–2127, 2003.

64. **What causes a prolonged QT interval?**
Congenital long QT syndrome
- Hereditary form: ion channelopathies (genetic defects in specific potassium and sodium channel genes), Jervell and Lange-Nielsen syndrome (associated with deafness), Romano-Ward syndrome
- Sporadic type

Acquired long QT syndrome
- Drug-induced (especially antiarrhythmics, tricyclic antidepressants, phenothiazines)
- Metabolic and electrolyte abnormalities (hypocalcemia, hypokalemia, very-low-energy diets)
- Central nervous system and autonomic nervous system disorders (especially after head trauma or stroke)
- Cardiac disease (myocarditis, coronary artery disease)

Behere SP, Shubkin CD, Weindling SN: Recent advances in the understanding and management of long QT syndrome, *Curr Opin Pediatr* 26:727–733, 2014.
Roden DM: Long QT syndrome, *N Engl J Med* 358:169–176, 2008.
SADS (Sudden Arrhythmia Death Syndromes) Foundation: www.sads.org. (Available is a list of drugs which should be avoided in patients with long QT syndrome.) Accessed on Mar. 31, 2015.

KEY POINTS: ELECTROCARDIOGRAMS

1. As compared with adults, newborns and infants normally have right ventricular dominance.
2. Premature atrial beats in children are usually benign.
3. QT intervals must be corrected for heart rates.

---

65. **What ECG features are found in the long QT syndromes?**
    These are disorders of repolarization with prolongation of the QT interval, corrected for heart rate (QTc). Other ECG findings are relative bradycardia, T-wave abnormalities, and episodic ventricular tachyarrhythmias, particularly torsades de pointes (Fig. 3-7).

Lead II   Lead V$_5$

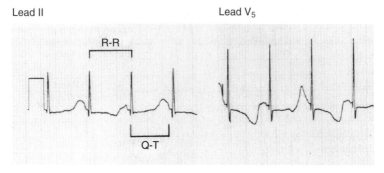

Bazett formula: $QTc = \dfrac{QT}{\sqrt{R\text{-}R}}$

Figure 3-7. Long QT syndrome, leads II and V5. Note long QT interval and T-wave alternans (alternating upright and downgoing T waves). *(From Towbin JA: Molecular genetic basis of sudden cardiac death,* Pediatr Clin North Am *51:1230, 2004, Fig. 1.)*

66. **What characterizes torsades de pointes?**
    From the French for "to turn on a point," this is a ventricular tachycardia of varying forms characterized by abrupt changes in amplitude and polarity (Fig. 3-8). It is a pathologic tachyarrhythmia seen in patients with prolonged QT syndromes and the use of certain drugs (e.g., cisapride, thioridazine).

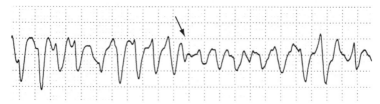

Figure 3-8. Torsades de pointes polymorphic ventricular tachycardia. Note the phase change (*arrow*) with change in QRS polarity. (From Samson RA, Atkins RA: Tachyarrhythmias and defibrillation, *Pediatr Clin North Am* 55:891, 2008.)

67. **When should amiodarone *not* be used as the first-line therapy in patients with ventricular tachycardia?**
    In patients with torsades de pointes (polymorphic ventricular tachycardia with a long QT interval) or with ventricular tachycardia and a long QT interval, amiodarone should not be used. Amiodarone is a class III antiarrhythmic agent and will lengthen the QT interval, predisposing the patient to further arrhythmias.

68. **What are the ECG findings in patients with complete heart block?**
The atrial and ventricular activities are entirely independent. P waves are regular, and QRS complexes are also regular, with a rate slower than the P rate (Fig. 3-9).

Figure 3-9. Complete heart block. Tracing demonstrates atrial activity *(arrows)* independent of slower ventricular rhythm. *(From Zitelli BJ, Davis HW:* Atlas of Pediatric Physical Diagnosis, *ed 4. St. Louis, 2002, Mosby, p 144.)*

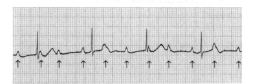

69. **How abnormal are premature atrial contractions?**
Premature atrial beats are usually benign, with the exception of patients with an electrical or anatomic substrate for supraventricular tachycardia (SVT) or atrial flutter.

70. **How does SVT in children differ from physiologic sinus tachycardia?**
SVT typically has the following features:
   • Sudden onset and termination rather than a gradual change in rate
   • Persistent ventricular rate of >180 beats/minute
   • Fixed or almost fixed RR interval on ECG
   • Abnormal P-wave shape or axis or absent P waves
   • Little change in heart rate with activity, crying, or breath holding

71. **When are isolated premature ventricular contractions (PVCs) usually benign in the otherwise healthy school-aged child?**
   • Structurally normal heart
   • ECG intervals, especially QTc, are normal
   • No evidence of myocarditis, cardiomegaly, or ventricular tumor
   • No history of drug use
   • Electrolytes and glucose are normal
   • Ectopy decreases with exercise

72. **Name the two most common mechanisms of SVT**
   • **WPW syndrome** (due to an accessory bypass tract)
   • **AV nodal reentry**

73. **What are the clinical settings in which SVT may occur?**
   • Structurally normal heart: Accessory bypass tract or AV nodal reentry
   • Congenital heart disease (preoperatively or postoperatively): Ebstein anomaly, L-TGA with VSD and pulmonic stenosis; after Mustard, Senning, Fontan procedures
   • Hypertrophic cardiomyopathy
   • Dilated cardiomyopathy
   • Drug-induced: Sympathomimetics (e.g., cold medications, theophylline, beta-agonists)
   • Infections: Myocarditis
   • Hyperthyroidism

74. **What are some of the causes of a wide QRS complex?**
   • Premature ventricular contraction
   • Ventricular tachycardia
   • Premature atrial contraction with aberrant conduction
   • SVT with aberrant conduction
   • Bundle branch blocks
   • Preexcitation syndromes (WPW syndrome)
   • Electrolyte abnormalities
   • Myocarditis
   • Cardiomyopathy
   • Electronic ventricular pacemaker

75. **What vagal maneuvers are used to treat paroxysmal SVT in children?**
Infants
- Place plastic bag filled with crushed ice over forehead and nose
- Induce gag with tongue blade

Older children and adolescents
- Above methods
- Unilateral carotid massage
- Valsalva maneuver (abdominal straining while holding breath)
- Doing a headstand
    In general, the Valsalva maneuver and carotid massage are not as effective for children younger than 4 years. Ocular pressure is not recommended because it has been associated with retinal injury. Vagal stimulation slows conduction and prolongs refractoriness of the AV node, thereby interrupting the reentrant circuit.

76. **In addition to vagal maneuvers, what treatments are used acutely for managing SVT?**
If a patient's clinical condition has deteriorated, synchronized direct-current **cardioversion** is indicated. In patients who are stable and for whom vagal maneuvers have failed, **adenosine** has replaced digoxin and verapamil as the first drug of choice. An initial bolus of 100 mcg/kg will exert an effect in 10 to 20 seconds by slowing conduction through the AV node. If this is ineffective, the dose can be increased in increments of 50 to 100 mcg/kg every 1 to 2 minutes to a maximum single dose of 300 mcg/kg. The usual starting dose in adults is 6 mg and then 12 mg if the tachycardia persists.

77. **Why should an electrographic tracing (preferably with multiple leads) be carried out while administering intravenous adenosine?**
Adenosine is used to convert reentrant SVT to sinus rhythm. During the conversion, observation of the termination of the arrhythmia on ECG can often reveal the mechanism of the tachycardia. If the tachycardia does not terminate other information can be obtained from the ECG including,
- The tachycardia is atrial in origin; one can observe varying degrees of AV block with the atrial tachycardia persisting (e.g., atrial flutter).
- The tachycardia is junctional or ventricular with 1:1 ventriculoatrial (VA) conduction; adenosine may induce VA block with VA dissociation.
- The tachycardia terminated and was immediately restarted by a premature atrial beat.

78. **In what settings should the dose of adenosine be modified for a suspected cardiac arrhythmia?**
Adenosine should not be routinely used in **post–cardiac transplantation patients**. Previous experience with adenosine in these patients has produced asystole with no underlying escape rhythm. Because the heart in these patients does not have normal sympathetic and parasympathetic innervation following transplantation, the response to catecholamines is typically blunted, and the heart rate is generally slower than normal. Additionally, many cardiac transplant recipients are taking dipyridamole (Persantine), which potentiates the effects of adenosine, thereby prolonging the duration of AV block. In patients with **working pacing wires**, it may be possible to use a lower dose of adenosine.
    Due to the abnormal flow patterns in patients with the **Fontan procedure**, these patients frequently require higher doses of adenosine for the treatment of cardiac arrhythmias.

79. **Which children are candidates for transcatheter ablation techniques for SVT?**
Ablation therapy is used most commonly in children with arrhythmias that are refractory to medical management and in those with life-threatening symptoms or possible lifelong medication requirements. Ablation is now commonly performed in children who are symptomatic from WPW or AV nodal reentrant tachycardia. Recommendations for transcatheter ablation are changing as evidence of increased safety and efficacy of the procedure is gathered. Recommendations vary with the age of the patient, the severity of the arrhythmia, the type of lesion, the difficulty with medical control of the rhythm disorder, and the skill of the operator.

McCammond AN, Balaji S: Management of tachyarrhythmias in children, *Curr Treat Options Cardiovasc Med* 14:490–502, 2012.

80. **What is the lethal arrhythmia of WPW syndrome?**

The lethal arrhythmia in patients with WPW is **atrial fibrillation with a rapid ventricular response that degenerates into ventricular fibrillation**. The rate of the ventricular response in these patients is dependent on the effective refractory period of the accessory pathway and not the AV node. This can result in ventricular rates of 250 to 300 beats per minute. Following ablation of the accessory pathway, these patients are no longer at risk for atrial fibrillation.

81. **How is WPW syndrome diagnosed on the baseline ECG?**

An accessory pathway bypasses the AV node, thereby resulting in early ventricular depolarization (preexcitation). It is the most common cause of SVT in children. In infants and younger children with rapid heart rates, the delta wave may not be as evident. Classic findings (Fig. 3-10) include:

- Slurring of the initial portion of the QRS (delta wave).
- PR interval of <100 msec
- QRS duration of >80 msec
- Nonspecific ST and T wave changes
- Additional clues that may be suggestive of WPW include the following:
  - No Q wave in left chest leads
  - Left axis deviation

Perry JC, Giuffre RM, Garson A Jr: Clues to the electrocardiographic diagnosis of subtle Wolff-Parkinson-White syndrome in children, *J Pediatr* 117:871–875, 1990.

Wolff-Parkinson-White Preexcitation

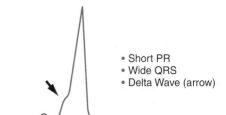

- Short PR
- Wide QRS
- Delta Wave (arrow)

Figure 3-10. Wolf-Parkinson-White preexcitation.
(From Goldberger AL, Goldberger AD, Shvikin A: Clinical Electrocardiography: A Simplified Approach, ed 8. Philadelphia, 2013 Elsevier Saunders, p 208.)

INFECTIOUS AND INFLAMMATORY DISORDERS

82. **How many blood cultures should be obtained in patients suspected of bacterial endocarditis?**

At least **three** separate blood cultures should be obtained. The use of multiple sites may decrease the likelihood of mistaking a contaminant for the true etiologic agent.

83. **Why might properly collected blood cultures be negative in the setting of clinically suspected bacterial endocarditis?**

- Prior antibiotic use
- Endocarditis may be right-sided
- Nonbacterial infection: fungal (e.g., *Aspergillus, Candida*) or unusual organisms (e.g., *Bartonella, Rickettsia, Chlamydia*)
- Unusual bacterial infection: slow-growing organisms (e.g., *Brucella, Haemophilus)* or anaerobes
- Lesions may be mural or nonvalvular (i.e., less likely to be hematogenously seeded)
- Nonbacterial thrombotic endocarditis (sterile platelet-fibrin thrombus formations following endocardial injury)
- Incorrect diagnosis

Starke JR: Infective endocarditis. In Cherry JD, Harrison GJ, Kaplan SL, et al editors: *Feigin and Cherry's Textbook of Pediatric Infectious Diseases*, ed 7. Philadelphia, 2014, Saunders Elsevier, p 358.

84. **When is antibiotic prophylaxis for a dental procedure recommended?**
    In 2007, the American Heart Association made significant changes in antibiotic recommendations for cardiac patients. Only those with the highest risk for adverse outcomes from endocarditis are advised to receive dental prophylaxis. Prophylaxis with dental procedures is recommended for the following:
    - Prosthetic cardiac valve
    - Previous endocarditis
    - Congenital heart disease (CHD): Unrepaired cyanotic CHD, including palliative shunts and conduits; repaired CHD with prosthetic material or device during the first 6 months after the procedure; repaired CHD with residual defects at the site of a prosthetic patch or prosthetic device (which inhibit endothelialization). Antibiotic prophylaxis is not recommended for any other forms of CHD.
    - Cardiac transplantation recipients who develop cardiac valvulopathy

    Wilson W, Taubert KA, Gewitz M, et al: Prevention of infective endocarditis: guidelines from the American Heart Association, *Circulation* 116:1736–1754, 2007.

85. **How reliable is the echocardiogram for diagnosing bacterial endocarditis (BE)?**
    Echocardiography can sometimes identify an intracardiac mass that is attached either to the wall of the myocardium or to part of the valve. Although the yield of echocardiography for diagnosing BE is low, the likelihood of a positive finding is increased under certain conditions (e.g., indwelling catheters, prematurity, immunosuppression, evidence of peripheral embolization). BE is a clinical and laboratory diagnosis (physical examination and blood cultures, respectively) and not solely an "echocardiographic" diagnosis. A negative study does not rule out BE.

    Starke JR: Infective endocarditis. In Cherry JD, Harrison GJ, Kaplan SL, et al editors: *Feigin and Cherry's Textbook of Pediatric Infectious Diseases*, ed 7. Philadelphia, 2014, Saunders Elsevier, p 359–360.

86. **When should myocarditis be suspected?**
    The presenting symptoms of myocarditis can be variable, ranging from subclinical to rapidly progressive CHF. It should be considered in any patient who experiences unexplained heart failure. Clinical signs include tachycardia out of proportion to fever, tachypnea, a quiet precordium, muffled heart tones, gallop rhythm without murmur, and hepatomegaly.

    Pettit MA, Koyfman A, Foran M: Myocarditis, *Pediatr Emerg Care* 30:832–835, 2014.

87. **What conditions are associated with the development of myocarditis?**
    Infections
    - *Bacterial:* Diphtheria
    - *Viral:* Coxsackie B (most common), coxsackie A, human immunodeficiency virus, echoviruses, rubella
    - *Mycoplasmal*
    - *Rickettsial:* Typhus
    - *Fungal:* Actinomycosis, coccidioidomycosis, histoplasmosis
    - *Protozoal:* Trypanosomiasis (Chagas disease), toxoplasmosis

    Inflammatory
    - Kawasaki disease
    - Systemic lupus erythematosus
    - Rheumatoid arthritis
    - Eosinophilic myocarditis

    Chemical and physical agents
    - Radiation injury
    - Drugs: Doxorubicin
    - Toxins: Lead
    - Animal bites: Scorpion, snake

88. **A child visiting from South America presents with symptoms including unilateral eye swelling and new-onset acute CHF. What is a likely diagnosis?**

Acute myocarditis as a result of **Chagas disease** (American trypanosomiasis) is likely. *Romaña sign* is unilateral, painless, violaceous, palpebral edema often accompanied by conjunctivitis. It is seen in 25% to 50% of patients with early Chagas disease in endemic areas. The swelling occurs near the bite site of the parasitic vector, the reduviid bug. Chagas disease, a protozoan infection due to *Trypanosoma cruzi*, is a common cause of acute and chronic myocarditis in Central and South America.

89. **What are the common clinical signs and symptoms of pericarditis?**
    - *Symptoms:* Chest pain, fever, cough, palpitations, irritability, abdominal pain
    - *Signs:* Friction rub, pallor, pulsus paradoxus, muffled heart sounds, neck vein distention, hepatomegaly

90. **What is the position of comfort in the patient with pericarditis?**

The typical patient with pericarditis prefers to sit up and lean forward.

91. **What is Kawasaki disease?**

Also called mucocutaneous lymph node syndrome, *Kawasaki disease* is a multisystem disease characterized by vasculitis of small and medium-sized blood vessels. If untreated, the condition can lead to coronary artery aneurysms and myocardial infarction. A high index of suspicion is important because Kawasaki disease has replaced acute rheumatic fever as the leading cause of identifiable acquired heart disease in the developed world.

Sundel RP: Kawasaki disease, *Rheum Dis Clin North Am* 41:63–73, 2015.
Kawasaki Disease Foundation: www.kdfoundation.org. Accessed on Jan. 6, 2015.

92. **What are the principal diagnostic criteria for Kawasaki disease?**

The presence of fever and at least four of five other features are needed for the classic diagnosis. The mnemonic **My HEART** may be helpful:
    - **M**ucosal changes, especially oral and upper respiratory; dry and chapped lips; "strawberry tongue"
    - **H**and and extremity changes, including reddened palms and soles and edema; desquamation from fingertips and toes is a later finding (second week of illness)
    - **E**ye changes, primarily a bilateral conjunctival infection without discharge
    - **A**denopathy that is usually cervical, often unilateral, and ≥ 1.5 cm in diameter
    - **R**ash that is usually a truncal exanthem without vesicles, bullae, or petechiae
    - **T**emperature elevation, often to 40 ° C (104°F) or above, lasting for >5 days

93. **What makes incomplete (or atypical) Kawasaki disease incomplete (or atypical)?**

Incomplete (or atypical) Kawasaki disease does not fulfill sufficient diagnostic criteria for classic Kawasaki disease. The clinical features are similar but differ in number. In incomplete disease, children have fever but fewer than four signs of mucocutaneous inflammation. About 15% to 20% of reported Kawasaki cases are of the incomplete variety, particularly in children younger than 1 year. Despite not meeting the classic criteria, children with incomplete Kawasaki disease remain at risk for the same coronary artery changes.

Manlhiot C, Christie E, McCrindle BW, et al: Complete and incomplete Kawasaki disease: two sides of the same coin, *Eur J Pediatr* 171:609–611, 2012.

94. **Which diagnostic manifestation of Kawasaki disease is most commonly absent?**

Cervical lymphadenopathy, in both complete and incomplete Kawasaki disease, is most commonly absent. Up to 90% of patients with incomplete disease and 40% to 50% of those who meet classic criteria for Kawasaki disease do not have adenopathy.

Fukushige J, Takahashi N, Ueda Y, Ueda K: Incidence and clinical features of incomplete Kawasaki disease, *Acta Paediatr* 83: 1057, 1994.

95. What laboratory tests are often abnormal in the first 7 to 10 days of the Kawasaki disease?
    - **Complete blood count:** Fifty percent of patients have an elevated white blood cell count (>15,000) with neutrophilia and a progressive normochromic, normocytic anemia. Platelet count increases and peaks in the second to third week of illness.
    - **Urinalysis:** Pyuria without bacteriuria (culture usually negative)
    - **Acute phase reactants:** C-reactive protein, erythrocyte sedimentation rate significantly elevated in 80%
    - **Blood chemistry:** Mild increase in hepatic transaminases, low serum sodium, protein, and/or albumin
    - **Cerebrospinal fluid:** Pleocytosis (usually lymphocytic) with normal protein and glucose

Harnden A, Takahashi M, Burgner D: Kawasaki disease, *BMJ* 338:1133–1138, 2009.

96. What is the typical age of children with Kawasaki disease?
    Eighty percent of cases occur between the ages of 6 months and 5 years. However, cases can occur in infants and teenagers. Both of these groups appear to be at increased risk for developing coronary artery sequelae. The diagnosis is often delayed, particularly in infants, because signs and symptoms of the illness may be incomplete or subtle. Of note, the condition is exceedingly rare in adults.

KEY POINTS: DIAGNOSTIC FEATURES OF KAWASAKI DISEASE

1. Erythema of oral cavity and dry, chapped lips
2. Conjunctivitis: Bilateral and without discharge
3. Edema and erythema and/or desquamation of hands and feet
4. Cervical lymphadenopathy
5. Polymorphous exanthem on trunk, flexor regions, and perineum
6. Fever, often up to 40 °C (104°F), lasting ≥5 days
7. No other identifiable diagnostic entity to explain signs and symptoms
8. Incomplete Kawasaki disease (fever but fewer than four of the other criteria) is common in children <1 year of age.

97. Why should all children with Kawasaki disease receive intravenous immunoglobulin (IVIG) therapy?
    IVIG has been demonstrated to decrease the incidence of coronary artery abnormalities in children with Kawasaki disease. Additionally, fever and laboratory indices of inflammation resolve more quickly after treatment. The most common dosing is a single infusion over 8 to 12 hours of 2 g/kg. In children who remain febrile 36 hours after the first infusion, a second dose of 2 g/kg is recommended.

    When administered 5 to 10 days after the start of fever, IVIG improves outcome, with coronary artery dilation developing in less than 5% of patients and giant coronary aneurysms developing in less than 1% of patients. At present, there is no reliable means of predicting which children with Kawasaki disease will develop coronary artery abnormalities. Therefore, all children with Kawasaki disease should receive parental immunoglobulin.

98. Is aspirin therapy of benefit for children with Kawasaki disease?
    By itself, high-dose aspirin (80 to 100 mg/kg per day divided into doses taken every 6 hours) is effective for decreasing the degree of fever and discomfort in patients during the acute stages of illness. It is unclear whether high-dose aspirin has an additive effect for decreasing the incidence of coronary artery abnormalities when used in conjunction with IVIG. Aspirin may be beneficial when administered in low doses after the resolution of fever because of its effects on platelet aggregation and prevention of the thrombotic complications seen in children with Kawasaki disease. Therefore, when fever has been absent for 48 hours, the patient is switched to aspirin in low doses (3 to 5 mg/kg/day) which is continued for about 6 to 8 weeks. If a follow-up echocardiogram at that time reveals no coronary abnormalities, therapy is usually discontinued. If abnormalities are present, therapy is continued indefinitely.

99. **What is the likelihood of a patient developing coronary artery pathology *with* and *without* treatment for Kawasaki disease?**
In 30% to 50% of patients, a mild diffuse dilation of coronary arteries begins 10 days after the start of fever. If untreated, 20% to 25% of these will progress to true aneurysms (Fig. 3-11). In about 1% of cases, giant aneurysms (>8 mm diameter) develop, which may heal with stenosis and lead to myocardial ischemia. With IVIG therapy, the incidence of aneurysms is reduced to less than 5%.

Harnden A, Takahashi M, Burgner D: Kawasaki disease, *BMJ* 338:1133–1138, 2009.

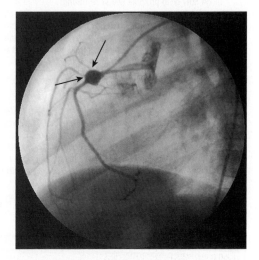

Figure 3-11. Lateral view of coronary angiogram showing right coronary artery with saccular aneurysm. *(From Vetter VL, editor: Pediatric Cardiology: The Requisites in Pediatrics. Philadelphia, 2006, Mosby, p 135.)*

PHARMACOLOGY

100. **How long before oral digoxin begins to work?**
Oral digoxin reaches peak plasma levels 1 to 2 hours after administration, but a peak hemodynamic effect is not evident until 6 hours after administration (versus 2 to 3 hours for intravenous digoxin).

101. **A child with WPW syndrome is given digoxin to prevent SVT. Why is the pediatric cardiologist concerned?**
Ventricular fibrillation has been reported in older children and adolescents with WPW who were treated with digoxin. Digoxin may shorten the effective refractory period of the bypass tract resulting in more rapid conduction through the accessory pathway. Digoxin also slows conduction through the AV node and this combination of effects may result in an increased risk of sudden death in patients with WPW who develop atrial fibrillation. For this reason, propranolol has replaced digoxin as the drug of choice for the treatment of children with WPW and SVT. Of note, verapamil may also both shorten the effective refractory period of the accessory pathway and raise the risk for sudden death in WPW patients should they develop atrial fibrillation.

102. **When should indomethacin be administered to newborns with a PDA?**
Indomethacin is effective for closing a PDA within the first 10 days of life. The drug is indicated for preterm infants with a hemodynamically significant PDA, which is defined as one in which there is deteriorating respiratory status (e.g., tachypnea, apnea, CO_2 retention, increased ventilatory support, failure to wean ventilatory support), poor cardiac output, or evidence of CHF.

Hamrick SEG, Hansmann G: Patent ductus arteriosus of the preterm infant, *Pediatrics* 125:1020–1030, 2010.

103. **What are the side effects of indomethacin in the neonate?**
- Mild but usually transient decreased renal function
- Hyponatremia

- Platelet dysfunction producing a prolonged bleeding time
- Occult blood loss from the gastrointestinal tract

104. **What are the contraindications for indomethacin therapy?**
Indomethacin is contraindicated if the creatinine level is >1.8 mg/dL, the platelet count is <60,000/mm^3, or there is evidence of a bleeding diathesis.

105. **What are the indications for prostaglandin E$_1$ (PGE$_1$) in the neonate?**
PGE$_1$ is indicated in cardiac lesions that depend on a PDA to maintain adequate pulmonary or systemic blood flow or to promote adequate mixing.
- Inadequate pulmonary blood flow (e.g., pulmonary atresia with intact ventricular septum, tricuspid atresia with intact ventricular septum, critical pulmonary stenosis)
- Inadequate systemic blood flow (e.g., critical coarctation of the aorta, interrupted aortic arch, HLHS)
- Inadequate mixing (e.g., transposition of the great vessels)

106. **What are the major side effects of PGE$_1$?**
Apnea, fever, cutaneous flushing, seizures, hypotension, and bradycardia or tachycardia are the major side effects of PGE$_1$.

107. **How do α, β, and dopaminergic receptors differ?**
α: In vascular smooth muscle, these receptors cause vasoconstriction.
β_1: In myocardial smooth muscle, these receptors increase myocardial contractility (inotropic effect), cardiac rate (chronotropic effect) and AV conduction (dromotropic effect).
β_2: In vascular smooth muscle, these receptors cause vasodilation.
Dopaminergic: In renal and mesenteric vascular smooth muscle, these receptors cause vasodilation.

108. **How do relative receptor effects differ by drug type?**
See Table 3-6.

Table 3-6. Relative Receptor Effects by Drug Type

DRUG	α	β_1	β_2	DOPAMINERGIC
Epinephrine	+++	+++	+++	0
Norepinephrine	+++	+++	+	0
Isoproterenol	0	+++	+++	0
Dopamine*	0 to +++ (dose related)	++ to +++ (dose related)	++ (dose related)	+++
Dobutamine	0 to +	+++	+	0

Effect of medication: 0 = none; + = small; ++ = moderate; +++ = large.
*For dopamine, at low doses (2 to 5 μg/kg/min), dopaminergic effects predominate. At high doses (5 to 20 μg/kg/min), increased α and β effects are seen. At very high doses (>20 μg/kg/min), a markedly increased α effect with decreased renal and mesenteric blood flow occurs. For dobutamine, β_1 inotropic effects are more pronounced than are chronotropic effects.

109. **How are emergency infusions for cardiovascular support prepared?**
See Table 3-7.

Table 3-7. Emergency Infusions for Cardiovascular Support

CATECHOLAMINE	MIXTURE	DOSE
Isoproterenol, epinephrine, norepinephrine	0.6 mg × body wt (in kg), added to diluent to make 100 mL	1 mL/hr delivers 0.1 μg/kg/min
Dopamine, dobutamine	6 mg × body wt (in kg), added to diluent to make 100 mL	1 mL/hr delivers 1 μg/kg/min

PHYSICAL EXAMINATION

110. **What causes the first heart sound?**
The *first heart sound* is caused by the closure of the mitral and tricuspid valves.

111. **What causes the second heart sound?**
The *second heart sound* is caused by the closure of the aortic and pulmonary valves.

112. **In what settings can an abnormal second heart sound be auscultated?**
Widely split S_2
- Prolonged RV ejection time
- RV volume overload: Atrial septal defect, partial anomalous pulmonary venous return
- RV conduction delay: Right bundle branch block

Single S_2
- Presence of only one semilunar valve: Aortic or pulmonary atresia, truncus arteriosus
- P_2 not audible: Tetralogy of Fallot, transposition of great arteries
- A_2 delayed: Severe aortic stenosis
- May be normal in a newborn

Paradoxically split S_2 (A_2 follows P_2)
- Severe aortic stenosis
- Left bundle branch block

Loud P_2
- Pulmonary hypertension

113. **What is the difference between pulsus alternans and pulsus paradoxus?**
- *Pulsus alternans* is a pulse pattern in which there is alternating (beat-to-beat) variability of pulse strength due to decreased ventricular performance. This is sometimes seen in patients with severe CHF.
- *Pulsus paradoxus* indicates an exaggeration of the normal reduction of systolic blood pressure during inspiration. Associated conditions include cardiac tamponade (e.g., effusion, constrictive pericarditis), severe respiratory illness (e.g., asthma, pneumonia), and myocardial disease that affects wall compliance (e.g., endocardial fibroelastosis, amyloidosis).

114. **How is pulsus paradoxus measured?**
To measure a pulsus paradoxus, determine the systolic pressure by noting the first audible Korotkoff sound. Then retake the blood pressure by raising the manometer pressure to at least 25 mm Hg higher than the systolic pressure, and allow it to fall very slowly. Stop as soon as the first sound is heard. Note that the sound disappears during inspiration. Lower the pressure slowly, and note when all pulsed beats are heard. The difference between these two pressures is the pulsus paradoxus. Normally, in children, there is an 8- to 10-mm Hg fluctuation in systolic pressure with different phases of respiration.

115. **What is the differential diagnosis for a systolic murmur in each auscultatory area?**
See Fig. 3-12.

116. **What are the most common innocent murmurs?**
See Table 3-8.

117. **What is the effect of sitting up on the typical innocent murmur?**
Sitting up usually brings out or increases the intensity of the murmur of a venous hum.
In contrast, the typical vibratory innocent murmur along the lower left sternal border is loudest in the supine child and will diminish in intensity and sometimes disappear while sitting upright.

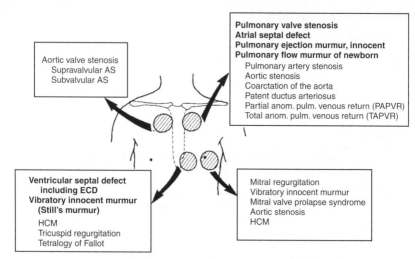

Figure 3-12. Systolic murmurs audible at various locations. Many may radiate to other areas. Less common conditions are shown in smaller type. *AS,* aortic stenosis; *ECD,* endocardial cushion defect, *HCM,* hypertrophic cardiomyopathy. *(From Park MK: Pediatric Cardiology for Practitioners, ed 4. St. Louis, Mosby, 2002, p 32.)*

Table 3-8. Most Common Innocent Murmurs

TYPE (TIMING)	DESCRIPTION OF MURMUR	COMMON AGE GROUP
Classic vibratory murmur; Still's murmur (systolic)	Maximal at MLSB or between LLSB and apex Low-frequency vibratory, "twanging string," or musical Grade 2-3/6 in intensity	3-6 years old; occasionally in infancy
Pulmonary ejection murmur (systolic)	Maximal at ULSB Early to midsystolic Grade 1-2/6 in intensity	8-14 years old
Pulmonary flow murmur of newborn (systolic)	Maximal at ULSB Transmits well to left and right chest, axillae, and back Grade 1-2/6 intensity	Premature and full-term newborns; usually disappears by 3-6 months of age
Venous hum (continuous)	Maximal at right (or left) supraclavicular and infraclavicular areas Inaudible in supine position Intensity changes with rotation of head and compression of jugular vein Grade 1-2/6 in intensity	3-6 years old
Carotid bruit (systolic)	Right supraclavicular area and over carotids Occasional thrill over a carotid artery Grade 2-3/6 intensity	Any age

LLSB = Lower-left sternal border; MLSB = mid-left sternal border; ULSB = upper-left sternal border.

118. What features are suggestive of a pathologic murmur?
    - Diastolic murmurs
    - Late systolic murmurs
    - Pansystolic murmurs
    - Continuous murmurs
    - Murmurs associated with a thrill
    - Murmurs at the aortic area (right-upper sternal border) and tricuspid area (left-lower sternal border)
    - Harsh quality
    - Associated cardiac abnormalities (e.g., asymmetrical pulses, clicks, abnormal splitting)

McCrindle BW, Shaffer KM, Kan JS, et al: Cardinal clinical signs in the differentiation of heart murmurs in children, *Arch Pediatr Adolesc Med* 150:169–174, 1996.
Rosenthal A: How to distinguish between innocent and pathologic murmurs in childhood, *Pediatr Clin North Am* 31:1229–1240, 1984.

119. If a murmur is detected, what other factors suggest that the murmur is pathologic?
    - Evidence of growth retardation (most commonly seen in murmurs with large left-to-right shunts)
    - Associated dysmorphic features (e.g., valvular disease in Hurler syndrome, Noonan syndrome)
    - Exertional cyanosis, pallor, or dyspnea, especially if associated with minor exertion such as climbing a few stairs (may be a sign of early CHF)
    - Short feeding times and volumes in infants (may be a sign of early CHF)
    - Syncopal or presyncopal episodes (may be seen in hypertrophic cardiomyopathy)
    - History of intravenous drug abuse (risk factor for endocarditis)
    - Maternal history of diabetes mellitus (associated with asymmetrical septal hypertrophy, VSD, D-transposition), alcohol use (associated with pulmonic stenosis and VSD), or other medications
    - Family history of congenital heart disease

Etoom Y, Ratnapalan S: Evaluation of children with heart murmurs, *Clin Pediatr* 53:111–117, 2014.

KEY POINTS: PATHOLOGIC MURMURS

1. Diastolic
2. Pansystolic
3. Late systolic
4. Continuous
5. Thrill present on examination
6. Additional cardiac abnormalities (e.g., clicks, abnormal splitting, asymmetric pulses)

SURGERY

120. What are shunt operations?
    Arterial shunts are connections between a systemic artery and the pulmonary artery and are used to improve oxygen saturation in patients with cyanotic CHD and diminished pulmonary blood flow. Venoarterial shunts connect a systemic vein and the pulmonary artery and are also used for similar purposes.

121. Name the major shunt operations (Fig. 3-13) for CHD.
    - The **Blalock-Taussig (BT)** shunt consists of an anastomosis between a subclavian artery and the ipsilateral pulmonary artery. The subclavian artery can be divided and the distal end anastomosed to the pulmonary artery (classic BT shunt), or a prosthetic graft (Gore-Tex) can be interposed between the two arteries (modified BT shunt). It allows for pulmonary blood flow in children with severe pulmonary stenosis or atresia.
    - The **Sano** shunt (not pictured) is a conduit from the right ventricle to the pulmonary artery and is often used as an alternative to the Blalock-Taussig shunt in the Norwood procedure for HLHS.
    - The **Waterston** shunt is an anastomosis between the ascending aorta and the right pulmonary artery. This procedure is rarely performed today.
    - The **Potts** shunt is an anastomosis between the descending aorta and the left pulmonary artery. This procedure is rarely performed today.

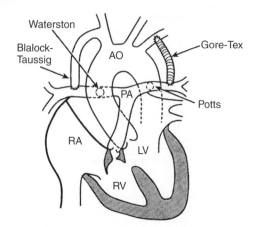

Figure 3-13. Major shunt operations. *AO,* aorta; *LV,* left ventricle; *PA,* pulmonary artery; *RA,* right atrium; *RV,* right ventricle. *(From Park MK:* Pediatric Cardiology for Practitioners, *ed 4. St. Louis, 2002, Mosby, p 194.)*

122. What is the purpose of the Fontan procedure?

The *Fontan procedure* (or operation) is designed to reroute systemic venous blood from the superior and inferior vena cava directly to the pulmonary arteries, thus bypassing the ventricle. It is most commonly used for any cardiac lesion with a single functional ventricle. A common current approach is anastomosis of the superior vena cava to the right pulmonary artery and redirection of flow from the inferior vena cava to the right pulmonary artery through either an intracardiac baffle or an extracardiac conduit. This deoxygenated blood flows passively to the lungs and returns to the ventricle to be pumped to the systemic circulation.

Tsai W, Klein BL: The postoperative cardiac patient, *Clin Pediatr Emerg Med* 6:216–221, 2005.

123. What are the most common rhythm disturbances after the Fontan procedure?

Because of the extensive atrial surgery in the Fontan procedure, there are two major cardiac rhythm issues.

- **Loss of sinus rhythm** with either a nonsinus atrial rhythm or junctional rhythm. Atrial pacing may be required in these patients to either increase heart rate or restore AV synchrony.
- **Intra-atrial reentrant tachycardia** was more common following the old-style Fontan procedure because of the incisional scars and size of the atrium. Although less common with the newer surgical techniques, it remains a major clinical problem in these patients; it is often drug resistant and requires either catheter or surgical ablation.

124. In what type of cardiac surgery is the complication of protein-losing enteropathy more common?

Fontan procedure. Protein-losing enteropathy, which occurs in 2% to 10% of cases, is a condition manifested by variable degrees of ascites, peripheral edema, diarrhea, malabsorption of fat, and hypoalbuminemia. The cardiac function is often normal in these patients, and the cause is attributed to abnormal flow dynamics in the mesenteric vasculature secondary to high pressures in the Fontan circulation.

125. What are some of the reasons to surgically close a VSD?

- Chronic respiratory failure secondary to heart failure
- Chronic heart failure
- Prevention of pulmonary vascular obstructive disease
- Growth failure secondary to chronic heart failure
- Persistent left heart volume load with chronic cardiomegaly
- Aortic valve prolapse with aortic valve insufficiency
- Recurrent endocarditis

126. **What are the indications for closure of an atrial septal defect?**
Asymptomatic children with a secundum atrial septal defect associated with RV dilation and increased pulmonary blood flow typically undergo elective closure between 3 and 5 years of age. Children with a typical secundum atrial septal defect can usually be closed with catheterization techniques. A primum or sinus venosus atrial septal defect is closed with surgery. In addition, a very large secundum defect or associated lesions are typically closed at surgery. The rare infant with a symptomatic atrial septal defect should undergo surgery at the time of diagnosis.

127. **What is the typical timing for the three operations for children with HLHS?**
- **Newborn**: *Norwood procedure*—reconstruction of the new aorta, atrial septectomy, and pulmonary shunt
- **4 to 8 months**: *Glenn shunt* (hemi-Fontan)—superior caval to pulmonary artery connection
- **2 to 4 years**: *Fontan procedure*—inferior vena cava to pulmonary artery connection

Barron DJ, Kilby MD, Davies MD, et al: Hypoplastic left heart syndrome, *Lancet* 374:551–564, 2009.

128. **What are long-term survival rates for children who undergo surgery for HLHS?**
Before the advances of the Norwood procedure in the 1980s, children with HLHS invariably died in the first weeks of life. Following the introduction of the Norwood procedure, survival rates have steadily increased. In the multicenter randomized Single Ventricle Reconstruction trial of infants with HLHS, 3-year survival was 67% for Norwood procedure with a right ventricle-to-pulmonary artery shunt (Sano) versus 61% for infants with Norwood procedure with a modified BT shunt.

Newburger JW, Sleeper LA, Frommelt PC, et al: Transplantation-free survival and interventions at 3 years in the single ventricle reconstruction trial, *Circulation* 129:2013–2020, 2014.

129. **What is the long-term prognosis for heart transplantation during infancy and childhood?**
Survival statistics have improved dramatically during the past 10 years with the use of newer and safer immunosuppressive agents such as cyclosporine and FK506. However, children who receive transplanted hearts are at increased risk for cardiac rejection, infection, accelerated coronary artery disease, and lymphoproliferative syndromes. Recent estimated 5-year survival rates vary between 65% and 80%.

130. **A 5-year-old girl, 2 weeks after an uncomplicated repair of a secundum atrial septal defect, presents with fever, respiratory distress, and a history of the need to sleep sitting up since discharge. What is the diagnosis of immediate concern?**
Post-pericardiotomy syndrome (PPCS) and **pericardial effusion**. PPCS typically occurs between 7 to 21 days after any surgical procedure which opens the pericardial space. Symptoms may include fever, chest pain, irritability, dyspnea, and a preference for sitting up. Physical examination may show fever, tachycardia, increased respiratory rate, hypotension with decreased pulse pressure, muffled heart tones, distended neck veins, hepatomegaly, and pulsus paradoxus.
The differential diagnosis includes residual cardiac lesions, cardiomyopathy, pneumonia, sepsis, and pleural effusions.

131. **What is the etiology of postoperative hypertension following repair of coarctation of the aorta?**
Postoperative hypertension is believed to be due to baroreceptor trauma secondary to surgery, an increase in circulating catecholamines, and an exaggerated renin-angiotensin system response. Treatment with sedation, analgesia, esmolol, nitroprusside, and propranolol has been successful. These drugs can be changed to enalapril or captopril when oral feedings are resumed.

132. **A 5-year-old boy, 6 days after an uncomplicated surgical repair of a coarctation of the aorta, presents with respiratory distress; a left pleural effusion is noted on a chest x-ray. What is the likely appearance and composition of the pleural fluid?**
Turbid, milky white, high in triglycerides and lymphocytes is consistent with a **chylothorax**. Following surgical repair of a coarctation of the aorta, patent ductus arteriosus or a vascular ring,

patients are at risk for chylous pleural effusions secondary to trauma to the thoracic duct. Injury to the thoracic duct can result in leakage of lymphatic/chylous fluid (of intestinal origin) into the pleural space. This typically starts after feedings are resumed and the patient starts to increase fat intake, which increases chyle formation. Children usually respond to a nonfat diet, but sometimes will need surgical ligation of the thoracic duct.

Acknowledgment

The editors gratefully acknowledge the contributions by Dr. Bernard J. Clark III that were retained from the first three editions of *Pediatric Secrets*.

CHAPTER 4

DERMATOLOGY

Kimberly D. Morel, MD, Christine T. Lauren, MD and
Maria C. Garzon, MD

ACNE

1. **When is acne most likely to develop?**
   The development of micro comedones is typically the earliest sign of acne. Studies have shown that comedones occur in three fourths of premenarchal girls at an average age of 10 years and in about half of 10- to 11-year-old boys. They may herald (or predate) the onset of puberty.

2. **When are pimples precocious?**
   Acne vulgaris that begins before age 7 years should warrant further investigation for endocrine abnormalities such as androgen excess or precocious puberty.

   Eichenfield LF, Krakowski AC, Piggott C, et al: Evidence-based recommendations for the diagnosis and treatment of pediatric acne, *Pediatrics* 131:S163–S185, 2013.

3. **Which skin structure is involved in acne pathogenesis?**
   The pilosebaceous unit. It consists of a vellus hair follicle in association with sebaceous glands, which secrete sebum into the lumen of the follicle.

4. **What are the four key factors in acne pathogenesis?**
   1. Androgen–dependent sebum production
   2. Abnormal follicular keratinization, which leads to follicular plugging
   3. Proliferation of *Propionibacterium acnes* bacteria that live in the lumen of the follicle and thrive in an anaerobic environment; *P. acnes* is lipolytic and breaks down sebum, releasing mediators of inflammation
   4. Inflammation

5. **Are blackheads caused by dirty skin?**
   No. The black color of a "blackhead," or open comedone, is caused by the mass of sebum and compact keratin debris that has oxidized at the follicular opening. Whiteheads, also called closed comedones, occur when the contents tent the overlying skin but are not exposed to the atmosphere.

6. **What is the difference between neonatal acne and infantile acne?**
   Neonatal or "baby" acne occurs in up to 20% of newborns and typically presents during the first 4 weeks after birth. Erythematous papulopustules develop on the face, especially the cheeks. It has been attributed to the transient elevation of androgenic hormones (both maternally derived and endogenous) that are present in a newborn infant. The lesions typically resolve within 1 to 3 months as androgen levels fall. *Neonatal cephalic pustulosis* is a term that has been proposed to replace *neonatal acne.* Because lesions have been shown to contain *Malassezia* species, neonatal "acne" may actually represent an inflammatory reaction to this yeast flora and not true acne at all.
   Infantile acne is uncommon and usually presents on a delayed basis (3 to 6 months). Histologically, the lesions are similar to true acne vulgaris as seen in older children: open and closed comedones; inflammatory papules; and rarely, nodules may be present. An examination for signs of androgen excess is indicated although most patients with this condition have no evidence of precocious puberty or increased hormonal levels. Systemic therapy may be required to minimize scarring.

[a]Disclaimer: Although off-label use of medications is discussed in this chapter, it is not designed to provide specific treatment guidelines.
[b]Conflict of interest: Dr. Kimberly Morel: Galderma, Scientific Advisory Board Meeting, July 2013. Pierre Fabre, Scientific Advisory Board Meeting, September 2013. Drs. Kimberly Morel, Christine Lauren and Maria Garzon, Astellas Pharma, Inc., grant support to University.

KEY POINTS: MORPHOLOGIC DESCRIPTIONS OF PRIMARY CUTANEOUS LESIONS

1. **Macule**: A circumscribed, flat area, recognizable by color variation from surrounding skin, ≤1 cm
2. **Patch**: A large macule, >1 cm
3. **Papule**: A circumscribed elevation, ≤1 cm
4. **Plaque**: A large superficial papule, >1 cm
5. **Nodule**: A circumscribed solid elevation, ≤1 cm
6. **Vesicle** (small blister): A clear, fluid-filled elevation, ≤1 cm
7. **Bulla** (large blister): A fluid-filled elevation, >1 cm
8. **Pustule**: A circumscribed elevation of skin filled with pus

7. **Which disorders resemble neonatal and infantile acne?**
   - **Miliaria rubra** or **pustulosa**, often in areas of occlusion and skin folds
   - **Milia**, white papules without surrounding erythema
   - **Sebaceous hyperplasia**, yellowish papules typically on the nose
   - **Seborrheic dermatitis**, erythematous scaly patches rather than pustules.

8. **Is an infant with acne more likely to be a teenager with acne?**
   The presence or severity of acne in an infant who is <3 months old is not believed to correlate with an increased likelihood of adolescent acne. However, delayed acne between 3 and 6 months of age (especially if persistent and severe) is associated with a higher likelihood of more severe adolescent disease. Family history of severe acne also increases the likelihood of future problems.

Herane MI, Ando I: Acne in infancy and acne genetics, *Dermatology* 206:24–28, 2003.

9. **Which factors exacerbate acne?**
   - Vigorous scrubbing or picking of lesions
   - Use of comedogenic makeup or other facial products
   - Medications: anabolic steroids and corticosteroids, lithium, barbiturates, and some oral contraceptives
   - Sweating and tight-fitting clothes or sports equipment
   - Hormone dysregulation, such as polycystic ovarian syndrome
   - Studies are evaluating the influence of high glycemic index diets and insulin resistance

KEY POINTS: MAIN FACTORS IN ACNE PATHOGENESIS

1. Androgen–dependent sebum production
2. Abnormal follicular keratinization
3. Proliferation of *Propionobacterium acnes*
4. Inflammation

10. **What are the most severe forms of acne?**
    Acne fulminans is a rare but severe disorder that has also been called acute febrile ulcerative acne. It occurs mainly in teenage boys as extensive, inflammatory, ulcerating lesions on the trunk and chest that are usually associated with fever, malaise, arthralgia, and leukocytosis. The etiology remains unclear, but immune complexes are thought to be involved. Treatment is systemic and includes the following: antibiotics, glucocorticoids, and retinoids.

    Acne conglobata is a severe form of acne that presents with comedones, papules, pustules, nodules, and abscesses. It is associated with significant scarring. It often arises in early adulthood, more typically in females. Systemic retinoid therapy is the treatment of choice.

James WD: Acne, *N Engl J Med* 352:1463–1472, 2005.

11. **What is the therapeutic approach to acne?**

Acne therapies, including comedolytics, antibacterial agents, and hormonal modulators, target various factors involved in the pathogenesis of acne.

- **Topical antibiotics** including erythromycin and clindamycin should be used in combination with benzoyl peroxide (BPO) to decrease the risk of *Propionibacterium acnes* antibiotic resistance. BPO itself is bactericidal against *P. acnes*.
- **Systemic antibiotics** (e.g., tetracycline and its derivatives) are most frequently used for moderate-to-severe papulopustular acne.
- **Topical retinoids** tretinoin, tazarotene (pregnancy category X), and adapalene are comedolytic agents that prevent the formation of new keratin plugs.
- **Systemic retinoids** (isotretinoin) are used in cases of severe acne vulgaris. The exact mechanism of action of isotretinoin is not known but affects all four factors in acne pathogenesis: keratinization/follicular plugging, inhibition of sebaceous gland activity, reduced *P. acnes,* and inflammation.
- **Hormonal modulation** is most commonly accomplished with oral contraceptives. Select oral contraceptives are Food and Drug Administration (FDA) approved to treat moderate to severe acne in menstruating females over age 14 years. Antiandrogenic agents such as spironolactone have been used in some teenage females with premenstrual flares, hirsutism, and male-pattern alopecia.

Eichenfield LF, Krakowski AC, Piggott C, et al: Evidence-based recommendations for the diagnosis and treatment of pediatric acne, *Pediatrics* 131:S163–S185, 2013.

12. **When is the use of oral isotretinoin indicated in teenagers with acne?**

Isotretinoin, which is 13-cis-retinoic acid, is most appropriately used for **nodulocystic acne**, **acne conglobata**, or **scarring acne** that has been unresponsive to standard modes of treatment (e.g., oral/topical antibiotics, topical retinoids). Given the known side effect of teratogenicity if even one dose of isotretinoin is taken during pregnancy or if a female becomes pregnant within 30 days of the last dose, rigorous monitoring and definitive contraceptive counseling are mandatory. The FDA and the manufacturers of isotretinoin created a registry, called iPLEDGE (www.ipledgeprogram.com), in an effort to reduce the risk of fetal exposure to isotretinoin. This program monitors patients on isotretinoin with monthly lab tests and verification of contraception and knowledge of risks.

Eichenfield LF, Krakowski AC, Piggott C, et al: Evidence-based recommendations for the diagnosis and treatment of pediatric acne, *Pediatrics* 131:S163–185, 2013.
Merritt B, Burkhart CN, Morrell DS: Use of isotretinoin for acne vulgaris, *Pediatr Ann* 38:311–320, 2009.

13. **What serious side effects may be associated with systemic minocycline therapy for acne?**

Tetracyclines, including the derivative minocycline, are widely prescribed oral antibiotics for acne and have been used safely over long periods of time. They are contraindicated for patients <8 years old because of the potential for permanent dental staining. Rare reactions—particularly to minocycline—have included skin discoloration, pneumonitis, autoimmune hepatitis, drug-induced lupus, serum-sickness-like reactions, and severe hypersensitivity reactions.

Brown RJ, Rother KI, Artman H, et al: Minocycline-induced drug hypersensitivity syndrome followed by multiple autoimmune sequelae, *Arch Dermatol* 142:862–868, 2009.

14. **Which combination of acne products will cause a yellow-orange skin and hair discoloration?**

The use of topical dapsone 5% gel (Aczone a off-label under age 12 years) plus BPO will lead to a yellow-orange skin discoloration. Patients should be warned to avoid applying these medications at the same time. Topical sulfacetamide applied at the same time as BPO will also cause this reaction. If alternating application morning and night, a gentle cleansing should occur between each step. Once the reaction occurs, it may take from a few days up to 2 months to resolve.

Dubina MI, Fleischer AB Jr; Interaction of topical sulfacetamide and topical dapsone with benzoyl peroxide, *Arch Dermatol* 145:1027–1029, 2009.

15. **What other topical acne products should not be used in combination?**
The combination of topical tretinoin plus BPO applied at the same time is known to cause oxidation and inactivity of the tretinoin. Tretinoin is also inactivated by sunlight, so it is recommended to apply it in the evening. BPO may be used by the patient the next morning. A topical combination product (Epiduo[b]) has been developed that contains adapalene in a stable combination with 2.5% BPO. It is FDA approved to treat acne in patients who are ≥9 years of age.

16. **What color will your red towel become after you wipe your BPO-covered face with it?**
Pink or even white! The oxidizing effect of BPO has a bactericidal effect on *P. acnes*; the downside is the oxidizing effect will bleach or fade clothing, towels, and bedsheets. Patients should be warned of this effect and to use caution when applying clothing after recent application of BPO.

CLINICAL ISSUES

17. **What skin findings in the midline lumbosacral region are suggestive of occult spinal dysraphism?**
    - Lipoma
    - Hypertrichosis
    - Pits: Sinuses or large dermal dimples (>0.5 cm) that are located >2.5 cm from the anal verge (particularly with lateral deviation of the cleft)
    - Vascular lesions (hemangioma (Fig. 4-1), port wine stain, telangiectasias)
    - Pigmentation variants (both hyperpigmentation, including lentigo and melanocytic nevus, and hypopigmentation)
    - Aplasia cutis congenita
    - Appendages (skin tags, tail)

Drolet BA, Chamlin SL, Garzon MC, et al: Prospective study of spinal anomalies in children with infantile hemangiomas of the lumbosacral skin, *J Pediatr* 157:789–794, 2010.
Drolet B: Birthmarks to worry about. Cutaneous markers of dysraphism, *Dermatol Clin* 16:447–453, 1998.

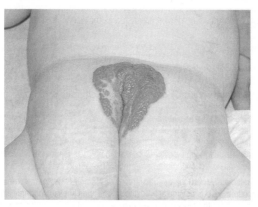

Figure 4-1. Lumbosacral hemangioma with underlying tethered cord. *(From Drolet BA, Garzon MC, editors: Birthmarks of medical significance,* Pediatr Clin North Am *57:1077, 2010.)*

KEY POINTS: MIDLINE LUMBOSACRAL LESIONS ASSOCIATED WITH OCCULT SPINAL DYSRAPHISM OR TETHERED CORD

1. Sacral pits (particularly with lateral deviation of the gluteal cleft)
2. Hairy patches
3. Appendages (skin tag or tail)
4. Sacral lipoma

5. Vascular lesions (hemangioma, port wine stain, telangiectasias)
6. Pigmentation variants (hyperpigmentation, including lentigo and melanocytic nevus, and hypopigmentation)
7. Aplasia cutis congenita

18. **What is the significance of accessory tragi?**
Accessory tragi are fleshy papules or nodules that are typically anterior to the normal tragus, or less commonly on the cheek or jawline. They contain variable amounts of cartilage. In most cases, accessory tragi are isolated cutaneous findings. Extensive defects may be associated with hearing loss. Newborns with accessory tragi should have their hearing tested. Less commonly, they are associated with other first branchial arch abnormalities (e.g., cleft lip and palate) or rare syndromes such as Treacher Collins, VACTERL or oculoauriculovertebral syndrome. Accessory tragi are treated by surgically excising the papule and its cartilaginous stalk.

19. **What conditions cause ringlike rashes on the skin?**
Not all rings are ringworm. Annular (ringlike) skin lesions can be seen in a wide variety of skin diseases in children. Common causes of these lesions include the following:
- Tinea corporis
- Dermatitis (especially nummular)
- Psoriasis
- Urticaria
- Granuloma annulare (often composed of small papules without overlying scale)
- Erythema migrans
- Systemic lupus erythematosus

KEY POINTS: DIFFERENTIAL DIAGNOSES OF RINGLIKE SKIN RASHES

1. Tinea corporis
2. Dermatitis (atopic, nummular, or contact)
3. Psoriasis
4. Granuloma annulare (often composed of small papules without overlying scale)
5. Erythema migrans
6. Systemic lupus erythematosus

20. **What is the appearance and natural history of molluscum contagiosum?**
Molluscum contagiosum is a common skin infection caused by a poxvirus. Lesions are small pinkish-tan, dome-shaped papules that often have a dimpled or umbilicated center. They are usually asymptomatic, but they may be associated with an eczematous dermatitis and itch. Superinfection may complicate the course, require antibiotic therapy, and increase the likelihood of scarring after resolution. In healthy children, the course is self-limited but may last for 2 years. In some cases, persistent and widespread molluscum may require screening for congenital or acquired immunodeficiencies.

21. **What is the best way to eradicate molluscum contagiosum?**
If watchful waiting is not desired, therapeutic options are primarily destructive methods. Curettage (with core removal), cryotherapy, and peeling agents (topical retinoids applied sparingly) can be used. A popular method involves the use of the blistering agent cantharidin,[a] which is applied to individual lesions in the physician's office. Immunomodulating (e.g., imiquimod,[a] cimetidine[a]) and antiviral therapies remain unproved in children.

Moye VA, Cathcart S, Morrell DS: Safety of cantharidin: a retrospective review of cantharidin treatment in 405 children with molluscum contagiosum, *Pediatr Dermatol* 31:450–454, 2014.

22. **What are the common causes of acute urticaria in children?**
Acute urticaria may last for several weeks. If it persists beyond that period, it is typically characterized as chronic urticaria. In children, the most common causes of acute urticaria include the five "I's":
- Infection (viral and bacterial are the most frequent, but fungal pathogens may also cause urticaria)
- Infestation (parasites)

- Ingestion (medication and foods)
- Injections or infusions (immunizations, blood products, and antibiotics)
- Inhalation (allergens such as pollens and molds)

Weston W, Orchard D: Vascular reactions. In Schachner LA, Hansen RC, editors: *Pediatric Dermatology*, ed 3. St. Louis, 2003, Mosby, pp 801–831.

KEY POINTS: COMMON CAUSES OF URTICARIA—THE FIVE I'S

1. Infection (viral and bacterial are the most frequent, but fungal pathogens may also cause urticaria)
2. Infestation (parasites)
3. Ingestion (medications and foods)
4. Injections or infusions (immunizations, blood products, and antibiotics)
5. Inhalation (allergens such as pollens and molds)

23. What is the characteristic clinical picture of erythema nodosum?
A prodrome of fever, chills, malaise, and arthralgia may precede the typical skin findings. Crops of red to blue tender nodules appear over the anterior shins. Lesions may be seen on the knees, ankles, thighs, and, occasionally, the lower extensor forearms and face. They may evolve through a spectrum of colors that resemble a bruise. Often the changes are misdiagnosed as cellulitis or secondary to a traumatic event. This condition is associated with a variety of infectious (e.g., group A beta hemolytic streptococcus, tuberculosis) and noninfectious (e.g., ulcerative colitis, leukemia) causes.

24. What, technically, are warts?
Benign epidermal tumors caused by multiple types of human papillomaviruses.

25. How are plantar warts distinguished clinically from calluses?
Plantar warts are warts on the soles of the feet that can be painful. They are flat or slightly raised areas of firm hyperkeratosis with a collarette of normal skin (Fig. 4-2). Unlike *calluses*, with which they can be confused, plantar warts cause obliteration of the normal skin lines (dermatoglyphics). Pinpoint-sized dark red dots (thrombosed capillaries) may be seen within the wart.

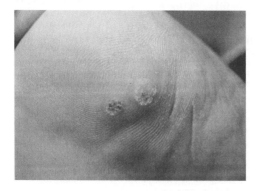

Figure 4-2. Plantar warts. Note disruption of skin lines. Characteristic black dots in the warts are thrombosed capillaries. *(From Cohen BA: Pediatric Dermatology, ed 2. London, 1999, Mosby, p 115.)*

26. How can common warts be treated?
The mode of therapy depends on the type and number of warts, the location on the body, and the age of the patient. No matter what treatment is used, warts can always recur; there are no absolute cures. The major goal is to remove warts without residual scarring. Of course, another option is no treatment at all because most warts self-resolve, but they may take years to do so. A variety of therapies are used. The most commonly used therapy is salicylic acid with regular paring and occlusion. The second is cryotherapy (topical liquid nitrogen) in combination with salicylic acid. Other therapies including topical tretinoin, duct tape application, electrodessication, pulsed dye laser, topical imiquimod, and contact immunotherapy have been used to treat recalcitrant warts in children.[a] In some case reports, oral cimetidine has been

reported to be effective, perhaps because of its immunomodulatory activity, although an evidence base is lacking.[a] Candida antigen injection as an immunotherapy has also been reported to be efficacious.[a]

Lynch MD, Cliffe J, Morris-Jones R: Management of cutaneous viral warts, *BMJ* 348:g3339, 2014.
Swanson A, Canty K: Common pediatric skin conditions with protracted courses: a therapeutic update, *Dermatol Clin* 31:239–249, 2013.

27. **An 8-year-old has a hard, nontender, freely mobile nodule of the neck with a slightly bluish hue of the skin. What is the most likely diagnosis?**
    Pilomatricoma (pilomatrixoma). Also called the benign calcifying epithelioma of Malherbe, it is a benign tumor that often arises in children and adolescents on the face and neck. It is usually not confused with a malignant condition, but excision is often recommended because these nodules increase in size or may become inflamed or infected.

28. **What is the "teeter-totter sign"?**
    A clue to the diagnosis of pilomatricomas. Like children playing on a see-saw, when one side goes up, the other goes down. Pilomatricomas are firm to rock hard, and when one end is pressed down, the other lifts.

29. **What are the most common causes of lumps and bumps in the skin of children?**
    Although most parents fear malignancy, nodules and tumors in the skin are rarely malignant. Epidermal inclusion cysts are one of the most common causes and are often recognized by their central punctum. Pilomatricomas are another common pediatric cause (see questions 27 and 28). Even though benign, they should be removed because they may continue to enlarge over time and may become inflamed or infected. Deep infantile hemangiomas may develop in early infancy; they are soft and partially compressible but may be difficult to recognize if they not associated with the superficial red component of the hemangioma. Imaging may be indicated if there are no external cutaneous clues. Any rapidly progressive or firm, tender lumps should be evaluated promptly because a pediatric surgery referral may be required to assist with a definitive diagnosis and to rule out the rare cases of malignancy.

Wyatt AJ, Hansen RC: Pediatric skin tumors, *Pediatr Clin North Am* 47:937–963, 2000.

30. **Why is a pyogenic granuloma neither pyogenic nor a granuloma?**
    A *pyogenic granuloma*, which is also called a lobular capillary hemangioma, is a common acquired lesion that develops typically at the site of obvious or trivial trauma on any part of the body. Local capillary proliferation occurs, often rapidly, and bleeding may develop (Fig. 4-3). Curettage and electrodessication of the base are curative. The lesion is neither an infectious pyoderma nor a granuloma on biopsy.

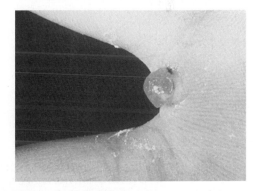

Figure 4-3. Pyogenic granuloma in the web space between fingers. *(From Cohen BA: Pediatric Dermatology, ed 2. London, 1999, Mosby, p 127.)*

31. **What condition is classically diagnosed by the Darier sign?**
    Mastocytoma. This is a benign lesion composed of mast cells that arises at birth or during early infancy. It appears as a pink/tan plaque or nodule, often with a peau d'orange surface. Darier sign refers to the eliciting of erythema and an urticarial wheal by stroking or rubbing the lesion. The skin changes are caused by the release of histamine from the mechanically traumatized mast cells.

32. **What disorder can present as "freckles" associated with hives?**
   Urticaria pigmentosa (mastocytosis). Presenting at birth or during early infancy, multiple mastocytomas appear as brown macules, papules, or plaques (vesicle formation can also occur) and are often mistaken for freckles or melanocytic nevi. Lesions are usually only cutaneous but infrequently they may affect other organ systems (e.g., lungs, kidney, gastrointestinal tract, central nervous system). The Darier sign is a key feature of diagnosis.

33. **What is impetigo?**
   Impetigo is a superficial skin infection that is caused by *Staphylococcus aureus* or group A streptococcus. Historically, streptococcus was the most prevalent agent. However, over the last few decades, *S. aureus* appears to be the predominant organism, although mixed infections may also occur. Bullous impetigo is usually caused by *S. aureus.*

34. **Is topical or systemic therapy better for impetigo?**
   Treatment usually requires an antibiotic that is active against both streptococci and staphylococci. Topical antibiotics can be used in localized disease. The components of over-the-counter triple antibiotic ointment (usually bacitracin-neomycin-polymyxin B) do have some activity against the pathogenic bacteria of impetigo, but mupirocin is more effective as a topical agent although resistance to mupirocin is on the rise. Systemic antibiotics, with activity against both *S. aureus* and group A streptococcus, are usually indicated for extensive involvement, outbreaks among household contacts, schools, or athletic teams, or if topical therapy has failed. Cephalosporins (e.g., cephalexin, cefadroxil), amoxicillin–clavulanate, and dicloxacillin are most effective. Erythromycin is unlikely to be useful because increasing numbers of staphylococci are resistant; local resistance patterns should determine if erythromycin can be used. Methicillin-resistant *S. aureus* (MRSA) is cultured as the causative agent of infections with more frequency. Most MRSA strains remain sensitive to trimethoprim-sulfamethoxazole and clindamycin.

Jungk J, Como-Sabetti K, Stinchfield P, et al: Epidemiology of MRSA at a pediatric healthcare system, *Pediatr Infect Disease J* 26:339–344, 2007.
Sladden MJ, Johnston GA: Common skin infections in children, *BMJ* 329:95–99, 2004.

35. **What dermatologic sign starts from a scratch?**
   Dermographism (dermatographism) occurs when susceptible skin is stroked firmly with a pointed object. The result is a red line that is followed by an erythematous flare, which is eventually followed by a wheal (Fig. 4-4). This "triple response of Lewis" usually occurs within 1 to 3 minutes. Dermographism

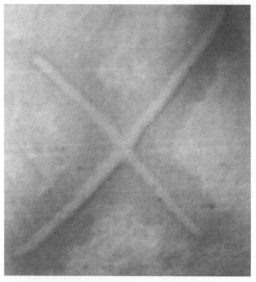

Figure 4-4. Dermographism. An urticarial response is elicited by firm stroking of the skin. *(From Goldbloom RB: Pediatric Clinical Skills, ed 4. Philadelphia, 2011, Elsevier Saunders.)*

(or skin writing) is an exaggerated triple response of Lewis and is seen in patients with urticaria. The tendency to be dermographic can appear at any age and may last for months to years. The cause is often unknown. White dermographism is seen in patients with an atopic diathesis, in whom the red line is replaced by a white line without a subsequent flare and wheal.

36. **Does a geographic tongue occur as a result of global travel?**
No, so there is no need to stay home. *Geographic tongue* refers to the benign condition in which denudations of the filiform papillae on the lingual surface occur, giving the tongue the appearance of a relief map (Fig. 4-5). The patterns may change over hours and days, and the histopathology resembles that of psoriasis. The patient is usually asymptomatic. No treatment is effective or necessary because self-resolution is the rule.

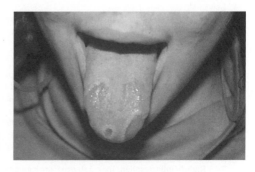

Figure 4-5. Geographic tongue. *(From Sahn EE: Dermatology Pearls. Philadelphia, 1999, Hanley & Belfus, p 162.)*

37. **What diseases are associated with a strawberry tongue?**
Scarlet fever caused by group A beta hemolytic streptococcus and Kawasaki disease are the most common disorders associated with a strawberry tongue. The "strawberry-like" surface characteristics are caused by prominent lingual papillae. A white strawberry tongue is caused by fibrinous exudate overlying the tongue. Red strawberry tongues lack the fibrinous exudate.

38. **What should parents look for in a sunscreen label?**
The FDA has mandated updated language regarding sunscreen labeling. Parents should look for a sunscreen that is described as broad spectrum, which indicates that it will be effective against both ultraviolet A (UVA) and ultraviolet B (UVB) rays. A product with a sun protection factor (SPF) of 30 to 50 is preferred; the maximum allowable labeling is SPF 50 because higher does not afford significantly greater protection. The words *sunblock* and *waterproof* are no longer allowed on the label. Parents should look for water-resistant sunscreen; however, 80 minutes is the maximum time that a sunscreen will remain on the skin during water-based activities or with sweating. Advice should also include physical protection including wearing sun-protective clothing, hats, and sunglasses. Of note, a vitamin D supplement should be considered when practicing cautious sun protection, especially if insufficient vitamin D is being derived from a fortified diet.

ECZEMATOUS DISORDERS

39. **What is the difference between eczema and atopic dermatitis?**
The term *eczema* derives from the Greek word *ekzein*, which means to erupt: *ek (ex)* (out) plus *zein* (to boil). To most physicians, eczema is synonymous with atopic dermatitis, a chronic skin disease manifested by intermittent skin eruptions. **Eczema** is primarily a *morphologic term* used to describe an erythematous, scaling, inflammatory eruption with itching, edema, papules, plaques, vesicles, and crusts. There are other "eczematous eruptions" (nummular eczema, allergic contact dermatitis), but "garden variety" eczema is certainly the most common.
Atopic dermatitis is a broader allergic tendency with multiple dermal manifestations that are mostly secondary to pruritus. Atopic dermatitis has been called an "itch that rashes, not a rash that itches." Its manifestations are dry skin, chronic and recurrent dermatitis, low threshold to pruritus, hyperlinear palms, eyelid pleats (Dennie-Morgan folds), pityriasis alba, and keratosis pilaris, among others.

40. What is the usual distribution of rash in atopic dermatitis?
    - *Infantile:* Cheeks; chin; trunk; and extensor surfaces of extremities, knees, and elbows
    - *Childhood (age 2 to puberty):* Neck; feet; wrists; and periorbital, antecubital, and popliteal fossae
    - *Adult:* Neck, hands, feet, and antecubital and popliteal fossae

KEY POINTS: MAIN FEATURES OF ATOPIC DERMATITIS

1. Extensor surface involvement in infancy
2. Flexural surface involvement in older children
3. Lichenification with chronic scratching
4. Dennie-Morgan folds under eyes
5. Part of atopic triad: atopic dermatitis, asthma, and allergic rhinitis
6. Decreased innate immunity in skin leads to increased susceptibility to bacterial and viral skin infections

41. Describe the five key battle plans to treat atopic dermatitis
    1. **Reduce pruritus.** Topical corticosteroids and bland emollients help reduce pruritus. Oral antihistamines may also be used for their sedative effect at night and may reduce pruritus.
    2. **Hydrate the skin.** Emollients (petrolatum and fragrance-free ointments and creams) prevent the evaporation of moisture via occlusion and are best applied immediately after bathing, when the skin is maximally hydrated, to "lock in" moisture. A "soak and smear" protocol is advisable in refractory cases.
    3. **Reduce inflammation.** Topical steroids[a] are invaluable as anti-inflammatory agents and can hasten the clearing of eruptions that are erythematous (inflamed). Medium-strength corticosteroids can be used on areas other than the face and occluded regions (diaper area); low-strength steroids (e.g., 1% hydrocortisone) may be used in these thin-skinned areas for limited periods of time. Topical immunomodulators, such as topical tacrolimus[b] and pimecrolimus, are approved for the intermittent treatment of moderate to severe atopic dermatitis in children 2 years old and older. However, their long-term side effects have not been fully evaluated.
    4. **Control infection.** Superinfection with *Staphylococcus aureus* is extremely common. First-generation cephalosporins such as cephalexin are the usual antibiotics of choice for infected atopic dermatitis. Dilute bleach baths are sometimes recommended 2 to 3 times per week to reduce staphylococcal colonization.
    5. **Avoid irritants.** Gentle fragrance-free soaps and shampoos should be used; wool and tight synthetic garments should be avoided; tight nonsynthetic garments may help minimize the "itchy" feeling; consider furniture, carpeting, pets, and dust mites as possible irritants and/or trigger factors.

Eichenfield LF, Tom WL, Chamlin SL, et al: Guidelines of care for the management of atopic dermatitis: section 1. Diagnosis and assessment of atopic dermatitis, *J Am Acad Dermatol* 70:338–351, 2014.
Eichenfield LF, Tom WL, Berger TG, et al: Guidelines of care for the management of atopic dermatitis: section 2. Management and treatment of atopic dermatitis with topical therapies, *J Am Acad Dermatol* 71:116–132, 2014.
Sidbury R, Davis DM, Cohen DE, et al: Guidelines of care for the management of atopic dermatitis: section 3. Management and treatment with phototherapy and systemic agents, *J Am Acad Dermatol* 71:327–349, 2014.

42. Why is there a black box warning on topical calcineurin inhibitors?
    The long-term side effects of chronic use are still under investigation. A black box warning is in place based on concerns regarding systemic absorption and the associated increased cancer risk in patient populations in which long-term systemic administration has occurred, such as organ transplant recipients. Patients should be instructed about the importance of sun protection while using topical immunosuppressive medications such as topical calcineurin inhibitors.

Thaçi D, Salgo R: Malignancy concerns of topical calcineurin inhibitors for atopic dermatitis: facts and controversies, *Clin Dermatol* 28:52–56, 2010.

43. Why shouldn't fluorinated (halogenated) and other potent topical steroids be used on the face?
    - Facial skin is thinner and therefore percutaneous absorption is higher.
    - Telangiectasias or spider veins can occur.
    - Cutaneous atrophy can occur.
    - Perioral dermatitis or poststeroid rosacea can occur with rebound symptoms that are worse than the original rash.

44. Is there a genetic basis for atopic dermatitis?
    It is likely that both genetic and environmental factors play a role. Susceptibility to atopic dermatitis is found in patients with mutations in *filaggrin*, an epithelial protein that cross-links keratin and serves to waterproof the epidermis, or outer layer of skin. Many children with atopic dermatitis have a family history of atopy. If one parent has an atopic diathesis, 60% of offspring will be atopic; if two parents do, 80% of children are affected. Monozygotic twins are often concordant for atopic disease.

Palmer CN, Irvine AD, Terron-Kwiatkowski A, et al: Common loss-of-function variants of the epidermal barrier protein filaggrin are a major predisposing factor for atopic dermatitis, *Nat Genet* 38:441–446, 2006.

45. Are there consistent immunologic alterations in children with atopic dermatitis?
    Humoral changes include elevated immunoglobulin E levels and a higher-than-normal number of positive skin tests (type I cutaneous reactions) to common environmental allergens. Cell-mediated abnormalities have been found only during acute flares of the dermatitis; these include mild to moderate depression of cell-mediated immunity, a 30% to 50% decrease in lymphocyte-forming E-rosettes, decreased phagocytosis of yeast cells by neutrophils, and chemotactic defects of polymorphonuclear and mononuclear cells. Innate immunity of the skin is altered with lower levels of antimicrobial peptides and increased susceptibility to bacterial and viral cutaneous infections.

Eichenfield LF, Tom WL, Chamlin SL, et al: Guidelines of care for the management of atopic dermatitis: section 1. Diagnosis and assessment of atopic dermatitis, *J Am Acad Dermatol* 70:338–351, 2014.

46. What is the role of filaggrin mutations in the development of atopic dermatitis?
    The filaggrin gene encodes for an epidermal protein (filaggrin, short for filament-aggregating protein) that is abundantly expressed in the outer layer of the epidermis. Filaggrin is essential for epidermal homeostasis and maintenance of skin barrier functions, as well as retention of water. About 10% of individuals of European ancestry are at least heterozygous carriers for the gene, which results in a 50% decrease in the expressed filaggrin protein. This group is more likely to develop eczema of increased severity.

Irvine AD, McLean WHI, Leung DYM: Filaggrin mutations associated with skin and allergic diseases, *N Engl J Med* 365:1315–1327, 2011.

47. What other skin conditions mimic atopic dermatitis?
    - Seborrheic dermatitis
    - Scabies
    - Psoriasis
    - Tinea capitis
    - Lichen simplex chronicus
    - Acrodermatitis enteropathica
    - Contact dermatitis
    - Langerhans cell histiocytosis
    - Xerotic eczema (dry skin)
    - Immunodeficiency disorders (e.g., Wiskott-Aldrich syndrome, hyperimmunoglobulin E syndrome, severe combined immunodeficiency)
    - Nummular eczema
    - Metabolic disorders (e.g., phenylketonuria, essential fatty acid deficiency, biotinidase deficiency)

48. What is the "atopic march"?

Approximately half of infants with atopic dermatitis will develop asthma, and two thirds will develop allergic rhinitis. Thus, the one condition in infancy marches toward others. Currently under study are ways to interrupt this progression.

Spergel JM, Paller AS: Atopic dermatitis and the atopic march, *J Allergy Clin Immunol* 112: S118–S127, 2003.

49. What features help differentiate seborrheic from atopic dermatitis during infancy?

See Table 4-1.

Table 4-1. Seborrheic Dermatitis Versus Atopic Dermatitis

CHARACTERISTICS	SEBORRHEIC DERMATITIS	ATOPIC DERMATITIS
Color	Salmon	Pink or red (if inflamed)
Scale	Yellowish, greasy	White, not greasy
Age	Infants <6 months or adolescents	May begin at 2-12 months and continue through childhood
Itching	Not present	May be severe
Distribution	Face, postauricular scalp, axillae, and groin	Cheeks, trunk, and extensors of extremities
Associated features	None	Dennie-Morgan folds, allergic shiners, hyperlinear palms
Lichenification	None	May be prominent
Response to topical steroids	Rapid	Slower

50. How should parents cope with cradle cap?

Seborrheic dermatitis of the scalp, also known as "cradle cap," occurs during infancy and presents as a yellow, greasy, scaling adherent rash on the scalp that may extend to the forehead, eyes, ears, eyebrows, nose, and the back of the head. It appears during the first few months of life and generally resolves in several weeks to a few months. Treatment includes the application of mineral oil followed by shampooing with a mild antidandruff shampoo containing selenium sulfide.[a] Parents should be cautioned to take extra care when washing the scalp because these shampoos may irritate the infant's eyes. A mild-potency topical steroid[a] such as hydrocortisone (1% to 2.5%) may be needed for persistent areas. Families should be advised not to scrub or pick off the scale because the underlying skin is often tender and inflamed.

51. What condition causes bumps on the cheeks, upper arms, and thighs?

Keratosis pilaris. Associated both with atopic dermatitis and ichthyosis vulgaris, this condition runs in families and is asymptomatic. It is characterized by spiny follicular papules, giving involved areas a "chicken skin" or "gooseflesh" feel. Usual treatment is with bland emollients or emollients that contain a mild peeling agent, such as lactic acid,[a] salicylic acid,[a] or an alpha hydroxy acid preparation.[a]

52. What are the causes of irritant contact diaper rash?

A variety of local factors are involved. Diapers contribute to the chafing of the skin and the prevention of moisture evaporation, thus increasing epidermal hydration and permeability to irritants and mechanical injury. Proteolytic enzymes in urine and stool and ammonia generated from urine irritate chafed skin. Seasoned pediatricians will advise that alcohol-based diaper wipes also feed the flames of diaper rash.

53. What features of diaper rash suggest more sinister diseases?

- Marked tenderness, rapid onset (staphylococcal scaled skin syndrome)
- Deep ulcerations, vesicles (herpes simplex)

- Beefy red, erosive, extensive lesions (particularly intertriginous) that are poorly responsive to topical steroids and antifungals (Langerhans cell histiocytosis, acrodermatitis enteropathica, immunodeficiency states)
- Extensive and severe lesions with pungent odor (abuse or neglect with infrequent changing)

Boiko S: Making rash decisions in the diaper area, *Pediatr Ann* 29:50–56, 2000.

54. **Are topical steroid/antifungal preparations useful for treating children with diaper dermatitis?**
Most diaper dermatitis is usually diagnosed as either irritant contact dermatitis or candidal dermatitis. Irritant diaper dermatitis responds well to very-low-potency topical corticosteroids[a] (as a result of their anti-inflammatory properties) and a topical barrier such as zinc oxide ointment. Candidiasis of the diaper area responds well to topical antifungal preparations; rarely, an oral anticandidal medication is necessary.[a] In both types of diaper dermatitis, frequent diaper changes, exposure to air, and avoidance of excessive moisture are helpful. Combination preparations containing both antifungal and corticosteroid medications are not recommended to treat diaper dermatitis because the strength of the steroid component in these products is usually too high for use in the diaper area.

Kazaks EL, Lane AT: Diaper dermatitis, *Pediatr Clin North Am* 47:909–920, 2000.

55. **Which dietary deficiencies may be associated with an eczematous dermatitis?**
Deficiencies in zinc, biotin, essential fatty acids, and protein (kwashiorkor) may be associated with eczematous dermatitis.

56. **What are the two main types of contact dermatitis?**
Irritant and **allergic**. Irritant contact dermatitis arises when agents such as harsh soaps, bleaches or acids have direct toxic effects when they come into contact with the skin. Allergic contact dermatitis is a T-cell mediated inflammatory immune reaction that requires sensitization to a specific antigen.

57. **What type of agents can cause allergic contact dermatitis in children?**
Allergic contact dermatitis can occur in all age groups, but it is often underrecognized in pediatric patients. Sensitizers include plant resins (poison ivy, sumac, or oak); nickel in jewelry, metal snaps, and belts; topical neomycin ointment; preservatives (formaldehyde releasers); fabric dyes; and materials used in shoes, including adhesives, rubber accelerators, and leather tanning agents. Of note, allergic contact dermatitis due to metals in mobile phones and other portable electronic devices, especially nickel and chromium, has been on the rise in recent years.

Jacob SE, Admani S: iPad-increasing nickel exposure in children, *Pediatrics* 134:e580–e582, 2014.
Richardson C, Hamann CR, Hamann D, et al: Mobile phone dermatitis in children and adults: a review of the literature, *Pediatr Allergy Immunol Pulmonol* 27:60–69, 2014.

58. **When does the rash in poison ivy appear relative to exposure?**
Poison ivy, or rhus dermatitis, is a typical delayed hypersensitivity reaction. The time between exposure and cutaneous lesions is usually 2 to 4 days. However, the eruption may appear as late as a week or more after contact in individuals who have not been previously sensitized (this explains why lesions continue to erupt after the initial "outbreak" of rash).

59. **Are the vesicles in poison ivy contagious?**
No. The contents of blisters do not contain the allergen. Washing the skin removes all surface oleoresin and prevents further contamination.

60. **What is the "id" reaction?**
Your superego will be stroked if you identify the "id" reaction in a confusing dermatologic case. This reaction is the generalization of a local inflammatory dermatitis (e.g., contact dermatitis, tinea capitis following treatment) to sites that have not been directly involved with the offending agent. The exact mechanism remains unclear, but it may be immune-complex mediated.

61. **How does the vehicle used in a dermatologic preparation affect therapy?**

In general, acute lesions (moist, oozing) are best treated with aqueous, drying preparations. Chronic, dry lesions fare better when a lubricating, moisturizing vehicle is used. As a rule, any vehicle that enhances hydration of the skin enhances the percutaneous absorption of topical medications (most of which are water soluble). Thus, in preparations of equal concentration, the potency relationship is ointment > cream > gel > lotion. See Table 4-2.

Table 4-2. Vehicles Used in Dermatologic Preparations

Drying Vehicles

Lotion: A suspension of powder in water; therapeutic powder remains after aqueous phase evaporates; useful in hairy areas, particularly the scalp

Gel: Transparent emulsion that liquifies when applied to skin; most useful for acne preparations and tar preparations for psoriasis

Pastes: Combination of powder (usually cornstarch) and ointment; stiffer than ointment

Moisturizing Vehicles

Creams: Mixture of oil in a water emulsion; more useful than ointments when environmental humidity is high and in naturally occluded areas; less greasy than ointment

Ointments: Mixture of water in an oil emulsion; also has an inert petroleum base; longer lubricating effect than cream

---

FUNGAL INFECTIONS

62. **What are useful methods for diagnosing tinea infections?**

Although the microscopic examination of potassium hydroxide (KOH) preparations is employed in the search for hyphae, the use of dermatophyte test medium (DTM) is reliable, simple, inexpensive, and more definitive. Samples from hair, skin, or nails are obtained by scraping with a scalpel, cotton-tipped applicator, or toothbrush (the latter especially for tinea capitis), and these are inoculated directly onto the test medium. After approximately 1 to 2 weeks, a color change from yellow to red in the agar surrounding the dermatophyte colony indicates positivity. If the most definitive diagnosis is needed, culture on Sabouraud medium is the test of choice.

KEY POINTS: MAIN FEATURES OF TINEA CAPITIS

1. Scaly alopecia
2. Black-dot hairs often observed
3. Associated with posterior cervical adenopathy
4. Potassium hydroxide test often positive
5. Diagnosis confirmed by positive fungal culture
6. Most common cause: *Trichophyton tonsurans*

---

63. **How does one differentiate between irritant diaper dermatitis and candidal diaper dermatitis?**

Both types of dermatitis often present together. Classic irritant diaper dermatitis involves the skin, which contacts the diaper with sparing of the protected skin folds. Candidal dermatitis, on the other hand, favors skin folds such as the inguinal folds and intragluteal cleft. In clinical practice, candidal infection is a common infection that can be precipitated by the compromise of the cutaneous barrier seen in irritant dermatitis. With candida infection, one typically sees confluent, beefy red plaques involving the groin creases. Scale and satellite papules or pustules are commonly seen at the periphery of the plaque. The diagnosis can be made clinically and with a KOH preparation and yeast culture. Treatment comprises a topical anticandidal agent, such as clotrimazole[a] and use of a thick barrier cream, such as zinc oxide. A few days of a low potency corticosteroid ointment may reduce the erythema significantly. Remember to consider other causes such as seborrheic dermatitis, psoriasis, acrodermatitis enteropathica, Langerhans cell histiocytosis or immunodeficiency for chronic and refractory diaper dermatitis.

64. **Does a scaly scalp and swollen glands qualify a patient to initiate griseofulvin?**
    No. In one study, scalp scaling and cervical adenopathy were more often caused by seborrheic or atopic dermatitis than tinea capitis.

Williams JV, Eichenfield LF, Burke BL, et al: Prevalence of scalp scaling in prepubertal children, *Pediatrics* 115:e1–e6, 2005.

65. **Why is it necessary to culture for tinea capitis?**
    Tinea capitis can be caused by a variety of dermatophyte fungal organisms, and over the last decade, resistance to commonly used treatments (griseofulvin) has been noted. Children with tinea capitis are requiring longer courses of treatment and higher doses of medication to eradicate the fungal infection. Moreover, other conditions (e.g., alopecia areata, psoriasis of the scalp) may be confused with tinea capitis. Therefore, just like for other pediatric infections, it is important to document the type of infection with a culture so that proper treatment may be administered.

66. **How can a culture be obtained if fungal culture medium is not available in the office?**
    The simplest method is to take a cotton swab culturette and moisten it with water. Then, take the swab and rub it over the affected areas and all four quadrants of the scalp. The cotton swab can be used to directly inoculate the fungal culture media if you have it in the office or transported back to the laboratory for inoculation.

Friedlander SF, Pickering B, Cunningham BB, et al: Use of the cotton swab method in diagnosing tinea capitis, *Pediatrics* 104:276–279, 1999.

67. **What are the clinical presentations of tinea capitis?**
    Tinea capitis occurs more commonly in preadolescent children, boys, and in African-American children in the United States. It can present with a variety of morphologic characteristics including scalp scaling, alopecia, erythema, papules, pustules, "black dot" tinea, or a kerion (a boggy, tender mass). The "black dot" presentation occurs when the infected hair shaft breaks at the surface of the scalp, leaving a bald patch with black dots (or lighter dots, depending on hair color) (Fig. 4-6). Regional adenopathy is very common with inflammatory tinea.

Hubbard TW: Predictive value of symptoms in diagnosing childhood tinea capitis, *Arch Pediatr Adolesc Med* 153:1150–1153, 1999.

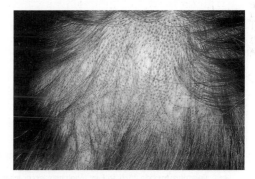

Figure 4-6. Black dot tinea. *(From Schachner LA, Hansen RC, editors:* Pediatric Dermatology, *ed 3. Edinburgh, 2003, Mosby, p 1096.)*

68. **How should children with tinea capitis be treated?**
    The dermatophytes (i.e., fungi) that cause tinea thrive deep in the hair shaft, beyond the reach of topical therapy alone. Recommended therapy includes systemic courses of griseofulvin or terbinafine. The choice of medication should be individualized based on culture results (griseofulvin remains treatment of choice for *Microsporum* species), cost, duration of therapy, and consideration of compliance. Oral griseofulvin (microsize or ultramicrosize preparation) has a long-term safety profile in children. It is given with fatty foods such as milk or ice cream to facilitate absorption. Terbinafine granules, which may be sprinkled onto nonacidic food, are FDA approved for the treatment of tinea capitis in children 4 years of age and older.

Moriarty B, Hay R, Morris-Jones R: The diagnosis and management of tinea, *BMJ* 345:e4380, 2012.

69. How should children who are receiving systemic medication for tinea capitis be monitored?

    The incidence of hepatitis or bone marrow suppression from *griseofulvin* in children is rare. Children who are undergoing an acute course of treatment (6 to 8 weeks) do not need obligatory blood counts or liver function tests. However, a history of hepatitis or associated symptoms would warrant a pretreatment evaluation of liver function and intermittent monitoring. Resistance by tinea to griseofulvin is increasing, and higher, longer dosing may be needed to achieve clinical cure. For those rare cases in which griseofulvin is going to be used for >2 months, one should consider obtaining complete blood counts and liver function tests on an every-other-month basis. When using *terbinafine*, a complete blood count and hepatic function panel are recommended to be performed at baseline and patients should be warned/monitored for evidence of side effects such as hepatotoxicity. Rare cases of hepatic failure and bone marrow suppression have been reported.

70. What is a kerion?

    A *kerion* is a fluctuant and tender mass that occurs in some cases of tinea capitis. It can be associated with alopecia, pustules, and purulent drainage. It is believed to be primarily an excessive inflammatory response to tinea, and thus, initial treatment consists of systemic antifungal agents, principally griseofulvin (>2 years) or terbinafine (> age 4 years), and selenium sulfide shampoo.[a] Prompt diagnosis and management is important to minimize the potential for permanent scarring. Short courses of oral steroids can be considered in those lesions that are exquisitely painful.[a]

    Honig PJ, Caputo GL, Leyden JJ, et al: Microbiology of kerions, *J Pediatr* 123:422–424, 1993.

71. What puts the "versicolor" in tinea versicolor?

    A very common superficial disorder of the skin, tinea versicolor (also known as pityriasis versicolor) is caused by the yeast form of *Malassezia furfur*, known as *Pityrosporum orbiculare* and *Pityrosporum ovale*. It appears as multiple macules and patches with fine scales over the upper trunk; arms; and occasionally, the face and other areas (Fig. 4-7). Lesions are "versatile" in color (i.e., light tan, reddish, or white) and may be "versatile" by season (i.e., lighter in summer and darker in winter as compared with surrounding skin). The yeast interferes with melanin production, possibly by the disruption of tyrosinase activity, at the involved sites. Diagnosis can be confirmed with a KOH preparation of a scraping from the involved skin, which has characteristic fungal hyphae and a grapelike spore pattern referred to as a "spaghetti and meatball" appearance. Dyspigmentation may persist for months after treatment.

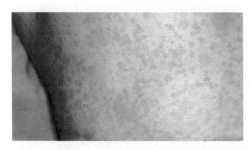

Figure 4-7. Tinea versicolor on the chest. *(From Gawkrodger DJ: Dermatology: An Illustrated Colour Text, ed 3. London, 2002, Churchill Livingstone, p 38.)*

72. How is tinea versicolor treated?

    - **Selenium sulfide 2.5% lotion:**[a] The shampoo or lotion is applied over the affected area overnight nightly during the first week, with decreasing frequency over the ensuing weeks. Monthly application may decrease recurrences.
    - **Ketoconazole 2% shampoo:**[a] The shampoo is applied to wet skin and lathered. Patients are instructed to let the shampoo remain in place without washing for 3 to 5 minutes. Treatment is repeated for 1 to 3 days in a row. Monthly prophylactic treatments are suggested to prevent recurrence.
    - **Topical antifungal creams:**[a] May be applied once to twice daily to limited areas. This is generally less favored in diffuse disease, which is commonly seen.
    - **Oral antifungal agents:**[a] These treatments, which are sometimes effective after a single one-time dose, may be considered off label in severe diffuse or recalcitrant tinea versicolor in older children and adolescents. However, side effects, including liver toxicity, should be considered.

73. Which rashes resemble tinea pedis (athlete's foot) in children?
    - *Dyshidrotic eczema*: Erythema with microvesicles of interdigital spaces and lateral feet
    - *Contact dermatitis*: Typically involves dorsum of feet and spares interdigital spaces
    - *Juvenile plantar dermatosis*: Glazed erythema and fissuring of toes and distal soles; often pruritic
    - *Pitted keratolysis*: Small pits that may converge to superficial erosions on sole of foot; hyperhidrosis and malodor is common; associated with *Corynebacterium* species or *Micrococcus sedentarius* infections

HAIR AND NAIL ABNORMALITIES

74. How fast does hair grow?
    Hair grows about 1 cm per month.

75. On what parts of the skin is hair not normally found?
    Hair is not normally found on the palms, soles, genitalia, and medial/lateral aspects of toes and fingers.

76. What causes sparse or absent hair in children?
    - **Congenital localized**: Nevus sebaceous (or sebaceous), aplasia cutis, incontinentia pigmenti, focal dermal hypoplasia, intrauterine trauma, infection (e.g., herpes)
    - **Congenital diffuse**: Loose anagen syndrome, Menkes syndrome, trichoschisis, genetic syndromes (e.g., ectodermal dysplasia, lamellar ichthyosis, Netherton syndrome)
    - **Acquired localized**: Tinea capitis, alopecia areata, traction alopecia, traumatic scarring (e.g., trichotillomania), androgenic alopecia, Langerhans cell histiocytosis, lupus erythematosus
    - **Acquired diffuse**: Telogen effluvium, anagen effluvium, acrodermatitis enteropathica, endocrinopathies (e.g., hypothyroidism)

Datloff J, Esterly NB: A system for sorting out pediatric alopecia, *Contemp Pediatr* 3:53–56, 1986.

77. Which kind of alopecia simply requires a change in hairstyle as the treatment?
    Traction alopecia. This condition is due to styling with tight braids or ponytails that create tension on the hair shaft. This process damages the area, which serves as the source of new cells for the hair follicle. An erythematous papular or papulopustular reaction may be seen. Treatment involves loose hair styles, avoiding chemical processing or heat treatments. With appropriate changes in hairstyling early on, the prognosis is excellent. However, if the process continues, it may result in scarring alopecia.

Castrelo-Soccio, L: Diagnosis and management of alopecia in children, *Pediatr Clin North Am* 61:427–442, 2014.

78. How can alopecia areata be differentiated clinically from tinea capitis?
    In *tinea capitis*, the fungal organism invades the hair shaft but is also present in the epidermis (the top layer of the skin). There are usually changes of scaling and inflammatory lesions that are intermingled with black dots representing broken hairs. In *alopecia areata*, the scalp is smooth, although patches may be pink to peach colored (Fig. 4-8). Some hairs within the patch may have a tapered appearance, with

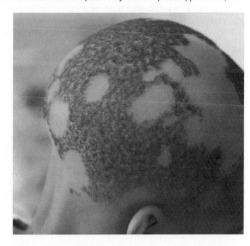

Figure 4-8. Well-demarcated, hairless patches of alopecia areata.

the wider end distally and a thinner end at the base of the scalp (i.e., the "exclamation point hair"). There is no lymphadenopathy in patients with alopecia areata, but this is not uncommon in patients with tinea capitis. The gold standard for diagnosis of tinea is a positive fungal culture.

79. **What are reported as poor prognostic indicators for recovery of hair in patients with alopecia areata?**
    - Atopy
    - Presence of other immune-mediated disease (e.g., thyroid disease, vitiligo)
    - Family history of alopecia areata (about 25% of patients)
    - Young age at onset
    - Longer duration of active disease

Gilhar A, Etzioni A, Paus R: Alopecia areata, *N Engl J Med* 366:1515–1525, 2012.
Uchiyama M, Egusa C, Hobo A, et al: Multivariate analysis of prognostic factors in patients with rapidly progressive alopecia areata, *J Am Acad Dermatol* 67:1163–1173, 2012.

80. **What are treatments for alopecia areata?**
    Treatment is based on the extent of disease: patchy, totalis (loss of all scalp hair), or universalis (loss of all body hair). Although the cause is unknown, alopecia areata is generally considered to be a T-cell-mediated autoimmune disorder. Therefore, treatments are directed at suppressing the immune response around the hair follicle. Topical or intralesional corticosteroids are the mainstays of therapy.[a] Systemic corticosteroids are rarely used chronically because of side effects.[a] Anthralin, as an irritant, or other topical sensitizers are designed to cause a mild dermatitis and theoretically alter local immunity to promote hair regrowth.[a] Other systemic immunosuppressive treatments have been tried in adult patients with alopecia areata; however, because of the potential for side effects, they are not typically employed in children. The option of not treating must be reviewed with the family. Support groups should be offered, and many patients have had improved self-esteem after being fitted with a hair prosthesis.

Castrelo-Soccio, L: Diagnosis and management of alopecia in children, *Pediatr Clin North Am* 61:427–442, 2014.
Children's Alopecia Project: www.childrensalopeciaproject.org. Accessed Nov. 17, 2014.
National Alopecia Areata Foundation: www.naaf.org. Accessed Nov. 17, 2014.

81. **Are most hairs growing or resting?**
    Most infants and children have about 90% of scalp hair in the **growing** (anagen) state and about 10% in the resting (telogen) state. On average, a single scalp hair will grow for about 3 years, rest for 3 months, and then, upon falling out, be replaced by a new growing hair.

82. **You are evaluating a healthy 4-year-old with fine, sparse hair who has never had a haircut. What condition do you suspect?**
    Loose anagen syndrome is typically seen in 2- to 5-year-old blond girls, but may also present in children with darker hair. The hair is of variable lengths and is easily pulled from the scalp. A microscopic examination of a few pulled hairs reveals predominance of anagen hair bulbs with ruffled cuticles. There are no associated nail, skin, or teeth findings in loose anagen syndrome. There is no treatment, but gentle hair styling should be encouraged. Fortunately, the condition tends to improve over time.

Dhurat RP, Deshpande DJ: Loose anagen hair syndrome, *Int J Trichology* 2:96–100, 2010.

83. **What is the likely diagnosis in a child who develops diffuse hair loss 3 months after major surgery?**
    Telogen effluvium. This is the most common cause of acquired diffuse hair loss in children. In a healthy individual, most hairs are present in a growing (anagen) phase. After a physical or emotional stress such as a significant fever, illness, pregnancy, birth, surgery, or large weight loss, a large number of scalp hairs can convert to the resting (telogen) phase. About 2 to 5 months after the stressful event, the hair begins to shed, at times coming out in large clumps. The condition is temporary and usually does not produce a loss of more than 50% of the hair. When the hair roots are examined, there is a characteristic lighter-colored root bulb, which characterizes a telogen hair. The hair loss can continue for 6 to 8 weeks, at which time new, short, regrowing hairs should be visible. The differential diagnosis for telogen effluvium includes nutritional deficiencies and abnormal thyroid function.

Anagen effluvium, the loss of growing hairs, is most commonly seen during radiation and chemotherapy treatments for cancer.

84. **What puzzling cause of asymmetric hair loss in a child will sometimes cause an intern to pull his or her hair out?**

Trichotillomania is hair loss as a result of self-manipulation, such as rubbing, twirling, or pulling. Hair loss is asymmetric. The most common physical finding is unequal hair lengths in the same region without evidence of epidermal changes of the scalp. Parents often do not observe the causative behavior, and convincing them of the likely diagnosis may take some effort. Behavior modification is often the first line of treatment. In younger children, the hair pulling behavior usually resolves; in older children it may persist and require psychiatric referral for additional management. Rarely, a child will swallow the hair and develop vomiting because of the formation of a gastric trichobezoar (hairball).

85. **What causes green hair?**

Children with blond or light-colored hair can develop green hair after long-term exposure to chlorinated swimming pools. It is the result of the incorporation of copper ions into the hair matrix. Over-the-counter chelating shampoos are available for prevention and treatment.

86. **How should ingrown toenails be managed?**

Soaks, open-toed sandals, properly fitting shoes, topical or systemic antibiotics, incision and drainage, or surgical removal of the lateral portion of the nail may all be used. Control is best obtained by letting the nail grow beyond the free end of the toe. Proper instruction on nail care, including straight rather than arc trimming, is mandatory.

87. **Which pathogens are responsible for paronychia?**

Acute paronychia (inflammation of the nail fold, usually with abscess formation) is most commonly caused by *Staphylococcus aureus*. The proximal or lateral nail fold becomes intensely erythematous and tender. If a collection of pus develops at this site, it should be incised and drained. The treatment of acute paronychia includes the oral administration of antistaphylococcal antibiotics.

Chronic paronychia is most often caused by *Candida albicans* and often involves a history of chronic water exposure (e.g., dishwashing, thumb sucking). Although rarely inflamed, there is edema of the nail folds and separation of the folds from the nail plate. The nails may become ridged and develop a yellow-green discoloration. A bacterial culture may reveal a variety of gram-positive and gram-negative organisms. Therapy includes topical antifungal agents and avoidance of water. There is no place for griseofulvin in the treatment of chronic paronychia.

88. **A healthy 7-year-old child who develops progressive yellowing and increasing friability of all nails over a period of 12 months likely has what condition?**

Twenty-nail dystrophy (trachyonychia). The progressive development of rough nails with longitudinal grooves, pitting, chipping, ridges, and discoloration occurring in isolation in school-aged children has been given this name, although not all nails need be involved. The etiology remains unclear, and a majority of cases resolve spontaneously without scarring. The nail changes, however, may be associated with other conditions, such as alopecia areata, lichen planus, psoriasis, and atopic dermatitis.

89. **What nail change may follow hand, foot, and mouth disease (HFMD) several weeks after the other hand and foot changes have resolved?**

Onychomadesis is separation of the proximal nail plate from the nail bed, which is believed to be caused by arrest of nail growth. It is most commonly associated with illness and appears several weeks afterwards. There are now numerous reports of onychomadesis following HFMD caused by Coxsackie virus.

Chu DH, Rubin AI: Diagnosis and management of nail disorders in children, *Pediatr Clin North Am* 61:293–308, 2014.

INFESTATIONS

90. **How do lice differ?**

- **Pediculosis capitis** (head lice): *Pediculus capitis*, the smallest and most common of the three human lice, is an obligate human parasite. Spread occurs directly by contact with an infected individual or indirectly through the use of shared combs, brushes, or hats. Infestation is more common in fine versus coarse hair types.

- **Pediculosis corporis** (body lice): *Pediculus humanus*, the largest (2 to 4 mm) of the three types, is usually associated with poor hygiene. It does not live on the body but instead in the seams of clothing. It can be a vector for other diseases, such as epidemic typhus, trench fever, and relapsing fever.
- **Pediculosis pubis** (pubic lice): *Phthirus pubis* is also known as the crab louse because it is a broad insect with legs that look like claws. It is sometimes mistaken for a brown freckle. Acquisition is primarily through sexual contact.

91. What are the clinical findings of head lice infestation?

    Scalp pruritus is most common, but many children are **asymptomatic.** A search for lice should be made in any school-aged child presenting with scalp itching. Nits (lice eggs) are found in greatest density on the parietal and occipital areas.

92. How is the diagnosis of head lice made?

    On physical examination, an actual louse (wingless, grayish insect about 3 to 4 mm) may be difficult to find, although one should easily be able to find nits. The nits are first attached to the hair close to the surface of the scalp and are oval and flesh-colored (Fig. 4-9). They are not easily removed from the hair shaft (as compared with hair casts, dandruff, and external debris). Over-diagnosis of head lice is common. Microscopic evaluation of the suspected nit can confirm the diagnosis. When the louse emerges, the empty egg case, or nit, appears white in color and remains firmly attached to the hair shaft as the hair grows out (see Fig. 4-9).

Pollack RJ, Kiszewski AE, Spielman A: Overdiagnosis and consequent mismanagement of head louse infestations in North America, *Pediatr Infect Dis J* 19:689–693, 2000.

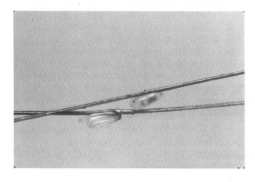

Figure 4-9. Viable head louse egg (right) and hatched empty nit (left) attached to a child's hair. *(From Schachner LA, Hansen RC, editors:* Pediatric Dermatology, *ed 3. Edinburgh, 2003, Mosby, p 1143.)*

93. What types of treatment are available for head lice?

    - **Permethrin:** 1% and 5% (Nix, Elimite)
    - **Pyrethrins:** (RID, A-200, R&C) (Resistance is increasing in these over-the-counter products.)
    - **Malathion:** 0.5% (Ovide is FDA-approved for the treatment of head lice in children 6 years and older; it is contraindicated in children under 2 years of age.)
    - **5% Benzyl Alcohol Lotion:** (Ulesfia is FDA-approved for treatment of head lice in children 6 months of age and older.)
    - **Asphyxiants:** Examples: petroleum jelly (Vaseline), mayonnaise, olive oil (These have questionable efficacy and are messy!)
    - **Ivermectin:** 0.5% lotion (Sklice is FDA-approved for treatment of head lice in children 6 months of age and older.)
    - **Lindane:** 1% (Kwell is not recommended given "black box warning" regarding serious neurotoxicity.)
    - **Nit picking:** (See question 95.)

Pariser DM, Meinking TL, Bell M, et al: Topical 0.5% ivermectin lotion for treatment of head lice, *N Engl J Med* 367:1687–1693, 2012.

Frankowski BL, Bocchini JA Jr, Council on School Health and Committee on Infectious Diseases: Head lice, *Pediatrics* 126:392–403, 2010.

94. **What precautions should be taken before prescribing malathion 0.5% lotion (Ovide) for head lice?**

Malathion, a weak organophosphate cholinesterase inhibitor, is an approved prescription topical treatment for resistant head lice and their eggs. It is approved for use in children ≥6 years of age. It is contraindicated for neonates and infants. Because it is flammable, malathion should never be used near an open flame or heat source. It should be used in a well-ventilated area given its odor, and precautions also include increased absorption through open sores.

95. **Should parents nit pick?**

Once an infestation of lice has been properly treated, the nits are not viable or contagious. Despite this, many schools will not allow children with nits to attend even though this nit-free policy has not been shown to be of benefit for controlling outbreaks. Increasing resistance to therapy may make removal more important to avoid diagnostic confusion. Manual removal (nit picking) is the most effective method; however, it is time consuming and tedious. Fine-toothed combs, such as the LiceMeister comb (available through the National Pediculosis Association [www.headlice.org]) or other fine-toothed veterinary combs, aid in the removal.

96. **How is a skin scraping for scabies or "scabies prep" done?**

Because the highest percentage of mites are usually concentrated on the hands and feet, the web spaces between digits are the best places to look for the characteristic linear burrows. Moisten the skin with alcohol or mineral oil, scrape across the area of the burrow with a small, rounded scalpel blade (e.g., No. 15 or blunt-edged Fomon blade), and place the scrapings on a glass slide with a drop of KOH (or additional mineral oil, if used) and a cover slip. Burrows, if unseen, can be more precisely localized by rubbing a washable felt-tip marker across the web space and removing the ink with alcohol (called the *burrow ink test*). If burrows are present, ink will penetrate through the stratum corneum and outline the site. Under the microscope, mites, eggs, and/or scybala (mite feces) may be seen (Fig. 4-10).

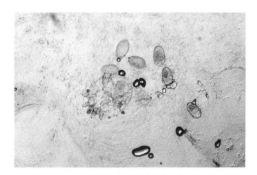

Figure 4-10. Scabies mite and eggs. *(From Gates RH, editor:* Infectious Disease Secrets, *ed 2. Philadelphia, 2003, Hanley & Belfus, p 356.)*

97. **What treatment eliminates the scabies' babies?**

The treatment of choice for treating scabies is permethrin 5% cream (Elimite, Acticin). It may be used in children as young as 2 months old with a low risk of neurotoxicity.[a] It is more effective and preferred over Lindane, which has a much higher potential risk of neurotoxicity.

Permethrin cream is applied from the neck to the toes at night with removal after 8 to 14 hours by bathing or showering. The scalp is also treated in infants and younger children without a full head of hair. Retreatment in 1 week is recommended. Physicians must make patients aware of the fact that lesions and pruritus may linger for at least 2 weeks after effective therapy. Antihistamines and low-potency topical steroids may help control symptoms.[a] It must be stressed that all family members and close contacts should be treated simultaneously.

Gunning K, Pippitt K, Kiraly B, et al: Pediculosis and scabies: treatment update, *Am Fam Physician* 86:535–541, 2012.

98. Which areas of the body are more commonly involved in scabies in younger children compared with adults?
Infants and children: axillae with nodules and scalp, face, soles, and dorsal foot
Adults: interdigital

Boralevi F, Diallo A, Miquel J, et al: Clinical phenotype of scabies by age, *Pediatrics 133*:e910–e916, 2014.

99. In what conditions is the "breakfast, lunch, and dinner" sign noted?
This is a tongue-in-cheek reference to the tendency of an insect to move from site to site for a meal. A typical appearance is a series of linear pink or urticarial papules each with a central pinpoint punctum that occur in response to the bite of a **bed bug** (*Cimex lectularius*) or other crawling insect (Fig. 4-11).

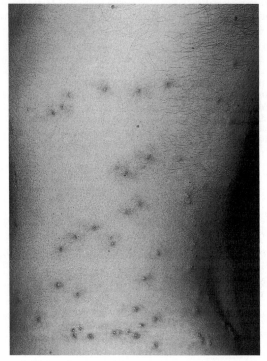

Figure 4-11. Bed bug bites with erythematous wheals or papules that may itch. They frequently attack exposed areas, especially at night. *(Callen JP, Greer KE, Paller AS, et al:* Color Atlas of Dermatology, *ed 2. Philadelphia, 2000, WB Saunders, p 67.)*

100. Will getting a new mattress ensure that the bed bugs won't bite?
No, infestations are not limited to the mattress. Other furniture, clutter in the room, and cracks and crevices in the wall or floor may also harbor bedbugs. They are then attracted to the warm moist carbon dioxide around the sleeping child in the dark of night.

NEONATAL CONDITIONS

101. What are the most common birthmarks?
- **Salmon patches** (nevus simplex, vascular stains) are faint, pink-red, macular patches composed of distended dermal capillaries that are found on the glabella, eyelids, and the nape of the neck. They are seen in 70% of white infants and 60% of black infants. Although they usually fade, they may persist indefinitely, becoming more prominent during crying.

- **Mongolian spots** (dermal melanosis) are blue-black macules that are found on the lumbosacral area and occasionally on shoulders and backs. They are seen in 80% to 90% of babies with darker skin types but ≤10% of white fair-skinned infants. Most of these spots fade by 2 years of age and disappear by age 10.

102. **How should pustular lesions be evaluated in the newborn period?**
It is very important to rule out infectious etiologies, because some may be life-threatening. The purulent material should be evaluated with a Gram stain, potassium hydroxide (KOH), Tzanck preparation, and bacterial and viral cultures. A Wright stain will reveal the presence of neutrophils or eosinophils. See Table 4-3.

Table 4-3. Common Neonatal Papular Lesions

CHARACTERISTICS	NEONATAL CEPHALIC PUSTULOSIS	MILIA	ERYTHEMA TOXICUM
Distribution	Face	Face and other areas	Face, trunk, and extremities
Appearance	Papule or pustule	Yellow or white papule	Yellow or white papule
Erythematous	Yes	No	Yes
Contents on smear	PMNs	Keratin + sebaceous material	Eosinophils
Incidence	Occasional	40-50% of term infants	30-50% of term infants
Course	Last several months	Disappear in 3-4 weeks	Disappear in 2 weeks

PMNs = Polymorphonuclear cells.

103. **What is the differential diagnosis of vesicles or pustules in the newborn?**
See Table 4-4.

Table 4-4. Differential Diagnosis of Vesicles in the Newborn

NONINFECTIOUS	INFECTIOUS
Miliaria	Candidiasis
Erythema toxicum	Staphylococcal folliculitis/impetigo
Transient neonatal pustular melanosis	Herpes simplex
Benign cephalic pustulosis (neonatal acne)	Congenital syphilis
Infantile acropustulosis	Varicella
Incontinentia pigmenti	Bacterial sepsis
Langerhans cell histiocytosis	Scabies

Adapted from: Frieden IJ, Howard R: Vesicles, pustules, bullae, erosions and ulcerations. In Eichenfield LF, Frieden IJ, Esterly NB, editors: Textbook of Neonatal Dermatology, *ed 2. Philadelphia, 2008, WB Saunders, pp 131–158.*

104. **What is the medical significance of cutis marmorata?**
Cutis marmorata is the bluish mottling of the skin often seen in infants and young children who have been exposed to low temperatures or chilling. The reticulated marbling effect is the result of dilated capillaries and venules causing darkened areas on the skin, which disappears with warming. Cutis marmorata is of no medical significance and no treatment is indicated. However, *persistent* cutis marmorata is associated with trisomy 21, trisomy 18, and Cornelia de Lange syndromes. There is also a congenital vascular anomaly called cutis marmorata telangiectatic

congenita (CMTC) that has persistent purple reticulate mottling of the skin. In addition capillary malformations (port wine stains) may have a reticulated appearance and be mistaken for cutis marmorata.

105. **A healthy infant with scattered reddish nodules on the back skin most likely has what condition?**

Subcutaneous fat necrosis consists of sharply circumscribed, indurated nodular lesions usually seen in healthy, term newborns and infants during the first few days to weeks of life. The stony hard areas of panniculitis are reddish to violaceous in color and are most often found on the cheeks, back, buttocks, arms, and thighs. Most lesions are self-limiting and require no therapy. However, occasionally they may extensively calcify and spontaneously drain with subsequent scarring. Remember that significant hypercalcemia may be present in a small number of patients. Therefore, a serum calcium level should be ordered whenever the disorder is suspected. It should be rechecked periodically until the condition resolves and for several months thereafter.

106. **What should the family of a newborn with a yellow, hairless patch with a cobblestone texture be advised to do?**

The lesion is likely a **nevus sebaceous**. This hamartomatous neoplasm usually presents as a yellow-pink hairless plaque on the scalp or face at the time of birth (Fig. 4-12) and is composed primarily of malformed sebaceous glands. Under the influence of androgens at puberty, the glands may hypertrophy and lead to the development of other neoplasms, most often benign adnexal tumors. The exact risk of basal cell carcinoma development is controversial but generally low. Some experts advise excision during the preteen, prepubertal years. Careful monitoring of the lesion for new growths or nonhealing ulcerations at all ages is advised, especially during adolescence.

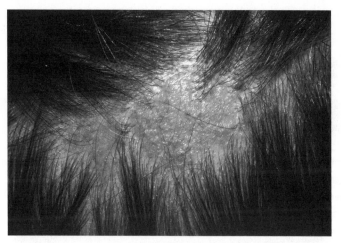

Figure 4-12. Orange-yellow nevus sebaceous of the scalp. *(From Kleigman RM, Stanton BF, Schor NF, et al:* Nelson Textbook of Pediatrics, *ed 19, Philadelphia, 2011, Elsevier Saunders, p 2235.)*

107. **What syndromes are associated with aplasia cutis congenita?**

Aplasia cutis congenita (congenital absence of the skin) presents on the scalp as solitary or multiple well-demarcated ulcerations or atrophic scars. Of variable depth, the lesions may be limited to epidermis and upper dermis or occasionally extend into the skull and dura (Fig. 4-13). When a "hair collar" is present, an underlying connection with the CNS must be considered. Although most children with this lesion are otherwise normal without associated anomalies, other associations include epidermolysis bullosa, placental infarcts, teratogens, sebaceous nevi, and limb anomalies. Aplasia cutis is a feature of trisomy 13, 4p-, oculocerebrocutaneous syndrome and Adams-Oliver syndrome.

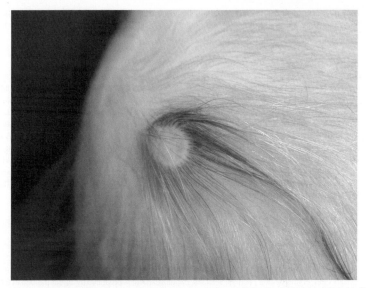

Figure 4-13. Healed aplasia cutis congenita with "hair collar sign." *(From Zitelli BJ, Davis HW:* Atlas of Pediatric Physical Diagnosis, *ed 5, Philadelphia, 2011, Mosby Elsevier, p 342.)*

108. **Describe the appearance and distribution of transient neonatal pustular melanosis.**
     Consisting of small vesicopustular lesions 2 to 4 mm in size, transient pustular melanosis occurs in almost 5% of black and <1% of white newborns. It may be present at birth or appear shortly after birth. The lesions most often cluster on the neck, chin, palms, and soles, although they may occur on the face and trunk. The pustules rupture easily and progress to brown, pigmented macules with a fine collarette of scale (Fig. 4-14). Microscopic examination of the

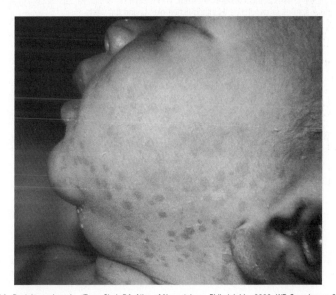

Figure 4-14. Pustular melanosis. *(From Clark DA:* Atlas of Neonatology. *Philadelphia, 2000, WB Saunders, p 261.)*

contents of the pustules reveals neutrophils with no organisms. There are no associated systemic manifestations, and the eruption is self-limited, although the hyperpigmentation may last for months.

109. Is erythema toxicum neonatorum really toxic?
Not in the least. *Erythema toxicum* is a common eruption composed of erythematous macules, papules, and pustules that occur in newborns, usually during the first few days of life. The lesions may start as irregular, blotchy, red macules, varying in size from millimeters to several centimeters. They often develop into 1- to 3-mm, yellow-white papules and pustules on an erythematous base, giving a "flea-bitten" appearance. They occur all over the body except on the palms and soles, which are spared because the lesions occur in pilosebaceous follicles, which are absent on the palmar and plantar surfaces. The rash is less common in premature infants, with incidence proportional to gestational age and peaking at 41 to 42 weeks. Although it may be seen at birth, it is most common during the first 3 to 4 days of life and is occasionally noted as late as 10 days of life. Erythema toxicum usually lasts 5 to 7 days and heals without pigmentation. Other than the rash, the newborn appears healthy.

110. For academic (and billing) purposes, is it possible to be more scientific about the diagnosis of "prickly heat"?
The scientific name for this condition is *miliaria rubra*. It is due to sweat retention, and its clinical morphology is determined by the level at which sweat is trapped. Sweat trapped at a superficial level produces clear vesicles without surrounding erythema (sudamina or crystallina). Miliaria rubra (prickly heat, erythematous papules, vesicles, papulovesicles) is produced by sweat trapped at a deeper level. Pustular lesions (miliaria pustulosa) and even abscesses (miliaria profunda) are produced with sweat retention at the deepest of levels (infants rarely develop these types). With the advent of air conditioning, miliaria rarely occurs in newborn nurseries.

PAPULOSQUAMOUS DISORDERS

111. What diseases are associated with the Koebner reaction?
Koebnerization is a response to local injury whereby skin lesions are found at the sites of trauma (e.g., linear lesions at the sites of scratching). This is seen in patients with psoriasis (Fig. 4-15), as well as those with other conditions including lichen planus and flat warts.

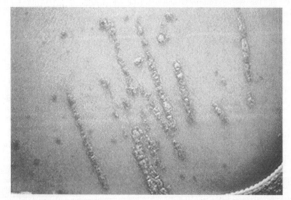

Figure 4-15. Koebner phenomenon in psoriasis with linear plaques at site of excoriations. *(From Cohen BA:* Pediatric Dermatology, *ed 2. St. Louis, 1999, Mosby, p 63.)*

112. **What is the typical pattern of lesions in childhood psoriasis?**

Psoriasis presents as well-circumscribed, erythematous plaques with overlying white scale in children and adults. These occur on the scalp, elbows, knees (Fig. 4-16), sacrum, and genitalia. Psoriasis may also present with guttate (droplike) lesions over the trunk and extremities. These children may have group A beta hemolytic streptococcus infection as an underlying precipitating factor.

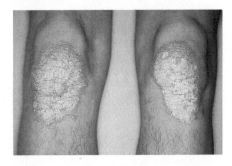

Figure 4-16. Plaques of psoriasis on the knees. *(From Gawkrodger DJ:* Dermatology: An Illustrated Colour Text, *ed 3. London, 2002, Churchill Livingstone, p 27.)*

113. **What percentage of children with psoriasis have nail involvement?**

Nail changes, most commonly pitting, may be the only manifestation of psoriasis (Fig. 4-17). The reported incidence of nail pitting in children with psoriasis is as high as 40%. In a recent study, boys were found to have nail involvement more often than girls. Other nail changes include onycholysis (separation of the nail plate from nail bed at the distal margin) and thickening of the nail plate, often with white-yellow discoloration.

Mercy K, Kwasny M, Cordoro KM, et al: Clinical manifestations of pediatric psoriasis: results of a multicenter study in the United States, *Pediatr Dermatol* 30:424–428, 2013.

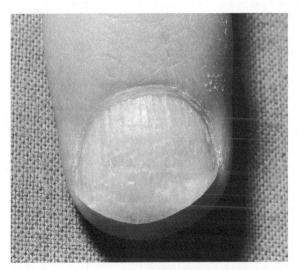

Figure 4-17. Nail pitting associated with psoriasis. *(From Goldbloom RB:* Pediatric Clinical Skills, *ed 4. Philadelphia, 2011, Elsevier Saunders, p 228.)*

114. **A skin scale that easily bleeds on removal is characteristic of what condition?**
The appearance of punctate bleeding points after removal of a scale is the *Auspitz sign*. It is seen primarily in **psoriasis** and is related to the rupture of capillaries high in the papillary dermis, near the surface of the skin.

115. **How is the increased prevalence of childhood obesity associated with psoriasis?**
Overweight and obesity are associated with higher likelihood of childhood psoriasis. In addition, adolescent patients with psoriasis have higher blood lipids. This highlights the importance of screening children with psoriasis for cardiovascular disease risk factors.

Koebnick C, Black MH, Smith N, et al: The association of psoriasis and elevated blood lipids in overweight and obese children, *J Pediatr* 159:577–583, 2011.

116. **What are treatment modalities for psoriasis?**
Various therapies have been used to treat psoriasis. The choice of treatment will depend on the extent of involvement, previous treatments, and the age of the patient. Topical treatments include topical corticosteroids, calcipotriene (a vitamin D analog), retinoids, and tar.[a] Other treatment modalities include UVB (typically narrow band UVB) phototherapy and, rarely, systemic retinoids and methotrexate.[a] Biologic agents such as etanercept have been used to treat widespread moderate-to-severe psoriasis in pediatric patients.[a]

Mercy K, Kwasny M, Cordoro KM, et al: Clinical manifestations of pediatric psoriasis: results of a multicenter study in the United States, *Pediatr Dermatol* 30:424–428, 2013.
Shah KN: Diagnosis and treatment of pediatric psoriasis, *Am J Clin Dermatol* 14:195–213, 2013.

117. **What are the eight Ps of lichen planus?**
- **Papules**: Usually 2 to 6 mm in diameter; often seen in a linear pattern as a result of the Koebner reaction
- **Plaques**: Commonly generated from a confluence of papules with exaggerated surface markings of the overlying skin (Wickham striae)
- **Planar**: Individual lesions, usually flat-topped
- **Purple**: Distinctly violaceous
- **Pruritus**: Often intensely itchy
- **Polygonal**: Borders of papules are often angulated
- **Penis**: Common site of involvement in children
- **Persistent**: Chronic, with remissions and exacerbations for up to 18 months

118. **How is pityriasis rosea distinguished from secondary syphilis?**
The distinction is often made with difficulty because both are primarily papulosquamous rashes. *Pityriasis rosea* classically consists of oval lesions that organize in parallel fashion on the trunk (the "Christmas tree" distribution) and are preceded in 40% to 80% of cases by a large annular erythematous lesion (herald patch). *Secondary syphilis* lesions occur 3 to 6 weeks after the chancre, and compared with pityriasis rosea, they may have more involvement of the palms, soles, and mucous membranes and accompanying lymphadenopathy. However, because atypical presentations are common, testing for syphilis should be performed in any sexually active individual who is diagnosed with pityriasis rosea.

119. **What is the treatment for pityriasis rosea?**
Pityriasis rosea is a self-limited condition that usually resolves in 6 to 12 weeks. Therefore, treatment is often not required, unless there is significant pruritus or cosmetic disfigurement. A wide range of treatments are reported. Topical corticosteroids[a] may help reduce pruritus, but they do not alter the course of the disease. UVB phototherapy results in clinical improvement in some individuals, and there are few reports to support the use of oral erythromycin[a] to shorten the course. However, overall evidence supporting the use of these therapies is lacking.

Drago F, Broccolo F, Rebora A: Pityriasis rosea: an update with a critical appraisal of its possible herpesviral etiology, *J Am Acad Dermatol* 61:303–318, 2009.

120. What is the likely diagnosis for a 5-year-old who presents with a linear array of recently acquired pink to hypopigmented papules on the arm?

Although the differential diagnosis may be broad, a common cause of this type of eruption is **lichen striatus**. This eruption is generally asymptomatic, does not require treatment, and lasts from weeks to a few years. Light spots following the acute rash may persist for longer.

Peramiquel L, Baselga E, Dalmau J, et al: Lichen striatus: clinical and epidemiological review of 23 cases, *Eur J Pediatr* 165:267–269, 2006.

PHOTODERMATOLOGY

121. Why is limiting excessive sun exposure in children important?

Many people experience a significant percentage of their lifetime sun exposure early in life. Years of unprotected sun exposure will lead to freckling, wrinkling, and skin cancer formation, including melanoma. In an era of rising rates of melanoma and squamous and basal cell carcinomas, the use of sun-protection strategies during the pediatric years could lower the risk to an individual.

122. Why should indoor tanning be addressed and discouraged in children?

Indoor tanning has become common among adolescent girls. In a recent study, 24% of high school girls reported indoor tanning use. Indoor tanning is associated with an increased risk of melanoma in adulthood. One study found that indoor tanning before the age of 35 years increases the risk of melanoma by 59%. Many, but not all, states now have legislation restricting tanning bed use among minors.

Guy GP Jr, Berkowitz Z, Tai E, et al: Indoor tanning among high school students in the United States, 2009 and 2011, *JAMA Dermatol* 150:501–511, 2014.

123. What are good strategies for protection against sun exposure?

- Seek shade when possible and remember that the sun's rays are strongest between 10 AM and 2 PM.
- Remember that water, snow, and sand reflect the sun's rays and may increase your chance of sunburn.
- Wear protective clothing, hats, and sunglasses.
- Apply sunscreen at least 30 minutes before sun exposure.
- Use a broad-spectrum sunscreen with an SPF of 30 or higher.
- Apply liberal amounts of sunscreen: about 1 oz (shot glass size or 30 mL) is enough to cover the exposed skin areas of an average sized adult; 15 mL is typically required for a 7-year-old child.
- Use a water-resistant sunscreen, and reapply sunscreen every 80 minutes during water-based activities or when sweating.
- Wear lip protection that contains sunscreen.

American Academy of Dermatology: www.aad.org/media-resources/stats-and-facts/prevention-and-care/sunscreens. Accessed on Mar. 14, 2015.

124. How is the SPF of a sunscreen determined?

SPF is the level of effectiveness of a sunscreen's ability to protect against UVB light. It is not a measurement of UVA light protection. The SPF rating is a ratio of the dose of ultraviolet light needed to produce minimal redness on sun-protected skin to the dose of ultraviolet light needed to produce minimal redness on unprotected skin.

125. Should sunscreens be avoided in infants?

This is controversial. There are concerns that the skin of infants <6 months of age has different absorptive characteristics and that biologic systems that metabolize and excrete drugs may not be fully developed. Therefore, clothing protection and sun protective behaviors are advised for children <6 months of age. Physical protection (e.g., clothing, hats, shade, sunglasses) is ideal, but if an infant's skin is not adequately protected, it may be reasonable to apply sunscreen to small areas, such as the face and the back of the hands. Physical sunscreens containing zinc oxide are preferred over chemical sunscreens for use on infant skin.

Committee on Environmental Health and Section on Dermatology: Ultraviolet light: a hazard to children and adolescents, *Pediatrics* 127:588–597, 2011.
American Academy of Pediatrics: www.healthychildren.org/English/ages-stages/baby/bathing-skin-care/Pages/Baby-Sunburn-Prevention.aspx. Accessed on Mar. 14, 2015.

126. **Do we risk developing vitamin D deficiency by using sun protection?**
Vitamin D synthesis is a beneficial effect of exposure to ultraviolet light and several studies suggest an association between low vitamin D levels and the development of cancer. This however should not be interpreted as a reason to seek a tan. In most people, adequate amounts of vitamin D can be obtained by ingesting a healthy diet including foods that naturally contain or are fortified with vitamin D. The American Academy of Pediatrics has increased their recommended daily intake of vitamin D to prevent rickets and vitamin D deficiency in children.

Wagner CI, Greer FR, AAP section on breastfeeding: Prevention of rickets and vitamin D deficiency in infants, children and adolescents, *Pediatrics* 122:1142–1152, 2008.

127. **Which "lime" disease is not transmitted by ticks?**
Limes contain psoralens that react with ultraviolet light and that can produce erythema, vesicles, and/or hyperpigmentation on areas of the skin that have come in contact with lime juice. This is known as **phytophotodermatitis** and is seen with other psoralen-containing plants, such as celery and figs. Additionally, berloque dermatitis (berloque is French for "pendant," which some lesions can resemble) is an irregularly patterned hyperpigmentation of the neck due to photosensitization by furocoumarins (i.e., psoralens) in perfumes. It is caused by fragrances that contain bergamot oil, an extract from the peel of a type of orange that is grown in southern France and Italy. Bergamot oil contains 5-methoxypsoralen, which enhances the erythematous and pigmentary response of UVA light.

128. **Which conditions are associated with marked sun sensitivity?**
    - **Inherited disorders**: Porphyrias, xeroderma pigmentosum, Bloom syndrome, Rothmund-Thomson syndrome, Hartnup disorder
    - **Exogenous agents**: Drugs (e.g., tetracyclines, thiazides), photoallergic contact dermatitis (associated with perfumes and para-aminobenzoic acid esters)
    - **Systemic disease**: Lupus erythematosus, dermatomyositis
    - **Idiopathic disorders**: Polymorphous light eruption, solar urticaria, actinic prurigo, hydroa vacciniforme

Chantorn R, Lim HW, Shwayder TA: Photosensitivity disorders in children: part I, *J Am Acad Dermatol* 67:1093.e1–e18, 2012.
Chantorn R, Lim HW, Shwayder TA: Photosensitivity disorders in children: part II, *J Am Acad Dermatol* 67:1113.e1–e15, 2012.

129. **What is the appearance of polymorphous light eruption?**
The most common pediatric photodermatosis, polymorphous light eruption is characterized by itchy red papules, plaques, or papulovesicles that appear several hours to days after ultraviolet light exposure. It can be diagnosed by phototesting (i.e., the induction of lesions by intentional ultraviolet light exposure) and by skin biopsy. It is usually suggested by the classic history and the exclusion of other photosensitivity disease.

Gruber-Wackernagel A, Byrne SN, Wolf P: Polymorphous light eruption: clinical aspects and pathogenesis, *Dermatol Clin* 32:315–334, 2014.

130. **Is a child with sun sensitivity protected by sitting behind a window?**
Yes and no, depending on the reason for the sensitivity. Ultraviolet light is divided into three wavelength groups: ultraviolet C (UVC), 200 to 290 nm; UVB, 290 to 320 nm; and UVA, 320 to 400 nm. UVC light is cytotoxic and can cause retinal injury, but fortunately it is almost completely absorbed by the ozone layer. UVB light causes sunburn; dermatologic flares (e.g., in patients with lupus erythematosus); and, with chronic exposure, skin cancer. UVA light (which is also emitted from the fluorescent lamps used in most schools) is responsible for psoralen and drug phototoxicity and porphyria flares. It can cause skin

cancer with chronic exposure. Windows block UVB light, but not UVA. Thus, children with UVA-sensitive disorders are not protected by sitting behind a window unless it has been pretreated with a UVA filter.

PIGMENTATION DISORDERS

131. **What disorders of childhood are associated with areas of hypopigmentation?**
    Hypopigmentation is caused by a decrease—not a total absence—of pigmentation or melanin. Conditions that feature hypopigmented lesions include tuberous sclerosis, tinea versicolor, pityriasis alba, nevus depigmentosus, hypomelanosis of Ito, leprosy, and postinflammatory hypopigmentation.

132. **Is treatment helpful for children with postinflammatory hypopigmentation?**
    In children with pityriasis alba, very-low-potency topical steroids, emolliation, and sun protection measures can make skin color more uniform. Treatment does not seem to help in other cases of postinflammatory hypopigmentation, such as those that occur after dermatitis, infection, abrasions, or burns, but sun protection is advisable.

133. **What treatments are available for vitiligo?**
    Vitiligo is a disorder of depigmentation (total absence of pigmentation with sharp demarcations; Fig. 4-18). The etiology is unknown but may be autoimmune in nature. There are rare associations with other autoimmune conditions, including thyroiditis and juvenile-onset diabetes. Treatment may be unsatisfactory. Potent topical steroids have been used for localized areas.[a] Off-label topical tacrolimus ointment[a, b] has been used with some success to treat facial vitiligo in children. Ultraviolet light therapy has been employed for some children with severe, extensive disease. More recently, excimer laser (308 nm) has been instituted as a potentially effective treatment for focal disease. Dyes (including self-tanning agents) and coverage cosmetics are often helpful for camouflaging skin lesions.

National Vitiligo Foundation: www.mynvfi.org. Accessed on Mar. 20, 2015.

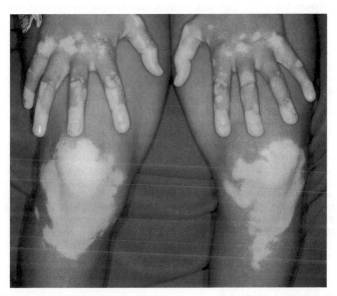

Figure 4-18. Vitiligo. Note well-demarcated areas of total depigmentation. *(From White GM, Cox NH: Diseases of the Skin: A Color Atlas and Text. London, 2002, Mosby, p 286.)*

134. **What conditions are associated with congenital depigmentation of the skin?**
    Congenital depigmentation, or albinism, constitutes a number of genetically inherited syndromes that are characterized by disorders of melanin synthesis and that may affect the skin, hair, and eyes.

Generalized (oculocutaneous) albinism is often complicated by ocular abnormalities, including visual impairment, photophobia, and nystagmus. *Piebaldism* is a distinct form of congenital depigmentation that affects segments of skin. Patients with this condition often have a forelock of white hair, which is caused by a genetic mutation that differs from generalized albinism. *Localized congenital depigmentation* associated with a white forelock, heterochromia irides, and congenital deafness characterizes Waardenburg syndrome.

135. **What is the likely diagnosis if a patient taking trimethoprim–sulfamethoxazole develops a single erythematous, sharply marginated, round lesion that leaves an area of hyperpigmentation upon resolution?**
    Fixed drug eruption. These 2- to 10-cm red to violaceous inflammatory plaques, are usually solitary and may blister. This hypersensitivity reaction occurs after medication ingestion (commonly antibiotics), especially trimethoprim–sulfamethoxazole and tetracycline. The resultant hyperpigmentation helps make the distinction.

Morelli JG, Tay YK, Rogers M, et al: Fixed drug eruptions in children, *J Pediatr* 134:365–367, 1999.

136. **Why are Spitz nevi and malignant melanoma often confused?**
    The Spitz nevus can appear suddenly and grow rapidly. Histologically, it has many features that can be mistaken for malignancy. It actually was previously referred to as benign juvenile melanoma. "Benign" is the key word for this red to brown, dome-shaped papule, which usually appears on the face or extremity. Clinicopathologic correlation is the key to making this diagnosis. It is essential that an experienced pathologist interpret the biopsy when a Spitz nevus is suspected. Melanoma in childhood has been misdiagnosed as Spitz nevi, and Spitz nevi have been misdiagnosed as melanoma.

Murphy ME, Boyer JD, Stashower ME, et al: The surgical management of Spitz nevi, *Dermatol Surg* 28:1065–1069, 2002.

137. **In children with pigmented nevi, what factors increase the risk of melanoma?**
    Melanoma is rare during childhood. If there is a family history of melanoma or atypical moles, a history of severe sunburns before the age of 18 years, or the child has a giant congenital nevus, the risk is greater. The risk increases with age and in those with fair skin (Fitzpatrick skin type), those children who tan poorly and freckle. Estimated risks vary for different-sized congenital nevi. The projected lifetime risk for a melanoma developing within a congenital nevus is controversial. For small congenital nevi, the risk is low. For giant congenital nevi, the risk is estimated to be 6% to 8%. Acquired nevi very rarely develop melanomas.

Gibbs NF, Makkar HS: Disorders of hyperpigmentation and melanocytes. In Eichenfield LF, Frieden IJ, Esterly NB, editors: *Textbook of Neonatal Dermatology*, ed 2. Philadelphia, 2008, WB Saunders, pp 397–421.

138. **How do the ABC's of pediatric melanoma differ from adult melanoma?**
    The conventional melanoma detection criteria in adults are based on the "ABCDE" rules, which stand for **A**symmetry, **B**order irregularity, **C**olor variegation, **D**iameter >6 mm, and **E**volution. In a recent retrospective review of pediatric melanoma, **A**melanosis, **B**leeding, "**B**umps," uniform **C**olor, variable **D**iameter, and **D**e novo development were also proposed additional descriptors for detecting melanoma in the pediatric population.

Cordoro KM, Gupta D, Frieden IJ, et al: Pediatric melanoma: results of a large cohort study and proposal for modified ABCD detection criteria for children, *J Am Acad Dermatol* 68:913–925, 2013.

VASCULAR BIRTHMARKS

139. **How are vascular birthmarks classified?**
    The updated biologic classification of vascular birthmarks is the most widely accepted classification of vascular birthmarks. It was first proposed in 1982 and was adapted recently to reflect new knowledge. Two broad categories of vascular birthmarks are described: **vascular tumors** and **vascular malformations**. There are many types of vascular tumors, but infantile hemangiomas are the most

common. These demonstrate cellular hyperplasia. Vascular malformations, which are composed of dysplastic, malformed vessels, are categorized on the basis of their flow characteristics and type of anomalous channels. The majority of vascular anomalies seen in childhood fit into these categories.

Vascular tumors (selected):
- Infantile hemangioma
- Congenital hemangioma
- Kaposiform hemangioendothelioma
- Tufted angioma
- Pyogenic granuloma

Vascular malformations:
- Capillary malformation (port wine stains, salmon patch)
- Lymphatic malformation (lymphangioma microcystic, macrocystic)
- Venous malformations
- Arteriovenous malformations
- Combined malformations

Wassef M and the Scientific Committee of the International Society for the Study of Vascular Anomalies: *Updated ISSVA classification.* Melbourne, Australia, April 2014.
Mulliken JB, Glowacki J: Hemangiomas and vascular malformations in infants and children, *Plast Reconstr Surg* 69:412–420, 1982.

140. **What is the natural history of untreated infantile hemangiomas?**
Hemangiomas or, more specifically, infantile hemangiomas, are common benign vascular tumors. They are rarely fully developed at birth, but precursor lesions (an area of pallor, telangiectasia, or "bruise") may be detected on close inspection within the first few days of life. They may have superficial and/or deep components. Hemangiomas undergo a growth phase until the child reaches the age of 6 to 12 months, at which time the tumors start to involute. Hemangiomas mark out their territory early and thereafter may grow in thickness or volume. Growth is nonlinear and often most dramatic in the first few months of life with many reaching 80% of their final size by 3 months of age. This process of involution occurs over several years. There still may be residual skin changes (e.g., skin redundancy, pallor, atrophy, telangiectasia) after the hemangioma has resolved. Management of infantile hemangiomas needs to be individualized because many factors are assessed in the decision to actively treat an infantile hemangioma.

Luu M, Frieden IJ: Haemangioma: clinical course, complications and management, *Br J Dermatol* 169:20–30, 2013.

141. **What are the major goals of the management of infantile hemangiomas?**
The decisions regarding which hemangiomas require treatment and the best therapeutic modalities may not always be easy ones. The major goals of management are as follows:
- Prevent or reverse life- or function-threatening complications.
- Treat ulcerated hemangiomas.
- Prevent permanent disfigurement caused by a rapidly enlarging lesion.
- Minimize psychosocial stress for the family and the patient.
- Avoid overly aggressive procedures that may result in scarring in lesions that have a good likelihood of involuting without significant residual lesions.

Luu M, Frieden IJ: Haemangioma: clinical course, complications and management, *Br J Dermatol* 169:20–30, 2013.

142. **What can patterns of hemangiomas on the skin surface tell us?**
The characteristics of hemangiomas on the skin surface can provide clues to underlying abnormalities and help predict outcomes. Hemangiomas are described as being superficial when they are located in the upper dermis and present as red papules and plaques ("strawberry"). Deep hemangiomas are located in the deeper dermis and subcutaneous tissue and are often blue-purple in color. Mixed hemangiomas have both superficial and deep components ("iceberg phenomenon"). Hemangiomas are also characterized based on their distribution on the skin surface. Hemangiomas that appear to arise from a single focus are called "localized" or "focal" hemangiomas, and lesions that cover a broad area on the skin surface, which might represent a developmental subunit, are called "segmental."

Multiple focal lesions (multifocal) may herald internal hemangiomas, and segmental hemangiomas may predict involvement with other anatomic and developmental disorders (PHACE syndrome).

Haggstrom AN, Lammer EJ, Schneider RA, et al: Patterns of infantile hemangiomas: new clues to hemangioma pathogenesis and embryonic facial development, *Pediatrics* 117:698–703, 2006.

143. Which hemangiomas are especially worrisome?
    - **Multiple cutaneous hemangiomas** may be associated with visceral hemangiomas (most commonly liver hemangiomas).
    - **Large/bulky hemangiomas** may cause significant disfigurement of underlying structures.
    - **Segmental hemangiomas** are associated with PHACE and LUMBAR syndromes.
    - **"Beard" hemangiomas** may be a marker for underlying laryngeal or subglottic hemangiomas that may impair respiratory function.
    - **Midline spinal hemangiomas** may be a marker for an underlying spinal cord abnormality.
    - **Head and neck hemangiomas,** usually segmental lesions >5 cm in diameter, may be associated with other congenital anomalies, including central nervous system, cardiac, ocular, and sternal defects (e.g., posterior fossa malformation, hemangioma, arterial abnormalities, coarctation, eye abnormalities, sternal defects [PHACE(S)] syndrome).
    - **Vulnerable anatomic locations** impair vital functions and cause disfigurement (e.g. periocular, neck, lip, nasal tip).
    - **Ulcerated hemangiomas** increase risk of superinfection, can bleed, cause pain, and lead to scarring.

Haggstrom AN, Drolet BA, Baselga E, et al: Prospective study of infantile hemangiomas: clinical characteristics predicting complications and treatment, *Pediatrics* 118:882–887, 2006.

144. When is treatment indicated for infantile hemangiomas?
    - Lesions that interfere with normal physiologic functioning (i.e., breathing, hearing, eating, vision), especially periocular hemangiomas (to prevent amblyopia)
    - Recurrent bleeding, ulceration, or infection
    - A rapidly growing lesion that distorts facial features or has the potential to result in a residual lesion that will cause disfigurement

Luu M, Frieden IJ: Haemangioma: clinical course, complications and management, *Br J Dermatol* 169:20–30, 2013.

145. What are the most commonly used treatments for problematic infantile hemangiomas?

In most cases, topical treatments are used for smaller superficial lesions that do not have a significant deep component; systemic medications are used for larger deeper infantile hemangiomas, those with an aggressive growth pattern, or those that require more aggressive therapy. Until recently, there were no FDA-approved treatments for infantile hemangioma. In March of 2014, a specific formulation of oral propranolol[b] received FDA approval for treatment of infants >5 weeks with problematic infantile hemangiomas. Other medications used for hemangioma remain "off label."

Beta blockers (topical timolol–gel forming solution[a] and oral propranolol[a]): Topical timolol–gel forming solution, an ophthalmologic preparation, has been reported to be effective for the treatment of superficial hemangiomas. Oral propranolol was first reported to be efficacious for halting the proliferation and speeding the regression of infantile hemangiomas in 2008. In many cases, it has become the first-line therapy for problematic hemangiomas.

Corticosteroids[a] (oral intralesional and topical): These were the mainstay of treatment for hemangiomas until several years ago. Their use has been largely supplanted by beta blockers.

Pulsed dye laser: This may be used with other modalities but is usually of little benefit in situations when systemic treatment with propranolol is indicated. Limited penetration restricts use to superficial lesions. It can be useful for painful ulcerated hemangiomas that fail to respond to other treatment modalities.

Surgery: Surgical excision is most commonly used to manage the residual lesions of hemangiomas. Facial lesions that leave a significant residual lesion are often managed around age 3 years before the child starts preschool.

Luu M, Frieden IJ: Haemangioma: clinical course, complications and management, *Br J Dermatol* 169:20–30, 2013.

KEY POINTS: WORRISOME HEMANGIOMAS

- **Multiple hemangiomas**: May be associated with visceral hemangiomas (most commonly liver hemangiomas)
- **Large/bulky hemangiomas**: May cause significant disfigurement of underlying structures
- **Segmental hemangiomas**: Associated with PHACE and LUMBAR syndromes
- **"Beard" hemangiomas**: May be a marker for underlying laryngeal or subglottic hemangioma that may impair respiratory function
- **Midline spinal hemangiomas**: May be a marker for underlying spinal cord abnormality
- **Head and neck hemangiomas**: Usually segmental lesions > 5 cm in diameter, may be associated with other congenital anomalies
- **Vulnerable anatomic locations**: Impair vital functions or cause disfigurement (e.g., periocular, neck, lip, nasal tip)
- **Ulcerated hemangiomas**: Increased risk of infection, cause pain and lead to scarring

146. **Why is an infant with a vascular tumor and new-onset thrombocytopenia so worrisome?**
This can indicate the development of the **Kasabach-Merritt syndrome** (or phenomenon), a life-threatening condition of rapidly enlarging vascular tumors and progressive coagulopathy. Platelets are sequestered within the lesion(s), forming thrombi and consuming coagulation factors. Ecchymoses may develop initially around the vascular tumor, but a disseminated coagulopathy with anemia can result. Aggressive therapy (often systemic steroids and/or vincristine, and surgery) is frequently needed. Kasabach-Merritt syndrome is not caused by common infantile hemangiomas but rather by two rare vascular tumors (Kaposiform hemangioendothelioma and tufted angioma).

147. **How do superficial hemangiomas differ from port wine stains?**
Superficial hemangiomas are superficial, palpable, vascular tumors that usually involute with time. In the past, they were called "strawberry" hemangiomas. A **port wine stain,** sometimes called nevus flammeus, is a type of capillary malformation that results in flat vascular malformations composed of capillary and postcapillary venule-sized vessels that do not involute. Some superficial hemangiomas may mimic port wine stains during the first few weeks of life; observation of their growth pattern is helpful for establishing the correct diagnosis (Table 4-5).

Table 4-5. Superficial Hemangiomas Versus Port Wine Stains

SUPERFICIAL HEMANGIOMAS	PORT WINE STAINS
Palpable	Flat, macular
Common (4–10% of children < 1 year old)	Less common (0.1–0.3%)
Often not apparent at birth (more visible at 2–12 weeks)	Present at birth
Bright red	Pale pink to blue-red (darkens with age)
Well-defined borders	Borders variable
Pathology: Proliferating angioblastic endothelial cells with variable blood-filled capillaries	Pathology: dermal capillary dilation
Majority involute spontaneously by age 9 years	No involution: may worsen with darkening and hypertrophy
Rapid growth phase	Proportionate growth (as child grows)
Suggested therapy: watchful waiting; active treatment for some lesions	Suggested therapy: Flash lamp pulsed-dye laser often used for facial lesions

148. What is "simple" about a nevus simplex?

Nevus simplex, also known as "stork bites" when they are on the nape of the neck and "angel's kiss" when located in the glabella and eyelids, are very common. Pink to red in color, they often fade without treatment in the first few years of life. Thus, reassurance and monitoring is usually the only treatment recommended, which is a "simple" solution. Their characteristic location helps differentiate them from true facial port wine stains, which do not fade with time and may require treatment.

149. When are port wine stains associated with other anomalies?

Sturge-Weber syndrome (Fig. 4-19) refers to the association of a facial port wine stain (typically affecting the skin innervated by the first branch of the trigeminal nerve), an ocular vascular anomaly linked with glaucoma, and a leptomeningeal vascular anomaly associated with seizures and developmental delay.

Klippel-Trenaunay syndrome refers to the association of a limb port wine stain (usually lower extremity) with ipsilateral soft tissue and bony overgrowth and venous/lymphatic anomalies.

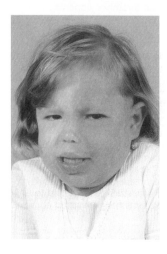

Figure 4-19. Sturge-Weber syndrome. The bilateral port wine stain involves the V_1, V_2, and V_3 regions and the right V_3. *(From Sahn EE: Dermatology Pearls. Philadelphia, 1999, Hanley & Belfus, p 225.)*

150. How are port wine stain–type capillary malformations treated?

Port wine stains are often pink to dark red in color during childhood. With maturity they often darken and take on their "port wine" color. Treatment of facial capillary malformations is generally recommended during infancy or early childhood when the lesions appear to be more amenable to therapy with the pulsed dye laser. The pulsed dye lasers that are used for treatment of port wine stains are designed to target oxyhemoglobin and lead to destruction of the blood vessels and subsequent lightening of the stain. Multiple treatments sometimes requiring general anesthesia or sedation are required to achieve lightening. It is important for patients and families to understand that this treatment often achieves cosmetically acceptable lightening but complete disappearance/removal of the birthmark is not yet possible with the current technologies. In some patients the stain will redarken after treatment, and touch-up treatments may be required.

VESICOBULLOUS DISORDERS

151. What is the Nikolsky sign?

This sign demonstrates **epidermal fragility.** Gentle lateral pressure placed on apparently intact skin causes an erosion, especially near preformed vesicles. This sign is positive in several autoimmune, infectious, and inherited blistering conditions, such as bullous pemphigoid, staphylococcal scalded skin syndrome (SSSS), and epidermolysis bullosa.

152. What are causes of skin blistering in childhood?
    - **Infectious:** Bacterial (bullous impetigo, SSSS), viral (herpes simplex virus, varicella)
    - **Contact dermatitis:** Poison ivy, phytophotodermatitis
    - **Inherited disorders:** Epidermolysis bullosa, bullous congenital ichthyosiform erythroderma
    - **Autoimmune disorders:** Linear immunoglobulin A disease, bullous pemphigoid, pemphigus vulgaris
    - **Other:** Erythema multiforme, toxic epidermal necrolysis, thermal injury (burns)

153. How is SSSS differentiated from toxic epidermal necrolysis (TEN)?
    Both are diffuse bullous diseases. **SSSS** commonly arises in young children <5 years old and develops after a localized staphylococcal infection with diffuse cutaneous disease caused by an exfoliative toxin. The level of blistering includes the superficial levels of the epidermis. **TEN** is believed to be a hypersensitivity reaction (often to a drug) and occurs in all age groups. The level of blistering in TEN is deep, and the entire epidermis is necrotic. (Table 4-6).

Table 4-6. Differentiation Between Staphylococcal Scalded Skin Syndrome and Toxic Epidermal Necrolysis

CHARACTERISTICS	STAPHYLOCOCCAL SCALDED SKIN SYNDROME	TOXIC EPIDERMAL NECROLYSIS
Etiology	Infectious; group II staphylococci	Immunologic; usually drug related
Morbidity/mortality	Low with treatment	High
Mucous membrane involvement	Rare	Frequent
Nikolsky sign	Present	Absent
Target lesions	Absent	Often present
Level of blister	Upper epidermis (below stratum corneum)	Subepidermal
Histopathology	No epidermal necrosis or dermal inflammation	Full-thickness epidermal necrosis; prominent perivascular dermal inflammation

Adapted from Roberts LJ: Dermatologic diseases. In McMillan JA, DeAngelis CD, Feigin RD, et al editors: Oski's Pediatrics, Principles and Practice, ed 3. Philadelphia, 1999, Lippincott Williams & Wilkins, p 379.

154. Why are neonates susceptible to SSSS?
    The answer lies in the fact that newborns share their susceptibility to SSSS with patients in renal failure. It is the **reduced clearance of the exfoliative toxin** by the newborn's immature kidneys that contributes to their increased susceptibility to SSSS.

155. Where can the *S. aureus* be found in patients with SSSS?
    S. aureus commonly colonizes the nasopharynx and the umbilicus. The source of infection may also be present in the urinary tract, a wound, conjunctiva, or blood. The bacteria are not usually present at the site of the skin lesions because they are the result of a systemic toxin-mediated effect.

156. What is the likely diagnosis for a 4-year-old child who develops a 1-week history of widespread painful and pruritic bullous lesions with crusted lesions around which vesicles are arranged in a string-of-pearls appearance?
    Chronic bullous dermatosis of childhood. This is the most common acquired autoimmune bullous disease of young children. It is characterized on biopsy by immunoglobulin A (IgA) and C3 deposition along the basement membrane (sometimes called linear IgA bullous dermatosis). Although the differential diagnosis of bullous diseases is large, the appearance of new vesicles or bullae in a string of pearls (or cluster-of-jewels) appearance around crusted or erythematous plaques is characteristic.

Sheehan M, Huddleston H, Mousdicas N: Chronic bullous dermatosis of childhood, *Arch Pediatr Adolesc Med* 162:581–582, 2008.

157. **What are the subtypes of epidermolysis bullosa (EB)?**

EB is a heterogeneous group of inherited disorders characterized by the formation of blisters and erosions at sites of friction or trauma. There are three subtypes of EB that are categorized based on the region of the dermal-epidermal junction (DEJ) that they affect: **simplex**, **junctional**, and **dystrophic**. The extent of blistering and the degree of scarring roughly correlate with the level of blister formation in the epidermis or dermis. A fourth subtype of EB has been added, **Kindler syndrome**, which affects multiple layers of the DEJ.

Dystrophic Epidermolysis Bullosa Research Association of America: www.debra.org. Accessed on Mar. 23, 2015.

158. **Should epidermolysis bullosa blisters be "popped"?**

Yes. Because patients with EB have a genetic abnormality of the proteins that hold their epidermis and dermis together, the pressure from simple accumulation of fluid within an intact blister can cause the blister to expand. The blister should be drained by a sterile needle or lancet after a gentle sterile alcohol prep of the site. The blister roof should be left intact.

159. **Which disorder is associated with "target lesions"?**

Erythema multiforme (EM). This is typically an acute, self-limited, but sometimes recurring skin condition (EM minor) believed to be a T cell–mediated immune reaction most commonly to certain infections (e.g., herpes simplex virus, streptococcal, Epstein-Barr virus [EBV]) but also to a variety of other triggers, particularly medications (e.g., sulfa drugs, penicillins, anticonvulsants). In EM major, erosions or bullae of the oral, genital, or ocular mucosa occur. Most mild cases resolve over 1 to 2 weeks. The characteristic target lesions occur as dusky, red papules that evolve into depressed, localized, damaged epithelium with spreading annular edema (pale) and inflammation on the periphery (erythema) (Fig. 4-20).

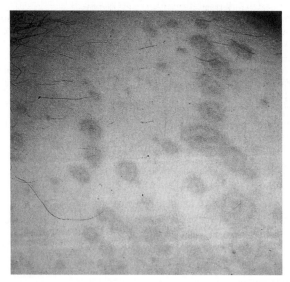

Figure 4-20. Erythema multiforme with typical target lesions. *(From Goldbloom RB: Pediatric Clinical Skills, ed 4. Philadelphia, 2011, Elsevier Saunders, Color plate 19-11.)*

160. **Is EM part of a continuum with Stevens-Johnson syndrome (SJS) and toxic epidermal necrolysis (TEN)?**

This is an area of controversy. Traditionally, these had been viewed as related disorders because they had some shared clinical and histologic features. However, the majority of EM cases are associated with infections, while SJS/TEN occurrences are believed to be drug-related in >90% of cases. There are also distinctions according to anamnesis (history), morphology, involved sites, extension of lesions, and pathogenic mechanisms. Current opinion favors these as distinct conditions, with SJS/TEN not being the end-stage result of some cases of EM.

Iwai S, Sueki H, Watanabe H, et al: Distinguishing between erythema multiforme major and Stevens-Johnson syndrome/toxic epidermal necrolysis immunopathologically, *J Dermatol* 39:781–786, 2012.
Roujeau JC: Stevens-Johnson syndrome and toxic epidermal necrolysis are severity variants of the same disease which differs from erythema multiforme, *J Dermatol* 24: 726–729, 1997.

161. **What distinguishes SJS from TEN?**
    Both are severe mucocutaneous disorders that are characterized by extensive necrosis and epidermal detachment. They are believed to be a continuum, usually triggered by medications, and are distinguished primarily based on the percentage of body surface that is involved. SJS is the less severe of the two, defined as <10% body surface involvement. TEN encompasses >30% of body area. Between 10% and 30% indicates a classification overlap.

162. **What medications are most commonly associated with SJS and TEN in children?**
    Sulfonamides and **anticonvulsants**, especially phenobarbital, carbamazepine, and lamotrigine. Less common causes are penicillins and NSAIDs. Very rarely, paracetamol (acetaminophen) may be involved.

Ferrandiz-Pulido C, Garcia-Patos V: A review of causes of Stevens-Johnson syndrome and toxic epidermal necrolysis in children, *Arch Dis Child* 98: 998–1003, 2013.

163. **Is steroid therapy[a] beneficial for the treatment of SJS or TEN?**
    This is a continuing area of controversy; studies are inconclusive. In SJS, treatment may be considered early during the course if multiple mucosal surfaces are involved, but skin denudation is limited. The potential for steroids[a] to increase medical complications (e.g., hemorrhage, infection) must be taken into account, but a large 2008 study found that it was lower than previously thought. If initiated, clinical response (or lack thereof) should be carefully followed, and steroids should be discontinued if the condition is worsening. Because the majority of cases of SJS will spontaneously resolve, other therapies are vital: skin care, nutritional support, ophthalmologic care, and the treatment of secondary bacterial infections. Steroids have been reported to be associated with an increased mortality rate among patients with TEN.

Koh MJ-A, Yay Y-K: An update on Stevens-Johnson syndrome and toxic epidermal necrolysis in children, *Curr Opin Pediatr* 21:505–510, 2009.
Schneck J, Fagot JP, Sekula P, et al: Effects of treatment on the mortality of Stevens-Johnson syndrome and toxic epidermal necrolysis: a retrospective study on patients included in the EuroSCAR study, *J Am Acad Dermatol* 58:33–40, 2008.

164. **What therapy should be considered for patients with rapidly progressive SJS or TEN?**
    Intravenous immune globulin[a] should be considered. Caution should be used, especially in patients with poor renal function, hypercoagulable states, or IgA deficiency.

Momin SB: Review of intravenous immunoglobulin in the treatment of Stevens-Johnson syndrome and toxic epidermal necrolysis, *J Clin Aesthet Dermatol* 2:51–58, 2009.

165. **What infection should be considered in a child with SJS and a cough?**
    Mycoplasma pneumonia induces mucosal erosions that mimic those of drug-induced SJS.

Bullen LK, Zenel JA: A 15-year-old female who has cough, rash and painful swallow, *Pediatr Rev* 26:176–181, 2005.

166. **In addition to hand-foot-mouth, which other body site is often affected in children with coxsackie virus infections?**
    Coxsackie viral infections often also cause skin lesions on the **buttocks,** prompting some clinicians to call the condition "hand-foot-mouth-butt syndrome."

Mohr MR, Sholtzow M, Bevan HE, et al: Exploring the differential diagnosis of hemorrhagic vesicopustules in a newborn, *Pediatrics* 127:e226–e230, 2011.

Acknowledgment

The editors gratefully acknowledge contributions by Dr. Robert Hayman, Dr. Leonard Kristal, and Dr. Vivian Lombillo that were retained from prior editions of *Pediatric Secrets*.

CHAPTER 5

EMERGENCY MEDICINE

Joan S. Bregstein, MD, Cindy Ganis Roskind, MD and F. Meridith Sonnett, MD

BIOTERRORISM

1. Why are children more vulnerable to biologic agents than adults?
   - **Anatomic and physiologic differences:** Thinner dermis, increased surface area-to-volume ratio, smaller relative blood volume, higher minute ventilation
   - **Developmental considerations:** Inability to flee dangerous situations, possible increased risk for post-traumatic stress disorder (PTSD)
   - **Some vaccines not licensed for children:** Anthrax (18 to 65 years), plague (18 to 61 years)
   - **Vaccines more dangerous in children:** Smallpox, yellow fever
   - **Antibiotics less familiar to pediatricians:** Tetracyclines, fluoroquinolones

---

Cieslak TJ, Henretig FM: Bioterrorism, *Pediatr Ann* 32:145–165, 2003.
Centers for Disease Control and Prevention Emergency Preparedness Response: http://www.bt.cdc.gov. Accessed 11-21-14.

2. What are the three routes of transmission of anthrax?
   - **Inhalation:** Most feared; can lead to multiorgan hemorrhagic necrosis
   - **Cutaneous:** Inoculated through wound, causing a black, painless ulcer
   - **Ingestion:** May cause gastrointestinal or upper respiratory symptoms
     Bacillus anthracis, which is a spore-forming gram-positive rod, can survive for extended periods before entering the body, when it will germinate and proliferate (Fig. 5-1).

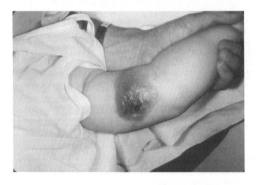

Figure 5-1. Cutaneous anthrax in a child. *(From Schachner LA, Hansen RC, editors:* Pediatric Dermatology, *ed 3. Edinburgh, 2003, Mosby, p 1033.)*

3. How are the lesions of smallpox distinguished from varicella (chickenpox)?
   - *Smallpox* lesions predominate on the face and extremities (centrifugal), whereas *varicella* lesions are typically heaviest on the trunk (centripetal).
   - Rash of *smallpox* progresses in similar stages (macules, papules, vesicles, crusting), whereas *varicella* is seen with multiple crops in differing stages.
   - *Smallpox* rash develops more slowly than *varicella* rash.

4. How can the presenting symptoms of bubonic plague be differentiated from those of plague resulting from bioterrorism?
   Bubonic plague—of "black death" fame—resulted from the bite of fleas, which led to large tender regional adenopathy (the "bubo") with subsequent hematogenous dissemination, multiorgan involvement, and septicemia. In bioterrorism, the organism *Yersinia pestis* could be aerosolized, and inhalation would result

in presentations more typical of pneumonic plague, with fever, chills, tachypnea, cough, and bloody sputum; lymphadenitis would likely be a later finding.

Dennis DT, Chow CC: Plague, *Pediatr Infect Dis J* 23:69–71, 2004.

5. **Why should families living near nuclear power plants keep potassium iodide (KI) in their medicine cabinets?**
   The American Academy of Pediatrics recommends that families living within 10 miles of a nuclear power plant (or 50 miles in densely populated areas, where evacuations may be more difficult) have KI on hand in the event of a nuclear radiation catastrophe. KI will inhibit the uptake of radioactive iodine (^{131}I) into the thyroid gland. Children are more susceptible than adults to the subsequent development of thyroid cancer if exposed. If KI is administered within 1 hour, 90% of ^{131}I is blocked, but after 12 hours, there is little effect.

Committee on Environmental Health, American Academy of Pediatrics: Radiation disasters and children, *Pediatrics* 111:1455–1466, 2003.

6. **Why are children particularly vulnerable to terrorism in the form of explosive and blast attacks?**
   - Smaller mass results in greater force per unit of body surface from energy released by explosion.
   - Children are more susceptible to fractures as a result of incompletely calcified growth plates.
   - The chest wall has greater pliability in children, resulting in greater chance of cardiac and pulmonary injury from blast explosives.

Garth RJN: Blast injury of the ear: an overview and guide to management, *Injury* 26:363–366, 1995.

7. **What categories of agents should be considered in the event of a chemical weapons attack?**
   - **Nerve:** Nerve agents are similar to organophosphate insecticides and include cholinesterase inhibitors, such as Sarin, Soman, and VX. Nerve agents inhibit the action of acetylcholinesterase at cholinergic neural synapses, where acetylcholine then accumulates. These agents are generally colorless, odorless, tasteless, and nonirritating to the skin. Nerve agent vapors are denser than air and tend to accumulate in low-lying areas, putting children at a higher risk than adults for exposure. The agents used in terrorist attacks are inhaled and absorbed through skin and mucous membranes.
   - **Asphyxiants:** Asphyxiants are toxic compounds that inhibit cytochrome oxidase, causing cellular anoxia and lactic acidosis (high anion gap). Hydrogen cyanide, the most commonly known toxicant in this class, is a colorless liquid or gas that smells like bitter almonds. Exposure to hydrogen cyanide produces rapid onset of tachypnea, tachycardia, and flushed skin, followed by nausea, vomiting, confusion, weakness, trembling, seizures, and death.
   - **Choking and pulmonary agents:** Choking agents include chlorine and phosgene. When inhaled, these agents produce massive mucosal irritation and edema, as well as significant damage to lung parenchyma.
   - **Blistering and vesicant agents:** Blistering agents include sulfur mustard and lewisite. Sulfur mustard is an alkylating agent that is highly toxic to rapidly reproducing and poorly differentiated cells; skin, pulmonary parenchyma, and bone marrow are frequently damaged. Lewisite is an arsenical compound that affects skin and eyes immediately on exposure.

8. **What should be the practitioner's initial management when a chemical weapons event occurs?**
   The single most important first step for treating all chemical exposures is the **initial decontamination strategy**. Immediate removal of patient clothing can eliminate about 90% of contaminants.

CHILD ABUSE: PHYSICAL AND SEXUAL

9. **What are important historical indicators of possible child abuse?**
   - Multiple previous hospital visits for injuries
   - History of untreated injuries
   - Cause of trauma not known or inappropriate for age or activity

- Delay in seeking medical attention
- History incompatible with injury
- Parents unconcerned about injury or more concerned about unrelated minor problem (e.g., cold, headache)
- History of abused siblings
- Changing or inconsistent stories to explain injury

Sirotnak AP, Grigsby T, Krugman RD: Physical abuse of children, *Pediatr Rev* 25:264–276, 2004.
Kottmeier P: The battered child, *Pediatr Ann* 16:343–351, 1987.

10. **What is the most common cause of severe closed head trauma in infants younger than 1 year?**

    Abusive head trauma. This is the terminology adopted by the American Academy of Pediatrics to replace the term *shaken baby syndrome*. It describes inflicted injury in infants and young children that results either from an impact to the head or violent shaking of the head, or a combination of both mechanisms. The term *shaken baby syndrome* was changed because it implied a knowledge on the part of the treating clinician of the mechanism of injury that was most often not known. Abusive head trauma is most common in infants <1 year of age and, compared with accidental head injury, has a much greater mortality rate. Male infants, and those from lower socioeconomic groups, tend to be at highest risk. Abusive head trauma manifests as subdural hematomas, subarachnoid hemorrhages, and cerebral infarcts. The diagnosis is suggested by the lack of a corroborating mechanism of injury in the face of a symptomatic child or, rarely, a confession by the perpetrator. In many cases, physical examination reveals retinal hemorrhages (Fig. 5-2); other signs of trauma are usually lacking. Diagnosis is confirmed by computed tomography (CT) or magnetic resonance imaging (MRI). If a lumbar puncture is performed, the fluid may be bloody or xanthochromic. The prognosis is grim for an infant who is in coma from this abuse: 50% die, and nearly half of the survivors have significant neurologic sequelae.

Niederkrotenthaler T, Xu L, Parks SE, et al: Descriptive factors of abusive head trauma in young children: United States, *Child Abuse Legl* 37:446–455, 2013.
Christian CW, Block R, Committee on Child Abuse and Neglect: Abusive head trauma in infants and children, *Pediatrics* 123:1409–1411, 2009.

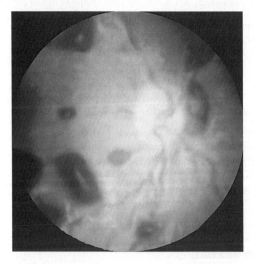

Figure 5-2. Retinal hemorrhages of victim of abusive head trauma. *(From Zitelli BJ, Davis HW: Atlas of Pediatric Physical Diagnosis, ed 4. St. Louis, 2002, Mosby, p 181.)*

11. **Why is the diagnosis of abusive head trauma often overlooked?**

    When an infant is unconscious with respiratory distress, apnea, and/or seizures, the diagnosis of abusive head trauma should be considered. However, depending on the degree of impact or shaking and the degree of resulting damage, the symptoms can be mild and nonspecific and may mimic symptoms of a viral illness, feeding disorder or dysfunction, or even colic. Victims may have a history of poor feeding, vomiting, lethargy, and/or irritability that may have gone on for days or weeks. Early identification of abusive injuries is critical because of the risk of increased mortality with each recurrent abusive event.

Schwartz, KA, Preer G, Mckeag H, et al: Child maltreatment: a review of key literature in 2013, *Curr Opin Pediatr* 26:396–404, 2014.
Jaspan T: Current controversies in the interpretation of nonaccidental head injury, *Pediatr Radiol* 38:S378–S387, 2008.

12. **What diagnostic tests may be contributory if abusive head trauma is suspected?**
    - **Head CT:** Good for demonstrating subarachnoid and large extra-axial hemorrhages and mass effect; may be falsely negative, especially early in the presentation
    - **MRI:** Good for diagnosing subdural and intraparenchymal lesions; may miss subarachnoid blood and fractures
    - **Spinal tap:** May yield bloody cerebrospinal fluid
    - **Skeletal survey:** May be normal or may reveal acute or healed rib or other fractures, which are suggestive of abuse
    - **Complete blood count:** May be normal or may show mild to moderate anemia
    - **Prothrombin time and partial thromboplastin time:** May show mild to moderate abnormalities or reveal frank disseminated intravascular coagulation (DIC)
    - **Amylase:** May show an increase, signifying possible pancreatic damage
    - **Liver function tests:** Abnormalities may signify occult liver injury

American Academy of Pediatrics, Section on Radiology: Diagnostic imaging of child abuse, *Pediatrics* 123:1430–1435, 2009.

13. **What physical examination findings are indicators of possible child abuse?**
    - Burns, especially cigarette or immersion burns on the buttocks or perineum or burns in a stocking-and-glove distribution
    - Genital trauma or sexually transmitted infection (STI) in a prepubertal child
    - Signs of excessive corporal punishment (welts, belt or cord marks, bites)
    - Frenulum lacerations in young infants or tongue bruising (associated with forced feeding)
    - Multiple bruises in various stages of resolution
    - Bruises in a premobile infant
    - Neurologic injury associated with retinal or scleral hemorrhages
    - Fractures suggestive of abuse (e.g., skull fractures in infants, metaphyseal fractures, posterior rib fractures, fractures in premobile infants, scapular fractures in infants beyond the immediate newborn period)

Sirotnak AP, Grigsby T, Krugman RD: Physical abuse of children, *Pediatr Rev* 25:264–276, 2004.
Kottmeier P: The battered child, *Pediatr Ann* 16:343–351, 1987.

14. **If retinal hemorrhages are noted in a child with seizures, how likely are the seizures to have caused the hemorrhages?**
    In theory, any seizure might cause retinal hemorrhages through a sudden rise in retinal venous pressure in conjunction with increased central venous and intrathoracic pressure. However, a prospective study of children with seizures who had ophthalmologic evaluation found no evidence of an association of seizures and retinal hemorrhages. Combining their data with some previous studies, the authors determined a prevalence of retinal hemorrhages with a seizure of only about 3 per 10,000—an extremely small likelihood. If retinal hemorrhages are found in a child with seizures, the possibility of nonaccidental injury must be explored.

Curcoy AI, Trenchs V, Morales M, et al: Do retinal haemorrhages occur in infants with convulsions? *Arch Dis Child* 94:873–875, 2009.

15. **In a suspected victim of child abuse, is an ophthalmology exam looking for retinal hemorrhages routinely indicated as part of the medical evaluation?**
    The answer used to be yes. In the past, all suspected child abuse victims of any sort were subjected to a screening eye exam for detection of retinal hemorrhages. However, recent research has convincingly

demonstrated that in the absence of positive neuroimaging, an eye exam will not reveal clinically significant retinal hemorrhages and is not necessary.

Greiner MV, Berger RP, Thackeray JD, et al: Dedicated retinal examination in children evaluated for physical abuse without radiographically identified traumatic brain injury, *J Pediatr* 163:527–531, 2013.

16. **When should child abuse be considered in the event of an unexplained death of a child?**
    Always. Sudden infant death syndrome (SIDS) should be a diagnosis of exclusion in any unexplained death. Deaths as a result of SIDS usually occur during the first year of life, most commonly (90%) in children <7 months old. All children who die suddenly of unclear causes should have a complete physical examination that looks for signs of external trauma (e.g., bruises, injury to the genitalia).

17. **Which conditions with ecchymoses (bruising) can be mistaken for child abuse?**
    - **Mongolian spots (dermal melanosis)** are commonly mistaken for bruises, especially when they occur elsewhere than the classic lumbosacral area; unlike bruises, they do not fade with time (Fig. 5-3).
    - **Coagulation disorders** include hemophilia or von Willebrand disease. In 20% of cases of hemophilia, there is no family history of disease; bruising may be noted in unusual places in response to minor trauma.
    - **Folk medicine** such as the Southeast Asian practices of spoon rubbing (quat sha) or coin rubbing (cao gio) can produce ecchymoses; the practice of cupping (the inversion of a heated cup on the back) produces circular ecchymoses.
    - **Moxibustion** is the Southeast Asian practice of burning an herbal substance on the child's abdomen to cure disease.
    - **Clothing** dyes, especially from jeans, sometimes mimic bruising; they are easily removed with topical alcohol.
    - **Vasculitis,** particularly Henoch-Schönlein purpura with a purpuric rash most commonly on the buttocks and lower extremities or idiopathic thrombocytopenic purpura (ITP), may be mistaken for signs of child abuse.
    - **Vitamin K deficiency**

Kaczor K, Pierce MC, et al: Bruising and physical child abuse, *Clin Pediatr Emerg Med* 7:153–160, 2006.

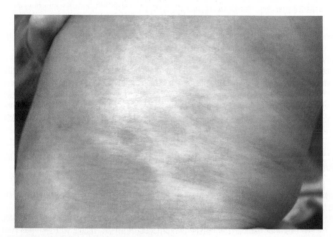

Figure 5-3. Mongolian spots (dermal melanosis) on an infant. *(From Jenny C, editor: Child Abuse and Neglect, Philadelphia, 2011, Elsevier Saunders, p 253.)*

18. How are fractures dated radiographically in children?

After a fracture, the following will be seen:

- **1 to 7 days:** Soft tissue swelling; fat and fascial planes blurred; sharp fracture line
- **7 to 14 days:** Periosteal new bone formation as soft callus forms; blurring of fracture line; occurs earlier for infants, later for older children
- **14 to 21 days:** More clearly defined (i.e., hard) callus forming as periosteal bone converts to lamellar bone
- **21 to 42 days:** Peak of hard callus formation
- **≥60 days:** Remodeling of bone begins with reshaping of the deformity (up to 1 to 2 years)

If the timing of an injury does not correlate with the dating of a fracture or if fractures at multiple stages of healing are present, child abuse should be suspected.

19. What fractures are suggestive of child abuse?

All fractures can be the result of child abuse, and a careful history will guide the clinician in the degree of suspicion indicated in each case. In infants and toddlers, physical abuse is the cause of up to 20% of fractures. This is an age group in which suspicion should be high. Some fractures have been shown to have a high specificity for abuse, and these are rib fractures in infants, particularly posteriomedially; classic metaphyseal lesions of long bones; and fractures of the scapula, spinous process, and sternum. Metaphyseal fractures (Fig. 5-4) require shearing forces not usually produced in accidental trauma, with an increased likelihood of mechanisms that involve shaking with limbs flailing, twisting, and jerking. The presence of multiple fractures, fractures of different ages and/or stages of healing, and complex skull fractures also have a good degree of specificity for abuse.

Flaherty EG, Perez-Rossello JM: Evaluating children with fractures for child physical abuse, *Pediatrics* 133: e477–e489, 2014.

Pierce MC, Bertocci G: Fractures resulting from inflicted trauma: assessing injury and history compatibility, *Clin Pediatr Emerg Med* 7:143–148, 2006.

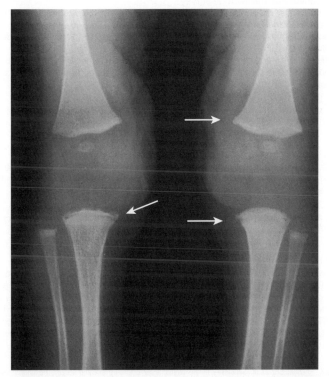

Figure 5-4. Radiograph of classic metaphyseal *(arrow)* lesions. *(From Jenny C, editor:* Child Abuse and Neglect, *Philadelphia, 2011, Elsevier Saunders, p 285.)*

20. **How certain can a clinician be in attributing a femur fracture in a nonambulatory child to nonaccidental trauma?**
    Femoral fractures in the nonambulatory child are most often the result of nonaccidental trauma. However, there are exceptions to this "rule." Certain femur fractures in young children may be accidental:
    - A short fall to the knee may produce a torus or impacted transverse fracture of the distal femoral metaphysis.
    - Children playing in a stationary activity center, like an Exersaucer, may sustain an oblique distal femur metaphyseal fracture.
    - Falls down a stairway in a nonambulatory child can sometimes cause one leg to become twisted underneath the child resulting in a spiral femoral fracture.

Haney SB, Boos SC, Kutz TJ, et al: Transverse fracture of the distal femoral metadiaphysis: a plausible accidental mechanism, *Pediatr Emerg Care* 25:841–844, 2009.
Pierce MC, Bertocci GE, Janosky JE, et al: Femur fractures resulting from stair falls among children: an injury plausibility model, *Pediatrics* 115:1712–1722, 2005.

21. **What is the purpose of the skeletal survey?**
    Skeletal injuries, particularly multiple healed lesions, are strong indicators of a pattern of abuse. The skeletal survey is a radiological evaluation of multiple bones in the body to:
    1. reveal fractures of additional bones (new or healing) other than the fractured bones already known to the clinician; and
    2. reveal fractures (new or healing) in a child suspected of abuse manifesting in ways other than fractures.

22. **What constitutes the skeletal survey?**
    The skeletal survey is a multiple-imaging series that includes x-ray views of the following:
    - **Appendicular skeleton:** Humeri, forearms, hands, femurs, lower legs, and feet
    - **Axial skeleton:** Thorax, pelvis (including mid- and lower lumbar spine), lumbar spine, cervical spine, and skull
    The series can include anywhere between 19 and 30 x-rays. "Body grams" (studies that encompass the entire child in one or two exposures) are not thought to be of sufficient sensitivity to be useful.

American Academy of Pediatrics, Section on Radiology: Diagnostic imaging of child abuse, *Pediatrics* 123: 1430–1431, 2009.

23. **Up to what age should a skeletal survey be ordered?**
    If physical abuse is suspected, the American Academy of Pediatrics recommends a mandatory study in children up to the age of 2 years. The yield diminishes after that age and is of little value after the age of 5 years.

American Academy of Pediatrics, Section on Radiology: Diagnostic imaging of child abuse, *Pediatrics* 123: 1432, 2009.

24. **What is the value of a follow-up skeletal survey?**
    Both the American Academy of Pediatrics and the American College of Radiology recommend follow-up skeletal surveys about 2 weeks after the initial study if the first was abnormal or equivocal or when abuse is suspected on clinical grounds despite a normal first study. The follow-up skeletal survey can demonstrate a previously-missed occult fracture by the presence of new callus formation. The yield can be substantial with studies demonstrating new findings ranging from 14% to 61%. Because of the additional radiation, research is also addressing the applicability of more limited views on the follow-up study.

Hansen KK, Keeshin BR, et al: Sensitivity of the limited view follow-up skeletal survey, *Pediatrics* 134: 242–248, 2014.

25. In addition to child abuse, what conditions must you consider as a cause of multiple unexplained long bone fractures in a young child?
    - **Osteogenesis imperfecta** (OI) is a rare congenital disorder that presents with bone fragility. In addition to frequent fractures, patients with this disorder often present with the following:
        - Blue sclera
        - Ligamentous laxity
        - Osteopenia
        - Wormian skull bones
        - Dentinogenesis imperfecta
        - Family history of OI (although not always because new cases can result from de novo mutations)
        - Hearing loss
    - Vitamin D deficiency rickets
    - Scurvy
    - Copper deficiency

26. When are burn injuries suspicious for child abuse?
    Burn injuries account for about 5% of cases of physical abuse. As with other injuries, the description of the incident causing the burn should be consistent with the child's development and the extent and degree of the burn observed. The following types are suspicious for abuse:
    - **Immersion burns:** Sharply demarcated lines on the hands and feet (stocking-and-glove distribution), buttocks, and perineum, with a uniform depth of burn; the immersion of a child in a hot bath is a classic example
    - **Geographic burns:** Burns, usually of second or third degree, in a distinct pattern, such as circular cigarette burns or steam iron burns
    - **Splash burns:** Pattern with droplet marks projecting away from the most involved area; splash marks on the back of the body usually require another person and may or may not be accidental

27. How do you recognize child abuse in a medical setting?
    In this form of child abuse, also called *Munchausen syndrome* or *pediatric condition falsification*, adult caregivers inflict illness on a child or falsify symptoms to obtain medical care for a child. Features include the following:
    - Recurrent episodes of a confusing medical picture
    - Multiple diagnostic evaluations at different medical centers ("doctor shopping")
    - Unsupportive marital relationship, often with maternal isolation
    - Compliant, cooperative, and overinvolved mother
    - Higher level of parental medical knowledge
    - Parental history of extensive medical treatment or illness
    - Conditions resolve with surveillance of the child in the hospital
    - Findings correlate with the presence of the parent

    Stirling J: Beyond Munchausen syndrome by proxy: identification and treatment of child abuse in a medical setting, *Pediatrics* 119:1026–1030, 2007.

28. How often is sexual abuse committed by an individual known previously by the child or adolescent?
    Between 75% and 80% of the time. Relatives are the perpetrators in about one third of cases.

29. In the case of suspected prepubertal sexual abuse, how critical is it to perform the physical exam immediately on presentation of the child to a medical facility?
    If no exchange of bodily fluids has occurred, and the child is not presenting with a medical emergency, such as vaginal bleeding, it is not necessary to perform a medical exam immediately in the office or emergency department (ED) setting. In fact, it is preferential to refer the child to a setting staffed by medical personnel familiar with the sexual abuse exam, such as a pediatric emergency department or a child advocacy center. If exchange of bodily fluids has occurred, then the timing of the exam is more critical. Guidelines vary from state to state with recommendations that forensic evidence be collected from 24 hours to 96 hours after an assault.

30. After the documentation of history and a careful physical examination, what evidence should be collected in cases of suspected sexual abuse in a *prepubertal* female?
Because sexually transmitted infections are not common in prepubertal children evaluated for abuse, culturing all sites (vaginal, rectal, and oral) for all organisms is not recommended if the child is not symptomatic. Each case should be treated individually. However, here are some considerations:
   - Whether the child was penetrated, either vaginally or anally
   - Whether the abuser was a stranger
   - Whether the abuser is known to have an STI or be at risk
   - Whether the child has a sibling or other relative in the household with an STI
   - Whether the child has signs or symptoms of an STI
   - Whether the child has already been diagnosed with a previous STI

   If the decision is made to collect specimens from a prepubertal child, the AAP recommends the use of a nucleic acid amplification test (NAAT) for detection of infection with *Chlamydia trachomatis* and *Neisseria gonorrhoeae*. Culture-based tests for these organisms are highly insensitive. However, it should be noted that the Food and Drug Administration (FDA) has not approved the use of the NAAT for cultures of the rectum and throat in pediatric patients.

Jenny C, Crawford-Jakubiak JE: The evaluation of children in the primary care setting when sexual abuse is suspected, *Pediatrics* 132:e558–e567, 2013.

31. After the documentation of history and a careful physical examination, what evidence should be collected in cases of suspected sexual abuse in a *postpubertal* female?
   - Pregnancy test, if postmenarchal
   - Evidence of sexual contact, including two to three swabbed specimens from each area of assault for the following substances: sperm (motile and nonmotile), acid phosphatase (secreted by the prostate; component of seminal plasma), P_{30} (prostate glycoprotein present in seminal fluid), blood group antigens
   - NAAT for STIs from all three sites
   - Evidence to document perpetrator: foreign material on clothing, suspected nonpatient hairs; DNA testing (controversial)

Jenny C, Crawford-Jakubiak JE: The evaluation of children in the primary care setting when sexual abuse is suspected, *Pediatrics* 132;e558-e567, 2013.
American Academy of Pediatrics, Committee on Child Abuse and Neglect: Guidelines for the evaluation of sexual abuse in children, *Pediatrics* 116:506–512, 2005.

32. After the initial ED evaluation for sexual assault, what kind of follow-up care should the ED physician offer?
   - Human immunodeficiency virus (HIV) follow-up counseling with infectious disease or HIV specialist in 3 to 5 days
   - Follow-up gynecologic examination at 1 to 2 weeks
   - Repeat serologic tests for syphilis and HIV in 6 weeks, 3 months, and 6 months
   - Psychiatric counseling

33. If a child who is not sexually active is diagnosed with an infection caused by an STI-associated organism, how likely is sexual abuse the reason for acquisition?
See Table 5-1.

Table 5-1. Likelihood of Sexual Abuse According to Organism

ORGANISM	LIKELIHOOD OF SEXUAL ABUSE
Neisseria gonorrhoeae	Diagnostic
Treponema pallidum (syphilis)	Diagnostic
Chlamydia trachomatis	Diagnostic
Human immunodeficiency virus	Diagnostic

Table 5-1. Likelihood of Sexual Abuse According to Organism (*Continued*)

ORGANISM	LIKELIHOOD OF SEXUAL ABUSE
Trichomonas vaginalis	Highly suspicious
Condyloma acuminata	Suspicious
Herpes (genital location)	Suspicious
Bacterial vaginosis	Inconclusive

Adapted from American Academy of Pediatrics: Sexually transmitted diseases. In Pickering LK, editor: 2006 Red Book, ed 27. Elk Grove Village, IL, 2006, American Academy of Pediatrics, p 172.

34. **Is the size of the hymenal opening an important finding in the diagnosis of sexual abuse?**

The hymenal opening is measured with a child in the supine, frog-leg position, and various studies have attempted to determine a size that most likely correlates with sexual abuse. The upper limit of normal had ranged from 4 to 8 mm, but variations in technique, positioning, and relative relaxation of the patient have rendered such measurements *generally unhelpful and nondiagnostic*. A more important part of the examination is inspection of the posterior hymen and surrounding tissues. Typically, a posterior rim of hymen measuring at least 1 mm is present unless there has been trauma. Complete transaction of the hymen leaves a permanent gap or defect. A full-thickness transaction through the posterior hymen (best visualized in the knee-chest position) is thought to be reliable evidence of trauma. Other variations of hymenal shape or size must be interpreted with caution because there is considerable overlap among abused and nonabused girls.

Berkoff MC, Zolotor AJ, Makoroff KL, et al: Has this prepubertal girl been sexually abused? *JAMA* 23:2779–2792, 2008.
Pillai M: Genital findings in prepubertal girls: what can be concluded from an examination? *J Pediatr Adolesc Gynecol* 21:177–185, 2008.

35. **What is the most common finding of the physical examination of a child who has been sexually abused?**

A **normal physical examination** is the most common physical finding, which is why, in the absence of vaginal bleeding or other medical emergency, the physical exam should be deferred to an experienced medical examiner in a pediatric ED or a child advocacy center. It is crucial to know that a normal examination does not rule out sexual abuse.

36. **What are the date-rape drugs?**

Date-rape drugs are substances that render a patient incapable of saying "no" or asserting herself or himself, which makes it easier for a perpetrator to commit rape. The term typically applies to three drugs—*flunitrazepam (Rohypnol)*, γ-*hydroxybutyrate (GHB)*, and *ketamine hydrochloride*—which go by a variety of street names. The effects of these drugs, including somnolence, muscle relaxation, and profound sedation and amnesia, are enhanced by the concurrent use of alcohol.

Kaufman M: Care of the adolescent sexual assault victim, *Pediatrics* 122:462–470, 2008.

37. **How can you tell whether a patient has been given a date-rape drug?**

Most of these drugs can be detected in blood and/or urine. However, because they are metabolized very quickly, it is important to screen early in your evaluation of the patient. For example, Rohypnol can be detected in blood for 24 hours and in urine up to 48 hours, GHB in urine only for up to 12 hours after ingestion, and ketamine in urine for up to 72 hours. None of these drugs is included in routine drug screen panels.

Kaufman M: Care of the adolescent sexual assault victim, *Pediatrics* 122:462–470, 2008.

KEY POINTS: FRACTURES OF ABUSE

1. Any fracture can be the result of nonaccidental trauma.
2. Critical in assessment: history, age of patient, developmental level of the patient, family history
3. Fractures with higher likelihood of abuse: rib, scapula, spinous process, sternum, long bone with metaphyseal lesions
4. Suspicious fractures: <18 months of age with humeral shaft fracture, complex or bilateral skull fractures, femoral fracture in nonambulatory child (without correlating history)
5. Skeletal surveys are indicated for suspected nonaccidental trauma in children <2 years of age.

KEY POINTS: RETINAL HEMORRHAGES

1. May be the only sign in an infant of a nonaccidental shaking injury
2. Almost never caused by seizures alone
3. Should always be assessed in an infant whose presenting symptoms include excessive irritability, lethargy, sepsislike appearance, seizures, or coma
4. Should always be confirmed by an ophthalmologist
5. If found, should be followed by a skeletal series and cranial neuroimaging (computed tomography scanning and/or magnetic resonance imaging)

KEY POINTS: SEXUAL ABUSE

1. The most common physical finding is a normal examination.
2. The perpetrator is known to the victim in 75% to 80% of cases.
3. Infections that are diagnostic of abuse are gonorrhea, syphilis, chlamydia, and HIV.
4. For a prepubertal victim of sexual assault, NAAT is the preferred test for gonorrhea and chlamydia because a culture is too insensitive.
5. Reasons for immediate medical examination include ongoing bleeding or evidence of acute injury.
6. Use of accepted or standardized protocols is important during the evaluative process.
   HIV, Human immunodeficiency virus; *NAAT,* nucleic acid amplification test.

ENVIRONMENTAL INJURY

38. How do fresh- and salt-water drownings differ?
    Fresh water injures the lung primarily by disrupting surfactant, thereby leading to alveolar collapse. Damage to the alveolar membranes leads to the transudation of fluid into the air spaces and pulmonary edema. **Salt water** pulls fluid into the air spaces directly by creating a strong osmotic gradient, and the accumulated water washes away surfactant, thereby leading to alveolar collapse. Both types result in abnormal surfactant function and increased capillary endothelial permeability. Patients develop ventilation-perfusion mismatch and hypoxemia, which may require aggressive mechanical support. Ultimately, management for either fresh- or salt-water drowning is the same.

Meyer RJ, Theodorou AA, Berg RA: Childhood drowning, *Pediatr Rev* 27:163–169, 2006.

39. How is the duration of submersion predictive of outcomes in drownings?
    Risk of death or severe neurologic impairment after hospital discharge increases with duration of submersion as follows:

    0 to 5 minutes: 10%
    6 to 10 minutes: 56%
    11 to 25 minutes: 88%
    >25 minutes: nearly 100%

Signs of brain-stem injury are also predictive of death or severe neurologic sequelae.

Szpilman D, Bierens JJLM, Handley AJ, et al: Drowning, *N Engl J Med* 366:2102–2110, 2012.

40. What cardiovascular changes occur as body temperature falls?
    - **31 °C to 32 °C:** Elevated heart rate, cardiac output, and blood pressure; peripheral vasoconstriction and increased central vascular volume; normal electrocardiogram (ECG)
    - **28 °C to 31 °C:** Diminished heart rate, cardiac output, and blood pressure; ECG irregularities include premature ventricular contractions (PVCs), supraventricular dysrhythmias, atrial fibrillation, and T-wave inversion
    - **<28 °C:** Severe myocardial irritability; ventricular fibrillation, usually refractory to electrical defibrillation; often absent pulse or blood pressure; J waves on ECG

41. What are the physiologic consequences of externally warming a severely hypothermic patient too rapidly?
    - **Core temperature "after-drop":** The body temperature drops because external rewarming causes peripheral vasodilation and the return of cold venous blood to the core.
    - **Hypotension:** Peripheral vasodilation increases total vascular space, thereby causing a drop in blood pressure.
    - **Acidosis:** Lactic acid returns from the periphery, thereby resulting in rewarming acidosis.
    - **Dysrhythmias:** Rewarming alters acid-base and electrolyte status in the setting of an irritable myocardium.

42. What are acceptable rewarming methods for the hypothermic child?
    For patients with mild hypothermia (32 °C to 35 °C), passive rewarming by removing cold clothing and placing the patient in a warm, dry environment with blankets is generally sufficient. Active external rewarming involves the use of heating blankets, hot-water bottles, and overhead warmers and can also be used for patients with acute hypothermia in the 32 °C to 35 °C range. Active external rewarming should not be used for chronic hypothermia (>24 hours). More aggressive core rewarming techniques should be considered for patients with temperatures lower than 32 °C. These techniques include gastric or colonic irrigation with warm fluids, peritoneal dialysis, pleural lavage, and extracorporeal blood rewarming with partial bypass. Intravenous and other fluids should be heated to 43 °C. Patients should be given warmed, humidified oxygen by facemask or endotracheal tube.

Brown DJA, Brugger H, Boyd J, Paal P: Accidental hypothermia, *N Engl J Med* 367:1930–1938, 2012.

43. What organ systems are affected in patients suffering from heat stroke?
    Heat stroke is a medical emergency of multisystem dysfunction that includes a very high body temperature (usually >41.5 °C). The systems that are affected include the following:
    - **Central nervous system (CNS):** Confusion, seizures, and loss of consciousness
    - **Cardiovascular:** Hypotension as a result of volume depletion, peripheral vasodilation, and myocardial dysfunction
    - **Renal:** Acute tubular necrosis and renal failure, with marked electrolyte abnormalities
    - **Hepatocellular:** Injury and dysfunction
    - **Heme:** Abnormal hemostasis, often with signs of DIC
    - **Muscle:** Rhabdomyolysis

Jardine DS: Heat illness and heat stroke, *Pediatr Rev* 28:249–258, 2007.

44. How quickly can temperature rise inside an enclosed automobile?
    The greatest rise in temperature in a closed vehicle occurs within the first 15 to 30 minutes. Leaving the window slightly open ("cracking the window") does not affect the rapid temperature elevation. In one observational study, the internal temperature of an automobile increased by ~40 °F compared with outside temperatures. Heat stroke is a significant cause of death in children who are left unattended in motor vehicles.

McLaren C, Null J, Quinn J: Heat stress from enclosed vehicles: moderate ambient temperatures cause significant temperature rise in enclosed vehicles, *Pediatrics* 116:e109–e111, 2005.

45. **What are characteristics of heat stroke?**
    - Heatstroke occurs when the body temperature exceeds 104 °F, resulting in thermoregulatory collapse.
    - Symptoms include: dizziness, disorientation, agitation, confusion, sluggishness, seizure, hot dry skin that is flushed but not sweaty, loss of consciousness, rapid heartbeat, and hallucinations.
    - A core body temperature of 107 °F or greater can be lethal as cells are damaged and internal organs begin to shut down.

McLaren C, Null J, Quinn J: Heat stress from enclosed vehicles: moderate ambient temperatures cause significant temperature rise in enclosed vehicles, *Pediatrics* 116:e109–e111, 2005.

46. **Why are children more vulnerable to effects of external temperature changes?**
    Children's thermoregulatory systems are not as efficient as an adult's and their body temperatures warm at a rate 3 to 5 times faster than an adult's.

47. **What are the signs and symptoms of significant upper airway heat exposure in a patient who has been in a house fire?**
    - Carbonaceous sputum
    - Singed nasal hairs
    - Facial burns
    - Respiratory distress
    One should not rely on the presence of respiratory distress as an indicator for prompt endotracheal intubation. The first three signs listed represent significant heat exposure to the airway, and progressive swelling can rapidly progress to upper airway obstruction.

48. **What are the signs and symptoms of impending respiratory failure as a result of mucosal injury and edema from heat exposure during a house fire?**
    - Hoarseness
    - Stridor
    - Increasing respiratory distress
    - Drooling and difficulty swallowing
    An endotracheal tube should be emergently considered for patients with the above signs and symptoms. Upper airway mucosal swelling may make intubation difficult, and the most experienced physician should perform this intervention.

49. **Which laboratory studies are needed for patients with suspected carbon monoxide (CO) poisoning?**
    - Blood carboxyhemoglobin (COHb) level
      0% to 1%: Normal (smokers may have up to 5% to 10%)
      10% to 30%: Headache, exercise-induced dyspnea, confusion
      30% to 50%: Severe headache, nausea, vomiting, increased heart rate and respirations, visual disturbances, memory loss, ataxia
      50% to 70%: Convulsions, coma, severe cardiorespiratory compromise
      70%: Usually fatal
    - **Hemoglobin level:** To evaluate correctable anemia
    - **Arterial pH:** To detect acidosis
    - **Urinalysis for myoglobin:** With CO poisoning, patients are susceptible to tissue and muscle breakdown with possible acute renal failure resulting from the renal deposition of myoglobin

50. **What are the key aspects of treatment for carbon monoxide poisoning in children?**
    - Treatment includes **100% oxygen** through non-rebreather mask until the COHb level falls to 5%. The half-life of COHb is 5 to 6 hours if the patient is breathing room air (at sea level). The half-life of COHb is reduced to 1 to 1½ hours if the patient is breathing 100% oxygen (at sea level). The half-life of COHb is reduced to under 1 hour with hyperbaric oxygen therapy.

- Refer for use of **hyperbaric oxygen** for the following conditions: a history of coma, seizure, or abnormal mental status at the scene or in the ED; persistent metabolic acidosis; neonate; pregnancy (the fetus is more vulnerable to hypoxic effects of CO); the HbCO level is more than 25%, even if the patient is neurologically intact.

51. Why is carbon monoxide such a deadly toxin?
    - CO is odorless and invisible and can overwhelm a patient without warning.
    - CO is ubiquitous as a product of partial combustion (car exhaust emissions, household heating equipment, burning charcoal).
    - In the absence of a clear history, early CO intoxication is often misdiagnosed as a flulike illness.

52. What is the pathophysiology of carbon monoxide poisoning?
    - CO develops a nearly irreversible bond with hemoglobin (with an affinity 200 to 300 times that of oxygen) that shifts the oxyhemoglobin dissociation curve to the left and changes its shape from sigmoidal to hyperbolic (with greatly diminished O_2 tissue release).
    - CO develops a strong bond with other heme-containing proteins, particularly in the mitochondria, thereby leading to metabolic acidosis and cellular dysfunction (especially in cardiac and CNS tissues).

53. What other serious exposure risk should one consider when managing a patient suffering from carbon monoxide poisoning?
    One of the most important considerations in managing a CO-poisoned patient is concomitant **cyanide** (CN) poisoning. In CO-exposed patients with persistent acidosis and high lactate levels, one should seriously consider CN poisoning and treat accordingly. Supplemental oxygen therapy is not adequate. If CN poisoning is suspected, treat the patient with sodium thiosulfate.

Weaver LK: Carbon monoxide poisoning, *N Engl J Med* 360:1217–1225, 2009.

54. What are the different degrees of burn injuries?
    See Table 5-2.

Table 5-2. Classification of Burn Wounds

DEGREE	DEPTH	CLINICAL APPEARANCE	CAUSE
Superficial	Epidermis	Dry, erythematous	Sunburn, scald
Partial	Superficial dermis	Blisters, moist, erythematous	Scald, immersion, contact
	Deep dermis	White eschar	Grease, flash fire
Full thickness	Subcutaneous	Avascular—white/dark, dry, waxy (yellow)	Prolonged immersion, flame, contact, grease, oil
	Muscle	Charred, skin surface cracked	Flame

Adapted from Coren CV: Burn injuries in children, Pediatr Ann 16:328–339, 1987.

55. How does the "rule of nines" apply in children?
    The *"rule of nines"* is a tool used to estimate the extent of burns in adults. For example, in adults, the entire arm is 9% of the total body surface area (TBSA), the front of the leg is another 9% of the TBSA, and so on. The resulting estimate of the extent of burns is particularly helpful for calculating fluid requirements. Correction for age is necessary with this formula because of differing body proportions. Therefore, for children, use the surface of a patient's palm, which represents about 1% of TBSA, as the tool for estimating the percentage of the TBSA affected by the burn (Fig. 5-5).

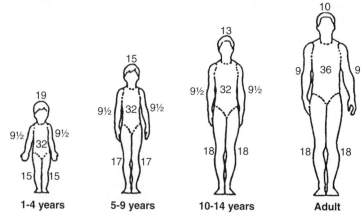

Figure 5-5. Rule of nines as applied to children. *(Carvajal HF: Burn injuries. In Behrman RE editor:* Nelson Textbook of Pediatrics, *ed 14. Philadelphia, 1992, WB Saunders, p 235.)*

56. **Which burn injuries are indications for hospitalization?**
    - Partial-thickness burns covering more than 10% of the TBSA
    - Full-thickness burns covering more than 2% of the TBSA
    - Significant burns involving the hands, feet, face, joints, or perineum
    - Burns resulting from suspected child abuse
    - Electrical burns
    - Circumferential burns (which may predispose the patient to vascular compromise)
    - Explosion, inhalation, or chemical burns (in which other organ trauma may be involved)
    - Significant burns in children younger than 2 years

Rodgers GL: Reducing the toll of childhood burns, *Contemp Pediatr* 17:152–173, 2000.

57. **Why are alkali burns worse than acid burns in the eye?**
    Alkali burns are caused by lye (e.g., Drano, Liquid-Plumr), lime, or ammonia, in addition to other agents; they are characterized by liquefaction necrosis. They are worse than acid burns because the damage is ongoing. When spilled in the eye, **acid** is quickly buffered by tissue and limited in penetration by precipitated proteins; coagulation necrosis results, which is usually limited to the area of contact. Alkali, however, has a more rapid and deeper advancement, thereby causing progressive damage at the cellular level by combining with membrane lipids. This underscores the importance of extensive irrigation of the burned eye, particularly in cases of alkali burns.

58. **How do the injuries produced by lightning and high-voltage wires differ?**
    - **Lightning:** Consists of direct current of extremely high voltage (200,000 to 2,000,000,000 volts) delivered over milliseconds. Lightning exposure causes massive electrical countershock with asystole, respiratory arrest, and minimal tissue damage.
    - **High-voltage wires:** Deliver alternating current of lower voltage (rarely exceeding 70,000 volts) over a longer period of time. High-voltage exposure causes ventricular fibrillation and deep tissue injury. The resultant muscle necrosis can lead to substantial myoglobin release and renal failure.

59. **In electrical injury, is alternating or direct current more hazardous?**
    At low voltages (e.g., those found in household electrical devices), **alternating current** is more dangerous than direct current. Exposure to alternating current can provoke tetanic muscle contractions so that the victim who has grasped an electrical source is unable to let go, thereby prolonging the exposure and producing greater tissue injury. Direct current or high-voltage alternating current typically causes a single forceful muscular contraction that will push or throw the victim away from the source.

60. **What agents are the most common causes of anaphylaxis seen in U.S. emergency rooms?**

Food. *Peanuts*, *tree nuts* (e.g., almonds, hazelnuts), and *seafood* head the list and are twice as common as bee stings as a trigger. Severe reactions occur 1 to 2 hours after exposure. Anaphylaxis may occur without a skin reaction, so a high index of suspicion is needed in a child with unexplained sudden bronchospasm, laryngospasm, severe gastrointestinal (GI) symptoms, or poor responsiveness. In some adolescents, certain foods (e.g., wheat, celery, shellfish), if ingested within 4 hours of exercise, can lead to food-dependent, exercise-induced anaphylaxis. Risk factors for fatal anaphylactic reactions include a history of asthma, delayed diagnosis, and delayed administration of epinephrine.

Rudders SA, Banerji A, Vassallo MF, et al: Trends in pediatric emergency department visits for food-induced anaphylaxis, *J Allergy Clin Immunol* 126:385–388, 2010.
Lack G: Food allergy, *N Engl J Med* 359:1252–1260, 2008.

61. **What are important considerations when treating frostbite in children?**
    - Rewarm the affected area in water with a temperature of 37 °C to 43 °C (99 °F to 109 °F) for 20 minutes.
    - Never attempt to rewarm if there is risk for refreezing.
    - Rubbing the affected area may cause further damage to tissue.

KEY POINTS: ENVIRONMENTAL INJURIES

1. Food (e.g., peanuts, tree nuts, seafood) is twice as common as insect stings as a cause of anaphylaxis in children.
2. Carbon monoxide poisoning is often misdiagnosed because the presenting symptoms can be flulike.
3. Consider cyanide poisoning in patients with CO exposure. If there is persistent acidosis and high lactate, initiate therapy with sodium thiosulfate.
4. Impending upper airway obstruction in house fires is more likely if there is the presence of carbonaceous sputum, singed nasal or facial hairs, or respiratory abnormalities (e.g., hoarseness, stridor).
5. Hospitalization is indicated for significant burns involving the hands, feet, joints, or perineum or if there are circumferential burns.
6. Alkali burns are worse than acid burns because of ongoing liquefaction necrosis.

RESUSCITATION

62. **What are common problems identified in cardiopulmonary resuscitation (CPR) done by professionals?**
    - Numerous studies have demonstrated rates of compression are often inadequate.
    - Chest wall decompression (the relaxation phase) is often incomplete.
    - Chest compressions are often too shallow.
    - Chest compressions are interrupted too frequently.
    - Ventilation is excessive.

Sutton RM, Niles D, Nysaether J, et al: Quantitative analysis of CPR quality during in-hospital resuscitation of older children and adolescents, *Pediatrics* 124: 494–99, 2009.

63. **What is the role for capnography during resuscitation?**

Capnography, the monitoring of carbon dioxide, has been shown to be beneficial during cardiopulmonary resuscitation because it may provide feedback on the effectiveness of chest compressions. When available, it should be utilized. However, the readings need to be interpreted cautiously because vasoconstrictive medications, lung disease, and minute ventilation can affect the results.

Kleinman ME, de Caen AR, Chameides L, et al: Part 10: Pediatric basic and advanced life support: 2010 international consensus on cardiopulmonary resuscitation and emergency cardiovascular care science with treatment recommendations, *Circulation* 122:S466–S515, 2010.

64. **Why is the airway of an infant or child more prone to obstruction than that of an adult?**
    - Infants have smaller airway diameters. Because airflow is inversely proportional to the airway radius raised to the fourth power (Poiseuille's law), small changes in the diameter of the trachea can result in very large drops in airflow.
    - The tracheal cartilage of an infant is softer and can collapse more easily if hyperextended.
    - In an infant, the lumen of the oropharynx is relatively smaller, owing to the larger size of the tongue and smaller size of the mandible.
    - Lower airways are smaller and less developed in children, thus putting them at risk for airway obstruction by small foreign bodies.

65. **How can the correct size of endotracheal tubes (ETTs) be estimated for a given patient?**
    Pediatric advanced life support guidelines now recommend that cuffed tubes be used in most children beyond the neonatal period. When choosing a *cuffed tube* the formula *[3.5 + (age in years/4)]* is most commonly used. Another guideline is that the child's pinky should approximate the internal diameter of the tube.

    When choosing an *uncuffed tube*, one should estimate one half size larger, and the formula *[4 + (age in years/4)]* is appropriate. Because these formulas are estimates, it is advisable to have tubes one-half size larger and smaller available and prepared before intubation.

Kleinman ME, de Caen AR, Chameides L, et al: Part 10: Pediatric basic and advanced life support: 2010 international consensus on cardiopulmonary resuscitation and emergency cardiovascular care science with treatment recommendations, *Circulation* 122:S466–S515, 2010.

66. **When should cuffed versus uncuffed ETTs be used?**
    In the past, uncuffed ETTs were recommended for children younger than 8 years because of concern that the cuff could place excessive pressure on the already narrow portion of the pediatric cricoid cartilage. However, the American Heart Association has advised that both cuffed and uncuffed tubes are acceptable for infants and children undergoing emergent intubation. Cuffed tubes may even be preferable in those at high risk of aspiration, burn victims, and those with lung diseases that may necessitate higher ventilation pressures. When using a cuffed tube, care should be taken to avoid excessive cuff pressures.

Kleinman ME, de Caen AR, Chameides L, et al: Part 10: Pediatric basic and advanced life support: 2010 international consensus on cardiopulmonary resuscitation and emergency cardiovascular care science with treatment recommendations, *Circulation* 122:S466–S515, 2010.

67. **How should the appropriate depth of an ETT be calculated?**
    After insertion of an ETT, the appropriate depth (measured from the gum line) may be approximated using the following formula for children older than 1 year:

    $$(\text{Age in years}/2) + 12 \text{ cm}$$

    These measurements should always be confirmed by clinical means and radiography.

68. **How should correct placement of an ETT be confirmed?**
    - Improvement or continued stability of vital signs including oxygen saturation
    - Bilateral chest wall rise
    - Bilateral symmetric breath sounds
    - Absence of gastric insufflation sounds over the stomach
    - Use of an exhaled CO_2 detector device and continuous waveform capnography
    - Direct laryngoscopy
    - Chest radiography

69. **What emergency drugs can be given through an ETT?**
    Lidocaine, Epinephrine, Atropine, Naloxone (LEAN). Vasopressin can also be administered through an ETT. However, if available, intraosseous or intravenous administration is always preferable because

absorption is more predictable. The optimal dose of most drugs through the endotracheal route is not known. However, recommendations for epinephrine are 10 times the intravenous dose, and for other drugs, 2 to 3 times the intravenous dose. If drugs are being given through the ETT, they should be followed with 5 mL of normal saline and positive-pressure ventilation.

Kleinman ME, de Caen AR, Chameides L, et al: Part 14: Pediatric basic and advanced life support: 2010 international consensus on cardiopulmonary resuscitation and emergency cardiovascular care science with treatment recommendations, *Circulation* 122:S876–S908, 2010.

70. What are the potential reasons for acute deterioration in an intubated patient?
    These can be remembered using the **DOPE** acronym:
    - **D**isplacement of the ETT
    - **O**bstruction of the ETT
    - **P**neumothorax
    - **E**quipment failure

American Heart Association: *PALS Provider Manual*, Dallas, 2006, American Heart Association, p 195.

71. When is atropine indicated during cardiopulmonary resuscitation?
    Atropine is recommended as a premedication before laryngoscopy in infants. It may be administered to the child with symptomatic bradycardia with a pulse after other resuscitative measures (i.e., oxygenation, ventilation, and epinephrine) have been initiated. Atropine may also be considered in cases of vagally induced bradycardia or anticholinergic poisoning.

Kleinman ME, de Caen AR, Chameides L, et al: Part 10: Pediatric basic and advanced life support: 2010 international consensus on cardiopulmonary resuscitation and emergency cardiovascular care science with treatment recommendations, *Circulation* 122:S466–S515, 2010.

72. When is the use of calcium indicated during cardiopulmonary resuscitation?
    Routine use of calcium is *generally not recommended* in resuscitation algorithms because it has not been shown to improve return of spontaneous circulation. Calcium use may be considered in the following specific situations:
    - Overdose of a calcium channel blocker
    - Hyperkalemia resulting in cardiac dysrhythmia
    - Documented hypocalcemia
    - Hypermagnesemia
    - Hyperkalemia

Kleinman ME, de Caen AR, Chameides L, et al: Part 10: Pediatric basic and advanced life support: 2010 international consensus on cardiopulmonary resuscitation and emergency cardiovascular care science with treatment recommendations, *Circulation* 122:S466–S515, 2010.

73. What are contraindications to the use of an intraosseous line?
    - Placement into a fractured bone
    - Placement through dirty or infected skin
    - Use in patients with bone disorders such as osteopetrosis or osteogenesis imperfecta
    - Repeat attempt into the same bone (owing to risk for extravasation through the initial puncture site)

Blumberg SM, Gorn M, Crain EF: Intraosseous infusion: a review of methods and novel devices, *Pediatr Emerg Care* 24:50–56, 2008.

74. Can laboratory tests be obtained from intraosseous lines?
    Compared with venipuncture, there appears to be a good correlation between serum and marrow electrolytes, hemoglobin, drug levels, blood group typing, and renal function tests. Correlation is poorer with liver function tests and arterial blood gas studies (P_{CO_2} and P_{O_2}). Additionally, the positive correlations

appear to worsen after 30 minutes of CPR and/or drug and fluid administration. The most reliable samples on which to base clinical decisions would be those obtained at the time of intraosseous line placement early in the resuscitation.

Blumberg SM, Gorn M, Crain EF: Intraosseous infusion: a review of methods and novel devices, *Pediatr Emerg Care* 24:51, 2008.

75. What are the complications of intraosseous lines?

Significant morbidity is very uncommon (<1%). The most common problems are extravasation of fluids and superficial skin infections. Osteomyelitis is rare (<0.6%) and typically only occurs with prolonged infusions. Other rare complications are skin necrosis, bone fractures, and compartment syndrome. Although there is the theoretical risk for significant bone growth arrest, growth plate damage, and fat embolism, these have not been reported. Obtaining venous access and discontinuing intraosseous infusions as soon as possible after stabilization have been recommended as means to further minimize complications.

Blumberg SM, Gorn M, Crain EF: Intraosseous infusion: a review of methods and novel devices, *Pediatr Emerg Care* 24:51, 2008.

76. What features indicate that an intraosseous needle has been correctly placed?

- A soft pop should be felt as you break through the cortex.
- The needle should be very stable.
- There should be free flow of intravenous fluids without infiltration of subcutaneous tissues.
- Bone marrow aspiration, although confirming placement, may not always be possible even when needle placement is correct. Therefore, if you cannot aspirate marrow, you should rely on other signs for determination of placement.

77. How can a child's weight be estimated?

Some rules of thumb:
- An average term neonate weighs 3 kg
- An average 1-year-old weighs 10 kg
- An average 5-year-old weighs 20 kg
  The following formula may also be used:

$$\text{Weight} = (3 \times \text{age}) + 7$$

New guidelines suggest that, in obese patients, medication doses should be calculated according to ideal body weight and should not be higher than recommended adult dosing.

Kleinman ME, de Caen AR, Chameides L, et al: Part 10: Pediatric basic and advanced life support: 2010 international consensus on cardiopulmonary resuscitation and emergency cardiovascular care science with treatment recommendations, *Circulation* 122:S466–S515, 2010.
Luscombe M, Owens B: Weight estimation in resuscitation: is the current formula still valid? *Arch Dis Child* 92:412–415, 2007.

78. Name the potentially reversible causes of cardiac arrest.

- H's: Hypoxemia, hypovolemia, hypothermia, hyper/hypokalemia, hypoglycemia, and hydrogen ion (acidosis)
- T's: Tamponade, tension pneumothorax, toxins, and thromboembolism

American Heart Association: *PALS Provider Manual*, Dallas, 2006, American Heart Association, p 178.

79. What are the typical clinical findings associated with supraventricular tachycardia (SVT)?

- Sudden onset
- Heart rate generally more than 180 beats per minute in children and more than 220 beats per minute in infants;
- Minimal heart rate variability

- Absent, abnormal, or inverted P waves
- Infants: Signs and/or symptoms that are nonspecific or, if SVT for hours or days, suggestive of congestive heart failure or shock (e.g., poor feeding, irritability, vomiting, cyanosis, pallor, cough, respiratory distress, lethargy)
- Verbal children: Palpitations and fluttering in the chest

Salerno JC, Seslar SP: Supraventricular tachycardia, *Arch Pediatr Adolesc Med* 163:268–274, 2009.

80. **If an infant develops SVT, how long before congestive heart failure (CHF) develops?**
It is rare for an infant to develop CHF from SVT in less than 24 hours. When SVT is present for 24 to 36 hours, about 20% develop CHF. At 48 hours, the number increases to 50%.

Salerno JC, Seslar SP: Supraventricular tachycardia, *Arch Pediatr Adolesc Med* 163:268–274, 2009.

81. **What factors may be predictive of outcomes after pediatric cardiac arrest?**
Factors associated with *improved likelihood* of return of spontaneous circulation including:
- Short time to initiation of adequate CPR
- High quality CPR
- Shorter overall duration of resuscitation
- Witnessed cardiac arrest

Factors associated with *poor outcomes* include:
- Infants
- Obesity
- Initial nonperfusing rhythm
- Out-of-hospital traumatic arrest

Kleinman ME, de Caen AR, Chameides L, et al: Part 10: Pediatric basic and advanced life support: 2010 international consensus on cardiopulmonary resuscitation and emergency cardiovascular care science with treatment recommendations, *Circulation* 122:S466–S515, 2010.

82. **Are fixed and dilated pupils a contraindication to resuscitation for a pediatric patient in cardiac arrest?**
No. Pupillary dilation begins 15 seconds after cardiac arrest and is complete after about 1 minute and 45 seconds. It may only be a sign of transient hypoxia. The only absolute contraindications to resuscitation are rigor mortis, corneal clouding, dependent lividity, and decapitation.

83. **When should a failing resuscitation be stopped?**
Although there are no definitive guidelines, some studies have suggested that when **more than two rounds of epinephrine** have been given and/or **more than 20 minutes** have elapsed since the initiation of resuscitation without clinical cardiovascular or neurologic improvement, the likelihood of death or survival with neurologic devastation greatly increases. Unwitnessed out-of-hospital arrests are almost always associated with a poor outcome. In settings of hypothermia, patients should be rewarmed to 36 °C before resuscitation is discontinued. In patients with acute, reversible conditions such as drug toxicity or cardiac disease, extracorporeal cardiac life support may be considered if available.

American Heart Association: *PALS Provider Manual.* Dallas, 2006, American Heart Association, p 182.
Schindler M, Bohn D, Cox PN, et al: Outcome of out-of-hospital cardiac or respiratory arrest in children, *N Engl J Med* 335:1473–1479, 1996.

84. **Why is resuscitation less successful in children than in adults?**
Adults more commonly experience collapse and arrest from primary cardiac disease and associated dysrhythmias—ventricular tachycardia and fibrillation. These are more readily reversible and carry a better prognosis. **Children**, however, have cardiac arrest as a secondary phenomenon from other processes, such as respiratory obstruction or apnea, often associated with infection, hypoxia, acidosis, or hypovolemia. Primary cardiac arrest is rare. The most common dysrhythmia associated with pediatric cardiac arrest is asystole. It is less frequently reversible, and by the time a child has cardiac arrest, severe neurologic damage is almost always present.

85. **Should family members be allowed to observe a resuscitation?**
This has been a controversial topic with family members historically being excluded from the setting of an ongoing resuscitation. However, data are accumulating that indicate that the presence of family members (1) does not interfere with medical efforts or result in increased stress for the medical team or increased medicolegal conflicts and (2) is associated with a lesser likelihood of PTSD-related symptoms, including anxiety and depression, for those who observe resuscitation compared with those who don't.

Jabre P, Belpomme V, Azoulay E, et al: Family presence during resuscitation, *N Engl J Med* 368:1008–1018, 2013.

SHOCK

86. **Are all children in shock hypotensive?**
No. Shock is an acute syndrome resulting from cardiovascular dysfunction that renders the circulatory system unable to provide oxygen and substrates to the body. In the initial stages of shock (*compensated shock*), blood pressure is often preserved. Physiologically, children will maintain a state of compensated shock until very late in the progression of illness.

87. **What are the signs and symptoms of early or compensated shock?**
   - Unexplained tachycardia
   - Mild tachypnea
   - Delayed capillary refill
   - Orthostatic changes in pressure or pulse
   - Irritability

88. **What are the signs and symptoms of late or uncompensated shock?**
   - Increased tachycardia
   - Increased tachypnea
   - Poor peripheral pulses
   - Capillary refill markedly delayed
   - Cool extremities
   - Hypotension
   - Altered mental status
   - Low urine output

89. **What external factors can affect the accuracy of measurement of capillary refill time in children and neonates?**
   - **Room temperature:** Children in a cool environment (19.4 °C) compared with those in a warmer environment (25.7 °C) will have a significantly prolonged (>2 seconds) capillary refill time (CRT). Seventy percent of healthy children in one study had prolonged CRT in the cooler environment but none had prolongation in the warmer environment.
   - **Ambient light:** Darker conditions do impact the ability to make accurate visual determinations.
   - **Site of measurement:** In neonates, CRT has been shown to be longer if it is measured in the heel compared with the head or sternum. Paradoxically, in older children, CRT was significantly faster when measured on the fingertip compared with the sternum.
   - **Pressure application:** In neonates, application of pressure for 3 to 4 seconds significantly increases CRT compared with briefer periods (1 to 2 seconds) of pressure application. Most guidelines call for pressure application between 3 to 5 seconds.
   - **Interobserver reliability:** When different observers measure CRT, studies have indicated agreement is not good, but improves with short (<1 second) or prolonged (>4 seconds) refill time.

King D, Morton R, Beran C: How to use capillary refill time, *Arch Dis Child Educ Pract Ed* 99:111–116, 2014.

90. **How much blood volume can be lost before hypotension may be seen in children?**
Some children can lose up to 30% of their blood volume before blood pressure noticeably declines. It is important to note that 25% of blood volume equals 20 mL/kg, which is only 200 mL in a 10-kg child. Losses >40% of blood volume cause severe hypotension that, if prolonged, may become irreversible.

91. What defines hypotension in children (i.e., systolic blood pressure <5th percentile for age)?
    See Table 5-3.

Kleinman ME, de Caen AR, Chameides L, et al: Part 14: Pediatric basic and advanced life support: 2010 international consensus on cardiopulmonary resuscitation and emergency cardiovascular care science with treatment recommendations, *Circulation* 122:S876–S908, 2010.

Table 5-3. Hypotension in Children

AGE	SYSTOLIC BLOOD PRESSURE (MM HG)
<1 month	≤60
1 month to 1 year	≤70
1 to 10 years	≤70 + (2 × age in years)
>10 years	≤90

92. What types of shock can occur in children?
    - **Hypovolemic:** Decreased circulating volume (blood loss; fluid loss from gastroenteritis, most common cause in children)
    - **Distributive:** Pooling of blood in peripheral vasculature (septic, anaphylactic, neurogenic)
    - **Cardiogenic:** Cardiac dysfunction with decreased cardiac output (e.g., congenital heart disease, myocarditis, dysrhythmia)
    - **Obstructive:** Mechanical obstruction of ventricular outflow tract (e.g., cardiac tamponade, tension pneumothorax)

93. What are the hallmarks of septic shock?
    - Fever or hypothermia
    - Metabolic acidosis
    - Vasodilation: widened pulse pressure and/or hypotension, bounding pulses

Angus DC, van der Poll T: Severe sepsis and septic shock, *N Engl J Med* 369:840–851, 2013.

94. What are the key initial management items for septic shock?
    Early recognition of sepsis and initiation of therapy is associated with improved outcome.
    - Control and/or maintain airway
    - Recognize poor perfusion and shock
    - Push 20 mL/kg up to 60 mL/kg of isotonic crystalloid solution as rapidly as possible and within the first hour.
    - If there is still evidence of shock or poor perfusion, begin vasoactive therapy at 1 hour

Dellinger RP, Levy MM, Rhodes A: Surviving sepsis campaign: international guidelines for management of severe sepsis and septic shock: 2012, *Crit Care Med* 41:580–637,2013.
Carcillo JA, Fields AI: Clinical practice parameters for hemodynamic support of pediatric and neonatal patients in septic shock, *Crit Care Med* 30:1370, 2002.

95. Are corticosteroids recommended for the treatment of septic shock?
    There have been some studies in adults suggesting that corticosteroids may be beneficial for the treatment of septic shock. Currently, corticosteroids are recommended only for children who may have *fluid-resistant* or *catecholamine-resistant septic shock* or who have a clear history or evidence of *adrenal insufficiency.* Even in these scenarios, use of steroids has not been convincingly shown to impart survival advantage in children.

Menon K, McNally JD, Choong K, et al: A systematic review and meta-analysis on the effect of steroids in pediatric shock, *Pediatr Crit Care Med* 14:474–480, 2013.

96. What is the most important pharmacologic therapy for anaphylactic shock?
    Epinephrine. Epinephrine should be administered intramuscularly as soon as possible. Plasma concentrations of epinephrine appear to be highest when given intramuscularly in the thigh compared with subcutaneously or intramuscularly in the arm. If the patient has severe refractory symptoms and hypotension, epinephrine may be given as a continuous intravascular infusion. Failure to administer epinephrine quickly increases the risk for death from anaphylaxis.

Liberman DB, Teach SJ: Management of anaphylaxis in children, *Pediatr Emerg Med* 24:861–866, 2008.

97. What are the possible causes of shock in the newborn period?
    The differential diagnosis is broad, but remember the mnemonic **THE MISFITS**:
    - **T**rauma (nonaccidental and accidental)
    - **H**eart disease and hypovolemia
    - **E**ndocrine (e.g., congenital adrenal hyperplasia)
    - **M**etabolic (electrolyte)
    - **I**nborn errors of metabolism
    - **S**epsis (e.g., meningitis, pneumonia, urinary tract infection)
    - **F**ormula mishaps (e.g., underdilution or overdilution)
    - **I**ntestinal catastrophes (e.g., volvulus, intussusception, necrotizing enterocolitis)
    - **T**oxins and poisons
    - **S**eizures

Brousseau T, Sharieff GQ: Newborn emergencies: the first 30 days of life, *Pediatr Clin North Am* 53:69–84, 2006.

98. A 4-day-old infant presents to the ED in shock with evidence of CHF and cyanosis. In addition to managing the airway and breathing, what is the first line of pharmacologic therapy?
    This baby likely has congenital heart disease with a ductal-dependent lesion such as hypoplastic left heart syndrome or coarctation of the aorta. The baby will require **prostaglandin E_1** infusion to maintain the patency of the ductus arteriosus until corrective surgery can be performed.

99. What are the four classes of medications that can be used to support cardiac output?
    - **Inotropes:** Increase cardiac contractility and often heart rate (e.g., dopamine, dobutamine, epinephrine)
    - **Vasopressors:** Increase vascular resistance and blood pressure (e.g., higher-dose dopamine, epinephrine, norepinephrine, vasopressin)
    - **Vasodilators:** Decrease vascular resistance and cardiac afterload and promote peripheral perfusion (e.g., sodium nitroprusside)
    - **Inodilators:** Increase cardiac contractility and reduce afterload (e.g., milrinone)

100. An 8-year-old presents to the ED after falling headfirst into an empty swimming pool. His heart rate is normal, yet despite aggressive fluid resuscitation he remains hypotensive. CT scans of the chest, abdomen, pelvis and head reveal only a small cerebral contusion. What is the likely cause of his hypotension?
    This patient is most likely suffering from **neurogenic shock**. Loss of sympathetic tone prevents the expected tachycardic response. The hallmarks of neurogenic shock are hypotension with either bradycardia or a normal heart rate despite fluid replenishment. If the hypotension cannot be corrected with fluid expansion, vasopressor therapy may be required, and within the first 8 hours, corticosteroids may be considered.

KEY POINTS: SIGNS AND SYMPTOMS OF SHOCK

1. Tachycardia
2. Poor peripheral pulses
3. Slow capillary refill
4. Cool extremities
5. Hypotension
6. Altered mental status

KEY POINTS: SHOCK IN PEDIATRIC TRAUMA

1. Shock in pediatric trauma patients is often masked because the inherent reserve in a child allows for the maintenance of vital signs for a long period of time, even in the presence of severe hemodynamic compromise.
2. Shock should be suspected in patients with tachycardia, a decrease in pulse pressure >20 mm Hg, skin mottling, cool extremities, delayed capillary refill (>2 seconds), and altered mental status.
3. The presence of hypotension in a child represents a state of uncompensated shock and indicates severe blood loss.
4. Shock is not explainable by head trauma alone, except in the case of an infant with open fontanels and unfused cranial sutures who may have a significant hemorrhage into the subgaleal or epidural space.
5. Shock may be associated with femur and/or pelvic fractures.
6. Shock should quickly prompt an evaluation of the child's abdomen for the source of blood loss.

TOXICOLOGY

101. What are the most common poisonings in children younger than 6 years?
See Table 5-4.

Table 5-4. Common Poisonings in Children

NONPHARMACEUTICALS	PHARMACEUTICALS
Cosmetics and personal care products	Analgesics
Cleaning substances	Cough and cold preparations
Plants, including mushrooms and tobacco	Topical agents
Battery, toys, and other foreign bodies	Vitamins
Insecticides, pesticides, and rodenticides	Antimicrobials

102. Which medications can kill a 10-kg toddler with 1 or 2 tablets, capsules, or teaspoonfuls?
   • **Tricyclic antidepressants** (amitriptyline, imipramine, desipramine)
   • **Antipsychotics** (thioridazine, chlorpromazine)
   • **Antimalarials** (chloroquine, hydroxychloroquine)
   • **Antiarrhythmics** (procainamide, flecainide)
   • **Calcium channel blockers** (nifedipine, verapamil)
   • **Oral hypoglycemics** (glyburide, glipizide)
   • **Opioids** (methadone, hydrocodone)
   • **Imidazolines** (clonidine, tetrahydrozoline)

Bar-Oz B, Levichek Z, Koren G: Medications that can be fatal for a toddler with one tablet or teaspoonful, *Paediatr Drugs* 6:123–126, 2004.

103. What medication causes the most overdose deaths in children each year in the United States?
Acetaminophen. Large numbers of accidental and suicidal intoxications occur each year in part because of its widespread availability.

Hanhan UA: The poisoned child in the pediatric intensive care unit, *Pediatr Clin North Am* 55:669–686, 2008.

KEY POINTS: ACETAMINOPHEN OVERDOSE

1. Significant ingestions may have no initial symptoms.
2. Assess for co-ingestions.
3. Administer charcoal if ingestion was within 4 hours of treatment.
4. Assess plasma acetaminophen level at 4 hours after ingestion (if possible) and apply nomogram.
5. Administer the antidote *N*-acetylcysteine within 8 to 10 hours of ingestion.

104. Name the toxicology "time bombs."

Time bombs are medications that lack symptoms early after ingestion but later have a profoundly toxic course.
- **Acetaminophen** (delayed hepatic injury)
- **Iron** (delayed cyanosis and profound metabolic acidosis)
- **Alcohols**—methanol (delayed acidosis), ethylene glycol (delayed nephrotoxicity)
- **Lithium**
- **Anticonvulsants**—phenytoin (Dilantin), carbamazepine
- **Time-release medications**

105. What empirical drug therapies are indicated for the poisoned child who presents with altered mental status?

All poisoned patients with depressed mental status should receive *oxygen* through a non-rebreather facemask. Blood glucose should be rapidly evaluated or empirical treatment for hypoglycemia with *intravenous glucose*, 0.5 g/kg, initiated. Hypoglycemia is associated with ingestion of ethanol, β-blockers, and oral hypoglycemic agents. *Naloxone* may be given as a diagnostic and therapeutic measure in the event of suspected or known opioid ingestion.

106. What is gastrointestinal decontamination?

Gastrointestinal decontamination refers to a variety of medications that may be administered and techniques that may be used to decrease the absorption of ingested poisons. Methods of gastrointestinal decontamination include activated charcoal, whole bowel irrigation, and gastric lavage. The effectiveness of these techniques is difficult to study, and much of the available evidence is based on animal and volunteer studies.

107. How does single-dose activated charcoal work and when should it be considered?

Single-dose activated charcoal is prepared as a liquid slurry and given orally to a poisoned patient. As it enters the stomach, it adsorbs toxins, thereby preventing absorption into the circulation. It is most efficacious when given within 1 hour of the time of ingestion. Single-dose activated charcoal may be considered in patients who have ingested a potentially toxic substance that is known to be adsorbed by charcoal within 1 hour of presentation. It is most likely to help children who may have ingested carbamazepine, dapsone, phenobarbital, quinine (Qualaquin), theophylline, salicylates, phenytoin, or valproic acid (Depakene). Charcoal is contraindicated in patients whose airway reflexes are compromised, and it should not be given through nasogastric tube unless the airway is protected with an ETT because of the risk for aspiration.

American Academy of Clinical Toxicology, European Association of Poisons Centres and Clinical Toxicologists: Position statement: single-dose activated charcoal, *J Toxicol Clin Toxicol* 43:61, 2005.

108. For what substances is charcoal not recommended?
- Hydrocarbons, because of possible increased risk for aspiration
- Others: acids, alcohols, alkalis, cyanide, iron, heavy metals, and lithium

American Academy of Clinical Toxicology, European Association of Poisons Centres and Clinical Toxicologists: Position statement: single-dose activated charcoal, *J Toxicol Clin Toxicol* 43:61–87, 2005.

109. When is gastric lavage indicated?

Gastric lavage involves the passage of a large orogastric tube (e.g., 24-Fr orogastric for a toddler, 36-Fr orogastric for a teenager) with sequential administration and aspiration of small volumes of normal saline (10 mL/kg in a child; 200 to 300 mL in an adult) with the intent of removing toxic substances present in the stomach. Efficacy remains unproved, and complications are significant (e.g., laryngospasm, esophageal injury, aspiration pneumonia); it should not be used routinely. A position paper by the American Academy of Clinical Toxicology (AACT) and European Association of Poisons Centres and Clinical Toxicologists (EAPCCT) indicates that there is no evidence showing that gastric lavage should be used routinely, if at all, in the management of poisonings. Evidence for use in special situations (e.g., lethal ingestions, recent exposures, substance not bound to activated charcoal) is weak. If performed by well-practiced physicians, it may be considered for patients with a life-threatening quantity of a poisonous ingestion occurring within 60 minutes of evaluation if the patient's airway is protected.

Benson BE, Hoppu K, Troutman WG, et al: Position paper update: gastric lavage for gastrointestinal decontamination, *Clin Toxicol* 51:140–146, 2013.

110. **What are the indications for whole bowel irrigation (WBI) in acute ingestions?**
This is a method of gastrointestinal decontamination using a large volume of polyethylene glycol–balanced electrolyte solution such as GoLYTELY given by mouth or nasogastric tube. These solutions are not known to cause electrolyte imbalance because they are neither significantly absorbed nor do they exert osmotic effect. WBI may be considered for toxic ingestions of sustained-release or enteric-coated medications. It may also be helpful in ingestions of large amounts of iron, or packets of illicit drugs. The most important contraindication to WBI is airway compromise. Although whole bowel irrigation may be helpful for those who have ingested heavy metals or long-acting or sustained-release medications, there are few clinical trials about the effectiveness of this procedure in children.

American Academy of Clinical Toxicology, European Association of Poisons Centres and Clinical Toxicologists: Position statement: whole bowel irrigation, *J Toxicol Clin Toxicol* 42:843–854, 2004.

111. **How is the manipulation of urinary pH used in treating poisonings?**
Acidification or *alkalinization* of the urine to enhance the excretion of weak acids and bases has been a traditional way to enhance the elimination of toxicologic agents. In recent years, its use has been limited because of the potential complications from fluid overload (e.g., pulmonary and cerebral edema), the risk for acidemia, and the use of other therapeutic advancements (e.g., hemodialysis). However, alkaline diuresis is still considered valuable in the management of acute overdoses of salicylates, barbiturates, or tricyclic antidepressants.

112. **What ingestions and exposures have available antidotes?**
See Table 5-5.

Table 5-5. Antidotes

INGESTION OR EXPOSURE	ANTIDOTE
Acetaminophen	N-acetylcysteine (Mucomyst)
Anticholinergics	Physostigmine
Benzodiazepines	Flumazenil
β-Blockers	Glucagon
Carbon monoxide	Hyperbaric oxygen chamber
Calcium channel blocker	Calcium, glucagon
Cyanide	Sodium nitrite, sodium thiosulfate
Digoxin	Digibind (antidigoxin antibody)
Ethylene glycol	Ethanol, fomepizole
Iron	Deferoxamine
Isoniazid	Pyridoxine (vitamin B_6)
Lead	EDTA, DMSA
Mercury	Dimercaprol, DMSA
Methanol	Ethanol
Methemoglobinemic agents	Methylene blue
Opiates	Naloxone, nalmefene
Organophosphates	Atropine, pralidoxime
Phenothiazines (dystonic reaction)	Diphenhydramine
Tricyclics	Bicarbonate
Warfarin (rat poison)	Vitamin K

DMSA = Dimercaptosuccinic acid; EDTA = Ethylenediaminetetraacetic acid.

113. For which kinds of ingestions is naloxone considered an antidote?

Naloxone (Narcan) is an antidote for opioid drugs. It reverses the CNS and respiratory depression of morphine and heroin and clears the depressed sensorium in overdoses due to many of the synthetic opioids, including propoxyphene, codeine, dextromethorphan, pentazocine, and meperidine. It is also a known antidote for clonidine.

114. Which ingestions are radiopaque on abdominal radiograph?

The mnemonic **CHIPS** indicates possible suspects.

- **C**hloral hydrate
- **H**eavy metals (arsenic, iron, lead)
- **I**odides
- **P**henothiazines, psychotropics (cyclic antidepressants)
- **S**low-release capsules, enteric-coated tablets

The likelihood of radiopacity depends on numerous factors, including weight of the patient, size of the ingestion, and composition of the pill matrix.

Barkin RM, Kulig KW, Rumack BH: Poisoning and overdose. In Barkin RM, Rosen P, editors: *Emergency Pediatrics*, ed 4. St. Louis, 1994, Mosby, p 335.

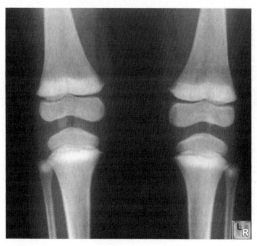

Figure 5-6. Long-bone radiograph of both knees of a child with lead poisoning showing dense metaphyseal bands involving the distal femurs, proximal tibias, and proximal fibulas. *(From Dapul H, Laraque D: Lead poisoning in children, Adv Pediatr 61:313–333, 2014.)*

115. What causes the radiographic "lead lines" of chronic lead poisoning?

Lead lines are transverse metaphyseal bands most prominent at the end of longer tubular bones which are seen in the later stages of chronic lead exposure (see Fig. 5-6). They represent **increased calcium** (not lead) **deposits.** Excessive lead interferes with bone metabolism and disrupts the resorption of primary spongiosa bone by disproportionately disrupting osteoclasts, which are involved in bone disassembling, compared with osteoblasts, which participate in calcium deposition. As a result of lead toxicity and relative increased osteoblastic activity, there is an exuberant calcium deposition that results in the dense metaphyseal bands corresponding to the zone of provisional calcification.

Raber SA: The dense metaphyseal band sign, *Radiology* 211:773–774, 1999.

116. What is a toxidrome?

A *toxidrome*, short for a toxic syndrome, is a clinical constellation of signs and symptoms that is very suggestive of a particular poisoning or category of intoxication. For example, patients with salicylate overdose commonly present with fever, hyperpnea and tachypnea, abnormal mental status (ranging from lethargy to coma), tinnitus, vomiting, and sometimes oil of wintergreen odor from methyl salicylate.

Koren G: A primer of paediatric toxic syndromes or "toxidromes", *Paediatr Child Health* 12:457–459, 2007.

117. **What is the toxidrome for anticholinergics?**
The classic description of anticholinergic toxicity is "mad as a hatter, fast as a hare, red as a beet, dry as a bone, blind as a bat, full as a tick, hot as Hades."
- The hatter: delirium, visual hallucinations
- The hare: tachycardia, hypertension
- The beet: flushed skin, facial flushing
- The bone: dry skin, dry mucous membranes
- The bat: dilated, sluggish pupils
- The tick: urinary retention, decreased GI motility, and hypoactive bowel sounds
- Hades: hyperpyrexia, inability to sweat

118. **What breath odors may be associated with specific ingestions?**
See Table 5-6.

Woolf AD: Poisoning in children and adolescents, *Pediatr Rev* 14:411–422, 1993.

Table 5-6. Breath Odors Associated with Specific Ingestions

CHARACTERISTIC ODOR	RESPONSIBLE TOXIN OR DRUG
Wintergreen	Methyl salicylate
Bitter almond	Cyanide
Carrots	Cicutoxin (of water hemlock)
Fruity	Ethanol, acetone (nail polish remover), isopropyl alcohol, chloroform
Fishy	Zinc or aluminum phosphide
Garlic	Organophosphate insecticide, arsenic, thallium
Glue	Toluene
Minty	Mouthwash, rubbing alcohol
Mothballs	Naphthalene, *p*-dichlorobenzene, camphor
Peanuts	Vacor rat poison (odor is from a flavoring agent)
Rotten eggs	Hydrogen sulfide, *N*-acetylcysteine, disulfiram
Rope (burned)	Marijuana, opium
Shoe polish	Nitrobenzene

119. **What are the limitations of the routine toxicology screen?**
Most toxicology screens are intended to detect drugs encountered in substance abuse. Even in larger pediatric hospitals, comprehensive toxicology screens generally include only a fraction of drugs available to children. Most blood screens analyze for acetaminophen, salicylates, and alcohols. Urine is often screened for substances of abuse and other common psychoactive drugs, including antidepressants, antipsychotics, benzodiazepines, sedative-hypnotics, and anticonvulsants. Other potential toxins that can cause mental status changes (carbon monoxide, chloral hydrate, cyanide, organophosphates) or circulatory depression (β-blockers, calcium channel blockers, clonidine, digitalis) may not be included but may be assayed through individual blood tests.

In clinical studies, toxicology screens are most valuable in quantitative settings (i.e., assessing drug levels). Additionally, treatment of the acutely poisoned patient must begin long before the results of many toxicology screens are available.

Archer JRH, Wood DM, Bargan PI: How to use toxicology screening tests, *Arch Dis Child Educ Pract Ed* 97, 194–199, 2012.
Moeller KE, Lee KC, Kissack JC: Urine drug screening: practical guide for clinicians, *Mayo Clin Proc* 83:66–76, 2008.

120. **After use of marijuana, how long does a urine screen remain positive?**
    After first-time single use, the drug screen can be positive for 3 days. A long-term heavy marijuana user can have a positive drug test that may persist 30 days or more after cessation. Two cautions: nonsteroidal medications, including ibuprofen and proton pump inhibitors, have been reported to cross-react with cannabinoid immunoassays. False-negative results can occur if a wise teen adds Visine to a urine specimen. The chemicals in Visine directly lower the concentrations of the cannabinoids in the urine.

Moeller KE, Lee KC, Kissack JC: Urine drug screening: practical guide for clinicians, *Mayo Clin Proc* 83:66–76, 2008.

121. **How do the types of alcohol ingestions vary?**
    All alcohols can cause CNS disturbances ranging from mild mentation and motor abnormalities to respiratory depression and coma. Each alcohol is associated with specific metabolic complications.
    - **Ethanol** (present in beverages, colognes and perfumes, aftershave lotion, mouthwash, topical antiseptic, rubbing alcohol) in infants and toddlers can cause the classic triad of coma, hypothermia, and hypoglycemia, and in adolescents, can cause intoxication and mild neurologic findings. At levels higher than 500 mg/dL, it can be lethal.
    - **Methanol** (present in antifreeze and windshield washer fluid) can cause severe, refractory metabolic acidosis and permanent retinal damage leading to blindness.
    - **Isopropyl alcohol** (present in jewelry cleaners, rubbing alcohol, windshield deicers, cements, paint removers) can cause gastritis, abdominal pain, vomiting, hematemesis, and CNS depression, moderate hyperglycemia, hypotension, and acetonemia without acidosis.
    - **Ethylene glycol** (present in antifreeze, brake fluid) causes severe metabolic acidosis. In addition, it is metabolized to oxalic acid, which can cause renal damage by the precipitation of calcium oxalate crystals in the renal parenchyma and can lead to hypocalcemia.

122. **Which alcohol is considered the most lethal?**
    Methanol. Deaths can arise from doses as little as 4 mL of pure methanol. Unique to methanol is that it becomes more toxic as it is metabolized. Methanol is broken down by alcohol dehydrogenase to formaldehyde and formic acid. It is the formic acid that causes the refractory metabolic acidosis and ocular symptoms.

123. **What is the treatment for methanol and ethylene glycol ingestions?**
    Both methanol and ethylene glycol require the enzyme alcohol dehydrogenase to create their toxic metabolites. Ethanol competitively inhibits the formation of these metabolites by serving as a substrate for the enzyme. However, it is inebriating, may cause hypoglycemia, and its kinetics are widely variable. Fomepizole is a safer and more effective blocker of alcohol dehydrogenase.

Brent J: Fomepizole for ethylene glycol and methanol poisoning, *N Engl J Med* 360:2216–2223, 2009.

124. **What is "MUDPILES"?**
    MUDPILES is a mnemonic for ingestions associated with a *high anion gap metabolic acidosis*.
    - **M**ethanol, metformin
    - **U**remia
    - **D**iabetic ketoacidosis
    - **P**araldehyde
    - **I**soniazid, iron, inborn errors of metabolism
    - **L**actic acidosis (seen with shock, CO, cyanide)
    - **E**thanol, ethylene glycol
    - **S**alicylates

125. How can pupillary findings assist in the diagnosis of toxic ingestions?
    - **Miosis** (pinpoint pupils): Narcotics, organophosphates, phencyclidine, clonidine, phenothiazines, barbiturates, ethanol
    - **Mydriasis** (dilated pupils): Anticholinergics (atropine, antihistamines, cyclic antidepressants); sympathomimetics (amphetamines, caffeine, cocaine, LSD, nicotine)
    - **Nystagmus:** Barbiturates, ketamine, phencyclidine, phenytoin

126. If a child has ingested an acetaminophen-containing product, when should the first acetaminophen level be obtained?
    A plasma level obtained **4 hours** after ingestion is a good indicator of the potential for hepatic toxicity. Nomograms are available for determining risk. As a rule, doses under 150 mg/kg are unlikely to be harmful.

127. When should a "NAC attack" begin?
    N-acetylcysteine (*NAC*) is a specific antidote for acetaminophen hepatotoxicity by serving as a glutathione substitute in detoxifying the hepatotoxic metabolites. It should be used for any acetaminophen overdose with a toxic serum acetaminophen level within the first 24 hours after ingestion. It is especially effective if used in the first 8 hours after ingestion. If acetaminophen levels are not available on a rapid basis or the time since ingestion is not clear, it is preferable to initiate NAC.

128. How does NAC prevent hepatotoxicity in acetaminophen overdose?
    Normally, 94% of acetaminophen is metabolized to glucuronide or sulfate form, and 2% is excreted unchanged in urine, both of which are nontoxic. The remaining 4% is conjugated with glutathione (with the help of cytochrome P-450) to form mercaptopuric acid, which is also not hepatotoxic. When a significant acetaminophen overdose occurs, cytochrome P-450 becomes the major system for metabolizing the acetaminophen, leading to depletion of hepatic stores of glutathione. When the glutathione is depleted to less than 70% of normal, a highly reactive intermediate metabolite binds to hepatic macromolecules, causing hepatocellular necrosis. It is presumed that NAC replenishes the glutathione, thus helping the cytochrome P-450 in converting the excess acetaminophen into mercaptopuric acid.

Heard KJ: Acetylcysteine for acetaminophen poisoning, *N Engl J Med* 359:285–292, 2008.

129. What arterial blood gas pattern is classic for salicylate poisoning?
    Metabolic acidosis and **respiratory alkalosis.** Salicylates directly stimulate the medullary respiratory drive center, causing tachypnea with diminished P_{CO_2} (respiratory alkalosis). They also cause lactic acidosis and ketoacidosis by inhibiting Krebs cycle enzymes, uncoupling oxidation phosphorylation, and inhibiting amino acid metabolism (metabolic acidosis).

130. What are hidden salicylates?
    These are salicylates that are found in over-the-counter products, such as Pepto-Bismol (bismuth salicylate). Salicylate absorption can be substantial, and in the setting of influenza or chickenpox, Pepto-Bismol use has been discouraged because of the potential for complications such as the development of Reye syndrome.

Szap MD: Hidden salicylates, *Am J Dis Child* 143:142, 1989.

131. What are the classic ECG findings associated with tricyclic antidepressants?
    Tricyclic antidepressants interfere with myocardial conduction and can precipitate ventricular tachycardias or complete heart block. A QRS interval >0.1 second is predictive of poor outcome in these patients. The presence of a large R wave in lead aVR is also associated with tricyclic antidepressants. If these findings are noted, treatment with sodium bicarbonate should be initiated. Sodium bicarbonate helps prevent the sodium channel blockade that is caused by these medications. Of note, diphenhydramine (Benadryl), if ingested in high doses, can mimic the ECG findings of tricyclic antidepressants.

132. **Which clinical and laboratory features correlate with an acutely elevated serum iron?**

Serum iron levels obtained 4 to 6 hours after ingestion correlate with severity of toxicity. Iron levels >300 µg/dL are associated with mild toxicity consisting of local GI symptoms, such as nausea, vomiting, and diarrhea. A serum iron level of 500 µg/dL is associated with serious systemic toxicity, and a level of 1000 µg/dL is associated with death. Other laboratory tests that correlate with an elevated iron level include leukocytosis (>15,000/mm^3) and hyperglycemia (>150 mg/dL). Sometimes, radiopaque tablets may be demonstrated on abdominal radiograph.

133. **What are the four clinical stages of iron toxicity and the correlating pathophysiology?**

- **Stage 1** (0.5 to 6 hours): During this stage, iron exhibits a direct corrosive effect on the small bowel. Symptoms include nausea, vomiting, abdominal pain, and/or GI hemorrhage.
- **Stage 2** (6 to 24 hours): Iron silently accumulates in the mitochondria; the patient is relatively symptom free.
- **Stage 3** (4 to 40 hours): This phase is characterized by systemic toxicity with shock, metabolic acidosis, depressed cardiac function, and hepatic necrosis.
- **Stage 4** (2 to 8 weeks): During this phase, pyloric stenosis and obstruction can develop as a result of earlier local bowel irritation.

134. **Which is more toxic, drinking dishwashing detergent or toilet bowl cleaner?**

You are better off with the *toilet bowl cleaner*, although both acid (toilet bowl cleaner) and alkali (dishwashing detergent) ingestions may cause severe esophageal burns. Alkalis cause injury by liquefaction necrosis, dissolving proteins and lipids, thereby allowing deeper penetration of the caustic substance and greater local tissue injury. With acids, coagulation necrosis of the tissue occurs. This results in the formation of an eschar that limits the penetration of the toxin into deeper tissues. Compared with acids, alkalis are more typically in solid and paste form, which increases tissue contact time and tissue injury.

135. **Which hydrocarbons pose the greatest risk for chemical pneumonitis?**

The household hydrocarbons with *low viscosities* pose the greatest aspiration hazard. These include furniture polishes, gasoline and kerosene, turpentine and other paint thinners, and lighter fuels.

136. **What is the differential diagnosis in a child who presents with confusion and lethargy?**

An altered state or level of consciousness can be due to many causes. The mnemonic **AEIOU TIPS** encompasses the many possible causes:

- **A**lcohol, abuse of substances
- **E**pilepsy, encephalopathy, electrolyte abnormalities, endocrine
- **I**nsulin, intussusception
- **O**verdose, oxygen deficiency
- **U**remia
- **T**rauma, temperature abnormality, tumor
- **I**nfection
- **P**oisoning, psychiatric conditions
- **S**hock, stroke, space-occupying lesion (intracranial)

Avner JR: Altered states of consciousness, *Pediatr Rev* 27:331–337, 2006.

137. **A patient receiving an antiemetic drug (e.g., promethazine) who develops involuntary, prolonged, twisting, writhing movements of the neck, trunk, and arms likely has what condition?**

Acute dystonia. This dystonic reaction is classically seen as an adverse side effect of antidopaminergic agents such as neuroleptics, antiemetics, or metoclopramide. In children, phenothiazines are the most common culprit. Treatment includes administration of diphenhydramine (Benadryl). Benztropine (Cogentin) is also used in adolescents.

138. **What do "SLUDGE" and "DUMBELS" have in common?**

Both are mnemonics used to remember the problems involved with *organophosphate poisoning*, lipid-soluble insecticides used in agriculture and terrorism ("nerve gas"). Organophosphates inhibit cholinesterase and cause all the signs and symptoms of acetylcholine excess.

- *Muscarinic effects* are increased oral and tracheal secretions, miosis, salivation, lacrimation, urination, vomiting, cramping, defecation, and bradycardia; may progress to frank pulmonary edema.
- *CNS effects* are agitation, delirium, seizures, and/or coma.
- *Nicotinic effects:* Sweating; muscle fasciculation; and ultimately, paralysis
- The mnemonic **SLUDGE** is **s**alivation, **l**acrimation, **u**rination, **d**efecation, **G**I cramps, and **e**mesis.
- The mnemonic **DUMBELS** is **d**efecation, **u**rination, **m**iosis, **b**ronchorrhea/bradycardia, **e**mesis, **l**acrimation, and **s**alivation.

139. **What metal intoxication can mimic Kawasaki disease?**

Mercury. *Acrodynia* is the term applied to one form of mercury salt intoxication that results in a constellation of signs and symptoms very similar to that currently recognized as Kawasaki disease. The classic presentation of acrodynia was described in children exposed to calomel, a substance used in teething powders, which was essentially mercurous chloride. The symptom complex included swelling and redness of the hands and feet, skin rashes, diaphoresis, tachycardia, hypertension, photophobia, and an intense irritability with anorexia and insomnia. Infants were often very limp, lying in a froglike position, with impressive weakness of the hip and shoulder girdle muscles. Similar symptoms have been described in children exposed to other forms of mercury, including broken fluorescent light bulbs or diapers rinsed in mercuric chloride.

140. **Why is cyanide so toxic?**

Cyanide ion binds to the heme-containing cytochrome as enzyme in the electron transport chain of mitochondria, which is the final common pathway in oxidative metabolism. Thus, with a significant exposure, virtually every cell in the body becomes starved of oxygen at the mitochondrial level and is unable to function. The body does have minor routes of cyanide detoxification, including excretion by the lungs and liver through rhodanese, a hepatic enzyme that combines cyanide with thiosulfate to form the less toxic thiocyanate for renal excretion. However, these mechanisms are inadequate in the face of a significant cyanide exposure. As with carbon monoxide poisoning, symptoms tend to be most prominent among the metabolically active organ systems. In particular, the CNS is rapidly affected, causing headache and dizziness, which may progress to prostration, convulsions, coma, and death. Less severe ingestions may be noted initially by burning of the tongue and mucous membranes, with tachypnea and dyspnea due to cyanide stimulation of chemoreceptors.

141. **In what settings should cyanide poisoning be suspected?**

- **Suicidal ingestion,** often involving chemists who have access to cyanide salts as reagents
- **Fires** causing combustion of materials such as wool, silk, synthetic rubber, polyurethane, and nitrocellulose, resulting in the release of cyanide
- Patients who are on **nitroprusside continuous infusion,** an antihypertensive agent that contains five cyanide moieties per molecule

142. **What kinds of plants account for the greatest percentage of deaths due to plant poisonings?**

Mushrooms account for at least 50% of deaths due to plant poisoning. The most dreaded variety is the *Amanita* species, which initially causes intestinal symptoms by one toxin (phallotoxin) and then hepatic and renal failure by a separate toxin (amatoxin). Other mushroom classes can cause a variety of early-onset (<6 hours) symptoms, including muscarinic effects (e.g., sweating, salivation, colic), anticholinergic effects (e.g., drowsiness, mania, hallucinations), gastroenteritis, and Antabuse-type effects if taken with alcohol.

143. **Is mistletoe toxic?**

Mistletoe, the popular Christmas plant, is an evergreen with small white berries. Ingestion of small amounts of the berries, leaves, or stems may result in GI symptoms, including pain, nausea, vomiting, and diarrhea. Rarely, large ingestions have resulted in seizures, hypertension, and even cardiac arrest. In some countries, extracts of mistletoe have been used for illegal abortifacients, brewed in teas that are particularly toxic. In the United States, the typical call to a poison center concerns a child who eats one or two mistletoe berries, which in general is unlikely to produce significant signs or symptoms.

144. **Should swallowed disc batteries be removed?**
Although the concern is that a disc battery may produce corrosive intestinal injury, most traverse the GI tract without incident. An initial radiograph for localization is indicated. If the disc battery is in the esophagus, removal is required. Otherwise, if the battery is in the stomach or beyond and the patient remains asymptomatic, watchful waiting is appropriate with follow-up imaging if the battery is not seen in the stool.

Litovitz T, Whitaker N, Clark L, et al: Emerging battery-ingestion hazard: clinical implications, *Pediatrics* 125:1168–1177, 2010.

145. **What are the available methods used to remove a foreign body from the esophagus?**
Three methods are used; local custom prevails regarding selection.
- **Esophagoscopy,** the most commonly used method, is done under general anesthesia.
- A **Foley catheter** can be inserted beyond the foreign body, inflated, and then pulled back to remove the object. This extraction method is used by various centers, particularly for coins if the ingestion is less than 24 hours old and no respiratory distress is present. Complications, such as airway obstruction by a displaced coin and esophageal perforation, are possible.
- In **bougienage,** the object is forced into the stomach.

146. **What recreational drug is most frequently associated with rave parties?**
Rave parties are large parties or festivals featuring live performances of electronic dance music, laser light shows, projected images, visual effects, and smoke machines. A number of drugs are associated with these events, including LSD and ketamine, but the drug that is most associated with rave parties is **MDMA** (popularly known as **ecstasy** or **Molly**), a psychoactive drug that has similarities to both the stimulant amphetamine and the hallucinogen mescaline.

147. **Why is ecstasy considered so dangerous?**
Ecstasy is rarely sold as pure ecstasy and often includes other drugs that the user may not be aware of; therefore, its effects are not predictable. The pure form (known as Molly for "molecular") can cause tachycardia, dry mouth, teeth grinding, and clenched jaw. Severe adverse reactions to the drug include pronounced hyperthermia, seizures, hypertensive crises, dysrhythmias, metabolic disturbances, DIC, rhabdomyolysis, acute kidney disease, liver toxicity, and stroke. It has also been known to be fatal in some cases. Care is supportive and usually involves some form of cooling.

KEY POINTS: TOXICOLOGY

1. Ipecac is no longer recommended for poisoning.
2. Activated charcoal is most efficacious if given within 1 hour of ingestion.
3. Gastric lavage has unproven efficacy for most ingestions.
4. Whole bowel irrigation is indicated for sustained-release or enteric-coated substances.
5. Alkalinization of urine is still considered valuable in the management of acute overdoses of salicylates, barbiturates, or tricyclic antidepressants.

TRAUMA

148. **What are the major signs of a blowout fracture?**
Traumatic force to the eye can result in a blowout fracture affecting either the orbital floor or the medial wall (Fig 5-7). The fracture may result from a sudden increase in intraorbital pressure or from a direct concussive force to the bony walls. Symptoms and signs can include the following:
- Pain and/or diplopia with upward gaze
- Compromised upward gaze on the affected side as a result of entrapment of the inferior rectus muscle
- Enophthalmos (i.e., posterior displacement of the globe of the eye)
- Loss of sensation over the upper lip and gums on the injured side
- Crepitus and tenderness over the inferior orbital ridge

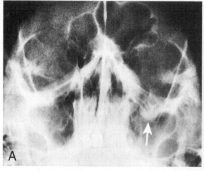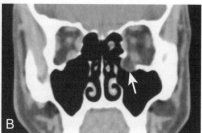

Figure 5-7. Waters view (**A**) shows polypoid soft-tissue mass in the roof of the left antrum *(arrow)*, which was a blowout fracture of the orbital floor. Coronal CT scan (**B**) shows the herniated soft tissues *(arrow)* of the blowout fracture. *(From Som PM, Curtin HD, editors:* Head and Neck Imaging, *ed 5. Philadelphia, 2011, Mosby, p. 513.)*

149. **When evaluating a patient with an eye injury, when should you suspect a ruptured globe and how should you handle it?**
Globe rupture denotes a full-thickness laceration of the cornea and/or sclera. This is an ophthalmologic emergency and must be recognized immediately. The hallmark clinical features include:
    * Tear drop pupil
    * 360-degree subconjunctival hemorrhage
    * Enophthalmos
    If globe rupture is suspected, an ophthalmologist should be emergently consulted and the acronym **SANTAS** should be followed:
    * **Shield** should be placed over the eye to protect from further damage.
    * **Antiemetics** should be given to protect against increased pressure.
    * **NPO** (nothing per oral, or by mouth) to prepare for surgery.
    * **Tetanus** shot should be given.
    * **Analgesics**, either parenteral or oral (avoid topical), should be administered.
    * **Sedation**, if not contraindicated by other injuries, should be given.

Levin AV: Eye trauma. In Fleischer GR, Ludwig S, editors. *Textbook of Pediatric Emergency Medicine*, ed 6. Philadelphia, 2010, Wolters Kluwer, pp 1448–1453.
Rahman WM, O'Connor TJ: Facial trauma. In Barkin RM, Caputo GL, editors: *Pediatric Emergency Medicine, Concepts and Clinical Practice*. St. Louis, 1997, Mosby, pp 252–253.

150. **When should an avulsed tooth be reimplanted?**
Avulsion is the complete displacement of the tooth from its socket. Primary teeth (i.e., baby teeth) should not be reimplanted because nerve root damage or dental ankylosis may result. Secondary teeth should be repaired as soon as possible to maximize the chance of tooth viability. An avulsed tooth may be stored in cold milk, saline, or placed under a cooperative patient's tongue and should be reimplanted as quickly as possible.

Bernius M, Perlin D: Pediatric ear, nose and throat emergencies, *Pediatr Clin North Am* 55:209–210, 2006.

151. **What are the three most important considerations when evaluating nasal trauma?**
    * **Bleeding:** If persistent, bleeding should be controlled with pressure, ice, topical vasoconstrictors, cauterization, and anterior or posterior nasal packing.
    * **Septal hematoma:** If the nasal septum is bulging into the nasal cavity, there is likely a hematoma that must be drained. If drainage is not performed, abscess formation or pressure necrosis can result and lead to a saddle-nose deformity.
    * **Watery rhinorrhea:** This may be a sign of cribriform plate, suborbital ethmoid, sphenoid sinus, or frontal sinus fracture with cerebrospinal fluid leak.

152. How long can you wait before a broken nose in a child must be reduced?

    If a nasal bone fracture causes asymmetry (which is noted as the swelling from acute trauma subsides), the fracture should be reduced **within 4 to 5 days**; a longer delay may result in mal-union.

153. After a motor vehicle collision, an 8-year-old presents with right-sided pain, a heart rate of 150 beats per minute, a blood pressure of 110/80 mm Hg, and capillary refill time of 3.5 seconds. How should his initial fluid therapy be managed?

    It is important to recognize that this child is in shock, despite a normal blood pressure for age. For children in shock, changes in blood pressure are often late and precipitous. Findings of tachycardia, prolonged capillary refill, and diminished pulses are indicative of intravascular *hypovolemia* in this patient, requiring aggressive fluid resuscitation. Isotonic crystalloid (saline or lactated Ringer solution) should be given in boluses of 20 mL/kg over 5 to 10 minutes. If, after 40 mL/kg of crystalloid, hemodynamic measures have not improved or have worsened, blood products should be given in 10 mL/kg boluses.

154. What are the signs and symptoms of a tension pneumothorax?

    A *tension pneumothorax* presents with hypotension, respiratory distress, diminished breath sounds on the affected side, and tracheal deviation. Treatment begins with emergent needle decompression in the second intercostal space at the midclavicular line followed by chest tube placement.

155. Which children with acute minor blunt head trauma require emergency CT scans?

    The largest prospective study of children younger than 18 years (>42,000 patients) with head trauma was designed to determine which patients are at very low risk for clinically important traumatic brain injury for whom CT is unnecessary. Derived prediction rules were developed based on age. Negative predictive values (i.e., the likelihood of something not being present, in this case significant brain injury) were 100% for the younger group and 99.95% for the older group (and thus CT was thought to be unnecessary) if the following characteristics were seen on evaluation:

    - **Younger than 2 years:** Normal mental status, no scalp hematoma except frontal, no loss of consciousness or loss of consciousness for less than 5 seconds, nonsevere injury mechanism (e.g., fall of less than 3 feet, motor vehicle collision without patient ejection or death of another passenger, no head injury by high-impact object), no palpable skull fracture, acting normally according to parents
    - **Aged 2 years and older:** Normal mental status, no loss of consciousness, no vomiting, nonsevere injury mechanism, no signs of basilar skull fracture, no severe headache

Kuppermann N, Holmes JF, Dayan PS, et al: Identification of children at very low risk of clinically important brain injuries after head trauma: a prospective cohort study, *Lancet* 374:1160–1170, 2009.

156. What is the risk associated with CT scans in children?

    The ionizing radiation of CT scans may be implicated as the cause of lethal malignancies. Using data from the cancer rates after the atomic bomb blasts in Japan in World War II and comparing that degree of radiation and sequelae with CT radiation, it is estimated that the potential rate of lethal malignancies from pediatric cranial CT may be between 1/1000 and 1/1500. This highlights the need to obtain CT studies with appropriate clinical indications and to limit the amount of radiation to be as low as possible during the procedure.

Brenner DJ, Hall EJ: Computed tomography—an increasing source of radiation exposure, *N Engl J Med* 35: 2277–2284, 2007.

157. When intracranial pressure is acutely elevated, how long is it before papilledema develops?

    Generally, 24 to 48 hours may pass before papilledema develops.

158. What are the components of the Glasgow Coma Scale (GCS)?

    Developed in 1974 by the neurosurgical department at the University of Glasgow, the scale was an attempt to standardize the assessment of the depth and duration of impaired consciousness and coma, particularly in the setting of trauma. The scale is based on eye opening, verbal responses, and motor responses, with a total score that ranges from 3 to 15 (Table 5-7).

Table 5-7. Glasgow Coma Scale

Best Verbal Response*
5 Oriented, appropriate conversation
4 Confused conversation
3 Inappropriate words
2 Incomprehensible sounds
1 No response

Best Motor Response to Command or to Pain (e.g., rubbing knuckles on sternum)
6 Obeys a verbal command
5 Localizes
4 Withdraws
3 Abnormal flexion (decorticate posturing)
2 Abnormal extension (decerebrate posturing)
1 No response

Eye Opening
4 Spontaneous
3 In response to verbal command
2 In response to pain
1 No response

*Children <2 years old should receive full verbal scores for crying after stimulation.

---

159. **How does the location of cervical spine fractures vary between younger children and older children and adults?**
Younger children tend to have fractures of the upper cervical spine, whereas older children and adults have fractures more often involving the lower cervical spine, for the following reasons:
- Changing fulcrum of the spine: In an infant, the fulcrum of the cervical spine is at approximately C2-C3; in a child who is 5 to 6 years old, the fulcrum is at C3-C4; from 8 to adulthood, it is at C5-C6. These changes are in large part the result of the relatively large head size of a child compared with that of an adult.
- Younger children have relatively weak neck muscles.
- Younger children have poorer protective reflexes.

Woodward GA: Neck trauma. In Fleisher GR, Ludwig S, editors: *Textbook of Pediatric Emergency Medicine*, ed 6. Philadelphia, 2010, Wolters Kluwer, pp 1379–1380.

160. **What is SCIWORA?**
SCIWORA stands for Spinal Cord Injury Without Radiographic Abnormality. SCIWORA is most commonly seen in children >8 years of age. These patients have signs and symptoms that are consistent with spinal cord injury, but radiographic and CT studies reveal no bony abnormalities. It is postulated that the highly malleable pediatric spine allows the cord to sustain injury from flexion-extension forces without causing bony disruption. MRI often reveals spinal cord injury in these cases. The initial neurologic complaints of these children should be taken seriously because onset of SCIWORA can be delayed up to 4 days. Even with normal radiographs, a patient with an altered sensorium or with neurologic abnormalities that are consistent with cervical cord injury (e.g., motor or sensory changes, bowel and bladder problems, vital sign instability) requires continued neck immobilization and more extensive evaluation.

161. Are single lateral cervical spine radiographs sufficient to "clear" a patient after neck injury?

No. In some studies, the sensitivity of a single view for fractures is only 80%. The American College of Radiology guidelines recommend at least three views: (1) anteroposterior (including the C7-T1 junction, C1-C7), (2) lateral, and (3) open mouth (odontoid). The last view is often difficult to obtain in younger children. CT and MRI are reserved for more extensive evaluation for spinal cord injury when the initial three views are negative in symptomatic patients. The use of oblique films is controversial.

Hutchings L: Clearing the cervical spine in children, *Trauma* 13:340–352, 2011.
Eubanks JD, Gilmore A, Bess S, et al: Clearing the pediatric cervical spine following injury, *J Am Acad Orthop Surg* 14:552–564, 2006.

162. Why is left shoulder pain after abdominal trauma a worrisome sign?

This may represent blood accumulating under the diaphragm, resulting in pain referred to the left shoulder (Kehr sign). The sign can be elicited by left upper quadrant palpation or by placing the patient in the Trendelenburg position. The finding is worrisome because it suggests possible solid organ abdominal injury—most commonly splenic injury—and requires surgical consultation and radiographic studies (usually CT or ultrasound) to grade the extent of injury.

Lee J, Moriarty KP, Tashjian DB: Less is more: management of pediatric splenic injury. *Arch Surg* 147:437–441, 2012.

163. A 5-year-old child has ecchymosis of the lower abdomen after a motor vehicle collision. What should you immediately suspect?

This child's injuries should immediately key you in to the possibility of a **lap-belt injury**. In children who are either too young (<8 years old) or too small, the lap belt of a car rests abnormally high on the child's body and, instead of crossing the lap at the hips, crosses the lap at the lower abdomen. The most common injuries to suspect are lumbar spine injuries, particularly a flexion disruption (Chance) fracture and bowel or bladder perforations or disruptions.

Santschi M, Echave V, Laflamme S, et al: Seat-belt in children involved in motor vehicle crashes, *Can J Surg* 48:373–376, 2005.

164. In a 7-year-old boy with a radiographically proven pelvic fracture, what diagnostic procedure should be done?

The urethra, as it passes through the prostate, is very close to the pubic bone and is thus susceptible to injury from a pelvic fracture. Urethral damage should be suspected in all patients with pelvic fractures, even those without hematuria. The recommended diagnostic procedure is a **retrograde urethrogram**.

165. In this same patient as in question 164, blood at the tip of the penis is noted. Why is catheterization contraindicated?

A boggy, high-riding prostate found on rectal examination and blood seen at the urethral meatus are clinical signs of **possible urethral disruption**; these two findings are contraindications for passing a Foley catheter. A partial urethral disruption could potentially be made into a complete one with the passing of the catheter.

166. What is the focus of the FAST examination?

FAST stands for *focused assessment with sonography in trauma*. It is used as a screen for abdominal and pericardial bleeding as blood appears black (hypoechoic) against the bright (hyperechoic) background of the internal organs. A FAST exam evaluates four principal areas for bleeding: the pericardial sac, the hepatorenal fossa (Morrison pouch), the splenorenal fossa, and the pelvis (pouch of Douglas). This noninvasive tool provides clinicians with rapid information about potentially life-threatening thoracic and abdominal injury. In victims of blunt abdominal trauma who are unstable, a positive FAST examination may be an indication that the patient needs urgent surgical intervention.

Levy JA, Bachur RG: Bedside ultrasound in the pediatric emergency department, *Curr Opin Pediatr* 20:235–242, 2008.

167. In children with blunt abdominal trauma, are there clinical findings that predict low risk of clinically important injury?

The PECARN research network prospectively enrolled 12,000 children following blunt abdominal trauma. If the following predictors were present, the rule correctly identified 99% of the children as low risk:

- No evidence of abdominal wall trauma or seat belt sign
- GCS score >13
- No abdominal tenderness
- No evidence of thoracic wall trauma
- No complaints of abdominal pain
- No decreased breath sounds
- No vomiting

Holmes JF, Lillis K, Monroe D, et al: Identifying children at very low risk of clinically important blunt abdominal injuries. *Ann Emerg Med* 62:107–116, 2013.

WOUND REPAIR

168. What advice should be given over the telephone regarding the transportation of an avulsed digit?

Wrap the severed piece in dry gauze (sterile, if possible). Place the wrapped piece in a small, sealed plastic bag to minimize its contact with water. Place this bag in a container filled with ice. It is incorrect to place the avulsed piece in any liquid because this causes tissue swelling. Direct contact with ice is to be avoided to prevent tissue necrosis.

169. Which lacerations should be referred to a surgeon or an ED physician who is familiar with wound repair?

- Large, complex lacerations
- Stellate or flap lacerations
- Lacerations with questions of tissue viability
- Lacerations involving lip margins (vermilion border)
- Deep lacerations with nerve or tendon damage
- Knife and gunshot wounds
- Strong concern about cosmetic outcome by either the patient or the family
- Lacerations involving open fractures or joint penetration
- Lacerations involving the inner eyelid, owing to the potential of damage to the tear ducts
- Deep lacerations involving the cheek, owing to potential damage to the parotid or facial nerve

170. How many days should sutures remain in place?

Blood supply dictates healing: the more blood, the better and the faster the healing. In general, as the site of laceration proceeds, from head to toe, the less blood supply there is and the greater the duration for suture placement: *eyelids*—3 days; *face, scalp*—5 days; *trunk, upper extremities*—7 to 10 days; and *lower extremities*—8 to 10 days.

171. When should a nerve injury be suspected in a finger laceration?

- **Abnormal testing of sensation** (diminished pain or two-point discrimination)
- **Abnormal autonomic function** (absence of sweat or lack of skin wrinkling after soaking in water)
- **Diminished range of motion of finger** (may also indicate joint, bone, or tendon disruption)
- **Pulsating blood emerging from the wound** (on the flexor aspect, the nerve is superficial to the digital artery, and arterial flow implies nerve damage)

172. What should be done if nerve damage is suspected?

For injuries to major nerves (e.g., the brachial plexus), immediate consultation is necessary. If the digital nerve is injured, immediate repair is not essential, and this is not a true emergency. Delayed nerve repair is very satisfactory, particularly in younger children. If an operating suite and personnel are not poised to proceed, skin closure can be done and the operation deferred (after surgical consultation). Care must be taken to avoid the use of a hemostat or clamp to stop arterial bleeding because this may cause further damage to the nerve. Simple pressure—often for extended periods—generally suffices.

173. **Which lacerations should not be sutured?**
Lacerations at high risk for infection should be considered for healing by secondary intention or delayed primary closure. As a general rule, these include cosmetically unimportant puncture wounds, human bites, lacerations involving mucosal surfaces (e.g., mouth, vagina), and wounds with a high probability of contamination (e.g., acquired in a garbage bin). Many authorities in the past recommended that wounds untreated for more than 6 to 12 hours on the arms and legs and for 12 to 24 hours on the face not be sutured. However, the type of wound and risk for infection are more important than any absolute time criterion. For example, a clean laceration of the face should be considered for suturing even 24 hours after the injury. A good rule of thumb is as follows: If you can irrigate and clean a wound to the point at which it looks "fresh," you are safe to close it primarily. Otherwise, you should let it heal by secondary intention.

KEY POINTS: LACERATIONS

1. The best defense against infection in the setting of wound closure is copious irrigation.
2. Irrigation can be painful and should be done *after* local anesthetic is applied or infiltrated.
3. Irrigation can be done with a number of different fluids, including sterile water, normal saline or tap water, but should not be done with betadine-containing fluids, which are abrasive to the tissue.
4. There is no one universal suture material that is good for all wounds. The material should be chosen based on location, size, and depth of the wound and the tensile strength that is required to easily appose the wound edges.
5. Suspect digital nerve injury if there is abnormal sensation, abnormal autonomic function, diminished range of motion of finger, or pulsating blood emerging from the wound.

---

174. **Which are at greater risk for infection, dog bites or cat bites?**
Generally, infection rates are higher in **cat bites** because of the greater likelihood of a puncture wound rather than a laceration injury. Additionally, *Pasteurella multocida*, which is the most common pathogen responsible for infection, is present in higher concentrations in cat bites. Wounds caused by cat and dog bites usually contain multiple other organisms, including *Staphylococcus aureus*; *Moraxella*, *Streptococcus*, and *Neisseria* species; and anaerobes.

Kannikeswaran N, Kamat D: Mammalian bites, *Clin Pediatr* 48:145–148, 2009.
Talon DA, Citron DM, Abrahamian FM, et al: Bacteriologic analysis of infected dog and cat bites, *N Engl J Med* 340:85–92, 1999.

175. **Should antibiotic prophylaxis be given for dog, cat, and human bites?**
This is a controversial topic. Although antibiotics are widely prescribed following mammalian bites, prophylactic antibiotics have been shown to significantly reduce infections in only two settings: bites to the hands and human bites. Some experts recommend treatment for other "high-risk" injuries such as cat bites, foot wounds, puncture wounds, wounds in immunocompromised patients, and wounds treated initially after 12 hours. It is important that all such wounds first be irrigated, cleaned, and débrided as necessary.

Singer AJ, Dagum AB: Current management of acute cutaneous wounds, *N Engl J Med* 359:1037–1046, 2008.

176. **Which animals most often carry the rabies virus?**
Although all species of animals are susceptible to rabies virus infection, only a few species are important as reservoirs for the disease. In the United States, rabies has been identified most commonly in **raccoons, skunks, foxes, coyotes,** and **bats**.

Center for Disease Control and Prevention Rabies Domestic Animal Surveillance: www.cdc.gov/rabies/location/usa/surveillance/domestic_animals.html. Accessed on Nov. 19, 2014.

177. Which are more likely to be rabid: cats or dogs?
During 2000 to 2004, more **cats** than dogs were reported rabid in the United States. This may be due to the facts that there are fewer cat vaccination laws, fewer leash laws with cats, and cats tend to roam more freely than dogs.

Center for Disease Control and Prevention Rabies Domestic Animals: www.cdc.gov/rabies/exposure/animals/domestic. html. Accessed Nov. 19, 2014.

178. If at a local petting zoo a playful 20-month-old child is bitten by a duck, scratched by a rabbit (breaking skin), spit on by a camel, and licked on the face by a horse, should rabies prophylaxis be given?
In general, no prophylaxis is needed for any of these animal wounds unless the animal is actively rabid. The local health department should be contacted if there is any question. Immediate rabies vaccination and rabies immune globulin are recommended for bites or scratches from bats, skunks, raccoons, foxes, and most other carnivores if these injuries break the skin. Bites from dogs and cats generally do not necessitate prophylaxis if the animal is healthy and can be observed closely for a 10-day period. No case in the United States has been attributed to a dog or cat that has remained healthy for the confinement period of 10 days.

American Academy of Pediatrics: Rabies. In Pickering LK, editor: *2012 Red Book*, ed 29. Elk Grove Village, IL, 2012, American Academy of Pediatrics, pp 600–607.

179. When is the use of lidocaine with epinephrine contraindicated as a local anesthetic?
Lidocaine with epinephrine is contraindicated when there is a question of tissue viability and in any instance in which vasoconstriction might produce ischemic injury to an end organ without an alternative blood supply (e.g., tip of the nose, margin of the ear, tip of the finger or toe).

180. What are methods for decreasing the pain of local lidocaine infiltration?
- Infiltration into the subcutaneous layer
- Infiltration at a slow rate
- Buffering the anesthetic (e.g., with bicarbonate; there is no magic formula, but one that works is 10 parts lidocaine and 1 part bicarbonate)
- Warming the anesthetic to body temperature
- Using a small-gauge needle (e.g., 30 gauge)
- Distraction techniques

181. What are some of the ingredients in the alphabet soup of topical anesthetics?
- **LET** (4% **l**idocaine, 0.1% **e**pinephrine, and 0.5% **t**etracaine)
- **TAC** (**t**etracaine, **a**drenaline, and **c**ocaine)
- **LMX** (4% and 5% lidocaine gel)
- **V-TAC** (**v**iscous TAC)
- **PLP** (**p**rilocaine, **l**idocaine, and **p**henylephrine)
- **EMLA** (**e**utectic **m**ixture of **l**ocal **a**nesthetics, typically lidocaine and prilocaine)
TAC was among the first of these to be developed, but its higher costs and safety concerns (as a result of the cocaine component) have resulted in others, particularly LET, replacing it as first-line therapy. The American Academy of Pediatrics recommends the use of topical anesthetics, such as LET, for simple lacerations of the head, neck, and extremities, or trunk <5 cm in length. Systemic toxicity can occur through excessive absorption of topical anesthetics; however, this can be minimized by avoiding mucosal membranes and large open wounds.

Zempsky WT: Pharmacologic approaches for reducing venous access pain in children, *Pediatrics* 122:S140–S153, 2008.

182. When should tissue adhesives be considered or avoided?
Consider tissue adhesives for the following:
- Wounds with good edge approximation and little wound tension
- Wounds that are clean and linear
- Wounds that ordinarily, if sutured, would require sutures 5-0 or smaller (i.e., wounds with little tension)

Avoid tissue adhesives for the following:
- Wounds where good edge approximation cannot be achieved (e.g., jagged wounds)
- Bite or puncture wounds
- Generally, wounds deeper than 5 mm
- Hands, feet, or joints, unless the affected area can be immobilized
- Oral mucosa or other mucosal surfaces, or areas with increased amounts of moisture as in the perineum or axilla
- Patients with conditions that may delay wound healing (e.g., diabetes mellitus or patients on long-term steroids)

183. **In which situations might you choose absorbable over nonabsorbable sutures when repairing a pediatric laceration?**
An absorbable suture is generally one that loses most of its tensile strength in 1 to 3 weeks and is fully absorbed within 3 months. Traditionally, absorbable sutures were used only for deep sutures. However, recently, the use of absorbable sutures for percutaneous closure of wounds in adults and children has been advocated. The advantages of absorbable sutures include the elimination of a follow-up visit to remove the patient's sutures and the possibility of decreased scarring and infection. Ideal wound candidates for absorbable sutures include the following:
- Facial lacerations, where skin heals quickly and prolonged intact sutures may lead to a suboptimal cosmetic result. (Fast absorbing sutures, which become absorbed in less than 1 week, are particularly good on facial wounds.)
- Percutaneous closure of lacerations under casts or splints
- Closure of lacerations of the tongue or oral mucosa
- Hand and finger lacerations
- Nail bed lacerations

184. **What is the proper fluid to use for wound irrigation?**
Normal saline, sterile water, or even tap water may be used. The key appears to be the flushing action, rather than the fluid. Some authors argue that for a number of reasons—availability, low cost, efficiency, and effectiveness—tap water should be strongly considered for wound cleansing in the ED. However, other cleansing solutions, antiseptics such as betadine and alcohol, remain controversial because of toxic effects on tissue and lack of significant clinical benefit.

Cooper DD, Seupaul RA: Is water effective for wound cleansing? *Ann Emerg Med* 60:626–627, 2012.

185. **How is conscious sedation best managed in children?**
There is no single best method for the conscious sedation of pediatric patients for diagnostic, radiologic, or minor surgical procedures. Surveys indicate that a wide variety of approaches are used in emergency rooms and radiology suites, including opioids (morphine, fentanyl), benzodiazepines (diazepam, midazolam), barbiturates (pentobarbital, thiopental), and nonbarbiturate anesthetic-analgesic agents (ketamine). Although conscious sedation, by definition, is a state of medically controlled depressed consciousness with a patent airway, maintained protective reflexes, and appropriate responses to stimulation on verbal command, the potential for rapidly developing problems should be anticipated. These can include hypoventilation, apnea, airway obstruction, and cardiorespiratory collapse. Consequently, pharmacologic agents used for conscious sedation should be administered under supervised conditions and in the presence of competent personnel who are capable of resuscitation, ongoing monitoring (especially pulse oximetry), and sufficient equipment for resuscitation (e.g., positive-pressure oxygen delivery system, suction apparatus). As a rule, few office settings are appropriate for conscious sedation.

Sury M: Conscious sedation in children. *Contin Educ Anaesth Crit Care Pain* 12:152–156, 2012.
Mandt MJ, Roback MG: Assessment and monitoring of pediatric procedural sedation, *Clin Pediatr Emerg Med* 8:223–231, 2007.

Acknowledgment

The editors gratefully acknowledge contributions by Drs. Jane Lavelle and Fred Henretig that were retained from previous editions of *Pediatric Secrets*.

CHAPTER 6

ENDOCRINOLOGY

*Mary Patricia Gallagher, MD, Marisa Censani, MD
and Sharon E. Oberfield, MD*

ADRENAL DISORDERS

1. What are the symptoms of adrenal insufficiency?
   - **Newborns:** Nonspecific findings of vomiting, irritability, and poor weight gain; may progress to cardiovascular shock
   - **Children:** Lethargy, easy fatigability, poor weight gain, and vague abdominal complaints; hyperpigmentation (primary insufficiency); symptoms of hypoglycemia (primary or secondary insufficiency); may also exhibit vascular collapse with intercurrent illness

2. What distinguishes primary and secondary adrenal insufficiency?
   - **Primary:** Abnormality of the adrenal gland, low cortisol accompanied by an elevated adrenocorticotropic hormone (ACTH) level; may also have mineralocorticoid deficiency
   - **Secondary:** Hypothalamic or pituitary dysfunction, low cortisol accompanied by an inappropriately normal or low ACTH level; normal mineralocorticoid production; often associated with multiple pituitary deficiencies

3. What is the differential diagnosis of primary adrenal insufficiency?
   - **Inherited enzymatic defects:** Congenital adrenal hyperplasia (multiple enzymatic defects are known), congenital adrenal hypoplasia
   - **Autoimmune disease:** Isolated, autoimmune polyendocrinopathy syndrome (APS) types 1 and 2; type 2 is also known as Schmidt syndrome
   - **Infectious disease:** Tuberculosis, meningococcemia, disseminated fungal infections
   - **Trauma:** Bilateral adrenal hemorrhage
   - **Adrenal hypoplasia:** Due to inherited defects in the adrenal ACTH receptors
   - **Iatrogenic:** Use of exogenous steroids

4. What are the most common causes of secondary adrenal insufficiency?
   Secondary causes can include failure of the hypothalamic and/or pituitary gland axis to develop in the embryonic stage or disruption of the axis as a result of tumor, central nervous system (CNS) trauma, irradiation, infection, or surgery. Prolonged treatment with exogenous glucocorticoids will also suppress the hypothalamic and pituitary parts of the axis.

5. What clinical clues suggest that adrenal insufficiency is a primary rather than a secondary problem?
   - **Primary adrenal insufficiency:** ACTH levels will rise as a result of disruption of the hormonal feedback loop, and these elevated levels often cause hyperpigmentation. Primary deficiency commonly leads to hyponatremia and hyperkalemia. This can present as salt craving or muscle cramping. Mild hypercalcemia may also be found.
   - **Secondary adrenal insufficiency:** ACTH levels are low; therefore, no hyperpigmentation occurs. Furthermore, in secondary insufficiency, function of the zona glomerulosa of the adrenal gland (responsible for aldosterone secretion) remains intact. Therefore, hyperkalemia and volume depletion are distinctly uncommon, but isolated hyponatremia may still occur as a result of decreased capacity to excrete a water load (dilutional hyponatremia). The most important clinical clues come from the history; that is, has the child been exposed to exogenous steroids, or is there a history of CNS insult? Additionally, are there deficiencies of other pituitary hormones?

6. What is the most common form of congenital adrenal hyperplasia (CAH)?
   CAH refers to a group of autosomal recessive disorders that result from various enzymatic defects in the biosynthesis of cortisol. Depending on the enzyme involved, the blockade can result in deficiencies and/or excesses in the other steroid pathways (i.e., mineralocorticoids and androgens). 21-Hydroxylase

deficiency accounts for more than 90% of cases; the complete (salt-losing, about two-thirds of cases) and partial (simple virilizing) forms occur in about 1 in 12,000 births and have an equal sex distribution. There are substantial differences in prevalence in various racial and ethnic groups. A late-onset or attenuated form (mild deficiency) manifests in adolescent girls with hirsutism and menstrual irregularities.

Zoltan A, Zhou P: Congenital adrenal hyperplasia: diagnosis, evaluation, management, *Pediatr Rev* 30:e49–e57, 2009.

7. **In newborns with CAH, why are girls likely to be diagnosed earlier than boys?**
The most common forms of CAH result in excess androgen production in the fetus; the effects of prenatal androgen excess on the development of the clitoris and labia majora can be easily identified in the newborn period. In boys, androgen excess does not cause any clearly abnormal appearance of the external genitalia. CAH should always be considered in the differential diagnosis of disorders of external sexual development, particularly in infants with a 46,XX karyotype.

8. **How do the major steroid preparations vary in potency?**
See Table 6-1.

Table 6-1. Potency of Common Steroid Preparations

NAME	RELATIVE GLUCOCORTICOID POTENCY	RELATIVE DOSING (MG)	RELATIVE MINERALOCORTICOID POTENCY
Cortisone	1	100	+
Hydrocortisone	1.25	80	++
Prednisone	5	20	+
Prednisolone	5	20	+
Methylprednisolone	6	16	0
9a-Fluorocortisol	20	5	+++++
Dexamethasone	50	1	0

Adapted from Donohoue PA: The adrenal cortex. In McMillan JA, DeAngelis CD, et al, editors: Oski's Pediatrics, Principles and Practice, ed 3. Philadelphia, 1999, JB Lippincott, p 1814.

9. **How do physiologic, stress, and pharmacologic doses of hydrocortisone differ?**
   - *Physiologic:* Careful studies have shown that adrenal glucocorticoid production in the normal individual is about 7 to 8 mg/m^2 per 24 hours. Because 50% to 60% of oral hydrocortisone is absorbed, the recommended oral physiologic replacement is about 12 to 15 mg/m^2 per 24 hours.
   - *Stress:* On the basis of studies performed before the development of high-quality radioimmunoassays, the consensus opinion was that production of glucocorticoid increased about threefold when individuals were physiologically stressed. Hence, when the term *stress dose* is used, it generally means that the dose is at least three times above physiologic replacement, that is, 50 to 100 mg/m^2 per 24 hours of hydrocortisone.
   - *Pharmacologic:* Glucocorticoids are extensively used in pharmacologic doses for the treatment of various inflammatory processes and in surgery or trauma to reduce or prevent swelling and inflammation. Doses of glucocorticoid higher than 50 mg/m^2 per 24 hours of hydrocortisone that are being used to treat these conditions are referred to as *pharmacologic doses*; that is, the medication is not being used for adrenal replacement or stress dosing.

10. **When does adrenal-pituitary axis suppression occur in prolonged glucocorticoid treatment?**
As a general rule, the longer the duration of treatment and the higher the dose of glucocorticoid, the greater the risk for adrenal suppression. If pharmacologic doses of glucocorticoids are used for less than

10 days, there is a relatively low risk for permanent adrenal insufficiency, whereas daily use for more than 30 days carries a high risk for prolonged or permanent adrenal suppression. The reason for glucocorticoid treatment must also be considered; that is, a child with severe head trauma may have initially been on treatment with glucocorticoids to reduce brain swelling but is also at significant risk for secondary pituitary deficiencies.

CALCIUM METABOLISM AND DISORDERS

11. **What are the causes of hypercalcemia?**
Remember the "High **5-Is**" mnemonic: **H** (**h**yperparathyroidism) plus the five **I**s (**i**diopathic, **i**nfantile, **i**nfection, **i**nfiltration, and **i**ngestion) and **S** (**s**keletal disorders).
Hyperparathyroidism:
- Familial
- Isolated
- Syndromic

Idiopathic:
- Williams syndrome

Infantile:
- Subcutaneous fat necrosis
- Secondary to maternal hypoparathyroidism and inadequate transfer of calcium across the placenta.

Infection:
- Tuberculosis

Infiltration:
- Malignancy
- Sarcoidosis

Ingestion:
- Milk-alkali syndrome
- Thiazide diuretics
- Vitamin A intoxication
- Vitamin D intoxication

Skeletal Disorders:
- Hypophosphatasia
- Immobilization
- Skeletal dysplasias

12. **An 8-year-old in a spica cast after hip surgery develops vomiting and a serum calcium concentration of 15.3 mg/dL. Has there been error in the order written for intravenous fluids and what should be done?**
This child's extreme hypercalcemia is likely due to immobilization from the full body cast and bone resorption. A serum calcium concentration of more than 15 mg/dL or the presence of significant symptoms (i.e., vomiting, hypertension) constitutes a *medical emergency* and requires immediate intervention to lower the calcium level. The initial approach of medical treatment is to increase urinary excretion of calcium. This is achieved with isotonic saline at two to three times maintenance rates with normal renal function. Once hydration is adequate, furosemide, 1 mg/kg intravenously every 6 to 8 hours, may be added until calcium decreases to 12 mg/dL. Furosemide and other loop diuretics are potent diuretic and calciuric agents. Meticulous monitoring of input and output and of serum and urinary electrolytes (including serum magnesium) is vital.

Electrocardiographic (ECG) monitoring is mandatory because hypercalcemia can be associated with conduction disturbances including premature ventricular contractions, ventricular tachycardia, prolonged PR interval, prolonged QRS duration, decreased QTc interval, and atrioventricular block. Additional treatment with glucocorticoids to decrease calcium absorption and antihypercalcemic agents to inhibit bone resorption may also be considered. Admission to an intensive care unit for careful monitoring of cardiac status, electrolyte levels, and fluid management may be necessary. If increased mobilization is possible, this will help correct the hypercalcemia.

Kirkland JL: Parathyroid glands. In Crocetti M, Barone MA, editors: *Oski's Essential Pediatrics*, ed 2. Philadelphia, 2004, Lippincott Williams & Wilkins, p 551.

13. **Is it the Chvostek or Trousseau sign that gets the tap?**

Both are clinical manifestations of neuromuscular irritability that occur when hypocalcemia or hypomagnesemia are present; normal extracellular calcium concentrations are necessary for muscle and nerve function.

- **Chvostek sign:** Tapping the parotid gland over the facial nerve in front of the ear results in facial muscle spasm with movement of the upper lip.
- **Trousseau sign:** Mild hypoxia induced by inflating a blood pressure cuff at pressures greater than systolic for 2 to 5 minutes results in carpopedal spasm in the setting of hypocalcemia.

Of these two signs, Trousseau sign is more specific. It is recommended that both clinical signs be confirmed with measurement with ionized calcium. An easy way to remember the difference is that the *Chvostek* sign affects part of the *cheek*.

Cooper M, Gittoes N: Diagnosis and management of hypocalcemia, *BMJ* 336:1298–1302, 2008.

14. **What is hypoparathyroidism?**

Parathyroid hormone (PTH) is a calcium regulatory hormone released by the parathyroid glands that increases serum calcium by increasing the resorption of Ca^{2+} from bone and by increasing gastrointestinal and urinary absorption of calcium through the increasing synthesis of calcitriol. Hypoparathyroidism can result from a developmental defect, destruction by surgery or autoimmune process, or from a biosynthetic defect in hormone production. The result can be acute or chronic hypocalcemia. An intact PTH level should be obtained in all children presenting with hypocalcemia. The result should be interpreted in light of the calcium level; that is, is the PTH appropriately elevated for the degree of hypocalcemia?

Shoback D: Hypoparathyroidism, *N Engl J Med* 359:391–403, 2008.

15. **In what clinical circumstances should hypoparathyroidism be suspected?**

- Manifestations of hypocalcemia (e.g., carpopedal spasm, bronchospasm, tetany, seizures)
- Lenticular cataracts (these can also occur with other causes of long-standing hypocalcemia)
- Changing behaviors, ranging from depression to psychosis
- Mucocutaneous candidiasis (seen in familial form)
- Dry and scaly skin, psoriasis, and patchy alopecia
- Brittle hair and fingernails
- Enamel hypoplasia (if hypocalcemia is present during dental development)

16. **What are the main causes of hypocalcemia in children?**

- **Nutritional:** Inadequate intake of vitamin D and, in rare instances, severely inadequate intake of calcium and/or excessive intake of phosphate may cause this condition.
- **Renal insufficiency:** This may be the result of the following: (1) increased serum phosphorus from a decreased glomerular filtration rate with depressed serum calcium and secondary hyperparathyroidism or (2) decreased activity of renal α-hydroxylase, which converts 25-hydroxyvitamin D into the biologically active form, $1,25\text{-}(OH)_2$ D.
- **Nephrotic syndrome:** With lowered serum albumin, total calcium levels are reduced. Additionally, intestinal absorption of calcium is decreased, urinary losses of cholecalciferol-binding globulin are increased, and urinary losses of calcium are increased with prednisone therapy (standard treatment for minimal change nephrotic syndrome). In patients with hypoalbuminemia, there will be a decrease in total calcium but no decrease in ionized calcium. The corrected calcium is estimated by adding 0.8 mg/dL to the total calcium for every 1-mg decrease in the serum albumin below 4 mg/dL.
- **Hypoparathyroidism:** In infants, this may result from a developmental defect during embryogenesis (parathyroid gland aplasia or hypoplasia) and may occur in the context of a syndrome such as DiGeorge syndrome caused by a deletion in chromosome 22q11. In older children, it may occur in the context of autoimmune polyglandular syndrome (type 1) or mitochondrial myopathy syndromes.
- **Pseudohypoparathyroidism:** This is a group of peripheral resistance syndromes in which resistance to PTH results in elevated PTH levels in the setting of normal renal function and subsequent hypocalcemia due to blunted or absent PTH effect in the setting of high serum concentrations of PTH.
- **Disorders of calcium sensor genes:** Activating mutations of the calcium sensing receptor gene (CaSR) result in calcium being sensed as normal at subphysiologic levels and PTH secretion switched off inappropriately causing hypoparathyroidism.

Moe SM: Disorders involving calcium, phosphorus, and magnesium, *Prim Care* 35:215–237, 2008.
Umpaichitra V, Bastian W, Castells S: Hypocalcemia in children: pathogenesis and management, *Clin Pediatr* 40:305–312, 2001.

17. **What is the most likely diagnosis in a child with hypocalcemia who has abnormally shaped fingers?**

   Albright hereditary osteodystrophy (AHO), a type of pseudohypoparathyroidism, is characterized by short stature, obesity, developmental delay, and brachydactyly, specifically a shortening of the fourth and fifth metacarpals (Fig. 6-1).

Desai N, Kalra A: Short fourth and fifth metacarpals, *JAMA* 308:1034–1035, 2012.

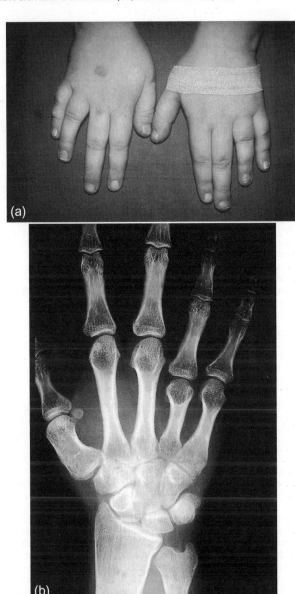

Figure 6-1. Short fourth and fifth metatarsals of a child (**A**), which are more readily appreciated on the radiograph (**B**). *(From Moshang T Jr: Pediatric Endocrinology: The Requisites in Pediatrics. Philadelphia, 2005, Elsevier Mosby, p 8.)*

CLINICAL SYNDROMES

18. **How does the syndrome of inappropriate secretion of antidiuretic hormone (SIADH) develop?**

    Antidiuretic hormone (ADH) is released from the posterior pituitary gland and serves as a regulator of extracellular fluid volume. The secretion of ADH is regulated by changes in osmolality sensed by the hypothalamus and alterations in blood volume detected by carotid and left atrial stretch receptors. By definition, the secretion of ADH in SIADH is *inappropriate*; therefore, the person cannot be given this diagnosis if dehydrated.

    Intracranial pathology can increase the secretion of ADH directly by local CNS effects, and intrathoracic pathology can increase secretion by stimulating volume receptors. Medications can directly promote ADH release and enhance its renal effects. SIADH is usually asymptomatic until symptoms of water intoxication and hyponatremia develop. Nausea, vomiting, irritability, personality changes, progressive obtundation, and seizures can result. An individual with hyponatremia that has developed over a prolonged period of time is less likely to have symptoms than one in whom the hyponatremia has developed acutely.

19. **What is cerebral salt wasting and how is it separated from SIADH?**

    Cerebral salt wasting (CSW) is defined as excessive urinary sodium losses in individuals with intracranial disease that result in hyponatremia and dehydration. The mechanism is still not clear. CSW typically develops in the first week after brain injury and generally resolves over time. Both CSW and SIADH are associated with hyponatremia. However, individuals with CSW have signs of intravascular volume depletion (e.g., rapid pulse, low blood pressure), whereas children with SIADH have evidence of intravascular volume overload. In SIADH, fluid restriction often leads to an increase in the serum sodium. In contrast, fluid restriction in CSW will not increase serum sodium but will further impair intravascular volume; therefore, it can be dangerous and may result in cardiovascular compromise.

20. **What are the five criteria for the diagnosis of SIADH?**
    1. Hyponatremia with reduced serum osmolality
    2. Urine osmolality elevated compared with serum osmolality (a urine osmolality <100 mOsm/dL usually excludes the diagnosis)
    3. Urinary sodium concentration excessive for the extent of hyponatremia (usually >20 mEq/L)
    4. Normal renal, adrenal, and thyroid function
    5. Absence of volume depletion

21. **What clinical features suggest diabetes insipidus (DI)?**

    Because DI is caused by an insufficiency of ADH or the inability to respond to ADH, the signs and symptoms tend to be directly related to excessive fluid loss. The clinical spectrum may vary depending on the child's age. The infant may present with symptoms of failure to thrive as a result of chronic dehydration, or there may be a history of repeated episodes of hospitalizations for dehydration. There may also be a history of intermittent low-grade fever.

    Often, caretakers report a large volume of intake or an inability to keep a dry diaper on the infant. The higher absorbency of disposable diapers may delay the diagnosis in infants. In the young child, DI may appear as difficulty with toilet training. In the older child, the reappearance of enuresis, increasing frequency of urination, nocturia, or dramatic increases in fluid intake may be noted. Frequent urination with large urinary volumes should lead to the suspicion of DI.

22. **How is the diagnosis of DI made?**

    Deprivation of water intake for a limited time and judicious monitoring of physical and biochemical parameters may be required. The diagnosis of DI rests on the demonstration of the following: (1) an inappropriately dilute urine in the face of a rising or elevated serum osmolality; (2) urine output that remains high despite the lack of oral input; and (3) changes in physical parameters that are consistent with dehydration (weight loss, tachycardia, loss of skin turgor, dry mucous membranes). A child who, with water deprivation appropriately concentrates urine (>800 mOsm/L) and whose serum osmolality remains constant (<290 mOsm/L) is unlikely to have DI. When DI is considered, a pediatric endocrinology consultation is strongly recommended.

    If a child meets the criteria for the diagnosis of DI, the water-deprivation test is usually ended with the administration of some form of ADH, such as desmopressin, and the provision of fluids. If the urine subsequently becomes appropriately concentrated, this confirms the diagnosis of ADH deficiency (central DI). Failure to concentrate suggests renal resistance to ADH (nephrogenic DI). DI may often be the first clinical sign of tumor of the hypothalamus or base of the skull (e.g., Wegener granulomatosis). Brain magnetic resonance imaging (MRI) is recommended if a diagnosis of DI is confirmed.

Ranadive SA, Rosenthal SM: Pediatric disorders of water balance, *Endocrinol Metab Clin North Am* 38:663–672, 2009.
Linshaw MA: Congenital nephrogenic diabetes insipidus, *Pediatr Rev* 28:372–379, 2007.

DIABETIC KETOACIDOSIS

23. What is diabetic ketoacidosis (DKA)?

DKA is a state of severe metabolic derangement that results from both severe insulin deficiency and increased amounts of counter-regulatory hormones (catecholamines, glucagon, cortisol, and growth hormone). The main features are hyperglycemia (glucose > 200 mg/dL), ketone production, and acidosis (venous pH < 7.30 or serum $HCO_3 < 15$ mEq/L).

24. What percentage of newly diagnosed diabetic patients present with symptoms of DKA?

This is extremely variable from location to location (13% to 80%) depending on access to care; economic status of the community; and other factors, including family history. The early symptoms of DKA are more likely to be missed or misinterpreted in very young children.

Klingensmith GJ, Tamborlane W, Wood J, et al: Diabetic ketoacidosis at diabetes onset: still an all too common threat in youth, *J Pediatr* 162:330.e1–334.e1, 2013.
Usher-Smith JA, Thompson M, Ercole A, et al: Variation between countries in the frequency of diabetic ketoacidosis at first presentation of type 1 diabetes in children: a systematic review, *Diabetologia* 55(11):2878–2894, 2012.

25. What are the mainstays of therapy for DKA?

- Adequate initial supportive care (airway maintenance if necessary, supplemental oxygen as needed)
- Volume resuscitation (which should begin before starting insulin therapy)
- Insulin administration (Initial dose of 0.05 to 0.1 unit/kg/hour)
- Frequent monitoring of vital signs, electrolytes, glucose, and acid-base status

Olivieri L, Chasm R: Diabetic ketoacidosis in the pediatric emergency department, *Emerg Med Clin North Am* 31:755–773, 2013.

26. What should be the initial fluid management in DKA?

The association of the rate of sodium and fluid administration in DKA and the development of cerebral edema remains controversial. The concern is that falling osmolarity might contribute to cerebral edema. The International Society for Pediatric and Adolescent Diabetes (ISPAD) recommends the following:

Initial:
- In the rare patient who presents in **shock,** circulatory volume should be rapidly restored with isotonic saline (or lactated Ringer solution) in 20 mL/kg boluses with reassessment after each bolus.
- In patients who are severely volume depleted but not in shock, the initial volume is typically 10 mL/kg given over 1 to 2 hours.

Subsequent:
- Once a patient is hemodynamically stable, fluid replacement is given more slowly. Replacement of the remainder of the fluid deficit (after subtracting the volume of the boluses that were received) is given over the next 48 hours at a rate not to exceed 1.5 to 2 times the maintenance rate. Generally, DKA is associated with an initial weight loss of 7% to10%.
- Choice of fluid tonicity should be made based on each patient's clinical status (degree of hyperosmolarity, CNS status, serum sodium trend, etc.). ISPAD guidelines state that "no treatment strategy can be definitively recommended as being superior to another based on evidence."

Wolfsdorf J, Craig ME, Daneman D, et al: Diabetic ketoacidosis in children and adolescents with diabetes, *Pediatr Diabetes* 10(Suppl 12):118–133, 2009.

27. **Why is a falling serum sodium concentration during the treatment of DKA of concern?**
Most patients with DKA have a significant sodium deficit of 8 to 10 mEq/kg, which needs to be replaced. After initial fluid boluses, fluids containing 0.5% normal saline or greater are generally required. As a general rule, the serum sodium concentration is low at the outset and rises throughout the course of treatment. An initial sodium concentration of more than 145 mEq/L suggests severe dehydration or hyperosmolarity.

The "corrected" serum sodium should be followed throughout treatment. This value can be calculated using the equation: Corrected sodium = Measured sodium (mEq/L) + 0.016 × [serum glucose (mg/dL) − 100]. A corrected serum sodium that begins to fall with treatment merits prompt attention because it indicates either inappropriate fluid management or the onset of SIADH and can signal impending cerebral edema.

Katz MA: Hyperglycemia-induced hyponatremia—calculation of expected serum sodium depression, *N Engl J Med* 289 (16):843–844, 1973.

28. **What is the typical potassium status in children with DKA?**
In almost all children with DKA, there is a depletion of intracellular potassium and a **substantial total body potassium** deficit of 3 to 6 mmol/kg, although the initial measured serum potassium value may be normal or high, in large part because of acidosis. Replacement therapy will be needed. If the patient is hypokalemic, potassium should be given with the initial volume expansion and before insulin administration. Insulin administration results in potassium transport into cells with a further decrease in serum levels. If the initial potassium level is within a normal range, begin potassium replacement (with the concentration in the infusate at 40 mEq/L) after the initial volume expansion and concurrent with starting insulin therapy, provided that urine output can be documented. If the initial potassium measurement is significantly elevated, defer potassium replacement until urine output has been documented and the hyperkalemia abates. Of note, if rapid serum potassium levels are not available, an electrocardiogram (ECG) to look for changes of hypokalemia or hyperkalemia (e.g., T-wave changes) can be valuable in guiding management.

Wolfsdorf J, Craig ME, Daneman D, et al: Diabetic ketoacidosis in children and adolescents with diabetes, *Pediatr Diabetes* 10(Suppl 12):118–133, 2009.

29. **Why do potassium levels fall during the management of DKA?**
Correction of acidosis (less K^+ exchanged out of cell for H^+ as pH rises)
- Insulin administration (increases cellular uptake of K^+)
- Dilutional effects of rehydration
- Ongoing urinary losses
Most patients are potassium depleted, although the serum K^+ is usually normal or elevated. A low K^+ is particularly worrisome because it suggests severe potassium depletion.

30. **Should bicarbonate be used for the treatment of children with DKA?**
The pros and cons of using sodium bicarbonate are shown in Table 6-2.

Table 6-2. Factors Determining Use of Bicarbonate Treatment in Diabetic Ketoacidosis

PROS	CONS
Improved pH enhances myocardial contractility problems rare in children and response to catecholamines	Cardiac function problems rare in children
Ventilatory response to acidosis blunted when pH is <7.0	Ventilatory response well-maintained in children
No adverse effect of bicarbonate on oxygenation has been demonstrated clinically	May alter oxygen-binding of hemoglobin, potentially decreasing tissue oxygenation

Table 6-2. Factors Determining Use of Bicarbonate Treatment in Diabetic Ketoacidosis (*Continued*)

PROS	CONS
Questionable relevance of central nervous system acidosis	Paradoxical central nervous system acidosis documented in humans
May be useful in the rare patient with hyperkalemia	Hypokalemia may result from uptake of K^+ as acidosis is corrected; low serum K is six times more common after bicarbonate treatment May be associated with increased hyperosmolarity and cerebral edema

31. **Are there any indications for the use of bicarbonate?**

Bicarbonate administration for the acidosis in DKA has not been shown to be beneficial in controlled trials. The establishment of an adequate intravascular volume and the provision of sufficient quantities of insulin are far more important in the treatment of DKA than bicarbonate. The decision to initiate bicarbonate therapy should be based on an arterial blood gas level and not a venous blood gas level. Two possible indications include:

- **Profound metabolic acidosis** (arterial pH < 6.9), which may be compromising cardiac contractility and/or adversely affecting the action of epinephrine during resuscitation
- **Life-threatening hyperkalemia** with bradycardia, severe muscle weakness

Wolfsdorf J, Craig ME, Daneman D, et al: Diabetic ketoacidosis in children and adolescents with diabetes, *Pediatr Diabetes* 10(Suppl 12):125, 2009.

Green SM, Rothrock SG, Ho JD, et al: Failure of adjunctive bicarbonate to improve outcome in severe pediatric diabetic ketoacidosis, *Ann Emerg Med* 31:41–48, 1998.

32. **When should glucose be added to the intravenous fluids in patients with DKA?**

This will depend on the rate at which the serum glucose level is decreasing. Generally, when the glucose level approaches 300 mg/dL, glucose should be added to the intravenous fluid. It is usually wise to order the appropriate glucose-containing fluid in advance to avoid hypoglycemia. Many centers now use the *"two-bag"* method: they order two bags of intravenous fluid, with identical electrolyte content except for the glucose concentration. One contains 10% or 12.5% glucose, and the other contains no glucose. As the blood sugar approaches 300 mg/dL, glucose is added to the infusate (through a Y tube). With the two-bag system, it is possible to alter the concentration of glucose anywhere between 0% and 12.5%, with a goal of maintaining the blood sugar in the 100- to 200-mg/dL range, thereby avoiding hypoglycemia. It is important to note that if the blood glucose concentration is decreasing too quickly or is too low before the resolution of acidosis, it is preferable to increase glucose levels by adding glucose to the infusate rather than decreasing the rate of insulin infusion.

Poirier MP, Greer D, Satin-Smith M: A prospective study of the "two-bag system" in diabetic ketoacidosis management, *Clin Pediatr* 43:809–813, 2004.

KEY POINTS: DIABETIC KETOACIDOSIS

1. The triad of metabolic derangement includes hyperglycemia, ketosis, and acidosis.
2. Abdominal pain can mimic appendicitis; hyperventilation can mimic asthma or pneumonia.
3. Initial bolus of insulin is no longer recommended.
4. Total-body potassium is usually significantly diminished.
5. Cerebral edema is the most common cause of morbidity and mortality in children with DKA.
6. If the sodium level begins to fall with fluid replenishment, beware of secretion of antidiuretic hormone and possible cerebral edema.
7. Bicarbonate therapy is usually not indicated for acidosis.

33. **In the past, a bolus of insulin was given at the start of therapy for DKA. Is that still recommended?**
   No. An initial bolus (traditionally 0.1 U/kg) was previously given before any subsequent insulin. This has been found to be unnecessary and may increase the risk for cerebral edema.

Wolfsdorf J, Glaser N, Sperling MA: Diabetic ketoacidosis in infants, children, and adolescents: a consensus statement from the American Diabetes Association, *Diabetes Care* 29:1150–1159, 2006.

34. **Is continuous or bolus insulin better for the initial treatment of DKA?**
   Extensive evidence demonstrates that **continuous** intravenous (IV) insulin (with an initial dose of 0.05 to 0.1 unit/kg/hr) should be the standard of care. The lower insulin dose may be more suitable for younger children, who are more insulin sensitive. Therapy should begin after the initial fluid bolus is complete. Beginning insulin at the start of fluid therapy increases the risk for severe hypokalemia and for decreasing the serum osmolarity too quickly. In general, this infusion should be maintained until the acidosis has significantly improved (pH >7.30, bicarbonate >15 mmol/L, and/or closure of the anion gap). If continuous IV administration of insulin is not possible, short- or rapid-acting insulin (insulin lispro or insulin aspart) can be given subcutaneously (SC) or intramuscularly (IM) every 1 to 2 hours if peripheral circulation is not impaired. A recommended initial dose is 0.3 unit/kg SC followed 1 hour later by SC insulin at 0.1 unit/kg every hour or 0.12 to 0.2 unit/kg every 2 hours.

Wolfsdorf J, Craig ME, Daneman D, et al: Diabetic ketoacidosis in children and adolescents with diabetes, *Pediatr Diabetes* 10(Suppl 12):123–124, 2009.
Wolfsdorf J, Glaser N, Sperling MA: Diabetic ketoacidosis in infants, children, and adolescents: a consensus statement from the American Diabetes Association, *Diabetes Care* 29:1153–1154, 2006.

35. **Which corrects sooner during continuous insulin administration: hyperglycemia or acidosis?**
   Hyperglycemia. Even though there may be normalization of the serum glucose, a persistent acidosis may be present. Thus, the continuous infusion of insulin should not be reduced until there is resolution of the ketoacidosis. Glucose may be added to the intravenous fluids to prevent hypoglycemia while the acidosis is being corrected.

36. **What is the main cause of mortality in DKA?**
   Cerebral edema. Clinically significant cerebral edema occurs in up to 1% of pediatric patients with high mortality rates.

37. **What risk factors are associated with the development of cerebral edema?**
   The pathogenesis of cerebral edema is incompletely understood. Computed tomography (CT) studies have demonstrated that *subclinical* cerebral edema may occur in a majority of pediatric patients with DKA. The escalation to life-threatening cerebral edema is unpredictable, often occurring as biochemical abnormalities are improving. It may be sudden in onset or occur gradually, but it typically occurs during the first 5 to 15 hours after therapy begins. Risk factors identified include the following:
   - Younger age
   - Newly diagnosed patients
   - More profound acidosis
   - Attenuated rise in serum sodium during therapy
   - Greater hypocapnia (after correcting for acidosis)
   - Increased blood urea nitrogen (BUN)
   - Bicarbonate therapy for acidosis
   - Administration of insulin in first hour of fluid treatment
   - Higher volumes of fluid given during the first 4 hours

Wolfsdorf J, Craig ME, Daneman D, et al: Diabetic ketoacidosis in children and adolescents with diabetes, *Pediatr Diabetes* 10(Suppl 12):126, 2009.
Levin DL: Cerebral edema in diabetic ketoacidosis, *Pediatr Crit Care Med* 9:320–329, 2008.
Glaser NS, Wootton-Gorges SL, Buonocore MH, et al: Frequency of sub-clinical cerebral edema in children with diabetic ketoacidosis, *Pediatr Diabetes* 7:75–80, 2006.

38. What signs and symptoms suggest worsening cerebral edema during the treatment of DKA?
    - Headache
    - Vomiting, recurrent
    - Change in mental status: increased drowsiness, irritability, restlessness
    - Change in neurologic status: cranial nerve palsy, abnormal pupillary responses, abnormal posturing
    - Incontinence (age inappropriate)
    - Rising blood pressure
    - Inappropriate heart rate slowing
    - Decreased oxygen saturation

Wolfsdorf J, Craig ME, Daneman D, et al: Diabetic ketoacidosis in children and adolescents with diabetes, *Pediatr Diabetes* 10(Suppl 12):126, 2009.

DIABETES MELLITUS

39. What are the risks of a child developing type 1 diabetes (T1D) if one sibling or parent is affected?
    Most people with T1D have no family history of the disorder, but having a first or second degree relative with T1D increases the risk of T1D. The human leukocyte antigen (HLA) gene cluster is responsible for 40-60% of a person's GENETIC risk, with many other genes and unknown environmental factors also playing a role. The major genetic determinants are polymorphisms of class II HLA genes encoding DQ and DR with specific haplotypes imparting the highest risk. Current approaches to assessing T1D risk use family history, measurement of T1D associated antibodies and HLA genotyping (DR and DQ).
    - Sibling with T1D: 6%
    - DR3/4-DQ8 *positive* HLA identical sibling with T1D: 55% to 80%
    - DR3/4-DQ8 *positive* HLA nonidentical sibling with T1D: 5%
    - DR3/4-DQ8 *negative* HLA identical sibling with T1D: 25%
    - Father with T1D: 4% to 6%
    - Mother with T1D: 2% to 4%

Baschal EE, Eisenbarth GS: Extreme genetic risk for type 1A diabetes in the post-genome era, *J Autoimmun* 31:1–6, 2008.

40. How long does the "honeymoon" period last in patients with newly diagnosed T1D?
    The honeymoon usually begins within 2 to 4 weeks after the initiation of insulin treatment. It is a period of decreased exogenous insulin requirements due to residual endogenous insulin production. The honeymoon period may last for a few weeks or months, but it is not predictable. Evidence is accumulating that endogenous insulin production may be preserved by the maintenance of "excellent control" and avoidance of hyperglycemia. Cessation of the honeymoon is often heralded by increasing insulin requirements. This is generally gradual but may be more acute, occurring with an intercurrent illness that increases insulin requirements.

41. How do the types of insulin vary in their onset and duration of action?
    See Table 6-3.

Table 6-3. Pharmacokinetics of Insulin and Insulin-Like Agents*

INSULIN	ONSET	PEAK	EFFECTIVE DURATION
Rapid Acting Aspart, glulisine, lispro (NovoLog, Apidra, Humalog)	5-15 min	30-90 min	3-5 hr
Short Acting Regular[†]	30-60 min	2-3 hr	4-8 hr

Continued on following page

Table 6-3. Pharmacokinetics of Insulin and Insulin-Like Agents (*Continued*)

INSULIN	ONSET	PEAK	EFFECTIVE DURATION
Intermediate Acting			
NPH	2-4 hr	4-10 hr	10-16 hr
(Humulin N, Novolin N)			
Detemir (Levemir)	2-4 hr	3-8 hr	10-24 hr
Long Acting			
Glargine (Lantus)	2-4 hr	No peak	20-24 hr

*Assuming 0.1 to 0.2 U/kg per injection. Onset and duration vary significantly by injection site.
†Regular insulin is available in different strengths; the standard is U-100 (100 units per mL) but U-500 is also available for those with extreme insulin resistance.

42. When should the Somogyi phenomenon be suspected?

The *Somogyi phenomenon* is rebound hyperglycemia after an incident of hypoglycemia. This rebound is secondary to the release of counterregulatory hormones, which is the natural response to hypoglycemia. As tighter glucose control is maintained, there is an increased likelihood of hypoglycemia and therefore of the Somogyi phenomenon. If the hypoglycemia is recognized and treated promptly, rebound hyperglycemia is less likely to occur. Thus, the Somogyi phenomenon is commonly reported more frequently at night because there is the greater likelihood of unrecognized and untreated hypoglycemia when the child is asleep. The Somogyi phenomenon should be suspected when a child whose blood sugar is in excellent control begins to have intermittent high blood glucoses in the morning. If that pattern is noted, blood glucose concentration should be checked between 2:00 and 3:00 AM on several nights to determine whether hypoglycemia is occurring. If hypoglycemia can be documented, the dose or type of evening insulin may need to be altered, or the time that the dose is given may need to be changed.

43. What causes the "dawn phenomenon"?

The term *dawn phenomenon* describes a rise in blood glucose concentration that occurs during the early morning hours (between 5:00 and 8:00 AM), particularly among patients who have normal glucose levels throughout most of the night. The rise in glucose is thought to be due to several factors, including the following:

- The cumulative effect of increased nocturnal growth hormone
- The normal increase in the morning cortisol level

Preventing morning hyperglycemia in someone with a pronounced "dawn phenomenon" may be difficult without the use of an insulin pump.

KEY POINTS: DIABETES MELLITUS TYPE 1

1. Destruction of pancreatic islet cells causes an absolute insulin deficiency.
2. Classic triad of symptoms includes polyuria, polydipsia, and polyphagia.
3. Tighter glucose control substantially lowers complication rates of retinopathy, nephropathy, and neuropathy.
4. Obtaining a hemoglobin A_1C (glycosylated hemoglobin) level is a standard way to assess average control during the previous 2 to 3 months.
5. Puberty is a time of increased insulin resistance, thereby requiring increased dosing.

44. How rapidly can renal disease develop after the onset of diabetes mellitus?

Microscopic changes in the glomerular basement membrane may be present by 2 years after the diagnosis of diabetes. Microalbuminuria often may be detected as early as 5 years after the diagnosis of T1D. Patients with diabetic nephropathy account for more than 25% of those receiving long-term renal dialysis in the United States. Progression can be substantially delayed by meticulous attention to glycemic control.

45. **How is hemoglobin A₁C (HbA₁C) helpful for monitoring glycemic control?**

The hemoglobin A_1C level (also known as glycosylated hemoglobin), is a hemoglobin-glucose combination formed nonenzymatically within the cell. Initially, an unstable bond is formed between glucose and the hemoglobin molecule. With time, this bond rearranges to form a more stable compound in which glucose is covalently bound to the hemoglobin molecule. The amount of the unstable form may rise rapidly in the presence of a high blood glucose level, whereas the stable form changes slowly and provides a time-average integral of the blood glucose concentration through the 120-day life span of the red blood cell. Thus, glycohemoglobin levels provide an objective measurement of averaged diabetic control over time.

Cooke DW, Plotnick L: Type 1 diabetes mellitus in pediatrics, *Pediatr Rev* 29:374–384, 2008.
Rewers M, Pihoker C, Donaghue K, et al: Assessment and monitoring of glycemic control in children and adolescents with diabetes, *Pediatr Diabetes* 8:408–418, 2007.

46. **What are the goals for hemoglobin A₁C?**

See Table 6-4.

Table 6-4. Hemoglobin A_1C Goals for Children and Adolescents with Type 1 Diabetes

AGE	HBA₁C GOAL*
<19 years	<7.5%
≥19 years	<7.0%

*According to 2013 International Society of Pediatric and Adolescent Diabetes and 2014 American Diabetes Association Recommendations.

47. **What pathophysiologic process characterizes type 2 diabetes (T2D)?**

T2D is characterized by a resistance to insulin action accompanied by a relative insulin secretory defect, in the absence of autoimmune markers.

48. **Is the prevalence of T2D in children increasing?**

Previously rare in pediatrics, T2D in children is increasing in incidence and prevalence. In the United States, there was a 30% increase in the prevalence of T2D in children less than 19 years of age between 2001 and 2009. It is most common in non-white children and adolescents with a strong family history of T2D. It is rarely seen before the onset of puberty.

Dabelea D, Mayer-Davis EJ, Saydah S, et al: Prevalence of type 1 and type 2 diabetes among children and adolescents from 2001 to 2009, *JAMA* 311:1778–1786, 2014.

49. **What historical and clinical features suggest type 2 rather than type 1 diabetes?**

- **Obesity** is very common in children with T2D; it is much less common in children with T1D at diagnosis.
- **Age of onset:** T2D only rarely presents before the onset of puberty; T1D commonly presents in prepubertal as well as pubertal children.
- **Racial and ethnic minority groups,** particularly black, Mexican Americans, and Native Americans, are at higher risk for T2D.
- **Family history** is usually strongly positive when a child develops T2D; more than 50% of affected children have at least one first-degree relatives with T2D.
- **Acanthosis nigricans,** a marker of insulin resistance, is present in 90% of T2D cases, most commonly on the posterior neck.
- **Hyperandrogenism** in girls is associated with insulin resistance and obesity. This is common in girls and young women with T2D.
- **Differing symptoms:** Unlike patients with T1D, most children and adolescents with T2D will present without ketonuria (although up to 33% of children with T2D will present with ketonuria).

Liu L, Hironaka K, Pihoker C: Type 2 diabetes in youth, *Curr Probl Pediatr Adolesc Health Care* 34:254–272, 2004.

50. **What laboratory features are helpful to distinguish T1D from T2D?**

Although classification can usually be made on the basis of clinical characteristics, measurement of levels of **fasting insulin** and **C-peptide** (low in T1D; normal or elevated in T2D) or **islet cell autoantibodies** (positive in T1D; absent in T2D) may be useful to distinguish T1D from T2D. Be mindful that there can be overlap in the laboratory evaluation.

51. **What is acanthosis nigricans?**

Acanthosis nigricans is hyperpigmented and often highly rugated patches that are found most prominently in intertriginous areas, especially on the nape of the neck (Fig. 6-2). This is a marker of insulin resistance.

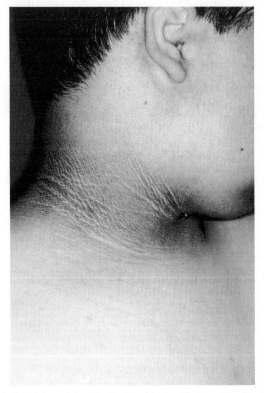

Figure 6-2. Acanthosis nigricans in an adolescent male. *(From Schachner LA, Hansen RC, editors:* Pediatric Dermatology, *ed 3. Edinburgh, 2003, Mosby, p 915.)*

52. **How is T2D diagnosed?**

The diagnosis of diabetes is based on blood glucose level cutoffs and the levels used are the same for T1D and T2D. The diagnosis is made when any of the following criteria are met:

- Random glucose concentration of 200 mg/dL or higher (if accompanied by classic symptoms: polyuria, polydipsia, weight loss)
- Fasting (>8 hours) glucose concentration of more than 125 mg/dL
- Abnormal oral glucose tolerance test defined as a glucose concentration of more than 200 mg/dL measured 2 hours after drinking 1.75 g/kg of glucose (with a maximum dose of 75 g)
- Hemoglobin $A_1C \geq 6.5\%$

American Diabetes Association: Standards of medical care in diabetes—2014, *Diabetes Care* 37(Suppl 1):S14–S80, 2014.

53. **Which pediatric patients should be screened for T2D?**
   The American Diabetes Association recommends screening beginning at 10 years of age (or earlier if puberty initiates before age 10 years). Screening should be performed using a fasting plasma glucose, oral glucose tolerance test, or hemoglobin A_1C for patients with the following risk factors:
   - Body mass index more than 85th percentile for age and sex, *plus*
   - Any two of following risk factors: positive family history in first- or second-degree relative; high-risk race/ethnicity (Native American, black, Hispanic, or Asian or Pacific Islander); presence of associated conditions (acanthosis nigricans, hypertension, dyslipidemia, polycystic ovarian syndrome)
   - Maternal history of diabetes or gestational diabetes during the child's gestation

American Diabetes Association: Standards of medical care in diabetes—2014, *Diabetes Care* 37(Suppl 1):S14–S80, 2014.

54. **What hemoglobin A_1C level is sufficient to diagnose diabetes?**
   A level $\geq 6.5\%$ on two occasions using a laboratory method is sufficient for the diagnosis. Levels between 5.7 and 6.4 place a person at increased risk for diabetes.

KEY POINTS: DIABETES MELLITUS TYPE 2

1. Pathophysiology includes progressive insulin secretory defect on the background of insulin resistance.
2. Incidence is rising rapidly in association with increased rate of pediatric obesity.
3. Acanthosis nigricans (altered skin pigmentation and texture) associated with insulin resistance is common (found in 90% of cases).
4. Diagnosis is based on detecting hyperglycemia: fasting (≥ 125 mg/dL), random with symptoms (≥ 200 mg/dL), or postprandial glucose challenge (≥ 200 mg/dL), or via HbA_1C of $> 6.5\%$.
5. Screen patients based on known risk factors (obesity, ethnicity, family history).

---

55. **When should oral hypoglycemic agents be considered as part of therapy?**
   If glucose control is not achieved with dietary adjustments and exercise within 2 to 3 months, oral hypoglycemic agents should be considered. Data on children and adolescents are limited. Metformin (Glucophage) is the best studied and is recommended as initial therapy by many experts. A daily multivitamin is required with metformin therapy because it can interfere with vitamin B_{12} and folic acid absorption. Insulin is often added to the regimen when patients are unable to meet glycemic targets using lifestyle and metformin alone.

Dileepan K, Feldt MM: Type 2 diabetes mellitus in children and adolescents, *Pediatr Rev* 34:541–548, 2013.

GROWTH DISTURBANCES

56. **How do the growth rates of boys and girls differ?**
   In both boys and girls, the rate or velocity of linear growth begins to decelerate right after birth. In girls, this deceleration continues until the age of about 11 years, at which time the adolescent growth spurt begins. For boys, the deceleration continues until the age of about 13 years. The peak rate of increase in boys occurs at 14 years of age. Growth and growth rate charts are readily available from the Centers for Disease Control and Prevention website (www.cdc.gov/growthcharts/).

57. **What is the best predictor of a child's eventual adult height?**
   Midparental height. This is an estimate of a child's expected genetic growth potential based on parental heights (preferably measured rather than by history).
   For girls: ([father's height − 13 cm] + [mother's height])/2.
   For boys: ([mother's height + 13 cm] + [father's height])/2.
   This gives the range (±5 cm) of expected adult height. The predicted height can be compared with the present height percentile, and any significant deviation can be a clue to an abnormal growth pattern in a child. It is important to remember that some forms of growth hormone deficiency are inherited, so one should not automatically assume that the short child with short parents has familial short stature.

58. **When have most children achieved the height percentile that is consistent with parental height?**
By the age of 2 years. Taking a boy's length at age 2 years and a girl's length at age 18 months and doubling them can obtain rough estimates of ultimate adult height.

59. **When is a detailed evaluation for short stature warranted?**
   - Severe height deficit (<1st percentile for age)
   - Abnormally slow growth rate (<10th percentile for bone age)
   - Predicted height is significantly different from midparental height
   - Body proportions are abnormal

Allen DB, Cuttler L: Short stature in childhood—challenges and choices, *N Engl J Med* 368:1220–1128, 2013.

60. **Name the major categories of causes of short stature**
   - *Familial* (for short children, ≤3 standard deviations, with very short parents, consider genetic forms of short stature)
   - *Constitutional delay* ("late bloomer")
   - *Chronic disease/treatment* (e.g., inflammatory bowel disease, chronic renal failure, renal tubular acidosis, cyanotic congenital heart disease)
   - *Chromosomal/syndromic* (e.g., Turner [45,X], 18q-, Down, achondroplasia)
   - *Endocrine* (e.g., hypothyroidism, growth hormone deficiency, hypopituitarism, hypercortisolism [endogenous and exogenous])
   - *Psychosocial* (e.g., chaotic social situation, orphanage)
   - *Intrauterine* (e.g., small for gestational age)
   Genetic patterns and constitutional delay account for the largest percentage of known causes.

61. **In a child with short stature, what rate of growth makes an endocrine abnormality unlikely?**
In general, heights should be measured over at least a 6-month interval to calculate an accurate rate because growth rates are not completely linear, and measurement is relatively imprecise. Rates of growth are also highly dependent on the age and pubertal status of the child. Growth velocity charts are available at http://www.cdc.gov/growthcharts. Growth rates that are consistently below the 25th percentile or crossing percentiles downward after the age of 2 years warrant careful consideration and possible investigation.

62. **When evaluating a short child, why should you ask when the parents reached puberty?**
The age at which puberty occurred in other family members may help identify children with constitutional delay because this entity tends to run in families. Most women will remember their age at menarche, and this age can be used as a reference for the age at which other pubertal events occurred. The strongest association for pubertal delay is between father and son. The most useful reference point for adult males is the age at which they reached adult height because almost all normal males will have reached their adult height by the age of 17 years (before high school graduation). Significant growth beyond this age suggests a history of pubertal delay.

63. **When does the pubertal growth spurt occur?**
For children with an average growth rate, pubertal growth begins earlier in girls. Mean age at the initiation of this spurt is 11 years for boys and 9 years for girls. Peak height velocity occurs at 13.5 years for boys and 11.5 years for girls. Peak velocity occurs at Tanner breast stage II to III for girls and Tanner testis stage III to IV for boys. Girls generally stop growing at an average of 14 years of age, but boys continue to grow until 17 years of age. The major hormone affecting growth cessation is estradiol in both girls and boys. The timing of the pubertal growth spurt may be earlier in certain ethnic groups and in very obese children. Assessment of short stature requires a determination of Tanner pubertal staging. On average, boys will grow 20 to 30 cm following the onset of puberty and girls between 15 and 25 cm.

Cheetham T, Davies JH: Investigation and management of short stature, *Arch Dis Child* 99:767–771, 2014.
Rogol AD, Roemmich JN, Clark PA: Growth at puberty, *J Adolesc Health* 31(Suppl):192–200, 2002.

64. **Are upper to lower body ratios helpful for the diagnosis of growth problems?**
Disproportionate short stature generally refers to an inappropriate ratio between truncal length and limb length (upper to lower segment ratio). Lower segment (limb length) is the distance from the superior border of the pubic bone to the floor surface. Height minus the lower segment gives the height of the upper segment (truncal length). In an infant, the head and trunk are quite long relative to the limbs, so the ratio of truncal length to limb length is about 1.7. Throughout childhood, this ratio declines, so that by 7 to 10 years of age this ratio is about 1.0. The adult ratio is 0.9.

An increased ratio is seen in bony dysplasias (e.g., achondroplasia, hypochondroplasia), hypothyroidism, gonadal dysgenesis, and Klinefelter syndrome (the patients are then tall in adolescence). Decreased ratios are seen in certain syndromes (e.g., Marfan syndrome), spinal disorders (e.g., scoliosis), and children who have been exposed to specific types of therapy (e.g., spinal irradiation).

Halac I, Zimmerman D: Evaluating short stature in children, *Pediatr Ann* 33:170–176, 2004.

65. **What laboratory studies should be obtained when evaluating short stature?**
Extensive laboratory tests are generally not indicated unless the growth velocity is abnormally low. Laboratory testing may include any or all of the following: complete blood count, urinalysis, chemistry panel, sedimentation rate, thyroxine, thyroid-stimulating hormone, insulin-like growth factor-1 (IGF-1), and IGF-binding protein-3 (IGFBP-3). Depending on the ethnic background of the child or the clinical history, testing might also be done for celiac disease, inflammatory bowel disease, renal tubular acidosis, or other occult conditions.

Random growth hormone levels are of little value because they are generally low in the daytime, even in children of average height. IGF-1 mediates the anabolic effects of growth hormone, and levels correlate well with growth hormone status. However, IGF-1 can also be low in nonendocrine conditions (e.g., malnutrition, liver disease).

IGFBP-3, which is the major binding protein for IGF-1 in serum, is also regulated by growth hormone. IGFBP-3 levels generally indicate growth hormone status and are less affected by nutritional factors than IGF-1. Most endocrinologists now use IGF-1 and IGFBP-3 as their initial screening tests for growth hormone deficiency.

Cheetham T, Davies JH: Investigation and management of short stature, *Arch Dis Child* 99:767–771, 2014.

66. **In a very obese child, how does height measurement help determine whether an endocrinopathy might be the cause?**
In children with simple obesity (e.g., familial), linear growth is typically enhanced; in children with endocrinopathies (such as Cushing's syndrome or hypothyroidism), it is usually impaired. If the height of a child is at, or greater than, the midparental height percentile, an endocrine cause of the obesity is unlikely. In some children with craniopharyngiomas, significant obesity with good linear growth can be seen despite documented growth hormone deficiency.

67. **How does a growth chart help determine the diagnosis of failure to thrive?**
If an infant is demonstrating deceleration of a previously established growth pattern or growth that is consistently less than the 5th percentile, the pattern of growth of head circumference, height, and weight can help establish the likely cause (Fig. 6-3). There are three main types of impaired growth:
- **Type I:** Retardation of weight with near-normal or slowly decelerating height and head circumference; most commonly seen in undernourished patients
- **Type II:** Near-proportional retardation of weight and height with normal head circumference; most commonly seen in patients with constitutional growth delay, genetic short stature, endocrinopathies, and structural dwarfism
- **Type III:** Concomitant retardation of weight, height, and head circumference; seen in patients with in utero and perinatal insults, chromosomal aberrations, and central nervous system abnormalities

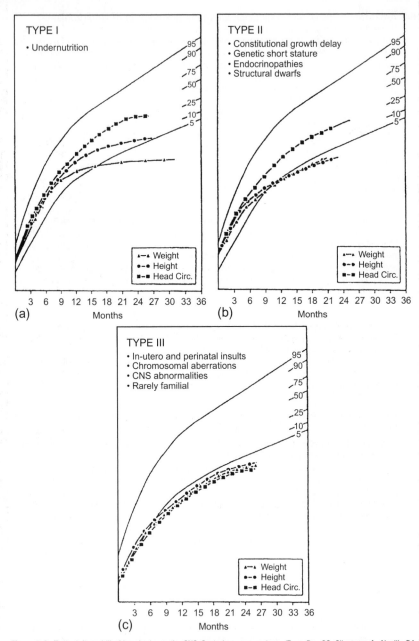

Figure 6-3. Types I, II, and III of impaired growth. *CNS,* Central nervous system. *(From Roy CC, Silverman A, Alagille DA: Pediatric Clinical Gastroenterology, ed 4. St. Louis, 1995, Mosby, pp 4–8.)*

68. **How can one track growth in children who have spinal cord abnormalities or severe scoliosis?**

    There is an excellent 1:1 correlation between span (longest fingertip to longest fingertip measured across the nape of the neck) and height. Thus, span is a useful proxy measure for height/length if it is not possible to get an accurate height. Height and rate of growth, when determined in this way, can be plotted on standard growth and velocity charts.

69. **What is bone age?**

    Bone age is a measure of *somatic maturity* and *growth potential.* Standards of normal skeletal radiographic maturation are available, and these are based on the progression of ossification centers that occur at particular ages. A radiograph of the left hand and wrist is taken and compared with those standards to determine a patient's bone age. This result can be compared with chronologic age to gauge the remaining potential for growth. The interpretation of bone ages can be somewhat difficult and dependent on the pediatric experience of the radiologist.

70. **Why is a bone age determination helpful for evaluating short stature?**

    A single bone age is of value for differentiating familial short stature and genetic diseases (in which bone age is normal) from other causes of short stature. A delayed bone age (>2 standard deviations below the mean) that correlates with the child's height age (age on growth chart at which child's height would be at the 50th percentile) is suggestive of constitutional delay, whereas a markedly delayed bone age is suggestive of endocrine disease. Serial bone ages determined every 6 to 12 months are often helpful because, in both the normal child and the child with constitutional delay, the bone age will advance in parallel with the chronologic age. In endocrine disease, the bone age falls progressively further behind the chronologic age. Bone age may be normal or delayed in patients with chronic disease, depending on the severity of disease, its duration, and the type of treatment used.

71. **What features suggest constitutional delay as a cause of short stature?**

    - No signs or symptoms of systemic disease
    - Bone age delayed up to 2 to 4 years but consistent with height age (age at which individual's height would plot on the 50th percentile)
    - Period of poorest growth often occurring between the ages of 18 and 30 months, with steady linear growth thereafter (i.e., normal rate of growth for bone age)
    - Parental or sibling history of delayed physical development
    - Height prediction consistent with family characteristics.

KEY POINTS: GROWTH DISTURBANCES

1. Bone age is used as a diagnostic key: genetically determined short stature (bone age = chronologic age) versus constitutional delay (bone age < chronologic age).
2. Midline defects (e.g., single maxillary incisor, cleft lip/palate) and short stature suggest hypopituitarism.
3. Random growth hormone levels are usually not helpful (due to pulsatile delivery during sleep); provocative testing is more reliable.
4. Family history is key. Use growth data about family to establish a pattern.
5. Short stature with overweight suggests endocrinopathy (adrenal, thyroid or growth hormone deficiency).
6. Growth hormone deficiency that appears during the first year of life is associated with hypoglycemia; after the age of 5 years, it is associated with short stature.

72. **How is constitutional delay managed?**

    If the results of history, physical examination, and clinical laboratory evaluation are unremarkable, the child is seen once every 3 to 6 months for accurate height measurements and determination of growth velocity. A bone age test may be done yearly to assess the progression of bony maturation. In patients with constitutional delay, the rate of bone maturation should keep pace with the chronologic age. In children who are of mid- to late pubertal ages (girls >13 years; boys >14 years) but showing minimal or no signs of puberty, selective use of estrogen or testosterone supplementation to initiate puberty or additional assessment may be indicated.

73. **Should growth hormone therapy be given to the normal short child?**

    This is an area of controversy in pediatric endocrinology. Human growth hormone is most effective when administered subcutaneously on a daily basis. It does increase growth rate and modestly improves adult height (1.2 to 2.8 inches). The safety profile has been good and the risk of short-term adverse events (such as intracranial hypertension or glucose intolerance) is very low. Long-term safety remains under study.

Opponents argue that short stature is not a disease and appropriate therapeutic goals are ill defined. The therapy is expensive, estimated in 2006 dollars to be about $35,000 to $50,000 per inch of height gained.

Allen DB, Cuttler L: Short stature in childhood—challenges and choices, *N Engl J Med* 368:1220–1128, 2013.
Allen DB: Growth hormone therapy for short stature: is the benefit worth the burden? *Pediatrics* 118:343–348, 2006.

74. **What are the clinical manifestations of growth hormone excess?**
    Before puberty, the cardinal manifestations are an increase in growth velocity with minimal bone deformity and soft tissue swelling—a condition called *pituitary gigantism*. Hypogonadotropic hypogonadism and delayed puberty often coexist with growth hormone excess, and affected children exhibit eunuchoid body proportions. If the growth hormone excess occurs after puberty (after epiphyseal closure), the more typical features of acromegaly occur, including coarsening of the facial features and soft tissue swelling of the feet and hands. Growth hormone excess is rare in children.

HYPOGLYCEMIA

75. **How is hypoglycemia defined?**
    A serum glucose concentration of less than 50 mg/dL is defined as hypoglycemia in childhood. Some argue for lower levels being used for term and preterm infants; however, these arguments are based on population sampling data rather than on physiology. Hypoglycemia is a laboratory finding, and its presence should always lead to a diligent search for the underlying pathology. A common cause of a falsely reported abnormal glucose is that the plasma is not quickly separated from the red blood cells. The red cells continue to metabolize glucose, thus lowering the glucose, often into an abnormal range. This should be suspected when the glucose result is reported as part of a chemistry panel, especially if the child was reported to be asymptomatic.

76. **What are the clinical findings associated with hypoglycemia?**
    Neuroglycopenic symptoms include irritability, headache, confusion, unconsciousness, and seizure. Adrenergic signs include tachycardia, tremulousness, diaphoresis, and hunger. Any combination of the above signs and symptoms should lead to the measurement of the blood glucose level.

77. **What are the causes of childhood hypoglycemia?**
    No single cause predominates in any age group. Therefore, the entire differential diagnosis must be considered in any child who presents symptoms of hypoglycemia. Hypoglycemia often occurs as a result of a combination of two or more of the problems listed in Table 6-5 (e.g., prolonged fasting during an

Table 6-5. Differential Diagnosis of Childhood Hypoglycemia

Decreased Glucose Utilization
Hyperinsulinism: focal (adenoma) or diffuse hyperplasia, oral hypoglycemic agents, exogenous insulin

Decreased Glucose Production
Inadequate glycogen reserves: Enzymatic defects in glycogen synthesis and glycogenolysis
Ineffective gluconeogenesis: Inadequate substrate (e.g., ketotic hypoglycemia), enzymatic defects

Diminished Availability of Fats
Depleted fat stores
Failure to mobilize fats (e.g., hyperinsulinism)
Defective use of fats: Enzymatic defects in fatty acid oxidation (e.g., medium-chain acyl CoA dehydrogenase deficiency)

Decreased Fuels and Fuel Stores
Fasting, malnutrition, prolonged illness, malabsorption

Increased Fuel Demand
Fever, exercise

Inadequate Counterregulatory Hormones
Growth hormone or cortisol deficiency, hypopituitarism

illness coupled with fever in medium-chain acyl-CoA dehydrogenase deficiency). Specific genetic testing is now available for a number of these entities.

78. **An unconscious 3-year-old girl is brought to the emergency department with a serum glucose concentration of 26 mg/dL. What other laboratory tests should be performed?**

Blood and urine samples are critically important. The first urine specimen obtained after the presentation of the child is of significant value, even if this cannot be gotten for several hours after the acute event. The blood sample, however, should be drawn before dextrose is administered. The principal laboratory evaluations should include the measurement of the following: (1) the metabolic compounds associated with fasting adaptation; (2) the hormones that regulate these processes; and (3) drugs that can interfere with glucose regulation. It is strongly recommended that an extra purple top and red top tube of blood be drawn, if at all possible. The extra tubes of blood should be kept for additional analyses once the first battery of tests described below is available or after specific recommendations by a metabolic specialist.

Blood can be sent for measurement of the following:
- Markers of the principal regulatory hormones: insulin, growth hormone, and cortisol
- Markers of fatty acid metabolism: ketones (β-hydroxybutyrate and acetoacetate), free fatty acids, and total and free carnitine
- Markers of gluconeogenic pathways: lactate, pyruvate, and alanine

Urine can be sent for measurement of the following:
- Ketones
- Metabolic by-products associated with known causes of hypoglycemia (e.g., organic acids, amino acids)
- Toxicology screen, especially for alcohol and salicylates

Taken together, these tests provide valuable clues as to the cause. For example, low levels of ketones and free fatty acids suggest that fat was not appropriately mobilized. As a consequence, ketones were not formed by the liver. Those biochemical abnormalities are seen in hyperinsulinemic states and can be confirmed by documenting a high level of circulating insulin. Low urinary ketones also suggest an enzymatic defect in fatty acid oxidation.

Josefson J, Zimmerman D: Hypoglycemia in the emergency department, *Clin Pediatr Emerg Med* 10:285–191, 2009.

79. **In patients with acute hypoglycemia, what are the treatment options?**

The principal acute treatment is the provision of glucose orally or intravenously. If the patient is alert, 4 to 8 ounces of a sugar-containing liquid (e.g., orange juice, cola) may be given. If the patient is obtunded, intravenous glucose (2 to 3 mL/kg of $D_{10}W$ or 1 mL/kg of $D_{25}W$) should be administered rapidly. If venous access cannot be achieved promptly, glucose can be provided through a nasogastric tube because glucose is rapidly absorbed. The risk for prolonged hypoglycemia far outweighs the risk associated with the passage of a nasogastric tube in an obtunded patient. Subsequently, the blood sugar should be monitored closely and, if necessary, maintained by the constant infusion of glucose (6 to 8 mg/kg/min). Ten percent dextrose and water in an electrolyte solution given at about 1.5 times maintenance dose approximates 6 to 8 mg/kg/min. Larger quantities may be necessary, and the blood sugar concentration should be closely followed.

Glucagon promotes glycogen breakdown. In settings in which glycogen stores have not been depleted (e.g., insulin overdose), 0.03 mg/kg (max dose of 1 mg) of glucagon IM or SC will raise blood glucose levels.

Glucocorticoids should not be used routinely. Their only clear indication is in known primary or secondary adrenal insufficiency. In other settings, they have little acute value and may cloud the diagnostic process. The decision to use glucocorticoids is somewhat dependent on the child's medical history (e.g., reasonable to use in the context of a history of prior central nervous system irradiation).

HYPOTHALAMIC AND PITUITARY DISORDERS

80. **What clinical signs or symptoms suggest hypothalamic dysfunction?**

The signs and symptoms of hypothalamic dysfunction are as variable as the processes controlled by the hypothalamus, ranging from disorders of hormonal production to disturbances of thermoregulation. Precocious or delayed sexual maturation represent the most common presentations of a hypothalamic endocrine abnormality in childhood. Diabetes insipidus, behavioral and cognitive disturbances, and excessive sleepiness are found in about one-third of all patients with hypothalamic dysfunction and may be the first manifestation of disease. Eating disorders (obesity, anorexia, bulimia) and convulsions are also reported. Dyshidrosis and disturbances of sphincter control (e.g., encopresis, enuresis) are occasionally seen.

81. **List the intracranial processes that can interfere with hypothalamic-pituitary function**
    - **Congenital:** Inherited deficiencies of gonadotropin-releasing factor, growth hormone–releasing hormone; syndromic (Laurence-Moon-Biedl and Prader-Labhart-Willi syndromes)
    - **Structural:** Craniopharyngioma, Rathke pouch cyst, hemangioma, hamartoma
    - **Infectious:** Meningitis and encephalitis
    - **Tumors:** Glioma, dysgerminoma, ependymoma, Wegener granulomatosis, histiocytosis X
    - **Idiopathic**

82. **Why is it bad to have a "Turkish saddle" that is too large?**
    The *sella turcica* derives its name from the Latin words for *Turkish saddle*. The name reflects the anatomic shape of the saddlelike prominence on the upper surface of the sphenoid bone in the middle cranial fossa, above which sits the pituitary gland. A variety of conditions can lead to sellar enlargement, including tumors of the pituitary or functional hypertrophy of the pituitary, which may occur in primary hypothyroidism or primary hypogonadism. Modern imaging techniques have supplanted the skull series as a tool for searching for pituitary or hypothalamic disease; however, an enlarged sella may be noted in children for whom skull series are obtained for other reasons (e.g., head trauma).

83. **Which tests are useful for studying suspected hypothalamic and pituitary malfunction?**
    Either MRI or CT is required to rule out structural pathology before searching for functional abnormalities. Studies of the pituitary-hypothalamus may include any or all of the following:
    - **Prolactin:** Random levels tend to be elevated in the presence of hypothalamic lesions. A normal level does not rule out CNS pathology. An elevated level may occur in an anxious or stressed child during venipuncture.
    - **Growth hormone production tests (see question 65):** These tests are generally indicated only if the child's growth rate is subnormal. Growth hormone–releasing factor is now available for testing pituitary responsiveness. It has proved useful, in some instances, for delineating pituitary causes of growth hormone underproduction from primary hypothalamic disease.
    - **Gonadotropin-releasing hormone analogue (GnRHa) provocative test:** Random levels of luteinizing hormone and follicle-stimulating hormone are not generally helpful if one is searching for pituitary hypofunction. The results of the GnRHa test must be correlated with the age of the child because there are developmental changes in the response to GnRHa.
    - **ACTH stimulation testing (Cortrosyn):** This test of adrenal production of cortisol is often used in determining whether there has been adrenal destruction or to demonstrate more subtle abnormalities in adrenal steroid hormonogenesis. The hypothalamic-releasing hormone, corticotrophin-releasing factor, is also available and can be used to examine the production of ACTH by the pituitary.
    - **Simultaneous urine and serum osmolalities:** A normal serum osmolality and a concentrated urine osmolality tend to rule out diabetes insipidus. If these results are equivocal, a water deprivation test may be required.
    - **Thyrotropin-releasing hormone (TRH)** is no longer available for provocative testing.

SEXUAL DIFFERENTIATION AND DEVELOPMENT

84. **An infant is born with "ambiguous genitalia." What features of the history and physical examination are key in the evaluation?**
    Of note, the term *ambiguous genitalia* is largely antiquated. The contemporary terminology is *disorder of sexual differentiation* (DSD). This term is thought to more accurately suggest causation rather than consequence and to be less pejorative in discussions with families and nonmedical lay people.

    History: One should search for evidence of maternal androgen excess (hirsutism during pregnancy) or androgen ingestion (rare now, but common in the 1960s with certain progestational agents), other hormonal use (e.g., for infertility or endometriosis), alcohol use, parental consanguinity, previous neonatal deaths, or a family history of previously affected children.

Physical examination: The presence of a gonadal structure in the labioscrotal fold strongly implies the presence of some form of testicular tissue. Gonads containing both ovarian and testicular components (ovotestes) have been found in the inguinal canal. However, it is rare to find an ovary in the inguinal canal. In the absence of a palpable gonad, no conclusions can be drawn regarding probable chromosomal sex. The size of the phallic structure and the location of the urethral meatus provide no information about genetic makeup. However, phallic size and function may be important considerations when determining the sex the child will be assigned.

The presence of *midline abnormalities* (e.g., cleft palate) suggests hypothalamic or pituitary dysfunction, whereas congenital anomalies such as imperforate anus suggest structural derangements. A digital rectal examination will confirm the patency of the anus and may allow palpation of the uterus. In infants and young children, ultrasound is the more definitive approach to exploring intra-abdominal structures and can often be helpful in confirming the presence or absence of müllerian structures and gonads. Other anomalies should be noted because disorders of genital development are often associated with other developmental disorders in syndromes.

Shomaker K, Bradford K, Key-solle M: Ambiguous genitalia, *Contemp Pediatr* 26:40–56, 2009.
Wolfsdorf J, Padilla A: Goodbye intersex. . .hello DSD, *Int Pediatr* 23:120–121, 2008.

85. What are the causes of a DSD?

Undervirilized male (XY karyotype):
- Androgen resistance: Complete (testicular feminization)
- Partial defects of androgen synthesis: 3-β-hydroxysteroid dehydrogenase deficiency, 5-α-reductase deficiency

Virilized female (XX karyotype):
- Excess androgen: Congenital adrenal hyperplasia, 21-hydroxylase deficiency, 3-β-hydroxysteroid dehydrogenase deficiency
- Maternal androgen exposure: Medication, virilizing adrenal tumor

Intersex (mosaic karyotypes; e.g., XO/XY)

Structural abnormalities

Houk CP, Lee PA: Consensus statement on terminology and management: disorders of sex development, *Sex Dev* 2:172–180, 2008.
MacLaughlin DT, Donahoe PK: Sex determination and differentiation, *N Engl J Med* 350:367–378, 2004.

86. Which studies are essential for the evaluation of a DSD?

- **Ultrasonography:** This test is the most helpful for identifying internal structures, particularly the uterus and occasionally the ovaries. The absence of a uterus suggests that testes were present early in gestation and produced müllerian-inhibiting factor, thereby causing regression of the müllerian-derived ducts and thus the uterus. The injection of contrast medium into the urethrovaginal openings will often demonstrate a pouch posterior to the fused labioscrotal folds. Occasionally, the cervix and cervical canal will be highlighted by this study as well.
- **Chromosomal analysis:** Obviously, this is useful for predicting gonadal content. There are a number of highly specialized and sensitive genetic tests to confirm the presence or absence of X or Y chromosomal material. A geneticist should always be consulted in infants with a DSD.
- **Measurement of adrenal steroids (17-hydroxyprogesterone, 11-deoxycortisol, 17-hydroxypregnenolone):** 17-Hydroxyprogesterone is the precursor that is elevated in the most common variety of congenital adrenal hyperplasia associated with a DSD (21-hydroxylase deficiency).
- **Measurement of testosterone and dihydrotestosterone:** It is very important to have input from staff with expertise in this area, including a geneticist, a pediatric endocrinologist, and a pediatric urologist. It is also essential that this group synthesize information after all data are available and that it be communicated to the family by a single spokesperson.

Hiort O, Bimbaum W, Marshall L, et al: Management of disorders of sex development, *Nat Rev Endocrinol* 10:520–529, 2014.
Lee PA, Houk CP, Ahmed SF, et al: Consensus statement on management of intersex disorders, *Pediatrics* 118: e488–e500, 2006.

87. **What major criteria are used to define a micropenis?**
To be classified as a micropenis, the phallus must meet two major criteria:
1. The phallus must be normally formed, with the urethral meatus located on the head of the penis and the penis positioned in an appropriate relationship to the scrotum and other pelvic structures. If these features are not present, then the term *micropenis* should be avoided.
2. The phallus must be more than 2.5 standard deviations below the appropriate mean for age. For a term newborn, this means that a penis less than 2 cm in stretched length is classified as a micropenis.

It is essential that the phallus be measured appropriately. This entails the use of a rigid ruler pressed firmly against the pubic symphysis, depressing the suprapubic fat pad as much as possible. The phallus is grasped gently by its lateral margins and stretched. The measurement is taken along the dorsum of the penis. Note should also be made of the breadth of the phallic shaft. Micropenis must be recognized early in life so that appropriate diagnostic testing can be done.

Lee PA, Mazur T, Danish R, et al: Micropenis. I. Criteria, etiologies and classification, *Johns Hopkins Med J* 146:156–163, 1980.

88. **What are the main concerns to be addressed during the initial evaluation of a 1-month-old infant with micropenis?**
1. **Is there a defect in the hypothalamic-pituitary-gonadal axis?** Specific tests include the measurement of testosterone, dihydrotestosterone, luteinizing hormone, and follicle-stimulating hormone. Because circulating levels of these hormones are normally quite high during the neonatal period, the measurement of random levels during the first 2 months of life may be useful for identifying diseases of the testes and pituitary. Beyond 3 months of age, the tests are generally not useful because the entire axis becomes quiescent and remains so until late childhood. Depending on the patient's age, provocative tests may be necessary, including the following: (1) repetitive testosterone injection to evaluate the ability of the penis to respond to hormonal stimulation; (2) the use of human chorionic gonadotropin as a stimulus for testosterone production by the testes; and (3) leuprolide administration to examine the responsiveness of the pituitary to stimulation. The trial of testosterone therapy is especially important because it indicates whether phallic growth is possible. If it is not, gender reassignment may become a consideration.
2. **Does a possible pituitary deficiency involve other hormones?** Isolated growth hormone deficiency, gonadotropin deficiency, and panhypopituitarism have been associated with micropenis. The presence of hypoglycemia, hypothermia, or hyperbilirubinemia (e.g., associated with hypothyroidism) in a child with micropenis should lead one to search for other pituitary hormone deficits and structural abnormalities of the CNS (e.g., septo-optic dysplasia).
3. **Is there a renal abnormality?** Because of the association of genital and renal abnormalities, it is prudent to obtain an abdominal and pelvic ultrasound to better define the internal anatomy.

89. **Discuss the terms that denote aspects of precocious sexual development.**
The terms used to describe precocious puberty reflect the fact that normal puberty is an orderly process by which female children are feminized and male children masculinized. The development of breast tissue without pubic hair is called *premature thelarche*. If pubic hair subsequently develops, the term *precocious puberty* is used. If pubic hair develops without breast tissue, it is *premature pubarche*. Because pubic hair development in the female is thought to be the result of adrenal androgens, the term *premature adrenarche* is commonly used. If the pubertal changes are early and appear to proceed in the orderly fashion of breast budding, pubic hair development, growth spurt, and, finally, menstruation, the term *true precocious puberty* is used. When some of the changes of puberty are present, but their appearance is isolated or out of normal sequence (e.g., menses without breast development), the term *pseudoprecocious puberty* is used.

90. **Boys or girls: Who is more likely to have an identifiable cause for precocious puberty?**
Although precocious puberty occurs much more frequently in girls (80% of cases are girls), **boys** are more likely to have identifiable pathology. As a general rule, the younger the child and the more rapid the onset of the condition, the greater the likelihood of detecting pathology.

91. **A 7 ½ -year-old girl develops breast buds and pubic hair. Is this normal or precocious?**

    Precocious puberty is the appearance of physical changes associated with sexual development earlier than normal. Traditionally this has been the development of feminine characteristics in girls who are younger than 8 years and masculine characteristics in boys who are younger than 9 years. In 1997, an office-based study of 17,000 healthy 3- to 12-year-old girls revealed that puberty was occurring on average 1 year earlier in white girls and 2 years earlier in black girls and suggested a revision of guidelines for the ages at which precocious puberty should be investigated. Many experts now recommend that an evaluation for precocious puberty of girls need not be undertaken for white girls older than 7 years or black girls older than 6 years with breast and/or pubic hair development. However, this remains controversial and a subject of ongoing debate and data collection. The recommendations for boys remain that investigations for pathologic etiologies be undertaken if pubertal changes begin before the age of 9 years.

    Euling SY, Herman-Giddens ME, Lee PA, et al: Examination of US puberty-timing data from 1940 to 1994 for secular trends: panel findings, *Pediatrics* 121(Suppl):S172–S191, 2008.

    Kaplowitz PB, Oberfield SE: Reexamination of the age limit for defining when puberty is precocious in girls in the United States: implications for evaluation and treatment, *Pediatrics* 104:936–941, 1999.

    Herman-Giddens ME, Slora EJ, Wasserman RC, et al: Secondary sexual characteristics and menses in young girls seen in office practice: a study from the Pediatric Research in Office Settings network, *Pediatrics* 99:505–512, 1997.

92. **Breast buds are noted on a 2-year-old girl. Is this worrisome?**

    Premature thelarche, or the development of breast buds, is the most common variation of normal pubertal development. A form of mild estrogenization, it typically occurs between the ages of 1 and 3 years. It is usually benign and should not be associated with the onset of other pubertal events. Precocious puberty, rather than simple premature thelarche, should be suspected if the following occur:
    - Breast, nipple, and areolar development reach Tanner stage III (i.e., continued progression is of concern).
    - Androgenization with pubic and/or axillary hair begins.
    - Linear growth accelerates.

    Ongoing parental observation and periodic reexamination are all that are required if there are no signs of progression.

93. **Which aspects of the physical examination are particularly important when evaluating a patient with precocious puberty?**
    - **Evidence of a CNS mass:** Examination of optic fundus for possible increased intracranial pressure; visual field testing for evidence of optic nerve compression by a hypothalamic or pituitary mass
    - **Evidence of androgenic influence:** Presence of acne and facial and axillary hair; increased muscle bulk and definition; extent of other body or pubic hair; in boys, increased scrotal rugation accompanied by thinning and pigmentation and penile elongation; in girls, clitoromegaly
    - **Evidence of estrogenic influence:** Size of breast tissue and nipple and areolar contouring; vaginal mucosa color (increased estrogen causes cornification of vaginal epithelium with a color change from prepubertal shiny red to a more opalescent pink); labia minor (become more prominent and visible between the labia majora as puberty progresses)
    - **Evidence of gonadotropic stimulation:** Testicular enlargement of greater than 2.5 cm in length or more than 4 mL in volume (preferably measured using a Prader orchidometer of labeled volumetric beads); pubertal development without testicular enlargement usually suggests adrenal pathology
    - **Evidence of other mass:** Asymmetrical testicular enlargement; hepatomegaly; abdominal mass

94. **Which radiologic and laboratory tests are indicated for the evaluation of precocious puberty?**

    Radiologic evaluation
    - *Bone age:* This study helps determine the duration of exposure to the elevated sex hormone. A significantly advanced bone age compared with the chronologic age suggests long-term exposure.
    - *Abdominal and pelvic ultrasound:* In boys, this test identifies possible adrenal or hepatic masses; in girls, it identifies adrenal masses, ovarian masses, or cysts. Increased uterine size and echogenicity suggest endometrial proliferation in response to circulating estrogen.
    - *Head CT or MRI:* This evaluation is useful in identifying pituitary or hypothalamic abnormalities.

    Laboratory evaluation
    - Obtain luteinizing hormone, follicle-stimulating hormone, estradiol, and testosterone levels.

- Adrenal steroid levels (17-hydroxyprogesterone, androstenedione, cortisol): More extensive testing may be needed in a virilized child if the initial studies are normal.
- Use provocative testing of the hypothalamic-pituitary axis (using a synthetic GnRHa) or of the adrenal gland (using a synthetic ACTH), especially in the child with slight but progressive pubertal changes.

95. **When does the male voice begin to crack?**
Voice "breaking" has traditionally been regarded as one of the harbingers of puberty. However, sequential voice analysis reveals that it is usually a late event in puberty, typically occurring between Tanner stages III and IV.

Harries ML, Walker JM, Williams DM, et al: Changes in the male voice at puberty, *Arch Dis Child* 77:445–447, 1997.

THYROID DISORDERS

96. **Which thyroid function tests are "standard"?**
Diseases of the thyroid represent a heterogeneous group of disorders. As such, there are no "standard" thyroid function studies that are appropriate for all children with suspected thyroid disease. The choice of laboratory tests is based on the results of a careful history and physical examination.
    Biochemical findings that suggest hyperthyroidism: A thyroid-stimulating hormone (TSH) level and a thyroxine level (total T_4 or free T_4) should be obtained. Compared to total T_4, the free T_4 is the biologically active component and theoretically is a better measure of thyroid function. TSH suppression is probably the most sensitive indicator of hyperthyroid status. If the patient is symptomatic and has a suppressed TSH level with a normal T_4 level, it will be necessary to obtain a triiodothyronine (T_3) radioimmunoassay because cases of T_3 thyrotoxicosis do occur. If the patient is asymptomatic but has an elevated T_4 level, some measure of binding capacity should be obtained (e.g., a T_3 uptake).
    Biochemical findings that suggest hypothyroidism: The laboratory evaluation consists of the quantitation of T_4 (total T_4 or free T_4) and TSH. A low T_4 level and an elevated TSH level are diagnostic of hypothyroidism.

97. **What signs and symptoms in an infant suggest congenital hypothyroidism?**
See Table 6-6.

Table 6-6. Symptoms and Signs of Hypothyroidism in Infancy

SYMPTOMS	SIGNS
Lethargy	Hypotonia, slow reflexes
Poor feeding	Jaundice (prolonged)
Constipation	Mottling
Poor weight gain	Distended abdomen
Cold extremities	Acrocyanosis
Hoarse cry	Coarse features
	Large fontanels, wide sutures

98. **What causes congenital hypothyroidism?**
- *Primary:* Agenesis or dysgenesis, ectopic, dyshormonogenesis
- *Secondary:* Hypopituitarism, hypothalamic abnormality
- *Other:* Transient, maternal factors (e.g., goitrogen ingestion, iodide deficiency)
    The most common cause of permanent primary congenital hypothyroidism is thyroid dysgenesis, or failure of the gland to develop properly. Ectopic thyroid gland location accounts for two-thirds of thyroid dysgenesis followed by aplasia or hypoplastic gland. The second most common cause is thyroid dyshormonogenesis, which is a defect in thyroid hormone production. Thyroid dysgenesis accounts for 85% of permanent primary congenital hypothyroidism; inborn errors of thyroid hormone biosynthesis comprise 10% to 15% of cases.

LaFranchi S: Approach to diagnosis and treatment of neonatal hypothyroidism, *J Clin Endocrinol Metab* 96:2959–2967, 2011.

99. **How effective are screening programs for congenital hypothyroidism?**
    Screening programs correctly identify 90% to 95% of children who are affected with congenital
    hypothyroidism. Screening programs are most likely to miss infants with large ectopic glands, those
    with partial defects in thyroidal hormone biosynthesis, and those with secondary (pituitary or
    hypothalamic) disease. If an infant presents with a clinical picture of hypothyroidism and has had a normal
    newborn screen, it is important to realize that the false-negative rate of the screening is up to 10%.

    Grüters A, Krude H: Detection and treatment of congenital hypothyroidism, *Nat Rev Endocrinol* 8:104–113, 2011.

100. **Discuss the risks of delaying treatment for congenital hypothyroidism.**
    Therapy should begin as early as possible because outcome is related to the time treatment is
    started. Because less than 20% of patients will have distinctive clinical signs at 3 to 4 weeks of
    age, screening is now performed on all newborns in the United States at 2 to 3 days of age, and
    most affected children are started on therapy before they are 1 month old. Many pediatricians
    and screening programs undertake a second screen at 2 weeks of age to ensure that children
    with treatable conditions are not missed. The prognosis for intellectual development is directly
    related to the amount of time from birth to the initiation of therapy, and there is an inverse
    relationship between age of diagnosis/treatment and intelligence quotient (IQ). In a literature
    review of 11 studies that evaluated starting treatment at an earlier age (12 to 30 days of life)
    compared with a later age (>30 days of life), infants started at an earlier age averaged 15.7
    IQ points higher than infants started at a later age.

    LaFranchi SH, Austin J: How should we be treating children with congenital hypothyroidism? *J Pediatr Endocrinol* 2007,
    (5):559–578.

101. **A suspected goiter (diffuse enlargement of the thyroid gland) is noted during a
    routine examination of an asymptomatic 7-year-old boy. What should be the
    course of action?**
    The evaluation of a child with goiter (Fig. 6-4) is generally straightforward. In the absence of signs of
    thyroidal disease, history should be obtained regarding recent exposure to iodine or other halogens.
    A family history should be obtained regarding thyroidal disease because thyroiditis tends to run in families.
    The initial laboratory evaluation typically includes T_4, TSH, and antithyroidal antibodies. If there is discrete
    nodularity within the thyroid or the gland is rock hard or tender, further diagnostic evaluation (ultrasound,
    CT) may be indicated. Parathyroid enlargement or lymphoma may be misdiagnosed as goiter.

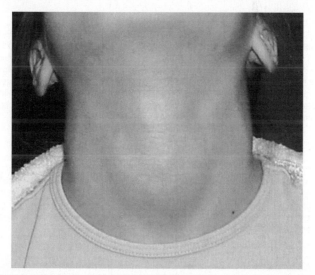

Figure 6-4. Goiter. Note the enlarged thyroid gland in a patient with Hashimoto thyroiditis, easily visualized with neck extension.
(From Zitelli BJ, McIntire SC, Nowalk AJ: Atlas of Pediatric Physical Diagnosis, ed 6. Philadelphia, 2012, Saunders, pp 369–400.)

102. **What is the most common cause of acquired hypothyroidism in childhood?**
The most common cause is chronic lymphocytic thyroiditis, also called *Hashimoto thyroiditis* or *autoimmune thyroiditis* and usually occurs early to mid puberty. Its incidence during adolescence is about 1% to 2%. The female-to-male ratio is 2:1.

Counts D, Varma SK: Hypothyroidism in children, *Pediatr Rev* 30:251–257, 2009.

103. **What is the most common clinical presentation of Hashimoto thyroiditis?**
Although symptoms of hypothyroidism or hyperthyroidism may be present, most pediatric patients are asymptomatic, and the condition is detected by the presence of goiter. The diagnosis of Hashimoto thyroiditis is primarily based on the demonstration of antithyroidal antibodies. Clinical manifestations may include a linear growth decline, fatigue, constipation, poor school performance, irregular menstrual periods, and cold intolerance.

Counts D, Varma SK: Hypothyroidism in children, *Pediatr Rev* 30:251–257, 2009.
Pearce EN, Farwell AP, Braverman LE: Thyroiditis, *N Engl J Med* 348:2646–2655, 2003.

104. **What should a parent be told about the prognosis of a child who has euthyroid goiter caused by chronic lymphocytic thyroiditis?**
About 50% of all children who present with symptoms of euthyroid goiter will have resolution of the goiter over several years, regardless of whether thyroxine replacement is given. It is difficult to predict which children will recover completely, which will remain euthyroid with goiter, and which will become hypothyroid. Large goiters and increased thyroglobulin at presentation, together with an increase in thyroid peroxidase antibody and TSH levels over time, are the most significant predictors for the development of hypothyroidism. Any child identified with thyroid disease should have T_4 and TSH values monitored every 4 to 6 months.

Radetti G: The natural history of euthyroid Hashimoto's thyroiditis in children, *J Pediatr* 149:827–832, 2006.

105. **What other autoimmune diseases are associated with chronic lymphocytic thyroiditis?**
Adrenal insufficiency, diabetes mellitus, juvenile idiopathic arthritis, systemic lupus erythematosus, rheumatoid arthritis, myasthenia gravis, idiopathic thrombocytopenia purpura, and autoimmune polyendocrine syndrome (type II)

106. **What does a normal T_4 and an elevated TSH suggest?**
The diagnosis of hypothyroidism is based on finding both a low T_4 level and an elevated TSH level. However, on occasion, the T_4 level can be maintained in a normal range by increased stimulation of the thyroid gland by TSH. This combination of laboratory values is suggestive of a failing thyroid and is referred to as *compensated hypothyroidism*. Because TSH is the most useful physiologic marker for the adequacy of a circulating level of thyroid hormone, an elevated TSH level is an indication for thyroid replacement therapy. If the TSH level is only minimally elevated and the child is asymptomatic, it is worthwhile to wait 4 to 6 weeks and repeat the T_4 and TSH tests before instituting therapy.

107. **What is the most common cause of hyperthyroidism in children?**
More than 95% of hyperthyroidism cases are due to Graves disease, a multisystem disease that is characterized by hyperthyroidism; infiltrative ophthalmopathy; and occasionally, an infiltrative dermopathy. The features of this disease may occur singly or in any combination. In children, the ophthalmopathy appears to be less severe, and the dermopathy is rare; the full syndrome may never develop. There has been a tendency to use the terms *Graves disease*, *thyrotoxicosis*, and *hyperthyroidism* interchangeably, but there are other causes of hyperthyroidism in childhood (e.g., factitious).

Léger J: Graves' disease in children, *Endocr Dev* 26:171–182, 2014.
Brown RS. Autoimmune thyroid disease: unlocking a complex puzzle. *Curr Opin Pediatr* 2009:21(4):523–528.

108. **In addition to Graves disease, what conditions may cause hyperthyroidism?**
    - *Excess TSH:* TSH-producing tumor (these are extraordinarily rare in children)
    - *Thyroid autonomy:* Adenoma, multinodular goiter, activating mutations of G proteins (e.g., McCune-Albright syndrome)
    - *Thyroid inflammation:* Subacute thyroiditis, Hashimoto thyroiditis
    - *Exogenous hormone:* Medication, ectopic production

109. **Describe the typical features of hyperthyroidism that occur as a result of Graves disease.**
    - **History:** The onset of symptoms is usually gradual, with increasing emotional lability, shortened attention span, and deteriorating school performance. Sleep disturbance, nervousness, headache, and weight loss despite increased appetite may be noted, as may easy fatigability and heat intolerance. Observation of the child's behavior while the history is being obtained from the parent is often instructive.
    - **Physical examination:** Weight may be low for height, and many children will be tall for age and genetic potential. Some children will have an acceleration in growth rate at the same time that their behavior begins to deteriorate. The pulse rate is usually inappropriately high for age. A widened pulse pressure or an elevated blood pressure is often noted, although this is a more variable finding in children than in adults.

110. **What causes Graves disease?**
    Graves disease is an autoimmune disorder in which TSH receptor antibodies bind to the TSH receptor, thereby resulting in the stimulation of thyroid hormone production and subsequent hyperthyroidism. Most thyroid receptor antibodies belong to the IgG class. The general name used for these antibodies is human thyroid-stimulating immunoglobulins (HTSI or TSI). These were formerly called long-acting thyroid stimulators (LATS).

KEY POINTS: THYROID DISORDERS

1. Midline neck masses usually involve the thyroid gland or thyroid remnants, such as a thyroglossal duct cyst.
2. Neck extension improves visualization and palpation of thyroid masses, especially with swallowing.
3. About 20% to 40% of solitary thyroid nodules in adolescents are malignant; expedited evaluation is needed.
4. Chronic lymphocytic thyroiditis is the most common cause of pediatric goiter in the United States.
5. Chronic lymphocytic thyroiditis most commonly appears as an asymptomatic goiter, thereby reinforcing the need for thyroid palpation (an often overlooked examination feature).
6. The best initial screening studies for hypothyroidism and hyperthyroidism are total T_4 and thyroid-stimulating hormone.

111. **Why does exophthalmos occur in Graves disease?**
    Exophthalmos is a bulging of the eye anteriorly (Fig. 6-5). The reason is unknown, but several facts suggest an autoimmune process:
    - Histologic studies reveal lymphocytic infiltration of the retrobulbar muscles.
    - Circulating lymphocytes are sensitized to an antigen that is unique to the retrobulbar tissues.
    - The thyroglobulin-antithyroglobulin antibody complexes found in patients with Graves disease bind specifically to the extraorbital muscles. There may be a separate class of antibodies that is responsible for changes in the retrobulbar muscles.

Bahn RS: Graves' ophthalmopathy, *New Engl J Med* 362:726–738, 2010.

112. **What treatment options are available for children with Graves disease?**
    The three types of therapy are antithyroid medication, radioactive (^{131}I) ablation, and subtotal thyroidectomy.

Léger J: Graves' disease in children, *Endocr Dev* 26:171–182, 2014.
Bauer AJ: Approach to the pediatric patient with Graves' disease: when is definitive therapy warranted? *J Clin Endocrinol Metab* 96:580–588, 2011.

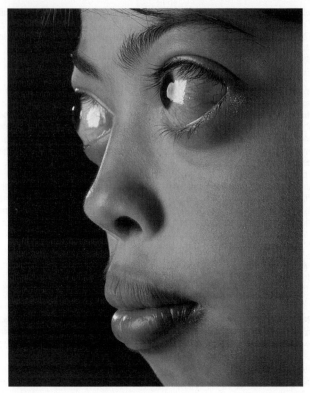

Figure 6-5. Exophthalmos in a young woman with Graves disease. *(From Moshang T Jr:* Pediatric Endocrinology: The Requisites in Pediatrics. *Philadelphia, 2005, Elsevier Mosby, p 7.)*

113. **Describe the principal modes of actions and the side effects of medications used to treat Graves disease.**

The thioamide derivatives—*propylthiouracil* and *methimazole*—have historically been the keystones of long-term management. However, their effective onset of action is slow because they block the synthesis but not the release of thyroid hormone. *Propranolol* is useful for treating many of the β-adrenergic effects of hyperthyroidism. It is used during the acute management of Graves disease but should be discontinued when the thyroid disease is controlled. *Iodide* (which can transiently block thyroid hormone release) and *glucocorticoids* are useful stopgap medications while awaiting the inhibitory effects of the thioamide; they are generally used only when the patient is acutely symptomatic (i.e., thyroid storm).

The thioamides are associated with side effects, the most serious of which have been a lupuslike syndrome involving the lungs or liver, thrombocytopenia, neutropenia, agranulocytosis, and hepatitis with elevated transaminase levels. The association of propylthiouracil and severe liver failure led to the issuing of a black box warning from the Food and Drug Administration in 2010, with methimazole now the preferred antithyroid medication option.

Rivkees SA: Pediatric Graves' disease: management in the post-propylthiouracil era, *Int J Pediatr Endocrinol* 2014:10, 2014.

114. **Has radioactive iodide fallen into disfavor as a treatment option for Graves disease?**

On the contrary, radioactive iodide (^{131}I) is increasing in popularity. In some pediatric endocrinology centers, this is now considered the first line of therapy. Concern had been voiced about the possible risk for thyroid carcinoma, leukemia, thyroid nodules, or genetic mutations, but as the individuals treated with ^{131}I during childhood have been followed for prolonged periods, experience suggests that children are not at a significantly increased risk for developing these conditions.

Rivkees SA: Pediatric Graves' disease: management in the post-propylthiouracil era, *Int J Pediatr Endocrinol* 2014:10, 2014.

115. **During a routine physical examination, a solitary thyroid nodule is palpated on an asymptomatic 10-year-old child. Can a wait-and-see approach be taken?**
Absolutely not. In children with a solitary nodule, about 20% to 40% have a carcinoma, 20% to 30% have an adenoma, and the remainder will have thyroid abscess, thyroid cyst, multinodular goiter, Hashimoto thyroiditis, subacute thyroiditis, or nonthyroidal neck mass. Given the relatively high incidence of carcinoma, a thyroidal mass demands prompt evaluation. Previous irradiation to the head or neck is associated with a significantly increased incidence of thyroid carcinoma. A family history of thyroid disease increases the likelihood of chronic lymphocytic thyroiditis or Graves disease. The presence of tenderness on palpation or high titers of antithyroid antibodies points away from a malignant process. However, in all cases, radiologic studies should be undertaken; in many cases, surgical exploration is required.

116. **How should this solitary thyroid nodule be investigated?**
The principal tools used in the investigation of a thyroid mass include ^{123}I scanning and ultrasound. Ultrasound is useful for delineating the size of the mass, its anatomic relationship to the rest of the thyroid, and the presence of cystic structures. [123]I imaging that reveals a single nonfunctioning mass ("cold" nodule) suggests a carcinoma or adenoma and is a clear indication for surgery. Patchy uptake is more characteristic of chronic lymphocytic thyroiditis, whereas a poorly functioning lobe may be found in a subacute thyroiditis. Fine-needle aspiration or biopsy is another approach to the investigation of a thyroid mass with current recommendations for aspiration of thyroid nodules ≥ 1 cm with ultrasound guidance improving diagnostic accuracy.

Gupta A, Ly S: A standardized assessment of thyroid nodules in children confirms higher cancer prevalence than in adults, *J Clin Endocrinol Metab* 98:3238–3245, 2013.
Mehanna HM, Jain A, Morton RP, et al: Investigating the thyroid nodule, *BMJ* 338:705–709, 2009.

117. **How is the euthyroid sick syndrome diagnosed?**
Euthyroid sick syndrome, also called *nonthyroidal illness syndrome*, is an adaptive response to slow body metabolism often seen in critical illness. It is also called the low T_3 syndrome because the most consistent finding is a depression of serum T_3. Reverse T_3, a metabolically inactive metabolite, is increased, although this is rarely measured. T_4 and thyroid binding globulin levels may be low or normal; free T_4 and TSH levels are normal. In sick preterm infants, the clinical picture is often confusing because levels of T_4, free T_4, and T_3 are naturally low. Infants and children with the euthyroid sick syndrome generally revert to normal as the primary illness resolves.

Marks SD: Nonthyroidal illness syndrome in children, *Endocrine* 36:355–367, 2009.

Acknowledgment

We would like to thank Dr. Daniel E. Hale for his significant contributions to this text as one of the original authors of the chapter.

CHAPTER 7

GASTROENTEROLOGY

Chris A. Liacouras, MD, Danielle Wendel, MD, Candi Jump, MD, Maire Conrad, MD, MS, Noah J.F. Hoffman, MD, Elizabeth C. Maxwell, MD, Amanda Muir, MD and Orith Waisbourd-Zinman, MD

CLINICAL ISSUES

1. What is the definition of failure to thrive?
   Failure to thrive (FTT) is a sign, not a diagnosis or a syndrome. It is a term that describes either weight loss or poor weight gain. In more severe cases linear growth and head circumference can be affected. Some specific FTT growth chart–based definitions for children <2 years of age include (1) weight below the 3rd and 5th percentile for age on more than one occasion, (2) weight declines two or more major percentile lines, (3) weight <80% of the ideal weight for age, and (4) a child below the 3rd or 5th percentile on the weight-for-length curve.

   Jaffe AC: Failure to thrive: current clinical concepts, *Pediatr Rev* 32:100–107, 2011.

2. What is the differential diagnosis of FTT?
   The causes of FTT can be divided into the following groups:
   *   **Inadequate nutritional intake**: not enough food offered, child not taking in enough, excessive juice, formula dilution
   *   **Malabsorption/loss**: gastrointestinal (GI) mucosal disease, pancreatic dysfunction, cholestatic liver disease, persistent vomiting
   *   **Increased metabolic demand**: congenital heart disease, chronic lung disease, chronic renal failure, acidosis, congenital or chronic infections, chronic systemic disease, genetic syndromes.

   Jaffe AC: Failure to thrive: current clinical concepts, *Pediatr Rev* 32:100–107, 2011.

3. How is FTT evaluated?
   The most important aspect of the evaluation for FTT is the history and physical examination. History should address feeding, stooling, developmental, psychosocial, and family history. The examination should also focus on any findings that suggest a malformation. Laboratory testing is rarely useful, but may include a complete blood count (CBC) basic metabolic profile (BMP), urinalysis, urine culture, and lead level.

4. What features of history or on physical examination suggest a medical condition leading to FTT?
   History: Recurrent vomiting, chronic diarrhea, frequent infections, and failure to gain weight despite adequate caloric intake
   Exam: Dysmorphic features, cardiac exam abnormalities, organomegaly or lymphadenopathy

5. How is the diagnosis of "pinworms" made?
   Direct visualization of larger adult worms in the perianal region of a child can sometimes be successful, with the best examination time 2 to 3 hours after the child is asleep. Additionally, **transparent adhesive tape** can be applied to the perianal region to collect eggs; the tape can be examined under low-power microscopy (Fig. 7-1). These specimens are best obtained in the morning. Because few pinworm ova are present in stool, examination of stool specimens for ova and parasites (for pinworms) is not recommended.

   American Academy of Pediatrics: Pinworm infection. In Pickering LK, editor: *2012 Red Book: Report of the Committee on Infectious Diseases*, ed 29. Elk Grove Park, IL, 2012, American Academy of Pediatrics, pp 566–567.

220

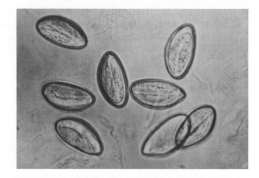

Figure 7-1. Pinworm eggs as collected on adhesive tape. *(From the Public Health Image Library, Centers for Disease Control and Prevention: http://phil.cdc.gov.)*

6. **What characterizes functional abdominal pain in children?**

   Previously called *recurrent abdominal pain*, this entity is common in pediatric practice and refers to children without evidence of inflammatory, anatomic, infectious, allergic, metabolic, or neoplastic processes that explain the symptoms. The cause is likely multifactorial, including abnormalities in the enteric nervous system with possible visceral hyperalgesia or a decreased threshold for pain in response to changes in intraluminal pressure secondary to physiologic stimuli. This combination of biopsychosocial mechanisms (physiologic, psychological, and behavioral) results in a broad range of management approaches.

7. **In children with abdominal pain, what historical features suggest a possible organic or serious cause?**

   - Involuntary weight loss
   - Deceleration of linear growth
   - GI blood loss
   - Significant vomiting (e.g., bilious emesis, hematemesis, protracted vomiting, cyclical vomiting, pattern concerning to physician)
   - Chronic severe diarrhea
   - Alarm signs on abdominal examination (right upper or lower quadrant tenderness, localized fullness or mass effect, peritoneal signs, hepatomegaly, splenomegaly, costovertebral angle tenderness)
   - Unexplained fevers
   - Family history of inflammatory bowel disease or other significant GI illnesses
   - Presentation of symptoms before 4 years or after 15 years of age

Rasquin A, DiLorenzo C, Forbes D, et al: Childhood functional gastrointestinal disorders: child/adolescent, *Gastroenterology* 130:1527–1537, 2006.
Di Lorenzo C, Colletti RB, Lehmann HP, et al: Chronic abdominal pain in children: a clinical report of the American Academy of Pediatrics and North American Society for Pediatric Gastroenterology, Hepatology, and Nutrition, *J Pediatr Gastroenterol Nutr* 40:245–248, 2005.

8. **What treatments are used for functional abdominal pain in children?**

   - **Dietary:** Low-lactose diets, dietary fiber, low-fructose diets, probiotics
   - **Pharmacologic:** Antidepressants, antispasmodics, prokinetic agents, H2-receptor antagonists, leukotriene-receptor antagonists
   - **Psychological:** Cognitive behavioral therapy, family intervention, relaxation and distraction techniques
   - **Complementary and alternative medicine:** Herbal medicine, peppermint oil, biofeedback, hypnotherapy, massage therapy, acupuncture

Whitfield KL, Shulman RJ: Treatment options for functional gastrointestinal disorders, *Pediatr Ann* 38:288–294, 2009.
Banez GA: Chronic abdominal pain in children: what to do following the medical evaluation, *Curr Opin Pediatr* 20:571–575, 2008.

9. **What is intractable singultus?**

   Persistent hiccups. Hiccups result from involuntary, spasmodic contracture of the diaphragm accompanied by a sudden closure of the glottis. Persistent hiccups can be a diagnostic and therapeutic challenge with a broad differential diagnosis including some central nervous system (CNS) possibilities, such as seizures and tumors.

Chang FY, Lu CL: Hiccup: mystery, nature and treatment, *J Neurogastroenterol Motil* 18:123–130, 2012.

10. **What is the most commonly ingested foreign body?**

    Coins account for more than 20,000 visits yearly to emergency departments in the United States. Symptomatic patients are more likely to have the coin lodged in the esophagus, although a significant portion of these patients may be asymptomatic. Coins lodged in the esophagus should be removed endoscopically within 24 hours because of the risk for ulceration and perforation.

11. **Which is potentially more dangerous after ingestion: a penny made in 1977 or one made in 1987?**

    The penny from 1987. In 1982, the composition of pennies changed. Coins minted after that date have higher concentrations of zinc, which is more corrosive and potentially more harmful after prolonged contact with stomach acid.

12. **What is the difference radiographically between a coin in the esophagus and a coin in the trachea?**

    A coin in the esophagus appears *en face* in the anteroposterior view (sagittal plane), whereas a coin in the trachea appears *en face* on the lateral view (coronal plane) (Fig. 7-2). This occurs because the cartilaginous ring of the trachea is open posteriorly, but the opening of the esophagus is widest in the transverse position.

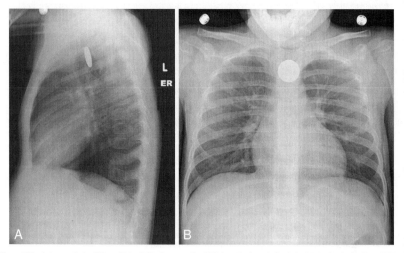

Figure 7-2. Anteroposterior (AP) and lateral chest x-rays of a child show the ingested coin in the proximal esophagus. *(From Ginsberg CG, Gostout CJ, Kochman M, Norton ID, editors:* Clinical Gastrointestinal Endoscopy, *ed 4. Philadelphia, Saunders/ Elsevier, 2012, p 231.)*

13. **Why is ingestion of a button battery more dangerous than ingestion of a coin?**

    Button batteries, like coins, often become lodged in the esophagus. If this happens they are capable of causing significant mucosal burns very quickly (sometimes in a matter of hours). In severe cases, batteries can erode through the wall of the esophagus and into surrounding structures including the aorta. This can lead to fatal hemorrhage. For this reason, if there is *any* suspicion that there is a button battery stuck in the esophagus, it must be removed emergently. Button batteries that reach the stomach do not pose as much risk but should be followed to ensure passage and removed if they do not pass out of the stomach within 2 to 3 days. It is also always important to determine the type of button battery ingested.

14. **Which is more dangerous, 2 magnets that are swallowed together or 2 magnets that are swallowed separately?**
Although swallowed magnets in any form always pose a significant risk, magnets that are swallowed **separately** pose greater risk. Magnets swallowed together usually attract (stick together) while magnets swallowed separately have the potential to migrate down the bowel separately and subsequently stick to each other across loops of bowel, leading to perforation.

Hussain SZ, Bousvaros A, et al: Management of ingested magnets in children, *J Pediatr Gastroenterol Nutr* 55:239–242, 2012.

15. **What are the indications for emergent foreign body removal?**
In general, any object(s) swallowed that may be "stuck in the esophagus" based on symptoms (chest pain, odynophagia, dysphagia, epigastric pain, drooling etc.), including meat impactions, should be removed emergently. Most sharp objects in the stomach should be emergently removed. Objects larger than 2.5 cm wide and 5 cm long are unlikely to pass through the pylorus and should be removed. Patients who report *any* symptoms (vomiting, pain, fever, dysphagia) need emergent evaluation even if the object is in the stomach or intestine.

16. **What is the grim news about Rapunzel syndrome?**
Rapunzel syndrome, which results from trichotillomania, is a trichobezoar (a bezoar formed from hair) that can form a cast outline of the stomach and small intestine and over time may extend into the small bowel. **Surgical removal** is typically the only therapeutic option for removing large trichobezoars such as those seen in the Rapunzel syndrome.

Gonuguntla V, Joshi D-D: Rapunzel syndrome: a comprehensive review of an unusual case of trichobezoar, *Clin Med Res* 7:99–102, 2009.

17. **What is the most common clinical presentation of juvenile polyps in children?**
Painless, rectal bleeding. Up to one-third of patients can have chronic blood loss with microcytic anemia. The peak prevalence in children is between 1 and 7 years of age. The polyps are most commonly found in the rectum. Large polyps can be the lead point for intussusception.

18. **What are the types of colonic polyps?**
- **Malignant:** Polyps with cells that have lost their normal differentiation (including adenomas, some of which have ability to become cancerous)
- **Hamartomatous:** Benign focal malformations composed of tissue elements normally found at that site but growing in a disorganized manner
- **Hyperplastic:** A serrated polyp without malignant potential
- **Inflammatory:** Polyps associated with inflammatory bowel diseases

19. **Why is it important to confirm a diagnosis of juvenile polyposis?**
Juvenile polyposis syndrome is defined by 5 or more polyps in the colon/rectum and 1 or more affected family members. This disorder is inherited in an autosomal dominant fashion. It is common (up to 12%) in patients with symptomatic polyps, especially with right colonic polyps, anemia, and adenomas rather than hamartomas. The importance of establishing a diagnosis of a polyposis syndrome is that some syndromes (e.g., Peutz-Jeghers and juvenile polyposis coli) are associated with a **risk for developing adenocarcinoma**, with an incidence as high as 30% in as

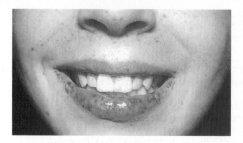

Figure 7-3. Macular pigmented lesions in patient with Peutz-Jeghers syndrome. *(From Kliegman RM, Stanton BF, St. Geme JW, et al, editors: Nelson Textbook of Pediatrics, ed 19. Philadelphia, 2011, Saunders, p 1362.e5.)*

few as 10 years after diagnosis. Another feature of Peutz-Jeghers syndrome is the presence of characteristic small, dark-colored spots (melanosis) on the lips, inside the mouth, and near the eyes and nostrils (Fig. 7-3).

Brosens LAA, Langeveld D, et al: Juvenile polyposis syndrome, *World J Gastroenterol* 17:4839–4844, 2011.

20. **How is ascites diagnosed by physical examination?**
    Severe ascites is commonly diagnosed by observation of the child in a supine and then an upright position. Bulging flanks, umbilical protrusion, and scrotal edema (in males) are generally evident. Three main techniques are used when the diagnosis is not obvious:
    - **Fluid wave:** This sign can be elicited in a cooperative patient by tapping sharply on one flank while receiving the wave with the other hand. The transmission of the wave through fatty tissue should be blocked by a hand placed on the center of the abdomen.
    - **Shifting dullness:** With the patient supine, percussion of the abdomen will demonstrate a central area of tympany at the top that is surrounded by flank percussion dullness. This dullness shifts when the patient moves laterally or stands up.
    - **"Puddle sign":** A cooperative and mobile patient may be examined in the knee-chest position. The pool of ascites is tapped while you listen for a sloshing sound or change in sound transmission with the stethoscope.

    Small amounts of ascites can be extremely difficult to detect with physical examination in children. Although ascites can be demonstrated on radiographs, the most sensitive and specific test is an abdominal-pelvic ultrasound, which can detect as little as 150 mL of ascitic fluid.

CONSTIPATION

21. **What constitutes constipation in childhood?**
    Constipation is defined as a delay or difficulty in defecation, present for 2 or more weeks and sufficient to cause distress in the patient. Normal stool frequency varies from several times a day to three stools per week. In children, constipation should be considered when the normal stooling pattern becomes more infrequent, when stools become hard or are difficult to expel, or when the child exhibits withholding patterns or behavioral changes toward moving his or her bowels. Soiling (encopresis) can be a sign of constipation.

Auth MKH, Vora R, Farrelly P, et al: Childhood constipation, *BMJ* 345:e7609, 2012.

22. **What features suggest an organic etiology for constipation?**
    - History of weight loss or inadequate weight gain
    - Lumbosacral nevi or sinus
    - Multiple café-au-lait spots
    - Abnormal neurologic examination (decreased tone, strength; abnormal reflexes)
    - Anal abnormalities (anteriorly displaced, patulous, or tight)

- Gross or occult blood in stool
- Abdominal distention with or without vomiting

Croffie JM, Fitzgerald JF: Constipation and irritable bowel syndrome. In Liacouras CA, Piccoli DA, editors: *Pediatric Gastroenterology: The Requisites in Pediatrics.* Philadelphia, 2008, Mosby Elsevier, p 33.

23. **What is the most important component of the physical examination when evaluating constipation?**

    The rectal examination. The presence of large amounts of stool in the rectal vault almost always indicates functional constipation. Lack of stool in the rectal vault could indicate recent evacuation; if expulsion of stool occurs after removal of the examining finger, Hirschsprung disease should be considered. Failure to perform a rectal examination is a common omission during the evaluation of children, and impaction in chronic constipation often goes undetected.

Safder S: Digital rectal examination and the primary care physicians: a lost art? *Clin Pediatr* 45:411–414, 2006.
Gold DM, Levine J, Weinstein TA, et al: Frequency of digital rectal examination in children with chronic constipation, *Arch Pediatr Adolesc Med* 153:377–379, 1999.

24. **What are some common triggers of constipation in healthy infants and children?**
    - **Introduction of solid foods or cow milk**: Diet may be low in fiber and not provide adequate fluid intake.
    - **Inadequate toilet training**: Toddlers may not respond appropriately to the need to defecate or may not have adequate foot support needed for effective evacuation of stool if using an adult-sized toilet. If passage of stool is painful, toddlers can begin to withhold stool. If stool is not made softer by increasing fiber and/or fluids in the diet or by stool softeners, this pattern can continue.
    - **School entry:** Children may be reluctant to use the toilet at school, leading to a pattern of stool withholding, painful stools, and constipation.

Borowitz SM, Cox DJ, Tam A, et al: Precipitants of constipation during early childhood, *J Am Board Fam Pract* 16:213–218, 2013.

KEY POINTS: CONSTIPATION

1. Ninety-nine percent of full-term infants pass stool less than 24 hours after birth. Failure to pass stool within the first 48 hours of life should be considered pathologic until proved otherwise.
2. The rectal examination is a common omission among patients undergoing an evaluation for constipation. Tone, the amount of stool, and the size of the rectal vault should be assessed.
3. Fecal soiling is almost always associated with severe functional constipation and not Hirschsprung disease.
4. Treatment of functional constipation is multimodal and includes medications.
5. Organic causes are suggested by weight loss, lumbosacral nevi, anal abnormalities, blood in stool, and abdominal distention.

25. **Which clinical features differentiate chronic retentive constipation from Hirschsprung disease?**

    See Table 7-1.

26. **How is Hirschsprung disease diagnosed?**

    Hirschsprung disease results from the failure of normal migration of ganglion cell precursors to their location in the GI tract during gestation. The diagnosis can be made by obtaining an unprepped **barium enema**, which will demonstrate a change in the caliber of the large intestine at the site where normal bowel meets aganglionic bowel (transition zone) (Fig. 7-4). An unprepped barium enema is required because the use of cleansing enemas can dilate the abnormal portion of the

Table 7-1. Clinical Distinctions Between Chronic Retentive Constipation and Hirschsprung Disease

CLINICAL FEATURE	FUNCTIONAL CONSTIPATION	HIRSCHSPRUNG DISEASE
Age of onset	>1 yr	<1 yr
Passage of meconium	Within 24 hr	Meconium passes after 24 hr
Abdominal pain	Frequent, colicky	Rare
Stool size	Large	Small, ribbonlike
Stool withholding behavior	Present	Absent
Encopresis (soiling)	Present	Very rare
Rectum	Filled with stool	Empty
Rectal examination	Stool in rectum	Explosive passage of stool
Growth	Normal	Poor

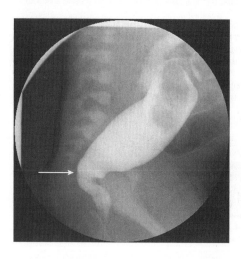

Figure 7-4. Contrast enema in a newborn with Hirschsprung disease. Note the transition zone *(arrow)* as the more dilated proximal colon tapers to a more narrow distal colon at the rectosigmoid junction. *(From Liacouras CA, Piccoli DA:* Pediatric Gastroenterology: The Requisites in Pediatrics, *Philadelphia, 2005, Elsevier Mosby, p 1170.)*

colon and remove some of the distal impaction, thereby resulting in a false-negative result. After the study, the retention of barium for 24 or more hours is suggestive of Hirschsprung disease or a significant motility disorder. This study is less reliable in a child younger than 6 months. **Rectal suction biopsies** or **full-thickness surgical biopsies** will confirm the absence of ganglion cells. Anal manometry is less reliable in children; in small infants, it requires specialized equipment.

27. What is the most common cause of encopresis?
    Encopresis, or fecal soiling, may be defined as the involuntary passage of fecal material in an otherwise healthy and normal child. The most common cause is **functional constipation with overflow incontinence.** Children with encopresis typically sense no urge to defecate. Fecal soiling is almost always associated with severe functional constipation.

28. How should children with chronic constipation and encopresis be managed?
    - The rectosigmoid colon should be **aggressively cleansed** of fecal material. Manual disimpaction is sometimes required. Multiple enemas over multiple days are commonly needed. Adult enemas should be used in children who are older than 3 years.

- Medications that act as an **osmotic laxative** by drawing fluid into the intestine to promote the passage of soft stools include polyethylene glycol powder and lactulose (a nonabsorbable sugar). Other osmotic agents, such as sorbitol and magnesium citrate, can be considered. For cases of long-standing functional constipation, osmotic laxatives should be continued for a minimum of several months while the dilated rectum returns to normal size.
- An **oral lubricant**, such as mineral oil, can help promote the continued passage of stool but can contribute to accidental soiling. In difficult cases, **stimulant medications**, such as bisacodyl or senna, can be substituted for short-term use.
- It is extremely important to **educate** patients and parents about the mechanics of the disorder. A high-fiber diet, possible limitation of dairy and complex carbohydrates, defined periods of toilet sitting (2 to 3 times daily for 10 minutes after meals), and a behavior modification system that rewards normal bowel movements are essential for eventual success. Integrative approaches of biofeedback, relaxation strategies, and mental imagery have been used for children who have severe "defecation anxiety." A goal is one to two soft bowel movements a day. Relapses are common.

Har AF, Croffie JM: Encopresis, *Pediatr Rev* 31:368–374, 2010.

DIARRHEA AND MALABSORPTION

29. **What time frame distinguishes acute and chronic diarrhea?**
Diarrhea is the frequent (>3 times per day) evacuation of liquid feces. *Acute* diarrhea is often self-limiting and lasts for a few days. Diarrhea is considered *chronic* when lasting >3 weeks.

30. **What is the most common cause worldwide of epidemic diarrhea?**
Norovirus. These single-stranded RNA viruses are believed to be responsible for at least 50% of all gastroenteritis outbreaks worldwide and a major cause of foodborne illness. With the widespread use of rotavirus vaccination, norovirus has become the most common cause of medically attended acute gastroenteritis in children <5 years in the United States.

Payne DC, Vinjé J, Szilagyi PG, et al: Norovirus and medically-attended gastroenteritis in the U.S. children, *N Engl J Med* 368:1121–1130, 2013.
Hall AJ, Vinjé J, Lopman B, et al: Updated Norovirus outbreak management and disease prevention guidelines, *MMWR* 60 (RR03):1–15, 2011.

31. **What are other common causes of acute diarrhea?**
- Viral (others include rotavirus, enterovirus)
- Bacterial (e.g., *Escherichia coli*, *Shigella*, *Salmonella*, *Yersinia*, *Campylobacter*, *Clostridium difficile*)
- Protozoal
- Allergic
- Medication side effect (e.g., antibiotic usage)
- Extra-intestinal infections (e.g., respiratory, urinary, sepsis)

32. **Which historical questions are key when seeking the cause of diarrhea?**
- Recent medications, especially antibiotics
- History of immunosuppression (e.g., recurrent major infections, history of malnutrition, acquired immunodeficiency syndrome, immunosuppressive medications)
- Illnesses in other family members or close contacts
- Travel outside of the United States
- Travel to rural or seacoast areas (i.e., involving the consumption of untreated water, raw milk, or raw shellfish)
- Attendance in day care
- Recent foods particularly focus on juice and fructose consumption
- Presence of family pets
- Food preparation and water source

Thielman NM, Guerrant RL: Acute infectious diarrhea, *N Engl J Med* 350:38–47, 2004.

33. **In what settings can diarrhea be a severe, life-threatening illness?**
    Severe diarrhea of any cause can lead to dehydration, which can cause significant morbidity and mortality. However, diarrhea can be a sign of a serious associated illness, which in itself can be life-threatening:
    - Intussusception
    - *Salmonella* gastroenteritis (neonatal or compromised host)
    - Hemolytic-uremic syndrome
    - Hirschsprung disease (with toxic megacolon)
    - Pseudomembranous colitis (classically due to *C. difficile*)
    - Inflammatory bowel disease (with toxic megacolon)

Fleisher GR: Diarrhea. In Fleisher GR, Ludwig S, editors: *Textbook of Pediatric Emergency Medicine*, ed 6. Philadelphia, 2010, Wolters Kluwer, p 213.

34. **Why is true diarrhea during the first few days of life especially concerning?**
    In addition to the greater potential for dehydration in a newborn, diarrhea in this age group is more commonly associated with major congenital intestinal defects involving electrolyte transport (e.g., congenital sodium- or chloride-losing diarrhea), carbohydrate absorption (e.g., congenital lactase deficiency), immune-mediated defects (e.g., autoimmune enteropathy), or those characterized by villous blunting (e.g., microvillus inclusion disease). Although viral enteritis can occur in the nursery, any newborn with true diarrhea warrants thorough evaluation and possible referral to a tertiary center.

Sherman PM, Mitchell DJ, Cutz E: Neonatal enteropathies: defining causes of protracted diarrhea in infancy, *J Pediatr Gastroenterol Nutr* 30:16–26, 2004.

35. **What are the most useful stool tests for diagnosing fat malabsorption?**
    Measurement of 72-hour fecal fat is the gold standard test for fat malabsorption. The patient must ingest a high-fat diet for 3 to 5 days (100 g daily for adults), and all stool is collected for the final 72 hours. A complete and accurate dietary history should be obtained concomitantly so the coefficient of fat absorption can be calculated. Steatorrhea is present if more than 7% of dietary fat is malabsorbed. In normal infants, up to 15% of fat can be malabsorbed. Other tests include Sudan staining of stool for fat globules (a qualitative test that, if positive, indicates gross steatorrhea), the steatocrit, and monitoring absorbed lipids after a standardized meal.

36. **What stool test is most useful for helping diagnose GI protein loss?**
    Fecal α_1-antitrypsin measurement is the most useful stool marker of protein malabsorption. It is important to concomitantly measure serum α_1-antitrypsin to ensure that the patient does not have α_1-antitrypsin deficiency, which could result in a false-negative stool study.

37. **How do patterns of secretory or enterotoxigenic and inflammatory diarrhea vary?**
    Secretory or *enterotoxigenic disease* is characterized by watery diarrhea and the absence of fecal leukocytes. *Inflammatory disease* is characterized by dysentery (i.e., symptoms and bloody stools), as well as fecal leukocytes and red blood cells.

38. **What is the primary pathophysiologic difference between secretory and osmotic diarrhea?**
    In *osmotic diarrhea*, undigested nutrients increase the osmotic load in the distal small intestine and the colon leading to decreased water absorption. In *secretory diarrhea*, a noxious agent causes the intestinal epithelium to secrete excessive water and electrolytes into the lumen.

39. **How can osmotic diarrhea be distinguished from secretory diarrhea?**
    In true osmotic diarrhea, symptoms should cease when the patient is made NPO. In addition, a fecal osmotic gap can be calculated. In osmotic diarrhea, the fecal electrolyte content becomes lower than the serum. Stool electrolytes should be collected and compared with a normal serum osmolality, 290 mOsm/kg. The fecal osmotic gap is $[290 - 2(Na + K)]$.
    See Table 7-2.

Table 7-2. Osmotic Diarrhea Versus Secretory Diarrhea

STOOLS	OSMOTIC DIARRHEA	SECRETORY DIARRHEA
Electrolytes	Na^+ <70 mmol/L	Na^+ >70 mmol/L
	Cl^- <25 mEq/L	Cl^- >40 mEq/L
Osmotic gap*	>135 mOsm	<50 mOsm
pH	<5.6	>6.0
Response to fasting	Improvement	None

*The osmotic gap is the osmolality of the fecal fluid minus the sum of the concentrations of the fecal electrolytes.
From Guarino A, DeMarco G: Persistent diarrhea In Walker WA, Goulet O, Kleinman RE, et al, editors: Pediatric Gastrointestinal Disease, *4th ed. Hamilton, Ontario, 2004, BC Decker, pp 180–193.*

40. **How should children with secretory diarrhea be managed?**
    After the child is taken off feeds, a vigorous attempt must be initiated to maintain fluid and electrolyte balance. If this is successful, the child should be evaluated for proximal small bowel damage, enteric pathogens, and a baseline malabsorption workup. If abnormalities of the mucosal integrity are suspected, a small bowel biopsy is performed; if the findings are significantly abnormal, the patient may be given parenteral alimentation and gradual refeeding. Electron microscopy may reveal congenital abnormalities of the microvillus membrane and the brush border. Hormonal causes of secretory diarrhea (e.g., a VIPoma, hypergastrinoma, or carcinoid syndrome) must be considered if initial studies are negative.

41. **What rare tumors can cause true secretory diarrhea?**
    - **Gastrinoma**: Children present with typical ulcer pain, hematemesis, vomiting, and melena. High acid output into the proximal small bowel leads to precipitation of bile salts and steatorrhea.
    - **VIPoma:** Children present with profuse watery diarrhea with marked fecal losses (20 to 50 mL/kg/day) due to high levels of vasoactive intestinal peptide (VIP).

42. **What features characterize "toddler diarrhea"?**
    Toddler diarrhea, which is also known as *chronic nonspecific diarrhea*, is a clinical entity of unclear etiology that occurs in infants between 6 and 40 months of age, often following a distinct identifiable enteritis and treatment with an antibiotic. Loose, nonbloody stools (at least two per day but usually more) occur without associated symptoms of fever, pain, or growth failure. Malabsorption is not a key feature.
    Multiple causes may be present: overconsumption of fruit juices, relative intestinal hypermotility, increased secretion of bile acids and sodium, and intestinal prostaglandin abnormalities. The diagnosis is one of exclusion, and toddlers should be evaluated for disaccharide intolerance, protein hypersensitivity, parasitic infestation, and inflammatory bowel disease. Treatment consists of reassurance, careful growth assessment, and psyllium bulking agents (as initial therapy). Other agents used with success have been cholestyramine and metronidazole.

43. **What is primary lactose intolerance?**
    In more than 50% of the population, beginning at the age of 5 years, lactase levels decline progressively after having been normal in infancy. These levels decline at different rates for different people depending on their genetics. Most adults with primary lactose intolerance have lactase levels of about 10% of those seen during infancy. Symptoms of lactose intolerance (e.g., bloating, nausea, cramps, diarrhea after dairy foods) may develop if excessive lactose loads are ingested.

44. **How does late-onset lactase deficiency vary by ethnicity?**
    See Table 7-3.

Table 7-3. Approximate Percentage of Low Lactase Activity by Ethnic Group

UNITED STATES		WORLDWIDE	
White	20%	Dutch	0%
Hispanic	50%	French	32%
Black	75%	Filipino	55%
Native American	90%	Vietnamese	100%

45. **What conditions produce secondary lactose intolerance?**

Any disorder that alters the mucosa of the proximal small intestine may result in secondary lactose intolerance. For this reason, the lactose tolerance test is commonly used as a screening test for intestinal integrity, although this has the disadvantage of concomitantly identifying all primary lactose malabsorbers. Although a combination of factors is present in many disease processes, secondary lactose intolerance can be organized into lesions of the microsurface, total surface, transit time, and site of bacterial colonization in the small bowel.

Microvillus and brush border:
- Post-enteritis
- Bacterial overgrowth
- Inflammatory lesions (Crohn disease)

Level of the villus:
- Celiac disease
- Allergic enteropathy
- Eosinophilic gastroenteropathy

Bulk intestinal surface area:
- Short bowel syndrome

Altered transit with early lactose entry into colon:
- Hyperthyroidism
- Dumping syndromes
- Enteroenteral fistulas

46. **How is lactose intolerance diagnosed?**

The most common noninvasive method of diagnosing lactose intolerance is a **breath hydrogen test**. The fasted patient is fed 2 g/kg (up to 25 g) of lactose, and end-expired air is collected every 15 minutes for the next 2 to 3 hours for the purpose of measuring hydrogen concentration. Fermentation of carbohydrate by bacteria in the colon results in hydrogen expiration after lactose ingestion. A peak hydrogen level of 20 parts per million above the baseline after about 60 minutes in concert with a symptomatic response is considered a positive test. Because of the need for colonic bacteria to ferment carbohydrate and produce hydrogen gas, it is important that the patient not receive antibiotics immediately before the test.

Direct measurement of lactase levels, as well as the other disaccharidases, can be obtained by biopsy of the duodenum or jejunum during upper endoscopy.

Heyman MB: Lactose intolerance in infants, children and adolescents, *Pediatrics* 118:1279–1286, 2006.

47. **What is the role of stool elastase measurement?**

Measurement of fecal pancreatic elastase is a screen for **pancreatic insufficiency**, which can be a cause of fat malabsorption (e.g., cystic fibrosis). A decreased measurement of pancreatic elastase is associated with pancreatic insufficiency, although values can be falsely decreased when the sample is obtained from diarrheal specimen.

48. **What three individual clinical features are the most accurate for predicting 5% dehydration?**
- Abnormal capillary refill
- Abnormal skin turgor
- Abnormal respiratory pattern

Steiner MJ, DeWalt DA, Byerley JS: Is this child dehydrated? *JAMA* 291:2746–2754, 2004.

49. **How accurate are urine specific gravity and blood urea nitrogen (BUN) measurements as means of assessing dehydration in children?**

    Notoriously unreliable. Although a high urine specific gravity is commonly thought to be associated with dehydration, a prospective study of 75 dehydrated children found the correlation was poor. BUN does not begin to rise until the glomerular filtration rate falls to about one-half of normal; it then rises by about 1% each hour, and it may rise even less in a fasting child with disease. In a prospective study, Bonadio and colleagues found that 80% of patients judged to be 5% to 10% dehydrated by common physical findings may have a normal BUN.

Steiner MJ, Nager AL, Wang VJ: Urine specific gravity and other urinary indices: inaccurate tests for dehydration, *Pediatr Emerg Care* 23:298–303, 2007.

Bonadio WA, Hennes HH, Machi J, Madagame E: Efficacy of measuring BUN in assessing children with dehydration due to gastroenteritis, *Ann Emerg Med* 18:755–757, 1989.

50. **How do various oral rehydration solutions differ in composition from other liquids that are commonly used for rehydration?**

    Many home remedies are either very deficient or very excessive in electrolytes or sugar. Chicken broth has no carbohydrates and very high sodium. Sodas (such as colas) can have up to $8 \times$ the recommended sugar content with negligible sodium and potassium. Apple has very high sugar content and very high osmolality and negligible sodium. Tea has neither carbohydrate nor sodium. Commercially available oral rehydration solutions incorporate carbohydrates (25 to 50 g/L), sodium (45 to 90 mEq/L), and potassium (20 to 25 mEq/L) to maximize coupled transport.

51. **How can the World Health Organization (WHO) oral electrolyte (rehydration) solution be duplicated?**

    The WHO solution is 2% glucose, 20 mEq K^+/L, 90 mEq Na^+/L, 80 mEq Cl^-/L, and 30 mEq bicarbonate/L. This solution is approximated by adding ¾ tsp of salt, 1 tsp of baking soda, 1 cup of orange juice (for KCl), and 8 tsp of sugar to 1 L of water.

52. **What traditional approaches to feeding during diarrhea are no longer recommended and should be avoided?**

    - **Switching to lactose-free formula:** This is usually unnecessary because, for most infants, clinical trials have not shown an advantage. Certain infants with severe malnutrition and dehydration may benefit from lactose-free formula.
    - **Diluted formula:** Half- or quarter-strength formula has been shown in clinical trials to be unnecessary and associated with prolonged symptoms and delays in nutritional recovery.
    - **Clear liquids:** Foods high in simple sugars (e.g., carbonated soft drinks, juice drinks, gelatin desserts) should be avoided because the high osmotic load might worsen diarrhea.
    - **Avoid fatty foods:** Fat may have a beneficial effect of reducing intestinal motility.
    - **BRAT diet:** The **b**ananas, **r**ice, **a**pplesauce, and **t**oast diet is unnecessarily restrictive and can provide suboptimal nutrition.
    - **Avoid food for at least 24 hours:** Early feeding decreases the intestinal permeability caused by infection, reduces illness duration, and improves nutritional outcome.

King CK, Glass R, Bresee JS, Duggan C, Centers for Disease Control and Prevention: Managing acute gastroenteritis among children: oral rehydration, maintenance, and nutritional therapy, *MMWR Recomm Rep* 52:1–16, 2003.

53. **What is the role of antiemetic agents in children with gastroenteritis?**

    Published guidelines have not yet formally recommended the use of antiemetic medications, particularly domperidone, metoclopramide, prochlorperazine, and promethazine, because of concerns of increased emergency department (ED) revisits rates of misdiagnosis, and health care costs. Oral ondansetron, a centrally acting 5-hydroxytryptamine antagonist, has been found to be useful in decreasing the risk for persistent vomiting, lessening the need for intravenous therapy in ED settings and reducing the likelihood of hospitalization.

Freedman SB, Hall M, Shah SS, et al: Impact of increasing ondansetron use on clinical outcomes in children with gastroenteritis, *JAMA Pediatr* 168:321–329, 2014.

54. **What are non-antimicrobial drug therapies for diarrhea?**

    In older children, adolescents, and adults, the following categories are used. Pediatric data are limited, and these medications are not typically approved or recommended for children <3 years of age.

    - **Antimotility agents** (loperamide [Imodium], diphenoxylate and atropine [Lomotil], tincture of opium [Paregoric]): These can cause drowsiness, ileus, and nausea and potentiate the effects of certain bacterial enteritides (e.g., *Shigella, Salmonella*) or accelerate the course of antibiotic-associated colitis.
    - **Antisecretory drugs** (bismuth subsalicylate [Pepto-Bismol]): These involve the potential for salicylate overdose.
    - **Adsorbents** (attapulgite, kaolin-pectin [Donnagel, Kaopectate]): These can cause abdominal fullness and interfere with other medications.

55. **What is the role of probiotic organisms in the treatment of antibiotic-associated diarrhea?**

    Probiotics (which are the opposite of antibiotics) are living organisms that are believed to cause health benefits by replenishing some of the more than 500 species of intestinal bacteria that antibiotics can suppress and by inhibiting the growth of more pathogenic flora. Among children receiving broad-spectrum antibiotics, about 20% to 40% are likely to experience some degree of diarrhea. *Lactobacillus GG, Bifidobacterium bifidum,* and *Streptococcus thermophilus* have been shown to limit antibiotic-associated diarrhea in children.

Applegate JA, Fischer Walker CL, Ambikapathi R, et al: Systematic review of probiotics for the treatment of community-acquired acute diarrhea in children, *BMC Public Health* 13:S3–S16, 2013.

KEY POINTS: DIARRHEA AND MALABSORPTION

1. History is crucial to diagnosis and should include recent medications, ill family contacts, travel, attendance at school or day care, pets, and water sources.
2. Three keys to the assessment of dehydration are (1) capillary refill, (2) skin turgor, and (3) respiratory pattern.
3. *Salmonella* species infection is more concerning among infants who are younger than 1 year because of the increased risk for dissemination (e.g., bacteremia, meningitis).
4. Toddler diarrhea is a common cause of chronic diarrhea in children between the ages of 6 and 40 months.
5. Celiac disease (a sensitivity to gluten) is common (up to 1% of the general population) and can present with subtle and varied symptoms.
6. Allergic or nonspecific colitis is the most common cause of bloody diarrhea in infants younger than 1 year.

56. **Why is *Salmonella enteritis* so concerning in a child who is younger than 12 months?**

    In older children with *Salmonella* gastroenteritis, secondary bacteremia and dissemination of disease rarely occur. In infants, however, 5% to 40% may have positive blood cultures for *Salmonella*, and in 10% of these cases, *Salmonella* can cause meningitis, osteomyelitis, pericarditis, and pyelonephritis. Thus, in infants who are younger than 1 year, outpatient management of diarrhea assumes even greater significance, particularly if *Salmonella* is suspected.

57. **What are the clinical manifestations of typhoid fever?**

    Typhoid fever is caused by *Salmonella* species *typhi* and *paratyphi*. It is characterized by fever, abdominal pain, nausea, decreased appetite, and constipation over the first week. The fever is sometimes paradoxically associated with bradycardia (Faget sign or sphygmothermic dissociation). Leukopenia is common. Diarrhea begins after approximately a week. If untreated it can last for 2 to 3 weeks and cause significant weight loss and melena. Treatment of typhoid fever is necessary only in patients with sepsis or bacteremia with signs of systemic toxicity or a metastatic focus, which can include otitis, endocarditis, cholecystitis, or encephalitis.

58. **Who was Typhoid Mary?**
    In 1907, a *JAMA* article traced a series of outbreaks of *Salmonella*-triggered typhoid fever in 7 families over a 7-year period to the same cook, Mary Mallon, who had been employed by each family during that period. She was subsequently found to be a carrier of *Salmonella*, the first asymptomatic typhoid carrier identified in the United States. Much of the remainder of her life was spent in an imposed quarantine.

Marineli F, Tsoucalas G, Androutsos G: Mary Mallon (1869-1938) and the history of typhoid fever, *Ann Gastroenterol* 26:132–134, 2013.

59. **What is the most common cause of travelers' diarrhea?**
    Enterotoxigenic *E. coli* is clearly the most commonly identified cause of traveler's diarrhea. Depending on the location, however, other bacteria (such as *Campylobacter* in Southeast Asia), viruses (norovirus, rotavirus), or parasites (*Giardia, Cryptosporidium*) can be present.

60. **How can travelers' diarrhea be prevented?**
    - **Avoidance:** In high-risk areas of developing countries, avoid previously peeled raw fruits and vegetables and any foods or beverages or ice cubes prepared with tap water.
    - **Bismuth subsalicylate:** Prophylactic bismuth subsalicylate (Pepto-Bismol) has been shown to minimize diarrheal illness in up to 75% of adults. Although some authorities recommend its use in children, others argue against it because of the risk for salicylate intoxication. It can interfere with absorption of doxycycline used for malaria prevention.
    - **Anti-infective drugs:** Prophylactic use of antimicrobial agents such as trimethoprim-sulfamethoxazole, azithromycin, neomycin, doxycycline, and fluoroquinolones can decrease the frequency of travelers' diarrhea in children and adults. However, routine use of antibiotics is not recommended because of potential risks for allergic drug reactions, antibiotic-associated colitis, and the development of resistant organisms.
    - **Immunization:** Although potentially an ideal solution, at present it is not an alternative.

Hill DR, Ryan ET: Management of travelers' diarrhea, *BMJ* 337:863–867, 2008.

61. **Which bacterial gastroenteritides may benefit from antimicrobial therapy?**
    See Table 7-4.

Table 7-4. Benefits of Antimicrobial Therapy in Specific Bacterial Gastroenteritides

ENTEROPATHOGEN	INDICATION FOR OR EFFECT OF THERAPY
Shigella species	Shortens duration of diarrhea Eliminates organisms from feces
Campylobacter jejuni	Shortens duration Prevents relapse
Salmonella species	Indicated for infants <12 mo Bacteremia Metastatic foci (e.g., osteomyelitis) Enteric fever Immunocompromise
Escherichia coli	
Enteropathogenic	Use primarily in infants Intravenous use if invasive disease
Enterotoxigenic (ETEC)	Most illnesses brief and self-limited
Enteroinvasive	Mimics shigellosis with diarrhea and high fever
Yersinia enterocolitica	None for gastroenteritis alone but indicated if suspected septicemia or other localized infection
Clostridium difficile	10-20% relapse rate

62. What strains of *E. coli* are associated with diarrhea?
    - *Enterotoxigenic* (ETEC): responsible for travelers' diarrhea
    - *Enteropathogenic* (EPEC): similar mechanism as ETEC; adheres to epithelial cells and releases toxins that induce intestinal secretions and limit absorption; responsible for epidemics in daycare settings and nurseries
    - *Enteroinvasive* (EIEC): invades mucosa and causes bloody diarrhea
    - *Enterohemorrhagic* (EHEC): produces a Shiga-like toxin that is responsible for hemorrhagic colitis; usually associated with contaminated food and undercooked beef; usually a self-limited gastroenteritis

63. What clinical entity has been attributed to EHEC, specifically strain O157:H7?
    Hemolytic uremic syndrome (HUS), which is the triad of microangiopathic hemolytic anemia, thrombocytopenia, and renal failure.

64. What is the most common cause of antibiotic-associated colitis?
    Clostridium difficile (C. difficile). Fever, abdominal pain, and bloody diarrhea begin as early as a few days after starting antibiotics (especially clindamycin, ampicillin, and cephalosporins). Definitive diagnosis is made by sigmoidoscopy, which reveals pseudomembranous plaques or nodules (Fig. 7-5).

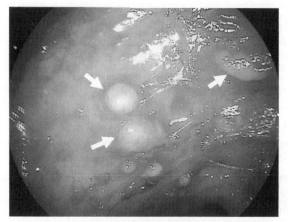

Figure 7-5. Flexible sigmoidoscopy showing adherent plaques *(arrows)* typical of pseudomembranous colitis. (From Barker HC, Haworth CS, Williams D: *Clostridium difficile* pancolitis in adults with cystic fibrosis, *J Cyst Fibros* 7(5):444–447, 2008.)

65. How is the diagnosis of *C. difficile* made?
    C. difficile causes diarrhea by producing two diarrheagenic toxins (A and B). Essay immunoassay for the toxins was previously the diagnostic test of choice. However, in 2013, the American College of Gastroenterology recommended that **nucleic acid amplification tests**, such as *PCR assays*, which detect toxin-encoding genes should be the standard diagnostic test because of superior sensitivity and specificity.

Surawicz CM, Brandt LJ, Binion DG, et al: Guidelines for diagnosis, treatment, and prevention of *Clostridium difficile* infections, *Am J Gastroenterol* 28:1219–1227, 2013.

66. How common is asymptomatic *C. difficile* carriage?
    Colonization rates in infants can be up to 70%, with percentages decreasing with age. By the second year of life, the rate declines to about 6%, and above age 2 years to 3%, which is the approximate rate in adults. These high colonization rates make the interpretation of positive tests in younger infants problematic. Toxin assays are more indicative of *C. difficile*–associated disease than culture. However, the toxin may be present without any symptoms, especially in infants, who

typically do not have the toxin receptors necessary for disease. Unless there is evidence of histologic colitis, asymptomatic carriers do not require treatment.

Bryant K, McDonald LC: *Clostridium difficile* infections in children, *Pediatr Infect Dis J* 28:145–146, 2009.

67. **Why are alcohol-based sanitizers insufficient when examining patients with *C. difficile*?**
    Typical alcohol-based hand hygiene products do not kill the spores of *C. difficile*. In addition to standard contact precautions (which include gloves at all times and gowns for direct contact with the patient or items in the room), handwashing with soap and water is recommended to more effectively remove spores from contaminated hands.

68. **What are the three most common presenting symptoms of giardiasis?**
    - Asymptomatic carrier state
    - Chronic malabsorption with steatorrhea and FTT
    - Acute gastroenteritis with diarrhea, weight loss, abdominal cramps, abdominal distention, nausea, and vomiting

69. **How reliable are the various diagnostic methods for detecting *Giardia*?**
    - Single stool examination for trophozoites or cysts: 50% to 75% (Fig. 7-6)
    - Three stool examinations (ideally 48 hours apart) for same: 95%
    - Single stool examination and stool enzyme-linked immunosorbent assay test for *Giardia* antigen: >95%
    - Duodenal aspirate or string test: >95%
    - Duodenal biopsy (gold standard): Closest to 100%

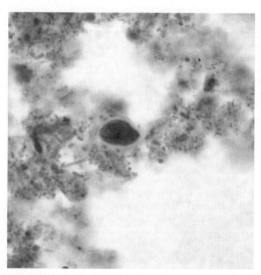

Figure 7-6. Trichrome stain of stool revealing cystic form of *Giardia* (in center). *(From Liacouras CA, Piccoli DA: Pediatric Gastroenterology: The Requisites in Pediatrics. Philadelphia, 2005, Elsevier Mosby, p 7.)*

70. **What are the potential complications of amebiasis?**
    The parasite *Entamoeba histolytica* disseminates from the intestine to the liver in up to 10% of patients and to other organs less commonly.
    - Liver abscess
    - Pericarditis

- Cerebral abscess
- Empyema

Haque R, Huston CD, Hughes M, et al: Amebiasis, *N Engl J Med* 348:1565–1573, 2003.

71. What is gluten?

After starch has been extracted from wheat flour, gluten is the residue that remains. This residue is made up of multiple proteins that are distinguished by their solubility and extraction properties. For example, the alcohol-soluble fraction of wheat gluten is wheat gliadin. It is this protein component that is primarily responsible for the mucosal injury that occurs in the small bowel in patients with celiac disease. The alcohol-soluble components of barley and rye are also toxic.

72. What classic clinical features suggest celiac disease?

Gluten-sensitive enteropathy (celiac disease) is a relatively common cause of severe diarrhea and malabsorption in infants and children. The classic presentation of celiac disease is a 9- to 24-month-old child with FTT, diarrhea, abdominal distention, muscle wasting, and hypotonia. After several months of diarrhea, growth slows; weight typically decreases before height. Often, these children become irritable and depressed and display poor intake and symptoms of carbohydrate malabsorption. Vomiting is less common. On examination, the growth defect and distention are commonly striking. There may be a generalized lack of subcutaneous fat, with wasting of the buttocks, shoulder girdle, and thighs. Edema, rickets, and clubbing may also be seen. Many patients with celiac disease, however, have a more subtle presentation rather than the classic constellation of symptoms and can present at an older age.

DiSabatino A, Corazza GR: Coeliac disease, *Lancet* 373:1480–1493, 2009.

73. What are possible nongastrointestinal manifestations of celiac disease?

- Dermatitis herpetiformis
- Iron deficiency anemia (unresponsive to treatment with oral iron supplements)
- Arthritis and arthralgia
- Dental enamel hypoplasia
- Chronic hepatitis
- Osteopenia and osteoporosis
- Pubertal delay
- Short stature
- Hepatitis
- Arthritis

Telega G, Bennet TR, Werlin S: Emerging new clinical patterns in the presentation of celiac disease, *Arch Pediatr Adolesc Med* 162:164–168, 2008.

74. What is the appropriate screening test for celiac disease?

Anti–tissue transglutaminase (TTG) immunoglobulin A (IgA) and **anti–endomysial antibodies (EMA) IgA** have been demonstrated to be highly sensitive and specific for celiac disease. Because of low cost, ease of test performance, and reliability, TTG is currently recommended for initial screening of celiac disease. Antigliadin antibodies, previously the most commonly employed screening test, are not as sensitive or specific for celiac disease and are currently not recommended as first-line screening. However, more advanced methods of measurement of antigliadin have shown promise. Antibodies found in patients with celiac disease are IgA antibodies. Selective IgA deficiency is the most common primary immunodeficiency in Western countries, with a prevalence of 1.5 to 2.5 per 1,000, and is even more common in patients with celiac disease. Therefore, a quantitative IgA level should be included when measuring screening antibodies.

Tran TH: Advances in pediatric celiac disease, *Curr Opin Pediatr* 26:585–589, 2014.
Guideline for the Diagnosis and Treatment of Celiac Disease in Children: Recommendations of the North American Society of Pediatric Gastroenterology, Hepatology, and Nutrition, *J Pediatr Gastroenterol Nutr* 40:1–19, 2005.

75. **What is the definitive way to diagnose celiac disease?**
Definitive diagnosis of celiac disease requires **multiple small bowel biopsies *via endoscopy*** while the patient is on a gluten-containing diet. Intestinal biopsies obtained on gluten may show a number of abnormalities including villous atrophy, elongated crypts, increased crypt mitoses, increased intraepithelial lymphocytes, plasma cell infiltrate in lamina propria, absence of brush border, and disorganization and flattening of the columnar epithelium ("villous blunting"). These abnormalities should resolve fully with repeat biopsies after a strict gluten-free diet. Recent European guidelines have recommended that the need for confirmatory biopsy can be omitted in children with clear symptoms of celiac disease, with high levels of transglutaminase antibody and with positive HLA typing. Celiac disease is strongly associated with HLA-DQ types 2 and 8.

Husby S, Koletzko S, Korponay-Szabó IR, et al: European Society for Pediatric Gastroenterology, Hepatology, and Nutrition guidelines for the diagnosis of coeliac disease, *J Pediatr Gastroenterol Nutr* 54:136–160, 2012.

76. **What is the mainstay of treatment for celiac disease?**
A strict **gluten-free diet** needs to be followed throughout life, although nearly one in four patients continues to experience gastrointestinal symptoms. Gluten-free diets should be without wheat, barley, and rye. Upon initial diagnosis, most recommend avoiding oats because of contamination, but eventually most patients with celiac can tolerate oats. Good substitutions are rice and corn flour products.

Paarlahti P, Kurppa K, Ukkola A, et al: Predictors of persistent symptoms and reduced quality of life in treated coeliac disease patients: a large cross-sectional study, *BMC Gastroenterol* 13:75, 2013.
Celiac Disease Foundation: www.celiac.org. Accessed Nov. 24, 2014.
Gluten Intolerance Group: www.gluten.net. Accessed on Nov. 24, 2014.

ESOPHAGEAL DISORDERS

77. **What is the likely diagnosis for an infant with excessive secretions and choking episodes in whom a nasogastric tube cannot be passed into the stomach?**
Esophageal atresia with tracheoesophageal fistula. This congenital anomaly is usually diagnosed during the newborn period, often when a chest radiograph reveals the intended nasogastric tube coiled in the upper esophageal pouch with the stomach distended with air. Treatment is surgical. The possible variations are shown in Figure 7-7.

78. **What underlying diagnoses should be considered in a patient who presents with a meat impaction in the esophagus?**
- Eosinophilic esophagitis
- Achalasia
- Esophageal stricture, congenital or acquired
- Prior esophageal surgery
Of note, in children with esophageal food impaction, endoscopy and biopsy reveal an underlying pathologic and potentially treatable etiology in the majority of patients.

Hurtado CW, Furuta GT, Kramer RE: Etiology of food impactions in children, *J Pediatr Gastroenterol Nutr* 52:43–46, 2011.

79. **What is the most common condition that might present as a food impaction in an *adolescent*?**
Eosinophilic esophagitis (EoE). Occurring in children and adults, EoE is characterized by multiple symptoms that are suggestive of gastroesophageal reflux (GER), including heartburn, emesis, regurgitation, epigastric pain, and feeding difficulties, which are typically unresponsive to acid suppression therapy. Pathologically, this is characterized by eosinophilic inflammation of the esophagus and is almost always related to food antigens. In adolescents and adults, EoE often presents with symptoms of dysphagia or, occasionally, food impaction.

80. **How is EoE diagnosed?**
The diagnosis of EoE requires **upper endoscopy**. According to the most recent EoE guidelines, EoE is a defined clinicopathologic diagnosis that consists of isolated esophageal dysfunction and

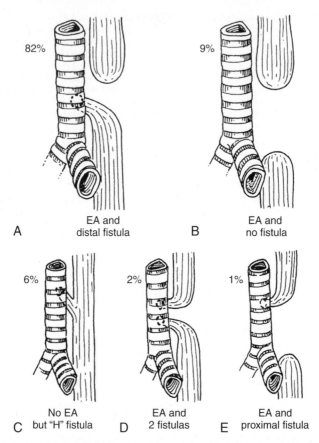

Figure 7-7. A, Esophageal atresia with distal esophageal communication with the tracheobronchial tree (most common type: 80%). **B,** Esophageal atresia without a distal communication. **C,** H-type fistulas between otherwise intact trachea and esophagus. **D,** Esophageal atresia with both proximal and distal communication with the trachea. **E,** Esophageal atresia with proximal communication. *(From Blickman H, editor: The Requisites: Pediatric Radiology, ed 2. Philadelphia, 1998, Mosby, p 93.)*

esophageal biopsies with greater than 15 eosinophils per high power field. Other causes of an isolated esophageal eosinophilia must be excluded, specifically GER and proton pump inhibitor responsive esophageal eosinophilia. Patients must be on an adequate dosage proton pump inhibitor for a period of 8 weeks before any biopsy.

Liacouras CA, Furuta GT, et al: Eosinophilic esophagitis: updated consensus recommendations for children and adults, *J Allergy Clin Immunol* 128:3–30, 2011.

81. What are common endoscopic findings in EoE?
    - Esophageal furrowing and edema
    - Esophageal rings or "trachealization" (Fig. 7-8)
    - White plaques
    - Esophageal strictures
    - Mucosal tearing

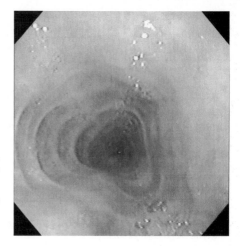

Figure 7-8. "Trachealization" or "felinization" of the midesophagus of a patient with EoE. The terms arise from the ringed appearance of the esophagus that cause it to resemble a human trachea or a cat esophagus, which has rings of cartilage. *(From Wyllie R, Hyams JS, editors:* Pediatric Gastrointestinal and Liver Disease, *ed 4. Philadelphia, Saunders, 2011, p 398.)*

82. What causes esophageal eosinophilia in EoE?

   EoE is an antigen-driven immune-mediated disease. Although aeroallergens have been implicated, specifically in mouse models, the **ingestion of food antigens** is responsible for greater than 98% of the disease. A pathological response induces a chronic inflammatory infiltrate in the esophagus with hyperplasia of the epithelia and muscular layers and fibrosis of the lamina propria.

   Virchow JC: Eosinophilic esophagitis: asthma of the esophagus? *Dig Dis* 32:54–60, 2014.

83. What are the symptoms of EoE?
   - *Infants/toddlers*: FTT, feeding issues, irritability, vomiting, regurgitation
   - *Children*: epigastric abdominal pain, vomiting, regurgitation, heartburn, and other gastroesophageal reflux disease (GERD) symptoms, and dysphagia
   - *Adolescents*: GERD symptoms, heartburn, dysphagia, and food impaction

   Liacouras CA, Spergel J, Gober LM: Eosinophilic esophagitis: clinical presentation in children, *Gastroenterol Clin North Am* 43:219–229, 2014.

84. What are the therapies for EoE?
   - **Oral steroids** are used when severe symptoms are present and can promote immediate histologic and symptomatic recovery; however, they are not used long-term for maintenance therapy.
   - **Topical swallowed steroids** are the most common pharmacologic medications used to treat EoE. These medications are used for both the initial treatment and for maintenance therapy.
   - **Dietary restriction** involves the removal of the offending food antigen(s).
     - Elemental formula is greater than 98% effective at inducing and maintaining disease remission; however, poor palatability and cost provide some limitations.
     - A six-food elimination diet (removing dairy, wheat, eggs, soy, nuts, fish/shellfish) has been shown to improve symptoms and esophageal histology in 65% to 75% of patients.
     - An allergy-directed diet using skin prick tests and atopy patch tests to determine offending foods has been shown to improve symptoms and esophageal histology in 60% to 70% of patients.

   Dellon ES, Liacouras CA: Advances in clinical management of eosinophilic esophagitis. *Gastroenterology* 147 (6):1238-1254, 2014.
   Liacouras CA, Furuta GT, et al: Eosinophilic esophagitis: updated consensus recommendations for children and adults, *J Allergy Clin Immunol* 128:3–30, 2011.

FOOD ALLERGIES

85. **What are the most common food allergies in children?**
   Cow milk, eggs, and **peanuts** account for 75% of abnormal food challenges. Soy, wheat, fish, and shellfish are also common allergens.

Lack G: Food allergy, *N Engl J Med* 359:1252–1260, 2008.
Food Allergy and Anaphylaxis Network: www.foodallergy.org. Accessed on Mar. 20, 2015.

86. **How are adverse food reactions characterized?**
   - **Food allergy:** Ingestion of food results in hypersensitivity reactions mediated most commonly by IgE.
   - **Food intolerance:** Ingestion of food results in symptoms not immunologically mediated, and causes may include toxic contaminants (e.g., histamine in scombroid fish poisoning), pharmacologic properties of food (e.g., tyramine in aged cheeses), digestive and absorptive limitations of host (e.g., lactase deficiency), or idiosyncratic reactions.

Guandalini S, Newland C: Differentiating food allergies from food intolerances, *Curr Gastroenterol Rep* 13:426–434, 2011.

87. **What can be the acute manifestations of milk protein allergy in childhood?**
   - Angioedema
   - Urticaria
   - Acute vomiting and diarrhea
   - Anaphylactic shock
   - Gastrointestinal bleeding

88. **What is the most common chronic manifestation of milk protein allergy?**
   Diarrhea of variable severity. Histologic abnormalities of the small intestinal mucosa have been documented, with the most severe form seen as a flat villous lesion. Protein-losing enteropathy may result from disruption of the surface epithelium. The stools of children with primary milk protein intolerance often contain blood.

Warren CM, Jhaveri S, Warrier MR, et al: The epidemiology of milk allergy in US children, *Ann Allergy Asthma Immunol* 110:370–374, 2013.

89. **What likely condition does a birch-allergic child have who develops tongue swelling when eating an apple?**
   Oral allergy syndrome. In this IgE-mediated condition, allergic children develop pruritus; tingling; and swelling of the lips, palate, and tongue when ingesting certain fresh fruits and vegetables because of cross-reactivity to proteins similar to those in pollen. In this case, birch shares allergens with raw carrots, celery, and apples. Symptoms generally are limited to the mouth but occasionally can progress to anaphylaxis. Most allergens are heat labile, so this patient should be advised to stick to baked apple pie for dessert.

Mansoor DK, Sharma HP: Clinical presentations of food allergy, *Pediatr Clin North Am* 58:315–326, 2011.

90. **Can dietary manipulation in the first few months of life reduce the risk for atopic dermatitis and food allergies?**
   This remains a heavily debated topic in pediatric medicine. Some observational studies have suggested that introducing complementary foods before 4 months of age might have a beneficial effect on the induction of immune tolerance. The debate will likely continue pending a large randomized, controlled intervention trial. In the meantime, infants who are at high risk for developing allergy (at least one parent or sibling with allergic disease) may benefit from certain approaches as recommended by the American Academy of Pediatrics (AAP) Committee on Nutrition.
   - Exclusive breastfeeding for at least 4 months decreases the incidence of atopic dermatitis and cow milk allergy during the first 2 years of life.

- Use of hydrolyzed formulas may delay or prevent atopic dermatitis.
- Solid foods should not be introduced before 4 to 6 months of age because there is no definitive evidence to support dietary intervention before this age.

Heinrich J, Koletzko B, Koletzko S: Timing and diversity of complementary food introduction for prevention of allergic diseases. How early and how much? *Expert Rev Clin Immunol* 10:701–704, 2014.
Greer FR, Sicherer SH, Burks AW: Effects of early nutritional interventions on the development of atopic disease in infants and children: the role of maternal dietary restriction, breastfeeding, timing of introduction of complementary foods and hydrolyzed formulas, *Pediatrics* 121:183–191, 2008.

91. **What are the symptoms of allergic proctocolitis or milk protein intolerance in an infant?**
    Infants, usually between birth and 4 months of age, develop frequent, mucus-streaked, bloody stools. Abdominal pain, irritability and vomiting may also be present.

92. **Does the diagnosis of allergic proctocolitis in infants usually require endoscopy?**
    No. The diagnosis is usually made based on **clinical history** and **physical examination** without the need for an endoscopy. Infants are usually being fed a milk-based formula. Proctocolitis is treated by removing the offending food antigen (milk or dairy). Switching to a soy-based formula is usually unsuccessful because of protein cross-reactivity, so it is recommended to switch to a partially hydrolyzed protein. If symptoms persist, an amino acid–based formula may be necessary. Breastfeeding mothers must abstain from milk and soy. Sometimes additional foods need to be excluded. It is important to council patients that it may take 3 to 6 weeks to see complete improvement in both clinical symptoms and GI bleeding.

GASTROINTESTINAL BLEEDING

93. **What features on physical examination can help identify an unknown cause of GI bleeding?**
    See Table 7-5.

Kamath BK, Mamula P: Gastrointestinal bleeding. In Liacouras CA, Piccoli DA, editors: *Pediatric Gastroenterology: The Requisites in Pediatrics.* Philadelphia, 2008, Mosby, pp 87–97.

Table 7-5. Features to Identify the Cause of Gastrointestinal Bleeding

Skin	Signs of chronic liver disease (e.g., spider angiomas, venous distention, caput medusae, jaundice)
	Signs of coagulopathy (e.g., petechiae, purpura)
	Signs of vascular dysplasias (e.g., telangiectasia, hemangiomas)
	Signs of vasculitis (e.g., palpable purpura on legs and buttocks suggests Henoch-Schönlein purpura)
	Dermatologic manifestations of IBD (e.g., erythema nodosum, pyoderma gangrenosum)
Head and neck	Signs of epistaxis (especially before placing a nasogastric tube, which can induce bleeding)
	Hyperpigmented spots on the lips and gums (suggests Peutz-Jeghers syndrome, which is associated with multiple intestinal polyps)
	Webbed neck (suggests Turner syndrome, which is associated with gastrointestinal vascular malformations and IBD)
	Lesions on buccal mucosa (suggests trauma)
Lungs	Hemoptysis (tuberculosis, pulmonary hemosiderosis)
Cardiac	Murmur of aortic stenosis (in adults, associated with vascular malformations of the ascending colon, although this association is not certain in children)
Abdomen	Splenomegaly or hepatomegaly (suggests portal hypertension and possible esophageal varices)

Continued on following page

Table 7-5. Features to Identify the Cause of Gastrointestinal Bleeding (*Continued*)

	Ascites (suggests chronic liver disease and possible varices)
	Palpable or tender loops of intestine (suggests IBD)
Joint	Arthritis (Henoch-Schönlein purpura, IBD)
Perianal	Perianal ulcerations and skin tags (suggest IBD)
	Perianal abscess (suggests IBD, chronic granulomatous disease immunodeficiency)
	Fissure (suggests constipation)
	Hemorrhoids (suggests constipation, portal hypertension)
	Rectal mass on digital examination (suggests polyp)
Growth	Failure to thrive (IBD, Hirschsprung disease)

IBD = Inflammatory bowel disease.

94. In patients with acute GI bleeding, how may vital signs indicate the extent of volume depletion?

    It is important to remember that when acute bleeding occurs in children, it may take 12 to 72 hours for full equilibration of a patient's hemoglobin to occur. Vital signs are much more useful for patient management in the acute setting (Table 7-6).

    Mezoff AG, Preud'homme DL: How serious is that GI bleed? *Contemp Pediatr* 11:60–92, 1994.

Table 7-6. Vital Signs and Blood Volume Loss

VITAL SIGNS	BLOOD VOLUME LOSS
Tachycardia without orthostasis	5-10% loss
Orthostatic changes Pulse increases by 20 beats/min Blood pressure decreases by 10 mm Hg	>10% loss
Hypotension and resting tachycardia	30% loss
Nonpalpable pulses	>40% loss

95. What is the simplest way of differentiating upper GI from lower GI bleeding?

    Nasogastric lavage. After the insertion of a soft nasogastric tube (12 Fr in small children, 14 to 16 Fr in older children), 3 to 5 mL/kg of room-temperature normal saline is instilled. If bright red blood or coffee-ground–like material is aspirated, the test is positive. A pink-tinged effluent is not a positive test because it can simply denote the dissolution of a clot and not active intestinal bleeding. By definition, upper GI bleeding occurs proximal to the ligament of Treitz. If the lavage is negative, it is unlikely that the bleeding is above this ligament, and this rules out gastric, esophageal, or nasal sources. However, bleeding from duodenal ulcers and duodenal duplications may sometimes be missed by these aspirates.

96. How does the type of bloody stool help pinpoint the location of a GI bleed?

    - **Hematochezia** (bright red blood): Normal stool spotting on toilet tissue likely suggests distal bleeding (e.g., anal fissure, juvenile colonic polyp). Mucous or diarrheal stools (especially if painful) indicate left-sided or diffuse colitis.
    - **Melena** (black, tarry stools) indicates blood denatured by acid and usually implies a lesion, likely before the ligament of Treitz. However, melena can be seen in patients with Meckel diverticulum as a result of denaturation by anomalous gastric mucosa.
    - **Currant jelly** (dark maroon) stools usually come from the distal ileum or colon and often are associated with ischemia (e.g., intussusception).

    Because blood is a cathartic, intestinal transit time can be greatly accelerated and makes defining the site of bleeding by the magnitude and color of the blood difficult. This difficulty underscores the importance of the initial nasogastric tube insertion.

97. What can cause false-negative and false-positive results when stool testing for blood?

Hemoglobin and its various derivatives (e.g., oxyhemoglobin, reduced hemoglobin, methemoglobin, carboxyhemoglobin) can serve as catalysts for the oxidation of guaiac (Hemoccult) or benzidine (Hematest) when a hydrogen peroxide developer is added, thereby producing a color change. Of note, iron does not cause false-positive results.

False negatives: Ingestion of large doses of ascorbic acid; delayed transit time or bacterial overgrowth, allowing bacteria to degrade the hemoglobin to porphyrin

False positives: Recent ingestion of red meat or peroxidase-containing fruits and vegetables (e.g., broccoli, radishes, cauliflower, cantaloupes, turnips)

98. How do the causes of *lower* GI bleeding vary by age group?

Newborn and infant:
- *Mucosal:* Peptic ulcer disease, necrotizing enterocolitis, infectious colitis, eosinophilic or allergic colitis, Hirschsprung enterocolitis, anal fissure
- *Structural:* Intestinal duplication, Meckel diverticulum, intussusception

Child:
- *Mucosal:* Anal fissure, juvenile polyp, infectious colitis, inflammatory bowel disease, solitary rectal ulcer, lymphonodular hyperplasia
- *Structural:* Intestinal duplication, Meckel diverticulum, intussusception, volvulus, Dieulafoy malformation (large tortuous arteriole in the stomach that erodes and bleeds)
- *Other:* Hemolytic-uremic syndrome, Henoch-Schönlein purpura, Munchausen syndrome by proxy, arteriovenous malformation, vascular malformation

Kamath BK, Mamula P: Gastrointestinal bleeding. In Liacouras CA, Piccoli DA, editors: *Pediatric Gastroenterology: The Requisites in Pediatrics.* Philadelphia, 2008, Mosby, pp 87–97.

99. A previously asymptomatic 18-month-old child has large amounts of painless rectal bleeding (red but mixed with darker clots). What is the likely diagnosis?

Although juvenile polyps can also cause painless rectal bleeding, the likely diagnosis is a **Meckel diverticulum**. This outpouching occurs from the failure of the intestinal end of the omphalomesenteric duct to obliterate. Up to 2% of the population may have a Meckel diverticulum, and about half contain gastric mucosa; most are usually silent throughout life. Meckel diverticulum is twice as common in males and usually appears during the first 2 years of life as massive painless bleeding that is red or maroon in color. Tarry stools are observed in about 10% of cases. A history of previous minor episodes may be obtained. The presentation can range from shock to intussusception with obstruction, volvulus, or torsion. Meckel diverticulitis, which occurs in 10% to 20% of cases, may be indistinguishable from appendicitis.

100. Worldwide, what is the most common cause of GI blood loss in children?

Hookworm infection. Caused by the parasites *Necator americanus* and *Ancylostoma duodenale*, this infection is often asymptomatic. Progressive microscopic blood loss often leads to anemia as a result of iron deficiency.

Crompton DW: The public health importance of hookworm disease, *Parasitology* 121:S39–S50, 2000.

101. How do the causes of upper GI bleeding vary by age group?
- **Newborns:** Swallowed maternal blood, vitamin K deficiency, stress gastritis or ulcer, vascular anomaly, coagulopathy, milk-protein sensitivity
- **Infants:** Stress gastritis or ulcer, acid-peptic disease, Mallory-Weiss tear, vascular anomaly, GI duplications, gastric or esophageal varices, duodenal or gastric webs, bowel obstruction
- **Children:** Mallory-Weiss tear, acid-peptic disease, varices, caustic ingestion, vasculitis, hemobilia, tumor

Gilgar MA: Upper gastrointestinal bleeding. In Walker WA, Goulet O, Kleinman RE, et al, editors: *Pediatric Gastrointestinal Disease*, ed 4. Hamilton, Ontario, 2004, BC Decker, pp 258–265.

102. What is the most likely cause of hematemesis in a healthy term infant?
     Swallowed maternal blood. The *Apt test* can be used to differentiate maternal from infant blood. Fetal hemoglobin resists denaturation with alkali better than adult hemoglobin does. Therefore, exposure of adult blood to sodium hydroxide will result in a brown color, whereas the newborn infant's blood will remain pink.

103. What are the two most likely causes of visible blood in the stool of an otherwise healthy infant?
     Anal/rectal fissure and **milk/soy protein allergy**. A physical exam and rectal exam are of particular importance in making the diagnosis.

KEY POINTS: GASTROINTESTINAL BLEEDING

1. Hemoglobin measurement is a much less reliable indicator of volume depletion than vital signs during the assessment of acute gastrointestinal bleeding.
2. Nasogastric lavage is a simple method for differentiating upper gastrointestinal bleeding from lower gastrointestinal bleeding and should always be performed in all patients suspected of having a significant gastrointestinal bleed.
3. The two most common causes of painless rectal bleeding in children are juvenile polyps and Meckel diverticulum.

---

104. What are the six most common causes of massive GI bleeding in children?
     1. Esophageal varices
     2. Meckel diverticulum
     3. Hemorrhagic gastritis
     4. Crohn disease with ileal ulcer
     5. Peptic ulcer (mainly duodenal)
     6. Arteriovenous malformation

Treem WR: Gastrointestinal bleeding in children, *Gastrointest Endosc Clin North Am* 5:75–97, 1994.

GASTROINTESTINAL DYSMOTILITY

105. How rapidly do infants outgrow GER?
     Forty percent of healthy infants have spitting or regurgitation more than once a day; mild reflux does not represent disease. As a rule, in those infants who have more significant primary GER (about 12% of total), 25% to 50% resolve by 6 months of age, 75% to 85% by 12 months of age, and 95% to 98% by 18 months of age. GER in older children may be more widespread than appreciated. Surveys of parents of children and adolescents (3 to 17 years) revealed that symptoms of heartburn regurgitation were relatively common (2% to 8% of patients).

Campanozzi A, Boccia G, Pensabene L, et al: Prevalence and natural history of gastroesophageal reflux: pediatric prospective study, *J Pediatr* 123:779–783, 2009.

106. When does GER become GERD (gastroesophageal reflux disease)?
     GERD occurs when physiologic GER (a variation of normal; "happy spitters") becomes pathologic with the onset of symptoms and complications. These could include feeding refusal, poor weight gain, painful emesis, chronic respiratory problems, and others. The delineation can be imprecise, and other medical conditions can present with symptoms similar to GERD or with secondary GERD.

Grossman AB, Liacouras CA: Gastrointestinal bleeding. In Liacouras CA, Piccoli DA, editors: *Pediatric Gastroenterology: The Requisites in Pediatrics.* Philadelphia, 2008, Mosby, pp 74–86.

107. **What are the diagnostic methods for GER?**

The diagnosis can be made either clinically or by diagnostic testing. Clinically, reflux should be suspected in any child who demonstrates frequent, effortless vomiting or regurgitation without evidence of GI obstruction. Clinical response to medical therapy can be diagnostic.

The **upper GI barium** study does not reliably indicate reflux but can assess for anatomic abnormalities, such as malrotation, which might contribute. **Nuclear scintigraphy**, a noninvasive test that uses radiolabeled milk ("milk scan") or a meal, can detect postprandial reflux and delay in gastric emptying but cannot distinguish between physiologic and pathologic reflux. The presence of histologic esophagitis on an endoscopic examination is suggestive but not diagnostic of reflux; the absence of esophagitis does not rule out reflux. The **24-hour pH probe,** traditionally thought to be the most reliable test for the diagnosis of GER, only detects acid reflux and cannot detect nonacid reflux. **Multichannel intraluminal impedance** is a newer technology that can be performed with a pH probe to assess all types of reflux: acid, weakly acid, and alkaline. It is often used in combination with pH probe testing to separate acid from nonacid reflux.

Shin MS: Esophageal pH and combined impedance-pH monitoring in children, *Pediatr Gastroenterol Hepatol Nutr* 17:13–22, 2014.

van der Pol RJ, Smits MJ, Venmans L, et al: Diagnostic accuracy of tests in pediatric gastroesophageal reflux disease, *J Pediatr* 162:983–987, 2013.

108. **How effective are nonpharmacologic agents as treatments for suspected GER?**

They can be quite effective clinically. In a study of infants with suspected GER, the following changes resulted in improvements after 2 weeks in reflux scores in three quarters and normalization in one quarter of patients:

- Switching formula-fed infants to semi-elemental formula thickened with rice cereal
- If breastfeeding, the mother should eliminate cow milk and soy products from her diet
- Avoiding seated and supine positioning as much as possible for the infant, especially after feeding
- Eliminating tobacco smoke because of its association with increased GERD

Orenstein SR, McGowan JD: Efficacy of conservative therapy as taught in the primary care setting for symptoms suggesting infant gastroesophageal reflux, *J Pediatr* 152: 310–314, 2008.

109. **How effective are H2 blockers and proton pump inhibitors (PPIs) in the treatment of GER?**

These medications, though widely prescribed, have very limited data on efficacy in the treatment of GER. Part of the lack of demonstrated clinical success may be that many symptoms blamed on GER (such as cough, gagging, desaturations, back arching, fussiness, and pain) and treated with H2 antagonists or PPIs are not associated with reflux events when studied with pH-multichannel intraluminal probes.

van der Pol R, Langendam M, Benninga M, et al: Efficacy and safety of histamine-2 receptor antagonists, *JAMA Pediatr* 168(10):947–54, 2014.

Chen I-L, Gao W-Y, et al: Proton pump inhibitor use in infants: FDA reviewer experience, *J Pediatr Gastroenterol Nutr* 54:8–14, 2012.

110. **An infant with known GER who periodically arches his or her back may have what syndrome?**

Sandifer syndrome is paroxysmal dystonic posturing with opisthotonus and unusual twisting of the head and neck (resembling torticollis) in association with GER. Typically, an esophageal hiatal hernia is also present.

111. **What is a Nissen fundoplication?**

Nissen fundoplication is the most commonly performed antireflux surgical procedure. It involves wrapping a portion of the gastric fundus 360 degrees around the distal esophagus in an effort to tighten the gastroesophageal junction.

112. **Which patients are candidates for fundoplication?**

Most infants with developmental GER do not require fundoplication. It is indicated in patients with **recurrent aspiration, refractory** or **Barrett esophagitis, reflux-associated apnea,** and **reflux-associated FTT** that is refractory to medical therapy. Patients with severe reflux and psychomotor retardation should be evaluated for fundoplication if a feeding gastrostomy is contemplated.

KEY POINTS: GASTROESOPHAGEAL REFLUX

1. More than 40% of healthy infants regurgitate effortlessly more than once per day. This does not represent significant gastroesophageal reflux.
2. Gastroesophageal reflux disease is usually a clinical diagnosis. Testing, such as upper gastrointestinal testing, nuclear scintigraphy, pH and impedance monitoring, and upper endoscopy, can be helpful in certain cases, but it usually is not necessary.
3. By the age of 12 months, the symptoms of 95% of infants with significant reflux have resolved.

113. **A teenage girl has symptoms of swallowing difficulties improved by positional head and neck changes, nocturnal regurgitation, and halitosis. What is the leading diagnosis?**

Achalasia, which is a motor disorder of the esophagus characterized by loss of esophageal peristalsis, increased lower esophageal sphincter (LES) pressure, and absent or incomplete relaxation of LES with swallowing. Most cases are sporadic, and patients can present at any age from birth until the ninth decade of life. Suspected causes include autoimmune, infectious, and environmental triggers.

114. **What are the key tests to diagnose achalasia?**

A **barium swallow/video-esophagram** will show a variable degree of esophageal dilatation with tapering at the gastroesophageal junction. Figure 7-9 shows the characteristic "birds beak" esophagus. Later in the disease process, the proximal esophagus can become widely dilated and tortuous and plain chest x-ray may show a widened mediastinum. **Esophageal manometry** (esophageal motility study) measures the pressure generated by the esophageal muscle. It can detect achalasia earlier in its course when a video-esophagram may be normal.

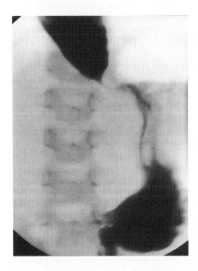

Figure 7-9. Barium swallow in a child with achalasia showing esophageal dilation and rapid tapering in a beaklike appearance. *(From Wyllie R, Hyams JS, Kay M, editors:* Pediatric Gastrointestinal and Liver Disease, *ed 3. Philadelphia, 2006, Saunders, p 330.)*

115. **What are treatment options for achalasia?**

Treatment options include pneumatic dilations (via therapeutic endoscopy), corrective laparoscopic surgery, botulinum toxin injection at the lower esophageal sphincter, and pharmacologic therapies. Pneumatic dilation is relatively well tolerated, but it often needs to be repeated if symptoms recur. Regardless of treatment modality used, patients continue to be at increased risk for aspiration secondary to pooling of food and saliva in the esophagus after meals. Many have complications of reflux esophagitis, which require ongoing surveillance.

Lee CW, Kays DW, Chen MK, et al: Outcomes of treatment of childhood achalasia, *J Pediatr Surg* 45:1173–1177, 2010.

116. **What are the common symptoms of gastroparesis?**
Gastroparesis is a disorder of gastric motility characterized by impairment of gastric contraction and emptying. Common symptoms include bloating, early satiety, nausea, vomiting (especially of undigested food eaten many hours before), and abdominal discomfort in the absence of mechanical obstruction.

117. **In what clinical settings should gastroparesis be suspected?**
- Preterm infants with immature GI tract
- Infants with cow milk protein allergy
- Postinfectious, including viral (rotavirus, Epstein-Barr virus [EBV], cytomegalovirus [CMV]) and *Mycoplasma* infection
- Postsurgical, including vagal nerve injury in upper abdominal surgery such as fundoplication or bariatric surgery
- Cystic fibrosis
- Type 1 diabetes mellitus
- Chronic intestinal pseudo-obstruction
- Muscular dystrophy
- Systemic autoimmune disorders, such as scleroderma

118. **How is postinfectious gastroparesis diagnosed?**
Patients will commonly present with persistent vomiting for days, weeks, or even months after a viral illness. Often the acute illness has passed, and the offending pathogen cannot be isolated. Diagnosis is mainly clinical, but can be confirmed with a delayed gastric emptying scan.

Saliakellis E, Fotoulaki M: Gastroparesis in children, *Ann Gastroenterol* 26: 204–211, 2013.

119. **How is gastroparesis treated?**
Dietary and behavioral modifications: Avoidance of carbonated beverages which can distend the stomach, drinking fluids throughout a meal, and walking 1 to 2 hours after a meal can promote better stomach emptying. In severe cases, a majority of calories can be provided in liquid form.

Pharmacotherapy: *Prokinetic agents* including (1) dopamine receptor antagonists (e.g., metoclopramide), which increase duration and frequency of antral and duodenal contractions, increase LES pressure, and relax the pyloric sphincter, and (2) erythromycin, a macrolide antibiotic with agonist activity of motilin receptors in smooth muscle cells of the GI tract (stomach and small bowel).

120. **A 12-year-old who presents with weight loss and a history of effortlessly and involuntarily regurgitating many meals has what likely diagnosis?**
Rumination syndrome. This is a functional gastrointestinal motility disorder characterized by repetitive effortless regurgitation of recently swallowed food from the stomach into the mouth within 30 minutes of ingesting the meal. When the stomach contents reach the mouth, it is either reswallowed or expelled. In infants and young children, rumination is commonly seen in patients with neurologic impairment or developmental delay. Adolescents are typically healthy. Children who have rumination typically do not retch and do not complain of dyspeptic/heartburn symptoms. Rumination syndrome can be difficult to diagnose. Differential diagnoses include bulimia nervosa and gastroparesis. The most effective treatments involve biofeedback and relaxation techniques.

Kessing BF, Smout AJ, Bredenoord AJ: Current diagnosis and management of the rumination syndrome, *J Clin Gastroenterol* 48:478-483, 2014.

HEPATIC, BILIARY AND PANCREATIC DISEASE

121. **What laboratory tests are commonly used to evaluate liver disease?**
See Table 7-7.

Table 7-7. Laboratory Tests Commonly Used to Evaluate Liver Disease

TEST	CLINICAL SIGNIFICANCE
Alanine aminotransferase (ALT, SGPT)	Increased with damaged hepatocytes
Aspartate aminotransferase (AST, SGOT)	Less sensitive than ALT for hepatic injury
Alkaline phosphatase (AP)	Increased in cholestatic disease; also comes from bone Higher in children because of bone growth (can identify source through isoenzyme)
γ-Glutamyltransferase (GGT)	More sensitive marker for cholestasis than AP
Bilirubin	Differential diagnosis different for conjugated versus unconjugated
Albumin	Low albumin can indicate chronic impairment in hepatic synthetic function
Prealbumin	Shorter half-life; may reflect more acute synthetic capabilities
Prothrombin time (PT)	Reflects synthetic function as a result of short half-life of factors
Ammonia	Impaired removal in patients with chronic liver disease; can lead to encephalopathy

122. **What conditions are associated with elevations of aminotransferases?**
    - Steatosis (fatty liver due to metabolic syndrome)
    - Hepatocellular inflammation (hepatitis)
    - Drug- or toxin-associated hepatic injury
    - Hypoperfusion or hypoxia
    - Passive congestion (right-sided congestive heart failure, Budd-Chiari syndrome, constrictive pericarditis)
    - Nonhepatic disorders (muscular dystrophy, celiac disease, macroenzyme of aspartate aminotransferase)

Teitelbaum JE: Normal hepatobiliary function. In Rudolph CD, Rudolph AM, editors: *Rudolph's Pediatrics*, ed 21. New York, 2003, McGraw-Hill, pp 1479.

123. **What is the most frequent cause of chronically elevated aminotransferases among children and adolescents in the United States?**
    Nonalcoholic fatty liver disease (NAFLD). The condition is most commonly associated with the metabolic syndrome in obese patients. Hepatic steatosis (abnormal lipid deposition in hepatocytes) occurs in the absence of excess alcohol intake. A main concern of the condition is that this simple benign fatty liver may progress to nonalcoholic steatohepatitis (or NASH) which involves inflammation of the liver and hepatocellular damage. This ultimately can lead to cirrhosis with possible liver failure and portal hypertension. It is unclear how and why certain children make that significant pathologic jump to marked liver disease.

Berardis S, Sokal E: Pediatric non-alcoholic fatty liver disease: an increasing public health issue. *Eur J Pediatr* 173:131–139, 2014.

124. **What is the main reason for the apparent increase in pediatric NAFLD?**
    The **growing obesity epidemic** is likely responsible. Some studies indicate that about half of obese children may have fatty liver. Children of Asian descent and of Hispanic (mostly Mexican) descent are also at increased risk compared with white and black American children.

Nieregarten MB, Freed GL: Pediatric nonalcoholic fatty liver disease, *Contemp Pediatr* 30:14, 2013.

125. What is the best way to screen for NAFLD?

Established screening guidelines are currently lacking. The most widely used test is **serum alanine aminotransferase (ALT),** which is the most common abnormal laboratory finding noted in the disease, but the sensitivity is low. In addition, the height of the measurement does not correlate with disease severity. Conversely, normal levels do not exclude possible fibrosis. Imaging studies, particularly ultrasound, have some diagnostic merit with potential detection of increased fatty echogenicity and hepatic enlargement. However, ultrasound is diagnostically most effective when hepatic steatosis is more advanced with a liver fat content of >30%. Computed tomography (CT) is a better study, but it has obvious radiation implications. The gold standard for diagnosis, liver biopsy, is too invasive as a screening test.

Berardis S, Sokal E: Pediatric non-alcoholic fatty liver disease: an increasing public health issue. *Eur J Pediatr* 173:131–139, 2014.

126. Why is it important to determine whether an elevated bilirubin is conjugated or unconjugated?

Bilirubin released from erythrocytes (unconjugated) is taken up by the liver and enzymatically converted (conjugated) to a more water-soluble form. On the basis of laboratory methodology, measurements of unconjugated bilirubin are referred to as *indirect reacting* and those of conjugated bilirubin as *direct reacting.* Elevated conjugated bilirubin is associated with obstruction of the biliary tract, intrahepatic cholestasis, or poorly functioning hepatocytes. Conjugated hyperbilirubinemia always requires further evaluation.

Harb R, Thomas DW: Conjugated hyperbilirubinemia: screening and treatment in older infants and children, *Pediatr Rev* 28:83–90, 2007.

127. When are levels of conjugated bilirubin considered abnormal?

Levels >20% of total bilirubin are considered abnormal. In significant indirect (unconjugated) hyperbilirubinemia, direct (conjugated) levels usually do not exceed 15%. The levels between 15% and 20% are thus somewhat indeterminate. Generally, direct bilirubin does not exceed more than 2 mg/dL.

128. What are the common causes of neonatal hepatitis and neonatal cholestasis?

See Table 7-8.

Table 7-8. Neonatal Conjugated Hyperbilirubinemia and Neonatal Hepatitis

Neonatal Hepatitis	**Metabolic**
Idiopathic	α_1-Antitrypsin deficiency
Viral	Tyrosinemia
Cytomegalovirus	Galactosemia
Herpesviruses	Cystic fibrosis
Hepatitis viruses	Bile acid synthetic disorders
Human immunodeficiency virus	Storage disorders
Enterovirus	Niemann-Pick disease
Rubella	Gaucher disease
Adenovirus	Lipidoses
Bacterial	Peroxisomal disorders
Bile Duct Obstruction	**Endocrine**
Biliary atresia	Hypothyroidism
Choledochal cyst	Panhypopituitarism
Neonatal sclerosing cholangitis	**Other Inherited Causes**
Congenital hepatic fibrosis	Alagille syndrome
Cholelithiasis	Familial intrahepatic cholestasis
Tumor or mass	Neonatal iron storage disease
	Toxic
	Parenteral nutrition
	Drugs
	Cardiovascular Disorders

Adapted from Suchy FJ: Approach to the infant with cholestasis. In Suchy FJ, Sokol RJ, Balistreri WF, editors: Liver Disease in Children, ed 3. New York, 2007, Cambridge University Press, pp 179–189.

129. What is the likelihood of chronic hepatic disease developing after acute infections with hepatitis viruses A to G?
     - **Hepatitis A:** 95% recover within 1 to 2 weeks of illness; chronic disease is unusual
     - **Hepatitis B:** >90% of perinatally infected infants develop chronic hepatitis B infection; 25% to 50% of children who acquire the virus between 1 and 5 years of age develop chronic infection; in older children and adults, only 6% to 10% develop chronic infection
     - **Hepatitis C:** 50% to 60% develop persistent infection
     - **Hepatitis D:** Occurs only in patients with acute or chronic hepatitis B infection; 80% develop viral persistence
     - **Hepatitis E:** Does not cause chronic hepatitis
     - **Hepatitis G:** Unknown

American Academy of Pediatrics: Hepatitis A-G. In Pickering LK, editor: *2012 Red Book, Report of the Committee on Infectious Diseases,* ed 29. Elk Grove Village, IL, 2012, American Academy of Pediatrics, pp 361–395.

130. Other than viral hepatitis, what are other common causes of acute and chronic hepatitis in children?
     - **Metabolic and genetic disorders:** Wilson disease, α_1-antitrypsin deficiency, cystic fibrosis, steatohepatitis
     - **Toxic hepatitis:** Drugs, hepatotoxins, radiation
     - **Autoimmune:** Autoimmune hepatitis, primary sclerosing cholangitis: anti–smooth muscle antibody positive, anti–liver-kidney-microsomal antibody positive
     - **Anatomic:** Cholelithiasis, choledochal cyst
     - **Other infectious:** CMV, EBV
     - **Toxic:** Ethanol, acetaminophen
     - **Other inherited:** Alagille syndrome, cystic fibrosis, familial intrahepatic cholestasis

131. How is α_1-antitrypsin deficiency most likely to present in infants and children?
     α_1-Antitrypsin deficiency is an autosomal recessive disorder that causes lung and liver disease. In the liver, injury results from intracellular accumulation of the mutant α_1-antitrypsin protein. In the lungs, the absence of functional α_1-antitrypsin leads to unchecked leukocyte elastase function, resulting in destruction of the alveolar walls and eventual emphysema. The pulmonary effects take years to evolve, so lung disease rarely is present in children. More common presenting symptoms are neonatal cholestasis, hepatomegaly, and chronic hepatitis. Although most patients do not have severe disease, this can progress to cirrhosis with liver failure.

Stockley RA: Alpha 1-antitrypsin deficiency, *Clin Chest Med* 35:39–50, 2014.

132. Why is measuring the level serum level of α_1-antitrypsin not enough to diagnose α_1-antitrypsin deficiency?
     α_1-Antitrypsin is an acute phase reactant and might not be decreased in all cases of α_1-antitrypsin deficiency. Pi typing (short for protease inhibitor typing) by electrophoresis is necessary to make the diagnosis. MM is the normal phenotype and has the highest activity; ZZ has the lowest activity and the most common association with liver disease. PiMM is the most common Pi type, with a distribution of about 87%; PiMS represents 8% and PiMZ 2%. The incidence of PiZZ ranges between 1 in 2000 and 1 in 5000.

Silverman EK, Sandhaus RA: Alpha₁-antitrypsin deficiency, *N Engl J Med* 360:2749–2757, 2009.

133. What is the metabolic defect in patients with Wilson disease?
     Wilson disease is an autosomal recessive **defect of copper metabolism** that results in markedly increased levels of copper in many tissues, most notably the liver, basal ganglia, and cornea (Kayser-Fleischer rings). The primary defect is a mutation in the transmembrane protein ATP7B, which is key to excreting excess copper into the biliary canalicular system. The combination of

markedly increased copper levels in a liver biopsy specimen, low serum ceruloplasmin, and increased urinary copper excretion strongly suggests Wilson disease.

Ala A, Walker AP, Ashkan K, et al: Wilson's disease, *Lancet* 369:397–408, 2007.

134. **What are the treatments of choice for Wilson disease?**
    Copper-chelating agents. *D-Penicillamine* has traditionally been the drug of choice, but another chelator, *trientine*, has been used successfully in patients who have discontinued penicillamine because of hypersensitivity reactions. Some advocate for trientine as an alternative agent to penicillamine because trientine has a better safety profile. Zinc sulfate, which inhibits intestinal copper absorption, has also been used. Patients require a low copper diet for life.

135. **A 3-year-old child who experiences mild fluctuating jaundice in times of illness "just like his Uncle Kevin" is likely to have what condition?**
    Gilbert syndrome, which is due primarily to a decrease in hepatic glucuronyl transferase activity. Normally, bilirubin is disconjugated to glucuronic acid. In patients with Gilbert syndrome, the defective total conjugation results in the increased production of monoglucuronides in bile and mild elevation in serum unconjugated (indirect) bilirubin. The syndrome is inherited in an autosomal dominant fashion with incomplete penetrance (boys outnumber girls by 4 to 1). Frequency of this gene in the population is estimated at 2% to 6%. Elevations of bilirubin are noted during times of medical and physical stress, particularly fasting.

136. **What are the clinical findings of portal hypertension?**
    Obstruction of portal flow is manifested by two physical signs: **splenomegaly** and **increased collateral venous circulations**. Collaterals are evident on physical examination in the anus and abdominal wall and by special studies in the esophagus. Hemorrhoids may suggest collaterals, but, in older patients, these are present in high frequency without liver disease, and thus their presence has no predictive value. Dilation of the paraumbilical veins produces a rosette around the umbilicus (the caput medusae), and the dilated superficial veins of the abdominal wall are visible. A venous hum may be present in the subxiphoid region from varices in the falciform ligament.

137. **How does autoimmune hepatitis (AIH) typically present?**
    There are three typical patterns of presentation: (1) *acute hepatitis*, with nonspecific symptoms of malaise, nausea and vomiting, anorexia, jaundice, dark urine, and pale stools; (2) *insidious,* with progressive fatigue, relapsing jaundice, headache, and weight loss; and (3) despite no history of jaundice, patients present with complications of *portal hypertension* (splenomegaly, GI bleeding from varices, and weight loss). Type I AIH is more common and characterized by antineutrophil antibodies and anti–smooth muscle antibodies. Type 2 AIH is characterized by anti–liver-kidney-microsomal antibodies.

138. **A patient with liver failure develops confusion. Why worry?**
    Hepatic encephalopathy can appear as either a rapid progression to coma or as mild fluctuations in mental status over an extended amount of time. A single underlying cause has not been established, but suspected toxins include ammonia, other neurotoxins, and relatively increased γ-aminobutyric acid activity. Management requires the limitation of protein intake, the use of lactulose to promote mild diarrhea, antibiotics to reduce ammonia production, intracranial pressure monitoring in advanced cases, and possible peritoneal dialysis for patients in severe coma and before liver transplantation.

139. **What is the most common indication for pediatric liver transplantation?**
    The most common indication is **extrahepatic biliary atresia** with chronic liver failure after a Kasai hepatoportoenterostomy. Other common indications include inborn errors of metabolism (e.g., α_1-antitrypsin deficiency, hereditary tyrosinemia, Wilson disease) and idiopathic fulminant hepatic failure.

140. **Calculous and acalculous cholecystitis: what are the differences?**
    Calculous cholecystitis: Gallstone impaction in the cystic duct results in gallbladder distention edema, biliary stasis, and bacterial overgrowth (e.g., *E. coli, Klebsiella,* enterococci). If untreated, this can lead to gallbladder infarction, gangrene, and perforation.

Acalculous cholecystitis: Gallbladder dysfunction results from a variety of conditions including major trauma, sepsis/hypotension, and diabetes. Bile stasis results, which can lead to an inflammatory response; ischemia; distention; and eventually, necrosis of gallbladder tissue.

141. **Which patients are at risk for cholelithiasis?**
See Table 7-9.

Table 7-9. Patients at Risk for Cholelithiasis

	PIGMENT STONE	CHOLESTEROL STONE
Race	—	Native American
Sex	—	Female
Age	—	Adolescence
Diet	—	Obesity
Total parenteral nutrition	+++	—
Hemolytic disease (especially sickle-cell disease, thalassemia, hereditary spherocytosis)	+++	—
Cystic fibrosis	—	+++
Ileal disease	—	+++
Defects in bile salt synthesis	—	+++
Hypertriglyceridemia	—	+++
Diabetes mellitus	—	+++

+++ = increased risk

142. **What are the possible causes of pancreatitis in children?**
In adults, the majority of cases of pancreatitis arise from gallstones or alcohol. In children, there is a much greater diversity in etiology.
- **33%: Systemic disorders** (sepsis and shock, vasculitis)
- **13% to 34%: Idiopathic**
- **10% to 40%: Trauma** (motor vehicle accidents, sports injuries, accidental falls, child abuse)
- **10% to 30%: Biliary disease** (gallstones, sludge)
- **<25%: Medications** (valproic acid, L-asparaginase, prednisone, 6-mercaptopurine)
- **<10%: Infections** (various viral, including mumps)
- **5% to 8%: Hereditary** (genetic mutations)
- **2% to 7%: Metabolic disorders** (diabetic ketoacidosis [DKA], hypertriglyceridemia, hypercalcemia)
- **<3%: Anatomic and structural anomalies** (pancreatic divisum, duct anomalies, sphincter of Oddi dysfunction)

Bai HX, Lowe ME, Husain SZ: What have we learned about acute pancreatitis in children? *J Pediatr Gastroenterol Nutr* 52:262–270, 2011.

143. **What is the typical presentation of acute pancreatitis in children?**
In children >3 years of age, the most common symptom is **abdominal pain**, which occurs in 80% to 95%. Pain is typically epigastric in location. Radiation to the back is uncommon. Nausea or vomiting occurs in 40% to 80%. Abdominal distention is also common. Infants and toddlers are less likely to complain of abdominal pain and nausea and are more likely to have fever.

Bai HX, Lowe ME, Husain SZ: What have we learned about acute pancreatitis in children? *J Pediatr Gastroenterol Nutr* 52:262–270, 2011.

144. **Which enzyme is a more sensitive marker of pancreatic injury in children: amylase or lipase?**
There is no clear winner. In a compilation of pediatric studies, the sensitivity of the amylase test in diagnosing pancreatitis has ranged from 50% to 85%, while lipase was only marginally more sensitive than amylase in most studies. Amylase values rise 2 to 12 hours after the onset of pancreatitis; lipase values rise at 4 to 8 hours. Because only one or the other may be elevated in individual patients, both lipase and amylase should be measured in suspected pancreatitis.

Srinath AI, Lowe ME: Pediatric pancreatitis, *Pediatr Rev* 34:79–89, 2013.
Bai HX, Lowe ME, Husain SZ: What have we learned about acute pancreatitis in children? *J Pediatr Gastroenterol Nutr* 52:262–270, 2011.

145. **What conditions may be associated with hyperamylasemia?**
Pancreatic: pancreatitis, pancreatic tumors, pancreatic duct obstruction, biliary obstruction, perforated ulcer, bowel obstruction, acute appendicitis, mesenteric ischemia, endoscopic retrograde cholangiopancreatogram (ERCP)
Salivary: infections (mumps), trauma, salivary duct obstruction, lung cancer, ovarian tumors or cysts, prostate tumors, DKA
Mixed or unknown: cystic fibrosis, renal insufficiency, pregnancy, cerebral edema, burns

KEY POINTS: HEPATIC AND BILIARY DISEASE

1. Portal hypertension manifests clinically as splenomegaly and increased collateral venous circulation.
2. Conjugated hyperbilirubinemia in any child is abnormal and deserves further investigation.
3. Extrahepatic biliary atresia is the most common pediatric indication for liver transplantation.
4. The younger the patient, the more likely it is that acute hepatitis B infection will become chronic.

INFLAMMATORY BOWEL DISEASE

146. **What is the epidemiology of pediatric inflammatory bowel disease (IBD)?**
The incidence and prevalence of IBD in general, and Crohn disease specifically, has increased over recent decades. The most significant increases have occurred in younger children with increases of 5% in those <4 years old and nearly 8% in children 5 to 9 years old. About 20% of all IBD cases are diagnosed before age 10 years. Mean age of diagnosis of pediatric IBD is 12½ years. About 10,000 new cases are diagnosed annually. Up to 25% of children who are diagnosed with IBD have a positive family history.

Glick SR, Carvalho RS: Inflammatory bowel disease, *Pediatr Rev* 32:14–24, 2011.

147. **How do ulcerative colitis and Crohn disease vary in intestinal distribution?**
Ulcerative colitis is limited to the superficial mucosa of the colon. It always involves the rectum and extends proximally to a variable extent. Ulcerative colitis more commonly involves the entire colon in children than in adults, who more commonly will have limited left-sided disease. Regional enteritis, or **Crohn disease**, is characterized by transmural inflammation of the bowel that may affect the entire tract from the mouth to the anus. Because of the transmural nature of the inflammation, patients can develop fistulas and abscesses more commonly with Crohn disease. The typical cobblestone appearance of Crohn disease is produced by crisscrossing ulcerations (Fig. 7-10). Crohn colitis, with no involvement of the small bowel, is more common in younger children and can be difficult to distinguish from ulcerative colitis.

Abraham C, Cho JH: Inflammatory bowel disease, *N Engl J Med* 36:2066–2078, 2009.
Bousvaros A, Antonioli DA, Colletti RB, et al: Differentiating ulcerative colitis from Crohn disease in children and young adults, *J Pediatr Gastroenterol Nutr* 44:653–674, 2007.

148. **What features differentiate ulcerative colitis from Crohn disease?**
See Table 7-10.

Crohn's and Colitis Foundation of America: www.ccfa.org. Accessed Nov. 24, 2014.

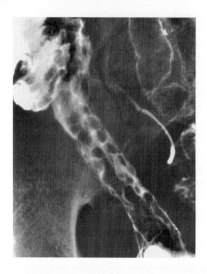

Figure 7-10. Crisscrossing ulcerations produce a cobblestone appearance in patients with Crohn disease. *(From Katz DS, Math KR, Groskin SA: Radiology Secrets. Philadelphia, 1998, Hanley & Belfus, p 150.)*

Table 7-10. Features that Differentiate Ulcerative Colitis from Crohn Disease

	ULCERATIVE COLITIS	CROHN DISEASE
Distribution	Colon only (gastritis recognized) Continuous	Entire gastrointestinal tract Skip lesions
Clinical presentation		
Bleeding	Very common	Common
Growth failure	Uncommon	Common
Weight loss	Less common	Common
Obstruction	Uncommon	Common
Perianal disease	Rare	Common
Endoscopic findings	Continuous inflammation 100% rectal involvement Erythema, edema, friability, ulceration on abnormal mucosa	Focal or segmental inflammation Rectal sparing Aphthous or linear ulcerations on normal-appearing mucosa Cobblestoning Abnormal terminal ileum: >50%
Histologic findings	Mucosa only No granulomas	Full-thickness granulomas

149. **What is the role of serologic panels in the diagnosis of IBD?**
Certain antibodies can help distinguish between Crohn disease and ulcerative colitis in patients with indeterminate colitis. These panels are not useful in population screening as false-positive results can create unwarranted anxiety and unnecessary testing. One-third of individuals with positive serology do not have IBD. Higher antibody titers are associated with more aggressive disease. Average positivity is as follows:
  - **ASCA** (anti-*Saccharomyces cerevisiae antibody*): CD (40% to 56%), UC (0% to 7%), Controls (<5%)

- **ANCA** (anti-neutrophil cytoplasmic antibody): CD (18% to 24%), UC (60% to 80%), Controls (<5%)
- **Anti-OmpC** (outer membrane protein C, *E. coli*): CD (25%), UC (6%), Controls (3%)

Glick SR, Carvalho RS: Inflammatory bowel disease, *Pediatr Rev* 32:18–19, 2011.

150. **What are the extraintestinal manifestations of pediatric IBD?**
In addition to the typical gastrointestinal involvement, other organ systems can become involved in IBD. These manifestations may become the major source of morbidity and presenting symptom(s) for some patients.
- Growth failure
- Arthralgias/arthritis
- Bone disease including osteopenia and osteoporosis
- Oral lesions, most commonly recurrent aphthous lesions
- Skin lesions: granulomatous, reactive, and secondary to nutritional deficiencies
- Eye lesions: episcleritis and uveitis
- Liver disease: hepatitis, fatty liver, cholelithiasis, amyloidosis, and primary sclerosing cholangitis
- Rare extraintestinal manifestations (<1% of pediatric IBD patients): hematologic abnormalities, venous thrombosis, pancreatitis, nephrolithiasis, pulmonary disease, neurologic disease

Rabizadeh S, Oliva-Hemkey M: Extraintestinal manifestations of pediatric inflammatory bowel disease. In Mamula P, Markowitz J, Baldassano R, editors: *Pediatric Inflammatory Bowel Disease*, Springer, 2007, Philadelphia, pp 87-92.

151. **What pharmacologic therapies are used in the treatment of ulcerative colitis and Crohn disease?**
Mild disease and remission: 5-Aminosalicylic acids (ASA) (mesalamine, mesalazine), oral and rectal, particularly for ulcerative colitis; antibiotics; extended-release budesonide;
Moderate disease: Metronidazole (for Crohn disease); prednisone
Severe and refractory disease: Azathioprine; 6-Mercaptopurine; intravenous steroids; methotrexate; anti-tumor necrosis factor agents (e.g., infliximab, adalimumab); cyclosporine

Jacobstein D, Baldassano R: Inflammatory bowel disease. In Liacouras CA, Piccoli DA, editors: *Pediatric Gastroenterology: The Requisites in Pediatrics*, Philadelphia, 2008, Mosby, p 138.

152. **How are therapies chosen for IBD?**
Traditionally, medications have been chosen in a "step-up" approach using medications with less severe side effects such as ASA or steroids before initiation of immunomodulators or biologic therapies. This is now being challenged with a "top-down" approach using more potent medications earlier in the course of the disease to induce mucosal healing, interrupt the natural history of the disease processes, and decrease potential for long-term complications including need for surgical intervention. Overall, the age, presenting symptoms and severity, and sex of the child must be taken into consideration when starting therapy.

153. **Is there a potential role for thalidomide in the treatment of Crohn disease?**
The use of thalidomide was one of the great medicinal tragedies of the twentieth century. Thalidomide was released initially in Germany in 1957 and marketed as a wonder drug for insomnia, anxiety, and nausea, especially morning sickness associated with pregnancy. Thousands of women who took the drug in the first trimester gave birth to infants with marked malformations of the extremities and other malformations. In 1998, it was resurrected as an anti-leprosy drug. In 2006, the Food and Drug Administration (FDA) approved a modified version of thalidomide for use in the treatment of multiple myeloma.
Thalidomide has properties of lowering tumor necrosis factor and inhibiting angiogenesis. Investigators in Italy found that, compared with placebo, treatment with thalidomide for children and adolescents with refractory Crohn disease resulted in improved clinical remission at 8 weeks, which was maintained in a long-term period of continued treatment.

Lazzerini M, Martelossi S, Magazzu G, et al: Effect of thalidomide on clinical remission in children and adolescents with refractory Crohn disease: a randomized clinical trial, *JAMA* 310:2164–2173, 2013.

154. **In a child who has been diagnosed with Crohn disease, what are potential long-term complications?**
- **Severe perianal disease** can be a debilitating complication. More prevalent in patients with Crohn disease, it may range from simple skin tags to the development of perianal abscesses or fistulas.
- **Enteroenteral fistulas** may occur and "short circuit" the absorptive process. The thickened bowel may obstruct or perforate, thus requiring operation. The recurrence rate is high after surgery, repeated operations are often necessary, and short bowel syndrome may result. In many cases, a permanent ostomy is placed, although pouch construction and continent ileostomies have become more common.
- **Growth retardation and delayed puberty** are seen extensively in patients with pediatric Crohn disease. The insidious onset may result in several years of linear growth failure before the correct diagnosis is made. With epiphyseal closure, linear growth is terminated, and short adult stature will be permanent.
- **Decrease in bone mineralization** (*osteopenia*) is a more commonly recognized complication of Crohn disease, secondary to growth failure and malnutrition, disease activity, and toxic effect of corticosteroids. All patients should have a bone densitometry scan to assess for this complication. Treatment includes increased weight-bearing activity, correction of nutritional deficits, vitamin D and calcium supplementation, and more aggressive medical treatment of disease.
- **Hepatic complications** of IBD include chronic active hepatitis and sclerosing cholangitis, which may require liver transplantation.
- **Nephrolithiasis** may occur in patients with resections or steatorrhea as a result of the increased intestinal absorption of oxalate.
- **Chronic reactive and restrictive pulmonary disease** has been noted.
- **Arthralgias** are common, but destructive joint disease is uncommon.

KEY POINTS: INFLAMMATORY BOWEL DISEASE

1. Ulcerative colitis is limited to the superficial mucosa of the large intestine, always involves the rectum, and demonstrates no skip lesions.
2. Crohn disease can occur anywhere in the gastrointestinal tract (from the mouth to the anus) and demonstrates transmural inflammation with skip lesions; noncaseating granulomas may be found on microscopic pathology. The transmural inflammation can result in the formation of abscesses or fistulas.
3. Potential long-term complications of inflammatory bowel disease include chronic growth failure, abscesses, fistulas, nephrolithiasis, and osteopenia.
4. Surgery can be curative for ulcerative colitis, but the incidence of postoperative recurrence is high in Crohn disease.

---

155. **Are children with IBD at increased risk for malignancy?**
The risk for malignancy has not been studied systematically among pediatric populations with IBD. The risk in adults depends both on the disease and its duration. After 10 years of ulcerative colitis, the risk rises dramatically (1% to 2% increased incidence of malignancy per year). The risk is thought to be higher in patients with pancolitis compared with those with limited left-sided disease. The carcinomas associated with ulcerative colitis are often poorly differentiated and metastasize early; they have a poorer prognosis and are more difficult to identify by radiographic and colonoscopic examinations. Most authors indicate that carcinoma of the bowel is much less common among patients with Crohn disease, although this has been disputed. The risk for lymphoma is increased in patients with Crohn disease. Immunosuppressive (e.g., 6-mercaptopurine) and biologic (e.g., infliximab) therapy may also increase the risk for neoplasia.

156. **When is surgery indicated for children with IBD?**
See Table 7-11.

NUTRITION

157. **What are various requirements for protein, fat, and carbohydrates?**
Protein should account for 7% to 15% of caloric intake and should include a balance of the 11 essential amino acids. Protein requirements range from 0.7 to 2.5 g/kg per day. **Fats** should provide 30% to 50% of caloric intake. Although most of these calories are derived from long-chain triglycerides, sterols,

Table 7-11. Indications for Surgery for Children with IBD

CROHN DISEASE	ULCERATIVE COLITIS
Perforation with abscess formation	*Urgent:*
Obstruction with or without stenosis	Hemorrhage
Uncontrolled massive bleeding	Perforation
Draining fistulas and sinuses	Toxic megacolon
Toxic megacolon	Acute fulminant colitis unresponsive to maximal
Growth failure in patients with localized	medical therapy
areas of resectable disease	
	Elective:
	Chronic disease with recurrent severe exacerbations
	Continuous incapacitating disease despite adequate
	medical treatment
	Growth retardation with pubertal delay
	Disease of >10 years' duration with evidence of
	epithelial dysplasia

From Hofley PM, Piccoli DA: Inflammatory bowel disease in children, Med Clin North Am 78:1293–1295, 1994.

medium-chain triglycerides, and fatty acids may be important in certain diets. Linoleic acid and arachidonic acid are essential for tissue membrane synthesis, and about 3% of intake must be composed of these triglycerides. The remaining 50% to 60% of calories should come from **carbohydrates**. About half of these are contributed by monosaccharides and disaccharides (e.g., sucrose, lactose) and the remainder by starches.

American Dietetic Association: www.eatright.org. Accessed on Mar. 20, 2015.

158. If recommended caloric intakes are maintained, what is normal daily weight gain of young children?
See Table 7-12.

Table 7-12. Normal Daily Weight Gain in Young Children*

AGE	WEIGHT GAIN RECOMMENDED (G)	CALORIC INTAKE (KCAL/KG/DAY)
0-3 mo	26-31	100-120
3-6 mo	17-18	105-115
6-9 mo	12-13	100-105
9-12 mo	9	100-105
1-3 yr	7-9	100
4-6 yr	6	90

*It should be noted that, when babies are primarily breastfed, growth during months 3 to 18 is less than that indicated by the table. On average, breastfed babies gain 0.65 kg less than formula-fed infants during the first year of life.
Data from Dewey KG, Heinig MJ, Nommsen LA, et al: Growth of breast-fed and formula-fed infants from 0 to 18 months: the DARLING Study, Pediatrics 89:1035–1041, 1992; and National Research Council, Food and Nutrition Board: Recommended Daily Allowances. Washington, DC, 1989, National Academy of Sciences.

159. What are the recommended bottle feedings by age?
See Table 7-13.

Table 7-13. Recommended Bottle Feedings by Age

AGE	NUMBER OF FEEDINGS	FLUID OUNCES PER FEEDING
Birth-1 week	6-10	1-3
1 week-1 month	7-8	2-4
1-3 months	5-7	4-6
3-6 months	4-5	6-7
6-9 months	3-4	7-8

160. Why should whole cow milk not be introduced until 1 year of age?
   Introduction of whole cow milk to infants <1 year of age is known to be detrimental to infants. It is associated with **iron deficiency anemia** because of its low iron content and occult intestinal blood loss, which occurs in 40% of normal young infants being fed cow milk. Early use of whole milk may contribute to weight acceleration and the development of **overweight/obesity**.

161. Why is honey not recommended for infants during the first year of life?
   Honey has been associated with infantile botulism as have some commercial corn syrups. *Clostridium botulinum* spores contaminate the honey and are ingested. In infants, intestinal colonization and multiplication of the organism may result in toxin production and lead to symptoms of constipation, listlessness, and weakness.

162. How is nutritional status objectively assessed in children?
   - **Growth chart:** Anthropometric data give an estimate of the height, weight, and head circumference of a child compared with a population standard. A change in the child's percentile months may signify the presence of a nutritional problem or systemic disease.
   - **Compare actual with ideal body weight** (average weight for height age): The ideal body weight is determined by plotting the child's height on the 50th percentile and recording the corresponding age. The 50th percentile weight for that age is obtained, and this ideal body weight is divided by the actual weight. The result is expressed as a percentage—the percent ideal body weight—that gives a better stratification of patients with significant malnutrition. An ideal body weight percentage of more than 120% is obese, 110% to 120% is overweight, 90% to 110% is normal, 80% to 90% is mild wasting, 70% to 80% is moderate wasting, and less than 70% is severe wasting.
   - **Measurement of midarm circumference:** This provides information about the subcutaneous fat stores, and the midarm-muscle circumference (calculated from the triceps skinfold thickness) estimates the somatic protein or muscle mass.
   - **Laboratory assessment:** Vitamin and mineral status can be directly assayed. Measurements of albumin (half-life, 14 to 20 days), transferrin (half-life, 8 to 10 days), and prealbumin (half-life, 2 to 3 days) can provide information about protein synthesis, but each may be affected by certain diseases. The ratio of albumin to globulin may decrease in patients with protein malnutrition.

163. What features on examination of the scalp, eyes, and mouth suggest problems of malnutrition?
   See Table 7-14.

164. How do marasmus and kwashiorkor differ clinically?
   - *Kwashiorkor* is edematous malnutrition as a result of low serum oncotic pressure. The low serum proteins result from a disproportionately low protein intake compared with the overall caloric intake. These children appear replete or fat, but they have dependent edema, hyperkeratosis, and atrophic hair and skin. They generally have severe anorexia, diarrhea, and frequent infections, and they may have cardiac failure.
   - *Marasmus* is severe nonedematous malnutrition caused by a mixed deficiency of both protein and calories. Serum protein and albumin levels are usually normal, but there is a

Table 7-14. Effects of Malnutrition on Scalp, Eyes, and Mouth

CLINICAL SIGN	NUTRIENT DEFICIENCY
Epithelial	
Skin	
Xerosis, dry scaling	Essential fatty acids
Hyperkeratosis, plaques around hair follicles	Vitamin A
Ecchymoses, petechiae	Vitamin K
Hair	
Easily plucked, dyspigmented, lackluster	Protein calorie
Mucosal	
Mouth, lips, and tongue	B vitamins
Angular stomatitis (inflammation at corners of the mouth)	B_2 (riboflavin)
Cheilosis (reddened lips with fissures at angles)	B_2, B_6 (pyridoxine)
Glossitis (inflammation of tongue)	B_6, B_3 (niacin), B_2
Magenta tongue	B_2
Edema of tongue, tongue fissures	B_3
Spongy, bleeding gums	Vitamin C
Ocular	
Conjunctival pallor due to anemia	Vitamin E (premature infants), iron, folic acid, B_{12}, copper
Bitot spots (grayish, yellow, or white foamy spots on the whites of the eyes)	Vitamin A

marked decrease in muscle mass and adipose tissue. Signs are similar to those noted in hypothyroid children, with cold intolerance, listlessness, thin sparse hair, dry skin with decreased turgor, and hypotonia. Diarrhea, anorexia, vomiting, and recurrent infections may be noted.

165. What vitamins and minerals are often deficient in strict vegans and some vegetarians?

    Vitamin B_{12}, iron, calcium, and zinc. The groups most at risk are infants, children, and pregnant and lactating women. Semivegetarian diets rarely lead to such deficiencies.

166. What two factors make vitamin D deficiency such a common problem?

    Changes in sun exposure/use of sunscreen and increases in obesity. Very few foods naturally contain vitamin D or are fortified with vitamin D. Exceptions are cod liver, tuna, fortified milk, and orange juice. The major source of vitamin D has been exposure to natural sunlight. If an individual wears a sunscreen with a protection factor of 30 or more, vitamin synthesis in the skin is reduced by >95%. If an individual has darker skin, which provides more natural sun protection, he or she requires 3 to 5 times longer exposure to make the same amount of vitamin D as a person with a white skin tone. Obesity is also a risk factor, because fat sequesters vitamin D. As sun exposure is reduced because of concerns about potential future malignancies and as obesity rates remain high, vitamin D deficiency is likely to remain a problem.

Holick MF, Binkley NC, et al: Evaluation, treatment and prevention of vitamin D deficiency: an Endocrine Society clinical practice guideline, *J Clin Endocrinol Metab* 96:1911–1930, 2011.

167. How much vitamin D should children receive on a daily basis?

    2015 recommendations are that children without risk factors should receive the following amounts of vitamin D at a minimum:

    Infants (<1 year): 400 IU/day
    Children (1 to 18 years): 600 IU/day

All exclusively breastfed infants should receive 400 IU/day of vitamin D supplement because breast milk is low in vitamin D. Some formula-fed infants also require supplementation if their intake is less than approximately 33 ounces of formula daily, which is the quantity needed to receive the recommended amount of vitamin D.

168. **What are the cutoffs for vitamin D deficiency and sufficiency?**
Levels <20 ng/mL are considered vitamin D deficient; a level >20 ng/mL is considered sufficient, but levels that are >30 ng/mL are more preferable.

OBESITY AND LIPID DISORDERS

169. **What are the weight status categories for children in terms of body mass index (BMI) percentile?**
    - **Underweight:** <5th percentile
    - **Healthy weight:** 5th to 85th percentile
    - **Overweight:** 85th to 95th percentile,
    - **Obese:** 95th to 98th percentile
    - **Severely (morbidly) obese**: ≥99th percentile

170. **What screening laboratory tests should be done for obese children?**
For children who are obese or severely obese, a basic laboratory evaluation to rule out the presence of obesity-related metabolic abnormalities should be considered. These would include:
    - **Liver function tests (AST and ALT):** to assess possible NAFLD
    - **Fasting lipid profile**: elevated triglycerides and reduced HDL is highly suggestive of significant insulin resistance
    - **CBC**: iron deficiency and iron deficiency anemia are common in obese children
    - **Fasting glucose**: sensitivity, however, is low to detect glucose intolerance. A standard oral glucose tolerance test should be considered for severe obesity, positive family history of type 2 diabetes or when acanthosis nigricans is present.
    - **Vitamin D level**: deficiency is common in obese children.
    - **Thyroid function tests**
    Other tests should be determined if comorbidities are suspected by history or exam.

Baker JL, Farpour-Lambert NJ, Nowicka A, et al: Evaluation of the overweight/obese child—practical tips for the primary health care provider: recommendations from the Childhood Obesity Task Force of the European Association for the Study of Obesity, *Obes Facts* 3:131–137, 2010.

171. **What are the different types of cholesterol?**
    Triglycerides: the major form of fat in the body
    LDL: low density lipoprotein; the "bad" cholesterol; formed from VLDL or chylomicrons; saturated and trans fats increase LDL; major carrier of cholesterol *into* the body tissues
    HDL: high density lipoprotein; "good" cholesterol; synthesized in the liver and gut; major carrier of cholesterol *away* from the body tissues
    VLDL: very low density lipoprotein; made by the liver; high in triglycerides
    Chylomicrons: transports dietary fat from intestines to liver and adipose tissues; high in triglycerides
    Non-HDL (total cholesterol − HDL): can be used if a nonfasting lipid profile is obtained or if triglycerides are >400

172. **Why is the promotion of cardiovascular health and the identification of specific risk factors important in *pediatric* medicine?**
    - Atherosclerotic changes originate in childhood.
    - Risk factors for the development of atherosclerosis can be identified in childhood.
    - The progression of atherosclerosis relates to the number and intensity of these risk factors.
    - Risk factors track from childhood to adult years.
    - Interventions exist for the management of identified risk factors.

Expert Panel on Integrated Guidelines: Expert panel on integrated guidelines for cardiovascular health and risk reduction in children and adolescents: summary report, *Pediatrics* 128: S217, 2011.

173. What are the screening guidelines for lipids?

Evidence-based guidelines from an expert panel from the National Heart Lung and Blood Institute (NHLBI) include the following:

Birth to 2 years: No lipid screening is recommended.

2 to 8 years: No universal screening is recommended unless there are risk factors for cardiovascular disease (see below)

9 to 11 years: Universal screening with nonfasting lipid panel is recommended. Obtain fasting lipid panel twice and average the results if non-HDL $\geq$145 mg/dL or HDL <40, or check fasting lipid panel and repeat if LDL $\geq$130 mg/dL, non-HDL $\geq$145 mg/dL, HDL <40, or triglycerides $\geq$100 mg/dL (if <10 years) or $\geq$130 mg/dL (if >10 years).

12 to 16 years: No routine screening is recommended unless there are risk factors for cardiovascular disease (see below). Universal lipid screening is not recommended in this age group because of decreased sensitivity and specificity for predicting adult values, particularly LDL.

17 to 19 years: Universal screening is recommended once in this age group with a nonfasting or fasting lipid profile; repeat in 2 weeks to 3 months if abnormal.

Risk factors: *parent with total cholesterol $\geq$240 mg/dL, early heart disease in a first or second degree relative, diabetes (type I or II), hypertension, BMI $\geq$95th percentile, smokes cigarettes, kidney disease, heart disease, chronic inflammatory disease, or HIV infection*

Expert Panel on Integrated Guidelines: Expert panel on integrated guidelines for cardiovascular health and risk reduction in children and adolescents: summary report, *Pediatrics* 128: S239, 2011.

174. What are the cutoffs for abnormal lipid levels?

See Table 7-15.

Table 7-15. Lipid Levels in Children and Adolescents

CATEGORY	ACCEPTABLE MG/DL	BORDERLINE MG/DL	HIGH MG/DL	LOW MG/DL
TC	<170	170-199	$\geq$200	
LDL-c	<110	110-129	$\geq$130	
Non HDL-c	<120	120-144	$\geq$145	
TG				
0-9 yr	<75	75-99	$\geq$100	
10-19 yr	<90	90-129	$\geq$130	
HDL-c	>45	40-45		<40

HDL-c = High-density lipoprotein cholesterol; LDL-c = Low-density lipoprotein cholesterol; TC = total cholesterol; TG = triglycerides.

175. What are the American Heart Association dietary strategies for all children older than 2 years?

- Balance dietary calories with physical activity to maintain normal growth.
- Engage in 60 minutes of moderate to vigorous play or physical activity daily.
- Eat vegetables and fruit daily, limit juice intake.
- Use vegetable oils and soft margarines low in saturated fat and *trans* fatty acids instead of butter or most other animal fats in the diet.
- Eat whole-grain breads and cereals rather than refined-grain products.
- Reduce the intake of sugar-sweetened beverages and foods.
- Use nonfat (skim) or low-fat milk and dairy products daily.
- Eat more fish, especially oily fish, broiled or baked.
- Reduce salt intake, including salt from processed foods.

American Heart Association: Dietary recommendations for children and adolescents: a guide for practitioners, *Pediatrics* 117:544–559, 2006.

176. How are the primary genetic hyperlipidemias classified?
See Table 7-16.

Table 7-16. Classification of Primary Genetic Hyperlipidemias

FREDERICKSON TYPE	LIPIDS INCREASED	LIPOPROTEINS INCREASED	PREVALENCE	CLINICAL FINDINGS
I	Triglyceride	Chylomicrons	Very rare	Eruptive xanthomas, pancreatitis, recurrent abdominal pain, lipemia retinalis, hepatosplenomegaly
IIa	Cholesterol	LDL	Common	Tendon xanthomas, PVD
IIb	Cholesterol, triglyceride	LDL + VLDL	Common	PVD, no xanthomas
III	Cholesterol, triglyceride	VLDL remnants (IDL)	Rare	PVD, yellow palm creases
IV	Triglyceride	VLDL	Uncommon	PVD, xanthomas, hyperglycemia
V	Triglyceride, cholesterol	VLDL + chylomicrons	Very rare	Pancreatitis, lipemia retinalis, xanthomas, hyperglycemia

IDL = Intermediate-density lipoprotein; LDL = low-density lipoprotein; PVD = peripheral vascular disease;
VLDL = very-low-density lipoprotein.

177. What is the most common hyperlipidemia in childhood?
Familial hypercholesterolemia, type IIA, with elevated cholesterol and LDL. This condition results from a lack of functional LDL receptors on cell membranes as a result of various mutations. When LDL cannot attach and release cholesterol to the cell, feedback suppression of hydroxymethylglutaryl coenzyme A reductase (the rate-limiting enzyme of cholesterol synthesis) does not occur, and cholesterol synthesis continues excessively. In the homozygous form of type IIa, xanthomas may appear before the age of 10 years and vascular disease before the age of 20 years. However, the homozygous form is very rare, with an incidence of 1 in 1,000,000 births. The heterozygous variety has a much higher incidence of 1 in 500, but it is less likely to produce clinical manifestations in children.

SURGICAL ISSUES

178. What is the natural history of an umbilical hernia?
Most umbilical hernias smaller than 0.5 cm spontaneously close before a patient is 2 years old. Those between 0.5 and 1.5 cm take up to 4 years to close. If the umbilical hernia is larger than 2 cm, it may still close spontaneously, but may take up to 6 years or more to do so. Unlike an inguinal hernia, incarceration and strangulation are rare with an umbilical hernia.

Barreto L, Khan AR, Khanbhal M, et al: Umbilical hernia, *BMJ* 347:f4252, 2013.
Yazbeck S: Abdominal wall developmental defects and omphalomesenteric remnants. In Roy CC, editor: *Pediatric Clinical Gastroenterology*, ed 4. St. Louis, 1995, Mosby-Year Book, pp 134–135.

179. Which umbilical hernias warrant surgical repair?
Because of the high probability of self-resolution, indications for surgery are controversial. Some authorities argue that a hernia larger than 1.5 cm at the age of 2 years warrants closure as a result of its likely persistence for years. Others argue that, because the likelihood of incarceration is small for

umbilical hernias, surgical closure is warranted before puberty only for persistent pain, history of incarceration, or associated psychological disturbances.

180. **When should an infant with inguinal hernia have it electively repaired?**
After the diagnosis of inguinal hernia is made, it should be repaired **as soon as possible**. In one large study of children with incarcerated hernia, 40% of patients had a known inguinal hernia before incarceration, and 80% were awaiting elective repair. Eighty percent of the children with incarceration of a hernia were infants younger than 1 year. Delay of repair should be minimized, especially in this age group. Another study found that if an infant presents with an incarcerated hernia, subsequently reduced in the ED, the potential for recurrent incarceration during a waiting period is increased 12-fold.

Chen LE, Zamakhshary M, Foglia RP, et al: Impact of wait time on outcome for inguinal hernia repair in infants, *Pediatr Surg Int* 25:225–232, 2009.
Stylianos S, Jacir NN, Harris BH: Incarceration of inguinal hernia in infants prior to elective repair, *J Pediatr Surg* 18:582–583, 1993.

181. **Does surgical repair of one hernia warrant intraoperative exploration for another on the opposite side?**
This is a controversial topic. Many surgeons opt to have pediatric patients undergo exploration of the contralateral side during a hernia repair because 60% of infants will have a patent processus vaginalis on the opposite side. By age 2 years, approximately 10% of these become clinical hernias, although a large percentage do spontaneously obliterate before that time. Other surgeons feel the potential risk of contralateral exploration (e.g., injury to the vas deferens, testes, and ilioinguinal nerve) mandates a watchful waiting approach. Surveys of pediatric surgeons indicate persistent widespread practice variability.

Palmer LS: Hernias and hydroceles, *Pediatr Rev* 34:457–463, 2013.
Ron O, Eaton S, Pierro A: Systematic review of the risk of developing a metachronous contralateral inguinal hernia in children, *Br J Surg* 94:804–811, 2007.

182. **How are incarcerated inguinal hernias reduced?**
Incarceration occurs most commonly during the first year of life. About one-third of infants <2 months of age with inguinal hernias will develop incarceration. Because the infant will likely need to be admitted, nothing should be given to eat or drink. Reduction is most easily accomplished if the infant is calm (preferably asleep), warm, and, if possible, in a slightly reverse Trendelenburg position. Analgesia (e.g., 0.1 mg/kg of intravenous morphine) may facilitate the relaxed state. With one hand, the examiner stabilizes the base of the hernia by the internal inguinal ring and, with the other hand, milks the sac distally to progressively force fluids and/or gas through the ring to eventually allow complete reduction. If unsuccessful, immediate surgery is indicated.

183. **Under what clinical settings should manual reduction of an inguinal hernia not be attempted?**
Reduction should not be attempted if the patient has clinical findings of shock, perforation, peritonitis, GI bleeding or obstruction, or evidence of gangrenous bowel (bluish discoloration of the abdominal wall).

184. **What is the significance of green vomiting during the first 72 hours of life?**
During the neonatal period, green vomiting should always be interpreted as a sign of potential intestinal obstruction potentially requiring surgical intervention. In one study of 45 infants with green vomiting, 20% had surgical conditions (e.g., malrotation, jejunal atresia, jejunal stenosis), 10% had nonsurgical obstruction (e.g., meconium plug, microcolon), and 70% had idiopathic vomiting that self-resolved. Plain radiographs frequently can be normal, particularly for malrotation, and thus falsely reassuring.

Williams H: Green for danger! Intestinal malrotation and volvulus, *Arch Dis Child Educ Pract Ed* 92:ep87–ep97, 2007.
Lilien LD, Srinivasan G, Pyati SP, et al: Green vomiting in the first 72 hours in normal infants, *Am J Dis Child* 140:662–664, 1986.

185. **What are the clinical findings of malrotation of the intestine?**

The lesion may display in utero volvulus, or it may be asymptomatic throughout life. Infants may display intermittent vomiting or exhibit signs compatible with complete obstruction. Any infant with bilious vomiting should be considered emergent and requires careful evaluation for volvulus and other high-grade surgical obstructions. Recurrent abdominal pain, distention, or lower GI bleeding may result from intermittent volvulus. Full volvulus with arterial compromise results in intestinal necrosis, peritonitis, perforation, and an extremely high incidence of mortality. Because of the extensive nature of the lesion, postoperative short gut syndrome is present in many patients who require resection. An upper GI contrast study is the examination of choice when the diagnosis is suspected.

186. **What causes the intestinal obstruction in malrotation?**

Malrotation of the intestine is the result of the abnormal rotation of the intestine in the tenth week of gestation around the superior mesenteric artery. Arrest of this counterclockwise rotation may occur at any degree of rotation. The cecum is unattached and located in the upper abdomen. One consequence of improper fixation of the mesentery allows for twisting (**volvulus**). Additionally, abnormal tissue (**Ladd bands**) connects the abnormally located cecum to the abdominal wall and may create a duodenal blockage (Fig. 7-11).

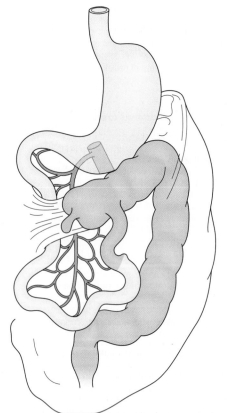

Figure 7-11. Incomplete intestinal rotation. Ladd bands are seen attaching the cecum to the right posterior abdominal wall. The duodenum can become compressed and possibly obstructed. *(From Holcombe GW, Murphy JP, Ostlie DJ:* Ashcraft's Pediatric Surgery, *ed 6. Philadelphia, 2014, Elsevier, pp 430–438.)*

187. **In an asymptomatic child with an incidental finding of malrotation, is surgery indicated?**

Because of the persistent possibility of acute volvulus and intestinal obstruction, surgery is always indicated when intestinal malrotation is diagnosed.

188. **What is the most common cause of intestinal obstruction in young children?**
Intussusception, which occurs when one portion of the bowel invaginates into the other is the most common cause of intestinal obstruction in young children. Intussusception usually occurs before the second year of life; half of all cases occur between the ages of 3 and 9 months.

189. **In what settings should intussusception be suspected?**
Colicky pain is seen in more than 80% of cases, but it may be absent. It typically lasts 15 to 30 minutes, and the baby usually sleeps between attacks. In about two-thirds of cases, there is blood in the stool (currant jelly stools). Other presenting symptoms include massive lower GI bleeding or blood streaking on the stools. The infant may appear quite toxic, dehydrated, or in shock; fever and tachycardia are common. A right lower quadrant mass may be palpable, or the area may feel surprisingly empty. Distention may accompany decreased bowel sounds.

190. **How commonly does intussusception appear with the classic findings?**
The classic triad of intussusception (colicky pain, vomiting, and passage of bloody stool) is the exception; overall, 80% of patients do not have this triad of symptoms. About 30% have blood in the stool, and this percentage may drop to about 15% if the abdominal pain was present for less than 12 hours. Palpation of a mass can suggest the diagnosis, but generally a high degree of suspicion is important. Delay in diagnosis is common.

Lochhead A, Jamjoom R, Ratnapalan S: Intussusception in children presenting to the emergency department, *Clin Pediatr* 52:1029–1033, 2013.
Klein EJ, Kapoor D, Shugerman RP: The diagnosis of intussusception, *Clin Pediatr* 43:343–347, 2004.

191. **What causes intussusception?**
Intussusception is caused by one proximal segment of the bowel being invaginated and progressively drawn caudad and encased by the lumen of distal bowel. This causes obstruction and may occlude the vascular supply of the bowel segment. There is commonly a lead point on the proximal bowel that initiates the process. Lead points have included juvenile polyps, lymphoid hyperplasia, hypertrophied Peyer patches, eosinophilic granuloma of the ileum, lymphoma, lymphosarcoma, leiomyosarcoma, leukemic infiltrate, duplication cysts, ectopic pancreas, Meckel diverticulum, hematoma, Henoch-Schönlein syndrome, worms, foreign bodies, and appendicitis.

Waseem M, Rosenberg HK: Intussusception, *Pediatr Emerg Care* 24:793–800, 2008.

192. **What is the most common type of intussusception?**
Ileocolic intussusception (Fig. 7-12) is most common, and it is also the most common cause of intestinal obstruction during infancy. Cecocecal and colocolic intussusceptions are less common. Gastroduodenal intussusception is rare and is usually associated with a gastric mass lesion such as a polyp or a leiomyoma. Enteroenteric intussusception is seen after surgery and in patients with Henoch-Schönlein syndrome.

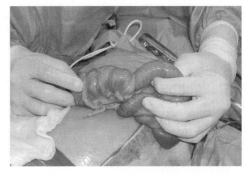

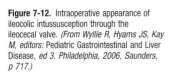

Figure 7-12. Intraoperative appearance of ileocolic intussusception through the ileocecal valve. *(From Wyllie R, Hyams JS, Kay M, editors: Pediatric Gastrointestinal and Liver Disease, ed 3. Philadelphia, 2006, Saunders, p 717.)*

193. How is intussusception diagnosed?

Radiographs can demonstrate a small bowel obstruction pattern, but the sensitivity is low (45%), so this is not typically used to diagnose intussusception. Ultrasound is increasingly being used to make this diagnosis and has a role in the evaluation of reducibility, potential pathologic lead point, and exclusion of residual intussusception after enema. Traditionally, the diagnostic study of choice is a barium enema because this can be both diagnostic and therapeutic. Air enema is now considered to be better at reduction, safer, faster, and result in less radiation compared with barium enemas. In 74% of cases, air enema under fixed hydrostatic pressure will reduce the intussusception. If this is unsuccessful, surgical reduction is necessary.

Applegate KE: Intussusception in children: evidence-based diagnosis and treatment, *Pediatr Radiol* 39: S140–S143, 2009.

194. How frequently does intussusception recur?

Overall recurrence rates for intussusception are about 13%. The recurrence rate during the first 24 hours is low, 2% to 4%, so the vast majority of recurrences will not be identified by overnight hospitalization.

Gray MP, Li S-H, Hoffman R, et al: Recurrence rates after intussusception enema reduction: a meta-analysis, *Pediatrics* 134:110–119, 2014.

195. Rotavirus vaccine and intussusception: how are they intertwined?

Rotashield, an oral rotavirus vaccine licensed in the United States in 1998, was suspended from use in 1999 when increased rates of intussusception were noted. Two new rotavirus vaccines, RotaTeq and Rotarix, were licensed in 2006 and 2008, respectively. International postlicensure studies and U.S. data have demonstrated a slightly increased risk for intussusception during the first 3 weeks after the first dose of both vaccines.

Yih WK, Lieu TA, Kulldorff M, et al: Intussusception risk after rotavirus vaccination in U.S. infants, *N Engl J Med* 370:503–512, 2014.

196. Duodenal or jejunoileal atresia: which is associated with other embryonic abnormalities?

Duodenal atresia. Duodenal atresia is caused by a persistence of the proliferative stage of gut development and a lack of secondary vacuolization and recanalization. It is associated with a high incidence of other early embryonic abnormalities. Extraintestinal anomalies occur in two-thirds of patients with this condition.

Jejunoileal atresia occurs after the establishment of continuity and patency as evidenced by distal meconium seen in these patients. The etiology is postulated to be a vascular accident, volvulus, or mechanical perforation. Jejunoileal atresias are usually not associated with any other systemic abnormality.

197. What is the classic radiographic finding in duodenal atresia?

The double bubble. Swallowed air distends the stomach and the proximal duodenum (Fig. 7-13).

198. How does the infant with biliary atresia classically present?

Biliary atresia is a condition in which the extrahepatic biliary system is obliterated, and bile flow is obstructed. In classic cases, an otherwise healthy-appearing term infant develops a recognizable jaundice by the third week of life, with increasingly dark urine and acholic stools. Usually, the child appears well, with acceptable growth. The skin color sometimes appears somewhat greenish yellow. The spleen becomes palpable after the third or fourth week, at which time the liver is usually hard and enlarged. In other cases, the jaundice is clearly present in the conjugated form during the first week of life. There is also a strong association between the polysplenia syndrome and earlier presentation of biliary atresia.

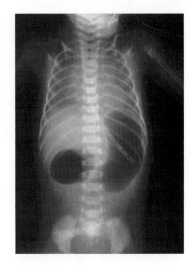

Figure 7-13. Duodenal atresia. *(From Zitelli BJ, Davis HW:* Atlas of Pediatric Physical Diagnosis, *ed 5. Philadelphia, 2007, Mosby, p 637.)*

199. **What is the surgical procedure for biliary atresia?**
The **Kasai procedure** (hepatoportoenterostomy). The remnants of the extrahepatic biliary tree are identified, and a cholangiogram is performed to verify the diagnosis. An intestinal limb (Roux-en-Y) is attached to drain bile from the porta hepatis.

200. **Which is accompanied by more complications: high or low imperforate anus?**
High-type imperforations. The distinction is based on whether the blind end of the terminal bowel or rectum ends above (high type) or below (low type) the level of the pelvic levator musculature. The patients with high-type imperforations will have ectopic fistulas (rectourinary, rectovaginal), urologic anomalies (hydronephrosis or double collecting system), and lumbosacral spine defects (sacral agenesis, hemivertebrae). The surgical repair in these patients is much more extensive, and future problems of incontinence, fecal impaction, and strictures are more likely.

201. **What is the classic presentation of pyloric stenosis?**
An infant 3 to 6 weeks old has progressive nonbilious projectile vomiting leading to dehydration with hypochloremic, hypokalemic, metabolic alkalosis. On physical examination, a pyloric "olive" is palpable, and peristaltic waves are visible.

202. **How is pyloric stenosis diagnosed?**
If the classic signs and symptoms are present in association with the typical blood chemistry findings (hypochloremia, hypokalemia, metabolic alkalosis) and a mass is palpated, the diagnosis can be made on **clinical** grounds. If the diagnosis is in doubt, **ultrasound** can be used to visualize the hypertrophic pyloric musculature (Fig. 7-14). **Upper GI contrast** studies demonstrate pyloric obstruction with the characteristic "string sign" and enlarged "shoulders" bordering the elongated and obstructed pyloric channel.

203. **What is the mechanism of hyperbilirubinemia in babies with pyloric stenosis?**
Unconjugated hyperbilirubinemia has been noted in 10% to 25% of babies with pyloric stenosis. Although an enhanced enterohepatic circulation for bilirubin probably plays a role in the pathogenesis of the hyperbilirubinemia, hepatic glucuronyl transferase activity is markedly depressed in these jaundiced infants. The mechanism of diminished glucuronyl transferase activity is not known, although inhibition of the enzyme by intestinal hormones has been suggested.

204. **In a patient with suspected pyloric stenosis, why is an acidic urine very worrisome?**
As vomiting progresses in infants with pyloric stenosis, a worsening hypochloremic metabolic alkalosis develops. Multiple factors (e.g., volume depletion, elevated aldosterone levels) result

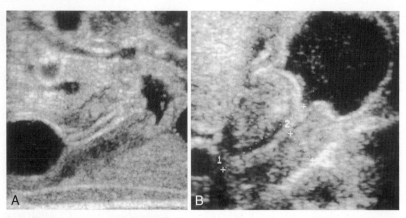

Figure 7-14. A, Ultrasound of pyloric stenosis. Note the elongated and curved pyloric channel with parallel walls and the thickened muscle with a "shoulder" projecting into the antrum. **B,** Longitudinal sonograph of the pylorus in a patient with pyloric stenosis. *1,* canal length = 1.7 cm; *2,* muscle wall thickness = 0.6 cm. *(From Glick PL, Pearl RH, Irish MS, Caty MG: Pediatric Surgery Secrets. Philadelphia, 2001, Hanley & Belfus, p 203.)*

in maximal renal efforts to reabsorb sodium. In the distal tubule, this is typically achieved by exchanging sodium for potassium and hydrogen. When total-body potassium levels are very low, hydrogen is preferentially exchanged, and a paradoxic aciduria develops (in the setting of an alkaline plasma). This acidic urine is an indication that intravascular volume expansion and electrolyte replenishment (especially chloride and potassium) are urgently needed.

205. **What is the connection between pyloric stenosis and macrolide antibiotics?**
The use of erythromycin during the first 2 weeks after birth is associated with an increased risk, up to 30-fold, for the development of pyloric stenosis. Azithromycin use increases the risk up to 8-fold. Use of erythromycin or azithromycin from 2 weeks to 4 months of age is also associated with an increased risk, albeit smaller. Speculation on a mechanism involves possible macrolide effects as a prokinetic agent on gastrointestinal smooth muscle, which could cause spasm of the pyloric muscle.

Eberly MD, Eide MB, Thompson JL, Nylund CM: Azithromycin in early infancy and pyloric stenosis, *Pediatrics* 135:483–488, 2015.
Lund M, Pasternak B, Davidsen RB, et al: Use of macrolides in mother and child and risk of infantile hypertrophic pyloric stenosis: nationwide cohort study, *BMJ* 348:1908–1918, 2014.

206. **What is the short bowel syndrome?**
The *short bowel syndrome* results from extensive resection of the small intestine. Normally, most carbohydrates, proteins, fats, and vitamins are absorbed in the jejunum and the proximal ileum. The terminal ileum is responsible for the uptake of bile acids and vitamin B_{12}. Short bowel syndrome results in FTT, malabsorption, diarrhea, vitamin deficiency, bacterial contamination, and gastric hypersecretion.

207. **Why are infants with short bowel syndrome prone to renal calculi?**
Chronic intestinal malabsorption results in an increase of intraluminal fatty acids, which saponify with dietary calcium. Thus, nonabsorbable calcium oxalate does not form, excessive oxalate is absorbed, and hyperoxaluria with crystal formation results.

208. **In extensive small bowel resection, how much is "too much"?**
Infants who retain 20 cm of small bowel as measured from the ligament of Treitz can survive if the ileocecal valve is intact. If the ileocecal valve has been removed, the infant usually requires a minimum of 40 cm of bowel to survive. The importance of the ileocecal valve appears to relate to its ability to retard transit time and minimize bacterial contamination of the small intestine.

KEY POINTS: SURGICAL ISSUES

1. Bilious (dark green) emesis in a newborn is a true gastrointestinal emergency; it is a sign of potential obstruction.
2. The classic triad of intussusception consists of the following: (1) colicky abdominal pain, (2) vomiting, and (3) bloody stools with mucus. However, it occurs in fewer than 20% of patients.
3. In patients younger than 2 years, intussusception is the most common abdominal emergency.
4. Pyloric stenosis typically presents with progressive, nonbilious, projectile vomiting and a hypochloremic, hypokalemic metabolic alkalosis in an infant between the ages of 3 and 6 weeks.
5. The classic picture of appendicitis is anorexia followed by pain followed by nausea and vomiting, with subsequent localization of findings to the right lower quadrant. However, there is a large degree of variability, particularly in younger patients.

209. Appendicitis in children: clinical, laboratory, or radiologic diagnosis?

The diagnosis of appendicitis has traditionally been a clinical one. The classic picture in children is a period of **anorexia followed by pain, nausea, and vomiting**. Abdominal pain begins periumbilically and then shifts after 4 to 6 hours to the right lower quadrant. Fever is low grade. Peritoneal signs are detected on examination. In unequivocal cases, experienced surgeons would argue that no laboratory tests are needed.

Laboratory studies have limited value in equivocal cases. White blood cell count of more than 18,000/mm^3 or a marked left shift is unusual in uncomplicated cases and suggests perforation or another diagnosis. A urinalysis with many white blood cells suggests a urinary tract infection as the primary pathology.

It is uncommon for children to undergo surgery for suspected appendicitis without imaging. CT has been considered the gold standard for diagnosis. Ultrasound has been studied as an alternative, but it is highly operator dependent with a wide reported sensitivity range. Magnetic resonance imaging (MRI) has been used in combination with ultrasound for the diagnosis of appendicitis in adults, but studies of its use in pediatric medicine are limited. The advantages of CT are less operator dependence; easier visualization of retrocecal appendix; and less interference with bowel gas, obesity, or the patient's pain. A major concern is the extent of radiation exposure, which is considerable particularly with the use of contrast studies.

Aspelund G, Fingeret A, Gross E, et al: Ultrasonography/MRI versus CT for diagnosing appendicitis, *Pediatrics* 133:1–8, 2014.
Acheson J, Banerjee J: Management of suspected appendicitis in children, *Arch Dis Child Educ Pract ED* 95:9–13, 2010.

210. How specific is the diagnosis of appendicitis if an appendicolith is noted on radiograph?

Although an appendicolith (or fecalith) on radiographic studies (plain film or CT scan) is significantly associated with appendicitis, it is not sufficiently specific to be the sole basis for the diagnosis. On CT scanning, these can be noted in 65% of patients with appendicitis and in up to 15% of patients without appendicitis. The positive-predictive value of finding an appendicolith is about 75%; in its absence, the negative-predictive value is only 26%.

Lowe LH, Penney MW, Scheker LE, et al: Appendicolith revealed on CT in children with suspected appendicitis: How specific is it in the diagnosis of appendicitis? *AJR Am J Roentgenol* 175:981–984, 2000.

211. Should a digital rectal examination be performed on all children with possible appendicitis?

Tradition says yes, but reviews of studies of the practice indicate that in children it can be emotionally and physically traumatic and associated with a high false-positive interpretation. It may be most helpful in equivocal cases involving pelvic or retrocecal appendicitis (about one-third of cases), suspected abscess formation, or for attempted palpation of adnexal or cervical tissues when vaginal examination is not indicated. Thus, many clinicians now view it as "investigatory" rather than "routine" and only when results will change management.

Brewster GS, Herbert ME: Medical myth: a digital rectal examination should be performed on all individuals with possible appendicitis, *West J Med* 173:207–208, 2000.

212. In children taken to surgery for suspected appendicitis, how often is perforation of the appendix present?

It depends to a large extent on the age of the child (and, of course, on the skill of the clinician). Unfortunately, as a result of the variable location of the appendix, the clinical presentation of pain in appendicitis is often very different from the classic case. The younger the child, the more difficult the diagnosis. In infants younger than 1 year, nearly 100% of patients who come to surgery have a perforation. Fortunately, appendicitis is rare in this age group because the appendiceal opening at the cecum is much larger than the tip, and obstruction is unusual. In children younger than 2 years, 70% to 80% are perforated; in those 5 years and younger, 50% are perforated. Particularly in younger children, a high index of suspicion is necessary, and rapid diagnosis is critical. If the onset of symptoms can be pinpointed (usually anorexia related to a meal), 10% of patients will have perforation during the first 24 hours, but more than 50% will perforate by 48 hours.

213. Should children with acute abdominal pain be given analgesia before a diagnosis?

A controversial question because a long-held fear has been that treating the pain may mask the symptoms, change the physical findings, and potentially delay the diagnosis of a possible surgical problem. However, there is growing evidence that the use of opiate analgesia in patients, including children, with acute abdominal pain does not result in increased mortality or morbidity.

Bailey B, Bergeron S, Gravel J, et al: Efficacy and impact of intravenous morphine before surgical consultation in children with right lower quadrant pain suggestive of appendicitis: a randomized controlled trial, *J Pediatr* 50:371–378, 2007.

Ranji SR, Goldman LE, Simel DL, et al: Do opiates affect the clinical evaluation of patients with acute abdominal pain? *JAMA* 296:1764–1774, 2006.

Acknowledgment

The editors gratefully acknowledge contributions by Drs. Douglas Jacobstein, Peter Mamula, Jonathan E. Markowitz, and David A. Piccoli that were retained from previous editions of *Pediatric Secrets*.

CHAPTER 8

GENETICS

Kwame Anyane-Yeboa, MD and Alejandro Iglesias, MD

CLINICAL ISSUES

1. Which disorders with ethnic and racial predilections most commonly warrant maternal screening for carrier status?
   See Table 8-1.

Table 8-1. Maternal Screening According to Ethnic and Racial Predilections

DISORDER	ETHNIC OR RACIAL GROUP	SCREENING TEST
Tay-Sachs disease	Ashkenazi Jewish, French, French Canadian	Decreased serum hexosaminidase A concentration, DNA studies
Familial dysautonomia	Ashkenazi Jewish	DNA
Gaucher disease	Ashkenazi Jewish	DNA
Canavan disease	Ashkenazi Jewish	DNA
Bloom syndrome	Ashkenazi Jewish	DNA
Fanconi anemia	Ashkenazi Jewish	DNA
Niemann-Pick disease (type A)	Ashkenazi Jewish	DNA
Mucolipidosis IV	Ashkenazi Jewish	DNA
Cystic fibrosis	Pan ethnic	DNA
Sickle cell anemia	Black, African, Mediterranean, Arab, Indian, Pakistani	Presence of sickling in hemolysate followed by confirmatory hemoglobin electrophoresis

DNA = Deoxyribonucleic acid.

2. Why are mitochondrial disorders transmitted from generation to generation by the mother and not the father?
   Mitochondrial deoxyribonucleic acid (DNA) abnormalities (e.g., many cases of ragged red fiber myopathies) are passed on from the mother because mitochondria are present in the cytoplasm of the egg and not the sperm. Transmission to males or females is equally likely; however, expression is variable because mosaicism with normal and abnormal mitochondria in varying proportions is very common.

McFarland R, Taylor RW, Turnbull DM: A neurological perspective on mitochondrial disease, *Lancet Neurol* 9:829–840, 2010.
Johns DR: Mitochondrial DNA and disease, *N Engl J Med* 333:638–644, 1995.

3. What is genetic imprinting?
   It is a genetic mechanism by which genes are selectively expressed from the maternal or paternal allele on a chromosome. As a consequence, depending on the gene, either the maternal or the paternal allele only is expressed. The inactive allele is epigenetically marked by histone modification, DNA (cytosine) methylation or both. The imprint is maintained throughout the life of the individual. However, imprints

are erased during early development of the male and female germ lines and then reset before germ cell maturation. Imprinted genes play crucial roles in growth, development, and tumor control. Imprinted genes can cause disease when the maternal/paternal gene that is usually expressed is mutated, silenced, or deleted. In humans about 50 genes are known to be imprinted. Classic examples of human diseases linked to imprinting defects are transient neonatal diabetes, Russell-Silver syndrome, Beckwith-Wiedemann syndrome, Prader-Willi syndrome, Angelman syndrome, and Albright hereditary osteodystrophy.

4. **What is uniparental disomy?**
   Uniparental disomy occurs when a fetus receives two copies of a chromosome, or portions of a chromosome, from only one parent with no copies from the other parent. In most instances, this is not significant. However, the concept of genetic imprinting does have a role here. Because some essential genes undergo genetic imprinting, if a fetus lacks those imprinted genes from one parent, there can be a loss of gene function, which can lead to the diseases noted in question 3.

Patten MM, Ross L, Curley JP, et al: The evolution of genomic imprinting: theories, predictions and empirical tests, *Heredity (Edinb)* 113:119–128, 2014.

5. **What is the etiology of arthrogryposis congenita?**
   Arthrogryposis congenita (AC) refers to nonprogressive, congenital joint contractures (single or multiple) that generally result from lack of fetal movements in utero.

   Any condition, intrinsic to the fetus or secondary to environmental/maternal factors, that decreases fetal movements can lead to arthrogryposis congenita. Decreased fetal movement leads to increased connective tissue around the joint(s), skin dimpling over the immobilized joint(s), and disuse atrophy of the muscles that mobilize the joint (Fig. 8-1). Etiologies include muscle disease, central nervous system (CNS) disorders, connective tissues disorders, maternal illness (e.g., myasthenia, myotonic dystrophy, hyperthermia (fever >39 °C), and a host of specific genetic disorders. Specific genetic conditions associated with arthrogryposis congenita are fetal akinesia syndrome, amyoplasia (classical arthrogryposis), distal arthrogryposis type 1, congenital contractural arachnodactyly (Beal syndrome), multiple pterygium syndromes, and cerebro-oculo-facial-skeletal syndrome (COFS). Inheritance varies depending on the specific type.

Hall JG: Arthrogryposis (multiple congenital contractures): Diagnostic approach to etiology, classification, genetics and general principles, *Eur J Med Gen* 57:464–472, 2014.

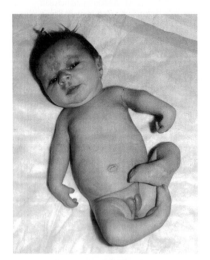

Figure 8-1. A 1-month-old girl with the quadrimelic form of arthrogryposis. *(From Staheli LT, Song KM: Pediatric Orthopedic Secrets, ed 3. Philadelphia, 2007, Elsevier, pp 494–498.)*

6. How common are genetic causes of hearing loss in childhood?

Hearing loss significant enough to affect speech and language development affects 2 to 3 of every 1000 births in the United States. **About 50%** of cases are due to genetic causes. Inheritance can be autosomal dominant, recessive, X-linked, or mitochondrial. More than 400 genetic syndromes include hearing loss as a feature including Waardenburg syndrome (pigmentary anomalies), Pendred syndrome (enlarged vestibular aqueduct), branchio-oto-renal syndrome (branchial arch and renal anomalies), Treacher-Collins syndrome, and Usher syndrome (retinitis pigmentosa).

Alford RL, Arnos KS, Fox M, et al: American College of Medical Genetics and Genomics guideline for the clinical evaluation and etiologic diagnosis of hearing loss, *Genet Med* 16:347–355, 2014.

7. What is the most common genetic mutation in infants with prelingual hearing loss?

Prelingual hearing loss is hearing loss detected before speech development. All congenital hearing loss, by definition, is prelingual. The *GJB2* gene (gap junction β-2) is the most common site for a mutation. In patients with congenital nonsyndromic deafness, about 75% are due to mutations in that gene. The *GJB2* gene encodes the protein connexin 26, which is critical for gap junctions between cochlear cells. Connexin mutations are usually autosomal recessive. Another mutation classified as 167delT is found exclusively in the Ashkenazi Jewish population.

Chan DK, Chang KW: GJB2-associated hearing loss: systematic review of worldwide prevalence, genotype, and auditory phenotype, *Laryngoscope* 124: e34–e53, 2014.

8. What are the genetic causes of microcephaly?

Microcephaly, defined as an occipital-frontal circumference below the 3rd percentile or 3 standard deviations below the mean, can be associated with more than 500 genetic syndromes. Chromosome defects, single gene disorders, or environmental causes can be responsible for microcephaly. Genetic diagnostic investigations can include karyotype, chromosomal microarray, and FISH testing. Research is focusing on the role of genetic disease associated with (and perhaps causative of) abnormalities in the centrosomes, the organelles that serve as the main microtubule organizing center of the cell. Centrosomal proteins control the mitotic spindle, which is essential for normal cell mitotic proliferation. Abnormalities of the centrosomes could be a central pathway in the development of microcephaly with abnormal neuronal production.

Gilmore EC, Walsh CA: Genetic causes of microcephaly and lessons for neuronal development, *Wiley Interdiscip Rev Dev Biol* 2:461–478, 2013.

9. Are older fathers at increased risk of having a child with a genetic disease?

Advanced paternal age is well-documented to be associated with **new dominant mutations.** The assumption is that the increased mutation rate is the result of the accumulation of new mutations from many cell divisions. The more cell divisions, the more likely an error (mutation) will occur. The mutation rate in fathers who are older than 50 years is five times higher than the mutation rate in fathers who are younger than 20 years. Autosomal dominant new mutations have been mapped and identified, including **achondroplasia, Apert syndrome**, and **Marfan syndrome**.

10. What is the most common genetic lethal disease?

Cystic fibrosis (CF). A genetic lethal disease is one that interferes with a person's ability to reproduce as a result of early death (before childbearing age) or impaired sexual function. CF is the most common autosomal recessive disorder in whites, occurring in 1 in 1600 infants (1 of every 20 individuals is a carrier for this condition) (Fig. 8-2). CF is characterized by widespread dysfunction of exocrine glands, chronic pulmonary disease, pancreatic insufficiency, and intestinal obstructions. Males are azoospermic. The median survival is about 29 years.

Cystic Fibrosis Foundation: www.cff.org. Accessed on Dec. 3, 2014.

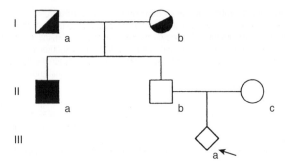

Figure 8-2. Risk for cystic fibrosis (CF) in offspring of a mother with no family history of CF and a healthy father whose brother has CF. (1) Because IIa is affected with CF, both his parents must be carriers. (2) The chance of IIb being a carrier is 2 out of 3 because we know that he is not affected by CF. (3) The risk of IIc being a carrier is 1 in 20 (the population risk). (4) The chance of IIIa being affected is calculated as follows: father's carrier risk × mother's carrier risk × chance that both will pass on their recessive CF gene to their child $= 2/3 \times 1/20 \times 1/4 = 1/120$.

11. What are the syndromes associated with macrosomia (large baby syndromes)?
    - **Prader-Willi** (obesity, hypotonia, small hands and feet)
    - **Beckwith-Wiedemann** (macrosomia, omphalocele, macroglossia, ear creases)
    - **Sotos** (macrosomia, macrocephaly, large hands and feet)
    - **Weaver** (macrosomia, accelerated skeletal maturation, camptodactyly)
    - **Bardet-Biedl** (obesity, retinal pigmentation, polydactyly)
    - **Infants of diabetic mothers**

12. What is the "H_3O" of Prader-Willi syndrome?
    Hyperphagia, hypotonia, hypopigmentation, and **obesity**. About 70% of Prader-Willi patients will have a deletion of an imprinted gene *SNPRN* on the long arm of paternally derived chromosome 15; in about 20% of these patients, both copies of the chromosome are maternally derived. The phenomenon in which a child inherits two complete or partial copies of the same chromosome from only one parent is referred to as *uniparental disomy*. The maternal uniparental disomy for chromosome 15 results in Prader-Willi syndrome, just as does a deletion of the paternal copy of the chromosome.

13. A child with supravalvular aortic stenosis, small and abnormally shaped primary teeth, low muscle tone with joint laxity, and elevated calcium noted on testing is likely to have what syndrome?
    Williams syndrome, also known as Williams-Beuren syndrome. The genetic abnormalities result from microdeletions on chromosome 7 in an area that codes for the gene elastin. The loss of this gene is thought to contribute to the cardiac and musculoskeletal features found in Williams syndrome. Other characteristic features include frequent ear infections, hyperacusis (sensitivity to loud noises), failure to thrive at a younger age, and personality traits of a strong social orientation ("cocktail party personality") combined with anxiety problems.

Prober BR: Williams-Beuren syndrome, *N Engl J Med* 362:239–252, 2010.
Waxler JL, Levine K, Pober BR: Williams syndrome: a multidisciplinary approach to care, *Pediatr Ann* 38:456–463, 2009.

14. What are the two most common forms of dwarfism that are recognizable at birth?
    - **Thanatophoric dwarfism:** This is the most common, but it is a *lethal* chondrodysplasia that is characterized by flattened, U-shaped vertebral bodies; telephone receiver–shaped femurs; macrocephaly; and redundant skinfolds that cause a puglike appearance. *Thanatophoric* means death loving (an apt description). The incidence is 1 in 6400 births.
    - **Achondroplasia:** This is the most common viable skeletal dysplasia, occurring in 1 in 26,000 live births. Its features are small stature, macrocephaly, depressed nasal bridge, lordosis, and a trident hand.

15. **What chromosomal abnormality is found in cri-du-chat syndrome?**
    Cri-du-chat syndrome is the result of a deletion of material from the short arm of chromosome 5 (i.e., 5p-), which causes many problems, including growth retardation, microcephaly, and severe mental retardation. Patients have a characteristic catlike cry during infancy, from which the syndrome derives its name. In 85% of cases, the deletion is a de novo event. In 15%, it is due to malsegregation from a balanced parental translocation.

16. **Is there a "Catch-22" to the Catch-22 syndrome?**
    Unlike the Heller novel, this puzzle does have solutions, both genetic and acronymal. The acronym has been used to describe the salient features of **DiGeorge/velocardiofacial syndrome**:
    - **C**ongenital heart disease (e.g., ventricular septal defect [VSD], truncus arteriosus, tetralogy of Fallot, aortic arch anomalies)
    - **A**bnormal face (e.g., ear anomalies, wide-set eyes, long face, nasal abnormalities; Fig. 8-3)
    - **T**hymic aplasia or hypoplasia
    - **C**left palate
    - **H**ypocalcemia (secondary to hypoparathyroidism)
    - **22:** Microdeletion of chromosome 22q11

    Kobrynski LJ, Sullivan KE: Velocardiofacial syndrome, DiGeorge syndrome: the chromosome 22q11.2 deletion syndromes, *Lancet* 370:1443–1452, 2007.

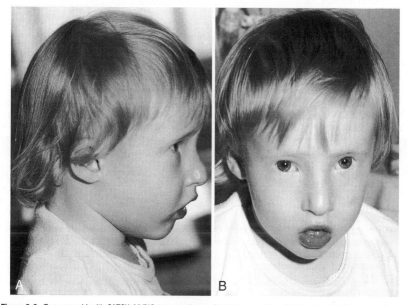

Figure 8-3. Two-year-old with CATCH-22/DiGeorge syndrome. Facial dysmorphisms include hypertelorism, low-set ears, micrognathia, small fishlike mouth, short philtrum, malformed nose and down-slanting palpebral fissures. Cardiac defect was truncus arteriosus. *(From Perloff JK: Clinical recognition of congenital heart disease,* Clinical Recognition of Congenital Heart Disease, *41:492–504, 2012.)*

17. **For what condition are patients with isolated limb hypertrophy at risk?**
    Embryonal cell tumors, including Wilms tumor, adrenal tumors, and hepatoblastoma. The risk in patients with isolated hemihypertrophy is about 6%; in patients with Beckwith-Wiedemann syndrome, it is 7.5%. Surveillance with abdominal ultrasound and α-fetoprotein measurements every 3 months is recommended until the child is at least **5** years old. In patients with Beckwith-Wiedemann syndrome, facial appearance is also affected (Fig. 8-4).

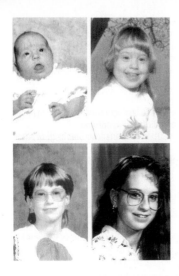

Figure 8-4. Facial shape in Beckwith-Wiedemann syndrome, illustrated from birth to adolescence in a single person. In infancy and early childhood, the face is round with prominent cheeks and relative narrowing of the forehead. Note that by adolescence the trend is toward normalization. *(From Allanson JE: Pitfalls of genetic diagnosis in the adolescent: the changing face,* Adolesc Med State Art Rev *13:257–268, 2002.)*

18. After Down syndrome, what are the next most common autosomal trisomies in live-born children?
    Trisomy 18 and **trisomy 13**. (See Table 8-2.)

Support Organization for Trisomy (SOFT) 18, 13 and Related Disorders: www.trisomy.org. Accessed on Dec. 3, 2014.
Trisomy 18 Foundation: www.trisomy18.org. Accessed on Dec. 3, 2014.

Table 8-2. Differences Between Trisomy 18 and Trisomy 13

TRISOMY 18	TRISOMY 13
Edwards syndrome (described in 1960)	Patau syndrome (described in 1960)
~1:8000 live births	~1:20,000 live births
Clinical features: IUGR, elfin appearance failure to thrive, cardiac and kidney defects severe mental deficiency, micrognathia, microcephaly, posterior heel prominence prominent occiput, overlapping fingers	*Clinical features*: CNS malformations (holoprosencephaly), heart defects, genitourinary anomalies, growth retardation, polydactyly, cleft lip/palate, nasal malformation
Poor prognosis: 40% survive to 1 month; 5% survive to 1 year	*Poorer prognosis*: Only 50% survive >1 week; 5% to 6 months
80% female	Slight female predominance
Advanced maternal age: ↑↑risk	Advanced maternal age: ↑risk

CNS = Central nervous system; IUGR = intrauterine growth restriction.

19. What are the reasons that a condition might be genetically determined but the family history would be negative?
    • Autosomal recessive inheritance
    • X-linked recessive inheritance

- Genetic heterogeneity (e.g., retinitis pigmentosa may be transmitted as autosomal recessive or dominant or X-linked recessive)
- Spontaneous mutation
- Nonpenetrance (i.e., not all disease-causing genes or genetic mutations exhibit clinical expression)
- Expressivity (i.e., variable expression)
- Extramarital paternity
  - Phenocopy (i.e., an environmentally determined copy of a genetic disorder)

Juberg RC: . . .but the family history was negative, *J Pediatr* 91:693–694, 1977.

20. **What online resources are available for a pediatrician who suspects a child has a genetic syndrome or would like additional information about a patient already diagnosed with a genetic problem?**

Two sites are particularly useful.

Online Mendelian Inheritance in Man (OMIM; www.omim.org): This site is a comprehensive compendium of human genes and genetic phenotypes. It is now edited primarily under the auspices of Johns Hopkins University School of Medicine.

GeneTests (www.ncbi.nlm.nih.gov/books/NBK1116): This site provides a wealth of genetic information, including peer-reviewed articles (*GeneReviews*) with disease descriptions, including diagnosis and management information. It is sponsored by the University of Washington at Seattle.

DOWN SYNDROME

21. **What are the common physical characteristics of children with Down syndrome?**
    - Upslanted palpebral fissures with epicanthal folds
    - Small, low-set ears with overfolded upper helices
    - Short neck with excess skinfolds in newborns
    - Prominent tongue
    - Flattened occiput
    - Exaggerated gap between first and second toe
    - Hypotonia
      See Fig. 8-5.

National Down Syndrome Society: www.ndss.org. Accessed on Mar. 24, 2015.

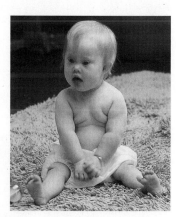

Figure 8-5. Characteristic facies seen in Down syndrome. The child's posture is due to hypotonia. *(From Lissauer T, Clayden G: Illustrated Textbook of Paediatrics, ed 4. Philadelphia, 2012, Elsevier, p 115–132.)*

22. **Are Brushfield spots pathognomonic for Down syndrome?**
    No. Brushfield spots are speckled areas that occur in the periphery of the iris (Fig. 8-6). They are seen in about 75% of patients with Down syndrome, but they also are found in up to 7% of normal newborns.

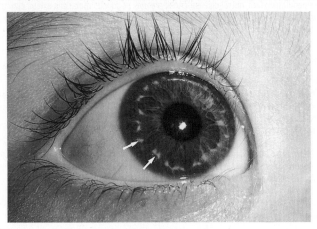

Figure 8-6. Brushfield spots *(arrows)* consisting of depigmented foci along the circumference of the iris in a child with Down syndrome. *(From Gatzoutis MA, Webb GD, Baubeney PEF, editors:* Diagnosis and Management of Adult Congenital Heart Disease, *ed 2. Philadelphia, 2011, Saunders, pp 29–47.)*

23. **What is the chance that a newborn with a simian crease has Down syndrome?**
    A single transverse palmar crease (Fig. 8-7) is present in 5% of normal newborns. Bilateral palmar creases are found in 1%. These features are twice as common in males as they are in females. However, about 45% of newborn infants with Down syndrome have a single transverse crease. Because Down syndrome occurs in 1 in 800 live births, the chance that a newborn with a simian crease has Down syndrome is only 1 in 60.

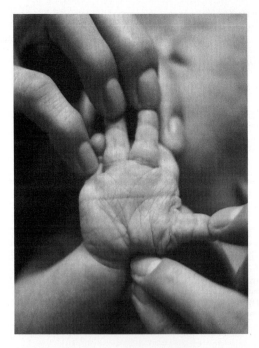

Figure 8-7. Simian crease. *(From Clark DA: Atlas of Neonatology, Philadelphia, 2000, WB Saunders, p 31.)*

24. **Why is an extensive cardiac evaluation recommended for newborns with Down syndrome?**
About 40% to 50% have congenital heart disease, but most infants are asymptomatic during the newborn period. Defects include atrioventricular canal (most common, 60%), VSD, and patent ductus arteriosus.

Down Syndrome: *Health Issues.* www.ds-health.com. Accessed on Mar. 23, 2015.

25. **What proportion of infants with Down syndrome has congenital hypothyroidism?**
About 2% (1 in 50), compared with 0.025% (1 in 4000) for all newborns, have congenital hypothyroidism. This emphasizes the importance of the state-mandated newborn thyroid screen. However, children with Down syndrome can become hypothyroid at any age.

26. **Infants with Down syndrome are at increased risk for a number of conditions during early infancy. What are they?**
- **Gastrointestinal malformations,** including duodenal atresia and tracheoesophageal fistula
- **Cryptorchidism**
- **Lens opacities and cataracts**
- **Strabismus**
- **Hearing loss,** both sensorineural and conductive

Down Syndrome Research Foundation: www.dsrf.org. Accessed on Mar. 23, 2015.

KEY POINTS: INCREASED RISKS FOR PATIENTS WITH DOWN SYNDROME DURING THE NEWBORN PERIOD AND EARLY INFANCY

1. Congenital heart disease: Atrioventricular canal defects, ventricular septal defects (VSD)
2. Gastrointestinal malformations: duodenal atresia, tracheoesophageal atresia
3. Congenital hypothyroidism
4. Lens opacities and cataracts
5. Hearing loss
6. Cryptorchidism

27. **What is the most common malignancy in an infant with Down Syndrome?**
Leukemia. Its frequency in these individuals is 50-fold higher for younger children (0 to 4 years old) and 10-fold higher for individuals 5 to 29 years old, for a 20-fold increase in lifetime risk. Before leukemia becomes apparent, children with Down syndrome are at increased risk for other unusual white blood cell problems, including *transient myeloproliferative disorder* (a disorder of marked leukocytosis, blast cells, thrombocytopenia, and hepatosplenomegaly that spontaneously resolves) and a *leukemoid reaction* (markedly elevated white blood cell count with myeloblasts without splenomegaly, which also spontaneously resolves).

Seewald L, Taub JW, Maloney KW, et al: Acute leukemias in children with Down syndrome, *Mol Genet Metab* 107:25–30, 2012.

28. **What is the genetic basis for Down syndrome?**
The syndrome can be caused by trisomy of all or part of chromosome 21:
- Full trisomy 21: 94%
- Mosaic trisomy 21: 2.4%
- Translocation: 3.3%

29. **What chromosomal abnormalities are related to maternal age?**
All trisomies and some sex chromosomal abnormalities (except 45,X and 47,XYY) are related to maternal age.

30. How does the risk for having an infant with Down syndrome change with advancing maternal age?

See Table 8-3. Most cases of Down syndrome involve nondisjunction at meiosis I in the mother. This may be related to the lengthy stage of meiotic arrest between oocyte development in the fetus until ovulation, which may occur as much as 40 years later.

Table 8-3. Approximate Risk for Down Syndrome (Live Births) by Maternal Age

MATERNAL AGE (YR)	APPROXIMATE RISK FOR DOWN SYNDROME
All ages	1 in 650
20	1:1500
30	1:1000
35	1:385
40	1:110
45	1:37

From Lissauer T, Clayden G: Illustrated Textbook of Paediatrics, ed 4. Philadelphia, 2012, Elsevier, pp 115–132.

31. Who was Down of Down syndrome?

John Langdon Down was a British physician. He originally described the condition that would later bear his name in 1866 based on measurements of the diameters of the head and palate and, in pioneering fashion, a series of clinical photographs taken in hospitals. His descriptions classified "mentally subnormal" patients on the basis of "ethnic classification" from which the widely used term "Mongolism" originated. It was not until 1961 that the term *Down's syndrome* came into vogue at the urging of genetic experts. Eponymous diseases no longer carry the possessive form and the condition is more properly referred to as *Down syndrome*.

Ward OC: John Langdon Down: the man and his message, *Downs Syndr Res Pract* 6:19–24, 1999.

DYSMORPHOLOGY

32. What is the clinical significance of a minor malformation?

The recognition of minor malformations in a newborn may serve as an indicator of altered morphogenesis or as a valuable clue to the diagnosis of a specific disorder. The presence of several minor malformations is unusual and often indicates a serious problem in morphogenesis. For example, when 3 or more minor malformations are discovered in a child, the risk for a major malformation also being present is >90%. The most common minor malformations involve the face, ears, hands, and feet. Almost any minor defect may occasionally be found as an unusual familial trait.

33. Do infants with the LEOPARD syndrome have spots?

This autosomal dominant condition is also known as *multiple lentigines* syndrome. Yes, infants with this syndrome have multiple lentigines (darkly pigmented macules). See Fig. 8-8. Other features include:

- **E**lectrocardiogram abnormalities
- **O**cular hypertelorism
- **P**ulmonic stenosis
- **A**bnormal genitalia
- **R**etarded growth
- **D**eafness

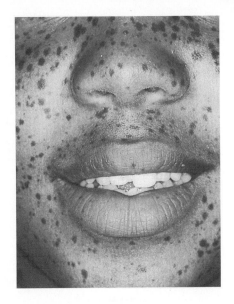

Figure 8-8. Multiple lentigines in a 13-year-old with LEOPARD syndrome. *(From Cohen BA: Pediatric Dermatology, ed 4. Philadelphia, 2013, Saunders Elsevier, p 151.)*

34. **Which is correct: CHARGE syndrome or CHARGE association?**

    CHARGE syndrome, formerly CHARGE association, is correct. A *syndrome* refers to a condition in which the underlying genetic cause has been identified. An *association* has signs and symptoms in combination greater than expected by chance alone, but without a known genetic etiology. It is now known that CHARGE syndrome is an autosomal dominant condition, and almost all cases are due to de novo mutations in the *CHD7* gene. Rare familial cases have been reported. *CHD7* (chromodomain helicase DNA-binding protein 7) is the only gene currently known to be affected in CHARGE syndrome. In 70% of CHARGE syndrome patients, a mutation can be identified in this gene.

35. **What is the proper way to test for low-set ears?**

    The designation is made when the upper portion of the ear (helix) meets the head at a level below a horizontal line drawn from the lateral aspect of the palpebral fissure. The best way to measure is to align a straight edge between the two inner canthi and determine whether the ears lie completely below this plane (Fig. 8-9). In normal individuals, about 10% of the ear is above this plane.

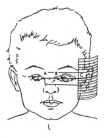
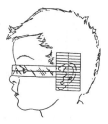

Figure 8-9. How to test for low-set ears. *(From Feingold M, Bossert WH: Normal values for selected physical parameters: an aid to syndrome delineation. In Bergsma D, editor: The National Foundation—March of Dimes Birth Defects Series 10:9, 1974.)*

36. **How is hypertelorism distinguished from telecanthus?**

    Hypertelorism is wide spacing of the eyes in which the interpupillary distance is increased. Hypertelorism can be a normal variant or may be seen in cranial abnormalities, DiGeorge syndrome, and multiple other syndromes. *Telecanthus* occurs when the inner canthi are laterally displaced but the interpupillary distance is normal. Telecanthus can be seen in fetal alcohol syndrome and Waardenburg

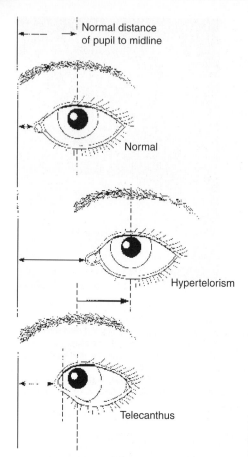

Normal distance
of pupil to midline

Normal

Hypertelorism

Telecanthus

Figure 8-10. Normal versus hypertelorism versus telecanthus. *(From Goldbloom RB:* Pediatric Clinical Skills, *ed 4. Philadelphia, 2011, Elsevier Saunders, p 63.)*

syndrome (Fig. 8-10). The eyes appear widely spaced but are not. *Hypotelorism* (not shown in figure) is a shortening of the interpupillary distance. Standard distances are found in various reference sources.

37. **What is the inheritance pattern of cleft lip and palate?**
Most cases of cleft lip and palate are inherited in a polygenic or multifactorial pattern. The male-to-female ratio is 3:2, and the incidence in the general population is about 1 in 1000. Recurrence risk after one affected child is 3% to 4%; after two affected children, it is 8% to 9%.

38. **Which syndromes are associated with colobomas of the iris?**
Colobomas (defects) of the iris (Fig. 8-11) are the result of abnormal ocular development and embryogenesis. They are frequently associated with chromosomal syndromes (most commonly trisomy 13, 4p-, 13q-) and triploidy. In addition, they may be commonly found in patients with the CHARGE syndrome, Goltz syndrome, and Rieger syndrome. Whenever iris colobomas are noted, chromosome analysis is recommended. The special case of complete absence of the iris (aniridia) is associated with the development of Wilms tumor and may be caused by an interstitial deletion of the short arm of chromosome 11.

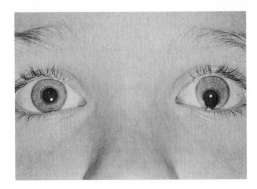

Figure 8-11. Left iris coloboma. *(From Zitelli BJ, Davis HW: Atlas of Pediatric Physical Diagnosis, ed 4. St. Louis, 2002, Mosby, p 674.)*

GENETIC PRINCIPLES

39. Identify the common symbols used in the construction of a pedigree chart
    See Fig. 8-12.

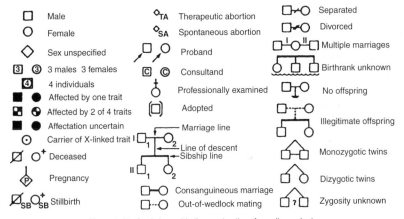

Figure 8-12. Symbols used in the construction of a pedigree chart.

40. How can the same genotype lead to different phenotypes?
    In *parental imprinting* (an area of the regulation of gene expression that is incompletely understood), the expression of an identical gene is dependent on whether the gene is inherited from the mother or the father. For example, in patients with Huntington disease, the clinical manifestations occur much earlier if the gene is inherited from the father rather than the mother. Modification of the genes by methylation of the DNA during development has been hypothesized as one explanation of the variability.

41. When a geneticist says they are going "FISH"ing, what does that mean?
    Fluorescence *in situ* hybridization (FISH) is a molecular cytogenetic technique that is used to identify abnormalities of chromosome number or structure using a single-stranded DNA probe (for a known piece of DNA or chromosome segment). The probe is labeled with a fluorescent tag and targeted to a single-strand DNA that has been denatured in place on a microscope slide. The use of fluorescent microscopy enables the detection of more than one probe, each of which is labeled with a different color. FISH is commonly used for the rapid prenatal diagnosis of trisomies with the use of amniotic fluid or chorionic villi using interphase cells from cultured specimens and probes for the most common chromosomal abnormalities (13, 18, 21, X, and Y). Although interphase FISH for prenatal diagnosis has low false-positive and false-negative rates, it is considered investigational and is used only in conjunction with standard cytogenetic analysis.

42. What is currently the best method for detecting small chromosome deletions and duplications?

Single nucleotide polymorphism microarray (SNP microarray) is currently the best method of detecting DNA copy number variations (CNVs). This test scans the whole genome for variations in DNA copy numbers. Standard chromosome analysis can detect chromosomal imbalances that are at least 5 Mb in size, whereas SNP-array is able to detect cryptic changes (deletions and duplications) that are not visible on standard chromosome analysis. It has become the method of choice for infants and children with multiple congenital anomalies and/or developmental delays. Five percent of such children have visible abnormalities on routine chromosome analysis, but an additional 10% to 15% will have an abnormality when screened with SNP array. It will eventually replace the current FISH analysis for detection of conditions such as DiGeorge syndrome and Williams syndrome. It is important to note that not all CNVs are deleterious; some are polymorphisms that are frequently carried by one parent. Parental studies are thus important in interpreting the comparative genomic hybridization, a molecular cytogenetic method for analyzing the CNV results, when the results are not clear.

Shaffer LG, Bejjani BA: Using microarray-based molecular cytogenic methods to identify chromosome abnormalities, *Pediatr Ann* 38:440–447, 2009.

Veltman JA: Genomic microarrays in clinical diagnosis, *Curr Opin Pediatr* 18:598–603, 2006.

INBORN ERRORS OF METABOLISM

43. What types of inherited metabolic conditions are routinely screened by most states?

Inherited metabolic disorders/inborn error of metabolism (IEM): organic acidemias, amino acid disorders, fatty acid oxidation defects, homocystinuria, galactosemia and biotinidase deficiency. Some states screen for Krabbe and X-linked adrenoleukodystrophy as well.

Endocrine disorders: congenital adrenal hyperplasia and hypothyroidism

Hemoglobinopathies: sickle cell disease and thalassemias

Congenital immunodeficiencies

Cystic fibrosis

Bennett MJ: Newborn screening for metabolic diseases: saving children's lives and improving outcomes, *Clin Biochem* 47:693–694, 2014.

Levy HL: Newborn screening conditions: what we know, what we do not know, and how we will know it, *Genet Med* 12(Suppl):S213–S214, 2010.

44. In what settings should inborn errors of metabolism be suspected?
   - Onset of symptoms correlating with dietary changes
   - Loss or leveling of developmental milestones
   - Patient with strong food preferences or aversions
   - Parental consanguinity
   - Unexplained sibling death, mental retardation, or seizures
   - Unexplained failure to thrive
   - Unusual odor
   - Hair abnormalities, especially alopecia
   - Microcephaly or macrocephaly
   - Abnormalities of muscle tone
   - Organomegaly
   - Coarsened facial features, thick skin, limited joint mobility, hirsutism

45. What are the main categories of specialized laboratory testing to detect an IEM?
   - Plasma amino acids
   - Plasma acylcarnitines
   - Urine organic acids

- Carnitine analysis
- Enzymatic assays for specific disorders
- Molecular testing for specific disorders

46. **What are the main principles of treatment for IEM?**
    - Removal of the offending compound
    - Use of special diets and supplements (medical foods) to provide appropriate nutrition, to keep offending compounds at minimum, and to avoid deficiencies
    - Use of medication that helps eliminate toxic compounds (i.e., ammonia scavengers) or to block the production of toxic compounds (such as in tyrosinemia type I)
    - Use of enzyme replacement therapies available for specific conditions (e.g., lysosome storage disorders)
    - Bone marrow/hematopoietic stem cell transplant for selected disorders

Saudubray JM, Berghe G, Walter JH, editors: *Inborn Metabolic Diseases: Diagnosis and Treatment*, ed 5. Berlin Heidelberg, 2012, Springer Verlag, pp 103–109.

47. **What are the main features of phenylketonuria (PKU)?**
    PKU is a defect in the hepatic enzyme phenylalanine hydroxylase, which results in an inability to metabolize one amino acid (phenylalanine) to another (tyrosine). Phenylalanine accumulates with toxic consequences. Untreated infants will develop microcephaly, early developmental delay, and later seizures. Clinical clues include musty-smelling infant sweat (due to phenylacetate, a phenylalanine breakdown product) and albinism (light colored skin and hair due to tyrosine deficits, a component of melanin. PKU is the most frequent IEM with an incidence of about 1:12,000. Inheritance is autosomal recessive. Carriers are asymptomatic. Treatment involves dietary manipulation to limit phenylalanine exposure, supplementation with other amino acids, and occasional pharmacotherapy to reduce serum phenylalanine levels. Early identification, as through newborn screening, and early treatment result in an excellent prognosis, but treatment is for life.

Greene CL, Longo N: National Institutes of Health (NIH) review of evidence in phenylalanine hydroxylase deficiency (phenylketonuria) and recommendations/guidelines from the American College of Medical Genetics (ACMG) and Genetics Metabolic Dietitians International (GMDI), *Mol Genet Metab* 112:85–86, 2014.

48. **What are the main characteristics of a patient with glycogen storage disease type 1 (GSD 1)?**
    Glycogen storage diseases, of which there are 11 types, involve defects in glycogen synthesis or breakdown in multiple organs, including muscles and liver. Type I (von Gierke disease), the most common, and others are listed in Table 8-4.
    - The cardinal feature of the disease is fasting hypoglycemia.
    - The main defect is in the enzyme glucose-6-phosphatase that allows glucose to be released from the glycogen molecule in the liver to other areas of the body.
    - Additional laboratory markers are lactic acidemia, increased uric acid, and triglycerides.
    - Clinical features include growth retardation, short stature, hepatomegaly, prominent abdomen, developmental delay/intellectual disability (if not treated) and acute symptoms associated with hypoglycemia (i.e., tremors, sweating, tachycardia, lethargy, seizures, coma, etc.).
    - Treatment is based on adequate supply of glucose: continuous feedings, frequent meals, uncooked cornstarch, and overnight feedings.
    - Outcome is good with proper treatment.

Vanier MT: Lysosomal diseases: biochemical pathways and investigations, *Handb Clin Neurol* 113:1695–1699, 2013.

49. **What are the main features of a patient with mucopolysaccharidosis?**
    Mucopolysaccharidoses are examples of storage diseases of lysosomes, which are intracellular organelles that degrade structural macromolecules. If enzymes are deficient, metabolites accumulate

Table 8-4. Most Common Glycogen Storage Disorders

TYPE Enzyme deficiency	MAIN FEATURES	LABORATORY	TREATMENT
I: Type Ia (Von Gierke) glucose-6-phosphatase	Truncal obesity, hepatomegaly, "doll face", nephromegaly, short stature, failure to thrive	Hypoglycemia after short fasting (3-4 hours), acidosis, elevated lactate, uric acid and triglycerides	Avoidance of fasting using frequent meals, overnight continuous feeds and uncooked cornstarch
I: Type Ib Glucose-6-phosphate transporter	Same as type Ia + neutropenia, leukocyte dysfunction, bacterial infections, diarrhea, immflamatory bowel disease (IBD)	Same as type Ia + neutropenia and leukocyte dysfunction	Same as type Ia + granulocyte colony growth factor
II (Pompe) α-glucosidase (acid maltase)	*Infantile:* cardiomyopathy, hypotonia, failure to thrive. *Juvenile/Adult:* progressive muscle weakness	No hypoglycemia	Enzyme replacement therapy (ERT): aglucosidase. High protein diet
III (Cori) debranching enzyme	Type IIIa: same as type Ia, but less hypoglycemia, normal kidneys, myopathy, cardiomyopathy Type IIIb: only liver	Hypoglycemia, normal lactate and uric acid	Avoidance of fasting using frequent meals, overnight continuous feeds and uncooked cornstarch
IV (Andersen) Branching enzyme	*Classic:* failure to thrive, hepatomegaly, progressive liver disease (liver failure, cirrhosis). *Neuromuscular form:* myopathy and cardiomyopathy	No hypoglycemia	Liver transplant
VI (Hers) Liver phosphorylase	Hepatomegaly, mild hypoglycemia, often asymptomatic	Mild hypoglycemia, elevated lactate and liver enzymes	Avoidance of fasting using frequent meals and uncooked cornstarch
IX Phosphorylase kinase (X-linked)	Hepatomegaly, mild hypoglycemia, often asymptomatic	Mild hypoglycemia, elevated lactate and liver enzymes	Avoidance of fasting using frequent meals and uncooked cornstarch

predominantly in the tissues that are primarily responsible for their degradation (e.g., heparin sulfate in the CNS, dermatan sulfate in bone and liver). All disorders are autosomal recessive except for type II (Hunter syndrome), which is X-linked recessive. Patients are normal at birth. Subsequent clinical features include progressive facial and skin changes ("connective tissue"), progressive skeletal deformities including growth restriction, bone dysplasia and contractures, and hepatomegaly. Depending on the type, there may be progressive psychomotor retardation with loss of acquired skills and intellectual disability. Treatment, when available, may involve enzyme replacement therapy and hematopoietic stem cell transplantation. Diagnosis is based on analysis of glycosaminoglycans (mucopolysaccharides) in urine, enzyme analysis, and molecular testing. See Table 8-5.

Vanier MT: Lysosomal diseases: biochemical pathways and investigations, *Handb Clin Neurol* 113: 1695–1699, 2013.

50. **An 8-month-old presents with vomiting, lethargy, hypoglycemia and no ketones on urinalysis. What condition is likely?**
    Medium-chain acyl-CoA dehydrogenase deficiency (MCAD). Disorders of fatty-acid oxidation or a deficiency of carnitine (the principal transporter of fatty acids into mitochondria) can result in maladaptation to the fasting stress that often accompanies an intercurrent illness. Hypoketotic hypoglycemia results from the inability to utilize fatty acids, which are the primary source of ketones. Screening for this condition, which is more common in families of Northern European ancestry, is included in most mandatory newborn screening panels. The clinical presentation varies, including no symptoms, but a presentation can be dramatic with severe vomiting, encephalopathy, coma, and death.

51. **What features should raise suspicion of mitochondrial disease?**
    Most mitochondrial diseases are *progressive* and *multisystemic*. Suspicion about a mitochondrial disorder should be raised if (1) the patient has either muscle disease and involvement of two additional organ systems (one of which may be the CNS) or (2) the CNS plus two other systems, or (3) multisystem disease (at least 3 systems) including muscle and/or the CNS. Organ systems affected are those with high energy demand such as skeletal and cardiac muscle, endocrine organs, kidney, retina, and the CNS. Any infant with unexplained failure to thrive, weakness, hypotonia, and a metabolic acidosis (particularly lactic acidosis) should be evaluated for a possible mitochondrial disorder.

Haas RH, Parikh S, Falk MJ, et al: Mitochondrial disease: a practical approach for primary care physicians, *Pediatrics* 120:1326–1333, 2007.
United Mitochondrial Disease Foundation: www.umdf.org. Accessed on Mar. 23, 2015.

52. **What is the most common presentation of childhood-onset mitochondrial disease?**
    Leigh syndrome. This is a progressive neurodegenerative condition that involves developmental regression, pyramidal signs, and brainstem dysfunction (e.g., dystonia, strabismus, nystagmus, swallowing problems), hypotonia, and lactic acidosis. It is also known as subacute necrotizing encephalomyelopathy. Etiology can be due to mutation in the mitochondrial DNA (mtDNA), autosomal recessive mutations (*SURF1*; a nuclear gene), or X-linked (*PDHA1*) mutations. The prognosis is poor.

Haas RH, Parikh S, Falk MJ, et al: Mitochondrial disease: a practical approach for primary care physicians, *Pediatrics* 120:1326–1333, 2007.

53. **When you are rounding in the well newborn nursery, one of the infants has an unusual odor. What are the typical body and urine odors associated with inherited metabolic disorders?**
    - *Musty, mildewy*: PKU
    - *Maple syrup*: maple syrup urine disease (MSUD)
    - *Sweaty feet*: isovaleric aciduria (IVA), glutaric aciduria type II

Table 8-5. Most Common Mucopolysaccharidoses

TYPE Enzyme deficiency	CLINICAL FEATURES	DIAGNOSIS	MANAGEMENT
Type I (Hurler: severe) α-L-Iduronidase	Onset first year of life; coarse facial features, corneal clouding, failure to thrive, recurrent upper respiratory infections, developmental delay, cardiac disease, hepatosplenomegaly	Increased dermatan and heparan sulfate in urine. Enzymatic assay. Molecular testing (IDUA gene)	Enzyme replacement (ERT) for non-SNC features. BMT/HSCT below 2½ years to treat ALL features including SNC
Type I (Sheie: milder) α-L-Iduronidase	Onset in adolescence and adulthood; normal intelligence, mostly normal height, mild skeletal deformities, degenerative joint disease, corneal clouding, cardiac valve disease	Increased dermatan and heparan sulfate in urine. Enzymatic assay. Molecular testing (IDUA gene)	Symptomatic; ERT
Type II (Hunter) Iduronate-2-sulphatase	Joint contractures, obstructive and restrictive airway disease, cardiac disease, skeletal deformities, cognitive decline. Mild form (adult onset).	X-linked. Normal corneas. Increased dermatan and heparan sulfates. Enzymatic assay. Molecular testing (IDS gene)	ERT for non-SNC features. Possible BMT or HSCT
Type III (Sanfilippo) 4 enzymes of the heparan sulphate metabolism	Encephalopathy with mild organ involvement; development/language delay, behavioral problems, sleep deprivation, hyperactivity, intellectual disability, seizures, neuro-degeneration.	Increased heparan sulphate in urine. Enzymatic assay. Molecular testing (4 different genes)	Symptomatic.
Type IV (Morquio) 2 enzymes of keratan sulphate metabolism	Normal intelligence. Short stature. Skeletal deformities, short neck, scoliosis, joint contractures, Atlanta-axial instability	Increased keratan sulphate in urine. Abnormal skeletal x-rays. Enzyme assays. Molecular testing for 2 genes.	Symptomatic. ERT
Type VI (Maroteaux-Lamy disease) arylsulphatase-B	Normal intelligence, skeletal deformities similar to Type I (Hurler). Often macrocephaly at birth.	Increased dermatan sulphate in urine. Enzymatic assay. Molecular testing (ARSB gene)	ERT

BMT = bone marrow transplant; HSCT = hematopoietic stem cell transplant.

- *Cat urine*: 3-methylcrotonylglycinuria, multiple carboxylase deficiency
- *Cabbage*: tyrosinemia type 1
- *Rancid butter*: tyrosinemia type 1
- *Sulphur*: cystinuria, tyrosinemia type 1
- *Fish-like*: trimethylaminuria, dimethylglycinuria

54. **Which inborn errors of metabolism can result in fetal hydrops?**
    - **Lysosomal disorders**: MPS type VII, sialidosis, mucolipidosis type II (I-cell disease), sphingolipidosis (Niemann-Pick type A, Gaucher, Farber, GM1, etc.), lipid storage disorders (Niemann-Pick type C), sialic storage disorders
    - **Sterol synthesis disorders**: Smith-Lemli-Opitz syndrome, mevalonic aciduria
    - **Peroxisomal disorders**: Zellweger
    - **Glycogen storage disease** type IV (Anderson disease)
    - **Glycosylation disorders**
    - Primary **carnitine** deficiency
    - **Mitochondrial disorders**
    - **Neonatal hemochromatosis**

55. **Which metabolic disorders can present as sudden unexpected death syndrome (SUDS)?**
    - Fatty acid oxidation defects
    - Some organic acidemias
    - Defects of aldosterone and glucocorticoid metabolism
    - McArdle syndrome (myophosphorylase deficiency)
    - Mitochondrial defects (e.g., Leigh syndrome)

56. **One of the infants in your care dies from a suspected IEM. What postmortem investigations are key?**
    - Serum and plasma: Centrifuge several milliliters immediately, freeze in separate fractions.
    - Dried blood spot: Obtain on filter paper card.
    - Urine: Freeze immediately; consider bladder wash with saline.
    - Bile: Obtain spot on filter card for acylcarnitine analysis.
    - DNA: Obtain 3 to 10 mL whole blood in EDTA tube; if necessary freeze without centrifuging.
    - Culture fibroblasts: skin biopsy, may be obtained up to 24 hours postmortem.
    - Cerebrospinal fluid (CSF): Obtain several 1-mL fractions; freeze immediately, if possible at -70 °C.
    - Muscle biopsy: DNA, histology, histochemistry, enzymatic studies (energy metabolism)
    - Liver biopsy: histochemistry, enzymatic assays

SEX-CHROMOSOME ABNORMALITIES

57. **Does the Lyon hypothesis refer to the "king of beasts"?**
    The *Lyon hypothesis* states that, in any cell, only one X chromosome will be functional. Any other X chromosomes present in that cell will be condensed, late replicating, and inactive (called the *Barr body*). The inactive X may be either paternal or maternal in origin, but all descendants of a particular cell will have the same inactive parentally derived chromosome.

58. **What are the features of the four most common sex-chromosome abnormalities?**
    See Table 8-6.

Table 8-6. Most Common Sex Chromosome Disorders

	47,XXY (KLINEFELTER)	47,XYY	47,XXX	45,X (TURNER)
Frequency of live births (males)	1 in 1000	1 in 1000	—	—
Frequency of live births (females)	—	—	1 in 1000	1 in 2000
Maternal age association	+	—	+	—
Phenotype	Tall, eunuchoid habitus, underdeveloped secondary sexual characteristics, gynecomastia (XXY)	Tall, severe acne, indistinguishable from normal males (XYY)	Tall, indistinguishable from normal females (XXX)	Short stature, webbed neck, shield chest, pedal edema at birth, coarctation of the aorta (45,X)
IQ and behavior problems	80-100; behavioral problems (XXY)	90-110; behavioral problems; aggressive behavior (XYY)	90-110; behavioral problems (XXX)	Mildly deficient to normal intelligence; spatial-perceptual difficulties (45,X)
Reproductive function	Extremely rare (XXY)	Common (XYY)	Common (XXX)	Extremely rare (45,X)
Gonad	Hypoplastic testes; Leydig cell hyperplasia, Sertoli cell hypoplasia, seminiferous tubule dysgenesis, few spermatogenic precursors (XXY);	Normal-size testes, normal testicular histology (XYY)	Normal-size ovaries, normal ovarian histology (XXX)	Streak ovaries with deficient follicles (45,X)

From Donnenfeld AE, Dunn LK: *Common chromosome disorders detected prenatally,* Postgrad Obstet Gynecol 6:5, 1986.

59. Of the four most common types of sex-chromosome abnormalities, which is identifiable at birth?

Only infants with Turner syndrome have physical features that are easily identifiable at birth (See Fig. 8-13).

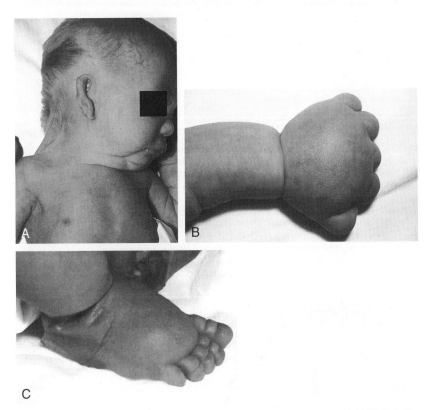

Figure 8-13. Newborn with Turner syndrome with (A) short, webbed neck with low posterior hairline, shield chest with widespaced nipples, micrognathia and (B and C) lymphedema of hands and feet, including toes. Lymphedema of the toes can lead to nail hypoplasia. (*From Zitelli BJ, McIntire SC, Nowalk AJ, editors:* Atlas of Pediatric Physical Diagnosis, *ed 6. Philadelphia, 2012, Saunders, p 15.*)

Loscalzo ML: Turner syndrome, *Pediatr Rev* 29:219–227, 2008.

KEY POINTS: TURNER SYNDROME

1. Majority: 45,X
2. Newborn period: Only sign may be lymphedema of feet and/or hands
3. Adolescence: Primary amenorrhea due to ovarian dysplasia
4. Short stature often prompts initial workup
5. Normal mental development
6. Classic features: Webbed neck with low hairline, broad chest with wide-spaced nipples
7. Increased risk for congenital heart disease: Coarctation of the aorta

60. What are the differences between Noonan syndrome and Turner syndrome?
See Table 8-7.

Table 8-7. Differences Between Turner Syndrome and Noonan Syndrome

TURNER SYNDROME	NOONAN SYNDROME
Affects females only	Affects both males and females
Chromosome disorder	Normal chromosomes
(45,X)	Autosomal dominant disorder
Near-normal intelligence	Mental deficiency
Coarctation of aorta is the most common	Pulmonary stenosis is the most common
Amenorrhea and sterility due to ovarian dysgenesis	Normal menstrual cycle in females

61. What is the second most common genetic form of mental retardation?
Fragile X syndrome (with Down syndrome being the most common). It affects an estimated 1 in 1000 males and 1 in 2000 females. About 2% to 6% of male subjects and 2% to 4% of female subjects with unexplained mental retardation will carry the full fragile X mutation.

FRAXA Research Foundation: www.fraxa.org. Accessed on Dec. 3, 2014.
National Fragile X Foundation: www.fragilex.org. Accessed on Dec. 3, 2014.

62. What are the characteristic facial features of fragile X syndrome?
Typical features include a long face, long everted ears, prominent mandible and large forehead. These tend to be more evident in affected adults. In younger children, the prominent features are prominent ears (Fig. 8-14).

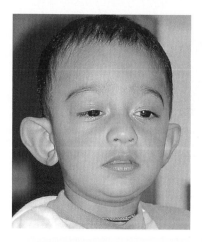

Figure 8-14. A child with Fragile X. At this age, the main feature is often the prominent ears. *(From Lissauer T, Clayden G: Illustrated Textbook of Paediatrics, ed 4. Philadelphia, 2012, Elsevier, p 115–132.)*

63. What is the nature of the mutation in fragile X syndrome?
Expansion of trinucleotide repeat sequences. When the lymphocytes of an affected male are grown in a folate-deficient medium and the chromosomes examined, a substantial fraction of X chromosomes demonstrate a break near the distal end of the long arm. This site—the fragile X mental retardation-1 gene (*FMR1*)—was identified and sequenced in 1991. At the center of the gene is a repeating trinucleotide sequence (CGG) that, in normal individuals, repeats 6 to 45 times. However, in carriers, the sequence expands to 50 to 200 copies (called a premutation). In fully affected individuals, it expands to 200 to 600 copies.

Bagni C, Oostra BA: Fragile X syndrome: from protein function to therapy, *Am J Med Genet A* 161A:2809–2821, 2013.

64. **What are the associated medical problems of fragile X syndrome in males?**
    Flat feet (80%), macroorchidism (80% after puberty), mitral valve prolapse (50% to 80% in adulthood), recurrent otitis media (60%), strabismus (30%), refractive errors (20%), seizures (15%), and scoliosis (>20%).

Lachiewicz AM, Dawson DV, Spiridigliozzi GA: Physical characteristics of young boys with fragile X syndrome: reasons for difficulties in making a diagnosis in young males, *Am J Med Genet* 92:229–236, 2000.

65. **What is the outcome for girls with fragile X?**
    Heterozygous females who carry the fragile X chromosome have more behavioral and developmental problems (including attention deficit hyperactivity disorder), cognitive difficulties (50% with an IQ in the mentally retarded or borderline range), and physical differences (prominent ears, long and narrow face). Cytogenetic testing is recommended for all sisters of fragile X males.

Visootsak J, Hipp H, Clark H, et al: Climbing the branches of a family tree: diagnosis of fragile X syndrome, *J Pediatr* 164:1292–1295, 2014.
Hagerman RJ, Berry-Kravis E, et al: Advances in the treatment of fragile X syndrome, *Pediatrics* 123:378–390, 2009.

KEY POINTS: FRAGILE X SYNDROME

1. Most common cause of inherited mental retardation
2. Prepubertal: Elongated face, flattened nasal bridge, protruding ears
3. Pubertal: Macroorchidism
4. Heterozygous females: 50% with IQ in the borderline or intellectually disabled range
5. First recognized trinucleotide repeat disorder

TERATOLOGY

66. **Which drugs are known to be teratogenic?**
    Most teratogenic drugs exert a deleterious effect in a minority of exposed fetuses. Exact malformation rates are unavailable because of the inability to perform a statistical evaluation on a randomized, controlled population. Known teratogens are summarized in Table 8-8.

Table 8-8. Known Teratogens

DRUG	MAJOR TERATOGENIC EFFECT
Thalidomide	Limb defects
Lithium	Ebstein tricuspid valve anomaly
Aminopterin	Craniofacial and limb anomalies
Methotrexate	Craniofacial and limb anomalies
Phenytoin	Facial dysmorphism, dysplastic nails
Trimethadione	Craniofacial dysmorphism, growth retardation
Valproic acid	Neural tube defects
Diethylstilbestrol	Müllerian anomalies, clear cell adenocarcinoma
Androgens	Virilization
Tetracycline	Teeth and bone maldevelopment
Streptomycin	Ototoxicity
Warfarin	Nasal hypoplasia, bone maldevelopment
Penicillamine	Cutis laxa
Accutane (retinoic acid)	Craniofacial and cardiac anomalies

67. Describe the characteristic features of the fetal hydantoin syndrome

Craniofacial: Broad nasal bridge, wide fontanel, low-set hairline, broad alveolar ridge, metopic ridging, short neck, ocular hypertelorism, microcephaly, cleft lip and palate, abnormal or low-set ears, epicanthal folds, ptosis of eyelids, coloboma, and coarse scalp hair

Limbs: Small or absent nails, hypoplasia of distal phalanges, altered palmar crease, digital thumb, and dislocated hip

About 10% of infants whose mothers took phenytoin (Dilantin) during pregnancy have a major malformation; 30% have minor abnormalities.

68. A pregnant female sommelier asks you what amount of Chateauneuf Du Pape is safe to ingest during pregnancy.

How much alcohol is safe to consume during pregnancy is unknown. The full dysmorphologic manifestations of fetal alcohol syndrome are associated with heavy intake. However, most infants will not display the full syndrome. For infants born to women with lesser degrees of alcohol intake during pregnancy and who demonstrate more subtle abnormalities (e.g., cognitive and behavioral problems), it is more difficult to ascribe risk because of confounding variables (e.g., maternal illness, pregnancy weight gain, other drug use [especially marijuana]). Furthermore, for reasons that are unclear, it appears that infants who are prenatally exposed to similar amounts of alcohol are likely to have different consequences. Because current data (including a 2014 meta-analysis) do not support the concept that any amount of alcohol is safe during pregnancy, the American Academy of Pediatrics recommends abstinence from alcohol for women who are pregnant or who are planning to become pregnant.

Sowell SR, Charness ME, Riley EP: Pregnancy: no safe level of alcohol, *Nature* 513(7517):172, 2014.

Flak AL, Su S, Bertrand J, et al: The association of mild, moderate, and binge prenatal alcohol exposure and child neuropsychological outcomes: a meta-analysis, *Alcohol Clin Exp Res* 38:214–226, 2014.

69. What are the frequent facial features of the fetal alcohol syndrome?

The three facial dysmorphisms found most characteristically are **short palpebral fissures, thin vermillion border,** and **smooth philtrum**. Additional features include:

- **Skull:** Microcephaly, midface hypoplasia
- **Eyes:** Epicanthal folds, ptosis, strabismus
- **Mouth:** Prominent lateral palatine ridges, retrognathia in infancy, micrognathia or relative prognathia in adolescence
- **Nose:** Flat nasal bridge, short and upturned nose (Fig. 8-15)

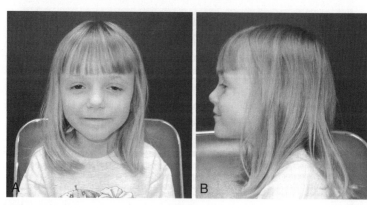

Figure 8-15. Patient with fetal alcohol syndrome. **A,** Note bilateral ptosis, short palpebral fissures, smooth philtrum, and thin upper lip. **B,** Short palpebral fissures are sometimes more noticeable in profile. Head circumference is second percentile. *(From Seaver LH: Adverse environmental exposures in pregnancy: teratology in adolescent medicine practice, Adolesc Med State Art Rev 13:269–291, 2002.)*

Hoyme HE, May PA, Kalberg WO, et al: A practical clinical approach to diagnosis of fetal alcohol spectrum disorders: clarification of the 1996 Institute of Medicine criteria, *Pediatrics* 115:39–47, 2005.

KEY POINTS: FETAL ALCOHOL SYNDROME

1. Growth deficiencies: Prenatal and postnatal
2. Microcephaly with neurodevelopmental abnormalities
3. Short palpebral fissures
4. Smooth philtrum
5. Thin upper lip

70. **What happens to children with fetal alcohol syndrome when they grow up?**
    Follow-up studies of adolescents and adults revealed that relative short stature, poorly developed philtrum, thin upper lip, and microcephaly persisted, but other facial anomalies became more subtle. Persistent mental handicaps (including intellectual disabilities), problematic academic functioning (particularly in mathematics), limited occupational options, and dependent living were major sequelae. Intermediate or significant maladaptive behavior was also a very common finding. Severely unstable family environments were common.

Spohr HL, Willms J, Steinhausen HC: Fetal alcohol spectrum disorders in young adulthood, *J Pediatr* 150: 175–179, 2007.

Streissguth AP, Aase JM, Clarren SK, et al: Fetal alcohol syndrome in adolescents and adults, *JAMA* 265: 1961–1967, 1991.

National Organization on Fetal Alcohol Syndrome: www.nofas.org. Accessed on Mar. 23, 2015.

Acknowledgment

The editors gratefully acknowledge contributions by Drs. Elain H. Zackai, JoAnn Bergoffen, Alan E. Donnenfeld, and Jeffrey E. Ming that were retained from the first three editions of *Pediatric Secrets*.

CHAPTER 9

HEMATOLOGY

Jennifer L. Webb, MD and Steven E. McKenzie, MD, PhD

BONE MARROW FAILURE

1. **What are the types of bone marrow failure?**
   Bone marrow failure is manifested by pancytopenia or, at times, by cytopenia of a single cell type.
   It can be **acquired** (acquired aplastic anemia) or **inherited/genetic** (e.g., Fanconi anemia, Kostmann syndrome, Diamond-Blackfan anemia, amegakaryocytic thrombocytopenia, thrombocytopenia-absent radius).

Chirnomas SD, Kupfer GM: The inherited bone marrow failure syndromes, *Pediatr Clin North Am* 60:1291–1310, 2013.
Hartung HD, Olson TS, Bessler M: Acquired aplastic anemia in children, *Pediatr Clin North Am* 60: 1311–1336, 2013.

2. **What are the causes of acquired aplastic anemia?**
   After careful exclusion of the known causes listed below, 80% of cases remain classified as **idiopathic**. A variety of associated conditions include the following:
   Radiation
   Immune diseases
   - Eosinophilic fasciitis
   - Hypogammaglobulinemia

   Drugs and chemicals
   - Regular: Cytotoxic (as in treatment for malignancy), benzene
   - Idiosyncratic: Chloramphenicol, anti-inflammatory drugs, antiepileptics, gold, nifedipine

   Viruses
   - Epstein-Barr virus (EBV)
   - Hepatitis (primarily B)
   - Parvovirus (in immunocompromised hosts)
   - Human immunodeficiency virus (HIV)

   Thymoma
   Pregnancy
   Paroxysmal nocturnal hemoglobinuria
   Preleukemia

Shimamura A, Guinana EC: Acquired aplastic anemia. In Nathan DG, Orkin SD, Ginsburg D, Look AT, editors: *Nathan and Oski's Hematology of Infancy and Childhood*, ed 6. Philadelphia, 2003, WB Saunders, p 257.

3. **What is the definition of severe aplastic anemia?**
   Severe disease includes a **hypocellular bone marrow biopsy** (<30% of the normal hematopoietic cell density for age) and **decreases in at least 2 out of 3 peripheral blood counts**: neutrophil count <500 cells/mm^3, platelet count <20,000 cells/mm^3, or reticulocyte count <1% after correction for the hematocrit. Categorization has important prognostic and therapeutic implications.

4. **What are the treatments and prognosis for children with aplastic anemia?**
   In the absence of definitive treatment, <20% of children with severe acquired aplastic anemia survive for >2 years. When bone marrow transplantation is performed using a human leukocyte antigen (HLA)-identical sibling donor, the 2-year survival rate exceeds 85%. The usual approach to the newly diagnosed child with severe acquired aplastic anemia is to perform bone marrow transplantation if there is an HLA-identical sibling to serve as the donor.

About 80% of children with severe aplastic anemia do not have a sibling donor for bone marrow transplantation. These children receive medical therapy, usually the combination of antithymocyte globulin, cyclosporine, and hematopoietic growth factors, such as granulocyte-macrophage colony-stimulating factor or granulocyte colony-stimulating factor. Two-year response and survival rates for combination medical therapy now exceed 80% in children.

Scheinberg P, Wu CO, Nunez O, et al: Long-term outcome of pediatric patients with severe aplastic anemia treated with antithymocyte globulin and cyclosporine, *J Pediatr* 153:814, 2008.

5. **What is the probable diagnosis of a 6-year-old child with pancytopenia, short stature, abnormal thumbs, and areas of hyperpigmentation?**
Fanconi anemia, or constitutional aplastic anemia, is a genetic disorder in which numerous physical abnormalities are often present at birth, and aplastic anemia occurs around the age of 5 years. The more common physical abnormalities include hyperpigmentation, anomalies of the thumb and radius, small size, microcephaly, and renal anomalies (e.g., absent, duplicated, or pelvic horseshoe kidneys). Patients with Fanconi anemia are also susceptible to leukemia and epithelial carcinomas.

6. **How is the diagnosis of Fanconi anemia made?**
Chromosomal breakage analysis, for example with diepoxybutane (DEB), can be used to make the diagnosis, and **molecular diagnosis** can confirm the diagnosis and be used to test relatives. In studies of peripheral blood lymphocytes, a high percentage of patients with Fanconi anemia will have chromosomal breaks, gaps, or rearrangements. Many genes causing the Fanconi anemia syndrome have now been identified, and molecular diagnosis has assumed increasing importance as studies linking genotype and phenotypes such as aplastic anemia and leukemia can be analyzed.

De Rocco D, Bottega R, Cappelli E, et al: Molecular analysis of Fanconi anemia: the experience of the Bone Marrow Failure Study Group of the Italian Association of Pediatric Onco-Hematology, *Haematol* 99:1022–1031, 2014.

7. **A 1-year-old child presents with pallor and lethargy and is found to have a normocytic anemia (hemoglobin 3.5 g/dL). The white blood cell (WBC) and platelet count are normal, and the exam is otherwise unremarkable. The reticulocyte count is 0.2%. What are two possible causes of this clinical scenario?**
Transient erythroblastopenia of childhood (TEC) and **Diamond-Blackfan anemia**. Both are disorders of red-cell production that occur during early childhood. Both disorders are characterized by a low hemoglobin level and an inappropriately low reticulocyte count. The bone marrows of patients with these conditions may be indistinguishable, showing reduced or absent erythroid activity in both cases.

8. **Why is distinguishing between the two conditions extremely important?**
TEC is a *self-limited disorder*, whereas Diamond-Blackfan syndrome usually *requires lifelong treatment.*

9. **How are the two conditions diagnosed?**
Age of presentation: Although there is an overlap in the age of presentation, Diamond-Blackfan syndrome commonly causes anemia during the first 6 months of life, whereas TEC occurs more frequently after the age of 1 year.
Red cells: The red cells in patients with Diamond-Blackfan syndrome have fetal characteristics that are useful for distinguishing this disorder from TEC, including increased mean cell volume, elevated level of hemoglobin F, and presence of i antigen.
Adenosine deaminase: The level of adenosine deaminase may be elevated in patients with Diamond-Blackfan syndrome but normal in children with TEC.
Mutations: Twenty-five percent of white patients with Diamond-Blackfan anemia have been found to have mutations in the gene for ribosomal protein S19, and molecular diagnosis for these mutations is very helpful when positive. Recently additional gene mutations have been identified in Diamond-Blackfan anemia. These also affect ribosomal proteins. In total, about three-fourths of Diamond-Blackfan patients can be identified by mutational analysis.

Viachos A, Ball S, Dahl N, et al: Diagnosing and treating Diamond Blackfan anemia: results of an international clinical conference, *Br J Hematol* 142:859–876, 2008.

10. **What is Kostmann syndrome?**
Kostmann syndrome is severe congenital neutropenia. At birth, or shortly thereafter, very severe neutropenia (absolute neutrophil count of 0 to 200/mm^3) is noted, often at the time of significant bacterial infection (e.g., deep skin abscess, pneumonia, sepsis). Even with antibiotic treatment, there is a high mortality during infancy unless granulocyte colony-stimulating factor (G-CSF) therapy is used to elevate the neutrophil count. Some recipients of G-CSF have survived the infection risk but have developed myelodysplastic syndrome or acute myeloid leukemia. Therefore, individualized judgment and monitoring are essential in G-CSF treatment of severe congenital neutropenia. An alternative treatment is bone marrow transplantation from an HLA-identical sibling donor. Patients with Kostmann syndrome may have mutations in *ELANE* or *HAX1* genes.

Boztug K, Klein C: Genetic etiologies of severe congenital neutropenia, *Curr Opin Pediatr* 23:21–26, 2011.

11. **You are asked to evaluate a 9-month-old male with eczema and recurrent respiratory infections who was found to be thrombocytopenic. What is the most likely diagnosis?**
Wiskott-Aldrich syndrome is an X-linked disease characterized by eczema, microthrombocytopenia, and combined B-cell and T-cell immunodeficiency. It is caused by mutations in the *WAS* gene.

Nurden P, Nurden A: Congenital disorders associated with platelet dysfunctions, *Thromb Haemost* 99:253–263, 2008.

12. **A 4-year-old with failure to thrive and chronic diarrhea has a normal sweat test but is noted to have neutropenia on a routine complete blood count (CBC). What is the most likely diagnosis?**
Shwachman-Diamond syndrome is characterized by exocrine pancreatic dysfunction (causing steatorrhea), skeletal abnormalities, growth retardation, and bone marrow insufficiency leading to neutropenia. It may initially be misdiagnosed as cystic fibrosis because of overlapping symptoms. Genetic testing for mutations in the *SBDS* gene is diagnostic.

Ganapathi K, Shimamura A: Ribosomal dysfunction and inherited marrow failure, *Br J Hem* 141:376–387, 2008.

CLINICAL ISSUES

13. **What is the hemoglobin value below which children are considered to be anemic (lower limit of normal)?**
    - Newborn (full term): 13.0 g/dL
    - 3 months: 9.5 g/dL
    - 1 to 3 years: 11.0 g/dL
    - 4 to 8 years: 11.5 g/dL
    - 8 to 12 years: 11.5 g/dL
    - 12 to 16 years: 12.0 g/dL

Dallman P, Siimes MA: Percentile curves for hemoglobin and red-cell volume in infancy and childhood, *J Pediatr* 94:26–31, 1979.

14. *When* **does the physiologic anemia of infancy occur?**
Physiologic anemia occurs at 8 to 12 weeks in full-term infants and at 6 to 8 weeks in premature **infants**. Full-term infants may exhibit hemoglobin levels as low as 9 g/dL at this time, and very premature infants may have levels as low as 7 g/dL.

15. *Why* **does the physiologic anemia of infancy occur?**
The mechanisms responsible for physiologic anemia are not completely understood. Red blood cell (RBC) survival time is decreased in both premature and full-term infants. Furthermore, the ability to increase erythropoietin production in response to ongoing tissue hypoxia is somewhat blunted, although the response to exogenous erythropoietin is normal.

16. In what settings of shortened RBC survival can the reticulocyte count be normal or decreased?

As a rule, the reticulocyte count is elevated in conditions of shortened RBC survival (e.g., hemoglobinopathies, membrane disorders, immune hemolysis) and decreased in anemias that are characterized by impaired RBC production (e.g., iron deficiency, aplastic anemia). The reticulocyte count may be unexpectedly low in a setting of shortened RBC survival in the following conditions:

- Aplastic or hypoplastic crisis is occurring at the same time, as is seen in patients with human parvovirus B19 infection.
- An autoantibody in immune-mediated hemolysis reacting with antigens that are present on reticulocytes leads to increased clearance of these cells.
- In patients in chronic states of hemolysis, the marrow may become unresponsive as a result of micronutrient deficiency (e.g., iron, folate) or because of a reduction in erythropoietin production, as is seen in patients with chronic renal failure.

17. How does the pathophysiology of anemia differ in chronic and acute infection?

Chronic infection and other inflammatory states impair the release of iron from reticuloendothelial cells, thereby decreasing the amount of this necessary ingredient that is available for RBC production. The lack of mobilizable iron may be the result of the action of proinflammatory cytokines (e.g., interleukin -1 [IL-1], tumor necrosis factor [TNF]-alpha). Giving additional iron under these circumstances further increases reticuloendothelial iron stores and does little to help the anemia.

Acute infection may cause anemia through a variety of mechanisms, including bone marrow suppression, shortened RBC lifespan, red-cell fragmentation, and immune-mediated RBC destruction.

18. Describe the differential diagnosis for children with splenomegaly and anemia.

Key question: Is the anemia the cause of the splenomegaly or is the splenomegaly the cause of the anemia?

Anemia-causing splenomegaly
- Membrane disorders
- Hemoglobinopathies
- Enzyme abnormalities
- Immune hemolytic anemia

Splenomegaly-causing anemia
- Cirrhotic liver disease
- Cavernous transformation of portal vessels
- Storage diseases
- Persistent viral infections

19. What is the significance of a leukemoid reaction?

A *leukemoid reaction* usually refers to a WBC count of >50,000/mm^3 and an accompanying shift to the left (i.e., the differential count shows an increase in immature cells). Causes include bacterial sepsis, tuberculosis, congenital syphilis, congenital or acquired toxoplasmosis, and erythroblastosis fetalis. Infants with Down syndrome may also have a leukemoid reaction that is often confused with acute leukemia during the first year of life.

20. Name the three most common causes of eosinophilia in children in the United States.

Eosinophilia, which is usually defined as more than 10% eosinophils or an absolute eosinophil count of 1000/mm^3 or greater, is most commonly seen in three atopic conditions: **atopic dermatitis**, **allergic rhinitis**, and **asthma**.

21. What conditions are associated with extreme elevations of eosinophils in children?

- Visceral larval migrans (toxocariasis)
- Other parasitic disease (trichinosis, hookworm, ascariasis, strongyloidiasis)
- Eosinophilic leukemia
- Hodgkin disease
- Drug hypersensitivity
- Idiopathic hypereosinophilic syndrome

22. A 14-month-old child presents symptoms including marked cyanosis, lethargy, and normal oxygen saturation by pulse oximetry after drinking from a neighbor's well. What is the likely diagnosis?

Methemoglobinemia should always be considered when a patient presents symptoms of cyanosis without demonstrable respiratory or cardiac disease. Methemoglobin is produced by the oxidation of ferrous iron in hemoglobin into ferric iron. Methemoglobin cannot transport oxygen. Normally, it constitutes <2% of circulating hemoglobin. Oxidant toxins (e.g., antimalarial drugs, nitrates in food or well water) can dramatically increase the concentration. Patients with cyanosis as a result of methemoglobinemia can have normal oxygen saturation as measured by pulse oximetry because the oximeter operates by measuring only hemoglobin that is available for saturation.

23. What is the treatment for methemoglobinemia?

In an acute situation in which levels of methemoglobin are >30%, treatment consists of 1 to 2 mg/kg of 1% methylene blue administered intravenously over 5 minutes and repeated in 1 hour if levels have not fallen to normal. Failure to respond to therapy should raise the possibility of glucose-6-phosphate-dehydrogenase (G6PD) deficiency, which prevents the conversion of methylene blue to the metabolite that is active in the treatment of methemoglobinemia. In these cases, hyperbaric oxygen therapy or exchange transfusion may be necessary.

24. Why are infants at greater risk for the development of methemoglobinemia?

- Antioxidant defense mechanisms (e.g., soluble cytochrome $b5$ and NADH-dependent cytochrome $b5$ reductase) are 40% lower in infants than teenagers.
- An infant's intestinal pH is relatively alkaline as compared with older children's. If nitrates are ingested (e.g., from fertilizer-contaminated well water), this higher pH more readily allows bacterial conversion of nitrate to nitrite, which is a potent oxidant.
- Infants are more susceptible to various oxidant exposures: nitrate reductase from foods such as undercooked spinach, menadione (vitamin K3) for the prevention of neonatal hemorrhage, over-the-counter teething preparations with benzocaine, and metoclopramide for gastroesophageal reflux.

Bunn HF: Human hemoglobins: Normal and abnormal. In Nathan DG, Orkin SH, editors: *Nathan and Oski's Hematology of Infancy and Childhood*, ed 5. Philadelphia, 1998, WB Saunders, p 729.

25. What are the critical steps in planning for a teenager with a chronic hematologic condition to transition to adult-oriented health care?

All teenagers with chronic conditions face challenges when transitioning to adult-oriented health care. There are several steps recommended to ease the transition for these potentially complex patients.

- Begin planning early! Collaborate with the patient and family to create a written health care transition plan by age 14 that includes what services will be needed, who will provide them, and how they will be financed. This should be updated annually until the patient successfully transitions.
- Encourage pediatric patients to begin to assume developmentally appropriate responsibilities for their care (scheduling appointments, calling for refills, etc.).
- Identify a health-care professional who assumes responsibility for care coordination and future planning and can partner with the patient and family through the transition to ensure care is uninterrupted.
- Maintain an up-to-date health-care summary to communicate the pertinent medical history of the patient to their new providers.

American Academy of Pediatrics, American Academy of Family Physicians, American College of Physicians-American Society of Internal Medicine: A consensus statement on health care transitions for young adults with special health care needs, *Pediatrics* 110:1304–1306, 2002.

COAGULATION DISORDERS

26. What features on history or physical examination help pinpoint the cause of a bleeding problem?

- **Platelet problems**: Although there can be considerable overlap, in general, platelet problems result in petechiae, especially on dependent parts of the body and mucosal surfaces. Additional manifestations of platelet disorders include epistaxis, hematuria, menorrhagia, and gastrointestinal (GI) hemorrhages.

- **Coagulation factor deficiencies or platelet problems**: Ecchymoses are suspicious for coagulation factor deficiencies or platelet problems when they occur in unusual areas, are out of proportion with the extent of described trauma (also seen in child abuse), or are present in different stages of healing. Delayed bleeding from old wounds and extensive hemorrhage (particularly into joint spaces or after immunizations) are also suggestive of coagulation protein disorders.

- **Disseminated intravascular coagulation (DIC)**: Bleeding from multiple sites in an ill patient is worrisome for DIC. If a patient has tolerated tonsillectomy and/or adenoidectomy or extraction of multiple wisdom teeth without major hemorrhage, a significant inherited bleeding disorder is unlikely.

27. What do the activated partial thromboplastin time (aPTT) and the prothrombin time (PT) measure in the basic clotting cascade?
    See Figure 9-1.

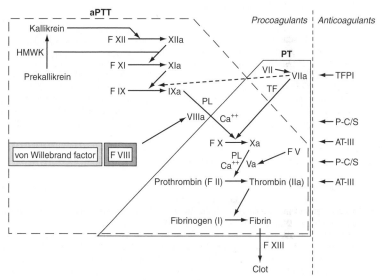

Figure 9-1. Simplified pathways of blood coagulation. The area inside the dotted line is the intrinsic pathway measured by the activated partial thromboplastin time (aPTT). The area inside the solid line is the extrinsic pathway, measured by the prothrombin time (PT). The area encompassed by both lines is the common pathway. *AT-III*, Antithrombin III; *F*, factor; *HMWK*, high-molecular-weight kininogen; *P-C/S*, protein C/S; *PL*, phospholipid; *TFPI*, tissue factor pathway inhibitor. *(Adapted from Montgomery RR, Scott JP: Hemostasis. In Behrman RE, Kliegman RM, Jenson HB, editors:* Nelson Textbook of Pediatrics, *ed 16. Philadelphia, 2000, WB Saunders, 2000.)*

28. What are the possible causes of a prolonged aPTT and PT?
    See Table 9-1.

29. What is the INR?
    The *international normalized ratio (INR)*, introduced in an attempt to standardize the PT, results from a calculation in which an individual patient's PT test value is divided by the laboratory's pooled normal plasma standard PT, then raised to an exponent applicable to each individual PT-initiating reagent available. Its utility is in monitoring Coumadin use in that the reported value has clinical utility regardless of which laboratory performed the PT test. The INR for individuals with normal coagulation proteins not receiving Coumadin therapy is 1.0 (+/−≈0.1 to 0.2 based on that lab's upper and lower range). For those receiving Coumadin therapy, the desired INR varies with the condition being treated, but it is often 2.0 to 3.0.

Table 9-1. Common Causes of Prolonged Prothrombin Time (PT) and Activated Partial Thromboplastin Time (aPTT)

SCENARIO	COMMON AND IMPORTANT CAUSES	COMMENTS
Prolonged PT	Vitamin K deficiency Liver disease Warfarin Factor VII deficiency Disseminated intravascular coagulation (DIC)	Isolated PT elevation is sensitive marker early in DIC development
Prolonged aPTT	Von Willebrand disease Hemophilia (factor VIII, IX, or XI deficiency) Heparin Antiphospholipid antibodies (associated with minor infections or, rarely, autoimmune or thromboembolic disease)	Rare deficiencies of factor XII, congenital abnormalities of the receptor for vitamin B_{12}-intrinsic factor complex Gastric mucosal defects that interfere with the secretion of intrinsic factor or phosphokinase may also elevate aPTT but are not clinically significant Half of children with prolonged aPTT do not have a bleeding disorder
Prolonged PT and aPTT	Heparin Warfarin Liver disease DIC	Fibrinogen measurement can help distinguish among liver disease and DIC (decrease in fibrinogen) and vitamin K (no decrease in fibrinogen)

From Savage W, Takemoto C: Bleeding and bruising, Contemp Pediatr *26:66, 2009.*

30. What are the frequency and the inheritance patterns of common bleeding disorders?
    - **von Willebrand disease:** This is the most common coagulopathy and it is autosomal dominant in the majority of cases. Frequency is estimated to be between 1 in 100 to 1 in 500.
    - **Factor VIII deficiency** (hemophilia A) and **factor IX deficiency** (hemophilia B): These conditions are inherited in an X-linked pattern so that females are carriers and males are affected. Inquiry about affected maternal male first cousins or uncles is appropriate. In general, heterozygotes for clotting factor deficiencies are not clinically affected. Factor VIII deficiency is more common (1 in 5000) than factor IX deficiency, affecting 80% to 85% of all patients with clinically diagnosed factor deficiency.

Journeycake JM, Buchanan GR: Coagulation disorders, *Pediatr Rev* 24:83–91, 2003.

31. Why is the lack of a family history of bleeding problems only moderate evidence against the likelihood of hemophilia A in a patient?
    The abnormal factor VIII gene responsible for hemophilia A exhibits marked heterogeneity, and **up to a third of cases** (either the immediate-carrier mother or the son himself) **may have developed a spontaneous mutation**. Molecular diagnosis of the most common mutation in severe factor VIII deficiency—a gene inversion in the distal portion of the gene in the affected male, the mother, and maternal relatives—may help the physician with understanding the family history.

32. What are the clinical classifications for hemophilia A and B?
    - **Severe:** <1% factor VIII or IX activity; spontaneous bleeding common; bleeding often involves joints, soft tissue, brain (intracranial hemorrhages in neonates), postcircumcision; most common type (50% to 70% of cases).
    - **Moderate:** 1% to 5% factor VIII or IX activity; bleeding after minor trauma, but not usually spontaneous; may involve joints and soft tissue, but less commonly central nervous system (CNS) or postcircumcision; least common type (10% of cases)

- **Mild:** 6% to 30% factor VIII or IX activity; bleeding only after major trauma or surgery; joint and soft tissue involvement, but uncommon after circumcision; more common than moderate type (30% to 40% of cases)

Sharathkumar AA, Pipe SW: Bleeding disorders, *Pediatr Rev* 29:121–129, 2008.
National Hemophilia Foundation: www.hemophilia.org. Accessed on Jan. 9, 2015.

33. What are the primary measures for achieving hemostasis in individuals with bleeding disorders?

Never forget anatomic or surgical technical causes and corrections for hemorrhage. As a result, primary measures are local measures ("push on it, put a stitch or staple in it"), supplemented occasionally with licensed topical prothrombotic agents. Replacement of the deficient blood component (s) is also important, but pharmacologic measures such as desmopressin acetate (DDAVP, which increases von Willebrand factor), antifibrinolytics such as epsilon aminocaproic acid (which stabilize clots), and topical hemostatic preparations such as fibrin glue can be useful.

34. To what degree should factor levels be raised for patients with hemophilia with or without life-threatening hemorrhage?

The following guidelines are applicable to patients with moderate (1% to 5% of normal factor levels) to severe (<1% of normal) hemophilia:

For *minor hemorrhages* (e.g., small muscle or oral), factor levels should be increased to 20% to 30% of normal.

For *major bleeding episodes* (e.g., hip bleeds, intracranial hemorrhage, bleeding around the airway), factor levels should be raised 70% to 100%, and repeat dosing should be strongly considered under close medical supervision.

35. How are doses of replacement factors calculated?

Recombinant factor VIII or factor IX concentrates are the treatments of choice. Each unit of factor VIII or factor IX is equivalent to the activity of 1 mL of normal plasma. With the recombinant products, a dose of 1 unit/kg should increase the factor VIII level by 1.5% to 2% and the factor IX level by 1%. Calculations can be made as follows:

$$\text{Factor VIII dose (units)} = (\text{Goal \% Increase}) \times (\text{kg}) \times 0.5$$
$$\text{Factor IX dose (units)} = (\text{Goal \% Increase}) \times (\text{kg})$$

For example: If you have a 28-kg patient with a head bleed and severe factor VIII deficiency that you wish to correct 100%, your goal dose is $100 \times 28 \times 0.5 = 1400$ units.

Another example: If you have a 50-kg patient with a minor bleed and severe factor IX deficiency that you wish to correct 30%, your goal dose is $30 \times 50 = 1500$ units.

Always round up to the nearest vial size so that there is no wastage of recombinant factor.

Of note, if there is an antibody inhibitor of the replacement factor, correction will not be achieved. Under these circumstances, alternate therapies are needed, such as porcine factor VIII, factor VIII inhibitor bypassing activity complexes, or recombinant factor VIIa.

Josephson N: The hemophilias and their clinical management, *Hematology* 2013:261–267, 2013.

36. In patients with severe hemophilia, can prophylaxis with factor replacement prevent severe hemorrhage?

In a study of boys with severe hemophilia A who were given regular recombinant factor VIII infusions up to 6 years of age, prophylaxis prevented joint damage and decreased the frequency of joint and other hemorrhages. Prophylaxis works. However, the cost was nearly $300,000 annually. How to reconcile the benefits and costs of effective expensive therapies remains a challenge for the health care system.

Manco-Johnson MJ, Abshire TC, Shapiro AD, et al: Prophylaxis versus episodic treatment to prevent joint disease in boys with severe hemophilia, *N Engl J Med* 357:535–544, 2007.
Roosendaal G, Lafeber F: Prophylactic treatment for prevention of joint disease in hemophilia—cost versus benefit, *N Engl J Med* 357:603–605, 2007.

37. **What are the half-lives of exogenously administered factors VIII and IX?**
The half-lives for the *first* doses of factors VIII and IX are 6 to 8 hours and 4 to 6 hours, respectively. With *subsequent* doses, factor VIII has a half-life of 8 to 12 hours, whereas factor IX has a half-life of 18 to 24 hours. Thus, for serious bleeding, the second dose of factor VIII should be given 6 to 8 hours after the first, whereas the second dose of factor IX should be given 4 to 6 hours after the first. Subsequent doses are usually given every 12 hours for factor VIII replacement and every 24 hours for factor IX replacement, but the measurement of actual factor levels may be necessary to guide therapy in life-threatening situations.

Gill JC: Transfusion principles for congenital coagulation disorders. In Hoffman R, Benz EJ, Shattil SJ, et al, editors: *Hematology: Basic Principles and Practice*, ed 3. New York, 2000, Churchill Livingstone, p 2282.

38. **Are longer-acting factors VIII and IX available?**
Both long-acting recombinant Factor IX and long-acting recombinant factor VIII were recently approved in the United States. They significantly affect the frequency of dosing for factor, especially because each is used for prophylaxis. The half-lives are extended by fusion with the Fc moiety of immunoglobulin G (IgG), which prevents lysosomal degradation of the factor. Other mechanisms to prevent degradation and prolong the half-life of factors VIII and IX, including PEGylation (the process of covalent attachment of polyethylene glycol (PEG) polymer chains to the recombinant factors) are being evaluated. Gene therapy also holds future promise for long-term cure.

Shapiro A: Long-lasting recombinant factor VIII proteins for hemophilia A, *ASH Education Program* 1:37–43, 2013.

39. **What can cause an elevation of the PT when other coagulation testing is normal?**
Factor VII deficiency. PT measures the function of the common pathway factors (including X, V, II, and fibrinogen) and the extrinsic pathway (tissue factor and factor VII). The aPTT measures the common pathway plus the function of the intrinsic pathway (including factors XII, XI, IX, and VIII). Isolated factor VII deficiency selectively elevates the PT. Other causes of elevated PT (e.g., liver disease, vitamin K deficiency, Coumadin toxicity) are not selective for lowering factor VII activity.

40. **Who gets hemophilia C?**
More commonly called *factor XI deficiency*, this is an uncommon type of hemophilia (<5% of total hemophilia patients). Unlike the X-linked nature of hemophilias A and B, it is an autosomal recessive disease that occurs most frequently in Ashkenazi Jews.

Asakai R, Chung DW, Davie EW, et al: Factor XI deficiency in Ashkenazi Jews in Israel, *N Engl J Med* 325:153–158, 1991.

41. **Why is factor IX deficiency also called "Christmas disease"?**
In 1952, investigators in England noted that, when blood from one group of hemophiliacs was added to the blood of another group of hemophiliacs, the clotting time was shortened. This provided the basis for the discovery of plasma substances in addition to what was then called "antihemophilic globulin" (and now called factor VIII), which is responsible for normal clotting. The name was derived because the first patient examined in detail with the unusual clotting deficiency (later designated as factor IX) was a boy named Christmas. The publication of the landmark article in fact occurred during the last week of December in 1952.

Biggs R, Douglas AS, Macfarlane RG, et al: Christmas disease: A condition previously mistaken for haemophilia, *Br Med J* 262:1378–1382, 1952.

KEY POINTS: HEMOPHILIA

1. X-linked recessive disorder
2. Hemophilia A: Factor VIII abnormalities (80% to 85% of total cases)
3. Hemophilia B: Factor IX abnormalities
4. Severity based on factor levels: Severe (<1%), moderate (1% to 5%), mild (5% to 30%)
5. Common initial presentation: Bleeding after circumcision

42. **What is the von Willebrand factor (vWF)?**

Synthesized in megakaryocytes and endothelial cells, vWF is a large multimeric protein that binds to collagen at points of endothelial injury. It serves as a bridge between damaged endothelium and adhering platelets, and it facilitates platelet attachment. It also serves as a carrier protein for factor VIII in circulation; it minimizes the clearance of factor VIII from plasma and accelerates its cellular synthesis.

43. **What are the coagulation abnormalities in von Willebrand disease?**

von Willebrand disease is actually a group of disorders caused by qualitative or quantitative abnormalities in vWF. Coagulation abnormalities in children with severe disease can include a prolonged bleeding time, prolonged PTT, decreased factor VIII coagulant activity, decreased factor VIII antigen, and decreased ability of patient plasma to induce aggregation of normal platelets in the presence of ristocetin (the so-called "ristocetin cofactor activity").

44. **What are initial diagnostic tests for suspected von Willebrand disease?**
   * Quantification of vWF antigen
   * Measurement of vWF function (either ristocetin-based platelet aggregation test, known as ristocetin cofactor assay) or vWF collagen-binding assay
   * Factor VIII clotting activity

   Screening tests for bleeding disorders (such as aPTT and bleeding time) can be normal in mild disease. Stress, pregnancy, or medications (e.g., oral contraceptives) can cause falsely elevated vWF levels in a patient. Once a diagnosis of vWF deficiency is suspected, vWF multimer analysis or genetic testing may assist in defining the subtype of vWF deficiency.

Cooper S, Takemoto C: Von Willebrand disease. *Pediatr Rev* 35:136–137, 2014.

45. **What does the ristocetin cofactor assay measure?**

vWF activity. vWF will bind to the glycoprotein IB receptor on platelets in the presence of the antibiotic ristocetin. A patient's plasma is serially diluted and mixed with platelets. The presence of vWF allows for platelet agglutination, which can then be quantified on the basis of the dilutions.

46. **How is von Willebrand disease treated?**

Treatment depends on the variant of von Willebrand disease that is identified:
   * *If protein is normal but diminished in quantity*, desmopressin acetate (DDAVP) is given to stimulate endogenous release. DDAVP is now available for intravenous use and for intranasal use (Stimate). It is important to test von Willebrand disease patients for the safety and efficacy of either form of DDAVP before clinical use. It is also important to distinguish the form of intranasal DDAVP used for vWF therapy from that used for enuresis management.
   * *If protein is abnormal but bleeding is mild*, desmopressin may also be of value.
   * *If protein is abnormal but bleeding is severe*, licensed vWF concentrates may be administered. A plasma-derived but highly purified product (trade name Humate P) provides both vWF and Factor VIII. The ristocetin cofactor activity is quantitated for each vial, which allows for more precise use.

Mannucci PM: Treatment of von Willebrand's disease, *N Engl J Med* 351:683–694, 2004.

47. **In an adolescent with menorrhagia, how likely is a bleeding disorder?**

Up to 20% may have a bleeding disorder, particularly von Willebrand disease. The American College of Obstetrics and Gynecology recommends screening for any patient under age 18 with menorrhagia.

Kulp JL, Mwangi CN, Loveless M: Screening for coagulation disorders in adolescents with abnormal uterine bleeding, *J Pediatr Adolesc Gynecol* 21:27, 2008.

48. **How does DDAVP work in the treatment of von Willebrand disease?**

DDAVP is a synthetic analog of vasopressin, the antidiuretic hormone. Within 1 to 2 hours of its administration (either intravenous, subcutaneous, or intranasal), plasma vWF levels increase by 2-fold to 8-fold. DDAVP appears to act by causing the release of vWF from the endothelial cells. Factor VIII levels also increase in part because of the increased stabilization of vWF/factor VIII complex by

DDAVP, which lessens proteolytic degradation. As a caution, DDAVP administration in the setting of von Willebrand disease type IIB may cause a dangerous drop in platelet count due to increased vWF binding and platelet clearance.

Robertson J, Lilicrap D, James PD: von Willebrand disease, *Pediatr Clin North Am* 55:377–392, 2008.

49. **Should children awaiting surgery undergo routine preoperative screening for potential abnormal bleeding?**
    This is controversial. A study from Philadelphia of 1600 pediatric patients scheduled for tonsillectomy who had a PT, aPTT, and bleeding time found only 2% with abnormal results, of which most were an isolated elevated aPTT. Of these patients, most had an antiphospholipid antibody, which was transient. A study of patients referred for isolated aPTT found that in the absence of symptoms and a negative family history, the diagnosis of a bleeding disorder was unlikely. Others argue that screening should be used despite the small yield to avoid missing an undiagnosed bleeding disorder.

Shah MD, O'Riordan MA, Alexander SW: Evaluation of prolonged aPTT values in the pediatric population, *Clin Pediatr* 45:347–353, 2006.
Burk CD, Miller L, Handler SD, et al: Preoperative history and coagulation screening in children undergoing tonsillectomy, *Pediatrics* 89:691, 1992.

50. **What is the role of vitamin K in coagulation?**
    Vitamin K is essential for the gamma-carboxylation of both procoagulants (including factors II, VII, IX, and X) and anticoagulants (proteins C and S). Gamma-carboxylation occurs in the liver and converts the proteins to their functional forms. Vitamin K is obtained in three ways: (1) as dietary fat-soluble K1 (phytonadione) from leafy vegetables and fruits; (2) as K2 (menaquinone) from synthesis by intestinal bacteria, and (3) as water-soluble K3 (menadione) from commercial synthesis.

51. **In what settings outside the newborn period can vitamin K abnormalities contribute to a bleeding diathesis?**
    - **Malabsorptive intestinal disorders** (e.g., cystic fibrosis, Crohn disease, short-bowel syndrome)
    - **Prolonged antibiotic therapy** (this diminishes intestinal bacteria)
    - **Prolonged hyperalimentation without supplementation**
    - **Malnutrition**
    - **Chronic hepatic disorders** (hepatitis, alpha1-antitrypsin deficiency) can diminish both the absorption of fat-soluble vitamin K (as a result of diminished bile salt production) and the use of vitamin K in factor conversion
    - **Drugs** that can disrupt vitamin K include phenobarbital, phenytoin, rifampin, and Coumadin

52. **What is the best test for distinguishing coagulation disturbances that result from hepatic disease, DIC, and vitamin K deficiency?**
    Factors II, V, VII, IX, and X are made in the liver, and all of these factors (except factor V) are vitamin K dependent. Therefore, the measurement of **factor V** is a useful test to distinguish liver disease from vitamin K deficiency because this factor is reduced in the former and normal in the latter disorder. Factor VIII is reduced in patients with DIC because of the consumptive process, but this factor is normal or increased in patients with liver disease and vitamin K deficiency. Therefore, the **factor VIII** level is a good test to distinguish DIC from the other two disorders (Table 9-2).

Table 9-2. Coagulation Abnormalities in Liver Disease, Vitamin K Deficiency, and Disseminated Intravascular Coagulation

	FACTOR V	FACTOR VII	FACTOR VIII
Liver disease	Low	Low	Normal or increased
Vitamin K deficiency	Normal	Low	Normal
Disseminated intravascular coagulation	Low	Low	Low

53. **What is DIC?**
DIC is an acquired syndrome that is precipitated by a variety of diseases and characterized by diffuse fibrin deposition in the microvasculature, consumption of coagulation factors, and endogenous generation of thrombin and plasmin. The process is uncontrolled, and the result can be significant microthrombus formation with ischemic injury to multiple organ systems.

54. **What tests are valuable for the diagnosis of suspected DIC?**
See Table 9-3.

Table 9-3. Tests for Diagnosis of Disseminated Intravascular Coagulation

TEST	USUAL RESULTS
Prothrombin time; activated partial thromboplastin time	Prolonged
Fibrinogen	<100 mg/dL*
Platelet count	Low
D-Dimer	>2 µg/mL
Factors II, V, and VIII	Usually low*

*These results may be normal, however, especially in patients with mild disseminated intravascular coagulation because synthesis increases with accelerated consumption.
Data from Nathan DG, Orkin SH, Ginsburg D, Look AT, editors: Nathan and Oski's Hematology of Infancy and Childhood, *ed 6. Philadelphia, 2003, WB Saunders, p 1524.*

55. **What is the treatment of choice for DIC?**
DIC occurs most commonly in the context of bacterial sepsis and hypotension. The best treatment is reversal of the underlying cause through treatment of the infection and appropriate fluid and pressor management. If bleeding is severe or if hemorrhage is occurring in a life-threatening location, platelets and fresh frozen plasma (FFP) should be given to make up for the loss of these elements, which is occurring from consumption. Heparin has not been proven to be effective for increasing survival in patients with sepsis and DIC. The replenishment of depleted antithrombin III levels with antithrombin III concentrate may decrease the risk of new thromboses.

Morley SL: Management of acquired coagulopathy in acute paediatrics, *Arch Dis Child Educ Pract Ed* 96:49–60, 2011.

56. **What are the common hereditary disorders that predispose a child to thrombosis?**
- **Factor V Leiden:** This is an abnormal factor V protein that is resistant to the normal antithrombotic effect of activated protein C.
- **Protein C deficiency:** Protein C inactivates factors V and VIII and stimulates fibrinolysis.
- **Protein S deficiency:** Protein S serves as a cofactor for the activity of protein C.
- **Antithrombin III deficiency:** Antithrombin III is involved in the inhibition of thrombin; factor X; and, to a lesser extent, factor IX.
- **Prothrombin variation:** Mutation at gene position 20210 increases prothrombin levels possibly through decreased mRNA degradation.
- **Hyperhomocysteinemia:** Often the result of a mutation of the *MTHFR* gene. Those with predisposition to hyperhomocystenemia due to thermolabile *MTHFR* variants benefit from folate supplementation, sometimes with vitamins B6 and B12 in addition.
- **Antiphospholipid antibodies:** These are passed from mother to infant prenatally. They can also be acquired, often in adolescence in the presence of systemic autoimmune diseases such as SLE.

Yang JY, Chan AK: Pediatric thrombophilia, *Pediatr Clin North Am* 60:1443–1462, 2013.

57. **What are the inheritance patterns of the hypercoagulable states?**
Factor V Leiden, protein C deficiency, and antithrombin III deficiency are all inherited in an autosomal dominant pattern. Factor V Leiden is transmitted with incomplete penetrance. Factor V mutation is present in 3% to 6% of white children, and evidence indicates that some of these

heterozygous individuals may have problems related to hypercoagulation (e.g., venous thrombosis). Nearly 200 pathogenic mutations have been described for protein C deficiency. Mutations in the *SERPINC1* gene are responsible for antithrombin III abnormalities.

58. **In an adolescent with an unprovoked deep vein thrombosis (DVT), what risk factors need to be assessed?**
In young patients with a spontaneous DVT (not line-associated), one main concern is an inherited thrombophilia. Adolescents with unprovoked DVTs may have an inherited condition; however, they may also have additional modifiable risk factors that predispose them to DVTs, such as the use of estrogen-containing birth control pills, smoking, driving/sitting for prolonged periods of time, excessive repetitive motions, and pregnancy. Autoimmune phenomena, including antiphospholipid antibody syndrome, also are increased in frequency in adolescents and should be evaluated.

59. **What anatomic variants will predispose individuals to venous thromboses?**
    - **May-Thurner syndrome** is an anatomic variant where the left common iliac vein is compressed by the right common iliac artery causing venous outflow tract obstruction predisposing patients to DVTs in the left lower extremity.
    - **Paget-Schroetter disease** is a form of upper extremity DVT in the axillary or subclavian veins due to extrinsic compression or repetitive injury as the subclavian vein passes by the junction of the first rib and the clavicle. This is also called "effort thrombosis" as athletes (particularly pitchers and violin players) are susceptible.

60. **What are the mechanisms for low molecular weight heparin and pentasaccharide as antithrombotic agents?**
Low molecular weight heparin (LMWH) is the sulfated oligosaccharide heparin, derived from natural sources such as beef lung and pig intestine, that has been subjected to heparinase treatment to reduce the average molecular weight. Dosing and bioavailability are standardized, with less frequent or no monitoring of the anti-Factor Xa activity, depending on clinical circumstances. LMWH still works by binding antithrombin to enhance its anti-Factor IIa and anti-Factor Xa activities.
Pentasaccharide (Fondaparinux) is a synthetic five sugar agent that binds antithrombin and primarily inhibits Factor Xa. It has a longer half-life and reduced monitoring advantages over heparin, but currently no antidote is available clinically.

61. **What are the direct thrombin inhibitors?**
Direct thrombin inhibitors (DTIs) are anticoagulant drugs that block the enzymatic activity of thrombin without binding to antithrombin. There are two classes of DTIs. The first class includes natural or synthetic derivatives of leech hirudin, usually cleared renally. The second class includes synthetic small molecule drugs such as dabigatran, which are usually cleared hepatically. Use in children is reserved for conditions in which heparin is contraindicated, such as heparin-induced thrombocytopenia (HIT).

DEVELOPMENTAL PHYSIOLOGY

62. **How do immunoglobulin (Ig) levels change during the first years of life?**
    - IgG levels in a full-term baby are equal or higher (5% to 10%) than maternal levels as a result of active placental transport. With an IgG half-life of 21 days, this transported maternal IgG reaches a nadir after 3 to 5 months. As the infant begins to make IgG, the level begins to rise slowly; it is 60% of adult level at 1 year of age, and it achieves the adult level by 6 to 10 years of age.
    - IgM concentrations are normally very low at birth, and 75% of normal adult concentrations are usually achieved by about 1 year of age.
    - IgA is the last immunoglobulin produced and approaches 20% of adult value by 1 year; however, full adult levels are not reached until adolescence. Because delays in the production of IgA are not unusual, the diagnosis of IgA deficiency is difficult to make with certainty in a child who is younger than 2 years.
    - IgD and IgE, both of which are present in low concentrations in the newborn, reach 10% to 40% of adult concentrations by 1 year of age.

63. **Why are antibodies not produced by the fetus in appreciable quantities?**
    - The fetus is in a sterile environment and is not exposed to foreign antigens.
    - The active transport of maternal IgG across the placenta may suppress fetal antibody synthesis.
    - Fetal and neonatal monocyte-macrophages may not process foreign antigens normally.

64. What is the role of the thymus?

The *thymus* is the primary lymphoid organ for the production and generation of T cells bearing the α/β T-cell antigen receptor. The thymus is responsible for the central selection of the T-cell repertoire, which allows for the establishment of tolerance toward self-antigens and responsiveness to nonself (i.e., foreign) antigens.

65. At what age does thymic function cease?

At birth, the thymus is at two-thirds of its mature weight, and it reaches its peak mass at about 10 years of age. Subsequently, thymic size declines, but substantial function (as measured by the output of new T cells) persists into very late adulthood (70 to 80 years of age).

Douek DC, McFarland RD, Keiser PH, et al: Changes in thymic function with age and during the treatment of HIV infection, *Nature* 396:690–695, 1998.

66. How does neutrophil function in the neonate compare with that of adults?

There is a diminished neutrophil storage in the neonate, and the cells display a reduced adhesion and migration capacity in response to chemotactic stimuli. By contrast, the efficiency for the ingestion and killing of bacteria is normal for these cells. Under suboptimal conditions, however, these effector functions may be diminished, and neutrophils from sick and stressed neonates can display a decreased microbicidal activity.

HEMATOLOGY LABORATORY

67. Of the seven red-cell parameters given by a Coulter counter, which are measured and which are calculated?

The Coulter counter, which is the most commonly used automated electronic cell counter, uses the impedance principle. A precise volume of blood passes through a narrow aperture and impedes an electrically charged field, and each "blip" is counted as a cell. The larger the red cell, the greater the electric displacement. In a separate chamber, the same volume is hemolyzed and colorimetrically analyzed to determine the hemoglobin concentration.

Measured values
- RBC count
- Mean corpuscular volume (MCV)
- Hemoglobin (Hb)

Calculated values
- Mean corpuscular hemoglobin (MCH, measured in pg/cell) = (10 × [Hb/RBC])
- Mean corpuscular hemoglobin concentration (MCHC, measured in g/dL) = (100 × [Hb/Hct])
- Hematocrit (Hct, given as a percentage) = (RBC × [MCV/10])
- Red-cell distribution width (RDW) = coefficient of variation in RBC size

68. How does the mean corpuscular volume help provide a quick screen of the possible causes of anemia?
- **Microcytic:** Iron deficiency, thalassemias, sideroblastic anemia
- **Normocytic:** Autoimmune hemolytic anemia, hemoglobinopathies, enzyme deficiencies, membrane disorders, anemia of chronic inflammation
- **Macrocytic:** Disorders of B12 and folic acid metabolism, bone marrow failure

69. What is a quick rule of thumb for approximating MCV?

70 + (age in years). This number (in mm^3) approximates the lower limit of MCV in children <12 years old, below which microcytosis is present. After the age of 12 years, the lower limit for normal MCV is 82 fL.

70. In addition to an elevated reticulocyte count, what laboratory studies suggest increased destruction (rather than decreased production) of RBCs as a cause of anemia?
- **Increased serum erythrocyte lactate dehydrogenase:** More commonly seen in patients with hemolytic diseases, it can be greatly elevated in patients with ineffective erythropoiesis (e.g., megaloblastic anemia).

- **Decreased serum haptoglobin:** When RBCs lyse, serum haptoglobin binds the released hemoglobin and is excreted. However, up to 2% of the population has congenitally absent haptoglobin.
- **Hyperbilirubinemia (indirect):** This is usually increased with RBC lysis. However, it may also be elevated in patients with ineffective erythropoiesis (e.g., megaloblastic anemia). Additionally, 2% of the population has Gilbert disease. In these patients, acute infection can cause a transient elevation of bilirubin as a result of liver enzymatic dysfunction rather than hemolysis.

71. **Why must the reticulocyte count sometimes be corrected?**
    Because the reticulocyte count is expressed as a percentage of total RBCs, it must be corrected according to the extent of anemia with the following formula: reticulocyte % × (patient Hct/normal Hct) = corrected reticulocyte count. For example, a very anemic 10-year-old patient with a hematocrit level of 7% (in contrast with an expected normal hematocrit of 36%) and a reticulocyte count of 5% has a corrected reticulocyte count of 1.0%: 5% × (7%/36%) = 1%. This is not appropriately elevated, as might be seen in patients with severe iron deficiency. The key concept is the appropriateness of the reticulocyte response to anemia. The corrected "retic count" should be elevated if the bone marrow is working properly and has all the right nutrients for making RBCs, including iron, folate, and vitamin B12.

72. **What is the significance of targeting on an RBC smear?**
    Red-cell targets on a peripheral smear are caused by excessive membrane relative to the amount of hemoglobin. Therefore, *target cells* are found when the membrane is increased (e.g., in patients with liver disease) or when the intracellular hemoglobin is diminished (e.g., in patients with iron deficiency or thalassemia trait). Target cells may also be found in patients with certain hemoglobinopathies (e.g., hemoglobins C and SC). In these instances, the target cells are caused by aggregation of the abnormal hemoglobin.

73. **In what conditions are Howell-Jolly bodies found?**
    Howell-Jolly bodies are nuclear remnants that are found in the red cells of patients with reduced or absent splenic function (e.g., sickle cell disease, heterotaxy) and in patients with megaloblastic anemias. They are occasionally present in the red cells of premature infants. These remnants are part of the process of normal red cell maturation but are typically removed by a normal spleen. Howell-Jolly bodies are dense, dark, and perfectly round, and their characteristic appearance makes them easily distinguishable from other red-cell inclusions and from platelets overlying red cells (Fig. 9-2).

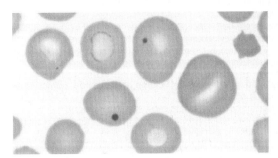

Figure 9-2. Red blood cells with Howell-Jolly bodies in a patient with hyposplenism. The cytoplasmic inclusions are nuclear remnants. *(From Hoffman R, Benz EJ Jr, Silberstein LE, et al, editors:* Hematology: Basic Principles and Practice, *ed 6. Philadelphia, 2013, Elsevier, p. 2259.)*

74. **What is the cause of Heinz bodies?**
    Heinz bodies represent precipitated denatured hemoglobin in the red cell. Heinz bodies occur when the hemoglobin is intrinsically unstable (e.g., hemoglobin Koln) or when the enzymes that normally protect hemoglobin from oxidative denaturation are abnormal or deficient (e.g., G6PD deficiency). These inclusions are not visible with a routine Wright-Giemsa stain but can be readily seen with methyl violet or brilliant cresyl blue stains.

75. What makes an "atypical lymphocyte" atypical?

Atypical lymphocytes (Fig. 9-3) are young lymphocytes (not lymphoblasts) that are characterized by an irregular plasma membrane with a large nucleus. Cytoplasm is typically basophilic. On a blood smear, where an atypical lymphocyte abuts an RBC, the shape of the lymphocyte will deform around it. Atypical lymphocytes are seen in a variety of illnesses, most commonly infectious mononucleosis.

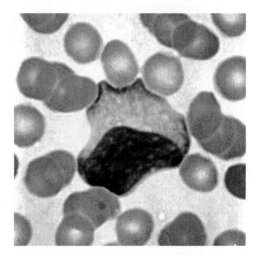

Figure 9-3. Atypical lymphocyte. Note the deformation of the lymphocyte by the adjacent red cells. *(From Zitelli BJ, Davis HW: Atlas of Pediatric Physical Diagnosis, 5th ed. Philadelphia, Mosby, 2007, p 421.)*

76. A patient with oculocutaneous albinism has repeated *Staphylococcus aureus* infections and the peripheral smear shown in Fig. 9-4. What is the likely diagnosis?

Chédiak-Higashi syndrome. This is an autosomal recessive disease with a defect in phagocytosis due to a mutation of a lysosomal trafficking regulator protein. Microtubules do not form normally and neutrophils do not respond to chemotactic stimuli. Giant lysosomal granules, which fail to function properly, are evident in a peripheral smear. Associated features include partial albinism, peripheral neuropathy, and a susceptibility to recurrent pyogenic infections.

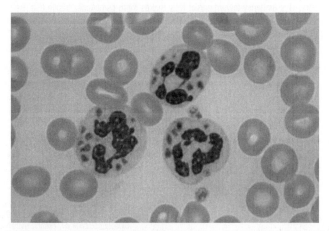

Figure 9-4. Chédiak—Higashi syndrome, microscopic peripheral blood smear. *(From Klatt EC: Robbins and Cotran Atlas of Pathology, ed 2, Philadelphia, 2010, Saunders Elsevier, p 67.)*

HEMOLYTIC ANEMIA

77. **What clinical features are suspicious for hemolytic anemia?**
    - Discolored urine (dark, brown, red)
    - Jaundice
    - Pallor
    - Tachycardia
    - Splenic and/or liver enlargement
    - If very severe, hypovolemic shock or congestive heart failure

78. **What two types of RBC forms are commonly seen on the peripheral smear in patients with hemolytic anemia?**
    - **Spherocytes or microspherocytes:** These forms can be seen in any hemolytic anemia that results from a loss of RBC membrane surface area (e.g., Coombs-positive hemolytic anemia, DIC, or hereditary spherocytosis).
    - **Schistocytes:** These various forms of fragmented RBCs can be seen in patients with microangiopathic hemolytic anemia, which is a form of intravascular hemolysis caused by mechanical disruption (e.g., prosthetic heart valves, hemolytic-uremic syndrome, thrombotic thrombocytopenic purpura, cavernous hemangioma).

79. **Name the two most common inherited disorders of red-cell membranes**
    Hereditary spherocytosis is characterized by hemolysis (anemia, reticulocytosis, jaundice, splenomegaly); spherocytosis; and, in most cases, a family history of hemolytic anemia, early gallstones, or splenectomy. The diagnosis can be made by establishing the presence of the clinical findings and by the finding of increased osmotic fragility of the RBCs. Hereditary spherocytosis is inherited as an autosomal dominant disorder about 75% of the time.

    Hereditary elliptocytosis is characterized by variable hemolysis, with a predominance of elliptocytes on the blood smear. It is usually inherited in an autosomal dominant pattern.

80. **Which disorder is most commonly associated with an elevated MCHC?**
    Hereditary spherocytosis. The hyperchromic appearance of spherocytes and microspherocytes is the result of the loss of surface membrane, an excess of hemoglobin, and mild cellular dehydration. In other hemolytic anemias that are associated with spherocytosis, the percentage of spherocytes is usually insufficient to raise the MCHC.

81. **What is the osmotic fragility test?**
    This is a test to confirm the diagnosis of hereditary spherocytosis. A normal RBC is discoid in shape as a result of its relative excess of surface area per cell volume from the redundancy of its cell membrane. In increasingly hypotonic solutions, more and more red cells will swell and burst at a standard rate. In spherocytosis, because there is less surface area to cell volume, more cells burst as compared with normal in these hypotonic solutions, particularly after incubating at 37 °C for 24 hours. This tendency toward earlier lysis makes them osmotically fragile (Fig. 9-5).

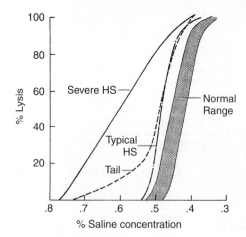

Figure 9-5. Osmotic fragility curves in hereditary spherocytosis (HS). *(From Nathan DG, Orkin SD, Ginsburg D, Look AT, editors:* Nathan and Oski's Hematology of Infancy and Childhood, *ed 6, Philadelphia, 2003, WB Saunders, p 610.)*

Novel tests utilizing flow cytometric techniques and the eosin 5-maleimide (EMA) binding assay have also proven useful in the diagnosis of HS.

Bolton-Maggs PHB, Langer JC, Iolascon A, et al: Guidelines for the diagnosis and management of hereditary spherocytosis—2011 update, *Br J Hem* 156:37–49, 2012.

82. **What is the difference between alloimmune and autoimmune hemolytic anemia?**
    - **Alloimmune hemolytic anemia:** Antibodies responsible for hemolysis are directed against another's RBCs; it may cause acute or delayed hemolytic reactions.
    - **Autoimmune hemolytic anemia (AIHA):** Antibodies are directed against the host's red cells.

83. **In which settings do alloimmune and AIHA most commonly appear?**
    Alloimmune: Red-cell antigen incompatibility between mother and fetus, transfusion of incompatible blood
    Autoimmune:
    - *Primary:* AIHA
    - *Secondary:*
      - Infections (e.g., *Mycoplasma pneumoniae*, EBV, varicella, viral hepatitis)
      - Drugs (e.g., antimalarials, penicillin, tetracycline)
      - Systemic autoimmune disorders (e.g., systemic lupus erythematosus, dermatomyositis)

84. **How does the cause of AIHA vary by age?**
    AIHA in children <10 years old is more likely to be *primary*. In children >10 years old, AIHA is more likely to be *secondary* to an underlying disease.

85. **What is the most important test to establish the diagnosis of AIHA?**
    The Coombs test or direct antiglobulin test (DAT). The diagnosis of AIHA requires the presence of autoantibodies that bind to erythrocytes and signs or symptoms of hemolysis. However, approximately 10% of patients with AIHA are Coombs negative. Thus, patients should be treated for AIHA if the disease is strongly suspected, even if the direct Coombs test is negative.

86. **What are the differences between autoimmune hemolytic anemias caused by "warm" and "cold" erythrocyte autoantibodies?**
    - **Warm** (usually IgG antibodies with maximum activity at 37 °C): These are most commonly directed against the Rh antigens and generally do not require complement for in vivo hemolysis. Hemolysis is predominantly *extravascular*—consumption occurs primarily in the spleen. Warm antibody-mediated hemolytic anemia is more likely to be associated with underlying disease (especially systemic lupus erythematosus in females) and to become chronic. Splenectomy and/or immunosuppression (e.g., with steroids) are often effective therapies.
    - **Cold** (IgM antibodies with maximum activity between 0 to 30 °C): These are most commonly directed against I or i antigen. Hemolysis is most commonly *intravascular* via complement activation. Extravascular hemolysis that does occur primarily involves hepatic consumption. Cold antibody-mediated hemolytic anemia is more commonly associated with acute infection (e.g., *Mycoplasma pneumoniae*, EBV, cytomegalovirus). Patients are less likely to develop chronic hemolysis, and therapy (e.g., splenectomy, immunosuppression) is often ineffective.

87. **A 6-year-old presents with acute anemia, fatigue, jaundice, and dark urine after an early spring swim in a local quarry. What is the likely diagnosis?**
    Paroxysmal cold hemoglobinuria is a transient autoimmune hemolysis due to a Donath-Landsteiner (D-L) antibody. This may be challenging to diagnose because the D-L antibody is a biphasic hemolysin that attaches to the RBC membrane at cold temperatures and initiates the complement cascade. Once the RBCs are warmed by the body, the D-L antibody falls off, but the cells continue to lyse. The Coombs test is often negative. Significant hemolysis occurs after exposure to cold (such as swimming in an unheated body of water). The antibody is often triggered by a preceding infection. Treatment consists of warming the patient and providing any blood products as needed.

88. **An 8-year-old black male developed jaundice and very dark urine 24 to 48 hours after beginning nitrofurantoin for a urinary tract infection. What is the likely diagnosis?**
    G6PD deficiency is the most common hemolytic anemia caused by an RBC enzymatic defect. The enzyme G6PD is a key component of the pentose phosphate pathway, which ordinarily generates

sufficient nicotinamide adenine dinucleotide phosphate hydrogen (NADPH) to maintain glutathione in a reduced state (and to make it available for combating oxidant stresses). The deficiency is inherited in an X-linked recessive fashion. In patients who are deficient (most commonly those of African, Mediterranean, or Asian ancestry), oxidant stresses (particularly certain drugs) can result in hemolysis.

89. **Why are "bite cells" seen in patients with G6PD deficiency"?**
Bite cells (Fig. 9-6) are abnormally shaped RBCs with semicircular portions removed from the cell margin that give the appearance of a "bite" having been taken from the cell. These cells are seen in hemolytic anemias and anemias involving an altered, denatured hemoglobin (Heinz bodies), such as G6PD deficiency. These are cleaved by macrophages in the spleen which results in the abnormal appearance.

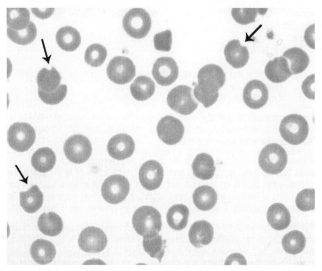

Figure 9-6. Bite cells in a patient with G6PD deficiency. *(From Naeim F, Rao PN, Song SX, Grody WW, editors:* Atlas of Hematopathology, *London, 2013, Academic Press/Elsevier, p 698.)*

90. **In a patient with G6PD deficiency, why is the initial diagnosis often difficult in the acute setting?**
The amount of G6PD enzymatic activity depends on the age of the RBC. Older RBCs have the least, and reticulocytes have the most. In an acute hemolytic episode, the older cells are destroyed first; younger ones may remain, and reticulocytes may increase. If erythrocytic G6PD levels are measured at this point, the result may be misleadingly near or above the normal range. If clinical suspicions remain, repeating the test when the reticulocyte count is reduced will give a more accurate measurement.

91. **What is favism?**
Favism refers to the clinical syndrome of acute hemolytic anemia from the ingestion of fava beans as an oxidative challenge in patients with G6PD deficiency. This is particularly common in portions of the Mediterranean and Asia, where fava beans are a dietary staple.

IMMUNODEFICIENCY

92. **How is neutropenia defined?**
Neutropenia is arbitrarily defined as an absolute neutrophil count (ANC) of $<1500/mm^3$. The ANC is determined by multiplying the percentage of bands and neutrophils by the total WBC count. An ANC of $<500/mm^3$ is severe neutropenia. Agranulocytosis is defined as an ANC of $<100/mm^3$. As a rule, the lower the ANC, the greater the risk for infectious complications.

KEY POINTS: INFECTIONS IN IMMUNODEFICIENCIES

1. Increased frequency
2. Increased and prolonged severity
3. Unusual organisms (frequently opportunistic microorganisms)
4. Unexpected or severe complications of infection
5. Repeated infections without a symptom-free interval

93. How do children with neutrophil disorders present?

Neutrophil disorders include those that affect quantity (e.g., various neutropenias) and those that affect function (e.g., chemotaxis, phagocytosis, bactericidal activity). These defects should be considered part of the differential diagnosis in patients with delayed separation of the umbilical cord, recurrent infections with bacteria or fungi of low virulence (but minimal problems with recurrent viral or protozoal infections), poor wound healing, and specific locales of infection (e.g., recurrent furunculosis, perirectal abscesses, gingivitis).

94. What is the most common cause of transient neutropenia in children?

Viral infections, including influenza, adenovirus, Coxsackie virus, respiratory syncytial virus, hepatitis A and B, measles, rubella, EBV, cytomegalovirus, and varicella. The neutropenia usually develops during the first 2 days of illness and may persist for up to a week. Multiple factors likely contribute to the neutropenia, including a redistribution of neutrophils (increased margination rather than circulation), sequestration in reticuloendothelial tissue, increased use in injured tissues, and marrow suppression. In general, otherwise healthy children with transient neutropenia as a result of viral infections are at low risk for serious infectious complications.

95. Excluding intrinsic defects in myeloid stem cells, what conditions are associated with neutropenia in children?

- **Infection:** Viral marrow suppression, bacterial sepsis-endotoxin suppression
- **Bone marrow infiltration:** Leukemia, myelofibrosis
- **Drugs**
- **Immunologic factors:** Neonatal alloimmune (secondary to maternal IgG directed against fetal neutrophils) and autoimmune (e.g., autoimmune neutropenia of childhood, systemic lupus erythematosus, Evans syndrome)
- **Metabolic factors:** Hyperglycinemia, isovaleric acidemia, propionic acidemia, methylmalonic acidemia, glycogen storage disease type IB
- **Nutritional deficiencies:** Anorexia nervosa, marasmus, B_{12}/folate deficiency, copper deficiency
- **Sequestration:** Hypersplenism

Segel GB, Halterman S: Neutropenia in pediatric practice, *Pediatr Rev* 29:12–23, 2008.

96. Which is the most common form of chronic childhood neutropenia?

Autoimmune neutropenia of infancy (ANI). This disorder displays a 3:2 female predominance and is caused by a chronic depletion of mature neutrophils. About 90% of all cases are detected within the first 14 months of life. The median duration of neutropenia is 20 months, and 95% of patients with this condition have fully recovered by the time they are 4 years old. The ANC of infants with ANI is usually below 500/mm³, and the bone marrow displays normal cellularity despite an arrest at late stages of metamyelocytes or at the band stage. Antineutrophil antibodies are occasionally detected, but their presence is not necessary for the diagnosis of ANI.

97. How common are primary immunodeficiencies?

- Primary immune deficiencies: 1:10,000 (excluding asymptomatic IgA deficiency)
- B-cell defects: 65%
- Combined cellular and antibody deficiencies: 15% (severe combined immunodeficiency: 1 in 100,000 newborns)
- Phagocytic disorders: 10%
- T-cell–restricted deficiencies: 5%
- Complement component disorders: 5%

In a survey study of 10,000 American households, the calculated prevalence of a diagnosed immunodeficiency was 1 in 2000 in children, 1 in 1200 in people of all ages, and 1 in 600 households.

Boyle JM, Buckley RH: Population prevalence of diagnosed primary immunodeficiency diseases in the United States, *J Clin Immunol* 27:497–502, 2007.
Immune Deficiency Foundation: www.primaryimmune.org. Accessed on Jan. 9, 2015.
International Patient Organization for Primary Immunodeficiencies: www.ipopi.org. Accessed on Jan. 9, 2015.

98. What are the typical clinical findings of the various primary immunodeficiencies?
See Table 9-4.

Table 9-4. Clinical Findings of Primary Immunodeficiencies

	PREDOMINANT B-CELL DEFICIENCY	PREDOMINANT T-CELL DEFICIENCY	PHAGOCYTIC DEFECTS	COMPLEMENT DEFECTS
Age at onset	After maternal antibodies have disappeared (usually >6 mo)	Early infancy	Early infancy	Any age
Type of infection	Gram-positive or gram-negative (encapsulated) bacteria, *Mycoplasma*, *Giardia*, *Cryptosporidium*, *Campylobacter*, enteroviruses	Viruses, particularly CMV-1 and CBV; systemic BCG after vaccination; fungal; *Pneumocystis carinii*	Gram-positive or gram-negative bacteria; catalase-positive organisms in CGD, especially *Aspergillus*	*Streptococcus*, *Neisseria*
Clinical findings	Recurrent respiratory tract infections, diarrhea, malabsorption, ileitis, colitis, cholangitis, arthritis, dermatomyositis, meningoencephalitis	Poor growth and failure to thrive, oral candidiasis, skin rashes, sparse hair, opportunistic infections, graft-versus-host disease, bony abnormalities, hepatosplenomegaly	Poor wound healing, skin diseases (e.g., seborrheic dermatitis, impetigo, abscess), cellulitis without pus, suppurative adenitis, periodontitis, liver abscess, Crohn disease, osteomyelitis, bladder outlet obstruction	Rheumatoid disorders, angioedema, increased susceptibility to infection

BCG = Bacille Calmette-Guérin; CBV = coxsackie B virus; CGD = chronic granulomatous disease; CMV-1 = cytomegalovirus type 1.

99. What is the single most important laboratory test if SCID is suspected?
A full blood count to document **lymphopenia** (2000/mm^3) is the single most important laboratory test during the initial evaluation of a patient for suspected SCID. However, a minority of patients with SCID (about 20%) may have a normal absolute lymphocyte count.

100. **Why are male children more likely to suffer from a primary immunodeficiency?**
Several primary immunodeficiency disorders are linked to the X-chromosome: agammaglobulinemia, hyper-IgM syndrome, severe combined immunodeficiency (the common cytokine receptor δ-chain deficiency), lymphoproliferative syndrome, Wiskott-Aldrich syndrome, one form of chronic granulomatous disease, and properidine deficiency. This fact accounts for the observation that the male-to-female ratio is 4:1 among patients with a primary immunodeficiency who are younger than 16 years.

101. **Which is the most common type of primary immunodeficiency?**
Selective IgA deficiency is the most common primary immunodeficiency. The prevalence of selective IgA deficiency has been calculated to range from 1 in 220 to 1 in 3000, depending on the population studied. However, most IgA-deficient subjects remain healthy, which has been attributed to a compensatory increase of IgM in bodily secretions. A minority of these patients demonstrate normal levels of secretory IgA and normal numbers of IgA-bearing mucosal plasma cells. Although IgA represents less than 15% of total immunoglobulin, it is predominant on mucosal surfaces. Therefore, most patients with symptoms have recurrent diseases involving mucosal surfaces, including otitis media, sinopulmonary infections, and chronic diarrhea. Systemic infections are rare.

102. **What are the diagnostic criteria for IgA deficiency?**
Serum concentrations of IgA lower than 0.05 g/L are diagnostic and almost invariably associated with a concomitant lack of secretory IgA. Serum levels for IgM are normal, and concentrations for IgG (particularly IgG1 and IgG3) may be increased in one-third of all IgA-deficient patients.

103. **What is the association of autoimmune disorders and IgA deficiency?**
Autoimmune disorders have been described in up to 40% of patients with selective IgA deficiency. These include systemic lupus erythematosus, rheumatoid arthritis, thyroiditis, celiac disease, pernicious anemia, Addison disease, idiopathic thrombocytopenic purpura, and AIHA.

104. **Why is immunoglobulin therapy not used as a treatment for selective IgA deficiency?**
Unless a patient has a concurrent IgG subclass deficiency (even in this setting, therapy is controversial), γ-globulin therapy is not indicated and is in fact relatively contraindicated because of the following:
- The short half-life of IgA makes frequent replacement therapy impractical.
- γ-Globulin preparations have insufficient IgA quantities to restore mucosal surfaces.
- Patients can develop anti-IgA antibodies with the potential for hypersensitivity complications, including anaphylaxis.

The Jeffrey Modell Foundation: www.info4pi.org. Accessed on Mar 20, 2015.

105. **In an infant with panhypogammaglobulinemia, how can the quantitation of B and T lymphocytes in peripheral blood help distinguish the diagnostic possibilities?**
- Normal numbers of T lymphocytes, no detectable B lymphocytes: X-linked agammaglobulinemia (Bruton disease)
- Normal numbers of T and B lymphocytes: Transient hypogammaglobulinemia of infancy, common variable immunodeficiency
- Decreased numbers of T lymphocytes, normal or decreased numbers of B lymphocytes: Severe combined immunodeficiency
- Decreased CD4 lymphocytes: HIV infection

KEY POINTS: WARNING SIGNS OF IMMUNODEFICIENCY

1. Eight or more new ear infections within 1 year
2. Two or more serious sinus infections within 1 year
3. Two or more months on antibiotics with little effect
4. Two or more severe pneumonia infections within 1 year
5. Failure of an infant to gain weight and grow normally
6. Recurrent deep skin or organ abscesses
7. Persistent thrush in mouth or elsewhere on skin after 1 year of age
8. Need for intravenous antibiotics to clear infections
9. Two or more deep-seated infections such as meningitis, osteomyelitis, cellulitis, or sepsis
10. A family history of primary immunodeficiency

106. **What is the underlying disorder in an 8-year-old girl with atypical eczema, pneumatoceles, and bouts of severe furunculosis?**

Hyper-IgE syndrome is the most likely diagnosis. This disease is clinically characterized by the following:
- Recurrent infections (almost invariably caused by *S. aureus*) of the skin, lungs (causing frequently persistent pneumatoceles), ears, sinuses, eyes, joints, and viscera
- Atypical eczema with lichenified skin
- Coarse facial features, especially the nose
- Osteopenia of unknown cause
- Delayed tooth exfoliation (i.e., prolonged retention of primary teeth)

The laboratory evaluation of the hyper-IgE syndrome reveals massively elevated IgE levels associated with IgG subclass and specific antibody deficiencies; variable dysfunctions of neutrophils; and an imbalance of cytokine production as a result of a Th2 predominance (IL-4, IL-5).

Grimbacher B, Holland SM, Gallin JI, et al: Hyper-IgE syndrome with recurrent infections—an autosomal dominant multisystem disorder, *N Engl J Med* 340:697–702, 1999.

107. **What are the proven indications for intravenous immunoglobulin (IVIG) therapy?**

More than 75% of IVIG used in the United States is for the treatment of autoimmune or inflammatory conditions. Dosing in those conditions is typically 4 to 5 times greater than replacement therapy in immunodeficiency disease. Among the FDA-approved indications for IVIG are the following:
- Primary immunodeficiency disease
- Chronic lymphocytic leukemia
- Pediatric HIV disease
- Kawasaki disease
- Allogeneic bone marrow transplantation
- AIHA
- Idiopathic thrombocytopenic purpura
- Guillain-Barré syndrome (acute inflammatory demyelinating polyradiculopathy)
- Chronic inflammatory demyelinating polyradiculoneuropathy
- Cytomegalovirus-induced pneumonia in solid organ transplant recipients
- Various dermatologic conditions (including toxic epidermal necrolysis)

Gelfand EW: Intravenous immune globulin in autoimmune and inflammatory diseases, *N Engl J Med* 367:2015–2025, 2012.

108. **What are the pharmacologic characteristics of IVIG?**

After the infusion, 100% of the IgG stays in the intravascular compartment. Over the course of the next 3 to 4 days, IgG equilibrates with the extracellular space, with 85% of the infused IgG still situated in the circulation. By the end of the first week, half of the IgG given has left the circulation, and by 4 weeks after the infusion, the serum levels have returned to baseline. However, these data apply to healthy individuals with a regular catabolism, and they have to be adjusted for both patients with a higher metabolic rate and for individuals transfused with increased IgG concentrations.

109. **What are the adverse reactions to IVIG?**

The common, infusion rate–related adverse events are chills, headache, fatigue and malaise, nausea and vomiting, myalgia, arthralgia, and back pain. Less frequent reactions are abdominal and chest pains, tachycardia, dyspnea, and changes in blood pressure. Serious but rare side effects include aseptic meningitis, thrombosis, DIC, renal and pulmonary insufficiency, and anaphylaxis in complete IgA-deficient individuals due to IgE antibodies specific for IgA. Subcutaneous therapy can reduce the occurrence of systemic adverse events in selected patients.

Orange JS, Hossny EM, Weiler CR, et al: Use of intravenous immunoglobulin in human disease, *J Allergy Clin Immunol* 117: S525–S553, 2006.

110. Which viral infections can result in hypogammaglobulinemia in the immunocompetent individual?

EBV, HIV, and congenital rubella. Single cases of hypogammaglobulinemia have also been described among children infected with cytomegalovirus and parvovirus B19.

111. What is the classic triad of Wiskott-Aldrich syndrome?

Thrombocytopenia with small platelets volume, eczema, and immunodeficiency. This syndrome is an X-linked disorder, and the initial manifestations are often present at birth and consist of petechiae, bruises, and bloody diarrhea as a result of thrombocytopenia. The eczema is similar in presentation to classical atopic eczema (antecubital and popliteal fossa). Infections are common and include (in decreasing frequency): otitis media, pneumonia, sinusitis, sepsis, and meningitis. The severity of immunodeficiency may vary but usually affects both T-cell and B-cell functions. It is important to note that this immunodeficiency is progressive and associated with a high risk for developing cancer; a teenager with this condition has a 10% to 20% statistical risk for developing a lymphoid neoplasm. Only about one-third of patients with Wiskott-Aldrich syndrome present with the classic triad.

Puck J, Candotti F: Lessons from the Wiskott-Aldrich syndrome, *N Engl J Med* 355:1759–1761, 2006.

112. What is the likely diagnosis of a patient presenting with a progressive ataxia, conjunctival abnormalities, and recurrent bacterial sinopulmonary infections?

Ataxia-telangiectasia. In patients with ataxia-telangiectasia, primarily progressive cerebella ataxia develops during infancy and is typically associated with other neurologic symptoms (e.g., the loss or decrease of deep tendon reflexes, choreoathetosis, apraxia of eye movements). The signs of telangiectasia occur usually after the onset of ataxia, generally between 2 and 8 years of age. The telangiectasias are primarily at the bulbar conjunctivae (Fig. 9-7). Recurrent infections (as a consequence of a humoral and cellular immunodeficiency) are observed in 80% of patients with ataxia-telangiectasia and are typically localized to the middle ear and the upper airways.

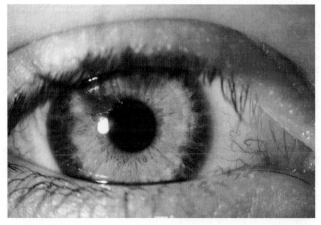

Figure 9-7. Telangiectasia of the conjunctiva. *(From Orth KAHM, Leung H, Andrews I, Sachdev R: Ataxia telangiectasia in a three-year-old girl, Pediatr Neurol 50:279, 2014.)*

KEY POINTS: SUSPECT IMMUNODEFICIENCY IN INFANTS WITH THESE CONDITIONS

1. Failure to thrive
2. Persistent cough
3. Persistent candidiasis
4. Absolute lymphocyte count $<2000/mm^3$

113. What disease did the "bubble boy" have?

    Adenosine deaminase (ADA) deficiency. In this form of SCID, the lack of ADA results in abnormalities of B- and T-cell function and increased susceptibility to infection. The bubble served as a means of minimizing contagion but also promoted social isolation. Although bone marrow transplantation has been curative as a treatment for this condition, ADA deficiency is the first disease to be treated by gene therapy (i.e., insertion of functional ADA genes into the patient's autologous cells and followed by infusion).

Aiuti A, Cattaneo F, Galimberti S, et al: Gene therapy for immunodeficiency due to adenosine deaminase deficiency, *N Engl J Med* 360:447–458, 2009.

114. Describe the molecular defect of chronic granulomatous disease (CGD)

    CGD is characterized by a profound defect in the oxygen metabolic burst in myeloid cells following the phagocytosis of microbes. The molecular mechanisms responsible for this disease are heterogenous because any defect of the four subunits that constitute the nicotinamide adenine dinucleotide phosphate hydrogen-oxidase can cause CGD. As a consequence, superoxide, oxygen radicals, and peroxide production are lacking, and patients with CGD cannot kill catalase-positive pathogenic bacteria and fungi (e.g., *S. aureus; Nocardia, Serratia,* and *Aspergillus* species).

115. Which laboratory tests are used for the diagnosis of CGD?

    Patients suspected to have CGD can be diagnosed as a result of their failure to generate reactive oxygen species during the respiratory burst or, alternatively, as a result of their inability to kill catalase-positive bacteria (*S. aureus, Escherichia coli*) in vitro with their phagocytes. The screening tests for the production of superoxide are the slide nitroblue tetrazolium reduction test and the flow cytometric 2',7'-dichlorofluorescein test.

116. What types of infections are commonly seen in children with CGD?

    Superficial staphylococcal skin infections, particularly around the nose, eyes, and anus, are common. Severe adenitis, recurrent pneumonia, indolent osteomyelitis, and chronic diarrhea are frequent. A male child with a liver abscess should be considered to have chronic granulomatous disease until it is proved otherwise.

117. Which disorder has to be considered in a newborn patient with delayed separation of the umbilical cord?

    Separation of the umbilical cord occurs normally on average by 10 days of life with a range of 3 to 45 days. Delayed separation can occur in patients with **leukocyte adhesion deficiency type 1** (LAD1), who suffer from a profound impairment of leukocyte mobilization into extravascular sites. The hallmark of this disorder is the complete absence of neutrophils at the site of infection and inflammation (e.g., wound healing).

118. Which potential life-threatening disorder of the complement system is associated with nonpruritic swelling and occasional recurrent abdominal pain?

    Hereditary C1 inhibitor deficiency. Angioedema of any part of the body—including the airway and the intestine—can occur as a consequence of failure to inactivate the complement and kinin systems. The condition has also been called hereditary angioneurotic edema. Infections, oral contraceptives, pregnancy, minor trauma, stress, and other variables have been noted to precipitate this autosomal dominant disease. Diagnosis is confirmed by direct assay of the inhibitor level. Clinical presentations include the following:

    • **Recurrent facial and extremity swelling:** Acute, circumscribed edema that is not painful, red, or pruritic, thereby clearly distinguished from urticaria; usually self-resolves in 72 hours
    • **Abdominal pain:** Recurrent and often severe, colicky pain as a result of interstitial wall edema with vomiting and/or diarrhea; may be misdiagnosed as an acute abdomen
    • **Hoarseness, stridor:** A true emergency because death by asphyxiation may occur as a result of laryngeal edema; epinephrine, hydrocortisone, and antihistamines are often of only limited benefit; and tracheostomy is needed if there is progression of symptoms

Bork K: An evidence-based therapeutic approach to hereditary and acquired angioedema, *Curr Opin Allergy Clin Immunol* 14:354-362, 2014.
Zuraw BL: Hereditary angioedema, *N Engl J Med* 359:1027–1036, 2008.

IMMUNOLOGY LABORATORY

119. **Which are the initial screening tests for a suspected immunodeficiency?**
The basic screening tests should include **CBC** (including hemoglobin, morphology, and absolute cellularity); **quantification of immunoglobulin levels** (IgM, IgG, IgE, and IgA); **antibody responses to previous antigen exposures** (e.g., vaccines, pathogen-defined infections); **determination of isohemagglutinin titers**; assessment of the classic complement pathway by determining the CH_{50}; and **workup of infections**, including determination of C-reactive protein, blood cultures, and appropriate radiography. The choice of the laboratory tests is generally dependent on the clinical findings and the immunodeficiency suspected, and the results have to be compared with age-matched controls. It is important to note that there is no justification for a blanket screening; tests should only be ordered if their results will affect either the diagnosis or management of the patient.

120. **Which laboratory tests allow for a broad evaluation of the humoral immune system?**
Serum immunoglobulin levels, quantitative: IgM, IgG, IgA, and IgE. A combined IgG, IgA, and IgM level of <400 mg/dL suggests immunoglobulin deficiency; >5000 IU/mL for IgE suggests hyper-IgE syndrome.

    IgG subclasses: These immunoglobulins should generally be measured primarily in patients >6 years old, in certain circumstances (e.g., in patients with selective IgA deficiency and normal to low IgG concentrations but demonstrated functional antibody deficiency), and in patients with recurrent sinopulmonary infections.
- Specific antibody titers: In response to documented infections and vaccinations
- Isohemagglutinin titer (anti-A, anti-B): 1:4 or less after the age of 1 year suggests specific IgM deficiency
- Tetanus, diphtheria (IgG1)
- Pneumococcal polysaccharide antigens (IgG2)
- Viral respiratory agents (IgG3)

    Determination of B-cell numbers: In the peripheral blood with the use of flow cytometry (CD19, CD20)

    B-cell proliferation and immunoglobulin production: With the use of in vitro assays

121. **Which diagnostic tests allow for the specific evaluation of T-cell functions?**
- **Total lymphocyte count:** Although most T-cell immunodeficiencies are not associated with a decreased lymphocyte count, a total count of <1500/mm^3 suggests a deficiency.
- **T-cell subpopulations:** Total T cells with <60% mononuclear cells, helper (CD4) cells <200/μL, or CD4/CD8 < 1.0 suggest T-cell deficiency.
- **Delayed-type hypersensitivity skin testing**
- **Proliferative responses** to mitogens, antigens, and allogeneic cells
- **Acquisition of activation markers** on T cells (using flow cytometry)
- **Cytotoxic assay**
- **Cytokine synthesis**
- **Adenosine deaminase** and **purine nucleoside phosphorylase** determination in RBCs
- **Molecular biologic studies** (including karyotyping and fluorescent in situ hybridizations)
- **Histology** of thymic and lymph-node biopsies

122. **What is the value of skin testing for the diagnosis of T-cell deficiencies?**
Skin tests for the assessment of delayed-type hypersensitivity are difficult to evaluate. A positive test is useful for eliminating the diagnosis of severe T-cell deficiency, whereas a negative test may reflect a T-cell defect, or it may result from the lack of an anamnestic response to the antigens used. Seventy-five percent of normal children between the ages of 12 and 36 months will respond to *Candida* skin testing at 1:10 dilution, and, by 18 months, about 90% of normal children will respond to one of a panel of recall antigens (tetanus toxoid, trichophyton, and *Candida*); the younger the child, the less likely the reactivity. The cell-mediated reaction may be obscured by a humoral (Arthus) reaction as a result of previous priming.

123. **What is the importance of the CD4/CD8 ratio?**
The CD4/CD8 ratio is an index of helper to suppressor and cytotoxic cells and may be significantly altered in patients with a variety of immunodeficiencies. In normal individuals, the ratio ranges from 1.4:1.0 to 1.8:1.0. In patients with viral infections (particularly HIV), the ratio can be reduced; in patients with bacterial infections, it can be increased.

124. Which laboratory tests appropriately evaluate the phagocytic system?

Absolute granulocyte count

Antineutrophil antibodies (however, antineutrophil antibodies are found in only one-half of the cases of autoimmune neutropenia of infancy)

Bone marrow biopsy (to differentiate increased consumption from decreased production)

Specific *in vitro* and *in vivo* assays:

- *Determination of chemotaxis*: in vivo (skin wounds) or in vitro (Boyden chambers): Measurements are not routinely used for diagnostic purposes
- *Quantification of neutrophil adherence*: Measurement of cell surface expression of leukocyte function antigen-1 (CD11/CD18) by flow cytometry; adherence to inert surfaces such as nylon, wool, or plastic
- *Determination of the respiratory burst*: (1) Nitroblue tetrazolium test (NBT) measures the ability of phagocytic cells to ingest and reduce a yellow dye to an intercellular blue crystal; (2) Dihydrorhodamine (DHR)—in activated granulocytes reactive oxygen intermediates reduce DHR 123 to rhodamine 123, which results in an increase in fluorescence that can be quantified by flow cytometry
- *Enzyme assays* (myeloperoxidase, glucose-6-phosphate dehydrogenase, glutathione peroxidase, NADPH-oxidase)
- *Test treatment with rHu granulocyte colony-stimulating factor*: Autoimmune forms of neutropenia in small children respond to minor doses (1 mcg/kg) within a couple of days, whereas congenital forms require larger doses with responses after 2 to 3 weeks of treatment
- *Mutational analysis*

125. How is the classic complement cascade evaluated?

The primary screening test is the CH_{50}. This test assesses the ability of an individual's serum (in varying dilutions) to lyse sheep RBCs after those cells are sensitized with rabbit IgM antisheep antibody. The CH_{50} is an arbitrary unit that indicates the quantity of complement necessary for 50% lysis of the RBCs in a standardized setting. Test results are usually expressed as a derived reciprocal of the test dilution needed for 50% lysis. The test is relatively insensitive because major reductions in individual complement components are necessary before the CH_{50} is altered. Therefore, determination **C3** and **C4 levels** are often included in the initial screening of a child with a suspected complement deficiency.

IRON-DEFICIENCY ANEMIA

126. What is the world's most common single-nutrient deficiency?

According to the World Health Organization, it is **iron**. It's estimated that 2 billion people, or over 30% of the world's population, are anemic, many due to iron deficiency. In developing countries, about 40% of preschool children are estimated to be anemic.

World Health Organization: www.who.int/nutrition. Accessed on Mar 18, 2015.

127. At what age do exclusively breast-fed infants become at risk for iron deficiency?

Healthy term infants who are exclusively breast-fed are at risk for iron deficiency after they are 4 to 6 months old. The AAP Committee on Nutrition has recommended that exclusively breast-fed infants be supplemented with iron (1 mg/kg per day) starting at 4 months of age and continued until appropriate iron-containing complementary foods have been introduced. The age of risk for exclusively breast-fed premature infants can be more complicated, particularly for the smaller and sicker infants. The lower iron stores of premature infants are more rapidly depleted as compared with term babies. The AAP Committee on Nutrition recommends that all preterm breast-fed infants receive an iron supplement (2 mg/kg per day) by 1 month of age and that it be continued until sufficient iron-containing foods or formula are being consumed.

Baker RD, Greer FR; Committee on Nutrition American Academy of Pediatrics: Diagnosis and prevention of iron deficiency and iron-deficiency anemia in infants and young children (0-3 years of age), *Pediatrics* 126:1040–1050, 2010.

128. **Why are infants who begin consuming cow milk at an early age susceptible to iron-deficiency anemia?**

Lower bioavailability. Although breast milk and cow milk contain about the same amount of iron (0.5 to 1.0 mg/L), nonheme iron is absorbed at 50% efficiency from breast milk but at only 10% from cow milk. In addition, cow milk may cause **microscopic GI bleeding** in younger infants as a result of mucosal injury, possibly from sensitivity to bovine albumin. In older infants, cow milk may interfere with iron absorption from other sources.

Thorsdottir I, Thorsdottir AV: Whole cow's milk in early life, *Nestle Nutr Workshop Ser Pediatr Program* 67: 29–40, 2011.
Sullivan P: Cow's milk-induced intestinal bleeding in infancy, *Arch Dis Child* 68:240–245, 1993.

129. **As iron becomes depleted from the body, what is the progression at which laboratory tests change?**

The left end of the line for each test indicates the point at which the result deviates from its baseline. As shown in Fig. 9-8, in general, the depletion of marrow, liver, and spleen reserves (as represented by ferritin) occurs first. This is followed by a decrease in transport iron (as represented by transferrin saturation) and finally a fall in hemoglobin and MCV. The figure illustrates that the absence of anemia does not exclude the possibility of iron deficiency and that iron depletion is relatively advanced before anemia develops. Tests of soluble transferrin receptor have become of interest in patients with iron-deficiency anemia because the elevated levels are very sensitive indicators.

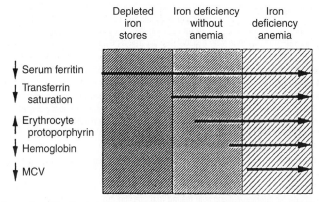

Figure 9-8. Progression of laboratory test changes with iron depletion. *MCV,* Mean corpuscular volume. *(From Dallman PR, Yip R,Oski FA: Iron deficiency and related nutritional anemias. In Nathan DG, Oski FA, editors:* Nathan and Oski's Hematology of Infancy and Childhood, *ed 4, Philadelphia, 1993, WB Saunders, p 427.)*

130. **How might the reticulocyte hemoglobin content be helpful for the diagnosis of iron deficiency?**

Because the reticulocyte is the most recently produced RBC in circulation, the earliest sign of iron deficiency may be a fall in the concentration of hemoglobin in reticulocytes. This number can be calculated from automated counting equipment and may be a reliable and inexpensive alternative to ferritin. Studies have indicated that patients with a concentration of ≥ 30 pg per cell have virtually no chance of iron deficiency.

Brugnara C, Zurakowski D, DiCanzio J, et al: Reticulocyte hemoglobin content to diagnose iron deficiency in children, *JAMA* 281:2225–2230, 1999.
Cohen AR: Choosing the best strategy to prevent childhood iron deficiency, *JAMA* 281:2247–2248, 1999.

131. **Why are tests for iron stores more difficult to interpret during acute inflammatory states?**
The *ferritin* level, which is used to monitor body iron stores, is exquisitely sensitive to inflammation, increasing even with mild upper respiratory infections. Elevations of ferritin may persist for some time. By contrast, *serum iron, transferrin level,* and *percent transferrin saturation* may decrease with infection or inflammation. *Free erythrocyte protoporphyrin* should not be affected by acute inflammation but may increase in chronic inflammatory states.

132. **What is the role of hepcidin in iron metabolism?**
Hepcidin is part of the system of iron regulatory proteins that have undergone an explosive increase in our understanding. The iron regulatory system controls intestinal iron absorption, blood transport, tissue deposition, and mobilization of stores for utilization. Hepcidin is synthesized in the liver and participates in the orchestration of uptake and utilization.

Collard KJ: Iron homeostasis in the neonate, *Pediatrics* 123:1208–1216, 2009.

133. **What are the common causes of microcytic anemia in children?**
   - **More common:** Iron deficiency (from nutritional insufficiency and/or blood loss), thalassemia (α- or β-; major, minor, or trait)
   - **Less common:** Lead toxicity, hemoglobinopathy (with or without thalassemia), chronic inflammation, copper deficiency, sideroblastic anemia

134. **How is the RDW useful for distinguishing causes of microcytic anemia?**
The *red blood cell distribution width (RDW)* is a quantification of anisocytosis (variation in red-cell size). It is derived from the RBC size histogram that is measured by automated cell counters, and it is reported as a percentage. In children, normal values range from about 11.5% to 14.5% but can vary among instruments. Statistically, it is the coefficient of variation of red-cell volume distribution. When elevated in a patient with microcytosis, it suggests that iron deficiency is a more likely cause of anemia than the thalassemia trait. Children with the thalassemia trait tend to have values that overlap with normal RDW values. The combination of an RDW above the normal range with a free erythrocyte protoporphyrin level of >35 µg/dL is more sensitive and specific for iron-deficiency anemia.

135. **What is the Mentzer index?**
MCV/RBC. This is one of the formulas used to distinguish the hypochromic, microcytic anemias of the thalassemia trait from iron deficiency. As a general rule, iron deficiency causes alterations in RBCs that tend to be variable, whereas thalassemia generally results in more uniformly smaller cells. In patients with the beta-thalassemia trait, the Mentzer index is usually <13; in patients with iron deficiency, it is usually >13.

136. **In a child with suspected iron-deficiency anemia, is a therapeutic trial with iron an acceptable diagnostic approach?**
Yes. If an infant or child is otherwise well, a therapeutic trial of 4 to 6 mg/kg/day of elemental iron can substitute for additional diagnostic testing (e.g., ferritin, transferrin saturation, free erythrocyte protoporphyrin), because dietary iron deficiency is the most likely cause of microcytic anemia. If the child is iron deficient, compliant with therapy, and there is not ongoing undetected blood loss, the hemoglobin should rise by >1 g/dL in about 2 weeks. If the hemoglobin does rise, therapy should be continued for an additional 2 months to replenish iron stores.

137. **After iron therapy is initiated, how early can a response be detected?**
2 to 5 days: Increase in reticulocyte count
7 to 10 days: Increase in hemoglobin level

For patients with mild iron-deficiency anemia, the hemoglobin level should be checked after several weeks of therapy. For patients with more severe anemia, it may be useful to check the hemoglobin and reticulocyte levels after several days to make certain that the hemoglobin has not declined to dangerous levels and that the reticulocyte response is beginning.

138. **What foods affect the bioavailability of nonheme iron?**
It is decreased by phosphates, tannates, polyphenols, and oxalates found in cereal, eggs, milk, cheese, tea, and complex carbohydrates. It is increased by fructose; citrate; and especially, ascorbic acid found

in red kidney beans, cauliflower, and bananas. In children with iron deficiency, the administration of replacement iron with a vitamin-C-fortified fruit juice 30 minutes before a meal makes physiologic sense.

139. **What are the options for use of parenteral iron therapy?**
When oral iron therapy has failed or cannot be used, there are several formulations of iron for intravenous use with generally good tolerance. These include formulations such as iron sucrose, sodium ferric gluconate, and ferric carboxymaltose. Usually repletion of iron stores requires multiple treatments over time; however, novel parenteral iron supplements (iron isomaltoside) may only require single dose administration. Care must be exercised in administration to avoid untoward side effects. Monitoring is required to ensure that anemia is reversed and that iron stores are restored.

140. **What are the differences between pica, geophagia, and pagophagia?**
All are clinical markers that suggest the diagnosis of iron deficiency. *Pica* is a more general term that indicates a hunger for material that is not normally consumed as food. *Geophagia* refers to the consumption of dirt or clay, and *pagophagia* refers to the excessive consumption of ice. These are distinguished from *cissa*, which is the physiologic craving during pregnancy for unusual food items or combinations.

141. **What is the derivation of the term *pica*?**
The condition comes from the Latin term for the magpie, *Pica hudsonia*. This bird is believed to eat almost anything, hence the term pica for the tendency to eat nonnutritional substances.

Borgna-Pignatti C, Marsella M: Iron deficiency in infancy and childhood, *Pediatr Ann* 37:332–333, 2008.

142. **Discuss the relationship between iron deficiency and development in infants and toddlers.**
Multiple studies have shown an association between iron deficiency in infants between 9 and 24 months old and lower motor and cognitive scores and increased behavioral problems as compared with nonanemic controls. Some longer-term studies suggest that the developmental impairments may be long lasting. Debate remains about whether this relationship is causal and, if so, whether the correction of anemia leads to a reversal of the problems.

Baker RD, Greer FR; Committee on Nutrition American Academy of Pediatrics: Diagnosis and prevention of iron deficiency and iron-deficiency anemia in infants and young children (0-3 years of age), *Pediatrics* 126:1040–1050, 2010.
Buchanan GR: The tragedy of iron deficiency during infancy and childhood, *J Pediatr* 135:413–415, 1999.

143. **What are the risk factors for iron deficiency or iron-deficiency anemia in a 1-year-old?**
- Low socioeconomic status (especially children of Mexican-American descent)
- Exposure to lead
- History of prematurity or low birth weight
- Exclusive breastfeeding beyond 4 months of age without supplemental iron
- Introduction of whole milk before 1 year of age
- Feeding problems
- Poor growth
- Inadequate nutrition (particularly seen in infants with special care needs)

Baker RD, Greer FR; Committee on Nutrition American Academy of Pediatrics: Diagnosis and prevention of iron deficiency and iron-deficiency anemia in infants and young children (0-3 years of age), *Pediatrics* 126:1040–1050, 2010.

144. **Why are iron-deficient children at increased risk for lead poisoning?**
- Pica associated with iron deficiency increases the likelihood of ingestion of lead-contaminated items.
- GI absorption of lead may be increased in patients who consume less iron-containing nutrients.

Watson WS, Morrison J, Bethel MI, et al: Food iron and lead absorption in humans, *Am J Clin Nutr* 44:248–256, 1986.

145. How and when should younger children be screened for iron deficiency?

This is controversial. AAP recommendations, which previously had advised selective screening only, began in 2010 to advocate universal screening at approximately 12 months of age with a hemoglobin measurement and an assessment of risk factors for iron deficiency/iron-deficiency anemia. Critics have argued that this type of screening process does not identify early enough those with iron problems, including by definition those with iron deficiency alone before the development of anemia. Other screening tests that have been suggested as better biomarkers of iron status include reticulocyte hemoglobin concentration, transferrin saturation, serum transferrin receptor 1 (TfR1) concentration, and zinc protoporphyrin. Zinc protoporphyrin is a red cell–specific intermediary metabolite required for the biosynthesis of hemoglobin.

Baker RD: Zinc protoporphyrin to prevent iron deficiency, *JAMA Pediatr* 167:393–394, 2013.
Baker RD, Greer FR; Committee on Nutrition American Academy of Pediatrics: Diagnosis and prevention of iron deficiency and iron-deficiency anemia in infants and young children (0-3 years of age), *Pediatrics* 126:1040–1050, 2010.

KEY POINTS: IRON-DEFICIENCY ANEMIA

1. The introduction of whole cow milk before the age of 1 year increases risk as a result of occult gastrointestinal bleeding.
2. Red-cell distribution width is increased because deficiency results in uneven red-cell size (anisocytosis).
3. Low levels of ferritin indicate diminished tissue iron stores.
4. This condition impairs cognitive development in infants.
5. Absence of anemia does not exclude the possibility of iron deficiency. Iron depletion is relatively advanced before anemia occurs.

MEGALOBLASTIC ANEMIA

146. What is megaloblastic anemia?

Megaloblastic anemia is a macrocytic anemia that is characterized by large red-cell precursors (megaloblasts) in the bone marrow and that is usually caused by nutritional deficiencies of either folic acid (folate) or vitamin B12 (cobalamin).

147. Is megaloblastic anemia the most common cause of macrocytic anemia?

No. Macrocytic anemia can be found in conditions associated with a high reticulocyte count (e.g., hemolytic anemia, hemorrhage), bone marrow failure (e.g., Fanconi anemia, aplastic anemia, Diamond-Blackfan anemia), liver disease, Down syndrome, and hypothyroidism.

148. What findings on a CBC are suggestive of megaloblastic anemia?

- **RBCs:** Elevated MCH and mean cell volume (often 106 fL or more), with normal MCHC; marked variability in cell size (anisocytosis) and shape (poikilocytosis)
- **Neutrophils:** Hypersegmentation (>5% of neutrophils with five lobes or a single neutrophil with six lobes)
- **Platelets:** Usually normal; thrombocytopenia in more severe anemia

149. What are the causes of vitamin B12 (cobalamin) deficiency in children?

Decreased intake
- May occur in vegetarians who consume no animal products
- Seen in exclusively breast-fed infants of B12-deficient mothers
- General malnutrition

Decreased absorption
- Ileal mucosal abnormalities (e.g., Crohn disease)
- Surgical resection of terminal ileum (e.g., infant with history of surgical necrotizing enterocolitis [NEC])
- Competition for cobalamin in bacterial overgrowth syndromes or infection with the fish tapeworm *Diphyllobothrium latum*
- Congenital abnormalities of the receptor for vitamin B12–intrinsic factor complex
- Gastric mucosal defects that interfere with the secretion of intrinsic factor

150. What are the best dietary sources of folate and B12?
- *Folate*: Folate-rich foods include liver, kidney, and yeast. Good sources also include green vegetables (particularly spinach) and nuts. Moderate sources include fruits, bread, cereals, fish, eggs, and cheese. Pasteurization or boiling destroys folate.
- *Vitamin B12*: Humans do not manufacture B12; bacteria and fungi do. Animals require it, whereas plants do not. Consequently, our major dietary source of vitamin B12 is the consumption of animal tissue, milk, or eggs. Seafood, which live on bacterial diets, are also a good dietary source. Of note is that B12 is required for normal folate metabolism.

151. What is pernicious anemia?
Pernicious anemia is a megaloblastic anemia that is caused by a **lack of intrinsic factor**. Intrinsic factor is a glycoprotein that is released from the gastric parietal cells that binds to vitamin B12 to form a complex that is ultimately absorbed in the terminal ileum.

152. A 10-month-old child who was exclusively fed goat milk is likely to develop what type of anemia?
Megaloblastic anemia as a result of folic acid deficiency. Goat milk contains very little folic acid compared with cow milk. Infants who are consuming large amounts of goat milk— especially if they are not receiving significant supplemental solid foods—are susceptible to this type of anemia. In addition, the diagnosis can be complicated by the higher risk of coexistent iron-deficiency anemia in this age group.

PLATELET DISORDERS

153. How can a platelet count be estimated from a peripheral smear?
As a rule, each platelet that is visible on a high-power microscopic field ($100 \times$ objective) represents 15,000 to 20,000 platelets/mm^3. If platelet clumps are observed, the count is usually $> 100,000$/mm^3.

154. What are the main pathophysiologic processes that can result in thrombocytopenia?
- Peripheral destruction
- Consumptive coagulopathy
- Splenic sequestration
- Bone marrow failure

155. A previously healthy 3-year-old child develops mucosal petechiae, multiple ecchymoses, and a platelet count of 20,000/mm^3 2 weeks after a bout of chicken pox. What is the most likely diagnosis?
Acute immune thrombocytopenic purpura (ITP). ITP is one of the most common bleeding disorders of childhood, and the presentation of symptoms occurs after infection in about 50% of cases.

156. What microscopic features would suggest a diagnosis other than ITP in a patient with a platelet count of 20,000/mm^3?
- Platelet clumps (in vitro phenomenon caused by ethylenediaminetetraacetic acid (EDTA) that results in artifactually low platelet counts)
- Leukemic blasts
- RBC fragments (suggest a microangiopathic etiology such as hemolytic-uremic syndrome or Kasabach-Merritt syndrome)
- Large platelets (seen in inherited platelet disorders such as Bernard-Soulier syndrome, MYH9 syndromes, DiGeorge syndrome)
- Atypical lymphocytes (thrombocytopenia rarely occurs as part of infectious mononucleosis)
- Uniformly small platelets (a feature of Wiskott-Aldrich syndrome)

Thachil J, Hall GW: Is this immune thrombocytopenic purpura? *Arch Dis Child* 93:76–81, 2008
Drachman JG: Inherited thrombocytopenia: when a low platelet count does not mean ITP, *Blood* 103:390–398, 2004.

157. What is the natural history of acute childhood ITP?
With or without medical treatment, 50% to 60% of patients with acute ITP will have normal platelet counts within 1 to 3 months of diagnosis, and 75% are well after 6 months. By 1 year, only 10% of

children with ITP remain thrombocytopenic, and some of the children with chronic ITP still improve as long as 5 to 10 years after diagnosis. About 5% of patients have recurrent ITP. Because of this predominantly benign natural course of ITP, careful consideration is necessary before instituting treatment that is hazardous or irreversible.

158. **In a toddler with suspected ITP, what is the significance of a palpable spleen on examination?**
Although patients with ITP may rarely have a palpable spleen tip, the presence of splenomegaly in a patient with thrombocytopenia warrants more aggressive evaluation for an associated problem (e.g., collagen-vascular disease, hypersplenism, leukemia, glycogen storage disorder).

159. **In patients with suspected ITP, should a bone marrow evaluation be done?**
Recent guidelines suggest that with classic ITP, there is no need for a bone marrow examination even in patients who have failed IVIG and may require steroids. However, if a patient has features that are potentially consistent with an alternative diagnosis, such as other cytopenias, organomegaly or an atypical history and physical exam, a bone marrow evaluation should be considered.

Neunert C, Lim W, Crowther M, et al: The American Society of Hematology 2011 evidence-based practice guideline for immune thrombocytopenia, *Blood* 117:4190–4207, 2011.

160. **When should medical treatment be given for acute ITP without active bleeding?**
Because the long-term prognosis of ITP does not appear to be influenced by medical treatment, the management of a newly diagnosed child with ITP and no serious bleeding is observation and specific instructions for thrombocytopenic precautions. Historically, the concern at very low platelet counts ($<$10,000/mm^3) was the risk of intracranial hemorrhage which was rare ($<$1% of affected patients), but had mortality rates that ranged from 30% to 50%. However, current data suggest that the risks of up-front therapy in a child with minimal or no bleeding outweighs the potential benefits. Up-front therapy should be considered for those patients who may fail to follow thrombocytopenic precautions (such as active toddlers) or those who already have significant bleeding.

Cooper N: A review of the management of childhood immune thrombocytopenia: how can we provide an evidence-based approach? *Br J Haematol* 165:756–767, 2014.

161. **What are thrombocytopenic precautions in children?**
The goal of thrombocytopenic precautions is to prevent significant trauma in children who may be at risk for bleeding as a result of their ITP. An easy rule of thumb for families is for the child to keep one foot on the ground at all times (no climbing, swinging, diving, etc.) as this limits the height of fall a child could take.

162. **How do treatments for ITP compare?**
- **IVIG:** 0.8 to 1.0 g/kg/day, raises the platelet count in approximately 85% of patients. The response usually occurs within 48 hours and persists for 3 to 4 weeks. Up to 75% of patients will have some degree of limited adverse reaction (e.g., nausea, vomiting, headaches, fever). IVIG is more expensive than steroids.
- **Corticosteroids:** Corticosteroids are similarly effective, but oral steroids take about twice as long (4 days) to raise the platelet count significantly. The steroid effect may be multifactorial because signs of hemorrhage tend to decrease before the increase in platelets occurs. This may include microvascular endothelial stability. Side effects of long-term frequent steroid use are multiple.
- **Anti-D immunoglobulin:** Anti-D immunoglobulin (immunoglobulin with antibody Rh [D]) should be given intravenously to individuals with adequate hemoglobin count, (Rh)D-positive RBCs, and intact splenic function. It is more rapidly given than IVIG, with a slightly smaller proportion of responders.
- **Splenectomy**: When done laparoscopically, splenectomy successfully restores the platelet count to safe ($>$50 k/μL) or normal ($>$150 k/μL) in 75% to 80% of patients who fail drug therapy. Preoperative immunization against encapsulated bacteria is necessary to minimize the risk of postsplenectomy sepsis; many also advocate oral antibiotic prophylaxis postoperatively.
- **Anti-CD20 (rituximab)**: In refractory severe cases, antibody therapy directed at B-lymphocyte CD20 has achieved some partial and complete responses that are sustained.

163. **Which children with ITP are candidates for splenectomy?**
Splenectomy improves the platelet count in up to 90% of patients. Because spontaneous remission is common in acute ITP, splenectomy is usually limited to bleeding that is life threatening and unresponsive to medical therapies. Patients with ITP lasting >1 year with continued bleeding, severe thrombocytopenia, or unacceptable restrictions may be reasonable candidates for splenectomy.

164. **What evaluations should be considered in a patient with persistent refractory thrombocytopenia?**
    * Antinuclear antibody, double-stranded DNA, C3, C4, p-ANCA (to rule out systemic lupus erythematosus and other collagen vascular diseases)
    * Quantitative immunoglobulin levels, pneumococcal titers (to rule out common variable immune deficiency)
    * Bone marrow aspiration or biopsy (to evaluate for possible myelodysplastic syndrome or marrow failure)
    * Viral studies (including polymerase chain reaction for HIV, hepatitis C, EBV, cytomegalovirus, parvovirus, and human herpesvirus 6 and 8)

Kalpatthi R, Bussel JB: Diagnosis, pathophysiology and management of children with refractory immune thrombocytopenic purpura, *Curr Opin Pediatr* 20:8–16, 2008.

165. **How is neonatal alloimmune thrombocytopenia diagnosed and treated?**
Neonatal alloimmune thrombocytopenia may occur when a fetus expresses platelet antigens inherited from the father that the mother lacks. Some mothers, especially those with "permissive" HLA types, form IgG antibodies that cross the placenta and cause moderate to severe thrombocytopenia in the fetus. Infants of mothers with first pregnancies can be affected, and there is a high recurrence risk. Both mother and father should have the common platelet alloantigens typed for incompatibility, and the mother should be tested for IgG antiplatelet antibodies recognizing that difference. In second and subsequent pregnancies at risk, especially for intracranial hemorrhage, maternal IVIG has been demonstrated to be of benefit. Affected infants should receive washed maternal platelets; antigen-matched platelets or in exceptionally dire circumstances, untyped platelets with or without concomitant treatment with IVIG and steroids. Under investigation is whether prenatal platelet typing is of benefit in prevention of the substantial proportion of cases in first pregnancies.

Bussel, JB, Sola-Visner, M: Current approaches to the evaluation and management of the fetus and neonate with immune thrombocytopenia, *Semin Perinatol* 33:35–42, 2009.

166. **In what conditions of children is thrombocytosis most commonly seen?**
    * Acute infections (e.g., upper and lower respiratory tract infections)
    * Chronic infections (e.g., tuberculosis)
    * Iron-deficiency anemia
    * Hemolytic anemia
    * Medications (e.g., vinca alkaloids, epinephrine, corticosteroids)
    * Inflammatory disease (e.g., Kawasaki disease)
    * Malignancy (e.g., chronic myelogenous or megakaryocytic leukemia)

Chiarello P, Magnolia M, Rubino M, et al: Thrombocytosis in children, *Minerva Pediatr* 63:507–513, 2011.
Yohannan MD, Higgy KE, al-Mashhadani SA, Santhosh-Kumar CR: Thrombocytosis. Etiologic analysis of 663 patients, *Clin Pediatr* 33:340–343, 1994.

167. **What level of thrombocytosis requires treatment?**
A high platelet count in most children does not appear to be a cause of significant morbidity because it is often transient. In some centers, aspirin in doses of 81 mg daily are administered when the platelet count exceeds $1.5 \times 10^6/mm^3$. The early introduction of aspirin therapy may be more important if the patient has other problems that might contribute to hyperviscosity, such as a high WBC count or hemoglobin level.

Denton A, Davis P: Extreme thrombocytosis in admissions to paediatric intensive care: no requirement for treatment, *Arch Dis Child* 92:515–516, 2007.

SICKLE CELL DISEASE

168. **What is the mutation that results in sickle cell disease?**
On the β-globin gene on chromosome 11, the seventeenth nucleotide is changed from thymine to adenine and thus the sixth amino acid in the β-globin chain becomes valine instead of glutamic acid. Thus, only a single nucleotide substitution is required (GTG for GAG), but the result is sickle hemoglobin (HbS), which polymerizes on deoxygenation, makes the RBC more rigid, and causes structural damage to the RBC membrane. This change leads to hemolytic anemia and contributes to vasoocclusion. The α-chain is normal.

NHLBI Evidence Based Management of Sickle Cell Disease: Expert Panel Report 2014. http://www.nhlbi.nih.gov/health-pro/guidelines/sickle-cell-disease-guidelines. Accessed on Mar. 18, 2015.
NHLBI Comprehensive Sickle Cell Centers: www.everythingsicklecell.com. Accessed on Mar. 20, 2015.
Sickle Cell Disease Association of America: www.sicklecelldisease.org. Accessed on Jan. 9, 2015.

169. **Why is sickle cell disease often asymptomatic during the first months of life?**
During the neonatal period, the presence of large amounts of fetal hemoglobin reduces the rate of polymerization of HbS and the sickling of RBCs that contain this abnormal hemoglobin. As the amount of fetal hemoglobin decreases after age 3 to 6 months, patients with sickle cell disease are increasingly likely to experience their first clinical manifestations.

170. **What are the various genotypes that can cause the clinical syndrome of sickle cell disease?**
Genotypes depend on which two genes make up the β chain component. In general, severity varies from $SS > S\beta^{0-}$ thalassemia $> SC > S\beta^+$ thalassemia $> S$-hereditary persistence of fetal hemoglobin (HPFH). Hemoglobin concentrations increase from an average of 6 to 8 g/dL with HbSS to 11 to 14 g/dL for HbS-HPFH, which contributes to the variation in clinical severity. Only $S\beta^+$ thalassemia has any hemoglobin A on electrophoresis (5% to 30%).

171. **What are the two major pathophysiologic mechanisms in sickle cell anemia that cause the morbidities associated with the disease?**
- **Hemolysis:** Sickled RBCs undergo both intravascular and extravascular hemolysis, which leads to anemia, reticulocytosis, jaundice, gallstones, and occasional aplastic crisis. It now appears that chronic hemolysis impacts on the utilization and bioavailability of NO (nitric oxide), a potent vasoactive agent. Long-term hemolysis has been associated with pulmonary hypertension and right-sided heart failure.
- **Vasoocclusion:** Intermittent and chronic vasoocclusion result in both acute exacerbations (e.g., painful crisis, stroke) and chronic disease manifestations (e.g., retinopathy, renal disease). The adhesion of sickled erythrocytes to inflamed vascular endothelium is a principal pathologic component. Activation of leukocytes and platelets, as well as components of the coagulation protein cascade, is also prominent.

172. **A 6-month-old black male has painful swelling of both hands. What is the most likely diagnosis?**
Hand-foot syndrome, or dactylitis. This common early manifestation of sickling disorders in infants and young children is characterized by painful swelling of the hands, feet, and proximal fingers and toes caused by symmetric infarction in the metacarpals, metatarsals, and phalanges (Fig. 9-9).

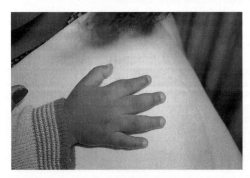

Figure 9-9. Swelling of the fingers from dactylitis. *(From Lissauer T, Clayden G:* Illustrated Textbook of Pediatrics. *London, 1997, Mosby, p 238.)*

A lack of systemic signs, the presence of symmetric involvement, and young patient age help distinguish hand-foot syndrome from the much less common osteomyelitis, which may also complicate sickle cell disease.

173. **When does functional asplenia occur in children with sickle cell disease?**
It may begin as early as 5 or 6 months of age, and it may precede the presence of Howell-Jolly bodies in the peripheral smear. Most children with HbSS who are >5 years old have functional asplenia, with a small, atrophied spleen. Clinical experience indicates that the period of increased risk for serious bacterial infection parallels the development of functional asplenia. Consequently, in addition to routine vaccinations, antibiotic prophylaxis with penicillin is recommended beginning at 2 months of age. Loss of splenic function usually occurs later in patients with HbSC or HbSβ$^+$ thalassemia or those receiving chronic transfusion therapy.

174. **What is the most common cause of death in children with sickle cell disease?**
Infection. Splenic dysfunction causes increased susceptibility to meningitis and sepsis (particularly pneumococcal). The incidence of infection can be reduced by 84% with daily penicillin taken orally and initiated early in infancy (before 4 months of age) and continued into childhood. Though studies demonstrated no further benefit after 5 years of age, many providers continue penicillin prophylaxis into the teenage years. Pneumococcal and meningococcal vaccines may provide further protection.

175. **What are the four main categories of acute events requiring intervention in patients with sickle cell disease?**
- **Aplastic crisis:** Hemoglobin may fall as much as 10% to 15% per day without reticulocytosis
- **Acute hemolytic crisis:** Acute hemolysis may be precipitated by infection or febrile illness. Hemoglobin may fall while total and indirect bilirubin levels are elevated. Reticulocyte count may be preserved or elevated. Patients present with jaundice and dark urine.
- **Vasoocclusive events:** Includes painful crises (most common), acute chest syndrome, acute central nervous system events (stroke), and priapism
- **Acute splenic sequestration:** May occur rapidly, with profound hypotension and cardiac decompensation

Dover GJ, Platt OS: Sickle cell disease. In Nathan DG, Orkin SD, Ginsburg D, Look AT, editors: *Nathan and Oski's Hematology of Infancy and Childhood*, ed 6, Philadelphia, 2003, WB Saunders, p 802.

176. **How should a child with a vasoocclusive (painful) event be managed?**
For outpatients with an acute painful crisis, ibuprofen or acetaminophen and codeine are reasonable choices. Patients with intensely painful crises require day unit or inpatient hospitalization for opioid (including morphine) analgesia, ideally given intravenously. Use of meperidine in this situation is no longer recommended unless the patient has a specific preference for the medication or allergy to other morphine derivatives. Patient-controlled analgesia offers the dual benefit of a constant infusion and intermittent boluses of an analgesic. Other supplementary agents, including nonsteroidal analgesics (e.g., ketorolac), and vasodilators/membrane active agents (e.g., arginine) are under study. For severe crises, blood transfusions to reduce the percentage of sickle cells to <30% may be beneficial as part of a multimodal pain approach.

177. **A 15-month-old with sickle cell disease presents with pallor and fatigue, but no jaundice. On exam, his spleen is palpable to his umbilicus. What is the diagnosis and how should it be managed?**
Acute splenic sequestration represents a true emergency and is the second leading cause of death in young children with sickle cell disease. The clinical problem is primarily one of hypovolemic shock as a result of the pooling of blood in the acutely enlarged spleen. The hemoglobin level may drop to as low as 1 to 2 g/dL. The major therapeutic effort should be directed toward volume replacement with whatever fluid is handy. In most instances, normal saline or colloid solutions will be adequate until properly cross-matched blood is available. Patients may experience "auto-transfusion" where, after a bolus of fluid, the spleen begins to shrink and formerly trapped RBCs reenter circulation, raising the hemoglobin beyond what

one would expect with transfusion or fluids alone. Close monitoring of hemoglobin and repeated assessment of spleen size are critical to ensure the patient does not become polycythemic. Splenectomy may be considered for patients with recurrent splenic sequestration.

Yawn BP, Buchanan GR, Afenyi-Annan AN, et al: Management of sickle cell disease: summary of the 2014 evidence-based report by expert panel members, *JAMA* 312:1033–1048, 2014.

178. What is "acute chest syndrome" in sickle cell patients?

Acute chest syndrome refers to the constellation of findings (e.g., fever, cough, chest pain, pulmonary infiltrates) that can resemble pneumonia or pulmonary infarction. The exact mechanism is unknown, and the cause is likely multifactorial. Various infections (e.g., viral, chlamydial, mycoplasmal) may initiate respiratory inflammation, which ultimately causes localized hypoxia; increased pulmonary sickling may then result. Rib and other bone infarcts can also occur, and hypoventilation may result from chest splinting. Pulmonary fat embolism has been seen to occur, particularly in the setting of a preceding bony painful crisis (e.g., the thigh).

Zar HJ: Etiology of sickle cell chest, *Pediatr Pulmon* 26:S188–S190, 2004.

179. How should the acute chest syndrome in sickle cell patients be treated?

- **Aggressively** because rapid progression to respiratory failure is possible.
- **Optimization of ventilation** is vital, including supplemental oxygen, analgesics adequate to minimize splinting, incentive spirometry, and other possible measures (e.g., bronchodilators, nitrous oxide).
- **Judicious hydration:** Overly vigorous hydration can lead to pulmonary edema.
- **Antibiotics:** These should typically be given to cover *Chlamydia, Mycoplasma,* and *Streptococcus pneumoniae.*
- **Blood transfusion,** including erythrocytapheresis (automated RBC exchange transfusion), has been shown to improve the status of patients with acute chest syndrome; this should be considered for patients with severe or worsening disease.

Rees DC, Williams TN, Gladwin MT: Sickle-cell disease, *Lancet* 376:2018–2031, 2010.
Graham LM: Sickle cell disease: Pulmonary management options, *Pediatr Pulmonol* 26:S191–S193, 2004.

180. How often is priapism a problem in children with sickle cell disease?

Priapism is an unwanted, painful erection that is usually unrelated to sexual activity. It is an underappreciated morbidity in adolescents with sickle cell disease, usually occurring at least once by the age of 20 years and typically by the age of 12 years. Most patients are unaware of the term and the consequences; early urologic intervention may prevent irreversible penile fibrosis and impotence.

Rachid-Filho D, Cavalcanti AG, Favorito LA, et al: Treatment of recurrent priapism in sickle cell anemia with finasteride: a new approach, *Urology* 74:1054–1057, 2009.
Maples BL, Hagemann TM: Treatment of priapism in pediatric patients with sickle cell disease, *Am J Health Sys Pharm* 61:355–363, 2004.

181. What are some long-term morbidities associated with sickle cell disease?

- Stroke
- Chronic lung disease
- Renal failure
- Congestive heart failure
- Retinal damage
- Leg ulcers
- Aseptic necrosis of the hip or shoulder
- Poor growth

182. How can stroke be prevented in children with sickle cell disease?

Children with sickle cell disease are at increased risk of stroke. The risk of stroke increases and peaks around 2 to 5 years of age then declines, only to increase again in the late teens and throughout adulthood. To prevent initial strokes, children (age 2 to 16 years old) should undergo annual screening with transcranial Doppler ultrasounds (TCDs) to assess flow velocities of the intracranial vessels. Elevated velocities are predictive of increased stroke risk. **Regular blood transfusions** are an effective primary prevention strategy to prevent strokes. The goal of transfusion therapy is to keep the HbS percent below 30%. Children who have already suffered an overt stroke also benefit from regular transfusions as a secondary prevention method.

Yawn BP, Buchanan GR, Afenyi-Annan AN, et al: Management of sickle cell disease: summary of the 2014 evidence-based report by expert panel members, *JAMA* 312:1033–1048, 2014.
Armstrong-Wells J. Grimes B. Sidney S, et al: Utilization of TCD screening for primary stroke prevention in children with sickle cell disease, *Neurology* 72:1316–1321, 2009.

183. **If initiated for either primary or secondary stroke prevention, when should blood transfusions be discontinued?**

    Currently, there is no clear recommendation as to when it is safe to discontinue routine transfusions for either primary or secondary stroke prevention. Patients may have normalization of their TCDs while on chronic transfusions; however, once a routine transfusion program has been stopped, they may quickly revert to their high-risk velocities. One large study tried to transition patients with a history of stroke from transfusions to hydroxyurea combined with phlebotomy in an effort to maintain the same level of stroke protection while also alleviating the transfusional iron burden. However, the study was closed early because investigators saw an increase in stroke events without a decrease in iron burden.

Ware RE and Helms RW: Stroke with transfusions changing to hydroxyurea, *Blood* 119:3925–3932, 2012.
Adams RJ and Brambilla D: Discontinuing prophylactic transfusions used to prevent stroke in sickle cell disease, *N Engl J Med* 353:2769–2778, 2005.

184. **What is the primary mechanism by which hydroxyurea is beneficial for sickle cell disease?**

    Hydroxyurea is a cytotoxic drug that has been used primarily to treat chronic myelogenous leukemia and polycythemia vera. However, its use was shown to **increase hemoglobin F (HbF) totals**. It is unclear if this is due to direct effects on γ chain transcription sites or due to preferential γ chain production during erythroid regeneration following cytotoxic insult. Increased concentrations of HbF (particularly >20%) are associated with decreased sickling of the RBCs and decreased hemolysis, which results in increased hemoglobin. Clinically, patients experience fewer vasoocclusive painful events, episodes of acute chest syndrome, transfusion requirements, and hospitalizations. It is unclear if hydroxyurea can prevent or reverse organ damage.

Platt OS: Hydroxyurea for the treatment of sickle cell anemia, *N Engl J Med* 358:1362–1369, 2008.
Strouse JJ, Lanzkron S, Beach MC, et al: Hydroxyurea for sickle cell disease: a systematic review for efficacy and toxicity in children, *Pediatrics* 122:1332–1342, 2008.

185. **Hydroxyurea treatment in young children: how early and how beneficial?**

    Infants (9 months to 18 months) have been started on hydroxyurea (maximum dose 20 mg/kg/day) with minimal toxicity and no increased rate of infection. In a recent Phase 3 randomized controlled trial comparing hydroxyurea to placebo, infants started on hydroxyurea had lower rates of recurrent vasoocclusive events, dactylitis, acute chest syndrome, transfusion, and hospitalization. TCD velocity rates were also lower, although it is unclear if this translates into decreased risk of stroke. There were no significant differences between the groups in their splenic or renal function.

Thornburg CD, Files BA, Luo Z, et al: Impact of hydroxyurea on clinical events in the BABY HUG trial, *Blood* 120:4304–4310, 2012.
Wang WC, Ware RE, Miller ST, et al: Hydroxycarbamide in very young children with sickle-cell anaemia: a multicenter, randomized, controlled trial (BABY HUG), *Lancet* 377:1663–1672, 2011.

186. How common is the sickle cell trait in the United States?

Heterozygosity for the sickle gene occurs in about 8% of blacks in the United States; 3% of Hispanics in the eastern United States; and a much smaller percentage of individuals of Italian, Greek, Arabic, and Veddah Indian heritage. Of note is that 2% of blacks in the United States have the hemoglobin C trait.

187. Does sickle cell trait have any significant morbidity?

Under normal physiologic conditions, no significant morbidity is associated with sickle cell trait. RBCs in individuals with sickle cell trait contain only 30% to 40% sickle hemoglobin, which is insufficient to cause sickling. However, in hypoxic settings, sickling may occur. Portions of the kidney may have physiologically low oxygen concentrations that can interfere with function and lead to an inability to concentrate urine (hyposthenuria) and hematuria (usually microscopic and asymptomatic). At high altitudes (e.g., when mountain climbing or in an unpressurized aircraft), splenic infarction is possible.

KEY POINTS: SICKLE CELL DISEASE

1. A genetic mutation leads to abnormal beta-globin chain that promotes polymerization of hemoglobin and sickling in the setting of hypoxia.
2. Eight percent of blacks have the sickle cell trait.
3. Acute events include aplastic, hemolytic, vasoocclusive, and sequestration.
4. The risk of serious bacterial infection is increased among these patients as a result of functional asplenia.
5. Dactylitis (painful hand/foot swelling) is often the earliest manifestation.

188. What is the second most common worldwide hemoglobin variant?

Hemoglobin E. This variant is particularly high in the Southeast Asian population (especially those of Laotian, Thai, and Cambodian heritage). Heterozygotes are asymptomatic; homozygotes can have a mild microcytic anemia. The most common abnormal findings on a peripheral smear are microcytosis and target cells.

THALASSEMIA

189. What are the thalassemias?

The *thalassemias* are a heterogeneous group of disorders of hereditary anemia due to *diminished* or *absent normal globin chain production*. Normally, four alpha-globin genes and two beta-globin genes are expressed to make the tetrameric globin protein, which then combines with a heme moiety to make the predominant hemoglobin that is found in red cells, HbA (sub-units $\alpha_2\beta_2$). Depending on the number of genes that are deleted, the production of polypeptide chains is diminished. In patients with alpha-thalassemia, alpha-globin production is lowered; in patients with beta-thalassemia, beta-globin production is lowered. When one class of polypeptide chains is diminished, this leads to a relative excess of the other chain. The result is ineffective erythropoiesis, precipitation of unstable hemoglobins, and hemolysis as a result of intramedullary RBC destruction.

190. Where was β-thalassemia first described?

Despite its incidence being highest in the Mediterranean region, β-thalassemia was first described by a hematologist, Dr. Denton Cooley, in 1925 in Detroit. Why Detroit and not Europe for the first recognition? Speculation is that the condition was thought to be malaria, endemic to that region and with similar clinical features of hemolysis, anemia, and splenomegaly.

Weatherall DJ, Clegg JB: Historical perspectives: the many and diverse routes to our current understanding of the thalassemias. In Weatherall DJ Clegg JB, editors: *The Thalassemia Syndromes*, ed 4. Oxford, 2001, Blackwell Science, p 3.

191. What accounts for the variability in the clinical expression of the thalassemias?

Clinical heterogeneity results from variability in the number of gene deletions (particularly in alpha-thalassemia). As a rule, the greater the number of deletions, the more severe the symptoms. A large number of point mutations have been identified in various populations; this can contribute to the phenotypic diversity. In addition, the inheritance of other thalassemia genes (e.g., delta-thalassemia) or the persistence of fetal hemoglobin can modify the clinical course.

192. **How is the diagnosis of thalassemia made in most clinical laboratories?**
Homozygous beta-thalassemia is detected by the absence (β^0) or reduction (β^+) of the amount of HbA ($\alpha_2\beta_2$) relative to HbF ($\alpha_2\gamma_2$ or fetal hemoglobin) on hemoglobin electrophoresis. The carrier state for beta-thalassemia is characterized by a low mean cell volume and, in most instances, an increased level of HbA2 ($\alpha_2\delta_2$) or HbF. The levels of these two hemoglobins are most accurately measured by column chromatography. Estimation or quantitation from electrophoretic patterns is frequently misleading. The alpha-thalassemia trait remains a diagnosis of exclusion (low mean cell volume in the absence of an identifiable cause) in the clinical laboratory, although the enumeration of missing alpha genes for the most common deletions in specific ethnic populations is accomplished by molecular techniques. Newer polymerase chain reaction-based DNA tests for the common variants have become very useful.

193. **Describe the clinical features of the alpha-thalassemia syndromes**
When all four alpha-globin genes are missing or nonfunctional, this results in severe intrauterine anemia and hydrops fetalis. Extraordinary therapy such as *in utero* transfusion may result in survival. Absence of three functional alpha-globin genes results in HbH disease, which is a chronic moderate to severe anemia with jaundice and splenomegaly that may necessitate RBC transfusion therapy. Absence of two alpha-globin genes is associated with mild microcytic anemia. Absence of one alpha-globin gene is clinically silent (Table 9-5).

Table 9-5. Clinical Features of α-Thalassemia

SYNDROME	USUAL GENOTYPE	α GENE NUMBER	CLINICAL FEATURES
Normal	$\alpha\alpha/\alpha\alpha$	4	Normal
Silent carrier	α-/$\alpha\alpha$	3	Normal
α-Thalassemia trait	α-/α-	2	Mild microcytic anemia
HbH disease	- -/$\alpha\alpha$	1	Moderate microcytic anemia Splenomegaly Jaundice

194. **What is hemoglobin Barts?**
Hemoglobin Barts is a tetramer of γ-chains often noted on the newborn screen due to α-chain deletions. It can be present, in varying degrees, in the setting of alpha thalassemia trait, HbH disease, or fetal hydrops.

195. **What are the clinical features of the beta-thalassemia syndromes?**
  - **Thalassemia minor:** Minimal or no anemia (hemoglobin 9 to 12 g/dL); microcytosis; elevated RBC count; no need for transfusion
  - **Thalassemia intermedia:** Microcytic anemia with hemoglobin usually >7 g/dL; growth failure; hepatosplenomegaly; hyperbilirubinemia; thalassemic facies (i.e., frontal bossing, mandibular malocclusion, prominent malar eminences due to extramedullary hematopoiesis) develop between the ages of 2 and 5 years; intermittent or variable transfusion requirements
  - **Thalassemia major** (Cooley's anemia): Severe anemia (hemoglobin 1 to 6 g/dl) usually during the first year of life; hepatosplenomegaly; growth failure; transfusion dependent

Olivieri NF: The beta-thalassemias, *N Engl J Med* 341:99–109, 1999.

196. **How can coexistent iron deficiency increase the difficulty of diagnosing beta-thalassemia?**
The beta-thalassemia trait is usually diagnosed by hemoglobin electrophoresis, with quantitative hemoglobins revealing elevated HbA2 and/or HbF levels. Iron deficiency can cause a lowering of HbA2, thereby masking the diagnosis. With iron replacement, the hemoglobin A2 will rise to the expected elevated levels seen in patients with the beta-thalassemia trait.

197. What are the adverse effects of chronic transfusional iron overload in children with thalassemia?
- **Cardiac effects** include congestive heart failure; dysrhythmias; and less frequently, pericarditis. Cardiac T2* MRI imaging is both diagnostic and prognostic. Significant cardiac iron deposition predicts rates of heart failure and arrhythmia over the subsequent year.
- **Endocrine effects** include delays in growth and sexual development, hypoparathyroidism, and hypothyroidism. Diabetes as a result of iron overload is irreversible, even with intensive chelation
- **Hepatic effects** include progressive liver fibrosis and cirrhosis. Monitoring with dedicated MRI imaging is recommended.

Kirk P, Roughton M, Porter JB, et al: Cardiac T2* magnetic resonance for prediction of cardiac complications in thalassemia major, *Circulation* 120:1961–1968, 2009.

198. What are the two most common diseases that are associated with transfusion-related iron overload?
Thalassemia major and sickle cell disease.

199. How do you reduce iron accumulation in children who require repeated transfusions?
- **Chelation therapy:** Subcutaneous or intravenous deferoxamine has been the standard therapy for transfusional overload; however, new oral iron chelators including daily deferasirox and three times daily deferiprone have demonstrated efficacy as single agents. Studies of combination chelation therapy demonstrate acceptable toxicity profiles with improved iron status.
- **Splenectomy:** This is used primarily in patients with thalassemia (and a small subgroup of sickle cell patients) who have hypersplenism, which results in the premature destruction of RBCs and increased transfusion requirements.
- **Diet:** Drinking tea with meals reduces dietary iron absorption and may be most helpful in patients with diseases such as thalassemia intermedia, in which the bulk of excessive iron is dietary in origin.
- **Erythrocytapheresis:** Automated erythrocytapheresis (red cell exchange) rather than repeated simple transfusions may markedly reduce transfusional iron loading in patients with sickle cell disease.

Lo L, Singer ST: Thalassemia: Current approach to an old disease, *Pediatr Clin North Am* 49:1165–1192, 2002.

200. In addition to iron loading, what are additional risks of chronic transfusion therapy?
Patients on chronic transfusion therapy are at risk of **alloimmunization to RBC antigens,** which may make transfusions a challenge going forward, or HLA antigens, which may make bone marrow transplantation (BMT) a challenge. With every transfusion, patients experience an ongoing risk of transfusion-related infection and a risk of experiencing a transfusion reaction.

KEY POINTS: THALASSEMIA

1. Normal hemoglobin (HbA): Tetramer of two alpha and two beta chains
2. Associated with quantitative reduction in globin synthesis
3. Homozygous beta-thalassemia is most severe form, with pallor, jaundice, hepatosplenomegaly, growth retardation
4. Expansion of facial bones resulting from extramedullary hematopoiesis
5. Severity of alpha-thalassemia depends on number of genes deleted (1 to 4)
6. Alpha-thalassemia: More common among people of Southeast Asian ethnicity
7. Beta-thalassemia: More common in people of Mediterranean ethnicity

TRANSFUSION ISSUES

201. What is the difference between the direct and indirect Coombs tests?
- **Direct test:** Coombs serum (antihuman globulin) is added directly to a patient's washed RBCs. The occurrence of agglutination means that the patient's RBCs have been coated in vivo by an antibody. Direct Coombs testing is vital for diagnosing AIHAs.

- **Indirect test:** This involves incubating a patient's serum with RBCs of a known type and adding Coombs serum. If in vitro sensitization occurs, agglutination will result, which indicates that antibodies in the serum are binding to the antigens on the RBCs. Indirect testing is key for blood cross-matching.

202. **What is the difference between forward and reverse blood typing?**
A *forward type* determines antigens on patient or donor RBCs. It uses reagent monoclonal antibodies against A or B or Rh(D) and tests for agglutination. A *reverse type* determines antibodies in patient or donor serum or plasma. It tests for agglutination with RBCs of a known phenotype, ensuring the patient has appropriate naturally forming antibodies (anti-A or anti-B isoagglutinins). Outside of the neonatal period (age > 4 months), both a forward and a reverse type must be performed for a patient to have a valid ABO type.

203. **What can cause a patient to be ABO indeterminate?**
Inconsistencies with either the forward or reverse type may cause a patient to be ABO indeterminate. A compatible, but out of group, transfusion may cause the patient to be ABO indeterminate in both the forward or reverse direction. Often, these will result in "mixed field" results where the laboratory notes two populations of cells. Infants <4 months old may not have developed the naturally forming isoagglutinins, so the reverse may be invalid, and therefore, is not required to result their specimens. Usually the reverse type resolves by 6 months to 1 year of age. Leukemia or a history of bone marrow transplantation may cause a patient to be ABO indeterminate. Hypogammaglobulinemia may cause a patient to lack their appropriate serum isoagglutinins, causing a discrepancy in the reverse type. In contrast, IVIG infusion, a cold autoantibody or a cold alloantibody may cause excessive reactivity in the reverse type, thus making the patient ABO indeterminate.

204. **What is a naturally forming RBC antibody?**
RBC alloantibodies are antibodies against RBC antigens that the patient lacks. These are usually only formed after exposure to those antigens through transfusion or pregnancy. However, there are some alloantibodies (such as anti-A and anti-B) that do not require such exposure. This is because similar antigens are widely expressed in nature (e.g., aeroallergens, gut flora) and thus the individual is exposed "naturally."

205. **What is the difference between a type and screen and a type and cross?**
When a *type and screen* is performed, both a forward and reverse type are performed on the patient sample. In addition, patient serum or plasma is then incubated with RBCs of a known phenotype to assess for the presence of any alloantibodies. When a *type and cross* is performed, the patient sample has all of the elements of a type and screen performed, but then the plasma or serum of the patient is tested with RBCs of potentially compatible units of blood. If compatible, those units are reserved for the patient.

206. **What are the indications for the use of leukoreduced RBCs?**
When packed red cells are prepared from whole blood and then filtered, most of the remaining white cells are removed from the product. Because febrile transfusion reactions are usually the result of leukocytes, filtered products should be used for patients who have experienced such reactions to previous blood transfusions. Filtered red cells are also effective for reducing the transmission of cytomegalovirus in at-risk individuals. In addition, the use of filtered blood components reduces the risk of HLA alloimmunization, which is desirable for patients who have undergone repeated transfusions and for those who may need stem cell or solid organ transplants.

207. **What is the estimated total blood volume of children?**
Estimation of blood volume is dependent on both age and weight. Older children have a lower proportion of their weight as blood compared with younger children. As a rule of thumb, blood volume is estimated as follows:

Children >3 months of age: 70 mL/kg
Premature infants: 90 to 100 mL/kg
Term infants: 80 to 90 mL/kg

Morley SL: Red blood cell transfusions in acute paediatrics, *Arch Dis Child Pract Ed* 94:65–73, 2009.

208. **What is the RBC transfusion threshold for infants <4 months of age?**

Transfusion thresholds vary significantly by gestational age, postnatal age, and clinical status because of the complex physiology of neonates and young infants. In an effort to limit the risks associated with transfusions, restrictive transfusion practices are being examined to determine if reduced transfusion requirements might be used without increased morbidity and mortality. One set of proposed guidelines is as follows:

- Hct <20% with low reticulocyte count and symptomatic anemia
- Hct <30% requiring oxygen support or significant symptoms including apnea, bradycardia, tachycardia, or tachypnea.
- Hct <35% on >35% oxygen hood or escalated ventilatory support.
- Hct <45% on extracorporeal membrane oxygenation (ECMO) or with congenital cyanotic heart disease.

Kirpalani H, Whyte RK, Andersen C, et al: The Premature Infants in Need of Transfusion (PINT) study: a randomized, controlled trial of a restrictive (low) versus liberal (high) transfusion threshold for extremely low birth weight infants, *J Pediatr* 149:301–307, 2006.
Roseff SD, Luban NLC, Manno CS: Guidelines for assessing appropriateness of pediatric transfusion, *Transfusion* 42:1398–1413, 2002.

209. **What is the packed red blood cell (PRBC) transfusion threshold for children >4 months of age?**

Transfusion thresholds vary significantly by age and clinical status in older children as well. Restrictive practices are also being evaluated in older children. One study involving 637 children in a pediatric ICU found no difference in outcome between using hemoglobin thresholds of 7 g/dL versus 9.5 g/dL as the threshold for transfusion. One set of proposed guidelines is as follows:

- Hct <24% with symptoms of anemia
- Acute blood loss (>15%) unresponsive to other interventions
- Hct <40% on ECMO or severe cardiopulmonary disease
- Sickle cell disease with stroke, acute chest, symptomatic anemia, splenic sequestration, preoperatively for general anesthesia with goal for Hb of 10 g/dL
- Chronic transfusion for patients with failure of RBC production (beta thalassemia, Diamond-Blackfan anemia, etc.) with goal for Hb of 10 to 12 g/dL

Lacroix J, Hebert PC, Hutchison JS, et al: Transfusion strategies for patients in pediatric intensive care units, *N Engl J Med* 356:1609–1619, 2007.
Roseff SD, Luban NLC, Manno CS: Guidelines for assessing appropriateness of pediatric transfusion, *Transfusion* 42:1398–1413, 2002.

210. **In patients with severe chronic anemia, how rapidly can transfusions be given?**

When anemia is chronic, there has been cardiovascular adaptation and a relatively normal blood volume. Excessively rapid transfusions can lead to congestive heart failure. For patients with a hemoglobin level of <5 g/dL who exhibit no signs of cardiac failure, a safe regimen is to transfuse PRBCs at a rate of 1 to 2 mL/kg per hour by continuous infusion until the desired target is reached. In most patients, 1 mL/kg will raise the hematocrit level by 1%. Judicious use of a diuretic such as furosemide (or automated erythrocytapheresis, in larger children) can be considered.

Jayabose S, Tugal O, Ruddy R, et al: Transfusion therapy for severe anemia, *Am J Pediatr Hematol Oncol* 15:324–327, 1993.

211. **At typical doses, what are the expected increases and likely average survival of packed RBCs, platelets, and fresh frozen survival?**

See Table 9-6.

Table 9-6. Quick Facts About Blood-Product Dosing

PRODUCT	DOSE	EXPECTED INCREASE	SURVIVAL
PRBCs	10-15 mL/kg	10 mL/kg increases Hb by 2-3 g/dL	May persist 60-90 days in circulation
Platelets	10 mL/kg or 0.1-0.2 unit/kg	40 k/μL	Hours to days
FFP	10-15 mL/kg	1 mL/kg increases factor levels by 1%	4-6 hours

FFP = Fresh frozen plasma; PRBCs = packed red blood cells.

212. **What are the components of cryoprecipitate?**
Cryoprecipitate is a plasma product of concentrated factors VIII, XIII, vWF and fibrinogen which precipitates as FFP is thawed and is collected by centrifugation. Indications for use include situations when specific factor concentrates are not available (e.g., hemophilia), reversal of anticoagulation or DIC. Fibrinogen concentrate is also available for children with congenital fibrinogen deficiencies, including afibrinogenemia and hypofibrinogenemia.

213. **What are the most common types of transfusion reactions?**
Transfusion reactions occur infrequently, with approximately 2 to 7 events per 1000 units transfused. However, these reactions can be serious and even fatal. The most common transfusion reactions are **febrile nonhemolytic transfusion reactions**. Patients experience fever and chills, without evidence of hemolysis, while receiving a transfusion or several hours later. Patients may be treated with antipyretics and meperidine if the chills are significant. **Allergic transfusion reactions** are the second most common type. Often occurring with plasma containing platelets or FFP, symptoms may range from mild urticaria and pruritus to significant anaphylaxis with hypotension and angioedema. Antihistamines, steroids, or epinephrine may be necessary depending upon the severity of the reaction.

214. **What is the most common cause of transfusion-related death in the United States?**
Transfusion-related acute lung injury (TRALI) is the most common cause of transfusion related death. TRALI is characterized as acute respiratory distress with bilateral lung infiltrates and hypoxia within 6 hours of transfusion. HLA and human neutrophil antigen (HNA) antibodies have been implicated in the pathogenesis of this syndrome.

215. **What is the difference between an acute hemolytic transfusion reaction and a delayed hemolytic transfusion reaction?**
Acute hemolytic transfusion reactions result in rapid hemolysis during or within 24 hours of an infusion of incompatible blood products. Often, these are due to ABO incompatible transfusions. Patients may experience fever, chills, back pain, and a sense of "impending doom." They may also have hemoglobinuria, which may result in renal failure. Fluids, mannitol, and other supportive care measures may be necessary to treat this type of reaction.
Delayed hemolytic transfusion reactions may occur from 24 hours up to 28 days after transfusion, though usually present 10 to 14 days after transfusion. These are often due to RBC alloantibody incompatibility. The symptoms may be similar to acute hemolytic reactions, although they are often milder.

216. **Why do some blood products require irradiation?**
Irradiation with either x-rays or gamma irradiation prevents transfusion-associated graft versus host disease (TA-GVHD). TA-GVHD is caused by a proliferation of donor T-cells within the transfusion recipient that then attack the host. Symptoms include rash, hepatitis, and GI symptoms similar to classic GVHD; however, the hallmark of this disease is pancytopenia. It is greater than 90% fatal when it occurs. Patients at risk for TA-GVHD include patients with known or suspected cellular immunodeficiency; significant immunosuppression due to chemotherapy or BMT; infants <1200 g at birth or those who received *in utero* transfusions; and any patient receiving HLA-matched components, granulocytes or blood components from directed donors.

217. **In what clinical settings is apheresis utilized?**

During *apheresis*, whole blood is removed from the patient and components are centrifugally separated by density: RBCs > WBCs > platelets > plasma. Components as desired are removed with the remaining components returned to the patient along with replacement fluid or replacement blood products.

- *Erythrocytapheresis:* Patient RBCs are removed and replaced with donor PRBCs; this is usually performed on patients with sickle cell disease who want to prevent iron accumulation or who require an acute reduction in their HbS percent such as in the setting of acute stroke or acute chest syndrome.
- *Leukapheresis:* WBCs are removed; patient's RBCs, platelets, and plasma are returned along with some fluid; usually this is performed in the setting of acute leukemia with elevated WBC and signs or symptoms of leukostasis (>100, 000/µL in acute myelogenous leukemia [AML], >200,000 to 250,000/µL in acute lymphoblastic leukemia [ALL], and >400,000/µL in chronic myelogenous leukemia [CML]).
- *Plasmapheresis:* Plasma is removed; all cellular components are returned to the patient often with 5% albumin and saline as replacement fluid; replacement with FFP can be used if patients have a coagulopathy or when plasmapheresis is performed for certain conditions such as thrombotic thrombocytopenic purpura or hemolytic-uremic syndrome.
- *Thrombocytapheresis:* Platelets only are removed; usually only performed after platelet count is >1,500,000/µL; not usually performed in pediatrics.

218. **How are transfusion-transmitted diseases prevented?**

Direct testing and **donor screening/deferral**. Direct testing of blood products includes serologic testing for the presence of antibodies to known pathogenic antigens and nucleic acid amplification testing (NAAT), which detects viral DNA/RNA. All blood products or donors are tested using either or both of the above methods for HIV, hepatitis B, hepatitis C, HTLV-I/II, syphilis, West Nile Virus, and *Trypanosoma cruzi*. With implementation of NAAT testing, the window period for HIV detection has been reduced to 9 days and the window period for hepatitis C to <8 days. Transfusion-transmitted diseases without an FDA-approved donor screening test, such as malaria and prion diseases, are prevented through donor screening questions and donor deferrals. For example, individuals are excluded from donating blood for 1 year after traveling to malaria-endemic areas, and for 3 years after long-term residence (5 years or more) in a malaria-endemic area.

Galel S: Infectious disease screening. In Roback JD, Grossman BJ, Harris T, Hillyer CD, editors: *Technical Manual*, ed 17. Bethesda, MD, 2011, American Association of Blood Banks, p 239.

219. **What role does molecular testing play in providing blood products to patients?**

Molecular phenotyping of RBC antigens, which currently uses PCR-based, microarray technology, is an exciting and expanding area of transfusion medicine. This technology is able to identify the expected phenotype of a patient's or donor's RBCs at multiple (>30) antigens from DNA. This can be used to identify donors with rare RBC phenotypes to be added to the American Rare Donor Program (ARDP). It can also be used in clinical practice to allow for better matching of RBC products and to clarify serologic ambiguities.

Acknowledgment

The editors gratefully acknowledge contributions from Dr. Anne F. Reilly, Dr. Greg A. Holländer, and Dr. Anders Fasth that were retained from previous editions of *Pediatric Secrets*.

INFECTIOUS DISEASES

Jennifer Duchon, MDCM, MPH, Lisa Saiman, MD, MPH and
Marc D. Foca, MD

CHAPTER 10

ANTI-INFECTIVE THERAPY

> ### KEY POINTS ANTI-INFECTIVE THERAPY
>
> 1. Formal allergy testing is frequently negative in patients who report a penicillin allergy.
> 2. Rashes seen with viral or bacterial illnesses may confound a history of antibiotic allergy.
> 3. Methicillin-resistant *Staphylococcus aureus* (MRSA) is becoming a prevalent pathogen in the community, and empiric therapy for certain infections may be broadened to include MRSA coverage.
> 4. Antibiotic resistance is emerging in all types of organisms, risking the use of drugs that are safe and approved for use in the pediatric population.

1. **What are the main features of penicillins?**

   Penicillins are among the earliest classes of antibiotics developed. They are derived from the fungus *Penicillium*, and share a core structural feature—a β-lactam ring—with other classes of antibiotics, such as cephalosporins and carbapenems. Penicillins interfere with the peptidoglycan cross-linking that is required to produce stable bacterial cell walls. They penetrate most tissue spaces well but do not cross the blood-brain barrier except in the case of inflamed meninges. However, they have a high therapeutic index, and thus doses can be escalated to increase tissue penetration. They are not active against organisms that are cell-wall deficient, such as *Chlamydia* and *Mycoplasma* species.

2. **What are the different classes and spectra of activity of penicillins?**

   - **Penicillins** (penicillins G [intravenous] and V [oral]):
     - These are natural penicillins that are derived directly from the *Penicillium* mold. These drugs are active against most nonpenicillinase producing gram-positive cocci and gram-positive anaerobic organisms.
     - Penicillin G is the drug of choice for *Treponema pallidum* infection (syphilis) and *Streptococcus agalactiae* (also known as group B strep).
     - Penicillins are also the treatment of choice for group A streptococcal pharyngitis and some anaerobic infections.
   - **Antistaphylococcal penicillins** are also called **penicillinase-resistant penicillins** (methicillin, oxacillin, nafcillin, and dicloxacillin [oral]):
     - These have side chains attached to the penicillin lactam ring that inhibit their inactivation by antistaphylococcal penicillinases.
     - They display excellent activity against sensitive strains of *Staphylococcus aureus* and should be used, whenever possible, instead of vancomycin, which has less staphylococcal activity.
     - The bulky side chains also limit penetration of these drugs through the cell membrane, giving them a narrow spectrum of action.
   - **Aminopenicillins** (ampicillin and amoxicillin):
     - The spectrum is similar to that of penicillin but includes additional activity against aerobic gram-negative bacteria (i.e., *Escherichia coli*, *Listeria*, and *Salmonella* spp.).
     - Many previously susceptible gram-negative organisms are now resistant to the aminopenicillins.
   - **Extended spectrum**, also described as "Anti-pseudomonal penicillins" (piperacillin and ticarcillin):
     - These have an expanded gram-negative spectrum and can be used to treat susceptible strains of *Pseudomonas aeruginosa* and *Proteus* spp.
   - **Combinations with β-lactamase inhibitors:** The spectrum of certain penicillins can be increased by the addition of a β-lactamase inhibitor. β-Lactamases are a common basis for penicillin resistance in some bacteria. Available combinations include amoxicillin-clavulanate, ampicillin-sulbactam,

piperacillin-tazobactam, and ticarcillin-clavulanate, which extend their activity to cover *Haemophilus influenza, Bacteroides fragilis,* and some *Enterobacteriaceae.*

3. **In patients for whom the history lists "penicillin allergy," how commonly is a true allergy present on testing?**
A true allergy is present on testing ≤10% of the time. In patients reporting a penicillin allergy, skin tests and radioallergosorbent tests are frequently negative (≤20% and ≤ 3%, respectively). Much of the confusion arises from the use of the term "*allergic reaction*" to describe a gamut of nonimmunologic adverse experiences that may be attributable to either the medication, the underlying disease process, or an interaction of the two.

Pichichero ME: A review of evidence supporting the American Academy of Pediatrics recommendation for prescribing cephalosporin antibiotics for penicillin-allergic patients, *Pediatrics* 115:1048–1057, 2005.

4. **If a 16-year-old male develops a pruritic, maculopapular rash 1 week after starting treatment with amoxicillin for an exudative pharyngitis, should he be designated as "amoxicillin allergic?"**
No! As previously alluded to, the immune response that is mounted to a viral pathogen may alter the immune response to antimicrobials, creating an "allergic reaction" that is unique to the organism and drug at hand. The classic example of this is the development of a rash following treatment with amoxicillin in patients with Epstein-Barr virus (EBV). Recent reports have implicated the virus itself in addition to the interaction of the virus and the antimicrobial. In addition, many herpes viruses (such as EBV and human herpesvirus 6), as well as enteroviruses, will cause a maculopapular eruption as part of the viral syndrome. These patients are not allergic to penicillins. This should also be taken as further incentive to avoid prescribing antimicrobials for viral illnesses.

5. **What are the similarities between penicillins and cephalosporins?**
Both cephalosporins and penicillin are derived from fungi: cephalosporins are from the fungus *Acremonium* (formerly *Cephalosporium*), and penicillin is from the *Penicillium* fungus. Furthermore, they both contain a β-lactam ring and interfere with bacterial cell wall synthesis by irreversibly inhibiting penicillin-binding protein peptidoglycan cross-linking.

6. **How do the "generations" of cephalosporins differ from one another?**
They are divided into four "generations" based on antimicrobial spectrum of action; in general, activity against gram-negative organisms increases with increasing generation, whereas activity against gram-positive organisms decreases with each generation. Third- and fourth-generation cephalosporins have good penetration in the cerebrospinal fluid (CSF).

7. **What are the differences among first-, second-, third-, and fourth-generation cephalosporins?**
   - **First-generation cephalosporins** (e.g., cefazolin, cephalexin, cefadroxil)
     - Good activity against gram-positive organisms (especially *Methicillin-susceptible S. aureus* and streptococci spp.)
     - Frequently used as prophylaxis for orthopedic, cardiovascular, head and neck, and many types of neurosurgical or general surgical procedures (i.e., herniorrhaphy)
     - May have activity against some *E. coli* and *Klebsiella* species, but lack efficacy against *Haemophilus influenza*
     - May be considered as alternatives to penicillins for the treatment of group A streptococcal pharyngitis and group B streptococcal prophylaxis during labor.
   - **Second-generation cephalosporins** (e.g., cefuroxime, cefotetan, cefoxitin)
     - Increased spectrum of activity, including many gram-negative organisms
     - Increased activity against *B. fragilis*
     - Prophylaxis for intra-abdominal (e.g., cefotetan, cefoxitin)
     - Treatment for nosocomial pneumonia
     - No antipseudomonal activity
   - **Third-generation cephalosporins** (e.g., ceftriaxone, cefotaxime, cefixime, cefdinir, ceftazidime)
     - Broad spectrum, excellent activity against gram-negative bacteria
     - Generally less activity against gram-positive organisms than earlier generations, such as *methicillin-susceptible S. aureus.*

- Very high blood and CSF levels achievable in relation to minimal inhibitory concentration for bacterial strains
- Wide therapeutic index with generally minimal toxicity (similar to previous generations)
- Some offer single-daily dosing
- Ceftazidime: the first cephalosporin with antipseudomonal coverage
- More expensive
- **Fourth-generation cephalosporins** (e.g., cefepime)
  - Broadest spectrum, with activity against most staphylococcal and streptococcal species (NOT methicillin-resistant *S. aureus*) and gram-negative organisms, including *Pseudomonas* spp.
  - Crosses into the CSF
  - No activity against anaerobic organisms

Harrison CJ, Bratcher D: Cephalosporins: a review, *Pediatr Rev* 29:264–272, 2008.

---

8. Can cephalosporins be safely given to patients who are allergic to penicillin?
   Previous estimates of cross-sensitivity to cephalosporins among penicillin-allergic patients were thought to be 8% to 18%, but these rates have been criticized as inaccurate and excessive. Side-chain–specific antibodies appear to be key in the immune response to cephalosporins. The incidence of allergic cross-reactivity varies with the chemical side-chain similarity of the cephalosporin to penicillin or amoxicillin. For first-generation cephalosporins, the attributable increased risk is thought to be only 0.4%. For certain second- and third-generation cephalosporins (e.g., cefuroxime, cefpodoxime, and cefdinir), the risk is thought to be close to zero. No evidence supports an increase of anaphylaxis with cephalosporins among penicillin-allergic patients. The American Academy of Pediatrics (AAP) guidelines do endorse the use of selected second-generation and third-generation cephalosporins for penicillin-allergic patients as long as the penicillin reaction is not severe.

Pichichero M: A review of the evidence supporting the American Academy of Pediatrics recommendation for prescribing cephalosporin antibiotics for penicillin-allergic patients, *Pediatrics* 115:1048–1057, 2005.

---

9. What are the two primary mechanisms of resistance to β-lactam antibiotics?
   - **Penicillin-binding proteins (PBPs)**
   - PBPs are enzymes responsible for the cross-linking between glycan chains and are the target proteins for β-lactam antibiotics. Mutational alterations in PBPs can confer resistance by reducing binding of a β-lactam antibiotic to the active site. This mechanism can be overcome by a higher dose of the antibiotic.
   - **β-Lactamase**
   These are enzymes that hydrolyze the β-lactam ring of the antibiotic. The genes encoding these enzymes may be inherently present on the bacterial chromosome or may be acquired via plasmid transfer. Certain β-lactamase gene expression may be induced by exposure to β-lactams; for example, the genes encoding these β-lactamases are found in the chromosomes of organisms such as *Serratia*, *Pseudomonas*, *Acinetobacter*, *Citrobacter*, and *Enterobacter* (often labeled the "SPACE" organisms). This mechanism of resistance, in general, cannot be overcome simply by using a higher dose of drug.

10. What are the main features of carbapenems?
    Carbapenems are β-lactam antibiotics that also bind PBPs, disrupting the growth and structural integrity of bacterial cell walls. They provide gram-positive as well as enhanced anaerobic and excellent gram-negative coverage as compared with other β-lactams. They are also resistant to most β-lactamases, including so-called extended-spectrum β-lactamases (ESBLs). They do not cover methicillin-resistant *S. aureus* (MRSA).

11. What is the role of "double antimicrobial coverage"?
    Synergy is when the combination of two antibiotics has a greater killing effect than the sum of the two drugs given separately (i.e., the effect is superadditive: $2+2=5$). In general, the use of two drugs has not been shown to be better than one drug that appropriately targets the causative organism and site of infection. One exception to this is in infective endocarditis, where the use of two or more drugs is recommended in most circumstances. Another role for the use of more than

one drug for a suspected causative organism is in an unstable patient for whom there is a high suspicion for an infection with an antibiotic-resistant organism. Empiric therapy with more than one drug to cover "gaps" in sensitivities is often appropriate. Therapy can then be narrowed if an organism is isolated or as the patient improves.

12. **What are the "ESKAPE" organisms?**

The bacteria *Enterococcus faecium, S. aureus, Klebsiella pneumoniae, Acinetobacter baumannii, P. aeruginosa,* and *Enterobacter* species are sometimes referred to as the "ESKAPE" organisms, which emphasizes that they are major causes of nosocomial (and increasingly community-acquired) infections and have developed mechanisms to "escape" the effects of many antimicrobials. In addition to MRSA, vancomycin-resistant *E. faecium* (VRE), *Acinetobacter* species, multidrug-resistant (MDR) *P. aeruginosa,* carbapenem-resistant *Klebsiella* species, and *E.coli* are emerging as significant pathogens in both the United States and other parts of the world.

Boucher HW, Talbot GH, Bradley JS, et al: Bad bugs, no drugs: no ESKAPE! An update from the Infectious Diseases Society of America. *Clin Infect Dis.* 48:1–12, 2009.

13. **How can the emergence of antibiotic-resistant pathogens be minimized?**
   - Appropriate hand hygiene, contact isolation, and environmental decontamination to reduce the transmission of resistant organisms to other patients
   - Use of the most potent, narrowest spectrum antibiotic possible for an appropriate length of time
   - Minimization of the empiric use of broad-spectrum antibiotics
   - Avoidance of antibiotic treatment of illnesses that are likely viral
   - Awareness of local antibiotic resistance patterns

14. **What is the distinction between community-associated methicillin-resistant *S. aureus* (CA-MRSA) and hospital acquired methicillin-resistant *S. aureus* (HA-MRSA)?**

MRSA was first reported in 1961, and was described for the next three decades as primarily a nosocomial pathogen. A report describing the deaths of four previously healthy children in the Midwestern United States in 1998 brought to attention the issue of MRSA infections in the general population, and CA-MRSA was recognized as a distinct clinical entity.

The most commonly accepted definition of CA-MRSA, as put forth by the Centers for Disease Control and Prevention (CDC), is the diagnosis of MRSA in the outpatient setting or within 48 hours of hospital admission and a lack of risk factors for chronic medical conditions. However, the source of the infection, the antibiotic phenotype, and the genotype of the organism have all been ways to differentiate CA-MRSA from HA-MRSA. Practically, these definitions and distinctions are becoming less relevant as the epidemiology of MRSA and its resistance patterns change and expand. In many locations, strains historically classified as CA-MRSA now cause a majority of nosocomial disease. As molecular typing methods advance, it is likely that the terms CA-MRSA and HA-MRSA will become obsolete and be replaced with more descriptive terms for both the local and global strains of MRSA.

Mediavilla J, Chen L, Mathema B, Kreiswirth BN: Global epidemiology of community-associated methicillin resistant *Staphylococcus aureus* (CA-MRSA), *Curr Opin Microbiol* 15:588–595, 2012.
Chua K, Laurent F, Coombs G, Grayson ML, et al: Antimicrobial resistance: Not community-associated methicillin-resistant *Staphylococcus aureus* (CA-MRSA)! A clinician's guide to community MRSA – its evolving antimicrobial resistance and implications for therapy, *Clin Infect Dis* 52:99–114, 2011.

15. **Why is the D-test done?**

The *D-test* is done with MRSA isolates that are susceptible to clindamycin and resistant to erythromycin to evaluate whether that isolate might have resistance not constitutively expressed (i.e., always produced) but *inducible by exposure to macrolides.* If patients with this type of MRSA are begun on clindamycin, they may have a higher likelihood of treatment failure or recrudescence. The test involves placing antibiotic disks for erythromycin and clindamycin in close proximity on the agar plate. A flattening of the clindamycin zone of bacterial growth adjacent to the erythromycin disk produces a "D" appearance and indicates the MRSA isolate has inducible resistance to clindamycin (Fig. 10-1).

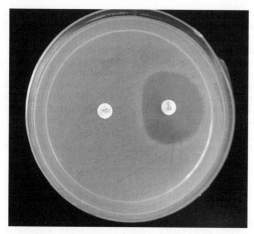

Figure 10-1. D-test showing flattened zone of clindamycin near the erythromycin disk, demonstrating erythromycin-induced clindamycin resistance. *(From Mohapatra TM, Shrestha B, Pokhrel BM: Constitutive and inducible clindamycin resistance in Staphylococcus aureus and their association with methicillin-resistant S. aureus (MRSA),* Int J Antimicrob Agents *33:188, 2009.)*

16. **Is mupirocin useful in the eradication of *S. aureus* in colonized children?**

Colonization of the nasal mucosa or skin is common in children. About 15% to 40% of healthy children are carriers of methicillin-sensitive *S. aureus* (MSSA). MRSA nasal carriage ranges from 1% to 24% in various studies involving day care, emergency room visits, or hospitalized children. The use of mupirocin applied twice to three times daily for 1 to 21 days was shown in some adult studies to significantly but variably decrease colonization and recurrent invasive disease. However, eradication is difficult and typically involves additional measures such as chlorhexidine baths, stringent cleaning of the home environment, and often decolonization of the family as well. Unfortunately, recolonization is common. Protracted use of mupirocin leads readily to increased rates of mupirocin resistance in both MSSA and MRSA isolates. Thus, mupirocin is not recommended for routine use in otherwise healthy children to decrease colonization. In certain special circumstances, such as patients with frequent skin and soft tissue infections and underlying medical conditions (e.g., severe eczema, acquired or congenital immunodeficiencies), decolonization may be warranted.

Marimuthu K, Harbarth S: Screening for methicillin-resistant *Staphylococcus aureus*... all doors closed? *Curr Opin Infect Dis* 27:356–362, 2014.

Abad CL, Pulia MS, Safdar N: Does the nose know? An update on MRSA decolonization strategies, *Curr Infect Dis Rep* 15:455–464, 2013.

Liu C, Bayer A, Cosgrove SE, et al: Clinical practice guidelines by the Infectious Diseases Society of America for the treatment of methicillin-resistant *Staphylococcus aureus* infections in adults and children: executive summary, *Clin Infect Dis* 52: 285–292, 2011.

17. **What is the "red man syndrome" and which antibiotic is it associated with?**

The *red man syndrome* is a frequent occurrence with the rapid infusion of **vancomycin** (although there are reports of red man syndrome from ciprofloxacin, rifampin, and amphotericin b) and is characterized by flushing of the neck, face, and thorax. Patients commonly complain of diffuse burning, itching, and dizziness and can develop fever and paresthesias around the mouth. Histamine release from degranulation of mast cells underlies this reaction; however, it is not mediated by IgE and therefore does not represent a true hypersensitivity reaction. Generally, the reaction appears in the first 10 minutes of administration and can be avoided by slowing the rate of drug infusion. Administration of an H_1-receptor antagonist (e.g., diphenhydramine) before vancomycin is given is also effective for preventing this reaction.

18. **How should infections with vancomycin-resistant enterococci be managed?**

Resistance to vancomycin has been observed in *Enterococcus faecium* and, less commonly, *Enterococcus faecalis*. These infections are acquired nosocomially, which reflects the fact that the organism can survive on inanimate surfaces (including medical equipment) for weeks. They occur more commonly with prolonged use of antibiotics. Basic tenets of anti-infective therapy apply: foreign bodies should be removed, infected fluid collections should be drained, and patients should be placed on contact isolation to prevent spread. The oxazolidinone antibiotic linezolid (Zyvox) has shown some effectiveness, but the data are limited. Combination streptogramin agent quinupristin-dalfopristin (Synercid) is approved for individuals ≥16 years of age, and dosing guidelines for children ≥12 years of age are available. It is noteworthy that quinupristin-dalfopristin has activity against *E. faecium* but not *E. faecalis*, and it has many drug interactions, which limits its use in certain situations. Daptomycin and newer cephalosporins, including ceftaroline, have direct or synergistic activity against these organisms as well, but there is less experience with their use in pediatric populations.

Patel R, Gallagher JC: Vancomycin-resistant enterococcal bacteremia pharmacotherapy, *Ann Pharmacother* 49:69–85, 2015.
Zirakzadeh A, Patel R: Vancomycin-resistant enterococci: colonization, infection, detection, and treatment, *Mayo Clin Proc* 81:529–536, 2006.

19. **Is vancomycin still effective against all staphylococci?**
   Within a few years of the emergence of VRE, isolates of *S. aureus* with reduced susceptibility and resistance to vancomycin were reported. In some of these isolates, acquisition of resistance genes from VRE has been demonstrated; in others, lower levels of resistance are conferred by a variety of mutations in a small number of staphylococcal regulatory genes. Fortunately, these isolates have retained susceptibility to a variety of other antibiotics. However, some recent reports indicate that methicillin-resistant, vancomycin-"heteroresistant" coagulase-negative staphylococci, mainly *Staphylococcus capitis*, could emerge as a significant pathogen in the neonatal intensive care unit (NICU). This is especially concerning because there are fewer safe and effective therapeutic options in this population. Appropriate use of vancomycin is key to preventing misuse and overuse and to limiting the likelihood of further emergence of vancomycin resistance.

Howden B, Peleg AY, Stinear TP: The evolution of vancomycin intermediate *Staphylococcus aureus* (VISA) and heterogenous-VISA, *Infect Genet Evol* 21:575–582, 2014.
Rasigade J, Raulin O, Picaud JC, et al: Methicillin-resistant *Staphylococcus capitis* with reduced vancomycin susceptibility causes late-onset sepsis in intensive care neonates, *PLoS One* 7:e31548, 2012.

20. **In what situations may treatment with vancomycin be considered appropriate?**
   - Serious infections (e.g., meningitis, endocarditis) attributable to β-lactam–resistant, gram-positive organisms (e.g., coagulase-negative *Staphylococcus* spp., MRSA, some enterococci spp.)
   - Neonates, immune-compromised or ill-appearing children with risk factors for invasive disease, such as the presence of an indwelling central venous device
   - Infections attributable to gram-positive microorganisms in patients with serious allergies to β-lactam antibiotics
   - Prophylaxis, as recommended by the American Heart Association, for endocarditis in certain high-risk patients
   - Prophylaxis for certain procedures (e.g., implantation of prosthetic materials or devices) at institutions with high rates of MRSA
   - Enterally administered vancomycin is indicated for antimicrobial-associated colitis (e.g., *Clostridium difficile,* especially the NAP-1 strain) that fails to respond to metronidazole or is life threatening

American Academy of Pediatrics: Antimicrobial agents and related therapy. In Pickering LK, editor: *2012 Red Book: Report of the Committee on Infectious Diseases*, ed 29. Elk Grove Park, IL, 2012, American Academy of Pediatrics, pp 805–806.

21. **Are fluoroquinolones safe to use in children?**
   Members of the fluoroquinolone class of antibiotics act against bacterial DNA gyrase and topoisomerase II, two enzymes that are required for bacterial DNA replication. No member of the class is approved by the U.S. Food and Drug Administration (FDA) for *routine* use in patients <18 years. Part of the basis for this recommendation is the occurrence of arthropathy in immature beagle dogs treated with ciprofloxacin or other quinolones. However, there is growing experience with the use of these antibiotics in adolescents and children, primarily those with cystic fibrosis in whom endogenous *P. aeruginosa* strains may display high-level resistance to other antibiotic classes (e.g., anti-pseudomonal penicillins, carbapenems,

aminoglycosides). FDA-approved pediatric indications for ciprofloxacin include postexposure treatment for inhalation anthrax and topical therapy for conjunctivitis. The AAP endorses the use of ciprofloxacin as oral therapy for urinary tract infection (UTI) and pyelonephritis caused by *P. aeruginosa* or other multidrug-resistant gram-negative bacteria in children aged 1 through 17 years. Fluoroquinolones may also be considered when parenteral therapy is not feasible and the infection is caused by multidrug-resistant organisms for which there are no other effective oral agents available, such as UTIs.

Bradley JS, Kauffman RE, Balis DA, et al: Assessment of musculoskeletal toxicity 5 years after therapy with levofloxacin, *Pediatrics* 134:e146–e153, 2014.
Bradley JS, Jackson mA: Committee on Infectious Diseases; American Academy of Pediatrics: the use of systemic and topical fluoroquinolones, *Pediatrics* 128:e1034–e1045, 2011.

22. What are the uses of ribavirin?
    Ribavirin is a guanosine analog that inhibits RNA polymerase and subsequently RNA synthesis. It was originally developed in 1972 and was used in the 1980s and 1990s as an inhaled therapy against respiratory syncytial virus (RSV). Both cohort and trial data failed to prove a benefit in mortality or ventilator days in mechanically ventilated infants who had been previously well. However, cohort data have shown that both the inhaled and the IV forms may be of use to prevent lower tract spread of upper tract disease and mortality in allogenic stem cell transplant patients. Most recently, it has shown activity against hepatitis C and is an approved therapy in children in combination with peginterferon gamma. Ribavirin also has activity against certain viral hemorrhagic fevers and is used to treat Lassa virus infections.

American Academy of Pediatrics: Hepatitis C. In Pickering LK, editor: *2012 Red Book: Report of the Committee on Infectious Diseases*, ed 29. Elk Grove Park, IL, 2012, American Academy of Pediatrics, p 393.
Moler F, Steinhart CM, Ohmit SE, Stidham GL: Effectiveness of ribavirin in otherwise well infants with respiratory syncytial virus-associated respiratory failure. Pediatric Critical Study Group, *J Pediatr* 128:422–428, 1996.

23. Why is chicken soup so helpful for upper respiratory infections (URIs)?
    The benefits of chicken soup have been of lore for hundreds of years, beginning in the twelfth century, when physician and philosopher Maimonides extolled its virtue. The precise mechanisms of its anecdotal therapeutic benefits remain elusive. A 2000 study at the University of Nebraska found that the nonparticulate component of chicken soup *in vitro* inhibited neutrophil migration in a concentration-dependent manner. A component of chicken soup, the dipeptide carnosine, may offer protection against reactive oxygen radical species-dependent injury. These anti-inflammatory effects may be some of the mechanisms by which chicken soup mitigates the symptoms of URIs. Of course, placebo effects should not be minimized.

Babizhayev MA, Deyev AI, Yegorov YE: Non-hydrolyzed in digestive tract and blood natural L-carnosine peptide ("bioactivated Jewish penicillin") as a panacea of tomorrow for various flu ailments, *J Basic Clin Physiol Pharmacol* 24:1–26, 2013.
Rennard BO, Ertl RF, Gossman GL, et al: Chicken soup inhibits neutrophil chemotaxis in vitro, *Chest* 118:1150–1157, 2000.

24. Is there any physiologic basis to the adage "starve a fever, feed a cold"?
    Some studies indicate that anorexia increases the number of type 2 T helper (Th2) cells, which are key in fighting bacterial infections. This would serve as a potentially useful behavioral adaptation, particularly in preantibiotic times. Eating, on the other hand, promotes type 1 T helper (Th1) cells by gastrointestinal (GI) stimulation of vagal and neurohormonal factors. The Th1 cells are essential components of the antiviral immune reaction, which might include rhinoviruses and others involved in the common cold.

Bazar KA, Yun AJ, Lee PY: "Starve a fever and feed a cold": feeding and anorexia may be adaptive behavioral modulators of autonomic and T helper balance, *Med Hypotheses* 64:1080–1084, 2005.

CLINICAL ISSUES

25. Name the three stages of pertussis infection (whooping cough)
    1. **Catarrhal** (may last 1 to 2 weeks): This stage is characterized by low-grade fever, URI symptoms, mild cough, and apnea in infants.

2. **Paroxysmal** (may last 1 to 6 weeks): Symptoms include severe cough occurring in paroxysms and onset of inspiratory "whoop."

3. **Convalescent** (may last 2 to 3 weeks): Resolution of symptoms occurs; however, coughing fits may persist. Because of the protracted nature of the disease, it is called the "hundred day cough" in China.

26. What is the most common cause of death in children with whooping cough?

Almost one quarter of infants and children will contract pneumonia, and approximately 2% will die from whooping cough. Ninety percent of deaths are attributable to **pneumonia**, which most often develops as a secondary bacterial infection. These cases can be easily missed during the paroxysmal phase, when respiratory symptoms are so prominent and usually attributed solely to pertussis. A new spiking fever should prompt a careful search for an evolving pneumonia.

27. Is antibiotic therapy of value in pertussis infection?

If used during the first 14 days of illness or before the paroxysmal stage, macrolide antibiotics such as erythromycin, clarithromycin, and azithromycin can decrease the severity of symptoms during the paroxysmal stage and help prevent transmission of the illness. If the diagnosis is established later in the course, these antibiotics should still be administered to eliminate the nasopharyngeal carriage of *Bordetella pertussis* and limit the spread of disease. Evidence suggests that treatment with macrolides is effective for eradicating carriage and preventing transmission.

28. What are ways on physical exam to help distinguish swelling as a result of mumps from swelling caused by lymphadenitis?

- Hatchcock sign: Upward pressure applied to the angle of the mandible produces tenderness with mumps; this maneuver produces no tenderness with adenitis.
- Have the patient sip on lemon juice or suck a lemon wedge. Stimulation of salivation will cause pain in mumps with enlargement of the parotid gland, but no change is noted in patients with adenitis.
- As swelling progresses, the angle of the jaw is obscured. In mumps, when the patient is viewed from behind, the ear lobe is commonly lifted upward and outward.
- With enlargement of the parotid gland, the parotid gland remains in its anatomic relationship with the long axis of the ear, but lymphoid enlargement typically is posterior (Fig. 10-2).

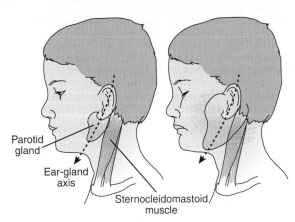

Parotid gland

Ear-gland axis

Sternocleidomastoid muscle

Figure 10-2. A parotid gland infected with mumps *(right)* is compared with a normal gland *(left)* in this schematic drawing. An imaginary line bisecting the long axis of the ear divides the parotid gland into 2 equal parts. In mumps, these anatomic relationships are not altered, but in lymphadenitis, an enlarged cervical lymph node is usually posterior to the imaginary line. *(From Kleigman RM, Stanton BF, Schor NF, et al: Nelson Textbook of Pediatrics, ed 19. Philadelphia, 2011, Elsevier Saunders, p 1079.)*

29. What is the empiric treatment of a skin and soft tissue infection (SSTI) in the setting of the increasing prevalence of CA-MRSA?

As with any SSTI, the principle of incision and drainage (I & D) of localized collections should prevail. In pediatric patients, data suggest that skin abscesses in the immunocompetent host will be adequately treated with I & D alone, without adjuvant antibiotic therapy. Whenever possible, specimens should be obtained for culture and susceptibility testing. For children with minor skin infections (such as impetigo), mupirocin 2% topical ointment can be used. Some authorities have suggested a change in empiric antibiotic therapy to include MRSA coverage is warranted when the patient-specific population prevalence of CA-MRSA infection exceeds 10% to 15%. However, in some communities, there is increasing resistance of both MRSA and methicillin-sensitive *S. aureus* (MSSA) to clindamycin and emerging resistance to trimethoprim-sulfamethoxazole. In hospitalized children with SSTI, empiric vancomycin is recommended. In patients who are clinically stable and do not have bacteremia and/or additional intravascular focus, empiric or step-down therapy with clindamycin may be started.

Singer AJ, Talan DA: Management of skin abscesses in the era of methicillin-resistant *Staphylococcus aureus*, *N Engl J Med* 370:1139–1047, 2014.
Liu C, Bayer A, Cosgrove SE, et al: Clinical practice guidelines by the Infectious Diseases Society of America for the treatment of methicillin-resistant *Staphylococcus aureus* infections in adults and children: executive summary, *Clin Infect Dis* 52:285–292, 2011.

30. What are the distinguishing features of staphylococcal scalded skin syndrome, staphylococcal toxic shock syndrome, and streptococcal toxic shock syndrome? See Table 10-1.

Table 10-1 Distinguishing Features of Staphylococcal Scalded Skin Syndrome, Staphylococcal Toxic Shock Syndrome, and Streptococcal Toxic Shock Syndrome

CLINICAL FEATURES	STAPHYLOCOCCAL SCALDED SKIN SYNDROME	STAPHYLOCOCCAL TOXIC SHOCK SYNDROME	GROUP A STREPTOCOCCAL TOXIC SHOCK-LIKE SYNDROME
Organism	*Staphylococcus aureus*	*Staphylococcus aureus*	Group A streptococci
	Usually phage group 11, type 71	Usually phage group 1, type 29	Usually type 1, 3, or 18
			Exotoxin A production
Site of infection	Usually focal	Mucous membranes	Blood, abscess, pneumonia, empyema, cellulitis, necrotizing fasciitis
	Mucocutaneous border: nose, mouth, diaper area	Infected wound or furuncle	
	Sometimes inapparent	Sometimes inapparent	Sometimes inapparent
Skin rash	Tender erythroderma: face, neck, generalized	Tender erythroderma: trunk, hands, feet	Erythroderma: trunk, extremities
	Bullae, no petechiae	Edema of hands, feet	
Desquamation	Early, first 1-2 days, generalized, feet	Late, 7-10 days, mostly hands and feet	Late, 7-10 days, mostly hands
		Hyperemia of oral and vaginal mucosa	Hyperemia of oral and vaginal mucosa
Mucous membranes	Normal	Hypertrophy of tongue papillae	Hypertrophy of tongue papillae

Continued on following page

Table 10-1 Distinguishing Features of Staphylococcal Scalded Skin Syndrome, Staphylococcal Toxic Shock Syndrome, and Streptococcal Toxic Shock Syndrome (*Continued*)

CLINICAL FEATURES	STAPHYLOCOCCAL SCALDED SKIN SYNDROME	STAPHYLOCOCCAL TOXIC SHOCK SYNDROME	GROUP A STREPTOCOCCAL TOXIC SHOCK-LIKE SYNDROME
Conjunctivae	Normal	Markedly injected	Injected
Course	Insidious, 4-7 days	Fulminant, shock with secondary multiorgan failure, 10% mortality	Fulminant, shock with early primary multiorgan failure, 30-50% mortality
	Benign, <1% mortality		

Adapted from Bass JW: Treatment of skin and skin structure infections, Pediatr Infect Dis J 11:152–155, 1992.

31. **Can antiviral medications be used to prevent or treat oral herpes simplex virus (HSV) infections?**

    In immunocompetent hosts, oral acyclovir or valacyclovir offers *significant therapeutic benefit* in primary HSV gingivostomatitis but has *limited efficacy* for the treatment of recurrent herpes labialis. Valacyclovir is the prodrug of acyclovir, meaning it is converted to acyclovir after absorption. Valacyclovir achieves higher plasma levels of acyclovir than oral preparations of acyclovir and is dosed less frequently, making it the agent of choice. Topical antivirals have not shown consistent benefit in either of these settings. Prophylaxis with valacyclovir can reduce the number of recurrences in adults (especially pregnant women) with herpes labialis, but it has not been well studied in children.

32. **What is the proper medical term for oral thrush?**

    Acute pseudomembranous candidiasis is the proper medical term for oral thrush—quite a mouthful. Although thrush is sometimes confused with residual formula in the mouth in infants, formula is more easily removed with a tongue blade. When thrush is scraped, small bleeding points often occur on the underlying mucosa.

33. **What is the most common specific etiology diagnosed in patients with systemic febrile illness after international travel?**

    Malaria, both in children and adults is the most common etiology. Next in frequency are dengue fever, typhoid fever, rickettsioses, and leptospirosis. Leishmaniasis should also be considered in travelers from endemic areas. Malaria, caused by the protozoan parasite of the genus *Plasmodium*, should be considered in the differential diagnosis in anyone with fever who has travelled to an endemic area in the previous year. More than half of the world's population lives in areas where malaria is endemic. Although there are more than 100 *Plasmodium* species, human infection is caused primarily by five: *P. falciparum, P. vivax, P. ovale, P. malariae,* and *P. knowlesi. P. falciparum* is responsible for the majority of malarial deaths globally.

Wilson ME, Weld LH, Boggild A, et al: Fever in returned travellers: results from the GeoSentinel surveillance network, *Clin Infect Dis* 44:1560–1568, 2007.

Freedman DO, Weld LH, Kozarsky PE, et al: Spectrum of disease and relation to place of exposure among ill returned travellers, *N Engl J Med* 354:119–130, 2006.

34. **What is the classic triad of malaria?**

    Spiking fevers, anemia, and splenomegaly. Malaria is caused by species of *Plasmodium* (transmitted by the *Anopheles* mosquito), which infect red blood cells (RBCs); certain species (particularly *P. vivax* and *P. ovale)* can have a dormant liver stage. The classic malarial fever involves a periodicity (typically 48 to 72 hours) associated with the rupture of RBCs. Chills, headache, abdominal pain, and myalgias are also common symptoms.

Cavagnaro CS, Brady K, Siegel C: Fever after international travel, *Clin Pediatr Emerg Med* 9:250–257, 2008.

35. How is malaria diagnosed?

Thick and thin blood smears. Thick smears are made by applying the blood film twice to a slide (and incorporating more RBCs). Giemsa stain is applied to both with an attempt to identify parasites in the cells. The thick smear is better for determining the presence of parasites, and the thin smear is better for species identification from the presence of specific cytologic characteristics (Fig. 10-3). A determination of parasite density (a rough gauge to severity of infection) can be made. Therapy depends on the species identified. If smears are negative and clinical suspicion remains strong, repeat smears should be obtained sequentially over a 3-day period; effort should be made to collect specimens when the patient is febrile, and parasitemia is heaviest.

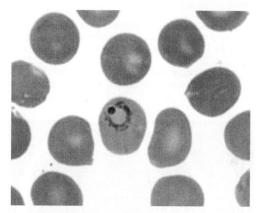

Figure 10-3. *Plasmodium malariae*, peripheral blood smear. The smear shows a red cell containing a *P. malariae* ring form trophozoite with one chromatin dot. The cytoplasm ring is thicker than that of *P. falciparum*, which also typically has two chromatin dots. *(From Morgan EA: Malaria. In Aster JC, Pozdnyakova O, Kutok JL:* Hematopathology: A Volume in the High Yield Pathology Series, *vol 33. Philadelphia, Elsevier, 2013, p 43.)*

36. Which illness is associated with the term "breakbone fever"?

Dengue fever. The term refers to the classic presentation of fever, severe headache, retro-orbital pain, fatigue, and severe myalgias or arthralgias. Most cases are less severe. The illness is caused by an arbovirus, transmitted by mosquitoes, that is endemic in tropical areas worldwide, including the Caribbean and Central and South America. Leukopenia, thrombocytopenia, and mild elevations of hepatic transaminases are common. Children, more commonly than adults, may develop *dengue hemorrhagic fever*, which encompasses fever, epistaxis, mucosal bleeding, and platelet counts lower than 100,000/μL. This may progress to *dengue shock syndrome* with significant mortality.

37. What causes leptospirosis?

Spirochetes of the genus *Leptospira* cause leptospirosis. These are typically acquired from animal contact, or water or soil contaminated by the urine of dogs, rats, or livestock in the course of recreation or work. Acquisition of illness is more common after heavy rainfall or flooding. The incubation period can be up to 1 month. In 90% of cases, the disease is self-limited.

38. What are the phases of leptospirosis?

- **Septicemic phase:** Initially, there are nonspecific symptoms of fever, chills, headache, and a transient rash. Conjunctivitis without purulent discharge occurs in about one-third of cases. Eighty percent of cases feature severe myalgias of the calves and lumbar area. Symptoms may last up to 1 week and improve for 1 to 4 days, when the second phase occurs.
- **Immune-mediated:** Fever returns, accompanied by potentially more severe findings, including aseptic meningitis and Weil syndrome (jaundice, nonoliguric renal failure, hemorrhage due to thrombocytopenia). Severe pulmonary hemorrhages with hemoptysis may develop. The protean manifestations are due to the pathophysiology as a generalized vasculitis.

American Academy of Pediatrics: Leptospirosis. In Pickering LK, editor: *2012 Red Book: Report of the Committee on Infectious Diseases*, ed 29. Elk Grove Park, IL, 2012, American Academy of Pediatrics, pp 469–471.

39. Which organisms are particularly dangerous to clinical microbiology laboratory workers?

The laboratory should be alerted when highly transmissible bacterial agents are suspected in specimens that have been submitted for culture. These bacteria include *Francisella tularensis* (the causative agent of tularemia), *Bacillus anthracis* (anthrax), and *Coxiella burnetii* (Q fever). In addition, the laboratory should process fungal cultures that contain molds and dimorphic fungi (e.g., *Histoplasma, Blastomyces*) in a biosafety cabinet to prevent exposure to spores.

CONGENITAL INFECTIONS

40. Which congenital infections cause cerebral calcifications?

Cerebral calcifications are most frequently observed in **congenital *Toxoplasma*** and **cytomegalovirus (CMV)** infections. They are seen occasionally in patients with congenital HSV infection and rarely in patients with congenital rubella infection or congenital varicella. The calcifications seen in CMV infections are typically found in the periventricular region (Fig. 10-4) because CMV has a predilection for the germinal matrix, as opposed to the calcifications of *Toxoplasma,* which are more generally seen in the brain parenchyma.

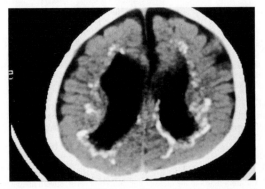

Figure 10-4. CT scan of infant with congenital CMV infection with periventricular calcification, hydrocephalus, and cerebral atrophy. *(From Shakoor A, Sy A, Acharya N: Ocular manifestations of intrauterine infections. In Pediatric Ophthalmology and Strabismus, ed 4. Philadelphia, Elsevier, 2013, p 81.)*

41. What are the late sequelae of congenital infections?

The late sequelae of chronic intrauterine infections are relatively common and may occur in infants who are asymptomatic at birth. Most sequelae present symptoms later in childhood rather than infancy.

- *CMV*: Hearing loss, minimal to severe brain dysfunction; motor, learning, language, and behavioral disorders. Longitudinal data from the National Health and Nutrition Examination Surveys (NHANES) have also implicated CMV as a risk factor for cardiovascular disease.
- *Rubella*: Hearing loss, minimal to severe brain dysfunction (motor, learning, language, and behavioral disorders), autism, juvenile diabetes, thyroid dysfunction, precocious puberty, progressive degenerative brain disorder
- *Toxoplasmosis*: Chorioretinitis, hydrocephalus, minimal to severe brain dysfunction, hearing loss
- *Neonatal herpes*: Recurrent eye and skin infection, minimal to severe brain dysfunction
- *Hepatitis B virus*: Chronic subclinical hepatitis, rarely fulminant hepatitis

Maldonado A, Nizet V, Klein J, et al: Current concepts of infections of the fetus and newborn infant. In Remington J, Klein J, Wilson C, Baker C, editors: *Infectious Diseases of the Fetus and Newborn Infant*, ed 7. Philadelphia, 2011, Elsevier Saunders, pp 2–23.

Plotkin SA, Alpert G: A practical guide to the diagnosis of congenital infections in the newborn infant, *Pediatr Clin North Am* 33:465–479, 1986.

42. **What is the most common congenital infection?**

   Congenital CMV infection is the most common; in some large screening studies, it occurs in up to 1.3% of newborns. However, the majority (80% to 90%) of infected neonates are asymptomatic at birth or in early infancy.

43. **How common is hearing loss from congenital CMV?**

   It's estimated that one third to two-thirds of children with symptomatic congenital CMV infection and 7% to 15% of asymptomatic newborns with CMV will develop hearing loss at a median age of 3½ years. There is debate regarding possible universal screening for newborn CMV infection, especially if the initiation of antiviral therapy could prevent or limit hearing loss. Postnatal exposure to CMV is not associated with hearing loss.

Johnson J, Anderson B: Screening, prevention, and treatment of congenital cytomegalovirus, *Obstet Gynecol Clin North Am* 41:593–599, 2014.

Misono S, Sie KCY, Weiss NS, et al: Congenital cytomegalovirus infection in pediatric hearing loss, *Arch Otolaryngol Head Neck Surg* 137:47–53, 2011.

44. **How is CMV transmitted from mother to infant?**

   CMV can be transmitted by the transplacental route and through contact with cervical secretions or breast milk. On occasion, transmission may occur by contact with saliva or urine.

45. **How should congenital CMV be treated?**

   The goals of treatment for congenital CMV have historically been to prevent the late sequelae of the disease, primarily sensory-neural hearing loss. However, the optimal treatment strategy (including choice of medication and duration of therapy) and which infants to treat are questions currently under investigation. Treatment is recommended for infants with life-threatening or vision-threatening disease, such as severe retinitis, interstitial pneumonitis, and active central nervous system infection. Whether treatment is indicated for isolated thrombocytopenia, mild hepatitis, viruria, or viremia without other symptoms is unclear. Treatments currently being studied include 6 weeks of IV ganciclovir and oral valganciclovir for 6 months or longer.

46. **What is the risk to the fetus if the mother is infected with parvovirus B19 during pregnancy?**

   Approximately 30% to 50% of pregnant women are susceptible to parvovirus infection. The risk of fetal loss after seroconversion is 5% to 10% and is greatest when maternal infection occurs during the first half of pregnancy. Fetal loss occurs as a consequence of hydrops, which develops as a result of parvovirus-induced anemia. The signs of parvovirus infection in adults are not very distinctive but may include fever; a maculopapular or lacelike rash, especially in a stocking-glove pattern; and joint pain. There are case reports of aplastic anemia persisting for weeks in surviving neonates.

47. **What are the consequences of primary varicella infection during the first trimester?**

   The congenital varicella syndrome consists of a constellation of features:
   - Limb atrophy, usually associated with a cicatricial (scarring) lesion
   - Neurologic and sensory defects
   - Eye abnormalities (chorioretinitis, cataracts, microphthalmia, Horner syndrome)
   - Cortical atrophy and mental retardation

   This syndrome usually follows maternal infection during the first trimester, although it may be seen after infection up to 20 weeks into gestation.

48. **What are the indications for postexposure prophylaxis for varicella in the newborn?**

   Prophylaxis should be given as soon as possible to a newborn whose mother develops varicella from 5 days before to 2 days after delivery. During this period of high risk, the fetus is exposed to high circulating titers of the virus without the benefit of maternal antibody synthesis. Currently, Varizig is the purified human immune globulin preparation licensed and available for use in the United States. It is most ideally given within 96 hours (4 days) for greatest effectiveness, but can be given up to 10 days after exposure. Other indications for use in the newborn include the following:
   - Premature infants ≥28 weeks of gestation who are exposed in the neonatal period and the mother has no history of chickenpox or positive varicella serology

- Premature infants ≤28 weeks of gestation or whose weight is 1000 g or less and who are exposed in the neonatal period regardless of maternal history, because little maternal antibody crosses the placenta before the third trimester of pregnancy

Centers for Disease Control and Prevention: Updated recommendations for use of VariZIG—United States, 2013, *Morb Mortal Wkly Rep* 62:574–576, 2013.

49. **Do urogenital mycoplasmas have a role in neonatal disease?**
    Ureaplasma urealyticum has been associated with low birth weight and bronchopulmonary dysplasia. This organism has been recovered from neonates with respiratory distress, pneumonia, and meningitis, but a causative role in these diseases has not been proven. Several reports of apparent *Mycoplasma hominis* meningitis and eye infection have been published.
    Vertical transmission occurs in up to 60% of newborns whose mothers have positive cultures for these organisms. Risk for transmission is higher in preterm and low-birth-weight infants and correlates with the prolonged rupture of membranes and maternal fever. Infants delivered by cesarean section over intact membranes have a very low rate of colonization compared with infants delivered vaginally.

50. **What are the features of congenital rubella syndrome (CRS)?**
    The most characteristic features of CRS are **congenital heart disease**, **cataracts**, **microphthalmia**, **corneal opacities**, **glaucoma**, and **radiolucent bone lesions**. The features of CRS can be divided into three broad categories:
    - **Transient:** Low birth weight, hepatosplenomegaly, thrombocytopenia, hepatitis, pneumonitis, and radiolucent bone lesions
    - **Permanent:** Deafness, cataracts, and congenital heart lesions (patent ductus arteriosus > pulmonary artery stenosis > aortic stenosis > ventricular septal defects)
    - **Developmental:** Psychomotor delay, behavioral disorders, and endocrine dysfunction
    Indigenous rubella transmission and CRS were declared eliminated in the United States in 2004 as a result of universal screening and vaccination policies in pregnant women. However, worldwide CRS remains a major health issue. The World Health Organization has targeted regional elimination of CRS by 2015.

51. **Should all pregnant women be screened for HSV infection during pregnancy?**
    Existing data indicate that antepartum cultures of the maternal genital tract fail to predict viral shedding at the time of delivery. Thus, **routine** antepartum cultures are **not** currently recommended. However, surveillance data have shown a decline in the overall seroprevalence of HSV in women of childbearing age from 2005 to 2010 compared with 2001 to 2004. About one fifth to one-third of women of childbearing age are seronegative for HSV-1 and HSV-2. This is in part driven by a significant reduction in the seroprevalence of HSV-1 in young people ages 14 to 19. Concern has been raised that this may lead to an increased incidence of primary HSV infection during pregnancy. Recent algorithms have been developed that incorporate maternal serologic status into the diagnosis and treatment strategies of infants born to mothers with active HSV lesions. Consequently, routine serologic screening (HSV-1 and HSV-2, IgG, and IgM) may be incorporated into antepartum screening in the future.

Bradley H, Markowitz LE, Gibson T, McQuillan GM: Seroprevalence of herpes simplex virus types 1 and 2—United States, 1999-2010, *J Infect Dis* 209:325–333, 2014.
Kimberlin DW: The Scarlet H, *J Infect Dis* 209:315–317, 2014.
Kimberlin D, Baley J; Committee on Infectious Diseases; Committee on Fetus and Newborn. Guidance on management of asymptomatic neonates born to women with active genital herpes lesions, *Pediatrics* 131:e635–e646, 2013.

52. **What are risk factors for the development of neonatal HSV disease?**
    HSV infection of the neonate infant may be acquired *before* delivery *(in utero), during* delivery (intrapartum or perinatal), and *after* delivery (postpartum or postnatal). The majority of illness, approximately 85%, is acquired during the intrapartum period. Classic risk factors for intrapartum or perinatal transmission include:
    - Primary, rather than recurrent, maternal infection, especially if acquisition is in the third trimester. (Women with primary genital HSV infections who are shedding HSV at delivery are 10 to 30 times more likely to transmit the virus than women with a recurrent infection.)
    - Negative maternal HSV IgG antibody status

- Prolonged rupture of membranes
- Violation of mucocutaneous barriers (e.g., use of fetal scalp electrodes)
- Vaginal rather than cesarean delivery

Stephenson-Famy A, Gardella C: Herpes simplex virus infection during pregnancy, *Obstet Gynecol Clin North Am* 41:601–614, 2014.

Kimberlin D, Baley J; Committee on Infectious Diseases; Committee on Fetus and Newborn. Guidance on management of asymptomatic neonates born to women with active genital herpes lesions, *Pediatrics* 131:e635–e646, 2013.

Corey L, Wald A: Maternal and neonatal herpes simplex virus infections, *N Engl J Med* 361:1376–1385, 2009.

53. What are the three forms of neonatal HSV disease?
- **Mucocutaneous disease** (localized to the skin, eye, or mouth [SEM])
- **Central nervous system** (CNS) disease
- **Disseminated disease**; multiple organ systems are involved and the clinical syndrome resembles bacterial sepsis

Up to 50% of infants will have CNS complications, from either primary CNS disease or disseminated disease with CNS involvement. It is important to note that infants with CNS or disseminated disease may not have visible skin lesions.

54. When should HSV disease be suspected in newborn or infants?
Current recommendations distinguish neonatal HSV *infection*, which is the asymptomatic period when viral replication is occurring, from HSV *disease*, when clinical signs and symptoms of HSV are present. In full-term infants <4 weeks and premature infants (<32 weeks of gestation) <8 weeks, HSV disease should be considered in the following cases:
- Skin lesions suspicious for HSV on the infant (may be single or grouped vesicles, pustules, bullae, or denuded skin)
- Ill-appearing infant with findings of poor feeding, irritability, lethargy, vomiting, and hypothermia or hyperthermia
- Seizures or encephalopathy associated with the current illness
- Abnormal liver function tests (elevated alanine aminotransferase [ALT] and/or aspartate aminotransferase [AST])
- Sterile CSF pleocytosis

In general, infants with SEM and disseminated disease present with clinical symptoms 10 to 14 days after infection and those with CNS disease 17 to 19 days after infection.

Kimberlin D, Baley J; Committee on Infectious Diseases; Committee on Fetus and Newborn. Guidance on management of asymptomatic neonates born to women with active genital herpes lesions. *Pediatrics,*131:e635–e646, 2013.

55. How should the neonate with suspected HSV disease be treated?
Progression from infection to disease is considered inevitable. One of the goals of therapy is to accurately identify infants with infection and intervene to prevent progression to disease. Intravenous acyclovir is the preferred drug and is administered pending definitive diagnosis. For confirmed mucocutaneous disease, treatment is continued for 14 days. For encephalitis and disseminated disease, treatment is continued for 21 days. For infants who have been recognized as having a high risk of progression to disease (e.g., infants born to mothers with primary HSV), 10 days of therapy with intravenous (IV) acyclovir is recommended even if cultures or polymerase chain reaction (PCR) testing of the infant is negative for HSV.

Kimberlin D, Baley J; Committee on Infectious Diseases; Committee on Fetus and Newborn. Guidance on management of asymptomatic neonates born to women with active genital herpes lesions, *Pediatrics,*131:e635 to e646, 2013.

56. In which groups of women is prenatal hepatitis B surface antigen (HBsAg) screening recommended?
In the past, women were screened for HBsAg if they fell into a high-risk group based on ethnic origin, immunization status, or history of exposure to blood products, IV drugs, or a high-risk partner. However, historic information revealed that at most 60% of HBsAg carriers were captured using these screening criteria. Thus, it is recommended that **all** pregnant women be screened for HBsAg.

57. What is the risk to the fetus if the mother is infected with hepatitis B virus?

Very significant. Ten percent to 20% of women who are HBsAg positive and 90% of women who are *both* HBsAg positive and seropositive for hepatitis B e antigen (HBeAg) will transmit the virus to their infants in the absence of hepatitis B vaccine at birth. Of women who are acutely infected during pregnancy, the risk of neonatal infection is greatest when maternal infection occurs during the third trimester; up to 90% of these neonates will be seropositive for HBsAg. Chronic hepatitis B virus infection with persistence of HBsAg occurs in 85% to 95% of infants who are infected by perinatal transmission, with a 25% to 30% lifetime prevalence of severe liver disease or liver cancer.

58. How should infants born to mothers with hepatitis B infection be managed?

For infants born to women who are HBsAg positive, hepatitis B immunoglobulin (0.5 mL intramuscularly) and the first dose of hepatitis B vaccine should be administered within 12 hours of delivery to reduce the risk for infection. Although breast milk is theoretically capable of transmitting the hepatitis B virus, the risk for transmission in HBsAg-positive mothers whose infants have received timely hepatitis B immunoglobulin and hepatitis B vaccine is not increased by breastfeeding.

American Academy of Pediatrics: Hepatitis B. In Pickering LK, editor: *2012 Red Book: Report of the Committee on Infectious Diseases*, ed 29. Elk Grove Park, IL, 2012, American Academy of Pediatrics, p 384.

59. How should infants born to mothers with hepatitis A infection be managed?

Neonates born to mothers with active hepatitis A infection are unlikely to contract the virus, and efficacy of postnatal prophylaxis with hepatitis A immunoglobulin has not been proven. Some experts recommend immunoglobulin if the mother's symptoms begin within 2 weeks before or 1 week after delivery, but this is controversial.

American Academy of Pediatrics: Hepatitis A. In Pickering LK, editor: *2012 Red Book: Report of the Committee on Infectious Diseases*, ed 29. Elk Grove Park, IL, 2012, American Academy of Pediatrics, p 368.

60. How should infants born to mothers with hepatitis C infection be managed?

The risk for vertical transmission of hepatitis C virus (HCV) is about 6% in mothers who demonstrate the presence of HCV RNA in the blood. This risk is increased in mothers who are coinfected with HIV. No preventive therapy exists. Nucleic amplification testing can be done at 1 to 2 months of age, if desired, to assess for neonatal infection. Antibody testing cannot be done until after 18 months because that is the expected duration of the passively acquired maternal antibody in infants. Mothers with hepatitis C infection should be advised that transmission of hepatitis C by breastfeeding has not been documented. Accordingly, maternal hepatitis C infection is not a contraindication to breastfeeding, although mothers with cracked or bleeding nipples should consider abstaining.

Wen JW, Haber BA: Maternal-fetal transmission of hepatitis C infection: what is so special about babies? *J Pediatr Gastroenterol Nutr* 58:378–382, 2014.
American Academy of Pediatrics: Hepatitis C. In Pickering LK, editor: *2012 Red Book: Report of the Committee on Infectious Diseases*, ed 29. Elk Grove Park, IL, 2012, American Academy of Pediatrics, p 395.

61. How do the clinical features of early and late congenital syphilis differ?

The manifestations of congenital syphilis are variable and may be divided into early and late findings. Early manifestations occur during the first 2 years of life, (e.g., "snuffles"); late manifestations, such as peg-shaped or notched central incisors, so-called "Hutchinson teeth" occur after 2 years of age (Fig. 10-5 and Table 10-2).

62. How is the diagnosis of congenital syphilis made?

- All pregnant women and infants should be screened for possible infection with a nontreponemal test for *Treponema pallidum*. Such tests include the rapid plasma reagin card test (RPR) and the Venereal Disease Research Laboratory (VDRL) slide test.
- If blood from the mother or infant yields a positive nontreponemal serologic test, a specific treponemal test should be performed on the infant's blood. Examples include the fluorescent treponemal antibody (FTA) absorption test and the microhemagglutination test for *T. pallidum*.

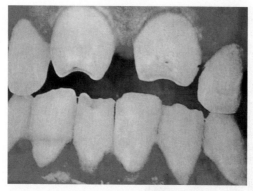

Figure 10-5. Hutchinson teeth. Note the notched, peg-shaped incisors with enamel defects and incipient caries. *(From Rodriguez-Cerdeira C, Silami-Lopes VC: Congenital syphilis in the 21st century, Actas Dermo-Sifiliográficas (English Edition) 103:687, 2011.)*

Table 10-2 Early and Late Manifestations of Congenital Syphilis

EARLY CONGENITAL SYPHILIS (310 PATIENTS)		LATE CONGENITAL SYPHILIS (271 PATIENTS)	
Hepatomegaly	32%	Pseudoparalysis of Parrot	87%
Skeletal abnormalities	29%	Short maxilla	84%
Splenomegaly	18%	High palatal arch	76%
Birth weight <2500 g	16%	Hutchinson triad	75%
Pneumonia	16%	Saddle nose	73%
Severe anemia, hydrops, edema	16%	Mulberry molars	65%
Skin lesions	15%	Hutchinson teeth	63%
Hyperbilirubinemia	13%	Higoumenakis sign	39%
Snuffles, nasal discharge	9%	Relative protuberance of mandible	26%
Painful limbs	7%	Interstitial keratitis	9%
Cerebrospinal fluid abnormalities	7%	Rhagades	7%
Pancreatitis	5%	Saber shin	4%
Nephritis	4%	Eighth nerve deafness	3%
Failure to thrive	3%	Scaphoid scapulae	0.70%
Testicular mass	0.30%	Clutton joint	0.30%
Chorioretinitis	0.30%		
Hypoglobulinemia	0.30%		

Adapted from Sanchez PJ, Gutman LT: Syphilis. In Feigin RD, Cherry JE, Demmler GJ, Kaplan SL (eds): Pediatric Infectious Diseases, 5th ed. Philadelphia, W.B. Saunders, 2004, pp 1730–1732.

- Evaluation of infants with suspected congenital syphilis should also include a complete blood count, analysis of the CSF (including a CSF VDRL), and long-bone radiographs (unless the diagnosis has otherwise been established) to look for characteristic findings (Fig. 10-6).

63. What are the pitfalls of RPR and VDRL testing?
    - Nontreponemal tests detect antibodies to cardiolipin and may yield false-positive results in a variety of maternal conditions, such as systemic lupus.

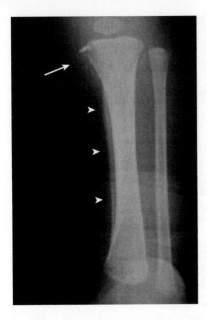

Figure 10-6. Radiograph of an infant with congenital syphilis shows periosteal reaction along the shaft of the left tibia *(arrowheads)* and a characteristic lucency of the medial proximal tibial metaphysis *(arrow)* called the Wimberger sign, which represents localized bony destruction. *(From Donnelly LF: Pediatric Imaging: The Fundamentals. Philadelphia, 2009, Saunders, p 171.)*

- False-negative tests may occur because of high titers of antibodies; this is termed the "prozone effect." It is recommended that the sample be diluted before testing to avoid this.
- A reactive serologic titer may persist after the initial decline (usually 4-fold) in response to treatment. This low level titer is usually <1:8 and may persist for life; this so-called "serofast" state can make interpretation of nontreponemal tests difficult.
- A mother who has been treated adequately for syphilis during pregnancy can still passively transfer antibodies to the neonate, which results in a positive titer in the infant in the absence of infection. In this circumstance, the infant's titer is usually less than the mother's and reverts to negative over several months.

64. If a pregnant woman is found to have *Chlamydia trachomatis* in her birth canal, what is the most appropriate course of action?
The U.S. Preventative Task Force recommends that all pregnant women <25 years of age or those with high risk behavior patterns be screened for *C. trachomatis*. Pregnant women with a known chlamydial infection should be treated with oral azithromycin to reduce the risk for neonatal chlamydial pneumonia and conjunctivitis because untreated mothers may transmit *Chlamydia* to babies born vaginally about 50% of the time. Simultaneous treatment of the male partners with doxycycline or azithromycin should also be undertaken.

U.S. Preventative Task Force: USPSTF Recommendations for STI Screening. www.uspreventiveservicetaskforce.org. Accessed on Mar. 20, 2015.

65. Should newborns of mothers with untreated chlamydial infection receive prophylactic antibiotic therapy?
Although these infants are at increased risk for infection, the efficacy of prophylactic antibiotics is not known and treatment is not indicated. Infants should be followed carefully for signs of conjunctivitis or pneumonia and treated if they are symptomatic.

American Academy of Pediatrics: *Chlamydia trachomatis*. In Pickering LK, editor: *2012 Red Book: Report of the Committee on Infectious Diseases*, ed 29. Elk Grove Park, IL, 2012, American Academy of Pediatrics, pp 276–277.

66. What is the risk to a fetus after primary maternal *Toxoplasma* infection?
The risk depends on the time during pregnancy that the mother becomes infected. Assuming that the mother is untreated, first-trimester infection is associated with a fetal infection rate of about 25%,

second-trimester infection with a rate of more than 50%, and third-trimester infection with a rate of roughly 70%. The severity of clinical disease in congenitally infected infants is inversely related to gestational age at the time of primary maternal infection.

67. **What is the typical presentation of congenital toxoplasmosis?**
At birth, 70% to 90% are asymptomatic. As with other congenital infections, the symptomatic neonatal presentations are varied, ranging from severe disease with hepatosplenomegaly, chorioretinitis, and/or neurologic features (e.g., seizures, hydrocephalus, microcephaly) in about 10% of infected infants to an asymptomatic infection. Among clinically asymptomatic infants, findings such as intracranial calcifications or retinal cysts may be present, and long-term risks include impaired vision, learning disabilities, mental retardation, and seizures.

68. **How can a woman minimize the chance of acquiring a *Toxoplasma* infection during pregnancy?**
Measures relate to personal hygiene, food preparation, and exposure to cats.
- Avoid raw meat. Using a food thermometer for confirmation, cook whole cuts of meat (excluding poultry) to at least 145 °F (63 °C), cook ground meat to at least 160 °F (71 °C) and cook all poultry to at least 165 °F (74 °C).
- Wash fruits and vegetables before consumption.
- Wash hands and kitchen surfaces thoroughly after contact with raw meat and unwashed fruits or vegetables, and wash thoroughly after gardening.
- Avoid changing cat litter boxes, or wear gloves while changing the litter and wash hands thoroughly afterwards. Changing the litter every 1 to 2 days will also reduce risk.
- Avoid untreated water in high-risk areas, such as developing countries.

EMERGING INFECTIOUS DISEASES

69. **Which mycobacterium may infect someone who has a home aquarium?**
Mycobacterium marinum. This atypical mycobacterial infection typically begins with clusters of superficial nodules or papules, which can become fluctuant. The condition can be misdiagnosed as a cellulitis. A detailed history can help establish the diagnosis.

70. **What are possible sources for an anthrax infection in a 17-year-old who lives on a cattle farm, makes and plays drums as a hobby, and works in a microbiology lab after school?**
- **Cutaneous anthrax** is the most common form of anthrax. It occurs when spores invade a violation in local skin integrity. Infection usually develops from 1 to 7 days after exposure. Without treatment, cutaneous anthrax is fatal 20% of the time, but it is curable with therapy. Cutaneous anthrax has been called "wool sorters disease," because the spores are found in animal hides (as well as other raw animal products), such as those used in wool processing or in making traditional hide drums. It can be contracted through improper handling of laboratory specimens. It was used as an agent of bioterror in the United States in 2001.
- **Inhalation anthrax** occurs when the spores are inhaled. Dissemination then occurs through lymphatic spread. Infection usually develops 7 to 14 days after exposure but may occur up to 60 days after exposure. Survival with treatment is ∼55%.
- **Gastrointestinal** anthrax occurs when spores are ingested, typically through raw or undercooked meat. Infection usually develops from 1 to 7 days after exposure. Survival with treatment is ∼60%.
Our patient could have contracted any form of the disease from a variety of his exposures. As with many infectious diseases, a careful history will often reveal the source of the infection.

71. **What are the novel coronaviruses?**
Coronaviruses are named for the crownlike spikes on their surface; they typically cause respiratory disease on the spectrum of the common cold. Two novel coronaviruses have been implicated in severe and sometimes fatal respiratory disease:
- **Severe acute respiratory syndrome (SARS)**, termed SARS-CoV, was first recognized in China in 2002. It spread to multiple countries and caused several hundred deaths from 2002 to 2003. Since 2004, there have not been any known cases of SARS-CoV infection reported anywhere in the world. The virus is felt to have originated in wild animals (civit cats and bats have been implicated) with transmission to humans who contacted them in markets in urban areas.

- **Middle East respiratory syndrome (MERS)**, termed MERS-CoV, was first recognized in Saudi Arabia in 2012. It has also spread to several countries. All cases to date have been linked to countries in and near the Arabian Peninsula. The true incidence of the disease is not known because there may be reporting bias of milder cases. The disease is thought to have a natural reservoir in camels.

72. **What viral etiology should be considered in a patient with acute, unexplained respiratory illness who is not febrile?**
Enterovirus D68 (EV-D68). This is a non-polio enterovirus first described in California in 1968. Symptoms range from mild respiratory illness with rhinorrhea, sneezing, cough and myalgia to severe symptoms such as wheezing, hypoxia and acute respiratory distress syndrome. However, even patients with serious illness due to EV-D68 may not have fever. Additionally, EV-D68 has been associated (although not causally substantiated) in a cluster of cases in 2014 of acute limb weakness. Most patients were found to have a distinctive pattern of abnormalities of the grey matter of the spinal cord on MRI.

Foster CB, Friedman N, et al: Enterovirus D68: a clinically important respiratory enterovirus. *Cleve Clin J Med* 82:26–31, 2015.

73. **What two diseases in particular should be in the differential diagnosis for a traveler returning from the Caribbean with a fever and rash?**
Dengue fever and Chikungunya virus infection. Dengue and Chikungunya viruses are both transmitted by the *Aedes aegypti* and *Aedes albopictus* mosquitoes and have overlapping clinical features and similar endemicity. **Dengue** has three clinical syndromes:
- **Undifferentiated fever** presents as a general febrile illness with fever, malaise, and other mild symptoms that overlap with a number of other viral syndromes. This is a typical presentation in children with their first infection.
- **Dengue fever with or without hemorrhage** presents with 2 to 7 days of high fever and ≥ 2 other symptoms such as severe headache, retro-orbital eye pain, myalgias, arthralgias, maculopapular rash, or petechial rash.
- **Dengue hemorrhagic fever or Dengue shock syndrome** presents initially as Dengue fever, but progresses to plasma leak and disseminated intravascular coagulation.
- Dengue fever or hemorrhagic fever usually occurs in older children or adolescents who have had previous infection.
   Chikungunya infection is characterized by acute onset of fever >39 °C (>102 °F) and joint pain that is usually severe, bilateral, and symmetric, as well as headache, myalgia, arthritis, nausea/vomiting, and a maculopapular rash, similar to dengue fever.
   Real-time PCR diagnosis is available for both Dengue and Chikungunya through the CDC and may be performed within 5 days of onset of symptoms. After that time frame, IgG and IgM serologic testing should be performed.

74. **What is the most common viral intestinal infection you can get from eating at a salad bar?**
Noroviruses are estimated to be responsible for up to 50% of foodborne outbreaks of viral gastroenteritis. Additionally, the majority (>90%) of diarrheal disease outbreaks on cruise ships are caused by noroviruses. The source of these outbreaks often stems from unsafe food handling practices from infected food service workers. Foods such as raw fruits and leafy green vegetables are often involved. Nausea, vomiting, and watery diarrhea with abdominal cramping have an acute onset 12 to 48 hours after exposure and resolve without treatment 24 to 72 hours later.

75. **When was the Ebola virus first discovered?**
1976. There were two simultaneous outbreaks, one in Sudan and one in the Republic of Congo. The name derives for a village in the Congo near the Ebola River where the outbreak occurred.

76. **What are the clinical features of an Ebola infection?**
Following an incubation period of 2 to 21 days, clinical disease begins with nonspecific signs and symptoms including fever, headache, myalgia, abdominal pain, and malaise, which overlap with many other viral and parasitic diseases in endemic regions. This is then followed several days later by vomiting and diarrhea. Conjunctival injection or subconjunctival hemorrhage, hepatic dysfunction (AST > ALT), and metabolic derangements also are common at this stage. In the most severe cases, microvascular instability and

subsequent hemorrhage, most commonly from the GI tract will occur. CNS manifestations can occur but are less common in children than in adults. Accompanying respiratory symptoms are more common in children.

Mortality is high (~50% to 70%), but this is likely confounded by low resource setting, age, baseline health, and comorbid conditions.

77. **What is the natural reservoir host of the Ebola virus?**
Although the reservoir remains unknown, many researchers believe the virus is animal-borne initially and **fruit bats** are the most likely natural reservoir. Primates (apes and monkeys) are also possibilities. Humans may contract the disease from exposure to infected bat excreta or saliva or by exposure to blood and bodily fluids from other infected sources, such as nonhuman primates that are consumed as food. Once the first human becomes infected through contact with an infected animal, person-to-person transmission (as well as spillover from continued contact with an animal reservoir or surface and material contaminated with infected fluids) allows an epidemic to promulgate.

THE FEBRILE CHILD

". . .since the advent of modern clinical thermometry by Wunderlich in 1871, the ritual of temperature taking has been surpassed only by Alexander Graham Bell's invention in 1874 as the major curse of pediatrics"

DS Smith: Fever and the pediatrician, *J Pediatr* 77:935, 1970.

78. **At what temperature does a child have fever?**
This is a simple question without a simple answer. Because body temperatures vary among individuals and age groups and vary over the course of the day in a given individual (lowest around 4:00 to 5:00 AM and highest in late afternoon and early evening), a precise cutoff point is difficult to determine. In children between the ages of 2 and 6 years, diurnal variation can range up to 0.9 °C (1.6 °F). Infants tend to have a higher baseline temperature pattern, with 50% having daily rectal temperatures higher than 37.8 °C (100.0 °F); after the age of 2 years, this elevated baseline falls. In addition, activity and exercise (within 30 minutes), feeding or meals (within 1 hour), and hot foods (within 1 hour) can cause body temperature elevations. Most authorities agree that, for a child <3 months, a rectal temperature higher than 38 °C (100.4 °F) constitutes fever. In infants between the ages of 3 and 24 months (who tend to have a higher baseline), a temperature of 38.3 °C (101 °F) or higher likely constitutes fever. In those >2 years, as the baseline falls, fever more commonly is defined as a rectal temperature higher than 38 °C (100.4 ° F).

79. **Where did the popular notion that a normal temperature is 98.6 °F originate?**
The temperature 98.6 °F was established as the mean healthy temperature in 1868 after >1 million temperatures from 25,000 patients were analyzed. Ironically, these were axillary temperatures, and the waters of what constitutes normal have been muddied since.

Mackowiak PA, Wasserman SS, Levine MM: A critical appraisal of 98.6 °F, the upper limit of the normal body temperature, and other legacies of Carl Reinhold August Wunderlich, *JAMA* 268:1578–1580, 1992.

80. **How does temperature vary among different body sites?**
There can be significant variability in the relationship between different sites, and conversions should be done with caution. As a general guideline:
- Rectal: Standard
- Oral: 0.5° to 0.6 °C (1 °F) lower
- Axillary: 0.8° to 1.0 °C (1.5° to 2.0 °F) lower
- Tympanic: 0.5° to 0.6 °C (1 °F) lower
There also is a great deal of variability in cutaneous (such as forehead or temporal artery) infrared thermometry, depending on a variety of conditions, including age.

81. **How accurate is parental palpation for fever in infants?**
It is common for parents to report a subjective fever by palpation without measuring a temperature by thermometry. Palpation by parents has a sensitivity and specificity of about 80% in children >3 months. In infants <3 months, the positive-predictive value of a parent reporting a palpable

fever is about 60%, with a negative-predictive value of 90%. For these younger infants, for whom identification of fever carries potentially greater clinical repercussions, parents seem to overestimate the presence of a fever, but they are more accurate determining when a child is afebrile.

Katz-Sidlow RJ, Rowberry JP, Ho M: Fever determination in young infants: prevalence and accuracy of parental palpation, *Pediatr Emerg Care* 25:12–14, 2009.

82. **How should the temperature of young infants be taken?**
    In infants who are <3 months (when fever can be more significant clinically), a rectal temperature is the preferred method. Tympanic recordings are much less sensitive in this age group because the narrow, tortuous external canal can collapse, thereby resulting in readings obtained from the cooler canal rather than the warmer tympanic membrane. Cutaneous infrared temporal artery thermometry may have reduced diagnostic accuracy in this age group. Axillary temperatures often underestimate fever. The oral route is typically not used until a child is 5 to 6 years of age.

83. **How do environmental factors affect an infant's temperature?**
    Studies in neonates and infants have found mixed results. One study of newborns in a warm environment of 80 °F (26 °C) found that rectal temperatures in bundled infants could be elevated to more than 38 °C, which is the "febrile range," although newborn infants may have a physiologically lower body temperature. Another study of infants 3-months-old and younger found that in room temperatures of 22.2° to 23.8 °C (72° to 75 °F), the bundling of infants for up to 65 minutes did not produce any rectal temperatures higher than 38 °C. Infants are also prone to hypothermia, especially in the hours following birth. Direct skin-to-skin contact in newborn infants has been shown to raise and sustain newborn temperatures. Smaller or preterm infants may be most susceptible to environmental factors such as cooler ambient temperatures.

Nimbalkar SM, Patel VK, Patel DV, et al: Effect of early skin-to-skin contact following normal delivery on incidence of hypothermia in neonates more than 1800 g: randomized control trial, *J Perinatol* 34:364–368, 2014.
Grover C, Berkowitz CD, Lewis RJ, et al: The effects of bundling on infant temperature, *Pediatrics* 94:669–673, 1994.

84. **What is occult bacteremia?**
    Occult bacteremia refers to the finding of bacteria in the blood of patients, usually between the ages of 3 and 36 months, who are febrile without a clinically apparent focus of infection.

85. **How has the pneumococcal vaccine (PCV) affected the incidence of occult bacteremia?**
    In trials done after the introduction of the *Haemophilus influenzae* type B (Hib) vaccine (1990) but before the introduction of the pneumococcal conjugate vaccine (2000), bacteremia rates for pneumococcus ranged from 1.6% to 3.1% in febrile ($\geq$39.0 °C), non–toxic-appearing children from ages 2 to 36 months. Since the introduction of the pneumococcal conjugate vaccine against 7 serotypes and 2 cross-reactive serotypes (PCV-7) of *S. pneumoniae*, bacteremia rates for *S. pneumoniae* have fallen to <1%. This benefit was sustained after the introduction in 2010 of the 13-valent PCV, which added coverage against 6 other serotypes. Other benefits, such as reduction in all types of invasive pneumococcal disease (e.g., community-acquired pneumonia) have also been noted, especially in children <2 years of age. Children who are incompletely immunized are at higher risk compared with those fully immunized, but this effect is mitigated somewhat by herd immunity in countries and communities with high vaccination rates.

Joffe MD, Alpern ER: Occult pneumococcal bacteremia: a review, *Pediatr Emerg Care* 26:448–454, 2010.
Wilkinson M, Bulloch B, Smith M: Prevalence of occult bacteremia in children ages 3 to 36 months presenting to the emergency department in the postpneumococcal conjugate vaccine era, *Acad Emerg Med* 16:220–225, 2009.

86. **What is meant by "serotype replacement"?**
    This is an increase in infections caused by serotypes not included in a vaccine. In the case of the initial conjugate pneumococcal vaccine in 2000, 7 vaccine serotypes and 2 cross-reactive serotypes were included in the vaccine and accounted for about 80% of invasive pneumococcal disease. Pneumococci have >90 serotypes, and after the introduction of that vaccine, there was a rise of infections caused

by nonvaccine serotypes, particularly 19A. The 13-valent conjugate vaccine (which added serotype 19A among others) was licensed in 2010 and early reports do indicate new serotype replacement patterns.

Angoulvant F, Levy C, Grimprel E, et al: Early impact of 13-valent pneumococcal conjugate vaccine on community-acquired pneumonia in children, *Clin Infect Dis* 58:918–924 2014.
Muñoz-Almagro C, Jordan I, Gene A, et al: Emergence of invasive pneumococcal disease caused by nonvaccine serotypes in the era of the 7-valent conjugate vaccine, *Clin Infect Dis* 46:183–185, 2008.

87. **What is the proper way to evaluate and manage febrile illness in neonates ≤28 days?**
    In general, patients <1 month with fever (≥38.0 °C) warrant urgent evaluation (including blood, urine, and CSF cultures) because of higher rates of bacteremia (including pathogens from the neonatal period such as group B streptococci) and greater difficulty in global assessment of wellness.

Jain S, Cheng J, Alpern ER, et al: Management of febrile neonates in US pediatric emergency departments, *Pediatrics* 133:187–195, 2014.

88. **What is the evaluation and management of febrile illness in infants >28 days to 90 days?**
    This remains controversial as the Hib and pneumococcal conjugate vaccines have altered the landscape of invasive bacterial disease. On average, up to 7% of febrile infants who are <3 months have serious bacterial infections (SBI), which can include bacteremia, meningitis, osteomyelitis, septic arthritis, UTI, or pneumonia. Of these, UTIs comprise the greatest percentage of bacterial infections. The incidence of bacterial meningitis and SBI due to *S. pneumoniae* has fallen; this is likely due in part to herd immunity secondary to vaccination of older infants. Consequently, in a well-appearing febrile infant, a previous emphasis on a comprehensive evaluation (i.e., urine, serum and CSF testing) has declined significantly. A 2014 study of 37 U.S. pediatric emergency departments (EDs) found that comprehensive evaluations were done in febrile infants (29 to 56 days) only 49% of the time and in older infants (57 to 89 days) only 13% of the time without a change in outcome compared with those without comprehensive evaluations. Thus, local institutional guidelines based on regional epidemiology, institutional experience, provider experience, and cohort data have become the norm in the absence of national guidelines. A urinalysis and urine culture are now the most important laboratory studies given the higher likelihoods of UTIs compared with other occult bacterial processes. Many centers also obtain a complete blood count and blood culture in this age group. Lumbar punctures (LPs) are commonly deferred in a smiling, well-appearing, febrile infant.

Aronson PL, Thurm C, Alpern ER, et al: Variation in care of the febrile young infant <90 days in US pediatric emergency departments, *Pediatrics* 134:667–677, 2014.
Hernandez DA, Nguyen V: Fever in infants <3 months old: what is the current standard? *Pediatr Emerg Med Rep* 16:1–15, 2011.

89. **How should older infants and toddlers (3 to 36 months old) with fever and no apparent source be managed?**
    Previously, much of the evaluation that centered on febrile children in this age group dealt with identifying possible occult bacteremia with the intent of using empiric antibiotic treatment to lessen the chance of dissemination to focal complications (particularly meningitis). However, rates of bacteremia and meningitis have fallen dramatically, particularly with the introduction of the conjugate pneumococcal vaccine. The most common cause of SBI in children with fever without a source in this age range is an occult UTI. Most pediatric infectious disease experts no longer recommend a complete blood count and/or blood culture or any laboratory tests (other than urinalysis and urine culture in certain settings) in the evaluation of a well-appearing febrile infant >90 days who has received Hib and pneumococcal vaccines because of the low risk for bacteremia and meningitis.

Hamilton JL, John SP: Evaluation of fever in infants and young children, *Am Fam Physician* 87:254–260, 2013.
Arora R, Mahajan P: Evaluation of child with fever without source: a review of literature and update, *Pediatr Clin North Am* 60:1049–1062, 2013.

90. When is a chest radiograph indicated for a febrile young infant?

Although some clinicians believe that chest radiographs should be performed for all febrile infants who are <2 to 3 months, in general it is appropriate to perform this study for neurologically normal infants who have respiratory symptoms or signs, including cough, tachypnea, irregular breathing, retractions, rales, wheezing, or decreased breath sounds. In a study done in the pre-PCV era of infants <8 weeks who were admitted with fever, 31% of patients with respiratory manifestations had an abnormal chest radiograph, compared with only 1% of asymptomatic infants. Leukocytosis (>20,000/mL) in febrile (>39 °C) patients <5 years increases the likelihood of an "occult pneumonia." In most cases, it is not possible to differentiate viral from bacterial pneumonias radiologically.

Hernandez DA, Nguyen V: Fever in infants <3 months old: what is the current standard? *Pediatr Emerg Med Rep* 16:1–15, 2011.

Murphy CG, van de Pol AC, Harper MB, et al: Clinical predictors of occult pneumonia in the febrile child, *Acad Emerg Med* 14:243–249, 2007.

Crain EF, Bulas D, Bijur PE, Goldman HS: Is a chest radiograph necessary in the evaluation of every febrile infant less than 8 weeks of age? *Pediatrics* 88:821–824, 1991.

91. What is the approach for a 2-week-old, otherwise healthy, afebrile, full-term female who presents to the ED with mastitis?

As the overall incidence of community-acquired *S. aureus,* including MRSA isolates, increases, this subject is controversial. Case series have shown that the majority of these lesions from which organisms are recovered are "community strains" of *S. aureus.* Included in the differential diagnosis is group B streptococcal (GBS) cellulitis-adenitis syndrome caused by serotype III. SSTIs are included in many algorithms as high risk for SBIs, but many of these infants are afebrile and without signs of disseminated infection, making their management unclear. Many providers will proceed with a full sepsis evaluation, including LP because of the age of the infant. As with the febrile infant, there is a diversity of practices both within and among institutions based on local epidemiology, provider experience, and patient demographics. Therapy should include coverage for *S. aureus*, including MRSA. One large case series found that a number of infants with localized *S. aureus* SSTIs who had an LP done had a sterile CSF pleocytosis, hypothesized to be an inflammatory reaction to bacterial toxins, further confounding treatment and diagnosis. GBS cellulitis-adenitis is a manifestation of late-onset GBS disease, and should be aggressively evaluated and treated if there is suspicion for this condition.

Nguyen R, Bhat R, Teshome G: Question 2: Is a lumbar puncture necessary in an afebrile newborn infant with localised skin and soft tissue infection? *Arch Dis Child* 99:695–698, 2014.

Fortunov RM, Hulten KG, Hammerman WA, et al: Evaluation and treatment of community-acquired *Staphylococcus aureus* infections in term and late-preterm previously healthy neonates, *Pediatrics.* 120:937–945, 2007.

92. What is a CLABSI?

A central line–associated blood stream infection (CLABSI) is defined as a BSI in a symptomatic patient with a central venous catheter that terminates at or close to the heart and who has had a hospital stay of at least 3 days. The line must be in place for >2 calendar days, and the BSI must occur while the line is in place or within 1 day of removal. There are multiple initiatives put forth by the National Healthcare Safety Network to reduce rates of CLABSIs because it is estimated that most of these infections may be preventable.

Hazamy P, Haley VB, Tserenpuntsag B, et al: Effect of 2013 National Healthcare Safety Network definition changes on central line bloodstream infection rates: Audit results from the New York State Department of Health, *Am J Infect Control* S0196-6553:1332–1337, 2014.

Beekmann SE, Diekema DJ, Huskins WC, et al: Diagnosing and reporting of central line–associated bloodstream infections, *Infect Control Hosp Epidemiol* 33:875–888, 2012.

93. How long should one wait before a blood culture is designated negative?

Bacterial growth is evident in most cultures of infected blood within 48 hours or earlier. With the use of continuous monitoring techniques, a study at Children's Hospital of Philadelphia of 200 cultures from central venous catheters found that the median time for a positive blood culture was 14 hours. In addition, 99.2% of cultures with gram-negative bacteria were positive by 36 hours, and 97%

of cultures with gram-positive bacteria were positive by 36 hours. A study from Australia of neonatal blood cultures found that the median time for positivity for group B *Streptococcus* was 9 hours, that for *E. coli* was 11 hours, and that for coagulase-negative staphylococci was 29 hours. Although 36 to 48 hours is generally sufficient time to isolate common bacteria present in the bloodstream, fastidious organisms may take longer to grow. Therefore, when one suspects anaerobes, fungi, or other organisms with special growth requirements, a longer time should be allowed before concluding that a culture is negative.

Shah SS, Downes KJ, et al: How long does it take to "rule out" bacteremia in children with central venous catheters? *Pediatrics* 121:135–141, 2008.
Jardine L, Davies MW, Faoagali J: Incubation time required for neonatal blood cultures to become positive, *J Paediatr Child Health* 42:797–802, 2006.

94. **What is the utility of so-called "rapid" pathogen testing?**
    Testing of antigens for influenza A and B and RSV was developed several years ago to provide rapid diagnosis of respiratory viruses known to cause severe disease in certain populations and for which some therapy exists. These generally had good specificity but lower sensitivity. More recently, PCR-based testing has a very high sensitivity and specificity for many common viruses and bacteria. These have been combined into panels of common respiratory viruses, pertussis, and bacteria causing atypical pneumonia, as well as a panel of common GI viruses, protozoa, and enteropathic bacteria. On one hand, some believe that the use of these tests may reduce antibiotic use in respiratory viral illnesses; others worry that the diagnosis of a common respiratory virus in a febrile young child may be falsely reassuring. Recommendations developed during the H1N1 influenza epidemic in 2009 discouraged outpatient and ED providers from testing patients for influenza who did not meet guidelines for antiviral therapy, but did recommend testing for patients ill enough to be hospitalized, for those with risk factors for severe disease, or patients with a suspected nosocomial illness. Initiation of antiviral therapy should not be delayed pending results of any viral testing in a child in whom treatment is indicated.

95. **When is a fever considered a fever of unknown origin (FUO)?**
    FUO is defined as the presence of daily (or nearly daily) fever (temperature of >38.3 °C [101 °F]) for at least 8 days in a single illness in a patient for whom a careful history, thorough physical examination, and preliminary laboratory data fail to reveal the probable cause.

96. **What is the eventual etiology of fever in children with FUO?**
    The differential diagnosis is extremely broad. The three major categories are **infectious**, **inflammatory** (e.g., vasculitis, rheumatoid arthritis), and **neoplastic**. Approximately half of cases have no identifiable cause, and the fever resolves without explanation. The largest category is *infectious*. As a general rule, in children <6 years, the most common causes involve respiratory or genitourinary tract infections; localized infections (e.g., abscess, osteomyelitis); juvenile rheumatoid arthritis; and, infrequently, leukemia. Adolescents, on the other hand, are more likely to have tuberculosis; inflammatory bowel disease; another autoimmune process; or, infrequently, lymphoma.

Marshall GS: Prolonged and recurrent fevers in children, *J Infect* 68:S83–S93, 2014.
Edwards KM, Halasa NB: Fever of unknown origin (FUO) and recurrent fever. In Bergelson JM, Shah SS, Zaoutis TE, editors: *Pediatric Infectious Diseases: The Requisites in Pediatrics.* Philadelphia, 2008, Mosby Elsevier, pp 266–273.

97. **How should a child with FUO be evaluated?**
    FUO is more likely to be an unusual presentation of a common disorder than a common presentation of a rare disorder. The diagnostic approach includes a meticulous fever diary with vigilance for the appearance of new signs and symptoms. A complete and detailed history is key, with particular attention to possible exposures, including animals, unpasteurized milk (*Yersinia* or *Campylobacter*), uncooked poultry, ticks, pica, or dirt ingestion (possible *Toxocara* or *Toxoplasma*), rabbits (*Tularemia*), mosquitoes, stagnant water, and reptiles (*Salmonella*). Travel history is also important. After performing a thorough physical examination, one should avoid indiscriminately ordering a large battery of tests. Initial tests may include a complete blood count, screen for inflammation (C-reactive protein or erythrocyte sedimentation rate), tests of renal function, liver enzymes, uric acid, LDH, urinalysis, urine and blood cultures, tuberculin skin test, and chest radiograph. Laboratory studies should subsequently be

targeted as much as possible toward the most likely diagnostic possibilities. The pace of the workup is determined by the severity of the illness.

Marshall GS: Prolonged and recurrent fevers in children, *J Infect* 68:S83–S93, 2014.
Tolan RW Jr: Fever of unknown origin: a diagnostic approach to this vexing problem, *Clin Pediatr* 49:207–213, 2010.

98. What is PFAPA?

PFAPA is the acronym for the syndrome of **p**eriodic **f**ever, **a**phthous stomatitis, **p**haryngitis, and cervical **a**denitis, a clinical syndrome of unclear etiology that is responsive to very short courses of corticosteroids for individual episodes and is perhaps the most common cause of regular, recurrent fevers in children. Despite the fear it instills in many parents, it is a benign, self-limited condition that resolves without therapy, and typically remits as children grow older. Tonsillectomy may provide benefit in protracted cases.

Feder HM, Salazar JC: A clinical review of 105 patients with PFAPA (a periodic fever syndrome), *Acta Paediatr* 99:178–184, 2010.

99. In addition to PFAPA, which syndromes are associated with periodic fevers?

Predictable periodic fever is a cardinal feature of a small number of *autoinflammatory disorders*, which are thought to be due to primary dysregulation of the innate immune system and may involve mutated proteins. Many are hereditary and have ethnic predilections. Periodic fever is uncommon in infectious diseases and malignancies. The most common periodic fever syndromes are summarized in Table 10-3.

Table 10-3 Characteristics of PFAPA Versus Other Selected Fever Syndromes

	PFAPA	FAMILIAL MEDITERRANEAN FEVER	HYPER-IGD SYNDROME (HIDS)	TNF-RECEPTOR-ASSOCIATED PERIODIC SYNDROME (TRAPS)
Age at onset	Childhood	<10 yr (80%)	Childhood	Variable
Length of fever episode	4 days	2 days	4-6 days	1-3 wk
Interval between fever episodes	2-8 wk	Irregular	Irregular	Irregular
Associated symptoms and signs	Aphthous stomatitis, pharyngitis, adenitis	Painful pleuritis, peritonitis, oligoarthritis, foot and ankle rash	Abdominal pain, cervical adenopathy, splenomegaly	Abdominal pain, pleuritis, rash, myalgias, orbital edema
Inheritance	Random	Autosomal recessive	Autosomal recessive	Autosomal dominant

IgD = Immunoglobulin D; PFAPA = syndrome of periodic fever, aphthous stomatitis, pharyngitis, and cervical adenitis; TNF = tumor necrosis factor.
Data from Goldsmith DP: Periodic fever syndromes, Pediatr Rev 30:e34–e41, 2009.

HUMAN IMMUNODEFICIENCY VIRUS INFECTION

100. How common is the maternal-to-infant transmission of HIV?

Virtually all infants born to mothers who are human immunodeficiency virus (HIV)-1 seropositive will acquire antibody to the virus transplacentally. Without any treatment, about 25% (range, 13% to 39%) of these infants will ultimately develop an active HIV infection. In nonbreastfeeding populations, about 30% of maternal-to-infant HIV transmission occurs *in utero*, and the remainder occurs intrapartum. Vertical transmission of HIV-2 is less common, occurring in 0% to 4% of cases.

DeCock KM, Fowler MG, Mercier E, et al: Mother-to-child transmission of HIV-1: timing and implications for prevention, *Lancet Infect Dis* 11:726–732, 2006.
Abrams EJ, Weedon J, Bertolli J, et al: New York City Pediatric Surveillance of Disease Consortium, Centers for Disease Control and Prevention: Aging cohort of perinatally human immunodeficiency virus-infected children in New York City. New York City Pediatric Surveillance of Disease Consortium, *Pediatr Infect Dis J* 20:511–517, 2001.

101. What drugs are recommended for reducing the maternal-to-infant transmission of HIV?

Currently, interventions to prevent transmission target the late intrauterine and intrapartum periods when the highest likelihood of transmission occurs. HIV-infected pregnant women in the United States are treated with combination antiretroviral therapy the same as nonpregnant adults. All HIV-exposed newborn infants should receive zidovudine (AZT) at a dose of 4 mg/kg orally every 12 hours for the first 6 weeks of life. Among infants born to mothers with high viral loads or those in whom antepartum and/or intrapartum prophylaxis was incomplete or not received, treatment with nevirapine is recommended (first dose at birth to 48 hours, second dose 48 hours after first dose, and third dose 96 hours after second dose). Nevirapine should be started as soon as possible after birth. Elective cesarean delivery is also recommended for women with high HIV loads.

AIDS Info: Recommendations for Use of Antiretroviral Drugs in Pregnant HIV-1-Infected Women for Maternal Health and Interventions to Reduce Perinatal HIV Transmission in the United States. http://aidsinfo.nih.gov. Accessed on Mar. 23, 2015.
Committee on Pediatric AIDS: HIV testing and prophylaxis to prevent mother-to-child transmission in the United States, *Pediatrics* 122:1127–1134, 2008.

102. What are the risk factors for perinatal transmission of HIV?
- AZT monotherapy during pregnancy (compared with combination antiretroviral therapy)
- High maternal viral load at or near delivery
- Rupture of membranes >4 hours before delivery
- Fetal instrumentation with scalp electrodes and forceps
- Vaginal delivery (especially with high maternal viral loads)
- Episiotomies and vaginal tears
- Prematurity and low birth weight (possible impaired fetal or placental membranes)
- Concurrent maternal HSV-2 infection (increased shedding of HIV in genital secretions)
- Breastfeeding
- Incidence of HIV during pregnancy and postpartum

Landesman SH, Kalish LA, Burns DN, et al: Obstetrical factors and the transmission of HIV, *Curr HIV Res* 11:10, 2013.
Paintsil E, Andiman WA: Update on successes and challenges regarding mother-to-child transmission of HIV, *Curr Opin Pediatr* 21:95, 2009.

103. Should HIV-infected women breast-feed?

No. HIV has been shown to be present in breast milk and also to be transmissible by breastfeeding. Worldwide, up to one-third to one-half of maternal-to-child transmission of HIV may occur through breastfeeding. This risk is increased when the infection is acquired after birth. Thus, in developed countries where alternative means of nutrition (i.e., formula) are readily available, breastfeeding is not recommended. In developing countries where breastfeeding may be protective against other causes of significant morbidity and mortality (e.g., diarrheal and respiratory illnesses) and alternative means of nutrition are less reliably available, recommendations remain controversial. The World Health Organization (WHO) recommends exclusive breastfeeding when replacement feeding is not acceptable, feasible, affordable, or safe. Exclusive breastfeeding appears to have lower rates of transmission than mixed (e.g., formula and solid foods) breastfeeding. It remains unclear what is the optimal duration of breastfeeding to balance its protective effect with the risk of HIV transmission. It is also unclear whether maternal antiretroviral treatment during lactation will reduce the risk for HIV-1 transmission during breastfeeding, and what the actual risk of an undetectable maternal viral load is to the breastfeeding infant.

AIDS Info: Recommendations for Use of Antiretroviral Drugs in Pregnant HIV-1-Infected Women for Maternal Health and Interventions to Reduce Perinatal HIV Transmission in the United States. http://aidsinfo.nih.gov/contentfiles/lvguidelines/perinatalgl.pdf. Accessed on Jan. 14, 2015.

Kuhn L, Reitz C, Abrams EJ: Breastfeeding and AIDS in the developing world, *Curr Opin Pediatr* 21:83–93, 2009.

Coovadia HM, Rollins NC, Bland RM, et al: Mother-to-child transmission of HIV-1 infection during exclusive breastfeeding in the first 6 months of life: an intervention cohort study, *Lancet* 369:1107–1116, 2007.

104. **How is an infection with HIV confirmed in the newborn infant?**
Because maternal antibody may persist in the infant well into the second year of life, enzyme-linked immunosorbent assay (ELISA) testing and Western blot testing are unreliable until about 18 months of age. Therefore, the diagnosis of HIV infection in the newborn usually relies on the direct detection of the virus or viral components in the infant's blood or body fluids by nucleic acid amplification testing (NAAT). The gold standard for diagnostic testing of infants and children <18 months is HIV-1 NAAT, which can directly detect HIV-1 deoxyribonucleic acid (DNA) or ribonucleic acid (RNA).
Infants born to HIV-infected women who have not taken antiretroviral therapy should be tested by HIV-1 NAAT during the first 48 hours of life to determine whether *in utero* acquisition has occurred. If a mother has been taking antiretroviral therapy since the second trimester and has an undetectable viral load the week before delivery, the risk for *in utero* transmission is low. An HIV-1 NAAT should be done within the first 14 to 21 days of life and at age 1 to 2 months and again at age 4 to 6 months. HIV can be *presumptively* excluded with 2 or more negative tests: one at age 14 days or older and the other at age 1 month or older. HIV is considered *definitively* excluded (in nonbreast-fed infants) on the basis of two negative virologic tests, with one test performed at age 1 month or older and the other test at age 4 months or older. A negative HIV-1 NAAT at 8 weeks also *presumptively* indicates disease exclusion. Any time a positive result is obtained, testing should be repeated on a second blood sample as soon as possible. The diagnosis of HIV infection is established if two separate samples are found to be positive by PCR testing. For children with negative testing, many experts recommend HIV-1 antibody assay testing at 12 to 18 months to confirm the absence of HIV infection.

AIDS Info: Recommendations for Use of Antiretroviral Drugs in Pregnant HIV-1-Infected Women for Maternal Health and Interventions to Reduce Perinatal HIV Transmission in the United States. http://aidsinfo.nih.gov/contentfiles/lvguidelines/perinatalgl.pdf. Accessed on Jan. 14, 2015.

Havens PL, Mofenson LM: Evaluation and management of the infant exposed to HIV-1 in the United States, *Pediatrics* 123:175–187, 2009.

Schutzbank WS, Steele RW: Management of the child born to an HIV-positive mother, *Clin Pediatr* 48:467–471, 2009.

105. **What are the earliest and most common manifestations of congenital HIV infection?**
    - Most infants with congenital HIV infection are asymptomatic at birth, although occasional patients have diffuse lymphadenopathy and hepatosplenomegaly.
    - Older infants with HIV infection commonly present symptoms of failure to thrive, loss of or failure to obtain normal developmental milestones, mucocutaneous candidiasis (especially after 1 year), hepatosplenomegaly, interstitial pneumonitis, or a combination of these features.
    - Toddlers and older children with HIV infection may have generalized lymphadenopathy, recurrent bacterial infections, recurrent or chronic parotitis, or progressive encephalopathy and loss of developmental milestones.

Simpkins EP, Siberry GK, Hutton N: Thinking about HIV infection, *Pediatr Rev* 30:337–348, 2009.

106. **When should *Pneumocystis* prophylaxis begin and end for an HIV-exposed infant?**
Historically, the peak incidence of *Pneumocystis* pneumonia in HIV-infected infants occurred at the age of 3 months (range, 4 weeks to 6 months). *Pneumocystis* prophylaxis should be initiated at the age of 4 to 6 weeks and continued until the infant is at least 4 months old unless the infant meets criteria for being *definitively or presumptively* HIV-uninfected. If the HIV status of the child is indeterminate

or confirmed positive, *Pneumocystis jiroveci* pneumonia prophylaxis should be continued until the child is 12 months old, at which time reassessment is done (based on CD4 T-lymphocyte counts).

AIDS Info: Guidelines for the Prevention and Treatment of Opportunistic Infections Among HIV-Exposed and HIV-Infected Children. http://aidsinfo.nih.gov/contentfiles/lvguidelines/oi_guidelines_pediatrics.pdf. Accessed on Jan. 14, 2015.

107. **Among patients <13 years of age with HIV infection, how is the severity of HIV illness classified?**
    According to the 1994 revised Pediatric HIV Classification System, for children 12 months of age and younger, three categories are used, which include CD4 count, percentage of total lymphocytes, and clinical staging (Table 10-4).

Terms, definitions and calculations used in CDC HIV surveillance publications: www.cdc.gov/hiv/statistics/recommendations/terms.html. Accessed on Mar. 23, 2015.

108. **What is the significance of the "viral load"?**
    Viral load refers to a quantification of HIV viral RNA as measured by various assays. It is a measure of the degree of infection; the lower limit of detection on ultrasensitive assays is 20 copies/mL, with an upper range of 20 to 50 million copies/mL. Higher levels are associated with increased likelihoods of rapid disease progression and poorer long-term prognosis. Viral loads are used as an ongoing measure of efficacy of treatment with the goal to achieve an undetectable level for as long as possible.

109. **What are the classes of antiretroviral agents (ARTs) used to treat HIV?**
    - **Nucleoside and nucleotide analogue reverse transcriptase inhibitors** (NRTIs) competitively inhibit the HIV reverse transcriptase (which converts HIV RNA into DNA) and terminate the elongation of viral DNA. They require intracellular phosphorylation for activation. NRTIs have little or no effect on chronically infected cells because their site of action is before the incorporation of viral DNA into host DNA. This class of drugs includes zidovudine, lamivudine, stavudine, zalcitabine, didanosine (ddI), tenofovir, emtricitabine, and abacavir.
    - **Nonnucleoside reverse transcriptase inhibitors** (NNRTIs) also inhibit the HIV reverse transcriptase, although they do so at a different site than do the NRTIs. They bind directly to the active site of HIV reverse transcriptase and do not require activation. This class of drugs includes efavirenz, nevirapine, etravirine, and rilpivirine.
    - **Protease inhibitors** (PIs) inhibit the HIV protease, which cuts HIV polyprotein precursors before viral budding. This class of drugs includes atazanavir, darunavir, fosamprenavir, nelfinavir, ritonavir, indinavir, saquinavir, tipranavir, and lopinavir/ritonavir (Kaletra).
    - **Integrase inhibitors** block the action of a viral enzyme that inserts the viral genome into the DNA of host cells. This class of drugs includes raltegravir, dolutegravir, and elvitegravir.
    - **Entry and fusion inhibitors** include enfuvirtide and maraviroc.

Guidelines for treatment of HIV-infected children and adolescents are regularly updated and available at http://www.aidsinfo.nih.gov/Guidelines. Accessed on Jan. 27, 2015. 5 Generally, triple-drug therapy (so-called potent combination antiretroviral therapy [c ART]) is recommended.
Patel K, Hernán MA, Williams PL, et al: Long-term effectiveness of highly active antiretroviral therapy on the survival of children and adolescents with HIV infection: a 10-year follow-up study, *Clin Infect Dis* 46:507–515, 2008.

110. **What are the common toxicities associated with antiretroviral therapy?**
    - Anemia occurs in up to 9% of children receiving AZT (compared with 4% to 5% of those on other regimens), and may be exacerbated in newborns because of the coincident physiologic nadir. Neutropenia occurs in 6% to 27% of children receiving antiretroviral therapy, particularly those taking AZT and ddI.
    - Thrombocytopenia occurs in 30% of untreated children with HIV infection and is more commonly an initial presentation of HIV infection than a complication of antiretroviral therapy. In initial trials, severe thrombocytopenia was seen in 2% of children receiving either ddI and AZT or lamivudine and AZT.

Table 10-4 Pediatric Human Immunodeficiency Virus (HIV) Classification for Children Younger Than 13 Years of Age

IMMUNOLOGIC DEFINITIONS	AGE-SPECIFIC CD4+ T-LYMPHOCYTE COUNT AND PERCENTAGE OF TOTAL LYMPHOCYTES						Immunologic Categories Clinical Classifications[a]			
	Younger Than 12 mo		1 Through 5y		6 Through 12y		N: No Signs or Symptoms	A: Mild Signs and Symptoms[b]	B: Moderate Signs and Symptoms	C: Severe Signs and Symptoms
	µL	%	µL	%	µL	%				
1: No evidence of suppression	≥1500	≥25	≥1000	≥25	≥500	≥25	N1	A1	B1	C1
2: Evidence of moderate suppression	750–1499	15–24	500–999	15–24	200–499	15–24	N2	A2	B2	C2
3: Severe suppression	<750	<15	<500	<15	<200	<15	N3	A3	B3	C3

[a]Children whose HIV infection status is not confirmed are classified by using this grid with a letter E (for perinatally exposed) placed before the appropriate classification code (eg, EN2).

[b]Lymphoid interstitial pneumonitis in category B or any condition in category C is reportable to state and local health departments as acquired immunodeficiency syndrome (AIDS-defining conditions).

AAP Committee on Infectious Diseases, Larry K. Pickering, Carol J. Baker, David W. Kimberlin. Red Book, 29th Edition (2012), American Academy of Pediatrics.

- Lipodystrophy can occur in children treated with NRTI, protease inhibitors (PIs), and efavirenz.
- GI side effects: Many children experience GI adverse effects such as nausea, vomiting, diarrhea, and abdominal pain, especially when AZT and PIs are initiated.
- CNS effects are encountered when initiating therapy with efavirenz. Commons symptoms include dizziness, drowsiness, vivid dreams, or insomnia. Rarely, seizures have been reported in children.
- Hepatitis can occur with almost all ARTs, but is seen less commonly in children than adults. Atazanavir and indinavir commonly cause indirect hyperbilirubinemia and for this reason are generally not used in neonates.
- Metabolic abnormalities such as dyslipidemia and insulin resistance can occur with most ART regimens.

http://aidsinfo.nih.gov/guidelines/html/1/adult-and-adolescent-arv-guidelines/31/adverse-effects-of-arv. Accessed on Mar. 20, 2015.

111. How should nonadherence to HIV medication be addressed?

Noncompliance with highly active antiretroviral therapy (HAART) regimens has been estimated as >50%, with the number being much higher for high-risk groups such as newly diagnosed teenagers and adolescents who acquired HIV perinatally. Close follow-up and simplification of medical therapy, when possible, are key. Recognizing and treating comorbid conditions such as depression and alcohol and drug abuse are also important. Intense follow-up (e.g., weekly) for some high-risk patients is recommended. Youth-friendly technology-based support interventions, such as cell phone and text message follow-up, are showing some promise in improving adherence.

Belzer ME, Naar-King S, Olson J, et al: The use of cell phone support for non-adherent HIV-infected youth and young adults: an initial randomized and controlled intervention trial, *AIDS Behav* 18:686–696, 2014.

112. Should a classroom teacher be told that a child is HIV positive?

There is no absolute requirement to inform a classroom teacher, a school principal, or childcare provider about a child's HIV status. It is not necessary for anyone except the child's physician to be aware of the diagnosis. In certain circumstances such as children with conditions that may lead to blood exposure, such as severe excoriated eczema or bleeding diathesis, it is advisable for a family to discuss this with the child's physician before starting any out-of-home program.

American Academy of Pediatrics: School health. In Pickering LK, editor: *2012 Red Book: Report of the Committee on Infectious Diseases*, ed 29. Elk Grove Park, IL, 2012, American Academy of Pediatrics, p 147.

113. What are the risk factors for HIV transmission after a needlestick injury?

In a case-controlled study that involved 33 health-care workers and 665 controls, the following risk factors were identified:

- High viral inoculum (patient with advanced disease)
- Large volume of blood (from a large-bore hollow needle)
- Deep puncture wound

Overall, the risk for transmission from needles contaminated with the blood of an HIV-infected patient is roughly 0.3%. Risk from a puncture wound in a random community setting is thought to be lower. There are no known transmissions from accidental nonoccupational (community) needlesticks.

American Academy of Pediatrics: Human immunodeficiency virus infection. In Pickering LK, editor: *2012 Red Book: Report of the Committee on Infectious Diseases*, ed 29. Elk Grove Park, IL, 2012, American Academy of Pediatrics, pp 438–439.
Cardo DM, Culver DH, Ciesielski CA, et al: A case-control study of HIV seroconversion in health care workers after percutaneous exposure. Centers for Disease Control and Prevention Needlestick Surveillance Group, *N Engl J Med* 337:1485–1490, 1997.

KEY POINTS: HUMAN IMMUNODEFICIENCY VIRUS INFECTION

1. Interventions to prevent maternal HIV transmission target the late intrauterine and intrapartum periods when the highest likelihood of transmission occurs.
2. Most infants with congenital HIV infection are asymptomatic at birth.
3. The gold standard for diagnostic testing of infants and children <18 months is HIV-1 nucleic acid amplification testing (NAAT), which can directly detect HIV-1 DNA or RNA.
4. Viral loads are used as an ongoing measure of treatment efficacy.
5. Triple-therapy (so-called potent combination antiretroviral therapy [cART]) is recommended for HIV-infected children.
6. Risk factors for increased HIV transmission after a needlestick injury include a high viral inoculum, large volume of blood, and deep puncture wound.

IMMUNIZATIONS

114. What is the derivation of the word "vaccination"?
    Edward Jenner, an eighteenth century British physician, had observed that dairymaids were protected naturally from smallpox, the infectious scourge of the world at that time, after they had developed cowpox, a milder blistering disease. In 1796, he inoculated a young boy with material from fresh cowpox lesions that had been taken from a dairymaid. Two months later, he again inoculated the boy, but with matter from a fresh smallpox lesion. No disease developed and the science of immunization was born. Because the Latin word for cow was *vacca* and for cowpox was *vaccinia*, Jenner called his new procedure *vaccination*.

Riedel S: Edward Jenner and the history of smallpox and vaccination, *Proc (Bayl Univ Med Cent)* 18:21–25, 2005.

115. Why are the buttocks a poor location for intramuscular (IM) injections in infants?
    The gluteus maximus is not a good choice for injections because of the following:
    - The gluteal muscles are incompletely developed in some infants.
    - There is a potential for injury to the sciatic nerve or the superior gluteal artery if the injection is misdirected.
    - Some vaccinations may be less effective if they are injected into fat (e.g., vaccines for rabies, influenza, and hepatitis B).

    If injections into the buttocks are given to older children, the proper site is the gluteus medius in the upper outer quadrant rather than the gluteus maximus, which is more medial.

Zuckerman JN: The importance of injecting vaccines into muscle, *BMJ* 321:1237–1238, 2000.

116. When administering an IM vaccination, is aspiration necessary before injection?
    Traditionally, the plunger has been withdrawn to verify that the needle tip is not in a vein. However, when vaccinations are given as recommended in the anterior lateral thigh in an infant or in the deltoid in toddlers >18 months, aspiration before injection is *not* required because no large blood vessels are located at those preferred sites. Additionally, the process of aspiration before injection is more painful and it takes longer to administer the vaccine.

Ipp M: Vaccine-related pain: randomized controlled trial of two injection techniques, *Arch Dis Child* 92:1105, 2007.
American Academy of Pediatrics: Acute immunization. In Pickering LK, editor: *2012 Red Book: Report of the Committee on Infectious Diseases*, ed 29. Elk Grove Park, IL, 2012, American Academy of Pediatrics, p 24.

117. Is there any risk associated with administering multiple vaccines simultaneously?
    Most vaccines can be administered simultaneously at separate sites without concern about effectiveness because the immune response to one vaccine generally does not interfere with immune responses to others. The immune system is capable of recognizing hundreds of thousands of antigens. However, some exceptions exist. For example, the simultaneous administration of cholera vaccine and yellow fever vaccine is associated with interference.

118. **Should premature babies receive immunization on the basis of postconception age or chronologic age?**

    In most cases, premature babies should be immunized in accordance with postnatal chronologic age. If a premature infant is still in the hospital at 2 months of age, the vaccines routinely scheduled for that age should be administered with the exception of the rotavirus vaccine, which should be deferred until the infant leaves the hospital because spread of this virus in patient units has been reported. Among premature infants who weigh <2 kg at birth, seroconversion rates to hepatitis B vaccine (HBV) are relatively low when immunization is initiated shortly after birth. Accordingly, in these infants, if the mother is HBsAg negative, immunization should be delayed until just before hospital discharge or until 30 days of age. If HBV is given at birth in infants < 2 kg, this should not be counted toward the primary series.

American Academy of Pediatrics: Immunization in special clinical circumstances and hepatitis B. In Pickering LK, editor: *2012 Red Book: Report of the Committee on Infectious Diseases*, ed 29. Elk Grove Park, IL, 2012, American Academy of Pediatrics, pp 69–71 and 384–384.

Saari TN, American Academy of Pediatrics Committee on Infectious Diseases: Immunization of preterm and low birth weight infants. American Academy of Pediatrics Committee on Infectious Diseases, *Pediatrics* 112:193–198, 2003.

119. **Which vaccines are egg-embryo–based vaccines?**

    Of the immunizations that are commonly administered to children, the **measles-mumps-rubella** (MMR) vaccine and certain **rabies** vaccine preparations are grown in chick embryo fibroblast culture. However, they do not contain significant amounts of egg protein. Children with egg allergy are at low risk for anaphylaxis to MMR and do not require skin testing or special precautions before or during the administration of this vaccine.

120. **What is the difference between whole-cell and acellular pertussis vaccines?**

    Whole-cell pertussis vaccines consist of whole bacteria that have been inactivated and are nonviable. These vaccines contain lipooligosaccharide and other cell wall components that result in a high incidence of adverse effects. This vaccine is no longer given in the United States.

    Acellular pertussis vaccines contain one or more *B. pertussis* proteins that serve as immunogens. All acellular pertussis vaccines contain at least detoxified pertussis toxin, and most contain other antigens as well, including filamentous hemagglutinin, fimbrial proteins, and pertactin. The acellular vaccines are associated with a much lower incidence of side effects and thus are given for all doses in the United States. Children <7 years of age who have received the whole-cell vaccine abroad should have the series continued with the acellular vaccine formulations.

American Academy of Pediatrics: Pertussis. In Pickering LK, editor: *2012 Red Book: Report of the Committee on Infectious Diseases*, ed 29. Elk Grove Park, IL, 2012, American Academy of Pediatrics, p 560.

121. **What are the absolute contraindications to pertussis immunization?**

    The adverse events after pertussis immunization that represent absolute *contraindications* to further administration of pertussis vaccine include the following:
    - Immediate anaphylactic reaction
    - Encephalopathy within 7 days of vaccination
    - Unstable or evolving neurologic conditions in children <1 year of age warrant postponement of the vaccine.

    The adverse events that represent *precautions* for further administration of pertussis vaccine include the following:
    - Moderate or severe acute illness with or without fever
    - Guillain-Barré syndrome within 6 weeks after a previous dose of tetanus toxoid-containing vaccine
    - History of arthus-type hypersensitivity reactions (local vasculitis associated with deposition of immune complexes and activation of complement) after a previous dose of tetanus or diphtheria toxoid–containing vaccine

Centers for Disease Control and Prevention: Vaccines and Immunizations. http://www.cdc.gov/vaccines/recs/vac-admin/contraindications-vacc.htm. Accessed on Jan. 14, 2015.

American Academy of Pediatrics: Pertussis. In Pickering LK, editor: *2012 Red Book: Report of the Committee on Infectious Diseases*, ed 29. Elk Grove Park, IL, 2012, American Academy of Pediatrics, pp 562–566.

122. **How long does protection against pertussis last after immunization?**
Vaccine-induced immunity to pertussis is relatively short-lived. On the basis of studies of patients who have been immunized with a whole-cell pertussis vaccine and exposed to a sibling with pertussis, protection against infection is about 80% during the first 3 years after immunization, dropping to 50% at 4 to 7 years and to near 0% at 11 years. Teenagers and adults thus become susceptible to pertussis and serve as vectors for infants, for whom morbidity and mortality are much higher. Because of the slow, steady resurgence of pertussis in the past two decades and the availability of an acellular pertussis vaccine combined with diphtheria and tetanus toxoid (Tdap), the Advisory Committee on Immunization Practices of the CDC has recommended that all adolescents >11 years of age should receive a booster dose. Anyone 19 years of age and older who has not received a dose of Tdap should also be vaccinated. This Tdap booster dose can replace 1 of the 10-year Td booster doses and is especially important for health-care workers. Additionally, all pregnant women should receive a Tdap booster during each pregnancy at 27 to 36 weeks.

Centers for Disease Control and Prevention: Pertussis: Summary of Vaccine Recommendations. http://www.cdc.gov/vaccines/vpd-vac/pertussis/recs-summary.htm. Accessed on Jan 14, 2015.
Halperin SA: The control of pertussis—2007 and beyond, *N Engl J Med* 356:110–113, 2007.

123. **What is cocooning?**
Pertussis vaccination in the United States has reduced annual pertussis-attributable morbidity and mortality by >90%. Despite this, the annual incidence of pertussis continues to rise. Some of the increase may be attributed to outbreaks in unvaccinated pockets of the country. Infants <6 months of age, who are too young to have completed the primary vaccination series, have up to a 20-fold higher incidence of pertussis than does the general population. Two-thirds of pertussis-infected infants in this age group require hospitalization, and pertussis-related deaths occur almost exclusively in young infants, the risk being inversely proportional to age and number of infant DTaP vaccine doses received. It is estimated that 75% of infants are infected by a household contact or caregiver. The Advisory Committee on Immunization Practices recommended Tdap vaccination of all adults, who come in close contact with children <1 year of age, especially health-care workers to help prevent pertussis-related complications and deaths. This circle of providing protected and protective caregivers is termed *cocooning*.
It is also recommended that all pregnant women should receive Tdap during *each* pregnancy at 27 to 36 weeks to facilitate transfer of passively acquired maternal IgG against pertussis to the infant and to ensure immunity.

American Academy of Pediatrics: Pertussis. In Pickering LK, editor: *2012 Red Book: Report of the Committee on Infectious Diseases*, ed 29. Elk Grove Park, IL, 2012, American Academy of Pediatrics, pp 562–566.
Grizas AP, Camenga D, Vázquez M: Cocooning: a concept to protect young children from infectious diseases, *Curr Opin Pediatr* 24:92–97, 2012.
Healy CM, Rench MA, Baker CJ: Implementation of cocooning against pertussis in a high-risk population, *Clin Infect Dis* 52:157–162, 2011.

124. **Which vaccines offer protection against cervical cancer?**
Vaccination for **human papillomavirus (HPV).** The first vaccine against HPV (Gardasil) was approved in 2006. It is a quadrivalent vaccine (HPV4) that prevents disease caused by HPV types 6, 11, 16, and 18. A bivalent vaccine (HPV2, Cervarix) was approved in 2009. HPV types 16 and 18 have been causally linked with cervical, vulvar, and vaginal cancers, as well as penile, anal, and oropharyngeal cancers. In December 2014, a new 9-valent HPV preparation (Gardasil 9) was approved by the FDA. The latest recommendations are that all boys and girls aged 11 or 12 years should get vaccinated. Catch-up vaccines are recommended for males through age 21 and for females through age 26, men having sex with men (MSM), and immunocompromised people through age 26 (including those with HIV and AIDS).

Human Papilloma Virus (HPV): http://www.cdc.gov/std/hpv/stdfact-hpv.htm#a4. Accessed on Jan. 14, 2015.
Jenson HB: Human papillomavirus vaccine: a paradigm shift for pediatricians, *Curr Opin Pediatr* 21:112–121, 2009.

125. **How effective is the pneumococcal conjugate vaccine?**
The pneumococcal conjugate vaccine is highly effective against invasive pneumococcal disease, reducing rates by up to 98% for vaccine-associated serotypes in children fully vaccinated during the first 2 years of

life. The greatest decline in invasive disease has been in the number of children experiencing bacteremia without a focus. This vaccine has a modest effect on pneumococcal otitis media, preventing about 35% of culture-confirmed cases in young children. Both of these effects were noted after the original heptavalent vaccine (PCV-7) was introduced in 2000. This reduction has continued at a more modest rate following the introduction of a 13-valent (PCV-13) vaccine, which includes serotype 19a, a serotype that has been noted to cause invasive disease but was not included in the PCV-7.

Angoulvant F, Levy C, Grimprel E, et al: Early impact of 13-valent pneumococcal conjugate vaccine on community-acquired pneumonia in children, *Clin Infect Dis* 58:918–924, 2014.

126. What is the "grandparent effect" of vaccination?

The rate of invasive pneumococcal disease has declined in people >65 years since the introduction of the conjugate pneumococcal vaccine in 2000. Meningitis rates have declined by 54%. Decreased nasopharyngeal carriage among vaccinated infants has likely reduced transmission to older individuals caring for them. This type of "herd effect" in elderly people is referred to as the *grandparent effect.*

Hsu HE, Shutt KA, Moore MR, et al: Effect of pneumococcal conjugate vaccine on pneumococcal meningitis, *N Engl J Med* 360:244–256, 2009.
Millar EV, Watt JP, Bronsdon MA, et al: Indirect effect of 7-valent pneumococcal conjugate vaccine on pneumococcal colonization among unvaccinated household members, *Clin Infect Dis* 47:989–996, 2008.

127. What serogroup capable of causing meningococcal infections is lacking in licensed polyvalent vaccines in the United States?

Serogroup B isolates account for about one-third of cases of meningococcal disease, but serogroup B polysaccharide is absent from these vaccines. Two quadrivalent meningococcal vaccines containing capsular polysaccharide from serogroups A, C, Y, and W135 are widely available in the United States, including a plain polysaccharide vaccine that is approved for use in children at least 2 years old and a polysaccharide diphtheria toxoid conjugate vaccine that is licensed for use in individuals 11 to 55 years old. A study in infants with the new tetravalent vaccine using a nontoxic mutant of diphtheria toxoid as the carrier protein has demonstrated good immunogenicity and may become part of the vaccination schedule for infants in the future.

All 11- to 12-year-olds should be routinely vaccinated with the conjugate vaccine. In addition, unvaccinated college freshmen living in dormitories should be offered either the plain polysaccharide vaccine or the conjugate vaccine. Vaccination is considered advisable for children at least 2 years old who are in high-risk groups, including those with functional or anatomic asplenia or complement deficiency. A meningococcal vaccine is given to all military recruits in the United States and should be considered for individuals traveling to areas of epidemic or hyperendemic disease. In addition, the current vaccines may be useful as an adjunct to chemoprophylaxis for the control of outbreaks caused by a vaccine serogroup.

Until recently, no vaccine was available in the United States with coverage of serogroup B. In October 2014, in response to recent outbreaks of serogroup B meningococcal disease on college campuses (with attributable fatalities), the first serogroup B meningococcal vaccine (Trumenba®) was approved for use in individuals 10 to 25 years of age as a 3-dose series. This vaccine does not provide coverage for serogroups A, C, Y, and W135.

Centers for Disease Control and Prevention: Meningococcal Disease. http://www.cdc.gov/meningococcal/outbreaks/vaccine-serogroupB.html. Accessed on Jan. 14, 2015.
Snape MD, Perrett KP, Ford KJ, et al: Immunogenicity of a tetravalent meningococcal glycoconjugate vaccine in infants: a randomized controlled trial, *JAMA* 299:173–184, 2008.
Bilukha OO, Rosentein N: Prevention and control of meningococcal disease: recommendations of the Advisory Committee on Immunization Practices, *MMWR* 54:1–21, 2005.

128. How effective is the varicella vaccine if given after exposure to the illness?

The varicella vaccine is highly effective (95% for the prevention of any disease, 100% for the prevention of moderate to severe disease) when used within 36 hours of exposure in an environment involving close contact. Ideally, it is given as soon as possible after the exposure but is recommended up to 5 days after exposure. The reason for the high efficacy is that naturally acquired varicella-zoster virus usually takes 5 to 7 days to propagate in the respiratory tract before primary viremia and dissemination occur, whereas vaccine virus may elicit humoral and cellular immunity in significantly less time.

Watson B, Seward J, Yang A, et al: Postexposure effectiveness of varicella vaccine, *Pediatrics* 105:84–88, 2000.

129. **Is the MMR vaccine effective in preventing measles if given after exposure to the illness?**
The measles vaccine, if given within 72 hours of measles exposure, will provide protection in some cases. In the case of a known measles exposure, such as during an outbreak, vaccination within 72 hours is recommended for all unvaccinated contacts, including children as young as 6 months. In children <1 year, this vaccine should not count as part of the primary series, which should continue as usual (with a minimum of 28 days separating vaccines).

130. **Of the vaccines included in the routine schedule, which ones contain live viruses?**
MMR, varicella, rotavirus, and influenza. Oral polio vaccine is a live attenuated virus vaccine, but it is no longer recommended for routine use. Other live virus vaccines include yellow fever virus vaccines.

KEY POINTS: IMMUNIZATIONS

1. Premature babies should be immunized in accordance with postnatal chronologic age.
2. Without a booster after age 5 years, protection against pertussis infection is about 80% during the first 3 years after immunization, dropping to 50% at 4 to 7 years and to near zero at 11 years.
3. Live vaccines include measles-mumps-rubella, varicella, cold-adapted, live-attenuated influenza, rotavirus, and yellow fever virus.
4. Vaccination of both boys and girls for human papillomavirus offers protection against cervical and other forms of cancer.
5. When administering an intramuscular vaccination, aspiration is not necessary before injection.

---

131. **What are the indications for palivizumab?**
Palivizumab is a humanized mouse monoclonal antibody that is directed against a RSV protein and that is approved for the prevention of RSV disease in selected children. It is typically administered intramuscularly for five doses, starting in November (or earlier if RSV infections are detected in the community). According to the AAP, updated recommendations for the consideration of palivizumab administration include the following:
- Infants born before 29 weeks in the first year of life
- Infants born before 32 weeks with chronic lung disease, defined as requirement for >21% oxygen for at least 28 days, also in the first year of life.
- Infants and children <2 years with chronic lung disease who are requiring ongoing medical therapy such as supplemental oxygen, chronic corticosteroid, or diuretic therapy
- Infants <12 months with hemodynamically significant congenital heart disease (i.e., not small ventricular septal defects [VSDs], atrial septal defects [ASDs], or infants with lesions adequately corrected by surgery unless they continue to require medication for congestive heart failure)
- Certain infants with neuromuscular disease or congenital abnormalities of the airways that compromise handling of respiratory secretions in the first year of life
- Infants and children <2 years who will be profoundly immunocompromised during the RSV season

Committee on Infectious Diseases and Bronchiolitis Guidelines Committee: Updated guidance for palivizumab prophylaxis among infants and young children at increased risk of hospitalization for respiratory syncytial virus infection, *Pediatrics* 134:415–420, 2014.

132. **What are the recommendations regarding the administration of live-virus vaccines to patients receiving corticosteroid therapy?**
Children receiving corticosteroid treatment can become immunosuppressed. Although some uncertainty exists, there is adequate experience to make recommendations about the administration of live-virus vaccines to previously healthy children receiving steroid treatment. In general, live-virus vaccines should not be administered to children who have received prednisone or its equivalent in a dose of 2 mg/kg/day or greater (or ≥20 mg per day for individuals whose weight is >10 kg) for more than 14 days. Treatment for shorter periods, with lower doses, or with topical preparations, local injections, or

inhaled corticosteroids should not contraindicate the use of these vaccines. However, immune suppression is possible with these medications and that should be taken into account at the time of vaccination.

American Academy of Pediatrics: Immunization in special clinical circumstances. In Pickering LK, editor: *2012 Red Book: Report of the Committee on Infectious Diseases*, ed 29. Elk Grove Park, IL, 2012, American Academy of Pediatrics, pp 81–82.

133. **What is thimerosal?**
    Thimerosal is a mercury-containing preservative that has been used as an additive to vaccines for decades because of its effectiveness for preventing contamination, especially in open, multidose containers. In an effort to reduce exposure to mercury, vaccine manufacturers, the FDA, the AAP, and other groups have worked to remove thimerosal from vaccines that contain this compound. By the end of 2001, all vaccines in the routine schedule for children and adolescents were free or virtually free of thimerosal, with the exception of some inactivated influenza vaccines.

134. **Does thimerosal or any vaccine or vaccine combination cause autism?**
    No. In the totality of studies to date, there is no compelling evidence that thimerosal or any vaccine combination causes autism, attention-deficit/hyperactivity disorder, or other neurodevelopmental disorders.

Taylor LE, Swerdfeger AL, Eslick GD: Vaccines are not associated with autism: an evidence-based meta-analysis of case-control and cohort studies, *Vaccine* 32:3623–3629, 2014.

135. **How should parents who refuse vaccinations be handled?**
    Many parents are aware about alleged controversial issues concerning routine childhood vaccines. A dialogue about specific parental concerns and beliefs should be undertaken calmly and without judgment because an ongoing discussion may be the most important step to eventual vaccine acceptance. The AAP recommends that generally, physicians should continue to care for children whose families reject immunization. However, if a physician truly believes that they cannot ethically provide care for a family, the professional relationship may be terminated after transfer of care to another physician has been ensured, and the parents have been given notice that the physician intends to terminate care. Parents who reject immunization should be advised of local laws restricting entry into school or childcare for unvaccinated or undervaccinated children. Documentation of such discussions in the medical record are advised, and sample "Refusal to Vaccinate" forms can be found on the AAP website; many states also have their form for providers generally available on individual state health department websites.

American Academy of Pediatrics: Immunization. http://www2.aap.org/immunization/pediatricians/refusaltovaccinate. html. Accessed on Jan. 14, 2015.
American Academy of Pediatrics: Active Immunization. In Pickering LK, editor: *2012 Red Book: Report of the Committee on Infectious Diseases*, ed 29. Elk Grove Park, IL, 2012, American Academy of Pediatrics, pp 10–11.
Gilmour J, Harrison C, Asadi L, et al: Childhood immunization: when physicians and parents disagree, *Pediatrics* 128:S167–S174, 2011.

INFECTIONS WITH RASH

136. What is the traditional numbering of the "original" six exanthemas of childhood, and when were they first described?
    - **First disease:** Measles (rubeola), 1627
    - **Second disease:** Scarlet fever, 1627
    - **Third disease:** Rubella, 1881
    - **Fourth disease:** Filatov-Dukes disease (described in 1900 and though to be a distinct scarlatiniform type of rubella, attributed more recently to exotoxin-producing *S. aureus*; term is no longer used)
    - **Fifth disease:** Erythema infectiosum, 1905
    - **Sixth disease:** Roseola infantum (exanthema subitum), 1910

Weisse ME: The fourth disease: 1900–2000, *Lancet* 357:299–301, 2001.

137. **What conditions are associated with fever and petechiae?**
The list is extensive because many viral and bacterial pathogens may cause a petechial rash as part of the syndrome or from associated thrombocytopenia or disseminated intravascular coagulopathy. Obviously, not all of these will be high on the differential diagnosis, but should be taken into account when evaluating the child returning from abroad.
- Human monocytic ehrlichiosis
- Drug hypersensitivity
- Meningococcemia
- Rocky mountain spotted fever
- Immune thrombocytopenic purpura
- Enteroviral infection
- Henoch-Schönlein purpura
- Staphylococcal sepsis
- Streptococcal infection
- Toxic shock syndrome
- "Infectious mononucleosis"
  - Cytomegalovirus
  - Epstein-Barr virus
  - Toxoplasmosis
- Kawasaki disease
- Adenovirus infection
- Dengue fever
- Typhus
- Arenavirus (e.g., Lassa)
- Arboviruses (e.g., yellow fever, Chikungunya)

Razzaq S, Schutze GE: Rocky mountain spotted fever, *Pediatr Rev* 26:125–129, 2005.

138. **What are the three Cs of measles?**
Cough, coryza, and conjunctivitis. After an incubation period of 4 to 12 days, these symptoms develop and are followed by a characteristic erythematous and maculopapular rash (typically on day 14 after exposure), which spreads from head to feet. The rash is described as morbilliform because it has both macular and papular features (Fig. 10-7).

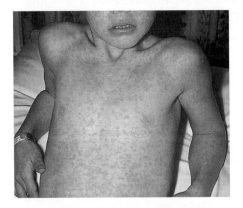

Figure 10-7. Morbilliform rash of measles. *(From Hobson RP: Infectious disease. In Walker BR, Colledge NR, Ralston SH, Penman ID: Davidson's Principles and Practice of Medicine, ed 22. Philadelphia, Elsevier, 2014.)*

139. **What do Koplik spots look like?**
Koplik spots are thought to be pathognomonic for measles. They are punctate white-gray papules that occur on a red background, initially opposite the lower molars, but they may spread to involve other parts of the mucosa (Fig. 10-8). However, they may be present for a day or less, are often difficult to appreciate, and should not be relied on to rule in or out the diagnosis.

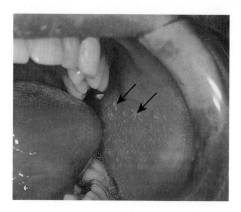

Figure 10-8. Koplik spots *(arrows). (From Hobson RP: Infectious disease. In Walker BR, Colledge NR, Ralston SH, Penman ID: Davidson's Principles and Practice of Medicine, ed 22. Philadelphia, Elsevier, 2014.)*

140. **What is "atypical" about atypical measles?**
   - Koplik spots are rarely present.
   - Conjunctivitis and coryza are not part of the prodrome.
   - Rash begins on the distal extremities and spreads toward the head (opposite what is seen in typical measles) or has a nondescript distribution and appearance.
   - Respiratory distress with clinical and radiographic signs of pneumonia and pleural effusions are increased in frequency.

   Atypical measles occurs primarily in patients who have received inactivated measles vaccine, which was used in the United States from 1963 to 1968 and is therefore more commonly seen in adults.

141. **How is measles diagnosed?**
   Measles IgM antibody requires only a single serum specimen and is diagnostic if positive. A capture IgM test is performed by the CDC. This test should be used to confirm every case of measles that is reported to have some other type of laboratory confirmation. It is important to note that in the first 72 hours after measles rash onset, up to 20% of tests for IgM may be negative. Tests that are negative in the first 72 hours after rash onset should be repeated. PCR-based testing is also available through the CDC. A high index of suspicion is warranted in identifying measles, whether typical or atypical because many providers, especially those in training, are not likely to have seen cases during their career. This may change as outbreaks in the United States and Canada are becoming more common in the era of vaccine refusal.

   CDC: Vaccines and Immunizations. http://www.cdc.gov/vaccines/pubs/pinkbook/meas.html#diagnosis. Accessed on Jan. 14, 2015.

142. **Why is postmeasles blindness so common in underdeveloped countries?**
   Up to 1% of patients with measles in underdeveloped regions experience the progression of measles keratitis to blindness. By contrast, measles keratitis in developed countries is usually self-limited and benign. There are two principal reasons for the progression to blindness among patients with measles in underdeveloped countries:
   - **Vitamin A deficiency:** Vitamin A is needed for corneal stromal repair, and a deficiency allows epithelial damage to persist or worsen. Many malnourished children have accompanying vitamin A deficiency, and vitamin A supplements are of benefit during active illness.
   - **Malnutrition:** Malnutrition may predispose a patient to corneal superinfection with HSV.

143. **How is measles treated?**
   No antiviral therapy exists for measles. Measles immune globulin has been shown to attenuate the disease if given within 6 days of exposure. It is recommended presently for infants <1 year of age (all infants <6 months or infants <1 year who have missed the window for vaccination), pregnant women without documentation of vaccination or immunity, and certain immunocompromised children. Although the incidence of postmeasles blindness is minimal in the United States, the WHO does

recommend that vitamin A be given to all children with acute measles, regardless of their country of residence. Vitamin A is administered once daily for 2 days:
- 200,000 IU for children 12 months of age or older
- 100,000 IU for infants 6 through 11 months of age; and
- 50,000 IU for infants <6 months of age

An additional age-specific dose should be given 2 through 4 weeks later to children with suspicion of vitamin A deficiency.

144. **What are the most feared neurologic complications of measles?**
- **Acute encephalitis:** Occurring in about 1 in every 1000 cases with permanent sequelae in a significant number of cases
- **Subacute sclerosing panencephalitis:** A rare progressive neurodegenerative CNS disease with seizures and intellectual deterioration that occurs on a delayed basis (average time of 11 years) following measles in unvaccinated children

Perry RT, Halsey NA: The clinical significance of measles: a review, *J Infect Dis* 189:S4–S16, 2004.

145. **Which viruses comprise the human herpesviruses (HHV)?**
HHV 1 & 2: herpes simplex virus (HSV-1 and HSV-2)
HHV 3: varicella-zoster virus (VZV)
HHV 4: Epstein-Barr virus (EBV)
HHV 5: cytomegalovirus (CMV)
HHV 6: human herpesvirus-6
HHV 7: human herpesvirus-7
HHV 8: Kaposi sarcoma herpesvirus

All human herpesviruses share characteristics of virion morphology, basic mode of replication, and capacity for latent and recurrent infections. HSV-1, HSV-2, and VZV are alpha-herpesviruses with short reproductive cycles that establish latent infections, primarily in sensory ganglia. CMV, HHV-6, and HHV-7 are β-herpesviruses with longer reproductive cycles with latency in white blood cells (WBCs) and other tissues. EBV and HHV-8 are gamma-herpesviruses with specificity for either T or B lymphocytes and latency in lymphoid tissue.

Gilden DH, Mahalingam R, Cohrs RJ, Tyler KL: Herpesvirus infections of the nervous system, *Nat Clin Pract Neurol* 3:82–94, 2006.

146. **What is the derivation of the word *herpes*?**
Herpes comes from the Greek *"herpein,"* which means "to creep." This describes the tendency of this group of infections both to have spreading cutaneous lesions and to have chronic, latent, or recurrent manifestations.

Beswick TSL: The origin and the use of the word herpes, *Med Hist* 6:214–232, 1962.

147. **What are the typical features of roseola (exanthema subitum)?**
Roseola occurs most commonly between ages 6 and 24 months. Most children have an abrupt onset of high fever (>39 °C) with no prodrome. Fever usually lasts 3 to 4 days but can range from 1 to 8 days. Within 24 hours of defervescence, a discrete erythematous macular or maculopapular rash appears on the face, neck, and/or trunk. Erythematous papules (Nakayama spots) may be noted on the soft palate and the uvula in two-thirds of patients. Other common findings on examination include mild cervical lymph node enlargement and edematous eyelids. A variety of symptoms can accompany the fever, including diarrhea, cough, coryza, and headache.

148. **What causes roseola?**
Multiple agents are implicated in the syndrome. Human herpesvirus 6 (HHV-6) was discovered in 1986, and in 1988, Japanese investigators isolated HHV-6 from four children with exanthema subitum. In 1994, HHV-7 was also isolated from children with the clinical features of roseola. *Roseola-like*

illnesses are also noted with various echoviruses (including coxsackieviruses A and B), parainfluenza virus, and adenoviruses.

Caserta MT, Hall CB, Schnabel K, et al: Primary human herpesvirus 7 infection: a comparison of human herpesvirus 7 and human herpesvirus 6 infections in children, *J Pediatr* 133:386–389, 1998.

149. How common is human herpesvirus type-6 (HHV-6) infection in children?

Infection with HHV-6 is ubiquitous and occurs with high frequency in infants, 65% of whom have serologic evidence of primary infection by their first birthday. Nearly all children are seropositive by age 4 years. HHV-6 infection results in typical cases of roseola and is also associated with a number of other common pediatric problems, including "fever without localizing findings," nonspecific rash, and EBV-negative mononucleosis. In a study by Hall and colleagues, up to one-third of all febrile seizures in children <2 years were the result of HHV-6 infections. On rare occasions, the virus has been associated with fulminant hepatitis, encephalitis, and a syndrome of massive lymphadenopathy called *Rosai-Dorfman disease*. These manifestations are more common in immune-suppressed children, such as those who have received a bone marrow transplant. Reactivation is common and can also lead to graft-versus-host disease in this population.

Fule Robles JD, Cheuk DK, Ha SY, et al: Human herpesvirus types 6 and 7 infection in pediatric hematopoietic stem cell transplant recipients, *Ann Transplant* 19:269–276, 2014.
Hall CB, Long CE, Schnabel KC, et al: Human herpesvirus-6 infection in children, *N Engl J Med* 331:432–438, 1994.

150. What is the spectrum of disease caused by parvovirus B19?

- Erythema infectiosum (most common; a childhood exanthem, also called *fifth disease* or "slapped-cheek disease" because of the classic appearance of the rash)
- Papular-purpuric gloves and socks syndrome (self-limited condition of edematous plaques with petechial purpura over the palms and soles)
- Arthritis and arthralgia (most common in immunocompetent adults)
- Intrauterine infection with *hydrops fetalis*
- Transient aplastic crisis in patients with underlying hemolytic disease
- Persistent infection with chronic anemia in patients with immunodeficiencies
- No symptoms

151. Describe the characteristic rash of Rocky Mountain spotted fever (RMSF) from *Rickettsia rickettsii*.

- Usually seen by day 3 of illness (5 to 11 days after tick bite), but may not appear until day 6
- Begins as blanching red macules and maculopapules, which evolve into petechiae in 1 to 3 days
- Begins on flexor surfaces of wrists and ankles and spreads to extremities, face, and trunk within hours
- As rash progresses, may become pigmented with areas of desquamation
- Involves palms and soles

Ten percent to 20% of patients do not develop a rash. Because of the relatively common lack of classic features and the importance of early treatment, RMSF should be considered in the differential diagnosis of any patient in an endemic area who presents with fever, myalgia, severe headache, nausea, and vomiting *without* rash. Presumptive empirical therapy can be begun pending diagnostic studies (biopsy or serology). The risk for death increases when therapy is delayed for more than 5 days.

Dantas-Torres F: Rocky Mountain spotted fever, *Lancet Infect Dis* 7:724–732, 2007.

152. Why is doxycycline recommended for *all* ages in patients with suspected RMSF?

Alternatives for older individuals could include tetracycline or a fluoroquinolone, but doxycycline is advised even in younger patients for the following reasons:

- Tetracycline at the recommended dose is associated with dental staining in children <8 years.
- Doxycycline at the recommended dose is unlikely to cause dental staining in younger children.
- Doxycycline is also effective against ehrlichiosis, which can mimic RMSF.

- Fluoroquinolones may cause cartilage damage in juvenile animal models, and their use is not recommended for children for this indication.
- Chloramphenicol, an alternative that has been used in the past, may have serious adverse effects (e.g., aplastic anemia), no oral preparation is available in the United States, and it may be less effective for RMSF than doxycycline.

American Academy of Pediatrics: Rickettsial diseases. In Pickering LK, editor: *2012 Red Book: Report of the Committee on Infectious Diseases*, ed 29. Elk Grove Park, IL, 2012, American Academy of Pediatrics, pp 620–625.
Lochary ME, Lockhart PB, Willliams WT Jr: Doxycycline and staining of permanent teeth, *Pediatr Infect Dis J* 17:429–431, 1998.

153. How long after exposure to chickenpox (varicella) do symptoms develop?
Ninety-nine percent of patients develop symptoms between 11 and 20 days after exposure.

154. What is the risk for varicella-associated complications in normal children 1 to 14 years old?
The most common complications of VZV infection include secondary bacterial skin infections (generally due to streptococci or staphylococci), neurologic syndromes (cerebellitis, encephalitis, transverse myelitis, and Guillain-Barré syndrome), and pneumonia. Thrombocytopenia, arthritis, hepatitis, and glomerulonephritis occur less commonly. Myocarditis, pericarditis, pancreatitis, and orchitis are described but are rare.

The frequency of these complications in normal children is not precisely known, but it is estimated to be low on the basis of hospitalization and mortality data. Before the introduction of the varicella vaccine in 1995, about 4 million cases of chickenpox occurred in the United States each year, resulting in roughly 10,000 hospitalizations and 100 deaths. Since the introduction of routine immunization against varicella, rates of infection have decreased by more than 95%.

Watson B: Varicella: a vaccine preventable disease—a review, *J Infect* 44:220–225, 2002.

155. How common are second episodes of varicella after natural infection?
About **1 in 500 cases** involve a second episode. These are more likely to occur in children who develop their first episode during infancy or whose first episode is subclinical or very mild.

Gershon A: Second episodes of varicella: degree and duration of immunity, *Pediatr Infect Dis J* 9:306, 1990.

156. What is herpes zoster?
Reactivated varicella-zoster virus infection (VZV). After the primary infection of chickenpox, the virus establishes a latent infection in the dorsal root ganglion. When reactivation occurs, the virus spreads to the skin through nerves, and a typical vesicular pattern along dermatomal lines occurs (Fig. 10-9). In its primary form, the infection is varicella; in its recurrent form, it is zoster and in common parlance is known as shingles. Varicella is also known as human herpesvirus 3 (HHV-3) and is one of 9 distinct herpes viruses known to cause disease in humans. This has led to the rather confusing name of herpes zoster for the reactivated varicella zoster virus.

157. In children with herpes zoster, what is the distribution of the rash?
Compared with adults, children have relatively more cervical and sacral involvement with resultant extremity and inguinal lesions:
- 50% thoracic
- 20% cervical
- 20% lumbosacral
- 10% cranial nerve

If there are lesions on the tip of the nose, herpes zoster keratitis is more likely because of possible involvement of the nasociliary nerve. When the geniculate ganglion is involved, there is risk for developing the Ramsay Hunt syndrome, which consists of ear pain with auricular and periauricular vesicles and facial nerve palsy.

Feder HM Jr, Hoss DM: Herpes zoster in otherwise healthy children, *Pediatr Infect Dis J* 23:451–457, 2004.

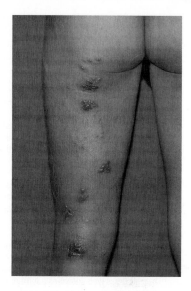

Figure 10-9. Herpes zoster with distribution along the S1 dermatome. *(From Lissauer T, Clayton G:* Illustrated Textbook of Pediatrics, *ed 2. London, 2001, Mosby, p 193.)*

158. **Is it possible to get herpes zoster after the varicella vaccine?**
Yes. Varicella is a live vaccine, and there was initial concern about how the live, attenuated vaccine strain would act in terms of development of subsequent zoster infection. Zoster is difficult to study because there is a long latent period between acquisition of varicella and development of zoster. However, cohort studies have shown a decreased risk in children of certain age groups, as well as adults, after childhood immunization with the varicella vaccine versus those infected with the wild-type virus. In adults, the use of a live-attenuated VZV vaccine has been shown to be effective in reducing the incidence and burden of herpes zoster and postherpetic neuralgia.

Adams EN, Parnapy S, Bautista P: Herpes zoster and vaccination: a clinical review, *Am J Health Syst Pharm* 67:724–727, 2010.
Civen R, Chaves SS, Jumaan A, et al: The incidence and clinical characteristics of herpes zoster among children and adolescents after implementation of varicella vaccination, *Pediatr Infect Dis J* 11:954–959, 2009.
Hambleton S, Steinberg SP, Larussa PS, et al: Risk of herpes zoster in adults immunized with varicella vaccine, *J Infect Dis* 197: S196–S199, 2008.

159. **Should chickenpox be treated with an antiviral medication?**
Neither oral acyclovir nor valacyclovir is recommended for routine use in otherwise healthy children with varicella. Early administration after onset of rash results in only a modest decrease in symptoms as antiviral drugs have a limited window of opportunity for efficacy. In immunocompetent hosts, most virus replication has stopped by 72 hours after onset of rash. By the time the disease is recognized, this window is usually passed. Oral acyclovir or valacyclovir may be considered for people at increased risk of moderate to severe varicella, such as unvaccinated people >12 years of age; children with severe eczema; children receiving long-term salicylate therapy; and people receiving short, intermittent, or inhaled courses of corticosteroids. IV acyclovir instead of oral acyclovir or valacyclovir is recommended for immunocompromised patients such as children receiving chemotherapy and patients being treated with chronic corticosteroids. Varicella-zoster immune globulin (or IVIG if this product is not available) can prevent or modify the course of disease if given up to 10 days after exposure and is indicated in certain situations such as
- Immunocompromised children without evidence of immunity
- Pregnant women without evidence of immunity
- Newborn infant whose mother had onset of chickenpox within 5 days before delivery or within 48 hours after delivery
- Hospitalized preterm infant (28 weeks or more of gestation) whose mother lacks evidence of immunity against varicella

- Hospitalized preterm infants (<28 weeks of gestation or birth weight 1000 g or less), regardless of maternal immunity

Treatment with immune globulin is not effective after clinical disease is diagnosed.

Updated Recommendations for Use of VariZIG — United States, 2013: www.cdc.gov/mmwr/preview/mmwrhtml/mm6228a4.htm. Accessed on January 14, 2015.
American Academy of Pediatrics: Varicella-zoster infections. In Pickering LK, editor: *2012 Red Book: Report of the Committee on Infectious Diseases*, ed 29. Elk Grove Park, IL, 2012, American Academy of Pediatrics, pp 777–782.

160. **Should healthy children with zoster be treated with antiviral medications?**
Routine antiviral therapy is **not indicated.** In general, the prognosis for children with herpes zoster is very good with extremely low probabilities of postherpetic neuralgia.

161. **Who gets herpes gladiatorum?**
Herpes gladiatorum is a term used to describe ocular and cutaneous infection with HSV-1, which occurs in wrestlers and rugby players. The infection is transmitted primarily by direct skin-to-skin contact and is endemic among high school and college wrestlers.

162. **What is eczema herpeticum?**
Eczema herpeticum (Fig. 10-10) is an extensive cutaneous vesicular eruption that arises from primary infection or reactivation of HSV in those with preexisting skin disease, usually atopic dermatitis (AD). HSV type 1 is the most common pathogen. To further confuse the herpes nomenclature, eczema herpeticum is also known as a form of Kaposi varicelliform eruption, which is a unique skin condition that occurs with viral infections such as HSV or coxsackievirus in those with AD or other underlying dermatologic disease. It is often difficult to distinguish from bacterial superinfection, and in fact, may coexist with a superficial *S. aureus* infection.

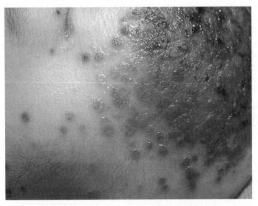

Figure 10-10. Eczema herpeticum. Note the monomorphic punched-out ulcers or vesicopustules within eczematous plaques. *(From Wolter S, Price HN: Atopic dermatitis, Pediatr Clin North Am 61:247, 2014.)*

163. **What is hand-foot-and-mouth disease?**
Hand-foot-and-mouth disease is an illness that is caused most commonly by coxsackie A viruses (especially A16) or enterovirus 71. It is associated with a petechial or vesicular exanthem involving the hands, the feet, and the oral mucosa in the posterior pharynx. Despite its name, it can also affect the buttocks in young children.

164. **What is the spectrum of disease caused by enterovirus?**
Besides the classic hand-foot-and-mouth disease, enterovirus may manifest as:
- Upper respiratory tract disease
  - Coryza, herpangina
- Lower respiratory tract illness
  - Pneumonia

- Gastrointestinal illness
  - Vomiting, diarrhea, and hepatitis
  - Rarely pancreatitis, orchitis
- Systemic disease
  - Noted especially in neonates, who may present with an overwhelming sepsislike syndrome
- Neurologic disease
  - Meningitis, encephalitis, limb paralysis
- Myocarditis

165. Why do real-time PCR positive test results indicate both "rhinovirus/enterovirus"?
Rhinovirus and enterovirus produce clinical syndromes that are distinct, although there generally may be some degree of overlap. However, both viruses are picornaviruses and are classified within the same genus. They share an identical genomic organization and have similar functional RNA secondary structures. As of now, commercially available diagnostics such as the RT-PCR are unable to distinguish between the two.

INFLUENZA

166. What is the difference between an epidemic, an outbreak, and a pandemic?
- *Epidemic:* Incident cases of an illness (or other health-related events, such as drownings) in a community or region, clearly in excess of normal expectancy
- *Outbreak:* An epidemic limited to a localized increase in the incidence of a disease (e.g., in a town or closed institution), also clearly in excess of normal expectancy
- *Pandemic:* An epidemic that has spread across a large region (e.g., multiple continents)

167. What are the types of influenza viruses?
- **Influenza A** infects many species, including humans, pigs, horses, and birds. It is subtyped on the basis of two surface glycoprotein antigens: *hemagglutinin* (H), of which there are 18 different subtypes, and *neuraminidase* (N), of which there are 11 different subtypes. The subtypes can be further divided into strains; for example, the H1N1 virus developed into a new strain in 2009, replacing the H1N1 strain that had previously caused disease in humans. This new strain was responsible for the 2009 H1N1 pandemic.
- **Influenza B** infects only humans. The disease is generally less severe than influenza A. The virus is not subtyped, but is broken down into lineages and strains.
- **Influenza C** causes very mild disease and has limited public health significance. The influenza vaccine does not protect against influenza C.

168. What are the functions of hemagglutinin and neuraminidase?
Hemagglutinin is a glycoprotein necessary for the initiation of infection because it allows viral binding to sialic acid residues on the respiratory epithelial cells. Progeny virions result after viral replication and bind to the epithelial cells. *Neuraminidase* cleaves sialic acid residues, which permits release of progeny virions into the respiratory tree.

169. What clinical features typically distinguish an infection with an influenza virus from the common cold?
See Table 10-5.

170. What is the difference between "antigenic shift" and "antigenic drift"?
- **Antigenic drift:** A subtle change in the hemagglutinin or neuraminidase gene caused by a point mutation or deletion results in a new strain that requires yearly reformulation of the seasonal influenza vaccine.
- **Antigenic shift:** This occurs much less frequently than antigenic drift (occurring only in influenza A) and involves a profound change in the virus with a new hemagglutinin or neuraminidase type produced, possibly from another species. For example, simultaneous infection of a host with a human and avian influenza strain can result in genetic reassortment and a novel virus.

171. What made the influenza A H1N1 pandemic strain of 2009 so novel?
The influenza A H1N1 strain caused a worldwide pandemic problem that began in early 2009. This strain was a quadruple reassortment of an influenza A virus involving two swine strains, one

Table 10-5 Influenza Versus Cold Symptoms

SIGNS AND SYMPTOMS	INFLUENZA	COLD
Onset	Sudden	Gradual
Fever	>38.3 °C (101 °F) lasting >3 days	Rare
Cough	Can become severe	Less common
Headache	Prominent	Rare
Myalgia	Severe	Slight
Fatigue	Fatigue lasting >1 wk	Mild
Extreme exhaustion	Early and prominent	Rare
Chest discomfort	Common	Mild
Stuffy nose	Sometimes	Common
Sneezing	Sometimes	Common
Sore throat	Sometimes	Common

From Meissner HC: Reducing the impact of viral respiratory infections in children, Pediatr Clin North Am *52:700, 2005.*

human strain, and one avian strain, which likely recombined through pigs as an intermediate mammalian host. Components of the 2009 pandemic virus are thought to have derived from the 1918 influenza pandemic. Transmissibility rates were extremely high.

Zimmer SM, Burke DS: Historical perspective—emergence of influenza A (H1N1) viruses, *N Engl J Med* 361:279–285, 2009.
Morens DM, Taubenberger JK, Fauci AS: The persistent legacy of the 1918 influenza virus, *N Engl J Med* 361:225–229, 2009.
Centers for Disease Control and Prevention: H1N1 Flu. www.cdc.gov/h1n1flu/cdcresponse.htm. Accessed on Jan 14, 2015.

172. **Which patients should not receive the *live-attenuated* influenza vaccine?**
   Contraindications are:
   - <2 years or >49 years
   - Pregnant women/teens
   - Children who have experienced severe allergic reactions to the vaccine or any of its components, or to a previous dose of *any* influenza vaccine
   - Children in close contact with severely immune suppressed persons
   - Patients taking salicylates
   - Those with a known or suspected immunodeficiency
   - Those with a history of egg allergy
   - Those who have received a live viral vaccine within past 4 weeks
   - Children aged 2 through 4 years who have asthma or who have had a wheezing episode by any history within the past 12 months

   Strong precautions to use include the following:
   - Children with other conditions considered high risk for severe influenza (chronic pulmonary or cardiac disorders, pregnancy, chronic metabolic disease, renal dysfunction, hemoglobinopathies, or immunosuppressive therapy)
   - Children ≥5 years of age with asthma
   - Nasal congestion that could impede vaccine delivery
   - A history of Guillain-Barré syndrome
   - Moderate to severe febrile illness

Prevention and Control of Seasonal Influenza with Vaccines: Recommendations of the Advisory Committee on Immunization Practices (ACIP) — United States, 2014–15 Influenza Season:

www.cdc.gov/mmwr/preview/mmwrhtml/mm6332a3.htm#Groups_Recommended_Vaccination_Timing_Vaccination. Accessed on Jan. 14, 2015.

American Academy of Pediatrics: *Influenza.* In Pickering LK, editor: *2012 Red Book: Report of the Committee on Infectious Diseases*, ed 29. Elk Grove Park, IL, 2012, American Academy of Pediatrics, pp 445–453.

173. What are the main antiviral medications used as treatment for influenza?

- **Neuraminidase inhibitors:** Oseltamivir (oral) and zanamivir (inhaled) prevent release of virions from the host cell. These agents are used against influenza B and A, including pandemic H1N1.
- **Adamantanes (M2 inhibitors):** Amantadine and rimantadine target the M2 protein of influenza A, which is involved in ion channels of viral membrane essential for viral replication.

Moscona A: Neuraminidase inhibitors for influenza, *N Engl J Med* 353:1363, 2005.

174. Does influenza display resistance to antiviral medications?

Yes. The adamantanes are not effective against influenza B viruses because of the difference in ion channel structure. These drugs are also not effective against the H3N2 and the 2009 H1N1 epidemic strain. The majority of these viruses contained a single amino acid substitution in the M2 protein, which conferred adamantane resistance. The H1N1 strain before 2009 (i.e., not the pandemic strain) did have a mutation causing a histidine to tyrosine substitution in neuraminidase, making a proportion of these strains resistant to neuraminidase inhibitors. However, this mutation (as are other resistance mechanisms) is sporadic and rare in the pandemic and other recent seasonal strains. Fortunately, the majority of influenza A and B isolates remain susceptible to oseltamivir.

Hurt AC: The epidemiology and spread of drug resistant human influenza viruses, *Curr Opin Virol* 8:22–29, 2014.

175. What are the indications for antiviral medications for influenza in children?

- Any child who is hospitalized or has severe or complicated illness
- Children <2 years of age
- Immunosuppressed children
- Children with conditions considered high risk for severe influenza: asthma, cardiac disorders, chronic metabolic disease, renal dysfunction, hemoglobinopathies
- Children who are taking salicylates
- Pregnant women/teens
- Residents of chronic care facilities
- Children with neurologic or neuromuscular disorders

  Ideally, antiviral therapy is initiated with 48 hours of symptom onset, but it may still be of some benefit if given at <5 days. An important point of emphasis is that initiation of therapy should not wait for confirmation of diagnosis, especially in high-risk or ill individuals. First-line therapy is oseltamivir.

Centers for Disease Control and Prevention: Antiviral drugs. www.cdc.gov/flu/professionals/antivirals/index.htm. Accessed on Mar. 24, 2015.

176. What complications can be associated with influenza infections?

Death due to exacerbation of an underlying medical condition or invasive coinfection from a secondary bacterial pathogen including bacterial pneumonia from *S. aureus*, including methicillin-resistant *S. aureus* (MRSA), *S. pneumoniae,* or group A streptococci.

Also:

- Otitis media
- Myositis (particularly with influenza B)
- Febrile seizures
- Encephalitis, encephalopathy
- Reye syndrome
- Guillain-Barré syndrome
- Transverse myelitis
- Myocarditis, pericarditis

Mistry RD, Fischer JB, Prasad PA, et al: Severe complications in influenza-like illnesses, *Pediatrics* 134:e684–e690, 2014.
Wong KK, Jain S, Blanton L, et al: Influenza-associated pediatric deaths in the United States, 2004–2012, *Pediatrics* 132:796–804, 2013.

177. **What bacterial coinfection is most commonly identified in influenza-associated pediatric deaths?**

     Methicillin-resistant *S. aureus* (MRSA). In children in the United States, most deaths associated with influenza tend to result either from an exacerbation of an underlying medical condition or invasive coinfection from another pathogen. As the percentage of children colonized with MRSA has increased, this bacterium has assumed a greater role in coinfecting lungs after the influenza virus has damaged the tracheobronchial tree. In a child with a suspected secondary pneumonia during influenza season, coverage for a possible MRSA infection should be considered.

Wong KK, Jain S, Blanton L, et al: Influenza-associated pediatric deaths in the United States, 2004–2012, *Pediatrics* 132:796–804, 2013.
Finelli L, Fiore A, Dhara R, et al: Influenza-associated pediatric mortality in the United States: increase of *Staphylococcus aureus* coinfection, *Pediatrics* 122:805–811, 2008.

LYMPHADENITIS AND LYMPHADENOPATHY

178. **What are the most common causes of acute and chronic lymphadenitis in normal, otherwise healthy children?**

     S. aureus and ***Streptococcus pyogenes* (group A streptococci)** account for more than 80% of cases of acute lymphadenitis, while **nontuberculous mycobacteria** and ***Bartonella henselae*** (cat-scratch disease) are the most common causes of chronic lymphadenitis.

179. **What infectious etiology should be considered in a toddler with an intensely erythematous but minimally tender submandibular or anterior-superior cervical node?**

     Nontuberculous mycobacterial infection (NTM) manifests as a group of nodes, which can increase in size, coalesce, and eventually spontaneously rupture to form sinus tracts.

180. **How is the diagnosis of NTM disease made?**

     Definitive diagnosis of NTM infection depends on **culture** and isolation of the organism from infected tissue. Cultures must be sent specifically for mycobacteria to ensure appropriate processing. Histopathologic examination of the tissue cannot adequately differentiate NTM infection from tuberculosis. PCR-based technology is being validated for NTM.

181. **How is NTM lymphadenitis treated?**

     Most experts recommend excision of the infected lymph node. Clarithromycin, rifampin, and ethambutol are effective against many strains of nontuberculous mycobacteria and are generally used when excision is incomplete because of nearby nervous tissue or vascular structures, when surgery is contraindicated, or for recurrent disease. Medical therapy is often prolonged. Organisms can display and develop resistance patterns that may be difficult to manage medically. Some experts have proposed "observation" therapy if this is tolerable to the family and patient because the majority of isolated lesions will regress without treatment.

Zeharia A, et al: Management of nontuberculous mycobacteria-induced cervical lymphadenitis with observation alone, *Pediatr Infect Dis J* 27:920–922, 2008.
Haverkamp M, et al: Nontuberculous mycobacterial infection in children: a 2-year prospective surveillance study in the Netherlands, *Clin Infect Dis.* 39:450–456, 2004.

182. **What infectious etiology should be considered in a child with swollen, tender axillary nodes?**

     Cat-scratch disease. This entity is caused by *B. henselae*, which is a fastidious, slow-growing, gram-negative bacillus rarely grown in culture. Thus, diagnosis is usually made by serologic or PCR tests. This organism is found in the oral flora of kittens, cats, and occasionally dogs.

183. **What is the typical course of the lymphadenitis in cat-scratch disease?**

     An otherwise healthy child or adolescent presents with **symptoms of regional lymphadenopathy** that begin 1 to several weeks after a scratch (unrecalled by many patients). The lymph nodes are usually moderately tender and are associated with overlying erythema and fluctuance. About 10% to 30% eventually suppurate. The lymph nodes most commonly involved are axillary and cervical, but epitrochlear, submandibular, inguinal, and preauricular nodes may be enlarged. Enlarged pectoral nodes are highly suggestive of cat-scratch disease. Fever is usually absent or low grade, but temperatures as high as 40°C have been described in 30% to 50% of cases. Infected nodes generally spontaneously resolve without specific therapy. Treatment with 5 days of antibiotics (including azithromycin, ciprofloxacin, trimethoprim-sulfamethoxazole, rifampin, or gentamicin) may speed recovery, and excision of the infected nodes is not recommended. Treatment with antimicrobial therapy is recommended for severely ill or immunocompromised individuals.

Klotz SA, Ianas V, Elliott SP: Cat-scratch disease, *Am Fam Physician* 83:152–155, 2011.
English R: Cat-scratch disease, *Pediatr Rev* 27:123–127, 2006.

184. What are other manifestations of cat-scratch disease in addition to lymphadenopathy?

In 20% to 25% of cases, other manifestations may occur including **Parinaud oculoglandular syndrome** (conjunctivitis, ipsilateral preauricular lymphadenopathy), **prolonged fever of unknown origin, encephalitis, osteolytic bone lesions, neuroretinitis, visceral organ involvement** (especially hepatosplenic), and **erythema nodosum**. This organism has also been associated with bacillary angiomatosis (a vascular proliferative disorder with cutaneous and visceral forms) and peliosis hepatitis (a vascular disorder with cystic blood-filled cavities in the liver parenchyma), both of which occur primarily in adults with HIV infection.

185. What are the presentations of Epstein-Barr virus (EBV) infection?

Young children with EBV infection are frequently **asymptomatic**. In adolescents and young adults, infection typically results in **infectious mononucleosis**, which is characterized as follows:

- *Clinical:* Fever, pharyngitis, lymphadenopathy (75% to 95%), splenomegaly (50%)
- *Hematologic:* More than 50% mononuclear cells, more than 10% atypical lymphocytes

A wide variety of symptoms (e.g., malaise, headache, anorexia, myalgias, chills, nausea) can occur. Neurologic presentations are rare but can include encephalitis, meningitis, myelitis, Guillain-Barré syndrome, and cranial or peripheral neuropathies.

EBV is also associated with posttransplant lymphoproliferative disorder, Burkitt lymphoma, nasopharyngeal carcinoma, and undifferentiated T- and B-cell lymphomas.

186. How was the monospot test developed?

In 1932, Paul and Bunnell observed that patients with infectious mononucleosis make antibodies that agglutinate sheep RBCs. These antibodies are referred to as *heterophil antibodies* and serve as the basis for the monospot test, which is a rapid slide agglutination test. Today, horse or beef RBCs are usually used because they are more sensitive to agglutination than are sheep RBCs. Heterophil antibodies can also occur in serum sickness and as a normal variant. If there is clinical confusion, differential absorption can pinpoint the cause. Heterophil antibodies in infectious mononucleosis do not react with guinea pig kidney cells, whereas those of serum sickness do. Normal variant heterophil antibodies do not react with beef RBCs.

Durbin WA, Sullivan JL: Epstein-Barr virus infections, *Pediatr Rev* 15:63–68, 1994.

187. What is the natural course of serologic responses to EBV infection?

Serologic responses to viral components, including viral capsid antigen (VCA), early antigen (EA), and Epstein-Barr nuclear antigen (EBNA), occur in a characteristic time frame (Fig. 10-11) and can assist in distinguishing possible acute from past infections. Acute infection is best characterized by the presence of high titers of VCA IgM or IgG with or without high titers of EA and with no or low titers of EBNA.

188. When are steroids indicated for children with EBV infection?

Among patients with acute EBV infection, steroids should NOT be considered for treatment of uncomplicated mononucleosis. Steroids are indicated for treatment of impending respiratory obstruction as a result of enlarged tonsils, autoimmune hemolytic anemia, aplastic anemia, neurologic disease, and severe life-threatening infection (e.g., liver failure).

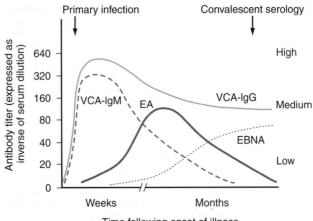

Figure 10-11. Idealized time course for antibody responses to various EBV antigens after primary infection with the virus. *EA*, Early antigen; *EBNA*, Epstein-Barr nuclear antigen; *IgG*, immunoglobulin G; *IgM*, immunoglobulin M; *VCA*, viral capsid antigen. *(From Katz BZ: Epstein-Barr virus (mononucleosis and lymphoproliferative disorders. In Long SS, editor: Principles and Practice of Pediatric Infectious Disease, ed 4. Philadelphia, 2012, Elsevier, p 1062.)*

189. **What are the clinical presentations of acquired CMV infection?**
    In normal hosts who develop symptomatic acquired CMV infection, clinical manifestations include fever, malaise, and nonspecific aches and pains. The peripheral blood smear reveals an absolute lymphocytosis and many atypical lymphocytes. In contrast with EBV-infectious mononucleosis, exudative pharyngitis is not prominent. Liver involvement is very common, and liver function tests are usually abnormal. Like EBV disease, CMV mononucleosis can persist for several weeks.

190. **What is the most common form of tularemia?**
    Ulceroglandular. Seventy-five percent of cases of tularemia are ulceroglandular. Three to 5 days (range, 1 to 21 days) after exposure, fever, myalgia, headaches, muscle soreness, and regional lymphadenopathy develop. The original lesion is a papule, which ulcerates. Bacteremia may result in multiorgan involvement.

Eliasson H, Broman T, Forsman M, et al: Tularemia: current epidemiology and disease management, *Infect Dis Clin North Am* 20:289–311, 2006.

191. **What vectors are commonly associated with tularemia?**
    Francisella tularensis (the causative agent of tularemia) is a zoonotic infection caused by contact with infected animals (rabbits, deer, and muskrats) or invertebrate vectors (ticks). Streptomycin, gentamicin, tetracyclines, chloramphenicol, and fluoroquinolones have been shown to be effective therapy for tularemia.

192. **Which other organisms can cause a mononucleosis-like clinical picture?**
    Toxoplasma gondii, HHV-6, adenovirus, acute HIV infection, group A streptococcal infection, hepatitis B, and rubella.

193. **Why is it called "mononucleosis"?**
    This refers to the tendency of certain infections, primarily EBV, to cause the development of morphologically abnormal lymphocytes (which may resemble monocytes), mainly from CD8+ T cells that respond to infection. These atypical cells can account for up to 30% of the WBC count. Atypical lymphocytes may also be present in a host of illnesses including *B. henselae,* babesiosis, tuberculosis, lymphoma and leukemia, and pertussis.

MENINGITIS

194. **What are the most common signs and symptoms of meningitis in infants <2 months?**
The findings of meningitis among neonates and young infants are often subtle. Temperature instability (fever is more common in full-term infants while hypothermia is more common in preterm infants) occurs in about 60% of infected infants. Neurologic symptoms including irritability, poor tone, and lethargy are noted in 60% of infants with meningitis. Seizures may be the presenting symptom in 20% to 50% of cases. Poor feeding or vomiting can occur as well. On physical examination, about 25% of newborns and young infants have a bulging fontanel. Only 13% have nuchal rigidity. Thus, the diagnosis of meningitis cannot be excluded in infants on the basis of the absence of these physical findings.

Pong A, Bradley JS: Bacterial meningitis and the newborn infant, *Infect Dis Clin North Am* 13:711–733, 1999.

195. **What percentage of neonates <30 days of age with bacterial sepsis and positive blood cultures have meningitis?**
As many as 20% of such infants will have culture-confirmed meningitis. Conversely, >30% of all infants evaluated for sepsis with negative blood cultures may have meningitis. This is especially notable in low-birth-weight infants.

Garges HP, Moody MA, Cotton CM, et al: Neonatal meningitis: what is the correlation among cerebrospinal fluid cultures, blood cultures, and cerebrospinal fluid parameters? *Pediatrics* 117:1094–1100, 2006.
Stoll BJ, Hansen N, Fanaroff AA, et al: To tap or not to tap: high likelihood of meningitis without sepsis among very low birth weight infants, *Pediatrics* 113:1181–1186, 2004.

196. **What is the most common cause of viral meningitis?**
More than 80% of infectious cases are caused by **enteroviruses** (i.e., coxsackievirus, enterovirus, and echovirus).

197. **What is the diagnostic test of choice for enteroviral meningitis?**
Enteroviruses can be diagnosed by **PCR testing,** which is rapid, sensitive, and specific.

198. **What are common arthropod-borne viral causes of meningoencephalitis in the United States?**
Several arboviruses can cause meningoencephalitis including the LaCrosse virus; Powassan virus; West Nile virus; and the St. Louis, Eastern, and Western equine encephalitis viruses; and the Japanese encephalitis virus. Human infections are most common in the summer and fall when mosquito and tick activity are highest. West Nile virus is an increasingly common cause of aseptic meningitis and meningoencephalitis, especially in the late summer and early fall. Mosquitoes are the primary vector, with a variety of birds (e.g., crows, jays, sparrows) known to serve as hosts. Significant avian mortality is often the first sign of significant West Nile virus activity in a locale. Non–vector-borne transmission (e.g., contaminated blood products, organ transplantation) has been described. Many state health departments and commercial laboratories have PCR-based tests to diagnose these infections.

Lanteri MC, Lee TH, Kaidarova Z, et al: West Nile virus nucleic acid persistence in whole blood months after clearance in plasma: implication for transfusion and transplantation safety, *Transfusion* 54:3232–3241, 2014.
American Academy of Pediatrics: Arboviruses In Pickering LK, editor: *2012 Red Book: Report of the Committee on Infectious Diseases*, ed 29. Elk Grove Park, IL, 2012, American Academy of Pediatrics, pp 232–235.

199. **Should computed tomography (CT) scans be performed before an LP during the evaluation of possible meningitis?**
Cranial imaging is not routinely indicated before LP, unless one of the following is present:
- Signs of herniation (rapid alteration of consciousness, abnormalities of pupillary size and reaction, absence of oculocephalic response, fixed oculomotor deviation of eyes)
- Papilledema
- Abnormalities in posture or respiration
- Generalized seizures (especially tonic), which are often associated with impending cerebral herniation

- Overwhelming shock or sepsis, possibly precluding the procedure
- Concern about a condition mimicking bacterial meningitis (e.g., intracranial mass, lead intoxication, tuberculous meningitis)

Tunkle AR, Hartman BJ, Kaplan SL, et al: Practice guidelines for the management of bacterial meningitis, *Clin Infect Dis* 39:1267–1284, 2004.
Haslam RH: Role of CT in the early management of bacterial meningitis, *J Pediatr* 119:157–159, 1991.

200. **What is the range of normal parameters for CSF in infants and children who do not have meningitis?**
   - **Term newborn infants:** WBC count, 0 to 20/mm^3; protein, 30 to 100 mg/dL; glucose, 30 to 120 mg/dL
   - **Infants and children:** WBC count, 0 to 9/mm^3; protein, 20 to 40 mg/dL; glucose, 40 to 80 mg/dL

Kestenbaum LA, Ebberson J, Zorc JJ, et al: Defining cerebrospinal fluid white blood cell count reference values in neonates and young children, *Pediatrics* 125:257–264, 2010.
Mann K, Jackson A: Meningitis, *Pediatr Rev* 29:425, 2008.

201. **If bloody CSF is collected during LP, how is CNS hemorrhage distinguished from a traumatic artifact?**
   Most often, the blood is a result of the traumatic rupture of small venous plexuses that surround the subarachnoid space, but pathologic bloody fluid can be seen in multiple settings (e.g., subarachnoid hemorrhage, herpes simplex encephalitis). Distinguishing features that suggest pathologic bleeding include the following:
   - Bleeding that does not lessen during the collection of multiple tubes
   - Xanthochromia of the CNS supernatant
   - Crenated RBCs noted microscopically

202. **How is a traumatic LP interpreted?**
   A "bloody tap" is a common result of an unsuccessful LP. Numerous formulas have been devised to adjust leukocyte totals in blood-contaminated CSF to determine whether CSF pleocytosis (and thus possible meningitis) is present. However, no formulas in neonates or older children have been useful to guide clinical decisions about bacterial meningitis.

Greenberg RG, Smith PB, Cotten CM, et al: Traumatic lumbar punctures in neonates, *Pediatr Infect Dis J* 27:1047–1051, 2008.
Bonsu BK, Harper MB: Corrections for leukocytes and percent of neutrophils do not match observations in blood-contaminated cerebrospinal fluid and have no value over uncorrected cells for diagnosis, *Pediatr Infect Dis J* 25:8–11, 2006.

203. **What is the best way to position the patient for an LP?**
   Some studies have shown increase in successful LPs in the **sitting position with flexed hips**, both in children and neonates, compared with the lateral flexed position (although the latter is more commonly practiced in the United States). Data obtained through measurements using ultrasound have shown that the interspinous space may increase in this position, leading to a higher likelihood of entering the appropriate space. Since the diameter of a 1.5 inch, 22-guage needle is 0.7 mm, even a small difference of 1 to 2 mm in those spaces could contribute to increased success. Data are conflicting whether differences occur in the subarachnoid space between the sitting and lateral flexed positions. Measurement of oxygenation levels via pulse oximetry for preterm infants in the sitting versus lateral knee-flexed positions during a LP have found better oxygenation in the sitting flexed position, which also suggests that this position might be better tolerated and potentially safer for the infant.

Hanson AL, Ros S, Soprano J: Analysis of infant lumbar puncture success rates: sitting flexed versus lateral flexed positions, *Pediatr Emerg Care* 30:311–314, 2014.
Oulego-Erroz I, Mora-Matilla M, Alonso-Quintela P, et al: Ultrasound evaluation of lumbar spine anatomy in newborn infants: implications for optimal performance of lumbar puncture, *J Pediatr* 165:862–865, 2014.
Gleason CA, Martin RJ, Anderson JV, et al: Optimal position for a spinal tap in preterm infants, *Pediatrics* 71:31–35, 1983.

204. How do the CSF findings vary in bacterial, viral, fungal, and tuberculous meningitis in children beyond the neonatal period?

A large overlap in parameters for meningitis caused by different pathogens is possible. For example, bacterial meningitis can be associated with a low WBC count early in the illness, or viral meningitis can be associated with a persistent dominance of neutrophils. The usual findings are summarized in Table 10-6.

Table 10-6 Typical Findings in Bacterial, Viral, Fungal, and Tuberculous Meningitis

CEREBROSPINAL FLUID FINDINGS	BACTERIAL	VIRAL	FUNGAL, TUBERCULOUS
White blood cells per mm^3	>500	<500	<500
Polymorphonuclear neutrophils	>80%	<50%	<50%
Glucose (mg/dL)	<40	>40	<40
Cerebrospinal fluid–to–blood ratio	<30%	>50%	<30%
Protein (mg/dL)	>100	<100	>100

205. What CSF indices help in the diagnosis of bacterial versus viral meningitis?

In the absence of culture data, there is no way one can differentiate bacterial from viral meningitis with certainty. In a study that derived prediction rules for children to determine which group of patients with CSF pleocytosis was most likely to have bacterial rather than viral meningitis, 5 high-risk criteria were defined. If all were **absent**, 100% of children did not have bacterial meningitis (100% negative-predictive value).

- CSF Gram stain positive
- CSF absolute neutrophil count (ANC) >1000 cells/μL
- CSF protein >80 mg/dL
- Peripheral blood ANC >10,000 cells/μL
- Seizure at or before presentation

Nigrovic LE, Malley R, Kuppermann N: Cerebrospinal fluid pleocytosis in children in the era of bacterial conjugate vaccines, *Pediatr Emerg Care* 25:112–120, 2009.

206. When is the best time to obtain a serum glucose level in an infant with suspected meningitis?

Because the stress of an LP can elevate serum glucose, the serum sample is ideally obtained just before the LP. When the blood glucose level is elevated acutely, it can take at least 30 minutes before the blood glucose equilibrates with that of the CSF.

207. Does antibiotic therapy before LP affect CSF indices?

Many children with presumptive meningitis are begun on antibiotic therapy before an LP often because a delay in performing the LP is anticipated. Prior administration of antibiotics does increase the likelihood of falsely negative CSF cultures in patients with bacterial meningitis. Similarly, the CSF Gram stain will still demonstrate bacteria with typical staining properties. Prior antibiotic use decreases the CSF protein concentration and increases the CSF glucose concentration. However, it does not substantially affect the CSF WBC or CSF ANC counts.

Nigrovic LE, Malley R, Macias CG, et al: Effect of antibiotic pretreatment on cerebrospinal fluid profiles in children with bacterial meningitis, *Pediatrics* 122:726–730, 2008.

Nigrovic LE, Kuppermann N, McAdam AJ, Malley R: Cerebrospinal latex agglutination fails to contribute to the microbiologic diagnosis of pretreated children with meningitis, *Pediatr Infect Dis J* 23:786–788, 2004.

208. How quickly is the CSF sterilized in children with meningitis?

Data are limited, and trial data are obviously not tenable. In successful therapy, the CSF is usually sterile within 36 to 48 hours of the initiation of antibiotics. In patients with meningococcal meningitis, CSF is typically completely sterile within 2 hours after starting treatment. With other organisms such as pneumococcus, the time until sterilization is generally at least 4 hours. In neonates the CSF may sterilize more slowly. Furthermore, absence of a positive culture in CSF obtained from the lumbar subarachnoid space does not exclude a positive culture from ventricles.

Kanegaye JT, Soliemanzadeh P, Bradley JS: Lumbar puncture in pediatric bacterial meningitis: defining the time interval for recovery of cerebrospinal fluid pathogens after parenteral antibiotic pretreatment, *Pediatrics* 108:1169–1174, 2001.

209. **What are the most common organisms responsible for bacterial meningitis in the United States?**
0 to <1 month old:
- GBS (*Streptococcus agalactiae*)
- *E. coli* (if presents after first week of life, galactosemia should be excluded)
- Miscellaneous Enterobacteriaceae
- *Listeria monocytogenes* (rare)
- *Streptococcus pneumoniae* (rare)
- *S. aureus* (in hospitalized preterm infants)
- Coagulase-negative staphylococci (in hospitalized preterm infants)

1 to <3 months old
- GBS
- Gram-negative bacilli
- *S. pneumoniae*
- *Neisseria meningitidis*

3 months to <3 years
- *S. pneumoniae*
- *N. meningitidis*
- GBS
- Gram-negative bacilli (including *E. coli* and *H. influenzae*)

3 to 10 years old
- *S. pneumoniae*
- *N. meningitidis*

10 to 18 years old
- *N. meningitidis*

   Before the development of conjugate vaccines for important bacterial pathogens, childhood bacterial meningitis was mostly due to *N. meningitidis*, *S. pneumoniae* and *H. influenzae* type b (Hib) in infants and children, and GBS and *E. coli* in neonates. Although the epidemiology of meningitis in young infants and neonates has remained fairly unchanged, the rate of meningitis due to *S. pneumoniae* has decreased following the introduction of the PCV-7 and PCV-13.

Angoulvant F, Levy C, Grimprel E, et al: Early impact of 13-valent pneumococcal conjugate vaccine on community-acquired pneumonia in children, *Clin Infect Dis* 58:918–924, 2014.

Nigrovic LE, Kuppermann N, Malley R, Bacterial Meningitis Study Group of the Pediatric Emergency Medicine Collaborative Research Committee of the American Academy of Pediatrics: Children with bacterial meningitis presenting to the emergency department during the pneumococcal conjugate vaccine era, *Acad Emerg Med* 15:522–528, 2008.

210. **What are the drugs of choice for the empiric treatment of bacterial meningitis in children >1 month?**
Empiric therapy for suspected bacterial meningitis should include both **vancomycin and a third-generation cephalosporin** agent (e.g., cefotaxime, ceftriaxone) because of increasing resistance to penicillin and cephalosporins among some *S. pneumoniae* isolates. These agents also provide excellent coverage against *N. meningitidis* and *H. influenzae*. Treatment failures have been reported when the dosage of vancomycin is <60 mg/kg per day. Vancomycin should not be used alone to treat *S. pneumoniae* meningitis because data from animal models indicate that bactericidal levels may be difficult to maintain in the CSF. The combination of vancomycin plus cefotaxime or ceftriaxone has been shown to produce a synergistic effect *in vitro*, in animal models, and in the CSF of children with meningitis. Empiric therapy may be expanded for children

with suspected bacterial meningitis who have immune deficiency, recent neurosurgery, penetrating head trauma, and anatomic defects.

Richard GC, Lepe M: Meningitis in children: diagnosis and treatment for the emergency clinician, *Clin Pediatr Emerg Med* 14:146–156, 2013.
Tunkle AR, Hartman BJ, Kaplan SL, et al: Practice guidelines for the management of bacterial meningitis, *Clin Infect Dis* 39:1267–1284, 2004.
Alter SJ: Pneumococcal infections, *Pediatr Rev* 30:155–164, 2009.

211. **What is the role of corticosteroids in the treatment of bacterial meningitis?**
The inflammatory response plays a critical role in producing the CNS pathology and resultant sequelae of bacterial meningitis. Several studies have demonstrated that treatment with dexamethasone reduces the incidence of hearing loss and other neurologic sequelae in infants and children with meningitis caused by *H. influenzae* type b when given before or at the same time as the first dose of antimicrobial therapy. However, a 2013 Cochrane review found no reduction in hearing loss in children with the use of steroids in meningitis due to non-*Haemophilus* species. For cases of meningitis caused by other pathogens, such as *N. meningitides* or *S. pneumoniae*, the current AAP recommendations are to "consider" the use of dexamethasone with or shortly before the first dose of antimicrobial therapy after considering the potential risks and benefits. The role of steroids in meningitis caused by other bacterial pathogens remains controversial. In adults, adjuvant corticosteroids decrease mortality in patients with pneumococcal meningitis, but this does not appear to be the case in children. Dexamethasone is not indicated for infants with early-onset sepsis/meningitis.

Brouwer MC, McIntyre P, Prasad K, van de Beek D: Corticosteroids for acute bacterial meningitis, *Cochrane Database Syst Rev* 6:CD004405, 2013.
American Academy of Pediatrics: Pneumococcal infections. In Pickering LK, editor: *2012 Red Book, Report of the Committee on Infectious Diseases*, ed 29. Elk Grove Village, IL, 2012, American Academy of Pediatrics, p 576.
Mongelluzzo J, Mohamad Z, Ten Have TR, Shah S: Corticosteroids and mortality in children with bacterial meningitis, *JAMA* 299:2048–2055, 2008.

212. **How long after treatment has been initiated must individuals with meningitis remain on droplet precautions?**
Droplet precautions, which mandate a single, closed room and that surgical masks be worn by the staff, are recommended for patients with suspected *H. influenzae* type b or meningococcal meningitis, but it can be discontinued after 24 hours of effective antimicrobial therapy.

213. **Should children receiving therapy for bacterial meningitis undergo repeat LP?**
Repeat LPs are not recommended for uncomplicated courses of meningitis. However, a repeat LP should be strongly considered for the following patients:
- Those with no clinical or poor clinical response to appropriate therapy within 24 to 36 hours
- Those with meningitis caused by penicillin-nonsusceptible or cephalosporin-resistant *S. pneumoniae*
- Those with *S. pneumoniae* who received dexamethasone because this agent might interfere with the ability to interpret clinical changes (e.g., fever)
- Those with prolonged or recurrent fever
- Those with recurrent meningitis
- Immunocompromised hosts
- Neonates with *Streptococcus agalactiae* and gram-negative meningitis should have a repeat LP after 2 to 3 days of treatment to determine appropriate duration of therapy.

Tunkle AR, Hartman BJ, Kaplan SL, et al: Practice guidelines for the management of bacterial meningitis, *Clin Infect Dis* 39:1267–1284, 2004.

214. **What is the accepted duration of treatment for bacterial meningitis?**
The duration of antibiotic treatment is based on the causative agent and clinical course. In general for **uncomplicated clinical courses**, a minimum of 7 days of therapy is required for meningococcal meningitis, 7 to 10 days for *H. influenzae* meningitis, and 10 days for pneumococcal meningitis. Meningitis caused by GBS or *L. monocytogenes* should be treated for 14 to 21 days, and meningitis caused by gram-negative

enteric bacilli should be treated for a minimum of 21 days or 21 days after the CSF is sterilized. Among patients with **complications** such as brain abscess, subdural empyema, delayed CSF sterilization, persistence of meningeal signs, or prolonged fever, the duration of therapy may need to be extended and should be individualized.

Repeat CSF cultures should be sterile. The duration of therapy should be extended if organisms are seen on Gram stain or isolated from CSF cultures from the repeat CSF examination. The duration of therapy should be extended if CSF examination at the conclusion of the standard duration of treatment shows >30% neutrophils, CSF glucose of <20 mg/dL, or CSF-to-blood glucose ratio of <20 percent, respectively.

Tunkle AR, Hartman BJ, Kaplan SL, et al: Practice guidelines for the management of bacterial meningitis, *Clin Infect Dis* 39:1267–1284, 2004.

215. In a patient with meningitis, what are the findings that suggest intracranial complications and provide indications for CT or magnetic resonance imaging (MRI)?
   - Prolonged obtundation
   - Prolonged irritability
   - Seizures developing after day 3 of therapy
   - Focal seizures
   - Focal neurologic deficits
   - Increasing head circumference
   - Persistent elevation of CSF protein or neutrophil count
   - Recurrence of disease

Oliveira CR, Morriss MC, Mistrot JG, et al: Brain magnetic resonance imaging of infants with bacterial meningitis, *J Pediatr* 165:134–139, 2014.
Wubbel L, McCracken GH: Management of bacterial meningitis, *Pediatr Rev* 19:78–84, 1998.

216. What are the most common causes of prolonged fever in patients with meningitis?
   - Inadequate treatment
   - Suppurative disease at other foci (e.g., pericarditis, arthritis, subdural empyema)
   - Healthcare-acquired infection (e.g., central line-associated bloodstream infection)
   - Thrombophlebitis (related to IV catheters and infusates)
   - Drug fever

217. What should the parents of a child with bacterial meningitis be told about long-term outcomes?
   Disease resulting from *S. pneumoniae* is associated with considerably more morbidity and mortality than is meningitis caused by *N. meningitidis* or *H. influenzae*. The mortality ranges from 8% to 15%. A 3-year multicenter surveillance study of invasive pneumococcal infections examined outcomes of meningitis caused by *S. pneumoniae* in 180 children. Twenty-five percent of children had evidence of neurologic sequelae at the time of hospital discharge, and 32% had unilateral or bilateral deafness. Predictors of mortality included coma on admission, requirement for mechanical ventilation, and shock. Hearing loss occurs in 5% to 10% of patients with meningitis caused by *H. influenzae* and *N. meningitidis*. Survivors of bacterial meningitis in the neonatal period often have much poorer neurodevelopmental outcomes. Survivors should be followed for hearing loss and other sequelae such as gross motor or cognitive impairment.

Oliveira CR, Morriss MC, Mistrot JG, et al: Brain magnetic resonance imaging of infants with bacterial meningitis, *J Pediatr* 165:134–139, 2014.
Koomen I, Grobbee DE, Roord JJ, et al: Hearing loss at school age in survivors of bacterial meningitis: assessment, incidence, and prediction, *Pediatrics* 112:1049–1053, 2003.
Arditi M, Mason EO Jr, Bradley JS, et al: Three-year multicenter surveillance of pneumococcal meningitis in children: clinical characteristics and outcome related to penicillin susceptibility and dexamethasone use, *Pediatrics* 102:1087–1097, 1998.

218. **How should contacts of children with *N. meningitidis* disease be managed?**
The attack rate of secondary cases among household contacts of an index patient with invasive disease caused by *N. meningitidis* is 500 to 800 times that of the general population. **Antibiotic prophylaxis is indicated for the following exposed individuals**:
- Household members, roommates, intimate contacts, contacts at childcare center, young adults exposed in dormitories, and military recruits exposed in training centers within the 7 days before the onset of the index patient's symptoms
- Airplane travelers seated next to an index patient on a flight lasting more than 8 hours or who were exposed to the index patient's respiratory secretions within the 7 days before the onset of the index patient's symptoms
- Medical personnel who were exposed to the index patient's respiratory secretions through intubation, endotracheal tube management, or mouth-to-mouth resuscitation
  Options for prophylaxis include:
- Rifampin given twice daily for 2 days
- IM ceftriaxone (1 dose)
- Oral ciprofloxacin (for those ≥18 years of age)
  Prophylaxis is not recommended for casual contacts at school, work, or hospital setting without direct exposure to the index patient's respiratory secretions.

American Academy of Pediatrics: Meningococcal infections. In Pickering LK, editor: *2012 Red Book: Report of the Committee on Infectious Diseases*, ed 29. Elk Grove Village, IL, 2012, American Academy of Pediatrics, pp 503–505.

219. **What is the most common parasitic infection of the CNS?**
Neurocysticercosis. This is a tapeworm disease that is most commonly initiated by the ingestion of undercooked pork containing *Taenia solium* larvae. After these larvae mature, eggs from adult tapeworms are then acquired by fecal-oral transmission among humans or by autoinoculation. If hematogenous spread of these eggs to the brain occurs, two types of complications can occur.
- Parenchymal cystic lesions can form a calcified granuloma that can result in seizures and/or headache.
- Extraparenchymal cysticerci can become trapped within the ventricles, foramina, or aqueduct and cause obstructive hydrocephalus manifesting as headache, nausea, vomiting, or change in mental status.

Garcia HH, Nash TE, Del Brutto OH: Clinical symptoms, diagnosis, and treatment of neurocysticercosis, *Lancet Neuro* 13:1202–1215, 2014.

OCULAR INFECTIONS

220. **Among neonates with conjunctivitis, what is the timing for the various etiologies?**
- Chemical: Onset in <2 days
- *Neisseria gonorrhoeae*: Onset in 2 to 7 days
- *C. trachomatis*: Onset in 5 to 14 days
- HSV: Onset in 10 to 14 days

221. **What is the best method of prophylaxis for ophthalmia neonatorum?**
Ophthalmia neonatorum is conjunctivitis in the first month of life. Historically, this referred to *N. gonorrhoeae* as the causative agent from acquisition at birth. Unrecognized and untreated maternal *N. gonorrhoeae* before delivery is now quite rare in the United States. *C. trachomatis* is now the more predominant etiology of neonatal conjunctivitis in the United States. Other bacterial microbes and HSV can be pathogens. As a consequence, erythromycin 0.5% ophthalmic ointment is now used routinely in nurseries in the United States to prevent conjunctivitis, although the efficacy for preventing chlamydial disease (primarily pneumonia) remains unclear. Worldwide, other methods are used, including gentamicin ointment, 2.5% povidone-iodine ophthalmic solution, and silver nitrate drops.

222. **Can newborns with chlamydial conjunctivitis be treated with topical therapy alone?**
No. Newborns diagnosed with chlamydial conjunctivitis should receive systemic therapy with oral erythromycin for 14 days. One study has suggested that oral azithromycin, 20 mg/kg/day for 3 days, is also effective. Topical

therapy will not eradicate the organism from the upper respiratory tract, and it fails to prevent the development of chlamydial pneumonia. Close follow-up evaluation is indicated to ensure the absence of relapse.

Hammerschlag M, Gelling M, Roblin PM, et al: Treatment of neonatal chlamydial conjunctivitis with azithromycin, *Pediatr Infect Dis J* 17:1049–1050, 1998.

223. **In children with conjunctivitis and otitis media, what are the most likely etiologic agents?**
     - *Bacterial:* Nontypeable *H. influenzae* is the most common cause of the so-called conjunctivitis-otitis syndrome, which is characterized by concurrent conjunctivitis and otitis media.
     - *Viral:* Adenovirus may also cause a conjunctivitis-otitis syndrome.

224. **Can bacterial conjunctivitis be distinguished from viral conjunctivitis on clinical grounds alone?**
     No. Classically, bacterial conjunctivitis is more common in infants and young children with the discharge being purulent or mucopurulent. A history of sticky eyelids with eyelash closure on awakening is predictive of a bacterial etiology. The most commonly implicated organism is nontypeable *H. influenzae.* Viral conjunctivitis is accompanied by a serous exudate in children of all ages, classically from adenovirus infections. Bacterial infections are commonly associated with otitis media, and otoscopy should be performed on all patients. However, clinical findings can overlap. Both bacteria and viruses can cause unilateral or bilateral symptoms.

Azari AA, Barney NP: Conjunctivitis: a systematic review of diagnosis and treatment, *JAMA* 310:1721–1729, 2013.
Richards A, Guzman-Cottrill JA: Conjunctivitis, *Pediatr Rev* 31:196–208, 2010.
Patel PB, Diaz MC, Bennett JE, et al: Clinical features of bacterial conjunctivitis in children, *Acad Emerg Med* 14:1–5, 2007.

225. **What is keratoconjunctivitis?**
     Keratoconjunctivitis is an inflammatory process that involves both the conjunctiva and the cornea. Superficial inflammation of the cornea (keratitis) occurs commonly in association with viral and bacterial conjunctivitis, particularly in adults. Hence, many cases of conjunctivitis are more correctly called *keratoconjunctivitis. Epidemic keratoconjunctivitis* is caused by adenovirus serotypes 8, 19, and 37. Some organisms, including measles virus, *P. aeruginosa, N. gonorrhoeae,* and HSV have a propensity to cause more severe infection of the cornea. Infection as a result of these pathogens must be recognized early to prevent corneal scarring with subsequent vision loss.

226. **What are the most common causative organisms of acute bacterial conjunctivitis?**
     - Neonate: *S. aureus, H. influenzae, C. trachomatis*
     - Child: *S. aureus, S. pneumoniae, H. influenzae, M. catarrhalis*
     - Adolescent/adult: *S. aureus, S. pneumoniae, Streptococcus* spp., *H. influenzae, M. catarrhalis, Acinetobacter* spp.

227. **How does the treatment vary by age for suspected acute bacterial conjunctivitis?**
     Topical therapy for *neonatal* chlamydial conjunctivitis should never be used as sole therapy because of the high likelihood of concomitant respiratory tract colonization (which can eventually progress to pneumonia). Infections resulting from *N. gonorrhoeae, P. aeruginosa, H. influenzae* type b, and *N. meningitidis* require systemic therapy to prevent the serious complications seen with these organisms. *Ophthalmic ointments* are usually preferred for infants and young children because they can be instilled more reliably and remain in the eye for a longer time. In older children, *ophthalmic solutions* may be preferred to prevent the blurring of vision that occurs with ointments. In general, the efficacy of ophthalmic ointments is presumed to be superior to that of solutions. However, several antibiotics are available in high-concentration solutions. These "fortified" formulations have not been compared prospectively with other preparations, but they are widely used because of their presumed enhanced efficacy.

228. **What should be the specific treatment for a 5-year-old diagnosed with infectious conjunctivitis in an outpatient setting?**
     This is controversial because viral and bacterial causes (and even allergic conjunctivitis) have clinical overlap, and cultures are not usually obtained on the initial evaluation to obtain a precise diagnosis. Two questions are paramount:

1. *Should empiric antibiotic therapy be started?* Topical antibiotics have been shown to decrease the duration of bacterial conjunctivitis, which does allow an earlier return to school and to work for parents. Treatment can thus reduce the socioeconomic costs of conjunctivitis and help prevent the spread of infection. However, the majority of cases of bacterial conjunctivitis are self-limiting and resolve without treatment. If the cause is indeed viral, antibiotic therapy is unnecessary and may contribute to resistance and unwarranted side effects. Given these options of treatment versus "watchful waiting," physician style and parental preferences hold large sway. Antibiotic treatment should be considered for purulent conjunctivitis, for those with significant discomfort, for contact lens wearers, for immunocompromised patients, and for any cases suspicious for either chlamydial or gonococcal conjunctivitis.

2. *If therapy is begun, which topical antibiotic is preferable?* Options are considerable, including newer (and expensive) therapies (e.g., fluoroquinolones) designed to counteract the growing resistance patterns of typical pathogens, such as *S. pneumoniae, H. influenzae,* and *Moraxella* spp. Once again, physician style, compliance considerations, and prescription coverage play a large role in choice of antibiotic therapy because clear-cut evidence-based guidelines are lacking.

Azari AA, Barney NP: Conjunctivitis: a systematic review of diagnosis and treatment, *JAMA* 310:1721–1729, 2013.
Williams L, Malhotra Y, Murante B, et al: A single-blinded randomized clinical trial comparing polymyxin B-trimethoprim and moxifloxacin for treatment of acute conjunctivitis in children, *J Pediatr* 162:857–861, 2013.

229. **What is Parinaud oculoglandular syndrome?**
Parinaud syndrome is characterized by granulomatous or ulcerating conjunctivitis and prominent preauricular or submandibular adenopathy. The most common cause is cat-scratch disease, but other causes include tularemia, sporotrichosis, tuberculosis, syphilis, and infectious mononucleosis. An important condition in the differential diagnosis to exclude is Kawasaki disease.

230. **How is orbital cellulitis distinguished from periorbital (or preseptal) cellulitis?**
Periorbital cellulitis involves the tissues anterior to the eyelid septum (Fig. 10-12), whereas *orbital cellulitis* involves the orbit and is sometimes associated with abscess formation and cavernous sinus thrombosis. Distinction between these processes requires assessment of *ocular mobility, pupillary reflex, visual acuity,* and *globe position* (e.g., proptosis), which are normal in periorbital cellulitis but may be abnormal in orbital cellulitis. An abnormality in any of these four areas mandates radiologic evaluation (usually CT scan of the orbit) and possible surgical drainage.

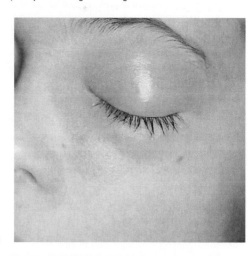

Figure 10-12. Periorbital cellulitis. *(From Zitelli BJ, Davis HW: Atlas of Pediatric Physical Diagnosis, ed 4. St. Louis, 2002, Mosby, p 848.)*

231. **What is the pathogenesis of periorbital and orbital cellulitis?**
- *Periorbital:* This cellulitis may result from **direct inoculation** in and around the eyelid, **trauma** (blunt or penetrating), and **spread of microorganisms** from the sinuses or nasopharynx into the preseptal space

- *Orbital:* Most cases originate in nearby paranasal sinuses (especially ethmoid) as a **complication of sinusitis.** The walls (lamina papyracea) of the ethmoid and sphenoid sinuses are paper thin with natural bony dehiscences that allow spread of infection. In addition, orbital and sinus veins anastomose and are valveless, which allows communicating blood flow and easier spread of infection.
- Complications of orbital cellulitis include subperiosteal orbital abscess, vision loss (from optic neuritis due to surrounding inflammation or thrombophlebitis in adjacent vessels), cavernous sinus thrombophlebitis, and brain abscess.

Sethuraman U, Kamat D: The red eye: evaluation and management, *Clin Pediatr* 48:588–600, 2009.

232. What are the most common organisms causing orbital cellulitis?
- **Staphylococci** are the most common organisms causing orbital cellulitis. They are implicated in both orbital and periorbital cellulitis because it is a colonizing organism of both the upper respiratory tract and the skin.
- **Streptococci**:
  - Group A *Streptococcus*
  - **S. pneumoniae and other alpha hemolytic strep such as S. anginosus**
  Anaerobic organisms and fungi, such as *Mucor* species and *Aspergillus*, should be considered in immunocompromised hosts.

233. What are treatment options for orbital cellulitis?
Treatment should be guided by the likely epidemiology of the disease. In this era of increasing MRSA colonization in the general population, empiric therapy often is comprised of coverage for MRSA, such as vancomycin combined with a third-generation cephalosporin, such as ceftriaxone. This choice also has the advantage of good CSF penetration, while an evaluation is being done for intracranial complications. Other choices include vancomycin and ampicillin/sulbactam or piperacillin/tazobactam, with the caveat that these latter agents do not have complete CNS penetration.

234. What is the difference between a hordeolum, a stye, and a chalazion?
- A **hordeolum** is a purulent infection of any one of the sebaceous or apocrine sweat glands of the eyelid, including the glands of Moll and Zeis, which drain near the eyelash follicle, and the meibomian glands, which drain nearer the conjunctiva. Clinically, a hordeolum is recognized as a red, tender swelling. It is usually caused by *S. aureus*.
- A **stye** is an external hordeolum, on the skin side of the eyelid.
- A **chalazion** is an internal hordeolum, on the conjunctival side of the eyelid.
  In all cases, these lesions are treated with warm compresses and topical antibiotic drops or ointment (although their value is debatable) and usually resolve within 7 days. Intralesional triamcinolone injection can be beneficial for a chalazion. A chalazion is more likely to become chronic and require surgical excision.

235. Why is the "ciliary flush" particularly worrisome when evaluating a patient with a pink or red eye?
Ciliary flush refers to circumcorneal hyperemia in which conjunctival redness is concentrated in the area adjacent to the cornea (limbus). This can be a sign of significant ocular pathology (e.g., keratitis, anterior uveitis, acute angle-closure glaucoma) and requires hastened referral to an ophthalmologist.

236. What organism should not be overlooked when treating ocular infections following penetrating trauma?
Bacillus cereus. This organism is a gram-positive, spore-forming rod, which is ubiquitous in soil. The spores can be very heat resistant. It may be a cause of severe ocular infection following penetrating trauma with contaminated foreign bodies, such as glass, metal, or sticks. Similar to its related bacillus of anthrax fame (*B. anthracis*), *B. cereus* is generally sensitive to and treated with ciprofloxacin.

OTITIS MEDIA

237. Is ear pulling a reliable sign of infection?
No. In the absence of other signs or symptoms (e.g., fever, URI symptoms), ear pulling alone is a very poor indicator of acute otitis media (AOM).

Baker RB: Is ear pulling associated with ear infection? *Pediatrics* 90:1006–1007, 1992.

238. What are the landmarks of the tympanic membrane?
See Fig. 10-13.

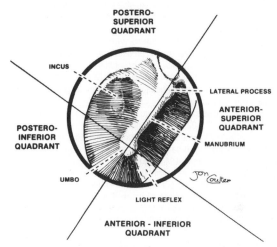

Figure 10-13. Right tympanic membrane. *(From Bluestone CD, Klein JO:* Otitis Media in Infants and Children. *Philadelphia, 1988, WB Saunders, p 76.)*

239. What are the most reliable ways, on physical examination, to accurately diagnosis AOM?
Good visualization of the tympanic membrane (TM) and the use of a pneumatic otoscope are key.
- **Visualization of position:** Bulging of the TM implies fluid under pressure, whereas retraction is more commonly seen with effusion rather than suppuration.
- **Color and translucence:** Normal TM color is pearly gray and translucent; cloudiness implies suppuration; distinct redness (especially if unilateral) can indicate infection, but can be seen in other settings, particularly with high fever. Marked redness without TM bulging is unusual in AOM.
- **Mobility:** Impaired mobility of the TM to positive pressure by pneumatic otoscopy implies a fluid-filled space.

Shaikh N, Hoberman A, Kaleida PH, et al: Otoscopic signs of otitis media, *Pediatr Infect Dis J* 10:822–826, 2011.
Rothman R, Owens T, Simel DL: Does this child have acute otitis media? *JAMA* 290:1633–1640, 2003.

240. What are the most common viral and bacterial agents that cause AOM?
Tympanocentesis is now rarely done except under the auspices of tympanostomy tube placement, but historically it has yielded bacteria and/or viruses in up to 96% of patients with AOM (66% bacteria and viruses together, 27% bacteria alone, and 4% virus alone).

The most common organisms that are recovered from patients with AOM (either from the nasopharynx or middle ear) are *S. pneumoniae,* nontypeable *H. influenzae,* and *M. catarrhalis.* The microbiology of AOM changed with the introduction of the initial 7-valent pneumococcal conjugate vaccine (PCV-7) with a shift towards increasing prevalence of *H. influenzae,* and serotypes of *S. pneumonia* that display antibiotic resistance or are not covered by PCV-7. The effect of PCV-13 on the microbiology of AOM remains under study.

Lieberthal A, Carroll AE, Chonmaitree T, et al: The diagnosis and management of acute otitis media, *Pediatrics* 131; e964–e999, 2013.
Ruohola A, et al: Microbiology of acute otitis media in children with tympanostomy tubes: prevalences of bacteria and viruses, *Clin Infect Dis.*43:1417–1422, 2006.

241. **What is the "watchful waiting" approach for otitis media?**
This is the observational option ("watchful waiting") for patients >2 years for whom the diagnosis of otitis media is certain, but the illness is not severe. Anticipating a high percentage of spontaneous improvement, clinicians defer antibiotic therapy. If the patient does not improve with observation for 48 to 72 hours, antibiotics are initiated. The intent is to reduce potentially unnecessary antibiotics. When using this option, reliable follow-up *must* be ensured.

242. **Should all children with AOM be treated with antibiotics?**
Observation as initial management for AOM in properly selected children does not increase the risk for serious complications, provided that follow-up is ensured and a rescue antibiotic is given for persistent or worsening symptoms. AAP guidelines published in 2013 endorse the following practices:
- Antibiotic therapy should be prescribed for AOM (bilateral or unilateral) in children 6 months and older with severe signs or symptoms
  - Severe AOM is defined as moderate or severe otalgia or otalgia for at least 48 hours or temperature 39 °C (102.2 °F) or higher
- Children 6 months to 23 months of age without severe signs or symptoms:
  - Antibiotic therapy should be prescribed for bilateral AOM in young children.
  - For nonsevere unilateral AOM in young children: it is reasonable to offer observation with close follow-up based on joint decision-making with caregivers, provided that follow-up can be ensured and there is a mechanism to begin antibiotic therapy if the child worsens or fails to improve within 48 to 72 hours of onset of symptoms.
- In children >23 months of age with AOM (unilateral or bilateral) without severe signs or symptoms, it is reasonable to offer observation with close follow-up.

Lieberthal A, Carroll AE, Chonmaitree T, et al: The diagnosis and management of acute otitis media, *Pediatrics* 131; e964–e999, 2013.
Spiro DM, Tay KY, Arnold DH, et al: Wait-and-see prescription for the treatment of acute otitis media: a randomized controlled trial, *JAMA* 296:1235, 2006.
Marcy M, Takata G, Chan LS, et al: Management of acute otitis media, *Evid Rep Technol Assess (Summ)* 15:1–4, 2000.

243. **What is the recommended therapy for children for whom treatment for AOM is indicated?**
High-dose (80 to 90 mg/kg/day) amoxicillin is recommended for children who have not taken amoxicillin in the previous 30 days and who do not have concurrent conjunctivitis (indicating *H. influenza* infection and the need for a β-lactamase inhibitor).

Lieberthal A, Carroll AE, Chonmaitree T, et al: The diagnosis and management of acute otitis media, *Pediatrics* 131; e964–e999, 2013.

244. **After an acute episode of otitis media (OM), how long does the middle ear effusion persist?**
About 70% of patients will continue to have an effusion at 2 weeks, 40% at 1 month, 20% at 2 months, and 5% to 10% at 3 months.

Teele DW, Klein JO, Rosner BA: Epidemiology of otitis media in children, *Ann Otol Rhinol Laryngol Suppl* 89:5, 1980.

245. **What are the indications for tympanostomy tubes?**
Tympanostomy tubes are most commonly inserted for the treatment of otitis media with effusion (OME) or for prophylaxis against recurrent otitis media. The newest AAP recommendations state that tympanostomy tubes may be offered for recurrent AOM (3 episodes in 6 months or 4 episodes in 1 year, with 1 episode in the preceding 6 months). This recommendation is based on limited trial data. For patients with recurrent otitis media, the benefit of tube placement is modest and must be weighed against the risk for complications, which include sclerosis, retraction, atrophy of the eardrum, and complication related to general anesthesia.

Lieberthal A, Carroll AE, Chonmaitree T, et al: The diagnosis and management of acute otitis media, *Pediatrics* 131; e964–e999, 2013.

Feldman HM, Paradise JL: OME and child development, *Contemp Pediatr* 26:40–41, 2009.
Paradise JL, Feldman HM, Campbell TF, et al: Tympanostomy tubes and developmental outcomes at 9 to 11 years of age, *N Engl J Med* 356:248–261, 2007.

246. **Should a child with tympanostomy tubes be allowed to swim?**
Otolaryngologists differ widely in their guidance to parents about issues of swimming and bathing. Controlled studies have shown that the rate of otorrhea is similar between nonswimmers (15%) and surface swimmers without earplugs (20%). Neither earplugs nor prophylactic eardrops appear to be necessary for most children who swim at the surface in the ocean or in a pool. If diving or underwater swimming is planned, fitted earplugs are often recommended. Bath water with shampooing can cause inflammatory changes in the middle ear, and thus, earplugs should be used if head dunking is anticipated during bathing. An *in vitro* study (using a head model) found water entry greatest with submersion in soapy water and with deeper swimming.

Wilcox LJ, Darrow DH: Should water precautions be recommended for children with tympanostomy tubes? *Laryngoscope* 124:10–11, 2014.
Hebert RL II, King GE, Bent JP III: Tympanostomy tubes and water exposure: a practical model, *Arch Otolaryngol Head Neck Surg* 124:1118–1121, 1998.

247. **A child with the acute onset of ear pain and double vision likely has what condition?**
Gradenigo syndrome is an *acquired paralysis* of the abducens muscle with *pain* in the area that is served by the ipsilateral trigeminal nerve. It is caused by inflammation of the sixth cranial nerve in the petrous portion, with involvement of the gasserian ganglion. The inflammation is usually the result of infection from otitis media or mastoiditis. Symptoms may include weakness of lateral gaze on the affected side, double vision, pain, photophobia, tearing, and hyperesthesia.

248. **What are differences between acute and chronic mastoiditis?**
- *Acute mastoiditis:* Presents as complication of acute otitis media with retroauricular inflammation (swelling and tenderness) and protrusion of the auricle; patients are younger; most likely causes are *S. pneumoniae* and *S. pyogenes* with MRSA increasing as a pathogen.
- *Chronic mastoiditis:* Typically with more extensive history of otitis media, including tympanostomy tubes; <50% with retroauricular swelling and tenderness; patients are older; most likely cause is *P. aeruginosa* with MRSA also increasing as a pathogen.

Lin HW, Shargorodsky J, Gopen Q: Clinical strategies for the management of acute mastoiditis in the pediatric population, *Clin Pediatr* 49:110–115, 2010.
Stähelin-Massik J, Podvinec M, Jakscha J, et al: Mastoiditis in children: a prospective, observational study comparing clinical presentation, microbiology, computed tomography, surgical findings and histology, *Eur J Pediatr* 167:541–548, 2008.

249. **What are the potential complications of mastoiditis?**
Epidural abscess, brain abscess, cervical abscess, sinus vein thrombosis, cervical vein thrombosis, and sensorineural hearing loss are potential complications.

250. **What famous playwright died of mastoiditis?**
Oscar Wilde died from CNS dissemination of mastoiditis, likely due to *S. pneumoniae*. This was especially ironic as his estranged father and Irish eye and ear surgeon, Sir William Wilde, introduced the retroauricular incision, which at the time was a novel surgical approach for the treatment of mastoiditis.

Bento RF, Fonseca ACO: A brief history of mastoidectomy, *Int Arch Otorhinolaryngol* 17:168–178, 2013.

PHARYNGEAL AND LARYNGEAL INFECTIONS

251. **Can group A β-hemolytic streptococcal (GAS) pharyngitis reliably be distinguished from viral causes?**
Streptococcal pharyngitis is a disease with variable clinical manifestations. Clues that suggest streptococcal disease include the abrupt onset of headache, fever, and sore throat with the

subsequent development of tender cervical lymphadenopathy, tonsillar exudate, and palatal petechiae in the winter or early spring. The presence of concurrent conjunctivitis, rhinitis, cough, or diarrhea suggests a viral process. The physical findings are by no means diagnostic and, when present, are more commonly found in children >3 years. Even the most skilled clinician cannot exceed an accuracy rate of about 75%. A throat culture or a rapid antigen test is essential for confirming streptococcal infection.

Neu J, Walker WA: Streptococcal pharyngitis, *N Engl J Med* 364:648–655, 2011.

252. What is the typical rash of scarlet fever?
The rash, which is caused by a streptococcal pyrogenic exotoxin, usually begins on the neck, face, and upper trunk and generalizes to the remainder of the body over 1 to 2 days. Palms and soles are usually spared. The rash has a sandpaper-like texture—pinpoint, erythematous, blanchable papules. The erythema (and some petechiae from fragile capillaries) may be prominent in skin folds (Pastia lines). Over 5 to 7 days, the rash fades and later is followed by desquamation, particularly on the hands, feet, axillae, and groin.

253. Why is a throat culture for GAS advised if a rapid antigen detection test is negative?
A variety of antigen detection tests are available. They have a high degree of specificity, but a lower sensitivity. Thus, a negative test does not exclude the possibility of GAS and a throat culture is recommended. In adults, however, because of the low incidence of GAS infections and the extremely low risk for acute rheumatic fever, the Infectious Disease Society of America recommends that the diagnosis can be made on the basis of antigen detection testing alone without confirmation of a negative antigen test by a negative throat culture.

Shulman S, Bisno AL, Clegg HW, et al: Clinical practice guideline for the diagnosis and management of group A streptococcal pharyngitis: 2012 update by the Infectious Diseases Society of America, *Clin Infect Dis* 55:e86–e102, 2012.

254. What is the rationale for the treatment of GAS pharyngitis?
- To prevent acute rheumatic fever (Even though there is a low incidence of acute rheumatic fever in the United States, worldwide rheumatic heart disease is the leading cause of cardiovascular death during the first five decades of life.)
- To shorten the course of the illness, including headache, sore throat, and lymph node tenderness
- To reduce the spread of infection
- To prevent suppurative complications

255. What is the recommended treatment for GAS pharyngitis?
Except in a patient with a history of penicillin allergy, the recommended therapy is IM benzathine G or oral penicillin V or amoxicillin for a duration of 10 days. Amoxicillin suspension is often prescribed rather than penicillin suspension because of better taste. First-line therapy for penicillin-allergic patients is narrow-spectrum cephalosporins (e.g., cephalexin, cefadroxil), clindamycin, or a macrolide (e.g., azithromycin, clarithromycin). Tetracyclines, trimethoprim-sulfamethoxazole, and older fluoroquinolones (e.g., ciprofloxacin) are not recommended.

Shulman S, Bisno AL, Clegg HW, et al: Clinical practice guideline for the diagnosis and management of group A streptococcal pharyngitis: 2012 update by the Infectious Diseases Society of America, *Clin Infect Dis* 55:e86–e102, 2012.

256. Why do some clinicians use treatments other than penicillins for GAS pharyngitis?
Although 100% of GAS cases have demonstrated *in vitro* susceptibility to penicillins, normal oropharyngeal flora (including *S. aureus* and *M. catarrhalis*) may produce β-lactamases that can inactivate penicillin and amoxicillin in the local oral environment. Other factors, including tolerability, cost, and prior responses to treatment, are also involved in the choice of antibiotics.

Brook I, Gober AE: Failure to eradicate streptococci and beta-lactamase producing bacteria, *Acta Paediatr* 97:193–195, 2008.

257. How does one differentiate a patient with a sore throat who is a streptococcal carrier with an intercurrent viral pharyngitis from one who is having repeated episodes of GAS pharyngitis?

Streptococcal carrier
- Signs and symptoms of viral infection (rhinorrhea, cough, conjunctivitis, diarrhea)
- Little clinical response to antibiotics (sometimes difficult to assess because of the self-resolving nature of viral infections)
- Group A *Streptococcus* present on cultures between episodes
- No serologic response to infection (i.e., anti-streptolysin O, anti-DNase B)
- Same serotype of group A *Streptococcus* in sequential cultures

Recurrent group A streptococcal pharyngitis
- Signs and symptoms consistent with group A streptococcal infection
- Marked clinical response to antibiotics
- No group A *Streptococcus* on cultures between episodes
- Positive serologic response to infection
- Different serotypes of group A *Streptococcus* on sequential cultures

Hill HR: Group A streptococcal carrier versus acute infection: the continuing dilemma, *Clin Infect Dis* 50:491–492, 2010.
Shaikh N, Leonard E, Martin JM: Prevalence of streptococcal pharyngitis and streptococcal carriage in children: a meta-analysis, *Pediatrics* 126:e557–e564, 2012.
Gerber MA: Diagnosis and treatment of pharyngitis in children, *Pediatr Clin North Am* 52:729–747, 2005.

258. When can children treated for positive streptococcal throat cultures return to school or day care?

Although clinical improvement often occurs promptly, most patients remain culture positive 14 hours after the initiation of antibiotics. However, by 24 hours, nearly all patients are culture negative. To minimize contagion, children should receive a full 24 hours of antibiotic therapy before returning to school or childcare.

American Academy of Pediatrics: Group A streptococcal infections. In Pickering LK, editor: *2012 Red Book: Report of the Committee on Infectious Diseases*, ed 29. Elk Grove Village, IL, 2012, American Academy of Pediatrics, p 677.
Snellman LW, Stang HJ, Stang JM, et al: Duration of positive throat cultures for group A streptococci after initiation of antibiotic therapy, *Pediatrics* 91:1166–1170, 1993.

259. How commonly do children <3 years of age develop GAS pharyngitis?

Traditional teaching has been that toddlers rarely develop streptococcal pharyngitis. However, studies indicate that the incidence of infection and the prevalence of carriage are greater than previously thought. In studies of patients <2 years with fever and clinical pharyngitis, 4% to 6% were positive for GAS; among well children, the carrier rate is about 6%. In young children, GAS infection is more commonly associated with a syndrome of fever, mucopurulent rhinitis, and diffuse adenopathy. The rate of rheumatic fever is exceedingly low in children <3 years.

Shulman S, Bisno AL, Clegg HW, et al: Clinical practice guideline for the diagnosis and management of group A streptococcal pharyngitis: 2012 update by the Infectious Diseases Society of America, *Clin Infect Dis* 55: e86–e102, 2012.
Berkovitch M, Vaida A, Zhovtis D, et al: Group A streptococcal pharyngotonsillitis in children less than 2 years of age—more common than is thought, *Clin Pediatr* 38:365–366, 1999.
Nussinovitch M, Finkelstein Y, Amir J, Varsano I: Group A beta-hemolytic streptococcal pharyngitis in preschool children aged 3 months to 5 years, *Clin Pediatr* 38:357–360, 1999.

260. How long after the development of streptococcal pharyngitis can treatment be initiated and still effectively prevent rheumatic fever?

Treatment should be started as soon as possible, but little is lost in waiting for throat culture results to establish the diagnosis. Antibiotic treatment prevents acute rheumatic fever even when therapy is initiated as long as **9 days** after the onset of the acute illness.

Catanzaro FJ, Stetson CA, Morris AJ, et al: The role of the streptococcus in the pathogenesis of rheumatic fever, *Am J Med* 17:749–756, 1954.

KEY POINTS: PHARYNGITIS

1. Clinical pictures of viral and streptococcal pharyngitis have significant clinical overlap.
2. Tetracyclines, trimethoprim-sulfamethoxazole, and older fluoroquinolones (e.g., ciprofloxacin) are not recommended for the treatment of group A β-hemolytic streptococcal pharyngitis.
3. Antibiotic treatment prevents acute rheumatic fever even when therapy is initiated as long as 9 days after the onset of acute illness.
4. Although the incidence of rheumatic fever is low in the United States, worldwide it is the leading cause of cardiovascular death during the first five decades of life.

261. **What diagnosis should be suspected in a teenager with pharyngitis followed by multifocal pneumonia and sepsis?**
Lemierre syndrome. This is a *septic thrombophlebitis* of the internal jugular vein that is typically caused by anaerobic organisms, such as the gram-negative rod *Fusobacterium necrophorum*. The illness begins as a pharyngitis or tonsillitis; once thrombophlebitis develops, it results in seeding of multiple organs with septic emboli. Pneumonia may lead to respiratory failure in untreated cases. Ultrasonography of the jugular vessels and CT scan of the chest are helpful for establishing the diagnosis. Anaerobic organisms may be difficult to capture with traditional cultures.

262. **What is the difference between herpangina and Ludwig angina?**
- *Herpangina* is a common viral infection during the summer and fall and is characterized by posterior pharyngeal, buccal, and palatal vesicles and ulcers. Coxsackieviruses A and B and echoviruses are the most common causative agents. In young children, it is often accompanied by a high temperature (39.4° to 40 °C [103° to 104 °F]). Herpangina is distinguished from HSV infections of the mouth, which are more anterior and involve the lips, tongue, and gingiva.
- *Ludwig angina* is an acute diffuse infection (usually bacterial due to mixed anaerobes) of the submandibular and sublingual spaces with brawny induration of the floor of the mouth and tongue. Airway obstruction can occur. The infections usually follow oral cavity injuries or dental complications (e.g., extractions, impactions).

Lin HW, O'Neill A, Cunningham MJ: Ludwig's angina in the pediatric population, *Clin Pediatr* 48:583–587, 2009.

263. **What is quinsy?**
Quinsy is a **peritonsillar abscess.** George Washington's death has traditionally been attributed to quinsy, but historians have debated whether an alternate pathologic explanation—epiglottitis—was more likely.

Morens DM: Death of a president, *N Engl J Med* 341:1845–1850, 1999.

264. **How is a peritonsillar abscess distinguished from peritonsillar cellulitis?**
A *peritonsillar abscess* is diagnosed when a discrete mass is noted, usually in school-age children and adolescents. The bulging abscess causes lateral displacement of the uvula. Trismus, due to spasm of masticator muscles, occurs more commonly in the setting of abscess than does simple cellulitis, which is characterized by signs of diffuse inflammation without a mass. Many patients have a "hot potato" voice, a muffled voice caused by palatal edema and spasm of the internal pterygoid muscle that elevates the palate.

Galioto NJ: Peritonsillar abscess, *Am Fam Physician* 77:199–209, 2008.

265. **What radiographic features suggest the diagnosis of a retropharyngeal abscess?**
When a patient's neck is extended, a measurement of the prevertebral space that exceeds two times the diameter of the C2 vertebra suggests an abscess (Fig. 10-14). Pockets of air in the

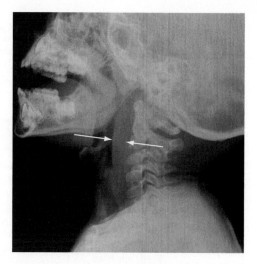

Figure 10-14. Thickening of the prevertebral soft tissues *(white arrows)* in a 3-year-old boy with neck stiffness due to a retropharyngeal abscess. *(From Taussig LM, Landau LI, editors: Pediatric Respiratory Medicine, ed 2. Philadelphia, 2008, Mosby, p 147.)*

prevertebral space also suggest abscess. The retropharynx extends to T1 in the superior mediastinum, so empyema or mediastinitis is also possible whenever a retropharyngeal abscess is identified. CT scanning can delineate the extent of these deep neck infections.

266. Which age group is most susceptible to retropharyngeal abscess?
This disease is most common in children **between the ages of 1 and 6 years**. There are several small lymph nodes in the retropharynx that usually disappear by the age of 4 or 5. These lymph nodes drain the posterior nasal passages and nasopharynx, and they may become involved if those sites are infected.

267. What are the indications for tonsillectomy in children 1 to 18 years old?
   • Obstructive sleep apnea syndrome due to adenotonsillar hypertrophy with comorbid conditions such as growth retardation, poor school performance, enuresis, and behavioral problems
   • Recurrent throat infection:
      • ≥7 episodes in the past year or
      • ≥5 episodes per year for 2 years or
      • ≥3 episodes per year for 3 years
      Each episode of sore throat must be accompanied by one or more of the following: temperature >38.3 °C, cervical adenopathy, tonsillar exudate, or positive test for GAS
      Other factors that may be considered in children who do not meet the criteria above that favor tonsillectomy are:
   • Multiple antibiotic allergies/intolerances
   • PFAPA (see question #98)
   • History of peritonsillar abscess

Baugh RF, Archer SM, Mitchell RM, et al: Clinical practice guideline: tonsillectomy in children, *Otolaryngol Head Neck Surg* 144:S1–S30, 2011.

268. How should children with epiglottitis be managed?
Acute epiglottitis is a medical emergency and all children should be assumed to have a critical airway (i.e., the potential for imminent occlusion exists). Because of the risk for airway obstruction with agitation of the patient, the patient should be allowed to remain with parents and free from restraint. Examination should be performed as cautiously as possible. Continuous observation regardless of the setting (e.g., radiology suite), avoidance of supine positioning, and arrangements for admission to an intensive care unit are mandatory. Ideally, the epiglottis is visualized directly in an operating room, and the child is intubated immediately afterward.

269. **What are the bacterial causes of epiglottitis?**
Previously, more than 90% of cases were caused by *H. influenzae* type b. However, because of the routine use of *H. influenzae* type b vaccines in infants beginning in 1989 and 1990, the incidence of epiglottitis has decreased dramatically. Pneumococci, staphylococci, and streptococci (group A), and nontypeable *H. influenzae* now account for a relatively large percentage of cases.

270. **How is epiglottitis distinguished clinically from croup?**
See Table 10-7.

Table 10-7 Clinical Distinctions Between Croup and Epiglottitis

	CROUP	EPIGLOTTITIS
Age	Younger (6 mo-3 yr)	Older (3-7 yr)
Onset of stridor	Gradual (24-72 hr)	Rapid (8-12 hr)
Symptoms	Prodromal upper respiratory infection Barking or brassy cough Hoarseness Slightly sore throat	Minimal rhinitis Little coughing Muffled voice Pain in throat
Signs	Mild fever Not toxic Variable distress Harsh inspiratory stridor Expiratory sounds uncommon	High body temperature (>39 °C) Toxic appearance Severe distress; sits upright; may drool Low-pitched inspiratory stridor May have a low-pitched expiratory sound
Radiology	Subglottic narrowing	Edema of epiglottis and aryepiglottic folds (positive thumb sign)

271. **What are the criteria for the admission of a child with viral croup?**
- Clinical signs of impending respiratory failure:
- Marked retractions, depressed level of consciousness, cyanosis, hypotonicity, and diminished or absent inspiratory breath sounds
- Laboratory signs of impending respiratory failure:
  - P_{CO_2} more than 45 mm Hg,
  - $Pa_{O_2} < 70$ mm Hg in room air
- Clinical signs of dehydration or inability to tolerate enteral fluids
- Failure of outpatient or emergency room management, such as dexamethasone and inhaled racemic epinephrine after appropriate monitoring interval
- Historic consideration:
  - High-risk infant with history of subglottic stenosis or prior intubations

Bjornson CL, Johnson DW: Croup, *Lancet* 371:329–339, 2008.

272. **Are steroids efficacious for the treatment of croup?**
The use of corticosteroids (including oral and IM dexamethasone and nebulized budesonide) has been shown to be beneficial in treating croup. In particular, corticosteroid treatment reduces the incidence of intubation and results in more rapid respiratory improvement. In addition, among patients with mild or moderate croup, corticosteroids appear to reduce the use of nebulized racemic epinephrine, the need for return visits, and the need for hospitalization. Optimal doses are not clearly established. Dosing of dexamethasone is often based on the severity of croup ranging from mild croup with oral dosing (0.3 to 0.6 mg/kg up to 10 mg) to severe croup with IV or IM dosing (0.6 mg/kg up to 15 mg).

Russell KF, Liang Y, O'Gorman K, et al: Glucocorticoids for croup, *Cochrane Database Syst Rev* 1:CD001955, 2011.
Baumer JH: Glucocorticoid treatment in croup, *Arch Dis Child Educ Pract Ed* 91:58–60, 2006.

273. If a child has received racemic epinephrine as a treatment for croup, is hospitalization required?

No. In earlier days, children treated with racemic epinephrine were routinely hospitalized to observe for potential "rebound" mucosal edema and airway obstruction, regardless of how they appeared clinically. However, a number of recent studies have shown that children who are free of significant stridor or retractions at rest 2 hours after the administration of racemic epinephrine can be safely discharged, provided that adequate follow-up is ensured. In most of these studies, oral or IM dexamethasone (0.6 mg/kg) was also administered.

Bjornson C, Russell K, Vandermeer B, et al: Nebulized epinephrine for croup in children, *Cochrane Database Syst Rev* 10: CD006619, 2013.
Cherry JD: Croup, *N Engl J Med* 358:384–391, 2008.
Baumer JH: Glucocorticoid treatment in croup, *Arch Dis Child Educ Pract Ed* 91:58–60, 2006.

274. Is a cool-mist vaporizer truly of benefit for patients with croup?

Probably not. The usual advice for the home management of croup includes the use of a cool-mist vaporizer. The theory is that the coolness serves as a vasoconstrictor and that the humidified mist serves to thin respiratory secretions. Although this therapy remains time honored, it is largely unproven. The calming effects of being held by a parent during the mist treatment may have greater impact. It certainly can't hurt.

Cherry JD: Croup, *N Engl J Med* 358:384–391, 2008.
Bjornson CL, Johnson DW: Croup, *Lancet* 371:329–339, 2008.

275. What are membranous croup and pseudomembranous croup?

Membranous croup is the historical term for **diphtheria**, and *pseudomembranous croup* is the historical term for **bacterial tracheitis**. Bacterial tracheitis is usually caused by *S. aureus* and may occur after trauma to the neck or trachea or after a viral respiratory tract infection such as croup. The presentation of bacterial tracheitis is similar to that of severe croup or epiglottitis, and consequently a lateral neck radiograph is frequently obtained. In bacterial tracheitis, this study often reveals narrowing of the tracheal lumen as the result of a thick, purulent exudate that can extend into both main stem bronchi.

Woodburn, FC: Is membranous croup diphtheria? Read before the Indiana State Medical Society at Indianapolis, May 17, 1894, *JAMA* 121:776–778, 1894.

SINUSITIS

KEY POINTS: PNEUMATIZATION OF THE PARANASAL SINUSES

1. Maxillary and ethmoid: Present at birth.
2. Sphenoid: Begins at 2 to 3 years of age, complete by age 6 years.
3. Frontal: Begins at 3 to 7 years of age, complete by age 12 years.
4. Front sinus pneumatization is absent in 1% to 4% of the population.

276. When do the sinuses develop during childhood?

The maxillary and ethmoid sinuses are present at birth. Pneumatization of the sphenoid sinuses begins at about 2 to 3 years of age and is usually complete by about age 5. Frontal sinus pneumatization varies considerably, beginning at about 3 to 7 years of age and finishing by age 12 years. Frontal sinus pneumatization is absent in about 1% to 4% of the normal population due to agenesis. About 15% have unilateral frontal sinus hypoplasia.

Adibelli ZH, Songu M, Adibelli H: Paranasal sinus development in children: A magnetic resonance imaging analysis, *Am J Rhinol Allergy* 25:30–35, 2011.

277. Does a thick, green nasal discharge on day 2 of a respiratory illness indicate a bacterial sinus infection?

No. The character of nasal secretions (e.g., purulent, discolored, tenacious) does not distinguish viral from bacterial. Mucopurulent rhinitis commonly accompanies the common cold. Early treatment (<7 to 10 days) of purulent nasal discharge is a common cause of antibiotic overuse.

278. What is the typical presentation of sinusitis in children?

Unlike adults who may present with fever and localized pain, children have **persistent nasal symptoms** (anterior or posterior discharge, obstruction, or congestion) without improvement for 10 to 14 days or worsening after 5 to 7 days with or without improvement ("second" or "double sickening") and daytime cough (which may worsen at night). A minority of children may present with a more acute disease accompanied by a temperature of 39 °C or higher and a persistent (≥3 days) purulent nasal discharge. These children generally appear ill. Headache and facial pain are uncommon in younger patients with sinusitis but are seen more commonly in older children and teenagers who have had increased sinus pneumatization.

Wald ER, Applegate KE, Bordley C, et al: Clinical practice guideline for the diagnosis and management of acute bacterial sinusitis in children aged 1 to 18 years, *Pediatrics* 132:e262 –e280, 2013.
Demuri GP, Wald ER: Acute bacterial sinusitis in children, *N Engl J Med* 367:1128–1134, 2012.

279. What is the role of sinus imaging in the diagnosis of sinusitis?

Both the AAP and Infectious Diseases Society of America (IDSA) guidelines discourage *routine* imaging to distinguish acute bacterial sinusitis from viral URI. Abnormal radiographs cannot distinguish bacterial or viral etiologies of sinusitis. Plain radiographs may have findings of diffuse opacification, mucosal swelling, and air-fluid levels. CT scans or MRI may also demonstrate abnormalities such as mucosal thickening or air-fluid levels even in children without complaints of upper respiratory symptoms.

Wald ER, Applegate KE, Bordley C, et al: Clinical practice guideline for the diagnosis and management of acute bacterial sinusitis in children aged 1 to 18 years, *Pediatrics* 132:e262–e280, 2013.
Chow AW, Benninger MS, Brook I, et al: IDSA clinical practice guideline for acute bacterial rhinosinusitis in children and adults, *Clin Infect Dis* 54:e72–e112, 2012.

280. What should be suspected in an adolescent male with a very severe frontal headache in the setting of sinusitis?

An **intracranial complication** of sinusitis, such as subdural or epidural empyema, venous thrombosis, brain abscess, or meningitis, should be suspected. For unclear reasons, previously healthy adolescent males with frontal sinusitis are noted to have an increased risk of intracranial complications.

Orbital complications, such as subperiosteal abscess, orbital cellulitis, orbital abscess, and cavernous sinus thrombosis, comprise the other major category of complications of acute sinusitis.

Wald ER, Applegate KE, Bordley C, et al: Clinical practice guideline for the diagnosis and management of acute bacterial sinusitis in children aged 1 to 18 years, *Pediatrics* 132:e262–e280, 2013.
Rosenfeld EA, Rowley AH: Infectious intracranial complications of sinusitis, other than meningitis, in children: 12 year review, *Clin Infect Dis* 18:750–754, 1994.

281. When should imaging be considered in cases of sinusitis?

A contrast-enhanced CT scan and/or an MRI with contrast is recommended when there is suspicion of orbital or CNS complications of acute bacterial sinusitis. The evidence for one imaging modality over the other is weak, but in general, CT is more readily available; faster (possibly obviating the need for sedation); will better visualize bony complications of the orbit (which are the most common types of complications); and in most cases, visualizes intracranial pathology. There are case reports of failure of CT to reveal intracranial complications of sinusitis, and so an MRI with contrast may be considered in the case of a negative CT with a high index of suspicion, or specific concern for soft tissue complications.

Wald ER, Applegate KE, Bordley C, et al: Clinical practice guideline for the diagnosis and management of acute bacterial sinusitis in children aged 1 to 18 years, *Pediatrics* 132:e262–e280, 2013.
Chow AW, Benninger MS, Brook I, et al: IDSA clinical practice guideline for acute bacterial rhinosinusitis in children and adults, *Clin Infect Dis* 54:e72–e112, 2012.

282. Which organisms are responsible for acute and chronic sinusitis in the pediatric age group?

In **acute, uncomplicated sinusitis**, the etiologic organisms closely parallel those associated with acute otitis media: *S. pneumoniae, H. influenzae,* and *M. catarrhalis.* There is some evidence that in the era of PCV-7 and PCV-13, β-lactamase-producing strains of *H. influenzae* may supplant *S. pneumoniae* as the most common organism. In patients with **chronic sinusitis**, the most common pathogens remain *S. pneumoniae, H. influenzae,* and *M. catarrhalis,* along with *S. aureus* and anaerobes. Fungal infection with zygomycosis (mucormycosis) is an important concern in immunosuppressed patients. *P. aeruginosa* or other colonizing gram-negative organisms must always be considered in patients with cystic fibrosis. *S. aureus,* both MRSA and MSSA, is emerging as a pathogen in acute and chronic sinusitis, particularly in cases of complicated disease.

Wald ER, Applegate KE, Bordley C, et al: Clinical practice guideline for the diagnosis and management of acute bacterial sinusitis in children aged 1 to 18 years, *Pediatrics* 132:e262–e280, 2013.
Chow AW, Benninger MS, Brook I, et al: IDSA clinical practice guideline for acute bacterial rhinosinusitis in children and adults, *Clin Infect Dis* 54:e72–e112, 2012.

283. What is the management of acute sinusitis?

Antibiotic therapy is designed to target the most common organisms. However, culture data from the postpneumococcal vaccine era are lacking because direct sampling from the sinuses is a procedure not commonly done. Amoxicillin, 45 mg/kg/day, is recommended by the AAP as first-line therapy for children ≥2 years of age with uncomplicated acute bacterial sinusitis. If there is a suspicion based on local epidemiology of resistant *S. pneumoniae,* high-dose (80 to 90 mg/kg/day) amoxicillin may be used. For children <2 years of age, children attending day-care facilities, or patients who have recently been treated with an antibiotic such as amoxicillin, amoxicillin-clavulanate with 80 to 90 mg/kg/day of the amoxicillin component is recommended. A 10- to 14-day course of therapy is typically advised.

Wald ER, Applegate KE, Bordley C, et al: Clinical practice guideline for the diagnosis and management of acute bacterial sinusitis in children aged 1 to 18 years, *Pediatrics* 132:e262–e280, 2013.
Chow AW, Benninger MS, Brook I, et al: IDSA clinical practice guideline for acute bacterial rhinosinusitis in children and adults, *Clin Infect Dis* 54:e72–e112, 2012.

284. List the predisposing factors for the development of chronic sinusitis

- Allergic rhinitis
- Anatomic abnormalities (e.g., polyps, enlarged adenoids)
- Impairment of mucociliary clearance (e.g., cystic fibrosis, primary ciliary dyskinesia)
- Foreign bodies (e.g., nasogastric tube)
- Abnormalities in immune defense (e.g., IgA deficiency)

TUBERCULOSIS

285. How effective is the Bacillus Calmette-Guerin (BCG) vaccination?

The BCG vaccines are among the most widely used in the world and are also perhaps the most controversial. The difficulties stem from the marked variation in reported efficacy of BCG against *M. tuberculosis* and *Mycobacterium leprae* infections. Depending on the population studied, efficacy against leprosy has ranged from 20% to 60% in prospective trials. The efficacy against tuberculosis has ranged from 0% to 80%. The highest protective effect is seen against meningeal and miliary tuberculosis in young children. In areas of high endemicity or in populations where morbidity and mortality is significant, the vaccine is used.

The vaccines were derived from a strain of *Mycobacterium bovis* in 1906 and were subsequently dispersed to several laboratories around the world, where they were propagated under nonstandardized conditions. Hence, the vaccines in use today cannot be considered homogeneous. This may explain the observed variation in efficacy.

286. When are the steps in screening for *M. tuberculosis*?

1. *Assessment of risk:* Primary care providers should assess patient risk factors for tuberculosis (TB) at the first visit, every 6 months for the first year of life, and then annually. Risk factors *include:* children with household contacts with confirmed or suspected TB, children

emigrating from countries with endemic TB or who have traveled to endemic countries and have had significant contact with persons at risk for TB. A validated screening questionnaire is available from the AAP.

2. For those children with a positive risk factor screen, the most common diagnostic test is the standard-strength PPD (Mantoux test); this contains 5 tuberculin units (TU) of purified protein derivative and is injected intradermally.

American Academy of Pediatrics: Tuberculosis. In Pickering LK, editor: *2012 Red Book: Report of the Committee on Infectious Diseases*, ed 29. Elk Grove Village, IL, 2012, American Academy of Pediatrics, pp 736–759.

287. **How is the Mantoux test interpreted in the context of clinical signs and symptoms and epidemiologic risk factors, such as a known exposure?**
Positive tests are defined as follows:
Palpable induration of ≥5 mm
- Children in close contact with confirmed or suspected cases of tuberculosis
- Children with radiographic or clinical evidence of tubercular disease
- Children receiving immunosuppressive therapy
- Children with immunodeficiency disorders, including HIV infection

Palpable induration of ≥10 mm
- Children <4 years
- Children with Hodgkin disease, lymphoma, diabetes mellitus, chronic renal failure, or malnutrition
- Children born in high-prevalence regions of the world, whose parents were born in such areas, or who have traveled to such areas
- Children frequently exposed to adults who are infected with HIV, homeless, incarcerated, illicit drug users, or migrant farm workers

Palpable induration of ≥15 mm
- Children 4 years or older with no risk factors

American Academy of Pediatrics: Tuberculosis. In Pickering LK, editor: *2012 Red Book Report of the Committee on Infectious Diseases*, ed 29. Elk Grove Village, 2012, IL, American Academy of Pediatrics, p 737.

288. **What are the reasons for a false-negative tuberculin skin test (TST)?**
About 10% to 40% of immunologically normal patients with culture-documented disease will have an initial TST that is negative. Reasons include:
- Testing during the incubation period (2 to 10 weeks)
- Young age
- Problems with the administration technique
- Severe systemic TB infection (miliary or meningitis)
- Concurrent infection: Measles, varicella, influenza, HIV, EBV, mycoplasma, mumps, rubella
Children who are on immunosuppressive medications, who suffer from malnutrition or an immunodeficiency may also have false-negative results.

289. **How does BCG immunization influence TB skin testing?**
Generally, the interpretation of PPD tests is the same in BCG recipients as it is in nonvaccinated children. If positive, consideration should be given to several factors when deciding who should receive antituberculous therapy. These factors include time since BCG immunization, number of doses received, prevalence of TB in the country of origin, contacts in the United States, and radiographic findings. As discussed below, interferon-γ release assay testing may be helpful in children who have received the BCG vaccine.

290. **What is the role of interferon-γ release assays (IGRAs) in the diagnosis of TB in children?**
IGRA assays rely on interferon-γ produced by lymphocytes sensitized by antigens specific to *M. tuberculosis*. These antigens are not found in the BCG vaccine or in nontuberculous mycobacteria, such as *M. avium* infection. A whole-blood ELISA can measure the interferon-γ concentration after incubation with antigen. IGRAs are preferable to TST in the following circumstances:
- Children ≥5 years of age who have received BCG vaccine
- Children ≥5 years of age who are unlikely to return for TST reading
The test is an acceptable but not preferable alternative to the TST in children <5 years of age. In children <2 years of age, there are limited data on the validity of the test.

American Academy of Pediatrics: Tuberculosis. In Pickering LK, editor: *2012 Red Book: Report of the Committee on Infectious Diseases*, ed 29. Elk Grove Village, IL, 2012, American Academy of Pediatrics, p. 744.

291. **How are IGRA results interpreted?**
    In general, the sensitivity of IGRAs is similar to TSTs in children ≥5 years. The specificity is higher because antigens found in the BCG vaccine and some nontuberculous mycobacteria do not react with the assay.
    - A child with a positive IGRA should be considered infected with *M. tuberculosis*.
    - A child with a negative IGRA result cannot be interpreted as definitively free of infection.
    - Indeterminate IGRA results do not exclude TB infection.
        - In the case of an indeterminate test, a repeat IGRA should be performed.
        - If the repeat is still indeterminate, a TST may be performed.

292. **How should a patient with a positive TST or IGRA be evaluated?**
    History should search for clues that are suggestive of active infection, such as recurrent fevers, weight loss, adenopathy, or cough. A history of recurrent infections in the patient or a family member may be suggestive of HIV infection, which is a risk factor for infection with *M. tuberculosis*. Information from previous tuberculin skin testing is invaluable. Epidemiologic information includes an evaluation of possible exposure to TB. A family history is obtained, including questions pertaining to chronic cough or weight loss in a family member or other contact. Travel history and current living arrangements should be elucidated. If the patient has immigrated to North America, a history of BCG vaccination should be ascertained.
    Physical examination should focus on pulmonary, lymphatic, and abdominal systems. Examination should corroborate a history of BCG vaccination.
    Laboratory evaluation, including a chest radiograph with a lateral film, is the next stage. Family members and close contacts should undergo skin testing. In certain circumstances, chest radiographs should be performed on the child's contacts. If any of the preceding evaluations suggests active infection, sputum, gastric aspirates, and other appropriate specimens (e.g., lymph node tissue) should be obtained for mycobacterial culture and NAAT.

293. **How common is HIV and TB coinfection?**
    Approximately 1 million people worldwide are coinfected with HIV and TB. In the United States, it is estimated that 10% of patients with active TB also have HIV. There is a 5% to 15% annual risk of acquiring TB in HIV-positive populations, and the risk of progression from latent to active disease is much greater. Children with HIV infection are considered at high risk for contracting TB, and annual TST beginning at 3 to 12 months of age, (or at the time of HIV diagnosis) is recommended. Children who are diagnosed with TB disease should be tested for HIV infection.

Zumla A, Ravliglione M, Hafner R, et al: Tuberculosis. *N Engl J Med* 368:745–755, 2013.

294. **What is latent tuberculosis infection (LTBI) and why is it treated?**
    A patient with a positive TST who has no clinical or radiographic abnormalities suggesting TB disease is thought to have LTBI. If a patient has never received antituberculous medication and has not had a known exposure to a person with isoniazid-resistant TB, treatment for LTBI has an efficacy near 100% in preventing progression to disease.

295. **In a younger child suspected of having TB disease, what is the utility of gastric aspirates?**
    In infants and young children, a cough may be absent or nonproductive. Hypertonic saline may be used in many children to successfully induce sputum for diagnosis. If this is not possible, gastric aspirates may be used as source for the culture or PCR identification of mycobacteria. The aspirate should be obtained early in the morning as the child awakens to sample the overnight accumulation of respiratory secretions. The first day's collection generally has the highest yield.

296. **What is the role of nucleic acid amplification testing (NAAT) in the diagnosis of TB?**
    NAAT/PCR-based technology is now commercially available for the detection of TB. The Xpert MTB/RIF assay also tests for rifampicin resistance. A recent Cochrane review indicates this assay has an overall sensitivity of 88% and a specificity of 98% in adults. Additionally, it has been shown to have a sensitivity of 68% in patients who are acid-fast bacilli (AFB) smear negative. Additional studies have shown a sensitivity of 80% in extrapulmonary specimens and a CSF sensitivity and specificity of 64% and 98%, respectively.

This is a hopeful development for timely diagnosis, given the limitation of obtaining cultures in children, as well as the generally low mycobacterial burden in many specimens in children.

Steingart KR, Schiller I, Horne DJ, et al: Xpert® MTB/RIF assay for pulmonary tuberculosis and rifampicin resistance in adults, *Cochrane Database Syst Rev* 1:CD009593, 2013.

297. **How do the manifestations of active pulmonary TB on chest radiograph differ between adults and children?**

Adults and adolescents more commonly present with *cavitary disease* and *pleural effusions*. The hallmark of pulmonary TB in children has classically been described as *hilar adenopathy*. Both adults and children, but more commonly adults, may present with lobar infiltrates. Classically, the right upper lobe has been implicated because the right main stem bronchus provides the most direct route for inhaled mycobacterium. A caveat is that TB may be heterogeneous in radiographic appearance and should never be "ruled out" given appropriate clinical suspicion based on x-ray alone, in either children or adults.

Janner D: *A Guide to Pediatric Infectious Disease*, Philadelphia, 2005, Lippincott Williams & Wilkins, p 126.
Agrons GA, Markowitz RI, Kramer SS: Pulmonary tuberculosis in children, *Semin Roentgenol* 28:158–172, 1993.

298. **How are children with active pulmonary TB treated?**

Recommendations for the treatment of active TB in children have evolved over the past several years. Previously, therapy for at least 9 months was suggested for uncomplicated pulmonary disease. Studies in adults and children have demonstrated that 6 months of combined antituberculous therapy (short-course therapy) is as effective as 9 months of therapy. To date, the combined results of multiple studies in pediatric patients have demonstrated the efficacy of 6 months of therapy to be more than 95%. The current standard regimen for active pulmonary TB in children consists of 2 months of daily isoniazid, rifampin, and pyrazinamide followed by 4 months of isoniazid and rifampin (daily or twice weekly). If drug resistance is a concern, either ethambutol or streptomycin is added to the initial three-drug regimen until drug susceptibilities are determined.

American Academy of Pediatrics: Tuberculosis. In Pickering LK, editor: *2012 Red Book: Report of the Committee on Infectious Diseases*, ed 29. Elk Grove Village, IL, 2012, American Academy of Pediatrics, p 745.
Perez-Velez CM, Marais BJ: Tuberculosis in children, *N Engl J Med* 367:348–361, 2012.

299. **Why are multiple antibiotics used for the treatment of TB disease?**

Compared with a patient with a positive test but no disease, two features of *M. tuberculosis* make the organism difficult to eradicate after infection has been established. First, mycobacteria replicate slowly and may remain dormant for prolonged periods, but they are susceptible to drugs only during active replication. Second, drug-resistant organisms exist naturally within a large population, even before the initiation of therapy. These features render the organism—when it is present in significant numbers—extremely difficult to eradicate with a single agent.

300. **What are the signs of TB meningitis?**

Tuberculous meningitis is a tragic form of the disease. It has a peak incidence in young children (<5 years of age) and is the most common extrapulmonary manifestation of TB in this age group, especially in HIV coinfected children. The symptoms are insidious and nonspecific. These include decreased level of consciousness and lethargy, cranial nerve palsies, poor weight gain, and low grade fever that persists, typically for >5 days. It can be difficult to clinically differentiate from other forms of meningitis once it is recognized because CSF AFB smears and cultures are often negative. Mortality approaches 30% and >50% of survivors have neurodevelopmental sequelae.

Chiang SS, Khan FA, Milstein MB: Treatment outcomes of childhood tuberculous meningitis: a systematic review and meta-analysis, *Lancet Infect Dis* 14:947–957, 2014.

301. **What is the importance of DOT in the treatment of TB?**

Directly observed therapy (DOT), administration of medication by a third party (either a health-care professional or a trained unrelated individual), has been found to be a valuable approach to the treatment of children and adolescents with TB disease. Failure to properly take chronic medications increases the likelihood of relapse and the development of resistance. DOT increases adherence and thus lowers rates of relapse, treatment failures, and drug resistance.

302. **Why is pyridoxine supplementation given to patients who are receiving isoniazid?**
Isoniazid interferes with pyridoxine metabolism and may result in peripheral neuritis or convulsions. The administration of pyridoxine is generally not necessary for children who have a normal diet because they have adequate stores of this vitamin. Children and adolescents with diets deficient in milk or meat, exclusively breast-fed infants, symptomatic HIV-infected children, and pregnant women should receive pyridoxine supplementation during isoniazid therapy.

303. **Why do children with TB rarely infect other children?**
TB is transmitted by infected droplets of mucus that become airborne when an individual coughs or sneezes. As compared with adults, children with TB have several factors that minimize their contagiousness:
- Low density of organisms in sputum
- Lack of cavitations or extensive infiltrates on chest radiograph
- Lower frequency of cough
- Lower volume and higher viscosity of sputum
- Shorter duration of respiratory symptoms

Starke JR: Childhood tuberculosis during the 1990s, *Pediatr Rev* 13:343–353, 1992.

304. **In addition to TB, what other airborne microbes can cause respiratory disease?**
See Table 10-8.

Table 10-8 Airborne Microbial Diseases

DISEASE	AIRBORNE SOURCE
Aspergillosis	Conidia spores from decaying vegetation and soil
Brucellosis	Aerosolized from carcasses of domestic and wild animals
Chickenpox	Aerosolized from respiratory secretions
Coccidioidomycosis	Arthroconidia from soil and dust
Cryptococcosis	Aerosolized from bird droppings
Histoplasmosis	Conidia spores from bat or bird droppings
Legionnaires disease	Aerosolized contaminated water, especially from air-conditioning cooling towers
Measles	Aerosolized respiratory secretions
Mucormycosis	Spores from soil
Psittacosis	*Chlamydia psittaci* from birds
Q fever	*Coxiella burnetii* from a variety of farm and other animals
Tularemia	Aerosolized from multiple wild animals, especially rabbits

305. **Which famous U.S. First Lady died of TB?**
Eleanor Roosevelt, for whom immunosuppressive therapy for aplastic anemia activated dormant TB, died of the disease. Historically, TB has been called "consumption" (as the disease "consumed" the individual with drastic weight loss). Other noteworthy historical and literary figures who died from TB include Thomas Wolfe, George Orwell, Fredrick Chopin, Anton Chekov, and the entire Brontë family (Maria, Elizabeth, Charlotte, Emily, Anne, and brother Branwell).

Acknowledgment

The editors gratefully acknowledge contributions by Drs. Alexis M. Elward, David A. Hunstad, and Joseph W. St. Geme III that were retained from previous editions of *Pediatric Secrets*.

CHAPTER 11

NEONATOLOGY

Kathleen G. Brennan, MD and Tina A. Leone, MD

CLINICAL ISSUES

1. **When does the ductus arteriosus (DA) close in well newborn infants?**
   The DA begins to constrict shortly after birth. At 24 hours of life, approximately 50% of term infants will no longer have detectable flow across the DA by echocardiography. At 72 hours of life the majority of newborn infants no longer have detectable flow across the DA. The DA initially closes functionally, meaning that blood no longer flows across the vessel, but it closes anatomically with fibrosis of the vessel at approximately 2 to 3 weeks of life. Therefore, if the DA closes despite significant congenital heart disease, it may be reopened with pharmacologic therapy using prostaglandin E1 before full anatomic closure.

2. **Why is it not always possible to auscultate a murmur in an infant with a ventricular septal defect (VSD) on the first day of life?**
   Murmurs are generated by high velocity or highly turbulent blood flow. The blood flow across a VSD increases in velocity over the first several days of life as the pulmonary arterial pressure decreases in the transition from fetal to postnatal life. The pulmonary artery pressure is higher than the systemic arterial pressure *in utero* and is approximately equal to the systemic pressure shortly after birth. However, the pulmonary artery pressure decreases dramatically over the first several days of life leading to a larger systemic to pulmonary pressure gradient. As the pressure gradient increases, the blood flow across the VSD increases in velocity, and the murmur becomes more apparent.

3. **What are the three main types of congenital heart disease, and how do they present in the newborn period?**
   - **Left-sided obstructive lesions** include diseases such as hypoplastic left heart syndrome, aortic stenosis, and coarctation of the aorta. The presentation for these diseases if they remain untreated is a shocklike syndrome due to inadequate systemic blood flow and excessive pulmonary blood flow. The infants will be pale or gray in appearance, hypotensive, tachycardic, and tachypneic. Pulses will be weak or undetectable, or in the case of coarctation of the aorta, will be strong in the upper extremities but weak/undetectable in the lower extremities. The infant may become oliguric or anuric and develop hepatomegaly. Signs of illness will often not be present until the DA closes.
   - **Right-sided obstructive lesions** are a group of diseases that lead to inadequate pulmonary blood flow and the main presenting feature is cyanosis. They include pulmonary atresia/stenosis, tricuspid atresia, tetralogy of Fallot, and some variations of truncus arteriosus. Deoxygenated blood on the right side of the heart will be shunted across the atrial septum or ventricular septum (through a VSD) leading to systemic hypoxemia. Providing oxygen to these infants will not significantly increase the systemic oxygen saturation values because the deoxygenated blood flowing from the right side of the heart to the left will not be influenced by the increased oxygen concentration in the lungs.
   - **Lesions of abnormal mixing of blood between the pulmonary and systemic circulations** include large septal defects, a large patent ductus arteriosus or abnormal pulmonary arterial connections (AP window). These diseases may not present until after the immediate newborn period but will result in tachypnea and respiratory distress followed by signs of congestive heart failure. The blood flow will be from the side with higher pressure (usually the left) to the side with lower pressure (the right). Therefore, oxygenated blood will flow from the systemic to pulmonary circulation causing excessive blood flow through the lungs leading to the tachypnea and respiratory distress.

4. **What is the chance that an extremely preterm infant will survive without significant impairment?**
   Survival rates for extremely preterm infants have improved dramatically as antenatal care and neonatal intensive care have improved over the last 30 to 40 years. In the United Kingdom, improvements in survival without disability were documented in two cohorts of extremely preterm infants in 1995 and 2006. In Victoria, Australia, rates of survival improved over time until the late 1990s when it plateaued; however, a decrease in severe disabilities lead to an improvement in quality adjusted survival. The most important

variable affecting immediate and long-term outcomes is gestational age. Additional factors such as gender, birth weight, use of antenatal steroids, and multifetal gestations all affect the chances of healthy survival among preterm infants. However, the course during the neonatal intensive care stay also influences the infant's long-term outcome. The NICHD Neonatal Research Network published outcome data for infants of 22 to 25 weeks of gestation at birth who were followed up to 18 to 22 months of age. The rates of death and death or profound impairment are shown in Table 11-1.

Moore T, Hennessy EM, Myles J, et al: Neurological and developmental outcome in extremely preterm children born in England in 1995 and 2006: the EPICure studies, *BMJ* 345:e7961, 2012.

Doyle LW, Roberts G, Anderson PJ, and the Victorian Infant Collaborative Study Group: Changing long-term outcomes for infants 500-999 g birth weight in Victoria, 1979-2005, *Arch Dis Child Fetal Neonatal Ed* 96:F44–F447, 2011.

Tyson JE, Parikh NA, Langer J, et al: Intensive care for extreme prematurity – moving beyond gestational age, *N Engl J Med* 358:1672–1681, 2008.

Table 11-1. Rates of Death and Death or Profound Impairment Among Infants Born at Extremely Low Gestational Ages

GESTATIONAL AGE (WEEKS)	DEATH (%)	DEATH OR PROFOUND IMPAIRMENT (%)
22	95	98
23	74	84
24	44	57
25	25	38

Data from Tyson JE, Parikh NA, Langer J, et al, and the NICHD Neonatal Research Network: Intensive care for extreme prematurity—moving beyond gestational age, N Engl J Med 358(16):1672–1681, 2008.

5. **What interventions are indicated in future pregnancies after a mother delivers a preterm infant?**
Women who have delivered preterm infants have an approximate 20% to 30% chance of delivering a preterm infant in subsequent pregnancies. These women are therefore considered high-risk and should be monitored closely in future pregnancies. Therapy with progesterone during subsequent pregnancies has been shown to decrease the rate of subsequent preterm birth, prolong the duration of pregnancy, and decrease perinatal/neonatal mortality and morbidity (necrotizing enterocolitis). Current guidelines by the Society for Maternal-Fetal Medicine recommend weekly intramuscular (IM) injections with 17-alphahydroxyprogesterone caproate starting at 16 to 20 weeks of gestation and continuing through 36 weeks.

Laughon SK, Albert PS, Leishear K, et al: The NICHD consecutive pregnancies study: recurrent preterm delivery by subtype, *Am J Obstet Gynecol* 210:131.e1–e8, 2014.

Dodd JM, Jones L, Flenady V, et al: Prenatal administration of progesterone for preventing preterm birth in women considered to be at risk of preterm birth, *Cochrane Database Syst Rev* 7:CD004947, 2013.

Society for Maternal-Fetal Medicine Publications Committee, with the assistance of Vincenzo Berghella: Progesterone and preterm birth prevention: translating clinical trials data into clinical practice, *Am J Obstet Gynecol* 206:376–386, 2012.

6. **Which infants require ophthalmologic evaluation for retinopathy of prematurity (ROP)?**
The American Academy of Pediatrics (AAP) recommends that an individual experienced in neonatal ophthalmology and indirect ophthalmoscopy examine the retinas of all neonates with a birth weight of <1500 g or a gestational age of <32 weeks, and selected infants weighing between 1500 and 2000 g who have had unstable clinical courses, including those requiring cardiorespiratory support.

American Academy of Pediatrics, American Academy of Ophthalmology, American Association for Pediatric Ophthalmology and Strabismus, American Association of Certified Orthoptists: Screening examination of premature infants for retinopathy of prematurity, *Pediatrics* 131:189–195, 2013.

Hartnett ME, Penn JS: Mechanisms and management of retinopathy of prematurity, *N Engl J Med* 367:2515–2526, 2012.

7. What are the stages of ROP?
   - **Stage I:** Line of demarcation separates vascular and avascular retina
   - **Stage II:** Ridging of line of demarcation as a result of scar formation
   - **Stage III:** Extraretinal fibrovascular proliferation present
   - **Stage IV:** Subtotal retinal detachment
   - **Stage V:** Complete retinal detachment
     The stage of ROP can be modified with the designation of "plus disease" if there is abnormal dilatation and tortuosity of the posterior retinal vessels.

8. What are the indications for treatment for ROP?
   Based on the results of the Early Treatment for Retinopathy of Prematurity randomized trial, treatment should be initiated for the following retinal findings:
   - **Zone I ROP:** Any stage with plus disease
   - **Zone I ROP:** Stage III with or without plus disease
   - **Zone II ROP:** Stage II or III with plus disease
     Standard treatment uses laser photocoagulation, which obliterates the retina peripheral to the area of vessel development. Improved short-term ophthalmologic outcomes have been demonstrated when intravitreal bevacizumab (Avastin) is used instead of laser therapy for ROP in zone 1 with plus disease.

American Academy of Pediatrics, American Academy of Ophthalmology, American Association for Pediatric Ophthalmology and Strabismus, American Association of Certified Orthoptists: Screening examination of premature infants for retinopathy of prematurity, *Pediatrics* 131:189–195, 2013.
Early Treatment for Retinopathy of Prematurity Cooperative Group: Revised indications for treatment of retinopathy of prematurity: results of the early treatment for retinopathy of prematurity randomized trial, *Arch Ophthalmol* 121:1684–1694, 2003.

9. When should hearing evaluations be repeated after neonatal intensive care unit (NICU) discharge?
   Any newborn infant who does not pass the universal newborn hearing screening evaluation should have a diagnostic hearing evaluation after hospital discharge. Even those who pass the universal newborn hearing screen should have a diagnostic hearing evaluation at 24 to 30 months of age if any risk factors for progressive sensorineural (SN) hearing loss are present, including a NICU stay of at least 5 days, the need for extracorporeal membrane oxygenation (ECMO) or assisted ventilation, use of ototoxic antibiotics such as aminoglycosides or loop diuretics, or exchange transfusion for hyperbilirubinemia.

Harlor AD Jr, Bower C: The committee on practice and ambulatory medicine, The section on otolaryngology-head and neck surgery, *Pediatrics* 124:1252–1263, 2009.

10. What are the manifestations of drug withdrawal in the neonate?
    The signs and symptoms of drug withdrawal in the neonate can be remembered by using the acronym **WITHDRAWAL**:
    - **W**akefulness
    - **I**rritability
    - **T**remulousness, temperature variation, tachypnea
    - **H**yperactivity, high-pitched persistent cry, hyperacusis, hyperreflexia, hypertonus
    - **D**iarrhea, diaphoresis, disorganized suck
    - **R**ub marks, respiratory distress, rhinorrhea
    - **A**pneic attacks, autonomic dysfunction
    - **W**eight loss or failure to gain weight
    - **A**lkalosis (respiratory)
    - **L**acrimation

Committee on Drugs: Neonatal drug withdrawal, *Pediatrics* 72:896, 1983.

11. **What is the recommended pharmacologic treatment for neonatal abstinence syndrome (NAS) from opioid withdrawal?**

Maternal antepartum opioid use has nearly quadrupled in the United States in the past decade with a resultant three-fold increase in NAS hospitalizations. Unfortunately there is no nationally accepted, evidence-based treatment protocol. There are some commonly utilized therapies—methadone or morphine as the initial drug of choice with phenobarbital or clonidine as second-line therapies—but there is no consensus about which initial treatment is best and what is the most ideal way to taper the medication. A 2014 survey of NICUs in Ohio found that adherence to an explicit weaning protocol appeared to be effective in reducing the total duration of opioid treatment and the hospital length of stay.

Hall ES, Wexelblatt SL, Crowley M, et al: A multicenter cohort study of treatments and hospital outcomes in neonatal abstinence syndrome, *Pediatrics* 134:e527–e534, 2014.
Kocherlakota P: Neonatal abstinence syndrome, *Pediatrics* 134:e547–e561, 2014.

12. **Should breastfeeding be initiated in infants with NAS?**

Yes. The AAP recommends that neonates prenatally exposed to maternal oral maintenance therapy medications, especially buprenorphine and methadone, be breast-fed because these infants have lower incidences of NAS and require shorter pharmacotherapy when the syndrome occurs when compared with infants who are not breastfed. Breastfeeding is contraindicated for mothers who are taking street drugs, are involved in polydrug abuse, or are infected with human immunodeficiency virus (HIV).

Kocherlakota P: Neonatal abstinence syndrome, *Pediatrics* 134:e547–e561, 2014.
Welle-Strand GK, Skurtveit S, Jansson LM, et al: Breastfeeding reduces the need for withdrawal treatment in opioid-exposed infants, *Acta Paediatr* 102:544–549, 2013.

13. **If maternal drug abuse is suspected, which specimen from the infant is most accurate for detecting exposure?**

Although urine has traditionally been tested when maternal drug abuse is a possibility, **meconium** has a greater sensitivity than urine and positive findings that persist longer. It may contain metabolites gathered over as much as 20 weeks, compared with urine, which represents more recent exposure. Recent studies show that umbilical cord tissue is as sensitive as meconium for the detection of fetal drug exposure.

Montgomery D: Testing for fetal exposure to illicit drugs using umbilical cord tissue vs. meconium, *J Perinatol* 26:11–14, 2006.

14. **Does *in utero* exposure to selective serotonin reuptake inhibitors (SSRIs) result in neonatal withdrawal?**

SSRIs are being prescribed with increasing frequency to pregnant women with depression. Recent data suggest that within days of birth, infants experience withdrawal symptoms, including irritability, crying, hypertonia, and seizures. The drug that figures most prominently is paroxetine (Paxil), but similar symptoms have been reported with fluoxetine (Prozac), sertraline (Zoloft), and citalopram (Celexa).

Alwan S and Friedman JM: Safety of selective serotonin uptake inhibitors in pregnancy, *CNS Drugs* 23:493–509, 2009.
Sanz EJ: Neonatal withdrawal symptoms after in utero exposure to selective serotonin reuptake inhibitors in pregnant women and neonatal withdrawal syndrome: a database analysis, *Lancet* 365:482–487, 2005.

15. **What is the difference between "sudden unexpected infant death (SUID)" and "sudden infant death syndrome (SIDS)"?**

SUID refers to an infant <1 year who dies suddenly and unexpectedly. In the United States, there are approximately 4000 such deaths per year. *SIDS*, a subset of SUID, is defined as the sudden death of an infant <1 year of age whose death cannot be explained after a thorough investigation (i.e., review of clinical history, examination of the death scene, complete autopsy). SIDS is the leading cause of death in the United States for infants ages 1 to 12 months.

16. **What is the "Back to Sleep" program?**

    This program, initiated in 1994, was an effort to promote recommendations for infants to be placed in a nonprone position as a strategy for reducing the risk of SIDS. This followed epidemiologic reports from Europe and Australia that demonstrated declines in the rate of SIDS for infants who did not fall asleep on their stomachs. It has more recently been renamed as the "Safe to Sleep" program following additional recommendations.

17. **What additional recommendations have been made regarding the most ideal sleep environment for infants?**

    In addition to supine positioning, recommendations to decrease the risk for SIDS or suffocation include use of a firm sleep surface; breastfeeding; room-sharing without bed-sharing; routine immunization; consideration of a pacifier; and avoidance of soft bedding, overheating, and exposure to tobacco smoke, alcohol, and illicit drugs.

Task Force on Sudden Infant Death Syndrome: SIDS and other sleep-related infant deaths: expansion of recommendations for a safe infant sleeping environment, *Pediatrics* 128:e1341–e1367, 2011.

18. **Do home apnea monitors help prevent sudden infant death syndrome (SIDS)?**

    Epidemiologic studies have not been able to demonstrate an impact of home monitoring on the incidence of SIDS. On that basis, the AAP recommends that home monitors not be prescribed to prevent SIDS. Indications for monitoring include the following:
    - Premature infants with persistent apnea and bradycardia
    - Technology-dependent infants
    - Infants with neurologic or metabolic disorders that affect respiratory control
    - Infants with chronic lung disease, especially those requiring O_2, continuous positive airway pressure (CPAP), and/or mechanical ventilation

---

Strehle EM, Gray WK, Gopisetti S, et al: Can home monitoring reduce mortality in infants at increased risk of sudden infant death syndrome? A systematic review, *Acta Paediatr* 101:8–13, 2012.

American Academy of Pediatrics: Apnea, SIDS and home monitoring, *Pediatrics* 111:914–917, 2003.

DELIVERY ROOM ISSUES

19. **When should the umbilical cord be clamped after birth?**

    Obstetric and midwifery practice has varied in the timing of umbilical cord clamping over the last 50 years from immediately clamping the cord after birth to clamping when the cord stops pulsating. Immediate cord clamping became common practice as a method aimed at preventing postpartum hemorrhage. However, this practice prevents the natural autotransfusion of fetoplacental blood into the newborn infant once the uterus begins contracting and the infant begins breathing. In preterm infants, delayed cord clamping (at least 30 to 60 seconds) has been shown to improve the hemodynamic transition after birth. Infants have less bradycardia after birth, less hypotension, receive fewer vasoactive medications, and have lower rates of intraventricular hemorrhage. Delayed cord clamping also increases early hemoglobin concentrations and improved iron stores at 4 months of age for term infants. The practice is now recommended by the American College of Obstetrics and Gynecology in preterm infants.

McDonald SJ, Middleton P, Dowswell T, Morris PS: Effect of timing of umbilical cord clamping of term infants on maternal and neonatal outcomes, *Cochrane Database Syst Rev* 7:CD004074, 2013.

Rabe H, Diaz-Rossello JL, Duley L, Dowswell T: Effect of timing of umbilical cord clamping and other strategies to influence placental transfusion at preterm birth on maternal and infant outcomes, *Cochrane Database Syst Rev* 8: CD003248, 2012.

Committee on Obstetric Practice, American College of Obstetricians and Gynecologists. Committee Opinion No. 543: timing of umbilical cord clamping after birth, *Obstet Gynecol* 120:1522–1526, 2012.

20. **How long has meconium been present in the amniotic fluid if an infant has evidence of meconium staining?**

    Gross staining of the infant is a surface phenomenon that is proportional to the length of exposure and meconium concentration. With heavy meconium, staining of the umbilical cord begins in as little as 15 minutes; with light meconium, it occurs after 1 hour. Yellow staining of the newborn's toenails requires 4 to 6 hours. Yellow staining of the vernix caseosa takes about 12 to 14 hours.

Miller PW, Coen RW, Benirschke K: Dating the time interval from meconium passage to birth, *Obstet Gynecol* 66:459–462, 1985.

21. **Is meconium staining a good marker for neonatal asphyxia?**
    No. Ten percent to 20% of all deliveries have *in utero* passage of meconium; therefore, meconium staining alone is not a good marker for neonatal asphyxia.

22. **If meconium is noted before or during the time of delivery, what is the recommended course of action?**
    Although intrapartum nasopharyngeal and oropharyngeal suctioning by the obstetrician before the delivery of the thorax has been advocated for many years to reduce the incidence of meconium aspiration syndrome, recent data suggest that this may not be efficacious. However, once the baby is delivered, the next steps depend on whether the baby is vigorous as defined by good cry, respiratory effort, muscle tone, and heart rate of more than 100 beats/minute. If the baby is not vigorous, a laryngoscope should be inserted into the mouth, and a large bore catheter should be used to suction the mouth and posterior pharynx so that the glottis can be visualized. An endotracheal tube is then inserted into the trachea, connected to a suction source, and slowly withdrawn. The procedure is repeated until the trachea is clear of meconium or the baby develops bradycardia, requiring initiation of resuscitative measures.

Velaphi S, Vidyasagar D: Intrapartum and postdelivery management of infants born to mothers with meconium stained amniotic fluid: Evidence based recommendations, *Clin Perinatal* 33:29–42, 2006.

23. **During asphyxia, how is primary apnea distinguished from secondary apnea?**
    A regular sequence of events occurs when an infant is asphyxiated. Initially, gasping respiratory efforts increase in depth and frequency for up to 3 minutes, and this is followed by cessation of breathing (*primary apnea*). If stimulation is provided during the period of primary apnea, respiratory function spontaneously returns. If asphyxia continues, gasping then resumes for a variable period of time, terminating with the "last gasp" and followed by secondary apnea. During *secondary apnea*, the only way to restore respiratory function is with positive-pressure ventilation (PPV). Thus, a linear relationship exists between the duration of asphyxia and the recovery of respiratory function after resuscitation. The longer the artificial ventilation is delayed after the last gasp, the longer it will take to resuscitate the infant. However, clinically, the two conditions may be indistinguishable.

24. **How should apnea be managed in the delivery room?**
    Any infant who has bradycardia (a heart rate < 100 beats/minute) or apnea that does not quickly respond to tactile stimulation should be treated with **assisted ventilation**. If the apnea does not improve with assisted ventilation provided via facemask, the infant will most likely require endotracheal intubation for continued respiratory support.

25. **What are the clinical signs of adequate ventilation?**
    During resuscitation, the adequacy of ventilation is determined clinically by observing chest rise with each inflation and by noting clinical improvement such as an increasing heart rate or onset of spontaneous respiratory effort. It is also possible to use an end tidal carbon dioxide detector with the facemask to visually see that gas exchange is occurring with each breath.

    When ventilation is not adequate, the clinician must make adjustments in order to deliver breaths more effectively. The Neonatal Resuscitation Program (NRP) suggests remembering the different adjustments that should be addressed by the pneumonic, **MR. SOPA:**

    M = Mask adjustment
    R = Repositioning
    S = Suctioning
    O = Open the mouth
    P = Increase the pressure
    A = Alternate airway

Kattwinkel J, editor: *Textbook of Neonatal Resuscitation*, ed 6. Dallas, 2011, American Heart Association and American Academy of Pediatrics, p 95.

26. What are the pros and cons of the T-piece resuscitator?
    The benefits of this device are that it provides the most consistent levels of pressure during assisted ventilation, and it can successfully provide positive end-expiratory pressure (PEEP) or CPAP if needed. The main drawback to the device is that the operator must intentionally increase the set pressure by turning a knob on the unit. An operator working alone may not be able to easily accomplish increasing the pressure with this device.

Bennett S, Finer NN, Rich W, Vaucher Y: A comparison of three neonatal resuscitation devices. *Resuscitation* 67:113–118, 2005.

27. How does one estimate the size of the endotracheal tube required for resuscitation?
    See Table 11-2.

Table 11-2. Endotracheal Tubes Needed for Resuscitation

TUBE SIZE (INTERNAL DIAMETER IN MM)	WEIGHT (G)	GESTATIONAL AGE (WK)
2.5	<1000	<28
3	1001-2000	28-34
3.5	2001-3000	34-38
3.5-4.0	>3000	>38

Data from Hertz D: Principles of neonatal resuscitation. In Polin RA, Yoder MC, Burg FD, editors: Workbook in Practical Neonatology, *ed 3. Philadelphia, 2001, WB Saunders, p 13.*

28. What is the "7-8-9" rule?
    The *7-8-9 rule* is an estimate of the length (in centimeters) that an oral endotracheal tube should be inserted into a 1-, 2-, or 3-kg infant, respectively. A variation of this rule is the tip-to-lip rule of adding 6 to the weight in kilograms of the infant to determine the insertion distance. With good visualization, the tube should be inserted 1 to 1.5 cm below the vocal cords. Tube placement should always be verified radiographically.

29. When should epinephrine be given during resuscitation in the delivery room?
    In a depressed infant with gasping or absent respirations and a heart rate <60 beats/minute, assisted ventilation should be initiated. If the heart rate remains <60 beats/minute despite adequate PPV, chest compressions should be initiated within 30 seconds. If there is no response to chest compressions (i.e., heart rate remains <60 beats/minute), epinephrine is indicated. Epinephrine (1:10,000) can be given intravenously or endotracheally, but the intravenous route is preferred because it is more likely to be effective. The recommended intravenous dose is 0.1 to 0.3 mL/kg. If given endotracheally, a larger dose of 0.3 to 1 mL/kg should be used.

Kattwinkel J, editor: *Textbook of Neonatal Resuscitation*, ed 6. Dallas, 2011, American Heart Association and American Academy of Pediatrics, pp 219–220.

30. Should sodium bicarbonate be given during resuscitation in the delivery room?
    No. Use of sodium bicarbonate is no longer recommended during neonatal resuscitation. The administration of bicarbonate may have adverse effects on cardiac and cerebral function, decrease systemic vascular resistance, and shift the oxyhemoglobin curve to the left, which further inhibits oxygen release. Furthermore, acute doses of sodium bicarbonate lead to rapid increases in osmolarity and increased risk of intracranial hemorrhage, particularly in premature infants.

Aschner JL, Poland RL: Sodium bicarbonate: basically useless therapy, *Pediatrics* 122:831–835, 2008.
Papile LA, Burstein J, Burstein R, et al: Relationship of intravenous sodium bicarbonate infusions and cerebral intraventricular hemorrhage, *J Pediatr* 93:834–836, 1978.

31. When should a laryngeal mask airway (LMA) be used in neonatal resuscitation?
    The LMA fits over the laryngeal inlet and may be used to effect ventilation when intubation is not
    feasible or is unsuccessful. The LMA should be considered when (1) anomalies of the lip, mouth, or
    palate make it impossible to achieve a good seal with the bag and mask; and (2) anomalies of the
    mouth, tongue, pharynx, mandible, or neck make visualization of the larynx with a laryngoscope
    impossible. Placement of the LMA does not require visualization and may be used to temporize
    while measures are taken to establish a more stable airway (Fig. 11-1).

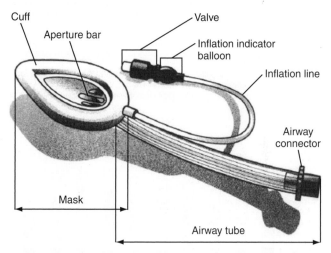

Figure 11-1. Laryngeal mask airway. *(From Asensio JA, Trunkey DD, editors:* Current Therapy of Trauma and Surgical Critical
Care. *Philadelphia, 2008, Mosby.)*

32. What is the role for CO_2 detectors in neonatal resuscitation?
    After intubation, visualization of passage of the tube through the vocal cords, auscultation of breath
    sounds, and observation of chest movement are often used to ensure proper placement of the
    endotracheal tube in the trachea. However, these signs may be misleading and must be confirmed
    by a rapid improvement in heart rate and detection of CO_2 in exhaled air following a few
    positive-pressure breaths. CO_2 detectors are available as either colorimetric devices or capnographs
    giving numeric CO_2 levels, with the former type being the most commonly used. Beware, however, that
    patients with very low cardiac output such as those in cardiac arrest may have markedly
    diminished pulmonary blood flow resulting in failure to detect CO_2 despite correct placement of
    the endotracheal tube.

33. What techniques are available to keep preterm infants warm in the delivery
    room?
    Immediately after birth, preterm infants can rapidly lose heat to the environment by evaporation
    (wet skin), conduction (cool blankets), convection (breezes), and radiation (cool air temperature).
    If preterm infants are treated with the standard warming methods used for term infants, the
    incidence of hypothermia with admission temperatures $< 35\ °C$ can be as high as 50% in the
    smallest infants. Several studies have shown that covering preterm babies (<29 weeks) with a
    thin plastic blanket immediately after birth without drying the skin (excluding the head) leads to
    higher admission temperatures and a lower incidence of hypothermia. Other interventions to
    maintain temperature in preterm infants include use of chemical heating mattresses, increasing the
    temperature of the delivery room, and use of a servo-controlled radiant warmer.

McCall EM, Alderdice F, Halliday HL, et al: Interventions to prevent hypothermia at birth in preterm and/or low birth weight
infants, *Cochrane Database Syst Rev* 3:CD004210, 2010.

34. **What amount of oxygen is recommended for neonatal resuscitation?**
The NRP recommends use of 21% O_2 when PPV is required in the resuscitation of full-term infants. A wide body of evidence shows that using 21% O_2 (room air) is just as effective as 100% O_2 and leads to a significant reduction in mortality rates. Therefore, current recommendations are to start with 21% O_2, but to be prepared to increase the inspired oxygen concentration to 100% if the infant has a sustained heart rate <60 beats/minute or is receiving chest compressions. Additionally the oxygen concentration should be increased if the oxygen saturation does not reach expected values over the first 10 minutes of life. In the case of preterm infants, many experts recommend 30% to 40% O_2 to start and adjusting the oxygen concentration to achieve normal oxygen saturations. Figure 11-2 shows normal Spo_2 values over the first 10 minutes of life.

Ten VS, Matsiukvich D, et al: Room air or 100% oxygen for resuscitation of infants with perinatal depression, *Curr Opin Pediatr* 21:188–193, 2009.
Saugstad OD, Ramji S, Soil RF, et al: Resuscitation of newborn infants with 21% or 100% oxygen: an updated systematic review and meta-analysis, *Neonatology* 94:176–182, 2008.
Richmond S, Goldsmith JP: Air or 100% oxygen in neonatal resuscitation? *Clin Perinatol* 33:11–27, 2006.

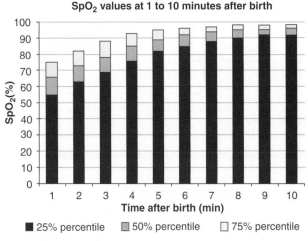

SpO_2 values at 1 to 10 minutes after birth

■ 25% percentile　　▨ 50% percentile　　☐ 75% percentile

Figure 11-2. Spo_2 values at each minute from 1 to 10 minutes of life.

35. **After a "traumatic" delivery, what are the possible injured systems?**
    - **Cranial injuries:** Caput succedaneum, subconjunctival hemorrhage, cephalhematoma, subgaleal hematoma, skull fractures, intracranial hemorrhage, cerebral edema
    - **Spinal injuries:** Spinal cord transection
    - **Peripheral nerve injuries:** Brachial palsy (Erb-Duchenne paralysis, Klumpke paralysis), phrenic nerve, and facial nerve paralysis
    - **Visceral injuries:** Liver rupture or hematoma, splenic rupture, adrenal hemorrhage
    - **Skeletal injuries:** Fractures of the clavicle, femur, and humerus

36. **What bone is the most frequently fractured in the newborn?**
The **clavicle**. This injury, which stems from excessive traction during delivery, generally results in a greenstick fracture (Fig. 11-3).

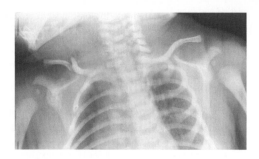

Figure 11-3. Radiograph of right clavicular fracture. *(From Clark DA:* Atlas of Neonatology. *Philadelphia, 2000, WB Saunders, p 8.)*

37. **Who was Virginia Apgar, and how does one remember her score?**
    Virginia Apgar, an anesthesiologist at Columbia Presbyterian Medical Center in New York City, introduced the Apgar scoring system in 1953 to assess the newborn infant's response to the stress of labor and delivery. A mnemonic to help remember the components of the score is as follows:
    - **A**ppearance (pink, mottled, or blue)
    - **P**ulse (>100, <100, or 0 beats/minute)
    - **G**rimace (response to suctioning of the nose and mouth)
    - **A**ctivity (flexed arms and legs, extended limbs, or limp)
    - **R**espiratory effort (crying, gasping, or no respiratory activity)
      Each category is assigned a rating of 0, 1, or 2 points, with a total score of 10 indicating the best possible condition.

38. **Is a low Apgar score alone sufficient to diagnose a neonate as asphyxiated?**
    No. It is not acceptable to label an infant as asphyxiated simply because of a low Apgar score. Asphyxiated infants demonstrate a constellation of findings including multiorgan system dysfunction and signs referable to the central nervous system (CNS). In addition, asphyxiated neonates typically have a profound metabolic acidosis. The cardinal features of hypoxic-ischemic encephalopathy include seizures, alterations of consciousness, and abnormalities of tone. Disorders of reflexes, respiratory pattern, oculovestibular responses, and autonomic function are less significant components of this entity.

American Academy of Pediatrics Committee on Fetus and Newborn, American Academy of Obstetricians and Gynecologists and Committee on Obstetric Practice: The Apgar score, *Pediatrics* 117:1444–1447, 2006.
Leuthner SR, Das U: Low Apgar scores and the definition of birth asphyxia, *Pediatr Clin North Am* 51:737–745, 2004.

39. **When should neonatal resuscitation be stopped?**
    Although each case should be considered individually, the discontinuation of efforts is generally appropriate after 10 minutes of absent heart rate despite adequate resuscitative measures. Current data suggest that asystole for longer than 10 minutes is highly unlikely to result in survival or survival without severe disability.

Kattwinkel J, editor: *Textbook of Neonatal Resuscitation*, ed 6. Dallas, 2011, American Heart Association and American Academy of Pediatrics, p 292.

FETAL ISSUES

40. **What is the most accurate method of pregnancy dating?**
    The combination of dating a pregnancy based on last menstrual period and a first trimester fetal ultrasound provides the most accurate method to date a pregnancy. A first trimester ultrasound provides an accurate gestational age assessment with a margin of error of 5 to 7 days. Ultrasound measurements in the second trimester provide a gestational age with a margin of error of 7 to 14 days. In the third trimester the margin of error for dating the pregnancy ranges between 21 to 30 days.

Committee on Obstetric Practice, American College of Obstetricians and Gynecologists: Committee opinion number 611: Method for estimating due date, *Obstet Gynecol* 124:863–866, 2014.

41. **What features constitute the biophysical profile?**
    The biophysical profile is a scoring system that assesses fetal well-being before birth. Five variables are assessed:
    1. Fetal breathing movements
    2. Gross body movements
    3. Fetal tone
    4. Reactive fetal heart rate
    5. Qualitative amniotic fluid volume
       Normal results equate to 2 points per variable, for a possible total of 10 points.

42. **What factors influence biophysical profile performance?**
    - Drugs (sedatives, theophylline, cocaine, and indomethacin)
    - Cigarette smoking, hyperglycemia, and hypoglycemia
    - Spontaneous premature rupture of membranes
    - Fetal arrhythmia
    - Periodic decelerations
    - Acute disasters (e.g., abruptio placentae)

43. **What are the increased risks of twin pregnancies?**
    - Premature delivery
    - Intrauterine growth restriction (IUGR), including discordant growth (which may occur in up to one-third of twin pregnancies)
    - Increased perinatal mortality, especially for premature, monozygotic, and discordant twins
    - Spontaneous abortion
    - Birth asphyxia
    - Fetal malposition
    - Placental abnormalities (abruptio placentae, placenta previa)
    - Polyhydramnios

44. **Why are monozygotic twins considered higher risk than dizygotic twins?**
    Monozygotic twins (identical twins) arise from the division of a single fertilized egg. Depending on the timing of the division of the single ovum into separate embryos, the amnionic and chorionic membranes can either be shared (if division occurs >8 days after fertilization), separate (if division occurs <72 hours after fertilization), or mixed (separate amnion, shared chorion if division occurs 4 to 8 days after fertilization). Sharing of the chorion and/or amnion is associated with potential problems of vascular anastomoses (and possible twin-twin transfusions), cord entanglements, and congenital anomalies. These problems increase the risk for IUGR and perinatal death.
    Dizygotic twins, however, result from two separately fertilized ova and, as such, usually have a separate amnion and chorion.

45. **What are the known benefits of antenatal corticosteroids and when are they indicated?**
    In multiple studies with large numbers of subjects, antenatal corticosteroid therapy has been shown to significantly improve newborn outcome with decreased rates of neonatal mortality, respiratory distress syndrome (RDS), intraventricular hemorrhage (IVH), and necrotizing enterocolitis (NEC).
    Antenatal corticosteroid treatment should be given to pregnant women with fetuses between 24 and 34 weeks at risk for delivery within the next week. Before 24 weeks the decision to provide steroid treatment should be individualized based on the plans for intervention after delivery at that gestational age. Beyond 34 weeks gestational age, there remains uncertainty about the benefit of antenatal corticosteroid therapy, and trials in this late preterm population are ongoing.

Brownfoot FC, Gagliardi DI, Bain E, et al: Different corticosteroids and regimens for accelerating fetal lung maturation for women at risk of preterm birth, *Cochrane Database Syst Rev* 8:CD006764, 2013.
Roberts D, Dalziel SR: Antenatal corticosteroids for accelerating fetal lung maturation for women at risk of preterm birth, *Cochrane Database Syst Rev* 3:CD004454, 2006.

46. **What are the potential fetal effects associated with diabetes during pregnancy?**
    Among the most significant of these problems is an increased risk for perinatal mortality. Congenital malformations constitute a significant risk for pregnancies complicated by pregestational diabetes mellitus. Physiologic and adaptational problems can also affect newborn infants exposed to diabetes

during pregnancy. Poor glycemic control is associated with most of the complications of diabetes during pregnancy but does not explain all possible problems. The most common congenital malformations seen in infants of diabetic mothers are congenital heart disease. Poorly controlled diabetes during pregnancy is associated with macrosomia, birth trauma, hypoglycemia, hypocalcemia, polycythemia, delayed surfactant development, and hypertrophic cardiomyopathy.

47. **How is hypertension in pregnancy classified?**
Hypertension complicates 2% to 3% of pregnancies and is divided into four categories:
- **Preeclampsia-eclampsia:** hypertension with systemic manifestations including proteinuria, thrombocytopenia, impaired liver function, and newly developed renal insufficiency (Eclampsia is the development of seizures in a woman with severe preeclampsia.)
- **Chronic hypertension:** hypertension before pregnancy
- **Chronic hypertension with superimposed preeclampsia**
- **Gestational hypertension:** elevated blood pressure during pregnancy without other systemic findings

48. **What are the clinical consequences for the fetus from maternal preeclampsia?**
- **Intrauterine growth restriction:** Preeclampsia is the most common cause of IUGR in infants without anomalies.
- **Preterm birth:** Preterm delivery is indicated when preeclampsia is severe and may be considered at lower levels of severity at the discretion of the obstetrician.
- **Hypoglycemia:** Hypoglycemia occurs as a consequence of poor intrauterine growth.
- **Neutropenia:** Neutropenia can be fairly significant but is usually self-limited.
- **Thrombocytopenia:** Thrombocytopenia is usually mild and is also self-limited.
- **Morbidities associated with prematurity:** Preterm infants born after preeclampsia have similar rates of morbidities as other preterm infants. However, the rates of bronchopulmonary dysplasia and neurodevelopmental impairment may be increased when compared with other infants of similar gestational ages.

American College of Obstetrics and Gynecologists: Executive summary: hypertension in pregnancy, *Obstet Gynecol* 122:1122–1131, 2013.
Backes CH, Markham K, Moorehead P, et al: Maternal preeclampsia and neonatal outcomes, *J Pregnancy* 2011:214365, 2011.

49. **How does postmaturity differ from dysmaturity?**
- **Postmature:** An infant born of a postterm pregnancy (>42 weeks of gestation)
- **Dysmature:** Features of placental insufficiency are present (e.g., loss of subcutaneous fat and muscle mass; meconium staining of the amniotic fluid, skin, and nails)

50. **What is the first bone in the human fetus to ossify?**
The **clavicle**. In the long bones, the process of ossification occurs in the primary centers of ossification in the diaphysis during the embryonic period of fetal development. Although the femora are the first long bones to show traces of ossification, the clavicles, which develop initially by intramembranous ossification, begin to ossify before any other bones in the body.

51. **What external characteristics are useful for estimating gestational age?**
See Table 11-3.

Table 11-3. External Gestational Age Charateristics

EXTERNAL CHARACTERISTICS	Gestational Age			
	28 WEEKS	**32 WEEKS**	**36 WEEKS**	**40 WEEKS**
Ear cartilage	Pinna soft, remains folded	Pinna slightly harder but remains folded	Pinna harder, springs back	Pinna firm, stands erect from head
Breast tissue	None	None	1-2 mm nodule	6-7 mm nodule

Continued on following page

Table 11-3. External Gestational Age Charateristics (*Continued*)

| EXTERNAL CHARACTERISTICS | Gestational Age | | | |
	28 WEEKS	32 WEEKS	36 WEEKS	40 WEEKS
Male genitalia	Testes undescended, smooth scrotum	Testes in inguinal canal, few scrotal rugae	Testes high in scrotum, more scrotal rugae	Testes descended, pendulous scrotum covered with rugae
Female genitalia	Prominent clitoris, small widely separated labia	Prominent clitoris, larger separated labia	Clitoris less prominent, labia majora covers labia minora	Clitoris covered by labia majora
Plantar surface	Smooth	1-2 anterior creases	2-3 anterior creases	Creases cover sole

From Volpe JJ: Neurology of the Newborn, ed 5. Philadelphia, 2008, WB Saunders, p 122.

52. At what gestational age does pupillary reaction to light develop?
   Pupillary reaction to light may appear as early as 29 weeks into gestation but is not consistently present until about 32 weeks.

53. At what gestational age does a sense of smell develop?
   Although earlier responses are inconsistent, normal premature infants respond to concentrated odor after 32 weeks of gestation.

54. When does the fetal heart begin to contract in utero?
   Contractions begin by the **twenty-second day of gestation**. These contractions resemble peristaltic waves and begin in the sinus venosus. By the end of the fourth week, they result in the unidirectional flow of blood.

55. How does fetal circulation differ from neonatal circulation?
   - Intracardiac and extracardiac shunts are present (i.e., placenta, ductus venosus, foramen ovale, and ductus arteriosus).
   - The two ventricles work in parallel rather than in series.
   - The right ventricle pumps against a higher resistance than the left ventricle.
   - Blood flow to the lung is only a fraction of the right ventricular output.
   - The lung extracts oxygen from the blood instead of adding oxygen to the blood.
   - The lung continually secretes a fluid into the respiratory passages.
   - The liver is the first organ to receive maternal substances (e.g., oxygen, glucose, amino acids).
   - The placenta is the major route of gas exchange, excretion, and acquisition of nutritional substances.
   - The placenta provides a low-resistance circuit.

Allen HD, Gutgesell HP, Clark EB, Driscoll DJ, editors: *Moss and Adams' Heart Disease in Infants, Children, and Adolescents*, ed 6, Baltimore, 2001, Williams & Wilkins, pp 41–63.

56. What is the normal rate of head growth in the preterm infant?
   The rate is about 0.5 to 1 cm/week during the first 2 to 4 months of life. An increase in the circumference of the head of about 2 cm in 1 week should raise a suspicion of CNS pathology, such as hydrocephalus. However, some premature infants may experience rapid "catch-up" head growth after significant early stress or illness. The ratio of body length to head circumference may be used to distinguish normal from abnormal head growth. A ratio of 1.42 to 1.48 is reportedly normal, whereas a low ratio of 1.12 to 1.32 indicates relative or absolute macrocephaly.

57. What morbidities (short-term and long-term) are known to occur more frequently in growth-restricted babies?

- **Short-term morbidities:** Perinatal asphyxia, meconium aspiration, fasting hypoglycemia, hyperglycemia with alimentation, polycythemia-hyperviscosity, and immunodeficiency
- **Long-term morbidities:** Poor developmental outcome and altered postnatal growth
  Most studies demonstrate normal intelligence and developmental quotients in infants who are small for gestational age (SGA), although there appears to be a higher incidence of behavioral and learning problems. The presence or absence of severe perinatal asphyxia is extremely important for predicting later intellectual and neurologic function. Recent population studies suggest that a complex interplay of genetics and the environment leads to an increased likelihood of hypertension, hypercholesterolemia, and diabetes mellitus in adulthood.

Tamashiro KL, Moran TH: Perinatal environment and its influences on metabolic programming of offspring, *Physiol Behav* 100:560–566, 2010.
Simmons R: Developmental origins of adult metabolic disease, *Endocrinol Metab Clin North Am* 35:193–204, 2006.

58. When do premature infants "catch up" on growth charts?
   Most catch-up growth takes place during the first 2 years of life, with maximal growth rates occurring between 36 and 40 weeks after conception. Little catch-up growth occurs after the chronologic age of 3 years. About 15% of infants born prematurely remain below normal weight at 3 years of age.

GASTROINTESTINAL ISSUES

59. When does the newborn infant's stomach begin to secrete acid?
   The pH of gastric fluid in newborns is usually neutral or slightly acidic and decreases shortly after birth. pH values are <3 by 6 to 8 hours of age and then increase again during the second week of life. Preterm infants frequently demonstrate gastric pH values >7 for many days depending on the degree of prematurity.

60. When is meconium usually passed after birth?
   Most infants pass some meconium during the first 12 hours of life. Overall, 99% of term infants and 95% of premature infants pass meconium by 48 hours of life. However, the smallest premature infants may have a delayed passage of meconium as a result of the relative immaturity of rectal sphincteric reflexes. A term newborn who does not pass stool by 48 hours of life should be evaluated for Hirschsprung disease.

61. How is gastroschisis differentiated from omphalocele in the newborn infant?
   Both are ventral wall defects, yet their pathogenesis and prognosis differ markedly (Table 11-4).

Table 11-4. Differences Between Gastroschisis and Omphalocele

	GASTROSCHISIS	OMPHALOCELE
Incidence	1 in 10,000 (now increasing)	1 in 5000
Defect location	Right paraumbilical	Central
Covering sac	Absent	Present (unless sac ruptured)
Description	Free intestinal loops	Firm mass including bowel, liver, etc.
Associated with prematurity	50%-60%	10%-20%
Necrotizing enterocolitis	Common (18%)	Uncommon
Common associated anomalies	Gastrointestinal (10%-25%) Intestinal atresia Malrotation Cryptorchidism (31%)	Trisomoy syndromes (30%) Cardiac defects (20%) Beckwith-Wiedemann syndrome Bladder exstrophy
Prognosis	Excellent for small defect	Varies with associated anomalies
Mortality	5%-10%	Varies with associated anomalies (80% with cardiac defect)

From Chabra S, Gleason CA: Gastroschisis: Embryology, pathogenesis, epidemiology, NeoReviews 6:e493–e499, 2005.

62. Which conditions are associated with intra-abdominal calcifications?

    Meconium peritonitis and **intra-abdominal tumors** are the most common disorders associated with intra-abdominal calcifications in the neonate. The calcifications of meconium peritonitis are streaky or plaquelike and occur over the abdominal surface of the diaphragm or along the flanks. Intra-intestinal calcifications appear as small round densities that follow the course of the intestine and occur in association with intestinal stenoses, atresias, and aganglionosis. Intra-abdominal calcifications have also been observed in infants with adrenal hemorrhages and congenital infections.

63. What is necrotizing enterocolitis (NEC)?

    NEC is a necrotizing, inflammatory intestinal disorder that is the most common acquired gastrointestinal emergency in newborns. Signs and symptoms include abdominal distention, increasing gastric residuals, stool with blood, erythema of the abdominal wall, and lethargy. A positive blood culture is found in 10% to 25% of cases at the time of diagnosis. Radiologic signs of NEC include dilated bowel loops, pneumatosis intestinalis, portal venous gas, and free intraperitoneal air if an intestinal perforation has occurred.

64. Is pneumatosis intestinalis pathognomonic for NEC?

    No. Pneumatosis intestinalis can be seen in various other conditions, including Hirschsprung disease, pseudomembranous enterocolitis, neonatal ulcerative colitis, and ischemic bowel disease. However, it is a characteristic finding in the majority of patients with NEC. Dark, concentric rings within the bowel wall represent hydrogen as a by-product of bacterial metabolism (Fig. 11-4).

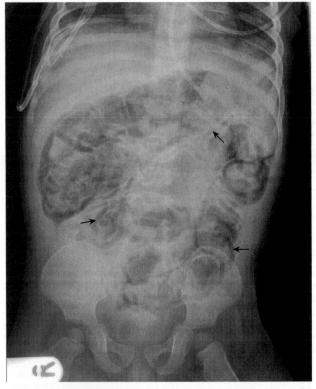

Figure 11-4. Pneumatosis intestinalis with intramural gas *(arrows). (From George S, Cook JV: Pneumatosis intestinalis,* J Pediatr *165:637, 2014.)*

65. What are the most important risk factors for NEC in preterm infants?

In an analysis of 15,072 neonates born at 98 centers over a 2-year period, the most important variables associated with NEC were **gestational age** and **birth weight**. Apgar score was not related. Other variables associated with an increased risk for NEC include the use of a ventilator on the first day of life, exposure to both glucocorticoids and indomethacin during the first week of life, and symptomatic patent DA requiring surgery. Cesarean delivery and the use of breast milk are associated with a lower risk for surgical NEC. The benefit of antenatal steroids has varied between studies.

Neu J, Walker WA: Necrotizing enterocolitis, *N Engl J Med* 364:255–264, 2011.

Guthrie SO, Gordon PV, Thomas V, et al: Necrotizing enterocolitis among neonates in the United States, *J Perinatol* 23:278–285, 2003.

66. Is it safe to feed infants with umbilical catheters?

The association of umbilical catheters with NEC is weak. In a 2006 survey of NICU directors, fellowship directors, and neonatologists, 93% of respondents felt it was safe to provide enteral feedings with an umbilical venous catheter in place and 75% with an umbilical artery catheter in place.

Hans DM, Pylipow M, Long JD, et al: Nutritional practices in the neonatal intensive care unit: analysis of a 2006 neonatal nutrition survey, *Pediatrics* 123:51–57, 2009.

67. How long should infants with NEC receive nothing by mouth?

Infants with true NEC (radiographic or surgical evidence) should continue to receive nothing by mouth for a minimum of 2 to 3 weeks. Infants in whom the diagnosis is suspected but not proved should be treated conservatively; many of these infants may be fed after 3 to 7 days.

68. Does the feeding of immunoglobulin to infants as prophylaxis prevent NEC?

The evidence does not support the administration of oral immunoglobulin for the prevention of NEC.

Foster J, Cole M: Oral immunoglobulin for preventing necrotizing enterocolitis in preterm and low birth-weight neonates, *Cochrane Database Syst Rev* 1:CD001816, 2004.

69. Is there a role for probiotics in the prevention of NEC?

Probiotics are nonpathogenic bacteria that promote health when allowed to multiply within the gastrointestinal tract. In human breast milk, they consist primarily of *Lactobacillus* and *Bifidobacterium* species. A systematic review of multiple studies revealed a reduction in the risk for NEC in infants >1,000 g. Elucidation of short-term and long-term effects such as systemic infection following exposure and alterations in immune and gastrointestinal function await further studies.

AlFaleh K, Anabrees J: Probiotics for prevention of necrotizing enterocolitis in preterm infants, *Cochrane Database Syst Rev* 4:CD005496, 2014.

Patel RM, Denning PW: Therapeutic use of prebiotics, probiotics and postbiotics to prevent necrotizing enterocolitis: what is the current evidence? *Clin Perinatol* 40:11–25, 2013.

Deshpande G, Rao, S, Patole S, et al: Updated meta-analysis of probiotics for preventing necrotizing enterocolitis, *Pediatrics* 125:921–930, 2010.

70. Are trophic feedings beneficial to preterm infants?

Trophic feedings, also called minimal enteral nutrition (MEN), are small quantity feedings considered an alternative to complete fasting before initiation of progressive feedings. Potential benefits include stimulation of motility of the GI tract and various hormonal secretions. A 2013 systematic review of studies that compared very low birth weight (VLBW) infants receiving no feedings to those given trophic feeds for at least 1 week after birth revealed no differences in the risk of developing NEC, time to achieve full feeds, and duration of hospital stay. A much larger, multicenter trial would be required to accurately assess the true impact of trophic feeds on NEC and help guide the decision to feed infants in this manner.

Ramani M, Ambalavanan N: Feeding practices and necrotizing enterocolitis, *Clin Perinatol* 40:1–10, 2013.

Morgan J, Bombell S, McGuire W: Early trophic feeding versus enteral fasting for very preterm or very low birth weight infants, *Cochrane Database Syst Rev* 3:CD000504, 2013.

HEMATOLOGIC ISSUES

71. When does the switch from fetal to adult hemoglobin synthesis occur in the neonate?

The switch from the production of hemoglobin F to hemoglobin A begins in a very programmed fashion in the fetus and neonate at **about 32 weeks of gestation**. At birth, about 50% to 65% of hemoglobin is type F.

72. Does the definition of anemia vary by gestational age?

For the term infant, most authorities consider a venous blood hemoglobin of <13 g/dL or a capillary hemoglobin of <14.5 g/dL as consistent with anemia. In preterm infants beyond 32 weeks of gestation, hematologic values differ only minimally from those of full-term infants, and therefore the same values may be used.

73. How does the hemoglobin concentration change during the first few days of life?

In all newborn infants, hemoglobin levels rise slightly during the first few hours of life (because of hemoconcentration) and then fall somewhat during the remainder of the first day. In healthy full-term infants, the hemoglobin concentration then stays relatively constant for the rest of the first week of life. However, appropriate-for-gestational-age infants of <1500-g birth weight may show a decline of 1 to 1.5 g/day during this same period, likely due to blood sampling.

74. When and at what dose should iron supplementation be initiated and for how long should it be maintained?

The timing for initiation of iron supplementation in preterm infants has been a subject of controversy for decades. Recommendations of the AAP, Canadian Pediatric Society, and European Society of Pediatric Gastroenterology and Nutrition suggest that doses of 2 to 4 mg/kg/day of iron be initiated at 4 to 8 weeks of age and maintained for 12 to 15 months.

Rao R, Georgieff MK: Iron therapy for preterm infants, *Clin Perinatol* 36:27–42, 2009.

75. Should erythropoietin be used in preterm infants?

Despite many earlier studies demonstrating reticulocytosis and increased hematocrit following treatment with erythropoietin, the modest effect of treatment on the number of transfusions and volume transfused in milliliters has raised questions regarding its efficacy. Because the smallest, most immature infants are frequently transfused before the onset of the effects of erythropoietin, the patients may not experience any decrease in the number of donors to which they are exposed. Furthermore, recent data have raised the question of whether the promotion of neovascularization by erythropoietin could result in an increased incidence of retinopathy of prematurity. Therefore, at the present time, there are no data supporting the routine use of erythropoietin in premature infants. Erythropoietin is currently being investigated as an adjunct therapy to prevent brain injury.

McPherson RJ, Juul SE: Erythropoietin for infants with hypoxic ischemic encephalopathy, *Curr Opin Pediatr* 22:139–145, 2010.

Von Kohorn I, Ehrankranz RA: Anemia in the preterm infant: erythropoietin vs erythrocyte transfusion—it's not that simple, *Clin Perinatol* 36:111–123, 2009.

76. How can Rh disease be prevented?

Pregnant women who are Rh negative should have antibody screening at the time of initial presentation and a repeat antibody screen at about 28 weeks of gestation. Unsensitized Rh negative women should receive 300 mg of Rh immunoglobulin (RhoGAM) prophylactically at 28 weeks of gestation and whenever an invasive procedure is performed. After delivery, if the infant is Rh positive, the mother should receive an additional dose of RhoGAM within 72 hours of delivery. At the time of delivery, the dose of RhoGAM may be increased if the fetomaternal hemorrhage is excessively large.

77. Why is the direct Coombs test frequently negative or weakly positive in infants with ABO incompatibility?

There are fewer A or B antigenic sites on the newborn red blood cell (RBC), and there is a greater distance between antigenic sites compared with adult RBCs. In addition, there is absorption of serum antibody by ABO antigens located on tissues throughout the body.

78. If fetomaternal hemorrhage is suspected as a cause of neonatal anemia, how is this diagnosed?

The **Kleihauer-Betke test** detects the presence of fetal cells in the maternal circulation. Because fetal hemoglobin is resistant to elution with acid, the treatment of a maternal blood smear with acid will result in darkly stained fetal cells among the maternal "ghost" cells. From the percentage of fetal RBCs and the estimated maternal blood volume, the size of the hemorrhage can be determined. One percent fetal cells in the maternal circulation indicate a bleed of about 50 mL.

79. If a gastric aspirate contains blood shortly after birth, what test can determine whether the blood is swallowed maternal blood or fetal hemorrhage?

The Apt test. This test relies on the increased sensitivity of adult hemoglobin to alkali as compared with fetal hemoglobin.

- **Method:** Mix the specimen with an equal quantity of tap water. Centrifuge or filter. Supernatant must have pink color to proceed. To five parts of supernatant, add one part of 0.25 N (1%) NaOH.
- **Interpretation:** A pink color persisting for more than 2 minutes indicates fetal hemoglobin. Adult hemoglobin gives a pink color that becomes yellow in 2 minutes or less, thereby indicating the denaturation of hemoglobin.

80. How is polycythemia defined?

Polycythemia is defined by a venous hematocrit of 65% because this exceeds the mean hematocrit found in normal newborns by two standard deviations. As the central venous hematocrit rises above 65%, there is an increase in viscosity. In neonates, some of the increase in viscosity with polycythemia is ameliorated by the lower viscosity of plasma. Because direct measurements of blood viscosity are not readily available in most laboratories, a high hematocrit level is thought to be the best indirect indicator of hyperviscosity.

81. What are the clinical manifestations of polycythemia?

The most common signs attributable to polycythemia include lethargy, hypotonia, tremulousness, and irritability. With severe CNS involvement, seizures can result. Hypoglycemia is common. Other organ systems can be involved, including the gastrointestinal tract (vomiting, distention, NEC), the kidneys (renal vein thrombosis, acute renal failure), and the cardiopulmonary system (respiratory distress, pulmonary hypertension and congestive heart failure). However, infants with polycythemia are often asymptomatic.

82. Which infants with polycythemia should be treated?

Because polycythemia results from a diverse array of etiologies, it is difficult to determine whether outcome depends more on etiology or the chronic elevation of viscosity. There is controversy regarding guidelines for treatment. Many authorities recommend a partial exchange transfusion, regardless of clinical signs, in infants with a central venous hematocrit level of at least 70% (because of the correlation with laboratory-measured hyperviscosity) or in those with a central hematocrit level of 65% or higher if there are signs and symptoms attributable to polycythemia.

Hopewell B, Steiner LA, Ehrenkranz RA, et al: Partial exchange transfusion for polycythemia hyperviscosity syndrome, *Am J Perinatol* 28:557–564, 2011.

83. What is the definition of thrombocytopenia in the neonate?

Based on numerous studies, a normal platelet count in neonates of any viable gestational age is defined as more than 150,000/mm^3. However, counts in the 100,000 to 150,000/mm^3 range are frequently seen in healthy newborns. Consequently, patients with counts in this latter category should have repeat counts, as well as further studies, if illness is suspected.

Roberts I, Stanworth S, Murray NA: Thrombocytopenia in the neonate, *Blood Rev* 22:173–186, 2008.

84. At what platelet count should platelet transfusion be considered?

Surveys of neonatologists reveal tremendous variability in the thresholds used for transfusion of platelets, especially because most are given prophylactically and not to treat active bleeding. Because the risk for bleeding is greatest in the first week of life, consensus opinion offers the guidelines shown in Table 11-5.

Table 11-5. Guidelines for Platelet Transfusion

PLATELET COUNT × 10⁹/L	NONBLEEDING NEONATE (1ST WEEK OF LIFE)	NONBLEEDING NEONATE (2ND WEEK AND ONWARD)	NEONATE WITH MAJOR BLEEDING
<30	Transfuse	Transfuse	Transfuse
30-49	Transfuse if <1000 g, clinically unstable, evidence of previous bleed, coagulopathy, and/or undergoing surgery	Do not transfuse	Transfuse
50-99	Do not transfuse	Do not transfuse	Transfuse

Adapted from Roberts I, Stanworth S, Murray NA: Thrombocytopenia in the neonate, Blood Rev *22:173–186, 2008.*

85. What features on physical examination suggest a specific cause of thrombocytopenia?
   - "Blueberry-muffin rash" (**to**xoplasmosis **r**ubella **c**ytomegalovirus **h**erpes [TORCH] or viral infection)
   - Absence of radii (thrombocytopenia **a**bsent **r**adii [TAR] syndrome)
   - Palpable flank mass and hematuria (renal vein thrombosis)
   - Hemangioma, large, often with bruit (Kasabach-Merritt syndrome)
   - Abnormal thumbs (Fanconi syndrome, albeit thrombocytopenia is less likely in newborns)
   - Markedly dysmorphic features (chromosomal abnormalities, particularly trisomy 13 or 18)

86. What is the most common cause of severe thrombocytopenia in the first day of life?
   Neonatal alloimmune thrombocytopenia (NAIT) occurs in 1/1000 newborn infants and is the most common cause of isolated severe thrombocytopenia in the first week of life. Transplacental passage of maternal alloimmune antibodies against paternally inherited human platelet antigens (HPA) found on fetal platelets result in NAIT. NAIT can occur with the first pregnancy, and it can result in thrombocytopenia severe enough to cause fetal intracranial hemorrhage. Identification of anti-HPA antibodies and HPA antigen typing of neonatal platelets confirm the diagnosis. Transfusion with random platelets may not be effective because the HPA antigens can be present on the transfused platelets. However, it is often possible to administer a specific HPA type to avoid continued destruction of the transfused platelets.

Bertrand G, Kaplan C: How do we treat fetal and neonatal alloimmune thrombocytopenia? *Transfusion* 54:1698–1703, 2014.

87. What treatment is available during subsequent pregnancies for mothers who have had a child affected with NAIT?
   NAIT recurs and increases in severity in subsequent pregnancies. With each subsequent pregnancy the risk for the fetus should be assessed with platelet typing of the fetus if possible. The mother can be treated with weekly infusions of intravenous immunoglobulin (IVIG) to minimize the incidence of thrombocytopenia and intracranial hemorrhage. Some experts recommend maternal treatment with corticosteroids (prednisone) in addition to IVIG later in gestation.

Kamphuis MM, Oepkes D: Fetal and neonatal alloimmune thrombocytopenia: prenatal interventions, *Prenat Diagn* 31:712–719, 2011.

88. When do the prothrombin time and partial thromboplastin time "normalize" to adult values?
   The *prothrombin* time reaches adult values at about **1 week** of age, whereas the *partial thromboplastin time* does not attain adult values until **2 to 9 months** of age.

89. **How is disseminated intravascular coagulation (DIC) diagnosed in the neonate?**
The laboratory findings of DIC include evidence of RBC fragmentation on peripheral smear; elevation of prothrombin time, partial thromboplastin time, and thrombin time; thrombocytopenia; decreased levels of factors V, VIII, and fibrinogen; and in some cases, the presence of fibrin split products.

90. **How should newborn infants with DIC be managed?**
Treatment should be directed primarily at the underlying disease rather than replacement of coagulation factors. In many cases, treatment of the former makes specific treatment of coagulation abnormalities unnecessary. However, in cases in which the stabilization of coagulopathy is not imminent, treatment with fresh-frozen plasma and platelets is recommended. In cases in which fluid overload is a major concern, exchange transfusion with fresh whole blood may be used. However, this second approach is not superior to the first with respect to the resolution of DIC. The use of heparin in patients with DIC should be reserved for infants with thrombosis of major vessels or purpura fulminans.

91. **What causes hemorrhagic disease of the newborn?**
For evolutionary reasons that are unclear, a newborn has only about 50% of the normal vitamin K–dependent cofactors. Unless vitamin K is given, these levels steadily decline during the first 3 days of life. In addition, breast milk is low in vitamin K. Early hemorrhagic disease can be observed during the first few days of life in infants who are exclusively breast-fed and who do not receive vitamin K prophylaxis at birth; they may bleed from various sites (e.g., umbilical cord, circumcision). Infants born to mothers who have received medications that affect the metabolism of vitamin K (e.g., warfarin, antiepileptic medications, antituberculous drugs) are at risk for developing severe life-threatening intracranial hemorrhages at or shortly after delivery.

92. **What are the risks and benefits of restrictive versus liberal transfusion criteria in preterm infants?**
There have been two large randomized trials in preterm infants to determine whether a liberal or restrictive transfusion policy is beneficial (Iowa and PINT trials). The thresholds for transfusion in the "restrictive transfusion groups" were similar in the two trials; however, the transfusion thresholds for the "liberal transfusion group" were significantly higher in the Iowa vs. the PINT trial. In the Iowa trial, the number of transfusions was reduced in the restrictive transfusion group, but the number of donors was not, likely related to a single donor transfusion policy at that center. In the PINT trial, the number of donor exposures was significantly decreased in the restrictive "transfusion" group, but only when red blood cell and platelet transfusions were both included in the analysis. In a secondary analysis, the number of infants with ultrasound abnormalities (periventricular leukomalacia or parenchymal brain hemorrhage) was significantly increased in the restrictive transfusion group. The NICHD is currently conducting a large randomized clinical trial to answer this question.

Crowley M and Kirpalani H: A rational approach to red blood cell transfusion in the newborn ICU, *Curr Opin Pediatr* 22:151–157, 2010.
Whyte, RK, et al: Neurodevelopmental outcome of extremely low birth weight infants randomly assigned to restrictive or liberal hemoglobin thresholds for transfusion, *Pediatrics* 123:207–213, 2009.
Kirpalani H, Whyte RK, Andersen C, et al: A randomized controlled trial of a restrictive vs. liberal transfusion threshold for extremely low birth weight infants: the PINT study, *J Pediatr* 149:301–307, 2006.

HYPERBILIRUBINEMIA

93. **What are the normal changes in bilirubin levels in full-term healthy newborns?**
All newborn infants exhibit a progressive rise in serum bilirubin concentrations following birth. Beginning with an average bilirubin concentration in cord blood of 2 mg/dL, serum levels rise and peak at 5 to 6 mg/dL between 48 and 120 hours of life. The 97th percentile for bilirubin in healthy full-term infants is 12.4 mg/dL for bottle-fed infants and 14.8 mg/dL for breast-fed infants. If untreated, at least 1% to 2% of newborns will develop bilirubin levels of 20 mg/dL.

94. **How should infants be assessed for jaundice before discharge?**
The AAP recommends two clinical options individually or in combination: a predischarge total serum bilirubin (or transcutaneous bilirubin) and/or assessment of clinical risk factors. Predischarge bilirubin values should be plotted on the chart in Figure 11-5 to assess risk.

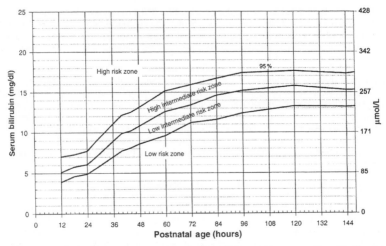

Figure 11-5. Assessment of jaundice. *(From Subcommittee on Hyperbilirubinemia: Management of hyperbilirubinemia in the newborn infant 35 or more weeks of gestation,* Pediatrics *114:297–316, 2004.)*

95. **How soon should infants be evaluated after discharge?**
    All infants discharged before the age of 24 hours should be seen by 72 hours of age by a qualified health care professional. Infants discharged between 24 and 47.9 hours should be evaluated by 96 hours of age, and those discharged after 48 hours should be seen by 120 hours of age.

Subcommittee on Hyperbilirubinemia: Management of hyperbilirubinemia in the newborn infant 35 or more weeks of gestation, *Pediatrics* 114:297–316, 2004.

96. **What is believed to be the fraction of bilirubin that is toxic to the CNS?**
    Routine clinical laboratory tests measure the total bilirubin and conjugated bilirubin concentrations. Of the total unconjugated bilirubin, most is bound to albumin and thus cannot cross the blood-brain barrier. Although the free bilirubin is believed to cause neurotoxicity, routine measurement in clinical practice is not available. Therefore, clinical decisions are commonly based on the total bilirubin concentration. It is unclear if monitoring the bilirubin/albumin ratio is of value.

Watchko JF, Tiribelli C: Bilirubin-induced neurologic damage—mechanisms and management approaches, *N Engl J Med* 369:2012–2030, 2013.
American Academy of Pediatrics: Clinical practice guideline: management of hyperbilirubinemia in the newborn infant 35 or more weeks of gestation, *Pediatrics* 114:297–316, 2004.

97. **Which infants are "set-ups" for ABO incompatibility?**
    Infants who are type A or B and whose mothers are type O are set-ups for ABO incompatibility. In individuals with type A or B blood, naturally occurring anti-A and anti-B isoantibodies are primarily IgM and do not cross the placenta. However, in type O individuals, isoantibodies are frequently IgG. These antibodies can cross the placenta and cause hemolysis. Although about 12% of maternal-infant pairs qualify as set-ups for ABO incompatibility, less than 1% of infants have significant hemolysis.

98. **What screening tests should pregnant women have to identify infants at risk for hyperbilirubinemia?**
    All pregnant women should be tested for ABO and Rh(D) blood types and have a serum screen for unusual isoimmune antibodies.

Subcommittee on Hyperbilirubinemia: Management of hyperbilirubinemia in the newborn infant 35 or more weeks of gestation, *Pediatrics* 114:297–316, 2004.

99. What are the clinical features of bilirubin toxicity?

The early clinical manifestations of bilirubin toxicity can be subtle. In addition, they can progress rapidly to severe and life-threatening manifestations. Acutely, toxicity is called *bilirubin-induced neurologic dysfunction* (BIND). For chronic cases, the term *kernicterus* is generally used. Using the BIND score, infants with subtle signs of bilirubin toxicity can be identified (Table 11-6).

Table 11-6. Clinical Features of Bilirubin-Induced Neurologic Dysfunction (BIND)

SIGNS	MILD	MODERATE	SEVERE
Behavior	Too sleepy Decreased feeding Decreased vigor	Lethargy and/or irritability (depending on arousal state) Very poor feeding	Semicoma Apnea Extreme irritability Seizures Fever
Muscle tone	Slight but persistent decrease in tone	Mild to moderate hypertonicity Mild nuchal or truncal arching	Severe hypotonia or hypertonia Atonic Opisthotonic posturing, bicycling

Cry pattern	High-pitched	Shrill and piercing (especially
		  when stimulated)
			Inconsolable, very weak, and
			  cries only with stimulation

100. When should phototherapy be instituted in infants who are at least 35 weeks of gestational age?

The AAP guidelines for instituting phototherapy in term and near-term infants are shown in Figure 11-6.

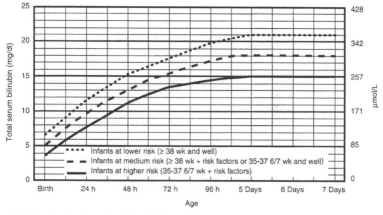

Figure 11-6. American Academy of Pediatrics guidelines for instituting phototherapy. *(From Subcommittee on Hyperbilirubinemia: Management of hyperbilirubinemia in the newborn infant 35 or more weeks of gestation, Pediatrics 114:297–316, 2004.)*

101. What distinguishes breastfeeding jaundice from breast milk jaundice?

Hyperbilirubinemia in breast-fed infants during the first week of life is called **breastfeeding jaundice** and is thought to be the result of poor caloric intake and/or dehydration. Hyperbilirubinemia in breast-fed infants after the first week of life is known as **breast milk jaundice**. The cause of breast milk jaundice is uncertain; however, possible etiologies include an increased enterohepatic circulation of bilirubin as a result of the presence of β-glucuronidase in human milk and/or the inhibition of the hepatic glucuronosyltransferase by substances found in some human milk samples (e.g., free fatty acids). The incidence and duration of these entities compared with physiologic jaundice are noted in Table 11-7.

Table 11-7. Comparison of Physiologic, Breastfeeding, and Breast Milk Jaundice

	PHYSIOLOGIC JAUNDICE	BREASTFEEDING JAUNDICE	BREAST MILK JAUNDICE
Time of onset (TSB >7 mg/dL)	After 36 hr	2-4 days	4-7 days
Usual time of peak bilirubin	3-4 days	3-6 days	5-15 days
Peak TSB	5-12 mg/dL	>12 mg/dL	>10 mg/dL
Age when total bilirubin <3 mg/dL	1-2 wk	>3 wk	9 wk
Incidence in full-term neonates	56%	12%-13%	2%-4%

TSB, Total serum bilirubin.
From Gourley G: Pathophysiology of breast milk jaundice. In Polin RA, Fox W, editors: Fetal and Neonatal Physiology. Philadelphia, 1992, WB Saunders, p 1174.

102. **Why should infants at risk for breastfeeding jaundice be fed more frequently?**
Breast-fed infants exhibit their maximal weight loss by day 3 of life and lose on average 6.1% ± 2.5% of their birth weight. Infants who are breast-fed an average of >8 times per day during the first 3 days of life have significantly lower serum bilirubin concentrations than those who are less frequently breast-fed. This practice accelerates and enhances the acquisition of milk supply. With increased milk available, dehydration is less likely to occur, and the excretion of bilirubin from the gastrointestinal tract is more rapid because of increased stooling. Infants with adequate intake should have 4 to 6 wet diapers per day.

103. **Where does bilirubin go when you turn on the lights?**
It becomes lumirubin (through a "cyclicization" reaction) and is rapidly excreted in bile, with a half-life of about 2 hours.

104. **What are the factors that affect the efficacy of phototherapy?**
- Spectrum of light emitted (blue-green is most effective)
- Spectral irradiance (intensive phototherapy = 30 to 50 W/cm^2 per nm)
- Spectral power (expose maximal surface area)
- Cause of jaundice (phototherapy is less effective with hemolysis and cholestasis)
- Total bilirubin at start (the higher the bilirubin, the greater the decline)

Subcommittee on Hyperbilirubinemia: Management of hyperbilirubinemia in the newborn infant 35 or more weeks of gestation, *Pediatrics* 114:297–316, 2004.

105. **What are the contraindications to phototherapy?**
Infants with a family history of light-sensitive porphyria should not receive phototherapy. The presence of direct hyperbilirubinemia is not considered a contraindication, but it will decrease the effectiveness of phototherapy and may result in bronze baby syndrome.

106. **What are the common adverse effects of phototherapy?**
Loose stools, increased insensible water loss, skin rashes, overheating, and the potential for burns if the lights are placed too close to the infant's skin. If direct hyperbilirubinemia is present, the bronze baby syndrome can result.

Maisels MJ, McDonagh AF: Phototherapy for neonatal jaundice, *N Engl J Med* 358:920–928, 2008.

107. **A newborn develops dark skin discoloration and dark urine after beginning phototherapy. What is the diagnosis?**
Bronze baby syndrome. Infants who develop the syndrome typically have an elevated direct serum bilirubin concentration. The bronze baby syndrome results from the retention of photoproducts (e.g., lumirubin) that cannot be excreted in the bile. Most infants appear to recover without complications. Direct hyperbilirubinemia is not a contraindication to phototherapy.

108. **What are the complications of exchange transfusions in the newborn?**
   Acute
   - Hypocalcemia (as a result of the binding of calcium by citrate)
   - Hypoglycemia
   - Thrombocytopenia (as a result of the removal of platelets and the use of stored blood that may be low in platelets)
   - Hyperkalemia (as a result of the higher potassium levels of stored blood)
   - Hypovolemia (if blood replacement is inadequate)

   Late
   - Anemia (for unknown reasons)
   - Graft-versus-host disease (as a result of the introduction of donor lymphocytes into a relatively immunocompromised neonatal host)

Patra K, Storfer-Isser A, Siner B, et al: Adverse events associated with neonatal exchange transfusion, *J Pediatrics* 144: 626–631, 2004.

109. **What is the relationship between neonatal hyperbilirubinemia and urinary tract infection (UTI)?**
   Unexplained jaundice developing between 10 and 60 days of age can be associated with a UTI in infants. The typical patient is usually afebrile (in two-thirds of cases) with hepatomegaly and minimal systemic symptoms. Hyperbilirubinemia is usually conjugated, and liver transaminases may be normal or mildly elevated. Treatment of the UTI (usually caused by *Escherichia coli*) results in reversal of the liver dysfunction, which is believed to be the result of endotoxins.

110. **Can transcutaneous bilirubin measurements be used in place of serum levels?**
   Numerous devices have been developed that accurately measure bilirubin levels that are highly correlated with serum bilirubin values. However, most studies show that the deviation of transcutaneous measurements is greatest (about 3 mg/dL) at the highest levels (>13 to 15 mg/dL). Therefore, many authorities recommend serum confirmation if the transcutaneous bilirubin is greater than the 75th percentile, more than 13 mg/dL, or if a level that is 3 mg/dL higher would be clinically meaningful.

O'Connor Mc, Lease MA, Whalen BL: How to use: transcutaneous bilirubinometry, *Arch Dis Child Educ Pract Ed* 98:154–159, 2013.
Grohmann K, Roser M, Rolinski B, et al: Bilirubin measurement for neonates: comparison of 9 frequently used methods, *Pediatrics* 117:1174–1183, 2006.

111. **What is the role of metalloporphyrins in the treatment of hyperbilirubinemia?**
   Metalloporphyrins are inhibitors of the rate-limiting enzyme, heme oxygenase, in the pathway of heme degradation leading to bilirubin production. Tin mesoporphyrin (SnMP) has been most extensively studied in human infants and has been shown to reduce the need for phototherapy. However, this compound is phototoxic, contains a foreign metal that may be released, induces the heme oxygenase,-1 promoter and can inhibit other enzymes such as nitric oxide synthase and soluble guanylate cyclase, whose products are required for important biologic functions. Thus, these compounds have not found widespread use in the treatment of hyperbilirubinemia. Advocates of "bloodless medicine" have promoted its use as a means of avoiding exchange transfusions.

Yaffe SJ, Aranda JV, editors: *Neonatal and Pediatric Pharmacology: Therapeutic Principles in Practice*, ed 3, Philadelphia, 2005, WB Saunders, pp 198–200.

112. **What is the role of IVIG use in the treatment of hyperbilirubinemia?**
   Several studies have demonstrated that in infants who are Coombs positive, high-dose IVIG decreased the need for exchange transfusion. Although these studies had design flaws, the AAP recommends that IVIG should be administered over 2 hours in infants with isoimmune hemolytic disease and a total bilirubin that is rising in spite of appropriate phototherapy.

Subcommittee on Hyperbilirubinemia: Management of hyperbilirubinemia in the newborn infant 35 or more weeks of gestation, *Pediatrics* 114:297–316, 2004.

INFECTIOUS DISEASE ISSUES

113. **What is the best method of umbilical cord care during the immediate neonatal period?**

No single method of cord care has been determined to be superior for preventing colonization and infections. Antimicrobial agents, such as bacitracin or triple dye, are commonly used, but there are no efficacy data (other than reduced colonization). Alcohol accelerates the drying of the cord, but it has not been shown to reduce the rates of colonization or omphalitis. The use of topical antibiotics has been shown to delay cord separation. Therefore, simply cleaning with normal saline and allowing the cord to dry naturally appears to be as safe and effective as using antibiotics.

Zupan J, Garner P, Omari AA: Topical umbilical cord care at birth, *Cochrane Database Syst Rev* 3:CD001057, 2004.
Mullany LC, Darmstadt GL, Tielsch J: Role of antimicrobial applications to the umbilical cord in neonates to prevent bacterial colonization and infection: a review of the evidence, *Pediatr Infect Dis J* 11:996–1002, 2003.

114. **Can sepsis be distinguished from other causes of respiratory distress in the neonate?**

Not reliably. Diagnosis is confirmed only by a positive blood, urine, or cerebrospinal fluid (CSF) culture.

115. **What is the single most important factor in determining whether an infant should be evaluated and treated for possible early-onset sepsis?**

The most important factor when considering treatment for sepsis is the presence of clinical signs of sepsis. An infant with signs of sepsis should be treated with antibiotics following a blood culture. If an infant has respiratory distress that is believed to be secondary to a noninfectious disease such as transient tachypnea of the newborn and has no other risk factors for sepsis, it may be reasonable to monitor the infant carefully without starting antibiotics. Risk factors for sepsis include maternal colonization with group B *Streptococcus* (GBS), signs and symptoms of chorioamnionitis in the mother, prematurity, and rupture of membranes for more than 18 hours.

Determining whether to evaluate asymptomatic infants with risk factors for sepsis is more difficult. Guidelines for the management of these infants have changed over recent years and continue to evolve. The goal of management is to identify infants with sepsis who require antibiotic therapy before they become symptomatic. However, it is also desirable to minimize treatment in infants who do not have infection. Unfortunately there is no perfect method to identify only infants with true infection, and clinicians must use sound judgment and familiarize themselves with the most current guidelines.

Benitz WE, Wynn JL, Polin RA: Reappraisal of guidelines for management of neonates with suspected early-onset sepsis, *J Pediatrics* 166:1070–1074, 2015.
Polin, RA, and the Committee on Fetus and Newborn: Management of neonates with suspected or proven early-onset bacterial sepsis, *Pediatrics* 129:1006–1115, 2012.

116. **Should a lumbar puncture (LP) be performed on all newborns as part of the sepsis evaluation?**

The need for LP as part of the sepsis evaluation of a newborn is controversial, with many authors suggesting it can be omitted in well-appearing infants. However, in symptomatic infants, an LP should be strongly considered because (1) bacterial meningitis can be present in newborns without CNS symptoms, and (2) a significant number of infants (15% to 30%) can have meningitis without bacteremia. An LP should be performed when sepsis is highly suspected based on clinical signs or laboratory data and in infants with positive blood cultures. The procedure should be postponed in an infant with cardiorespiratory instability or significant thrombocytopenia.

Stoll BJ, Hansen N, Fanaroff AA, et al: To tap or not to tap: high likelihood of meningitis without sepsis among VLBW infants, *Pediatrics* 113:1181–1186, 2004.
Wiswell TE, Baumgart S, Gannon CM, Spitzer AR: No lumbar puncture in the evaluation for early neonatal sepsis: will meningitis be missed? *Pediatrics* 95:803–806, 1995.

117. **List the contraindications to the performance of an LP.**

- Uncorrected thrombocytopenia or bleeding diathesis
- Infections in the skin or underlying structures adjacent to the puncture site
- Lumbosacral anomalies

- Cardiorespiratory instability
- Increased intracranial pressure: Although the presence of open sutures reduces the likelihood of herniation, this remains a possibility. In the presence of a rapidly deteriorating level of consciousness, cranial nerve palsies, abnormal posturing, abnormalities of vital signs without other cause and/or a tense fontanelle, brain imaging (computed tomography (CT) or magnetic resonance imaging [MRI]) should be obtained before performing an LP.

MacDonald MG, Ramasethu J: *Atlas of Procedures in Neonatology*, ed 4, Philadelphia, 2007, Lippincott Williams & Wilkins.

118. **What are normal CSF values for healthy neonates?**
    - More than 15 cells in a CSF sample should probably be considered suspect and more than 20 cells elevated; most cells should be mononuclear.
    - The CSF glucose concentration should be 70% to 80% of the blood glucose concentration.
    - Protein concentrations in excess of 100 mg/dL in a term infant should be viewed as suspect.
    - Protein concentrations in preterm infants often exceed 100 mg/dL, and there is an inverse correlation with gestational age.

119. **What is the preferred strategy for identifying women for intrapartum GBS prophylaxis?**
    The initial guidelines from the Centers for Disease Control and Prevention (CDC) recommended either late antenatal culture for GBS or a risk-based approach monitoring women with obstetric factors (e.g., maternal fever, rupture of membranes >18 hours). Despite a dramatic initial decline in the incidence of early-onset GBS disease, analysis revealed that the risk factor–based strategy identified <50% of affected infants' mothers compared with 85% to 90% with culture-based screening. On that basis, the universal late antenatal culture for GBS became the recommended approach, resulting in an overall decline of 81% in early-onset GBS to 0.25 cases/1,000 live births. GBS remains the leading infectious cause of morbidity and mortality among infants in the United States.

Verani JR, McGee L, Schrag S: Prevention of perinatal group B streptococcal disease: revised guidelines from the CDC, 2010, *MMWR Recomm Rep* 59:1–36, 2010.

120. **Which women should receive intrapartum antibiotic prophylaxis?**
    According to the 2010 CDC guidelines, antibiotic prophylaxis is recommended for women with a positive GBS screening culture within 5 weeks of delivery, GBS bacteriuria any time during pregnancy, or a previous infant with invasive GBS disease. For women with unknown GBS status, intrapartum antibiotic prophylaxis should be given if there is a prolonged rupture of membranes >18 hours or a temperature of >100.4 °F. Furthermore, given that preterm delivery is a key risk factor for early-onset GBS disease, the CDC guidelines recommend screening for GBS and antibiotic prophylaxis pending culture results for all women with unknown GBS status and onset of labor before 37 weeks of gestation.

    Intrapartum antibiotic prophylaxis is NOT recommended for routine, planned caesarean section deliveries before the onset of labor with intact amniotic membranes.

Verani JR, McGee L, Schrag S: Prevention of perinatal group B streptococcal disease: revised guidelines from the CDC, 2010, *MMWR Recomm Rep* 59:1–36, 2010.

121. **What is the typical clinical presentation of early-onset GBS disease?**
    Early-onset GBS sepsis is defined as GBS infection that presents within the first week of life. Infants typically become symptomatic in the first 24 to 48 hours of life with signs compatible with generalized sepsis (apnea, hypothermia, hypoglycemia, hemodynamic instability, vomiting, and lethargy) or respiratory distress (indicative of pneumonia). Localized infections such as meningitis, osteomyelitis, or septic arthritis are less common.

Koenig, JM, Keenan, WJ: Group B streptococcus and early-onset sepsis in the era of maternal prophylaxis, *Pediatr Clin North Am* 56:689–708, 2009.

122. **Do intrapartum antibiotics change the clinical presentation of early-onset GBS sepsis?**
No. While intrapartum antibiotic use reduces the incidence of early-onset GBS sepsis, it does not completely eliminate early-onset GBS sepsis. Furthermore, the presentation of early-onset GBS sepsis is unchanged by use of intrapartum antibiotic prophylaxis. In a study of 319 infants with early-onset GBS disease, the administration of intrapartum antibiotics to the mother did not affect the constellation and timing of clinical signs of disease. All infants born to pretreated mothers became ill during the first 24 hours of life (80% within the first 6 hours of life).

Bromberger P, Lawrence JM, Braun D, et al: The influence of intrapartum antibiotics on the clinical spectrum of early-onset group B streptococcal infection in term infants, *Pediatrics* 106:244–250, 2000.

123. **What are the most common pathogens that are responsible for late-onset sepsis in the newborn infant?**
   - Coagulase-negative staphylococci (48%)
   - *Staphylococcus aureus* (8%)
   - *Enterococcus* species (3%)
   - Gram-negative enterics (18%)
   - *Candida* species (10%)

Stoll BJ, Hansen N, Fanaroff AA, et al: Late-onset sepsis in very low birth weight neonates: the experience of the NICHD Neonatal Research Network, *Pediatrics* 110:285–291, 2002.

124. **What are the major risk factors for nosocomial sepsis?**
   - Prematurity
   - Use of parenteral alimentation and central lines
   - Intravenous fat emulsions
   - H_2 blockers
   - Steroids for bronchopulmonary dysplasia (BPD)
   - Prolonged duration of mechanical ventilation
   - Overcrowding
   - Heavy staff workloads

125. **Is methicillin-resistant *S. aureus* (MRSA) a significant pathogen in the NICU?**
Although *S. aureus* accounts for 8% of late-onset sepsis in the NICU, the percentage of MRSA is not well established. Recent data suggest that a higher proportion of hospitalized patients with MRSA disease have community-acquired rather than hospital-acquired strains. In fact, about 3% of pregnant women had vaginal colonization with MRSA, which could be transmitted to their infants at the time of birth. Other reports have shown transmission of MRSA through breast milk. In NICUs with evidence of high rates of MRSA nasal colonization, decolonization using nasal mupirocin is recommended but unproven.

126. **How is systemic candidiasis diagnosed in the neonate?**
Candidiasis is diagnosed by cultures of blood, urine, and CSF or other body fluids that are generally sterile. Because cultures are only intermittently positive, multiple blood cultures should be obtained. A urinalysis demonstrating budding yeasts or hyphae should raise suspicion of systemic infection. Gram stains of buffy coat smears may also demonstrate organisms. An ophthalmologic examination may indicate the presence of candidal endophthalmitis. Renal and brain ultrasounds should be performed to look for characteristic lesions. In addition, echocardiography should be performed in infants with central catheters to rule out cardiac vegetations.

127. **Should preterm infants receive prophylaxis for the prevention of *Candida* infections?**
A number of studies have examined the role of fluconazole prophylaxis in reducing mortality, infections, and colonization among infants with very low birth weight. Although reduced mortality was not a consistent finding, decreased colonization and invasive infections were consistently seen. A recent large trial of infants <750 g (the highest risk group) found no benefit to prophylactic fluconazole on the combined outcome of death or neurodevelopmental impairment. Concerns remain that use of

prophylactic fluconazole will increase fluconazole resistance and the emergence of *Candida glabrata* and *Candida krusei*, which are inherently less sensitive to the drug.

Benjamin DK, Hudak ML, Duara S, et al: Effect of fluconazole prophylaxis on candidiasis and mortality in premature infants: a randomized clinical trial, *JAMA* 311:1742–1749, 2014.
Carey AJ, Saiman L, Polin RA: Hospital-acquired infections in the NICU: epidemiology for the new millennium, *Clin Perinatol* 35:223–249, 2008.

128. What is the risk for prenatal viral transmission in infants born to mothers with hepatitis B?

If a mother is HBsAg and HBeAg positive, the risk for transmission is 70% to 90%. The risk is substantially lowered to 5% to 20% if the mother is HBsAg positive but HBeAg negative. Infants infected in the perinatal period have a greater than 90% chance of developing chronic hepatitis B infection, and of these, 25% go on to develop hepatocellular carcinoma.

129. Should preterm infants receive hepatitis B vaccine during their newborn stay in the hospital?

Because of the possibility of decreased immunologic response to vaccine at birth in preterm infants with birth weight of <2000 g, hepatitis B vaccine should be deferred until 1 month chronologic age. If medically stable, gaining weight consistently, and ready for discharge before 1 month of age, preterm infants may receive the first dose before discharge. Of course, if the infant's mother is HBsAg positive or status unknown, vaccine must be administered despite birth weight of <2000 g within 12 hours of birth along with HBIG.

130. What prophylactic medications should be given to infants born to HIV-positive mothers?

Women with HIV infection should be treated with antiretroviral therapy during pregnancy with a goal of achieving a minimal viral load. Newborn infants born to women treated for HIV during pregnancy (who achieved adequate viral suppression) should receive zidovudine for 4 weeks. For women who were untreated during pregnancy or only received intrapartum prophylaxis, the CDC recommends treatment of newborn infants with zidovudine for 6 weeks and nevirapine for 3 doses during the first week of life.

Panel on Treatment of HIV-Infected Pregnant Women and Prevention of Perinatal Transmission. Recommendations for use of antiretroviral drugs in pregnant HIV-1-infected women for maternal health and interventions to reduce perinatal HIV transmission in the United States. Available at http://aidsinfo.nih.gov/contentfiles/lvguidelines/Perinatal GL.PDF. Accessed on Dec. 18, 2014.

131. When is treatment for congenital cytomegalovirus (CMV) infection indicated?

Infants with signs of central nervous system CMV infection have improved hearing and neurodevelopmental outcomes following therapy with ganciclovir for 6 weeks. Longer treatment courses of up to 6 months with oral valganciclovir may be superior to shorter courses of therapy. Infants with signs of systemic infection even without CNS involvement may also benefit from antiviral treatment.

Gwee A, Curtis N, Garland SM, et al: Question 2: Which infants with congenital cytomegalovirus infection benefit from antiviral therapy? *Arch Dis Child* 99:597–601, 2014.

METABOLIC ISSUES

132. How frequently are the various metabolic disorders detected by newborn screening?

Although there is some variability in different populations, some of the commonly held frequencies are as follows:

- Biotinidase deficiency: 1 in 60,000
- Congenital adrenal hyperplasia: 1 in 16,000 (North America)
- Cystic fibrosis: 1 in 3500 (whites), 1 in 7000 (Hispanics), 1 in 15,000 (blacks).
- Galactosemia: 1 in 47,000

- Homocystinuria: 1 in 300,000
- Hypothyroidism: 1 in 3000 to 4000
- Maple syrup urine disease: 1 in 185,000
- Medium-chain acyl CoA dehydrogenase deficiency: 1 in 6400 to 46,000
- Phenylketonuria: 1 in 13,500 to 19,000
- Sickle cell disease: 1 in 2000 to 2500
- Tay-Sachs disease: 1 in 3000 (U.S. Jews)
- Tyrosinemia: 1 in 12,000 to 100,000

Kay CI: Committee on Genetics: Newborn screening fact sheets, *Pediatrics* 118:e934–e963, 2006.

133. **In what settings should inborn errors of metabolism be suspected?**
     - Onset of symptoms that correlates with dietary changes
     - Loss or leveling of developmental milestones
     - Lethargy
     - Patient with strong food preferences or aversions
     - Parental consanguinity
     - Unexplained sibling death, mental retardation, or seizures
     - Unexplained failure to thrive, vomiting, or poor feeding
     - Unusual odor
     - Hair abnormalities, especially alopecia
     - Microcephaly or macrocephaly
     - Abnormalities of muscle tone
     - Organomegaly
     - Coarsened facial features, thick skin, limited joint mobility, and hirsutism

Levy PA: Inborn errors of metabolism, *Pediatr Rev* 30:131–138, 2009.

134. **What key urine odors are associated with inborn errors of metabolism?**
     - Cabbage: Tyrosinemia, type I
     - Cat urine: Carboxylase deficiencies
     - Fish: Trimethylaminuria
     - Hops: Oasthouse urine disease
     - Maple syrup: Maple syrup urine disease
     - "Mousy" or musty: Phenylketonuria
     - Sweaty feet or cheesy: Isovaleric acidemia; glutaric aciduria, type II

135. **One of the key presenting features of inborn errors of metabolism is the presence or absence of metabolic acidosis. Which inborn errors of metabolism present with metabolic acidosis?**
     - Presenting with metabolic acidosis *and* lactic acidemia
       - Defects in gluconeogenesis, glycogenolysis or pyruvate metabolism: e.g., glycogen storage disease, fructose-1,6-diphosphatase deficiency, pyruvate carboxylase or dehydrogenase deficiency
       - Krebs cycle defects
       - Respiratory chain defects
     - Presenting with metabolic acidosis *without* lactic acidemia
       - Maple syrup urine disease
     - Presenting with metabolic acidosis and *variable* presence of lactic acidemia
       - Organic acidemias (proprionic acidemia, methylmalonic acidemia, isovaleric acidemia)
       - Fatty acid oxidation defects

Martin, RJ, Fanaroff, AA, editors: *Fanaroff and Martin's Neonatal-Perinatal Medicine: Diseases of the Fetus and Infant*, ed 9, 1659–1675, 2011.

136. **What is the definition and management of neonatal hypoglycemia?**
The definition of hypoglycemia during the first 24 hours of life varies with postnatal age because of the physiologic/metabolic transition that occurs during that time. Figure 11-7 represents guidelines established by the Committee on Fetus and Newborn of the American Academy of Pediatrics (Fig. 11-7).

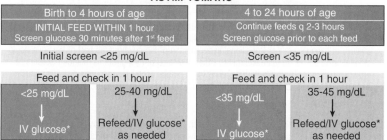

Screening and Management of Postnatal Glucose Homeostasis in Late Preterm and Term SGA, IDM/LGA Infants

[(LPT) infants 34-36⁶/⁷ weeks and SGA (screen 0-24 hrs); IDM and LGA ≥ 34 weeks (screen 0-12 hrs)]

Symptomatic and <40 mg/dL ────▶ IV glucose

ASYMPTOMATIC

Birth to 4 hours of age	4 to 24 hours of age
INITIAL FEED WITHIN 1 hour Screen glucose 30 minutes after 1ˢᵗ feed	Continue feeds q 2-3 hours Screen glucose prior to each feed
Initial screen <25 mg/dL	Screen <35 mg/dL

Feed and check in 1 hour		Feed and check in 1 hour	
<25 mg/dL ↓ IV glucose*	25-40 mg/dL ↓ Refeed/IV glucose* as needed	<35 mg/dL ↓ IV glucose*	35-45 mg/dL ↓ Refeed/IV glucose* as needed

Target glucose screen ≥45 mg/dL prior to routine feeds

*Glucose dose = 200 mg/kg (dextrose 10% at 2 mL/kg) and/or IV infusion at 5-8 mg/kg per min (80-100 mL/kg per d). Achieve plasma glucose level of 40-50 mg/dL.

Symptoms of hypoglycemia include: Irritability, tremors, jitteriness, exaggerated Moro reflex, high-pitched cry, seizures, lethargy, floppiness, cyanosis, apnea, poor feeding.

Figure 11-7. Algorithm for screening and management of postnatal glucose. (From Adamkin DH and Committee on Fetus and Newborn: Clinical report–postnatal glucose homeostasis in late-preterm and term infants, *Pediatrics* 127:576, 2011.)

137. **When is hypoglycemia most likely to occur in a neonate?**
During gestation, glucose is freely transferred across the placenta by the process of facilitated diffusion. However, after birth, the infant must adjust to the sudden withdrawal of this transplacental supply. In all infants, there is a nadir in blood sugar between 1 and 3 hours of life. During the first 12 to 24 hours of life, newborns are at increased risk for hypoglycemia because gluconeogenesis and especially ketogenesis are incompletely developed. These factors are accentuated in preterm infants, infants of diabetic mothers, infants with erythroblastosis fetalis, asphyxiated infants, and infants who are small or large for gestational age.

Sperling MA, Menon RK: Differential diagnosis and management of neonatal hypoglycemia, *Pediatr Clin North Am* 51:703–723, 2004.

138. **What is the prognosis of infants with hypoglycemia?**
There have been few studies looking at the long-term consequences of hypoglycemia in neonates, and many of the studies that do exist in the literature are complicated by confounders such as the lack of a uniform definition of hypoglycemia; incomplete follow-up; and the presence of other confounders such as hypoxemia, respiratory distress, and other medically complex conditions. Together these studies suggest that there are both clinical neurologic and MRI sequelae of **symptomatic** hypoglycemia in both term and preterm infants. There is no evidence that infants with "asymptomatic" hypoglycemia are at risk for neurodevelopmental impairment.

Tin W, Brunskill G, Kelly T, Fritz S: 15-year follow-up of recurrent "hypoglycemia" in preterm infants, *Pediatrics* 130: e1497–1503, 2012.
Lucas A, Morley R, Cole TJ, et al: Adverse neurodevelopmental outcome of moderate neonatal hypoglycaemia, *BMJ* 297:1304–1308, 1988.
Pildes RS, Cornblath M, Warren I, et al: A prospective controlled study of neonatal hypoglycemia, *Pediatrics* 54:5–14, 1974.

139. What features on physical examination suggest the etiology of hypoglycemia?
    - **Macrosomia:** This occurs in infants of diabetic mothers, infants with severe congenital hyperinsulinism, and infants with Beckwith-Wiedemann syndrome (recall that insulin is a growth factor and that hyperinsulinism leads to macrosomia).
    - **Midline defects:** Congenital pituitary deficiency can be associated with midline defects such as cleft lip, cleft palate, single central incisor, and microphthalmia.
    - **Micropenis:** This can be a sign of congenital hypopituitarism.
    - **Hepatomegaly:** This occurs in association with glycogen storage diseases and fatty acid oxidation disorders.
    - **Small for Gestational Age:** Infants who are SGA (<10th percentile) are at risk for both hypoglycemia and polycythemia (which is independently a risk factor for hypoglycemia).

140. What is the differential diagnosis for an infant with hypoglycemia?
    The differential diagnosis for hypoglycemia in the newborn period is broad. The most common etiology of hypoglycemia is transitional hypoglycemia of the newborn (as part of the physiologic adaptation to the *ex utero* environment). Other etiologies of hypoglycemia include disorders of growth (such as IUGR or infants who are SGA); perinatal asphyxia; endocrine disruption (such as hyperinsulinemia or abnormal cortisol production); hepatic dysfunction; and lastly, inborn errors of metabolism.

141. Should insulin be used to treat preterm infants with hyperglycemia?
    Studies comparing insulin treatment of hyperglycemia with reduction of glucose infusion rates showed no difference in mortality or morbidity, suggesting that the cause of hyperglycemia and not the blood sugar itself may determine the outcome.

Sinclair JC, Bottino M, Cowett RM, et al: Interventions for prevention of neonatal hyperglycemia in very low birth weight infants, *Cochrane Database Syst Rev* 10:CD007615, 2011.

142. What are the manifestations of hypocalcemia in the neonate?
    The major manifestations are **jitteriness** and **seizures**. Other nonspecific signs include lethargy, abdominal distention, and poor oral intake. Finally, infants with hypocalcemia may present with a high-pitched cry and laryngospasm. Chvostek sign (facial muscle twitching on tapping), and Trousseau sign (carpopedal spasm) may be present, but are rare during the neonatal period.

143. Which neonates are at highest risk to develop hypocalcemia?
    Early neonatal hypocalcemia (first 4 days of life)
    - Premature infants
    - Hypoxia-ischemia
    - IUGR
    - Infants of diabetic mothers
    - Maternal anticonvulsant use

    Late neonatal hypocalcemia (after the end of the first week of life)
    - High phosphate intake
    - Maternal hyperparathyroidism
    - Hypomagnesemia
    - Vitamin D deficiency
    - Intestinal malabsorption
    - Hypoparathyroidism
    - Decreased ionized fraction of calcium (with either normal or decreased total calcium)
        - Citrate (exchange transfusion)
        - Increased free fatty acid (Intralipid)
        - Alkalosis

144. When should hypocalcemia be treated in the neonate?
    Hypocalcemia should be treated when an infant is **symptomatic** or when the **total serum calcium level is <7.0 mg/dL.** Thresholds for treatment based on ionized calcium levels vary between medical centers because of different measurement technologies.

145. **How should symptomatic hypocalcemia be treated?**
The first line of therapy generally consists of increasing the amount of calcium in the intravenous infusion to achieve 20 to 75 mg/kg per day of elemental calcium and evaluating serum levels every 6 to 8 hours. After normal calcium levels are achieved, the intravenous dose can be weaned over 2 to 3 days. The infusion of a bolus of intravenous calcium (10% calcium gluconate, 2 mL/kg) over 10 minutes should be reserved for the infant with seizures. In the asymptomatic infant, hypocalcemia most frequently resolves spontaneously without the need for further therapy.

146. **What are the causes of neonatal hypomagnesemia?**
    - Hypercalcemia
    - Hyperphosphatemia
    - IUGR
    - Maternal diabetes
    - Intestinal malabsorption and urinary losses
    - Loop and thiazide diuretics

147. **In which neonates should the serum magnesium concentration be measured?**
    - Any hypocalcemic infant who is not responding to calcium therapy
    - Hypotonic infants born to mothers who received magnesium sulfate therapy before delivery
    - Infants with seizures of unknown etiology

148. **How is hypomagnesemia treated?**
Hypomagnesemic infants should be treated with 50% magnesium sulfate, 0.05 to 0.1 mL/kg, given IM or by slow intravenous infusion over 20 minutes. Magnesium levels are followed and the dosage repeated, if necessary.

NEUROLOGIC ISSUES

149. **After a difficult delivery, what three major forms of extracranial hemorrhage can occur?**
    - Caput succedaneum
    - Cephalhematoma
    - Subgaleal hemorrhage
    Figure 11-8 and Table 11-8 characterize the major forms of extracranial hemorrhages.

From Volpe JJ, editor: *Neurology of the Newborn*, ed 5, Philadelphia, 2008, WB Saunders, p 960.

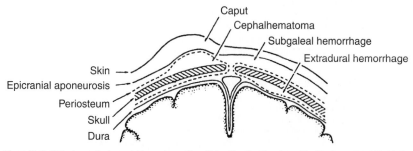

Figure 11-8. Major forms of extracranial hemorrhage. *(From Volpe JJ, editor:* Neurology of the Newborn, *ed 5. Philadelphia, 2008, WB Saunders, p 960.)*

Table 11-8. Major Varieties of Traumatic Extracranial Hemorrhage

LESION	FEATURES OF EXTERNAL SWELLING	INCREASES AFTER BIRTH	CROSSES SUTURE LINES	MARKED ACUTE BLOOD LOSS
Caput succedaneum	Soft, pitting	No	Yes	No
Subgaleal hemorrhage	Firm, fluctuant	Yes	Yes	Yes
Cephalhematoma	Firm, tense	Yes	No	No

From Volpe JJ, editor: Neurology of the Newborn, ed 5, Philadelphia, 2008, Saunders, p 960.

150. **If a cephalhematoma is suspected, should a skull radiograph be performed to evaluate for fracture?**
Cephalhematomas occur in up to 2.5% of live births. In observational studies, the incidence of associated fractures ranges from 5% to 25%. These fractures are almost always linear and nondepressed and do not require treatment. Thus, in an asymptomatic infant with a cephalhematoma over the convexity of the skull and without suspicion of a depressed fracture, radiographic imaging is not necessary. If the examination suggests cranial depression or neurologic signs are present, radiographic imaging is warranted.

151. **When screening for IVH, when is the best time to perform an ultrasound?**
In a series of infants studied by ultrasonography, about 50% had the onset of hemorrhage on the first day of life, 25% on the second day, and 15% on the third day. Thus, a single scan on the fourth day of life would be expected to detect more than 90% of IVHs. However, about 20% to 40% of hemorrhages show evidence of extension within 3 to 5 days after initial diagnosis, and thus a second scan is indicated to take place about 5 days after the first to determine the maximal extent of hemorrhage.

152. **What is the standard grading system for IVH?**
- **Grade I:** Germinal matrix hemorrhage only
- **Grade II:** IVH without ventricular dilation
- **Grade III:** IVH with ventricular dilation
- **Grade IV:** Grade III hemorrhage plus intraparenchymal involvement
 Some authorities have abandoned the grade IV classification in favor of "periventricular hemorrhagic infarction" to emphasize that these lesions have a different pathophysiology and are not simply extensions of germinal matrix or IVH into parenchymal tissue. As such, the extent of parenchymal involvement rather than the grade of hemorrhage is more important for determining prognosis.

153. **What is the cause of hydrocephalus after an intracranial hemorrhage?**
The acute hydrocephalus is believed to be a result of impairment of CSF absorption by the arachnoid membrane caused by the particulate blood clot. In subacute or chronic hydrocephalus, ventricular enlargement is the result of an obliterative arachnoiditis (likely a chemical inflammatory response from the continued presence of blood), which usually causes a communicating hydrocephalus. Less commonly, obstruction of the aqueduct of Sylvius can lead to a noncommunicating hydrocephalus.

154. **What factors predispose premature infants to the development of periventricular leukomalacia?**
Periventricular leukomalacia occurs primarily in the distribution of the end zones of deep penetrating arteries resulting in both focal (e.g., cysts) and more diffuse injury to white matter near the trigone of the lateral ventricles and around the foramen of Monro. Predisposing factors include the following:
- Cerebral hypoperfusion due to phenomena like hypotension and hypocarbia. They are more likely to occur in infants with impaired cerebrovascular autoregulation and a pressure-passive cerebral circulation.

- Infection and inflammation due to intrauterine infection and fetal inflammatory responses resulting in the production of cytokines, excitotoxic molecules, and reactive oxygen and nitrogen species
- Vulnerability of preoligodendroglia to free radicals and excitotoxic molecules (e.g., glutamate)

155. **What modalities should be used to detect periventricular leukomalacia?**
The most common imaging technique used in the NICU is ultrasound, which is capable of detecting cystic periventricular leukomalacia. However, because overt cysts, which represent focal necrosis, are seen in only 3% or less of preterm infants, MRI must be used to detect abnormal white matter signal, which may be seen in as many as 79% of preterm infants at term equivalent. What remains unclear is whether this observation represents noncystic periventricular leukomalacia or diffuse white matter gliosis. These entities may represent a spectrum of severity ranging from necrosis with cysts, to glial scars, to neither.

156. **What is the most common brachial plexus palsy?**
Erb palsy (Fig. 11-9). Neonatal brachial plexus injuries occur in less than 0.5% of deliveries and are often associated with shoulder dystocia and breech or forceps delivery.
- Involves upper plexus (C5, C6)
- In 50% of cases, C7 is affected
- Arm held limply adducted, internally rotated, and pronated with wrist flexed and fingers flexed ("waiter's tip" position)
- Biceps reflex absent, Moro reflex with hand movement but no shoulder abduction, palmar grasp present
- Ipsilateral diaphragmatic involvement in 5%

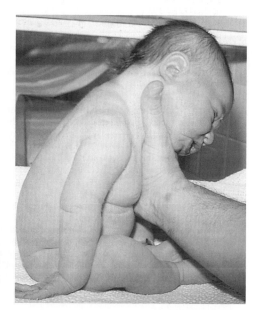

Figure 11-9. Erb palsy. Newborn demonstrating characteristic posture with the right arm limply adducted and internally rotated. *(From Zitelli BJ, Davis HW: Atlas of Pediatric Physical Diagnosis, ed 5. Philadelphia, 2007, Mosby, p 45.)*

157. **What is Klumpke paralysis?**
A brachial plexus palsy involving injury to the lower plexus (C8, T1). It is associated with weakness of the flexor muscles of the wrist and the small muscles of the hand ("claw hand"). Up to one-third of these patients have an associated Horner syndrome.

158. In newborns with facial paralysis, how is peripheral nerve involvement distinguished from central nerve involvement?
    - **Peripheral:** This usually results from compression of the peripheral portion of the nerve by prolonged pressure from the maternal sacral promontory. The use of forceps alone is not thought to be an important causative factor. Peripheral paralysis is unilateral. The forehead is smooth on the affected side, and the eye is persistently open.
    - **Central:** This type often results from contralateral CNS injury (temporal bone fracture and/or posterior fossa hemorrhage or tissue destruction). It involves only the lower half or two-thirds of the face; the forehead and eyelids are not affected.

    In both forms of paralysis, the mouth is drawn to the normal side when crying, and the nasolabial fold is obliterated on the affected side.

159. Is ankle clonus normal in the newborn infant?
    Bilateral ankle clonus of 5 to 10 beats may be a normal finding, especially in infants who are crying, hungry, or jittery. This is particularly true if the clonus is neither accompanied by other signs of upper motor neuron dysfunction nor asymmetric. Clonus should disappear at about 3 months of age.

160. What is therapeutic hypothermia?
    During *therapeutic hypothermia*, the core body temperature is decreased to 33.5 to 34.5 °C for duration of 72 hours with the intention to minimize brain injury after an insult. In term or near term (>36 weeks of gestation) newborn infants who have evidence of an hypoxic ischemic insult and encephalopathy at birth, the use of therapeutic hypothermia has been proven to decrease the incidence of death or neurodevelopmental impairment at 18 months of age from approximately 61% to 46%. The improvement in neurodevelopment has also been seen in mid-childhood with improved IQ scores in infants treated with hypothermia. The therapy is most effective when initiated as soon as possible after the insult. Because the timing of hypoxic-ischemic injury cannot be determined exactly, a somewhat arbitrary time frame of 6 hours from birth was used in most studies to begin cooling. There are two general methods of cooling: whole body cooling or selective head cooling using the "cool-cap." Neither method of cooling has been shown to be more effective.

Jacobs SE, Berg M, Hunt R, et al: Cooling for newborns with hypoxic-ischaemic encephalopathy, *Cochrane Database Syst Rev* 1:CD003311, 2013.

161. Which infants should be treated with therapeutic hypothermia?
    Therapeutic hypothermia is indicated for term or near term (>35 weeks of gestation) infants who show signs of encephalopathy (as evidenced by seizures or abnormal neurologic exam) after having an acute hypoxic ischemic event near the time of birth. Infants who meet these criteria must also have one of the following: a) a cord blood pH <7.0 (if available), a postnatal pH <7.1 or a base deficit >16, OR b) a 5-minute Apgar score of <5 or the need for ventilation at 10 minutes of life. These criteria should be considered in any infant >35 weeks' gestation who requires significant resuscitation at the time of birth.

162. How is neonatal encephalopathy evaluated and classified?
    In 1976, Sarnat and Sarnat developed a staging system for the neurologic findings seen after a perinatal hypoxic-ischemic insult. The system included three stages that were assigned based on findings in several categories: level of consciousness, neuromuscular control, complex reflexes, autonomic function, seizures, and EEG findings. A modified version of this staging system was used as the basis for the neurologic evaluation of infants enrolled in the therapeutic hypothermia trials. For details of a modified Sarnat score see Table 11-9.

Sarnat HB, Sarnat MS: Neonatal encephalopathy following fetal distress: a clinical and electrocardiographic study, *Arch Neurol* 33:696–705, 1976

163. What is the most common cause of a neonatal seizure?
    The most common etiology of neonatal seizures is **hypoxic-ischemic encephalopathy** with seizures beginning on the first day of life. Neonatal stroke is another frequent cause of seizure in the first days of life. Other causes of neonatal seizures may include: intracranial hemorrhage, infectious meningitis

Table 11-9. Characteristics of the Three Stages of Neonatal Encephalopathy

	STAGE 1	STAGE 2	STAGE 3
Level of Consciousness	Hyperalert	Lethargic or obtunded	Stupor
Neuromuscular Tone	Normal	Mild hypotonia	Flaccid
Posture	Mild distal flexion	Strong distal flexion	Intermittent decerebration
Primitive Reflexes	Weak suck Strong Moro	Weak or absent suck Weak or incomplete Moro	Absent suck Absent Moro
Deep Tendon Reflexes	Hyperactive	Hyperactive	Decreased or absent
Autonomic Function	Dilated pupils Tachycardia	Constricted pupils Bradycardia	Deviated, dilated or nonreactive Variable HR
Seizures	Absent	Common	Variable

HR, Heart rate.
Modified from Sarnat HB, Sarnat MS: Neonatal encephalopathy following fetal distress. A clinical and electroencephalographic study, Arch Neurol 33:696–705, 1976.

or encephalitis, and transient metabolic disturbances such as hypoglycemia, hyponatremia, and hypocalcemia. Inborn errors of metabolism, congenital anomalies of brain development, and neonatal epilepsy syndromes are rare causes of seizures that should be considered in the proper clinical setting.

Weeke LC, Groenendaal F, Toet MC, et al: The aetiology of neonatal seizures and the diagnostic contribution of neonatal cerebral magnetic resonance imaging, *Dev Med Child Neurol* 57:248–256, 2015.
Tekgul H, Gauvreau K, Soul J, et al: The current etiologic profile and neurodevelopmental outcome of seizures in term newborn infants, *Pediatrics* 117:1270–1280, 2006.

NUTRITION

164. How many calories are required daily for growth in a healthy, growing preterm infant?
    Preterm infants need about 120 cal/kg/day. About 45% of the caloric intake should be carbohydrate, 45% should be fat, and 10% should be protein. Infants who expend increased calories (e.g., those with chronic lung disease, fever, or cold stress) may need up to 150 cal/kg/day.

165. How should enteral feedings be started in the preterm infant?
    Initiation of feedings in preterm infants frequently depends on their cardiorespiratory stability. There is great variability from study to study on the definition of "early feedings," but most clinicians are starting enteral feedings no later than day 3 of life, unless the infant is critically ill or has reduced intestinal motility. Minimal enteral feeds (trophic feedings) generally consist of breast milk or preterm infant formula at a volume of 12 to 24 mL/kg/day.

Tyson JE, Kennedy KA, Lucke JF, Pedroza C: Dilemmas initiating enteral feedings in high risk infants: how can they be resolved? *Semin Perinatol* 31:61–73, 2007.

166. What are the medical benefits of breastfeeding?
    Proven benefits
    • Fewer episodes of otitis media and respiratory tract infections and gastrointestinal illness occur in breast-fed infants.
    • Decreased incidence of neonatal sepsis and necrotizing enterocolitis in preterm infants
    • Decreased risk of sudden infant death syndrome (SIDS)
    • Improved neurodevelopmental outcomes, especially in preterm infants

- Human milk facilitates the growth of beneficial, nonpathogenic flora compared with the pathogenic anaerobes and coliforms that predominate in infants who are fed formula.
- Formula-fed infants have reduced quantities of host-defense proteins in the gastrointestinal tract (e.g., lactoferrin, secretory IgA).
- Reduction in incidence of diabetes mellitus and obesity

American Academy of Pediatrics: Policy Statement: Breastfeeding and the use of human milk, *Pediatrics* 129: e827–e841, 2012.
Hoddinott P, Tappin D, Wright C: Breast feeding, *BMJ* 336:881–887, 2008.

167. **How does the composition of maternal breast milk differ for a full-term versus a premature baby?**
The composition of human milk for preterm infants differs from that for term infants in a number of ways. For every 100 mL, breast milk from women delivering preterm infants is higher in calories (67 to 72 kcal versus 62 to 68 kcal), higher in protein (1.7 to 2.1 g versus 1.2 to 1.7 g), higher in lipids (3.4 to 4.4 g versus 3.0 to 4.0 g), lower in carbohydrates, higher in multiple minerals and trace elements (especially sodium [Na], chloride [Cl], iron [Fe], Zinc [Zn], and copper [Cu]), and higher in vitamins (especially vitamins A and E). However, as breast milk becomes mature, many of these nutritional advantages are lost.

168. **How does colostrum differ from mature human breast milk?**
Colostrum is the thick, yellowish mammary secretion that is characteristic of the first postpartum week. It is higher in phospholipids, cholesterol, and protein and lower in lactose and fat than mature breast milk. Colostrum is particularly rich in immunoglobulins, especially secretory IgA.

169. **How do fore milk and hind milk differ?**
The caloric density of human milk increases in a nonlinear fashion while the infant is breastfeeding. Hind milk (produced at the end of the feeding) can have a fat content that is 50% higher than fore milk. In preterm infants with poor weight gain, hind milk may offer a nutritional advantage.

170. **What are contraindications to breastfeeding?**
   - **Inborn errors of metabolism:** Galactosemia, phenylketonuria, and urea cycle defects
   - **Infections:** Mothers with human T-cell lymphotropic virus (HTLV) types I and II should not breast-feed. For mothers with active tuberculosis (before treatment), peripartum development of varicella, and herpes simplex (when lesions are present on the breast), expressed breast milk can be used, but infants should not feed directly from the breast. In the industrialized world, it is not recommended that HIV-positive mothers breast-feed. However, in the developing world, the risks of malnutrition and infectious diseases may outweigh the risk of acquiring HIV from breastfeeding. A 2009 Cochrane review demonstrated that in areas endemic for HIV, infants who were exclusively breast-fed for 3 months had a lower risk of HIV acquisition than infants fed a combination diet of human milk and other foods.
   - **Substance abuse or use:** Cocaine, stimulants, and marijuana.
   - **Medications:** Sulfonamides (for infants with hyperbilirubinemia or glucose-6-phosphate dehydrogenase deficiency), radioactive medicines, chemotherapeutic agents (alkylating agents), bromocriptine (suppresses lactation), and lithium (in general, psychotropic drugs should be used with caution).
   Most other medications are compatible with breastfeeding, or suitable substitutes exist.

American Academy of Pediatrics: Policy statement: Breastfeeding and the use of human milk, *Pediatrics,* 129: e827–e841, 2012.
Horvath T, Madi BC, Iuppa IM, et al: Interventions for preventing late postnatal mother-to-child transmission of HIV, *Cochrane Database Syst Rev* 1:CD006734, 2009.

171. **What advice should be given to a mother who plans to express and save breast milk for later feedings?**
Ideally, the milk should be collected as cleanly as possible and stored rapidly at 3 ° to 4 °C or lower; the milk should be used within 5 days. Alternatively, breast milk can be stored in the freezer compartment of a refrigerator for about 6 months. If more prolonged storage is necessary (12 months), the milk should be kept frozen at a temperature of −20 °C or lower (usually in a separate freezer). After the milk has thawed, it should not be refrozen.

172. **What are the advantages of a 60/40 whey-to-casein ratio in infant formulas?**
The term 60/40 refers to the percentage of whey (lactalbumin) and casein in human milk or cow milk formulas. This ratio makes for small curds and therefore easy digestibility by the infant. The 60/40 ratio is of particular advantage to the preterm infant because it is associated with lower levels of serum ammonia and a decreased incidence of metabolic acidosis. Only human milk or formulas that supply protein in this ratio provide adequate amounts of the amino acids cystine and taurine, which may be essential for the preterm infant.

173. **"Low-iron" or "regular iron-fortified" formulas: which are preferred for infants?**
Generally, low-iron formulas have 4 to 6 mg/L of elemental iron, whereas regular iron-fortified formulas have 12 mg/L. Infants who are not breast-fed should be placed on regular iron-fortified formula. Although a greater percentage of iron is absorbed from the ingested low-iron formula, the quantity may not be sufficient to protect against the development of iron-deficiency anemia. In addition, despite anecdotal experiences, the incidence of colic, constipation, vomiting, and fussiness does not vary among infants fed the two formulas. The AAP recommends that all formula fed to infants be iron fortified.

American Academy of Pediatrics: Iron fortification of infant formulas, *Pediatrics* 104:119–123, 2009.

174. **Is vitamin supplementation necessary for exclusively breast-fed term infants?**
The following recommendations have been made by the AAP.
- Beginning in the first 2 months of life, all breast-fed infants should be supplemented with 400 IU/day of vitamin D to prevent the occurrence of rickets.
- Malnourished mothers may need to supplement their breast-fed babies with multivitamins.
- Mothers who are strict vegetarians may have low concentrations of B vitamins in their breast milk, and infants may need supplementation with vitamin B12.

AAP: *Pediatric Nutrition Handbook*, ed 6. Elk Grove Village IL, 2009.

175. **What is nonnutritive sucking?**
Nonnutritive sucking is a mode of sucking that is unique to humans and that is characterized by a highly regular, burst-pause pattern. Nonnutritive sucking occurs in all sleep and awake states, although it is seen less often during quiet sleep and crying. It assumes a recognizable rhythmic pattern after 33 weeks of gestation.

176. **Which fatty acids are essential for the neonate?**
Humans cannot synthesize fatty acids with double bonds in the omega-6 and omega-3 positions. Therefore, linoleic acid (omega-6) and linolenic acid (omega-3) must be provided in the diet to serve as precursors for fatty acids with these bonds. In infants weighing less than 1750 g who experience delay in achieving (or maintaining) full enteral feedings, arachidonic and docosahexaenoic acids may also be essential. These fatty acids are vital for normal brain development, myelination, cell proliferation, and retinal function. Fatty acids in human milk are composed of 12% to 15% linoleic acid.

177. **What are the proven advantages of supplementing formulas with long-chain polyunsaturated fatty acids?**
- Docosahexaenoic acid–supplemented infants transiently demonstrate higher behaviorally and electrophysiologically based measurements of visual acuity.
- The longer-term beneficial effects on visual function are inconsistent.
- The effects on cognitive development are controversial, but appear more compelling in preterm infants.

Simmer K, Patole S: Long chain polyunsaturated fatty acid supplementation in infants born at term, *Cochrane Database Syst Rev* 1:CD000376, 2008
Simmer K, Patole S: Long chain polyunsaturated fatty acid supplementation in preterm infants, *Cochrane Database Syst Rev* 1:CD000375, 2004.
SanGiovanni JP, Parra-Cabrera S, Colditz GA, et al: Meta-analysis of dietary essential fatty acids and long-chain polyunsaturated fatty acids as they relate to visual resolution acuity in healthy preterm infants, *Pediatrics* 105:1292–1298, 2000.

178. What are the manifestations of essential fatty acid deficiency?

Scaly dermatitis, alopecia, thrombocytopenia (and platelet dysfunction), failure to thrive, and increased susceptibility to recurrent infection. To prevent and treat fatty acid deficiency, 4% to 5% of caloric intake should be provided as linoleic acid and 1% as linolenic acid. This requirement can be met by 0.5 to 1.0 g/kg/day of intravenous lipids.

179. What are the manifestations of vitamin E deficiency in the neonate?

Hemolytic anemia (with reticulocytosis), **peripheral edema**, and **thrombocytosis**. Vitamin E is important for stabilizing the RBC membrane, and a deficiency can result in a mild hemolytic anemia. The AAP recommends that 0.7 IU (international unit) of vitamin E per 100 kcal be present in feedings for preterm infants. There is current consensus that infants weighing <1000 g require 6 to 12 IU of vitamin E per kilogram per day and that this can generally be met by preterm formulas that provide 4 to 6 IU per 100 kcal.

RESPIRATORY ISSUES

180. What causes infants to grunt?

Infants with respiratory disease tend to expire through closed or partially closed vocal cords to elevate transpulmonary pressure and to therefore increase lung volume. The latter effect results in an improved ventilation-to-perfusion ratio with better gas exchange. It is during the last part of expiration, when gas is expelled through the partially closed vocal cords, that the audible grunt is produced.

181. What do hyperpnea and tachypnea signify in the neonate?

- **Hyperpnea** refers to deep, relatively unlabored respirations at mildly increased rates. It is typical of situations in which there is reduced pulmonary blood flow (e.g., pulmonary atresia), and it results from the ventilation of underperfused alveoli.
- **Tachypnea** refers to shallow, rapid, and somewhat labored respirations, and it is seen in the setting of low lung compliance (e.g., primary lung disease, pulmonary edema).

182. Until what age are infants obligate nose breathers?

Although 30% of newborn infants breathe through their mouth or nose and mouth, the remaining 70% are obligate nose breathers until the third to sixth week of life.

183. What conventional mechanical ventilator settings are likely to affect Po_2 and Pco_2?

- **Pao_2 is *increased*** by raising the inspired oxygen concentration or the mean airway pressure, which can be accomplished with increases in PEEP, the peak inspiratory pressure (PIP), and the inspiratory-to-expiratory ratio.
- **Pco_2 is *decreased*** by increasing minute ventilation, which can be accomplished by increasing the ventilator rate or peak inspiratory pressure. An increase in PEEP without an increase in PIP may increase the $Paco_2$ by decreasing the tidal volume.

184. What factors determine the mean airway pressure on a conventional ventilator?

PIP, inspiratory time, PEEP, expiratory time, and ventilator rate.

185. What are the physiologic effects of PEEP?

PEEP can prevent alveolar collapse, maintain lung volume at end expiration, and improve ventilation-perfusion mismatch. However, an increase in PEEP may decrease tidal volume and impede CO_2 elimination. Elevations in PEEP to nonphysiologic values may decrease lung compliance, impair venous return, decrease cardiac output, and reduce tissue oxygen delivery.

186. What are the effects of severe hypercarbia ($Pco_2 \geq 100$ mm Hg) if there is no associated hypoxia?

There are few data about human newborns regarding the effects of isolated severe hypercarbia in the absence of hypoxia. However, results from animal studies and limited clinical observations in humans suggest that this condition can lead to a pressure-passive cerebral circulation and a possible increased risk for IVH. In addition, the high $Paco_2$ may disrupt the blood-brain barrier and enhance the deposition of molecules such as bilirubin in the CNS, thereby leading to kernicterus. Finally, on a cellular level, data in animal model systems demonstrate alterations in brain cell membrane lipid peroxidation and $Na+/K+$-ATPase activity. The significance of these latter findings remains undetermined. Moderate degrees of hypercarbia may be neuroprotective, and it may decrease lung injury in ventilated neonates.

187. **What are the most common causes of respiratory distress in term or late preterm infants?**

Respiratory distress after birth is usually identified by the presence of tachypnea (respiratory rate >65), nasal flaring, chest wall retractions, and hypoxemia. The most common causes of respiratory distress in term or late preterm infants include transient tachypnea of the newborn (TTN), pneumonia, and meconium aspiration syndrome. RDS can occur in late preterm or even term infants but its incidence decreases with advancing gestational age. Pneumothorax can occur in association with other respiratory diseases but can also occur spontaneously in up to 1% of newborn infants. Spontaneous pneumothorax is frequently asymptomatic and may resolve without any therapy.

188. **What are the risks and benefits of oxygen therapy in preterm infants?**

Preterm infants are thought to be at particular risk from excessive oxygen therapy due to immaturity of the antioxidant system. Hyperoxia may therefore lead to increased oxygen free radicals, which in turn lead to increased inflammation exacerbating the common morbidities associated with prematurity (e.g., bronchopulmonary dysplasia [BPD] and retinopathy of prematurity [ROP]). Historically, infants treated without or with lower amounts of oxygen did not survive as well as those treated with unrestricted oxygen. However, unrestricted oxygen therapy was found to be associated with ROP, sometimes leading to blindness. In recent years with the availability of pulse oximetry, large clinical trials have shown that attempting to maintain oxygen saturation at lower (85% to 89%) compared with higher (91% to 95%) levels was associated with higher rates of mortality but lower rates of ROP.

Saugstad OD, Aune D: Optimal oxygenation of extremely low birth weight infants: a meta-analysis and systematic review of the oxygen saturation target studies, *Neonatology* 105:55–63, 2014.
Stenson BJ, Tarnow-Mordi WO, Darlow BA, et al: Oxygen saturation and outcomes in preterm infants, *N Engl J Med* 368:2094–2104, 2013.
Schmidt B, Whyte RK, Asztalos EV, et al: Effects of targeting higher vs lower arterial oxygen saturations on death or disability in extremely preterm infants, *JAMA* 309:2111–2120, 2013.

189. **What is respiratory distress syndrome (RDS)?**

RDS is a pulmonary disease resulting from immature lung development and surfactant deficiency. Most frequently seen in preterm infants, the clinical presentation is characterized by signs of respiratory distress including nasal flaring, tachypnea, and grunting (an expiratory sound that is heard as the infant exhales against a partially closed glottis). Symptoms often present shortly after birth and can increase in severity over the first 48 to 72 hours of life. The radiologic findings of RDS consist of a homogenous ground glass appearance of the lung fields with visible air bronchograms (Fig. 11-10).

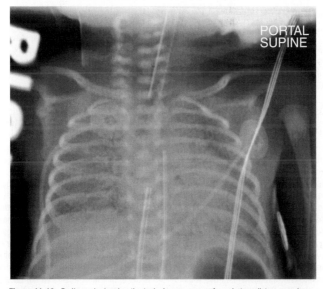

Figure 11-10. Radiograph showing the typical appearance of respiratory distress syndrome.

The pathophysiology of RDS involves insufficient surfactant stores leading to decreased compliance of the lungs and inability of the infant to maintain air in the lung at the end of expiration resulting in a tiny area of collapsed lung (microatelectasis). Due to poor lung compliance, the infant with RDS is also at risk for the development of air leak syndromes (pneumothorax and pulmonary interstitial emphysema).

190. **What is the composition and function of surfactant?**
   Surfactant is a surface-active lipoprotein complex comprised of a mixture of phospholipids (90%) (predominantly dipalmitoylphosphatidylcholine), proteins (10%), and a small portion of other neutral lipids. The main function of surfactant is to decrease surface tension of the alveoli allowing for maintenance of functional residual capacity preventing atelectasis and lung injury. The surfactant proteins also contribute to natural immunologic defenses and assist with the spreading of surfactant throughout the alveoli and the recycling of surfactant between cells and the airspaces.

191. **When is treatment with exogenous surfactant indicated in newborn infants?**
   Surfactant replacement therapy is indicated for preterm infants with RDS who have been intubated or who require a high oxygen concentration to maintain an oxygen saturation (Spo_2) >90% while on CPAP. Surfactant treatment may also be beneficial for infants with surfactant inactivation due to meconium aspiration syndrome, pneumonia, or pulmonary hemorrhage.

Polin RA, Carlo WA and Committee on Fetus and Newborn: Surfactant replacement therapy for preterm and term neonates with respiratory distress, *Pediatrics* 133:156–163. 2014.

192. **What is persistent pulmonary hypertension of the newborn (PPHN)?**
   PPHN is a clinical syndrome of severe hypoxemia resulting from failure of the fetal circulatory pattern to transition normally to the newborn circulatory pattern.
   The normal circulatory transition occurs as the infant is born and the umbilical cord is clamped removing the placenta from the circuit and increasing systemic vascular resistance. As the infant breathes, the lungs fill with air, the pulmonary vascular resistance falls leading to increased pulmonary blood flow, better oxygenation and increased pulmonary venous return to the heart. Following the fall in pulmonary arterial pressure (below systemic arterial pressure) blood flow through the DA transitions from a right to left (fetal pattern) to a left to right (newborn pattern).
   When the pulmonary vascular resistance does not decrease as expected, right-to-left shunting across the PDA and through the foramen ovale occurs. Therefore poorly oxygenated blood is shunted to the systemic circulation leading to significant hypoxemia.

193. **Is there a role for sildenafil (Viagra) in the treatment of PPHN?**
   Under normal conditions, vascular smooth muscle cGMP is degraded by phosphodiesterase-5 (PDE-5). As an inhibitor of PDE-5, sildenafil prolongs the half-life of cGMP and by so doing may prolong the vasodilating effects of nitric oxide (endogenous or exogenous). Trials to date assessing the effects of this drug, have demonstrated improved oxygenation and a possible reduction in mortality. Definitive data await trials with increased numbers of subjects and comparing sildenafil to other pulmonary vasodilators.

Nair J, Lakshminrusimha S: Update on PPHN: mechanisms and treatment, *Semin Perinatol* 38:78–91, 2014.
Kahveci H, Yilmaz O, Avsar UZ, et al: Oral sildenafil and inhaled iloprost in the treatment of pulmonary hypertension of the newborn, *Pediatr Pulmonol* 49:1205–1213, 2014.

194. **What is the pathophysiology and typical course of transient tachypnea of the newborn (TTN)?**
   TTN is the most common cause of respiratory distress in newborn infants and is caused by incomplete absorption of fetal lung fluid after birth. The fetal lungs are filled with fluid that is secreted by the pulmonary epithelial cells and is a critical component to lung development *in utero*. As the fetus approaches term gestation, the rate of secretion of lung fluid decreases and during labor the lung fluid is progressively absorbed into the interstitial spaces and lymphatics so that after birth the lungs can fill with air and any remaining lung fluid is cleared. When birth occurs before term, before labor, or by cesarean section the infant is more likely to retain enough fetal lung fluid to cause respiratory distress. Most frequently, the retained fetal lung fluid is reabsorbed after birth and the signs of respiratory distress (tachypnea and retractions) improve within 24-48 hours of life. Most infants do not need significant treatment during this time but some may need oxygen or CPAP to maintain adequate oxygenation and

decrease the work of breathing. A small number of infants may require more invasive respiratory support before the symptoms completely resolve. Chest radiographs of infants with TTN will show streaky parenchymal lung opacities and may have small pleural effusions but appear much improved within hours of birth.

195. **Why are fetuses with anhydramnios or severe oligohydramnios at risk for respiratory problems after birth?**

Appropriate lung development relies on the balance between fetal lung fluid secretion and drainage from the lung. The fluid is produced by lung cells and is passively drained from the lung into the amniotic fluid or is swallowed. When the amniotic fluid volume is markedly decreased, lung development will be impaired. Therefore, fetuses with anhydramnios due to renal disease or early rupture of membranes without re-accumulation of amniotic fluid are at risk for severe pulmonary hypoplasia. The severity of illness in these infants varies and is not always predictable prenatally.

196. **Has nasal prong CPAP been proven to decrease the risk for BPD?**

Retrospective studies evaluating the outcomes in different neonatal units suggested that the use of CPAP was associated with lower risk for BPD. However, it was not until recent years that this approach was prospectively tested in comparison with other standard therapeutic strategies to treat RDS. Several trials have now tested the hypothesis that early CPAP can decrease the risk for BPD when compared with ventilation and early surfactant therapy. The outcomes of these trials suggest that early CPAP decreases the need for mechanical ventilation. When the results of these trials are combined, the outcome of survival without BPD is somewhat improved with the early use of CPAP. The relative benefit of early CPAP depends on the comparison group, and each of the trials of early CPAP used somewhat different comparison groups. Therefore, when early CPAP is compared with ventilation as the primary treatment strategy, the benefit to early CPAP appears to be greater. However, when early CPAP is compared with early administration of surfactant followed by rapid extubation, the benefit of CPAP is not as clear.

Carlo WA: Gentle ventilation: the new evidence from the SUPPORT, COIN, VON, CURPAP, Colombian Network, and Neocosur Network trials, *Early Hum Dev* 88:S81–S83, 2012.

Dunn MS, Kaempf J, de Klerk A, et al: Randomized trial comparing 3 approaches to the initial respiratory management of preterm neonates, *Pediatrics* 128:e1069–e1076, 2011.

SUPPORT Study Group of the Eunice Kennedy Shriver NICHD Neonatal Research Network: Early CPAP versus surfactant in extremely preterm infants, *N Engl J Med* 362:1970–1979, 2010.

197. **What is the mechanism of action of inhaled nitric oxide (iNO) in the management of pulmonary hypertension?**

Nitric oxide (NO), produced endogenously in endothelial cells at the time of transition from fetal to neonatal life, diffuses to the vascular smooth muscle cell, where it increases the activity of soluble guanylate cyclase. This leads to the conversion of guanosine triphosphate to cyclic guanosine monophosphate (cGMP), which causes smooth muscle relaxation leading to pulmonary vasodilation. Similarly, when exogenous nitric oxide (iNO) is administered, it diffuses from the alveolus to the smooth muscle cells with similar effects. iNO is then rapidly bound and inactivated by reduced hemoglobin in the vascular space, thus avoiding concomitant reductions in systemic blood pressure.

198. **Which infants benefit most from extracorporeal membrane oxygenation (ECMO)?**

ECMO is prolonged cardiopulmonary bypass that is used to treat newborn infants with reversible pulmonary disease that has not adequately responded to conventional management. Although overall survival is about 70% to 80%, it varies by diagnosis, with survival rates of more than 90% for meconium aspiration syndrome, 75% for sepsis, and about 50% for congenital diaphragmatic hernia. Use of iNO has reduced the need for ECMO.

199. **What is the most common type of congenital diaphragmatic hernia (CDH)?**

Bochdalek hernia, which accounts for 90% of all CDHs, is the most common. This is a posterolateral hernia that most commonly (70% to 90%) occurs on the left side. Infants are usually symptomatic at birth and exhibit severe cardiorespiratory distress. Examination is characterized by a scaphoid abdomen and decreased breath sounds on the affected side. Radiographs reveal loops of bowel in the thoracic cavity (Fig. 11-11). Bag-mask ventilation should be minimized to avoid abdominal distention.

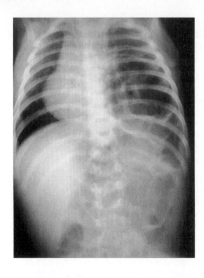

Figure 11-11. Chest radiograph of a newborn with a Bochdalek hernia. Note the absence of the left diaphragmatic shadow, gas-filled loops of bowel in the left chest, and heart and mediastinum shifted to the right. *(From Taussig LM, Landau LI, editors:* Pediatric Respiratory Medicine, *2008, Mosby, p 937.)*

200. What is bronchopulmonary dysplasia (BPD)?

BPD was first described in 1967 as a pulmonary disease identified following the acute phase of respiratory distress syndrome. The disease occurred after a period of treatment with mechanical ventilation using high pressures and oxygen concentrations. Clinical features included prolonged need for respiratory support and oxygen, and radiographs displayed alternating areas of lucency (bullae) and opacity (atelectasis) and cardiomegaly. The mortality rate associated with the disease was high, and pathologic findings discovered on autopsy revealed involvement of all tissues within the lung and included diffuse inflammatory changes, small airway disease, emphysematous alveolar changes, and extensive fibrosis. The pathogenesis of BPD has been attributed to ventilator and oxygen induced lung injury. However, the preterm immature lung is particularly susceptible to lung injury, and therefore lung immaturity itself plays a significant role in the development of lung disease. As respiratory care and survival rates of preterm infants have improved over the more recent years, BPD has been identified in a somewhat different form. The "new BPD" was described as a disease of lower gestational age premature infants that occurred despite fairly minimal levels of respiratory support and was seen pathologically as a disease of developmental arrest of the lung with alveolar simplification and reduced septation.

Jobe AJ: The new BPD: an arrest of lung development, *Pediatr Res* 46:641,1999.
Northway WH, Rosan RC, Porter DY: Pulmonary disease following respiratory therapy of hyaline-membrane disease, *N Engl J Med* 276:357–368, 1967.

201. In the current era of neonatal medicine, how is BPD or CLD (chronic lung disease) diagnosed?

BPD has traditionally been identified in maturing preterm infants by the ongoing need for respiratory support, specifically oxygen therapy. The names bronchopulmonary dysplasia and chronic lung disease have been used in different ways by different individuals and are sometimes used interchangeably. In previous eras of neonatology, BPD was diagnosed in infants treated with oxygen at 28 days of life. As more immature infants survived, the diagnosis shifted to describe infants treated with an oxygen need at 36 weeks adjusted gestational age. Because the indications for oxygen therapy vary by center with differing target oxygen saturation levels, an alternative "physiologic definition" of BPD was developed that involves performing a progressive room air challenge for infants treated with oxygen at 36 weeks adjusted age. In 2000 an NIH workshop developed a consensus definition for BPD that stratified the severity of disease and has been more predictive of later outcomes than previous definitions. Details of the consensus definition are outlined in Table 11-10.

Walsh MC, Szefler S, Davis J, et al: Summary proceedings from the bronchopulmonary dysplasia group, *Pediatrics* 117: S52–S56, 2006.
Ehrenkrantz RA, Walsh MC, Vohr BR, et al: Validation of the National Institutes of Health consensus definition of bronchopulmonary dysplasia, *Pediatrics* 116:1353–1360, 2005.

Table 11-10. NIH Consensus Definition of BPD for Infants <32 Weeks' Gestational Age

BPD Severity	Respiratory support at 36 weeks PMA or discharge to home, whichever comes first
Treatment with oxygen >21% for at least 28 days plus:	
Mild BPD	Breathing room air
Moderate BPD	Need for <30% oxygen
Severe BPD	Need for >30% oxygen and/or positive pressure (PPV or NCPAP)

PMA = postmenstrual age (gestational age in weeks + length of stay in weeks); PPV = positive-pressure ventilation; NCPAP = nasal continuous positive airway pressure.
Modified from: Jobe AH, Bancalari E: Bronchopulmonary dysplasia, Am J Respir Crit Care Med *163:1726, 2001.*

202. What are the respiratory benefits of caffeine therapy in preterm infants?

A large international multicenter trial showed that treatment of infants with a birth weight between 500 and 1250 g with caffeine reduced the incidence of chronic lung disease and led to weaning off positive pressure therapy 1 week sooner compared with placebo-treated controls. In addition, the incidence of death or disability was reduced in the caffeine group compared with the placebo group at 18 months but not at 5 years of age.

Schmidt B, Roberts RS, Davis P, et al: Caffeine therapy of apnea of prematurity, *N Engl J Med* 354:2112–2121, 2006.

Acknowledgment

The editors gratefully acknowledge contributions by Drs. Philip Roth, Mary Catherine Harris, Carlos Vega-Rich, and Peter Marro that were retained from the previous editions of *Pediatric Secrets.*

CHAPTER 12

NEPHROLOGY

Bernard S. Kaplan, MB BCh and Kevin E.C. Meyers, MB BCh

ACID-BASE, FLUIDS, AND ELECTROLYTES

1. **How is the cause of hyponatremia established?**
   The serum sodium concentration, even in states of volume depletion, reflects the extracellular water or volume status. In children presenting with *hyponatremia*, the **volume status** must always be evaluated. The causes of hyponatremia are
   Dilutional hyponatremia:
   - If the urine specific gravity is <1.003, look for causes of *excess free water* administration by taking a careful history: inappropriate oral or intravenous (IV) hypotonic fluid administration in a patient with acute or chronic renal failure who cannot excrete free water maximally; low-solute formulas or plain water in infants; excessive tap water use in infants with diarrhea or use as enemas; psychogenic polydipsia.

   If none of these causes is present, use the urinary sodium concentration to help categorize the cause of hyponatremia:
   Depletional hyponatremia with extrarenal losses:
   - If the patient is hypovolemic and the urinary sodium concentration is <20 mEq/L, the cause is likely to be gastrointestinal losses (vomiting, diarrhea, drainage tubes, fistulas, gastric drainage), skin losses (cystic fibrosis, heat stroke), or third spacing (burns, pancreatitis, muscle trauma, effusions, ascites, peritonitis).
   Depletional with renal losses:
   - If the urine sodium concentration is >20 mEq/L, the cause is likely to be diuretics, osmotic diuresis, salt-losing nephritis, mineralocorticoid deficiency, congenital adrenal hypoplasia, pseudohypoaldosteronism.
   - If the patient is euvolemic, and urine sodium concentration is >20 mEq/L, consider glucocorticoid or thyroid problems, syndrome of excessive antidiuretic hormone (SIADH), and the reset osmostat variant (a possible SIADH variant).
   - If the patient is hypervolemic and the urine sodium concentration is <20 mEq/L, consider edema-forming states: nephrotic syndrome, congestive heart failure, cirrhosis.
   - If the urine sodium concentration is >20 mEq/L, consider acute or chronic renal failure.

Avner ED: Clinical disorders of water metabolism: hyponatremia and hypernatremia, *Pediatr Ann* 24:23–30, 1995.

KEY POINTS: DIFFERENTIAL DIAGNOSIS OF HYPONATREMIA

- Hyponatremia with an elevated serum creatinine suggests renal disease.
- Hyponatremia with high urine osmolality and high urine sodium suggests SIADH.
- Hyponatremia with hyperkalemia and metabolic acidosis suggests renal tubular hyperkalemia or a corticosteroid disorder.
- Hyponatremia with proteinuria and hypoalbuminuria occurs in nephrotic syndrome
   SIADH, Syndrome of inappropriate antidiuretic hormone.

2. **What is the emergency treatment of symptomatic hyponatremia?**
   Patients with central nervous system symptoms, particularly seizures, should receive an initial urgent intravenous infusion of **hypertonic saline (3%)** at a dose of 3 mL/kg. This should raise the serum sodium concentration by approximately 3 to 4 mEq/L. The dose can be repeated every 10 to

20 minutes. Increasing the serum sodium concentration by only 4 to 6 mEq/L is usually sufficient to stop hyponatremic seizures.

Brenkert TE, Estrada CM, McMorrow SP, et al: Intravenous hypertonic saline use in the pediatric emergency department, *Pediatr Emerg Care* 29:71, 2013.

KEY POINTS: HYPONATREMIA

- Hyponatremia may reflect *appropriate* ADH stimulation as in cardiac decompensation and a non–steady state with arterial underfilling.
- Hyponatremia may reflect *inappropriate* ADH stimulation with euvolemia as in pneumonia, brain tumor, or severe pain.
- In children in intensive care and postoperatively, administration of hypotonic maintenance fluids increases the risk of hyponatremia when compared with administration of isotonic fluids.
- Isotonic fluids (normal saline) administered as maintenance should be avoided in children with ESRD, congestive heart failure, or hypertension.
    ADH, Antidiuretic hormone.

3. How is the cause of hypernatremia established?
   Hypernatremia is either due to **excess salt administration** or **excess free water loss**. A combination of history, clinical assessment of the patient's volume status, and measurement of urine sodium concentration measurement is required to establish the diagnosis.
   - *If the patient is **hypovolemic** and urine sodium concentration is <20 mEq/L,* consider extrarenal water losses—diarrhea, excessive perspiration.
   - *If the urinary sodium concentration is >20 mEq/L,* consider renal losses—renal dysplasia, obstructive uropathy, and osmotic diuresis.
   - *If the patient is **euvolemic** and the urine sodium concentration is variable,* consider extrarenal losses (insensible: dermal, respiratory) and renal losses (central diabetes insipidus, nephrogenic diabetes insipidus).
   - *If the patient is **hypervolemic** and the urine serum concentration is [usually] >20 mEq/L,* consider— improperly mixed formula in tube feeding, excess sodium bicarbonate administration, excess salt administration, salt poisoning, and primary hyperaldosteronism (rare in children).

Avner ED: Clinical disorders of water metabolism: hyponatremia and hypernatremia, *Pediatr Ann.*24:23–30, 1995

4. Why can correcting hypernatremia too rapidly cause seizures?
   Children with severe hyponatremia may seize before treatment is started, whereas those with hypernatremia may develop seizures in response to therapy. In patients with hypernatremic dehydration, increased extracellular osmolality draws fluid from the intracellular compartment, and cells, especially brain cells, shrink in size. However, the brain can generate idiogenic osmoles to minimize the loss of fluids. Idiogenic osmoles are principally amino acids and other organic solutes that allow brain cells to minimize cellular water loss. In fact, in chronic hypernatremia, brain size is almost normal. However, it takes about 24 hours to begin to generate or dissipate these idiogenic osmoles. Therefore, if correction of chronic hypernatremia of greater than 24 hours' duration is too rapid, water moves from the extracellular compartment back into the cerebral intracellular compartment, thereby causing cerebral edema. This can lead to seizures, cerebral hemorrhage, and even death. To prevent this in patients with chronic hypernatremia, the serum sodium concentration should not be allowed to decrease faster than 0.5 mEq/L per hour and ideally not more than 10 to 12 mEq/L/24 hr.

Schwaderer AL, Schwartz GJ: Treating hypernatremic dehydration, *Pediatr Rev* 28:148–150, 2005.

5. What is the differential diagnosis of nephrogenic diabetes insipidus (NDI)?
   - *Inherited NDI* may be due to arginine vasopressin (AVP) receptor (AVPR2 gene, X-linked) or aquaporin (AQP2 gene, recessive) abnormalities.
   - *Acquired NDI* may be due to electrolyte causes (hypokalemia, hypocalcemia), medications (diuretics, lithium, cisplatin), chronic kidney diseases, tubulointerstitial disease.
   - NDI can occur in renal Fanconi syndrome, renal tubular acidosis, and Bartter syndrome because of hypokalemia.

6. An infant boy presents with severe dehydration, polyuria, and hypernatremia. What is the first renal diagnosis that should come to mind?

Congenital NDI, which is caused by mutations in the aquaporin genes (AVPR2 or AQP2) is the first renal diagnosis that should come to mind. Aquaporins are membrane proteins involved in water transport. The genetic defect results in insensitivity in the distal nephron to AVP (ADH), so there is abnormal water reabsorption in the collecting ducts. This urine concentrating defect is present from birth, and symptoms of irritability, poor feeding, and poor weight gain begin in the first weeks of life. High fevers, dehydration and seizures, mental retardation, and psychological problems can occur. Persistent polyuria can cause megacystis, trabeculated bladder, hydroureter, and hydronephrosis.

Wesche D, Deen PM, Knoers NV: Congenital nephrogenic diabetes insipidus: the current state of affairs, *Pediatr Nephrol* 27:2183–2104, 2012.

7. What are the clinical and physiologic consequences of progressive hypokalemia (low potassium)?
   - Muscle weakness and paralysis, which can lead to hypoventilation and apnea
   - Constipation and ileus
   - Increased susceptibility for ventricular ectopic rhythms and fibrillation, especially in children receiving digitalis
   - Interference with the ability of the kidney to concentrate urine, leading to polyuria

8. What are the causes of hypokalemia?
   - Diuretics, occasionally laxatives
   - Metabolic alkalosis, especially in patients with pyloric stenosis
   - Severe diabetic ketoacidosis with dehydration
   - Diarrhea
   - Renal tubular acidosis, types I and II
   - Renal Fanconi syndrome
   - Bartter and Gitelman syndromes
   - Hypermineralocorticoid states: Primary hyperaldosteronism, Cushing syndrome, adrenal tumors, rare forms of congenital adrenal hyperplasia, dexamethasone-suppressible hypertension
   - Pituitary tumors producing adrenocorticotropic hormone
   - Hyperreninemic states such as renal artery stenosis

9. Which foods are high in potassium?

Raisins, baked potatoes, cocoa, oranges, bananas, French fries (especially supersized!), and carrots are high in potassium.

10. List the causes of hyperkalemia in children.
   - **Increased potassium intake:** Increased oral intake alone does not lead to hyperkalemia as long as the ability to excrete potassium is maintained. Increased intake is important when renal excretion is compromised in renal failure with oliguria-anuria or in patients taking angiotensin-converting enzyme (ACE) inhibitors. Rarely, an extremely high intake of potassium can lead to hyperkalemia (e.g., intravenous potassium, oral potassium penicillin, and blood transfusion using blood that has been stored a long time).
   - **Decreased renal excretion:** Impaired renal function leads to reduced potassium excretion, usually in patients with oliguric/anuric acute renal failure. Initially, potassium balance is maintained by increased excretion through the functioning nephrons, until the glomerular filtration rate (GFR) decreases to <15 mL/min/1.73 m^2.
   - **Redistribution of potassium** from the intracellular to extracellular compartment. *Metabolic acidosis* results in the movement of hydrogen ions into the intracellular space in order to buffer the intravascular pH. To maintain electroneutrality, potassium moves out of the cell resulting in hyperkalemia. Insulin promotes movement of potassium into cells. Therefore, insulin deficiency in diabetic ketoacidosis can lead to hyperkalemia. Intravascular hyperosmolality causes water movement out of cells, dragging potassium with it (solvent drag) followed by an increase in intracellular potassium concentration, creating a favorable gradient for potassium movement out of cells.

- **Tissue breakdown** can release potassium from the cells into the extracellular fluid. This occurs with trauma, rhabdomyolysis, chemotherapy (causing tumor lysis syndrome), massive hemolysis (e.g., transfusion reaction), strenuous exercise, and hyperkalemic periodic paralysis.
- **Medication-induced hyperkalemia:** β-blockers, potassium-sparing diuretics, ACE inhibitors, digoxin, succinylcholine, arginine, nonsteroidal anti-inflammatory drugs (NSAIDs), and calcineurin may induce hyperkalemia.
- **Pseudohyperkalemia** is defined as a rise in the serum potassium concentration with a concurrently normal plasma potassium concentration. The destruction of erythrocytes following venipuncture or capillary sampling is the most frequent reason for a raised serum potassium result in children. Pseudohyperkalemia is also seen with severe thrombocytosis due to release of potassium from platelet granules, severe polycythemia, or leukocytosis. In these instances, checking a *plasma* (as compared to a *serum*) potassium concentration will provide reassurance that the plasma concentration is normal.
- **Aldosterone deficiency or resistance (pseudohypoaldosteronism)** reduces potassium and hydrogen excretion and results in hyperkalemia and metabolic acidosis. Lack of aldosterone production occurs in primary adrenal insufficiency or with inborn errors of adrenal steroid metabolism (e.g., congenital adrenal hyperplasia, aldosterone synthase deficiency). Children with pseudohypoaldosteronism exhibit elevated aldosterone levels. Pseudohypoaldosteronism can occur with or without salt wasting.

Masilamani K, van der Voort J: The management of acute hyperkalemia in neonates and children, *Arch Dis Child.* 97:376–380, 2012.

11. When are calcium infusions indicated in a patient with elevated serum potassium?

If the **serum potassium level is >8 mEq/L** or there is a **cardiac dysrhythmia,** calcium infusions are indicated. A calcium infusion is the most rapid way to treat a dysrhythmia associated with hyperkalemia, but it does not reduce serum potassium concentrations. Hyperkalemia increases the cell's membrane potential, thereby making cells more dysrhythmogenic. Hypercalcemia increases the cell's threshold potential, restores the voltage difference between these two potentials, and decreases the likelihood of a dysrhythmia. The effect of a calcium infusion is transient.

12. What are key aspects in the treatment of hyperkalemia?
    1. **Stabilize membrane potentials:** Ten percent calcium gluconate is used, most typically when immediate action is required to improve an abnormal electrocardiogram (ECG).
    2. **Induce potassium transport into cells:** Therapies include glucose + insulin and sodium bicarbonate (in the setting of acidosis). The use of beta-2 agonists (both intravenous and inhaled) are recommended by some experts as another possible therapy.
    3. **Enhanced excretion of potassium:** This can be accomplished by a cation exchange resin (e.g., sodium polystyrene sulfonate); loop diuretic; and, as the ultimate therapy, dialysis.

13. What are the causes of periodic paralysis syndromes involving both high and low potassium levels?

Inherited channelopathies are disorders produced by abnormal ion channel function. In hypokalemic periodic paralysis, about 70% of patients have a mutation in a calcium channel gene. In hyperkalemic periodic paralysis, most cases are caused by mutations in the sodium channel SCN4A. Both diseases are characterized by intermittent weakness, usually in the morning. Of note, hyperkalemic period paralysis is a well-described and common malady in quarter horses, where it is called "Impressive syndrome" after the mutational source was found to have originated in a stallion named Impressive.

Saperstein DS: Muscle channelopathies, *Semin Neurol* 28:260–269, 2008.

14. What is the undetermined serum anion gap?

The undetermined serum anion gap is the difference between the serum sodium concentration and the sum of chloride plus bicarbonate. The anion gap represents anions that are not normally measured such as sulfate, organic anions, and charged albumin. The normal value is <15 mEq/L.

15. **How is the serum anion gap helpful in the evaluation of a metabolic acidosis?**
    In the presence of metabolic acidosis, the calculation of the anion gap determines which of two diagnostic pathways is more likely. If the anion gap is ***increased***, consider a cause listed under MUDPILES (see question 16). If the anion gap is ***normal***, consider diarrhea or renal tubular acidosis. Of note, always suspect an undetermined anion gap acidosis if the serum chloride and bicarbonate are both low.

16. **What are the causes of an elevated serum anion gap acidosis?**
    An increased anion gap reflects the addition of an acid with its anion that is not normally measured, such as salicylate but not hydrochloric acid. The mnemonic **MUDPILES** helps with remembering the causes of an elevated anion gap.
    - **M**ethanol (formic acid and formate)
    - **U**remia (guanidinosuccinic acid, phosphates, sulfates, and other acids)
    - **D**iabetic ketoacidosis (lactic acid, β-hydroxybutyrate, and acetoacetate)
    - **P**araldehyde, **P**henformin
    - **I**ron, **I**soniazid, **I**nborn errors of metabolism
    - **L**actic acidosis secondary to hypoxia, severe cardiorespiratory depression, shock, prolonged seizures or mitochondrial diseases
    - **E**thanol, **E**thylene glycol
    - **S**alicylate

17. **How limited is the respiratory response to metabolic alkalosis?**
    Metabolic alkalosis occurs when a net gain of alkali or loss of acid leads to a rise in the serum bicarbonate concentration and pH. In metabolic alkalosis (as in metabolic acidosis), there is a measure of respiratory compensation in response to the change in pH. This response, which is accomplished by alveolar hypoventilation, is limited by the overriding need to maintain an adequate blood oxygen concentration. Usually the P_{CO_2} will not increase >50 to 55 mm Hg despite severe alkalosis.

18. **What is the differential diagnosis in a child presenting with symptoms of primary metabolic alkalosis?**
    Metabolic alkalosis can be divided into two major categories on the basis of the *urinary chloride concentration* and the *response to volume expansion with a saline infusion.*

    Saline-responsive metabolic alkalosis: The urine chloride concentration is <10 mEq/L and there is significant volume depletion. Intravenously administered normal saline usually corrects the metabolic alkalosis; the classic example is pyloric stenosis.
    Causes include pyloric stenosis, profuse vomiting, excessive upper gastrointestinal suctioning, congenital chloride diarrhea, laxative abuse, diuretic use or abuse, cystic fibrosis, chloride-deficient infant formulas, post-hypercapnia syndrome, and administration of poorly reabsorbable anion. This can also occur after treatment of organic acidemias. Treatment of diabetic ketoacidosis with insulin leads to metabolism of acetoacetate, which results in the generation of bicarbonate.
    Saline-resistant alkalosis: The urine chloride is high and the patient is hypertensive. Administration of normal saline aggravates the metabolic alkalosis. In most of these cases, mineralocorticoid excess plays the central role in the generation of the alkalosis.
    Causes include hyperreninemic hypertension (renal artery stenosis, renin-secreting tumor), corticosteroid treatment, severe potassium deficiency, genetic block in steroid hormone synthesis (17α-OH deficiency, 11β-OH deficiency), Liddle syndrome, Bartter syndrome, Gitelman syndrome, primary hyperaldosteronism (extremely rare in children), and licorice-containing glycyrrhizic acid.

19. **Why is the urine pH often acidic (pH 5.0 to 5.5) in a child with metabolic alkalosis from severe vomiting?**
    Prolonged vomiting, such as is seen in pyloric stenosis, results in metabolic alkalosis because of loss of hydrogen ions and volume depletion (dehydration). There is also significant sodium, potassium, and chloride loss with a resultant hypokalemic, hypochloremic metabolic alkalosis. The volume depletion activates the renin-angiotensin-aldosterone response which results in increased distal reabsorption of sodium and water. To retain sodium, the kidney must release other cations (hydrogen in particular) into the urine. The hydrogen ions lower the urine pH. When volume is repleted, there will be suppression of aldosterone, the urine pH will become alkaline (pH 6.5 or more), and the metabolic alkalosis will lessen. The change of the urine from acidotic to alkalotic is one sign of adequate volume replenishment.

This scenario is sometimes referred to as the *"paradoxical aciduria of metabolic alkalosis,"* and your attending may use the term as well. If you are feeling courageous, you could respond that it is not paradoxical at all, once you understand the pathophysiology.

ACUTE KIDNEY INJURY

20. **Why has the term *acute kidney injury* replaced acute renal failure?**
    Acute kidney injury (AKI) reflects more appropriately the concept that smaller reductions in kidney function (short of complete organ failure) have significant clinical repercussions in terms of morbidity and mortality.

21. **What clinical and laboratory observations are useful for distinguishing prerenal oliguria (decreased effective circulating volume) from the oliguria of intrinsic AKI?**
    Clinical assessment of hydration, volume, and perfusion status is critical because these are more likely to be impaired in a prerenal state. In patients with intrinsic AKI there is more likely to be normal or excess volume; there may be evidence of edema or vascular congestion. If the assessment of the volume status suggests a volume deficit, a fluid bolus with normal saline can be both diagnostic and therapeutic. Laboratory studies that assist are summarized in Table 12-1.

Table 12-1. Laboratory Studies That May Distinguish Prerenal Oliguria From Acute Tubular Necrosis

PARAMETER	PRERENAL OLIGURIA	RENAL OLIGURIA
Random U_{Na} (mEq/L)	<20	>40
FE_{Na}*	<1%	>1%
Urine osmolality (mOsm/L)	>500	<300

$FE_{Na} = ([U_{Na} \times P_{Creat}]/[P_{Na} \times U_{Creat}]) \times 100\%$ (on a randomly collected, spot urine).

22. **What is the most common cause of AKI in young children in the United States?**
    This used to be the hemolytic uremic syndrome (HUS), which in most cases is caused by gastrointestinal infection with Shiga toxin–producing *E. coli*, especially the O157:H7 serotype. However, cases of acute tubular necrosis in infancy and childhood from **hypoxic, hypotensive, and/or hypovolemic insults,** or **drug-induced injury** now represent the largest group of causes. New observations indicate that the presence of proteinuria predicts the development of AKI independently of eGFR (estimated glomerular filtration rate based on creatinine level). The severity of AKI and duration are important predictors of chronic kidney disease and long-term mortality.
    The causes of AKI are listed in Table 12-2.

Siew ED, Furth SL: Acute kidney injury: a not-so-silent disease, *Kidney Int* 85:494–495, 2014.
Siew ED, Deger SM: Recent advances in acute kidney injury epidemiology, *Curr Opin Nephrol Hypertens* 21:309–317, 2012.

Table 12-2. Causes of Acute Kidney Injury (AKI)

Prerenal Causes of AKI	
Volume depletion	Severe diarrhea
	Protracted vomiting
	Osmotic diuresis
	Diuretics
	Extensive burns
	Hemorrhage
Decreased effective blood volume	Septic shock
	Anaphylaxis
	Nephrotic syndrome

Continued on following page

Table 12-2. Causes of Acute Kidney Injury (AKI) (*Continued*)

Cardiac failure	Anatomical malformation Arrhythmias Cardiomyopathy Tamponade Post-cardiac surgery
Intrinsic Causes of AKI	
	Postinfectious glomerulonephritis Lupus nephritis Henoch-Schönlein purpura nephritis IgA nephropathy Crescentic glomerulonephritis
Vascular	Renal venous thrombosis Vasculitis Nonsteroidal anti-inflammatory agents ACE inhibitors Hemolytic uremic syndrome
Tubular (ATN)	Severe prerenal failure Asphyxia/hypoxemia Crystal obstruction Medications Toxins Tumor-lysis syndrome
Interstitial nephritis	Allergic interstitial nephritis TINU syndrome Malignancy infiltrate Pyelonephritis Sarcoidosis
Postrenal Causes of AKI	
	Bilateral nephrolithiasis Neoplasm

ACE = angiotensin-converting enzyme; ATN = acute tubular necrosis; IgA = immunoglobulin A;
TINU = tubulointerstitial nephritis and uveitis.

23. What is the triad of clinical findings of HUS?
    - Acute renal failure with oliguria, anuria, and rarely polyuria
    - Acute hemolytic anemia: microangiopathic with fragmented red blood cells (RBCs) or schistocytes, nonimmune, Coombs negative
    - Thrombocytopenia

Kaplan BS, Drummond KN: The hemolytic-uremic syndrome is a syndrome, *N Engl J Med* 298:964–966, 1978.

24. What are the causes of HUS?
    Shiga toxin–producing *E. coli* OH157:H7 is the most frequent cause of HUS in the United States. Shiga toxin–producing *E. coli* O104:H4 infection caused a severe epidemic of HUS in Europe in 2011. Endothelial cell injury with secondary glomerular capillary microthrombi is central to the pathogenesis of HUS caused by Shiga toxin–producing *E. coli*. This is the most frequent cause of HUS, but there are other known causes of which atypical hemolytic uremic syndrome (aHUS) comprises about 10% of all causes. Genetic mutations increase the risk of aHUS and may lead to uncontrolled activation of the complement system when it is triggered.

25. Does the use of antibiotic therapy in children with diarrhea caused by *E. coli* OH157:H7 prevent HUS?

This is controversial. A study showed that children who received antibiotics (usually sulfa-containing or β-lactam antibiotics) during outbreaks had a higher rate (50% versus 7%) of HUS. A subsequent meta-analysis showed no protection and no association. Most specialists opt not to treat patients with *E. coli* OH157:H7 gastroenteritis with antibiotics because no benefit has been proven.

Safdar N, Said A, Gangnon RE, et al: Risk of hemolytic-uremic syndrome after antibiotic treatment of *Escherichia coli* O157:H7 enteritis: a meta-analysis, *JAMA* 288:996–1001, 2002.

26. Can anything be done to lessen the severity of the renal disease in children with HUS caused by *E. coli* OH157:H7?

About 15% of patients with *E. coli* O157:H7 gastroenteritis develop HUS within 2 to 14 days of onset of diarrhea. Intravenous volume expansion during this period, if indicated, may decrease the frequency of oligoanuric renal failure in patients with *E. coli* OH157:H7 at risk for HUS.

Additional therapies, such as plasma exchange, immunoadsorption, Shiga toxin–binding agents and complement inhibitors (e.g., eculizumab) are currently under study.

Keir LS, Marks SD, Kim JJ: Shigatoxin-associated hemolytic-uremic syndrome: current molecular mechanisms and future therapies, *Drug Des Devel Ther* 6:195–208, 2012.
Hickey CA, Beattie TJ, Cowieson J, et al: Early volume expansion during diarrhea and relative nephroprotection during subsequent hemolytic uremic syndrome, *Arch Pediatr Adolesc Med* 165:884–889,2011.

27. Why is Shiga toxin–associated HUS so terrifying for patients, family, and physicians?

Shiga toxin–associated HUS is terrifying because patients can die, intensive care is required for about 50% of cases, serious extrarenal complications can develop, and patients who recover may have chronic sequelae. Fortunately, about 70% of patients recover completely from the acute episode. The acute death rate is now <4%, and serious long-term complications are <15%. The kidneys bear the brunt of the long-term damage, which includes proteinuria (15% to 30% of cases), hypertension (5% to 15%), chronic kidney disease (CKD, 9% to 18%), and end-stage renal disease (ESRD) (3%). A smaller number have extrarenal sequelae, including colonic strictures, cholelithiasis, diabetes mellitus, or brain injury. Most of the patients who progress to ESRD do not recover normal renal function after the acute episode. The most important risk factors for both poor acute and long-term renal outcome are anuria for >10 days and prolonged need for dialysis >3 weeks. After the acute episode, all patients must be followed for at least 5 years and patients should be followed indefinitely if there is proteinuria, hypertension, or a reduced eGFR.

Spinale JM1, Ruebner RL, Copelovitch L, Kaplan BS: Long-term outcomes of Shiga toxin hemolytic uremic syndrome, *Pediatr Nephrol* 28:2097–2105, 2013.

28. What is meant by atypical hemolytic uremic syndrome (aHUS)?

This term describes a group of patients of all ages who present with the classic features of HUS but who *do not have Shigalike–toxin producing E. coli (STEC)* as the cause. Atypical HUS accounts for about 5% to 10% of HUS cases. Several genetic mutations have been identified that appear to cause excessive activation of the complement system. The classical distinctions between so-called typical and atypical HUS are starting to blur with new discoveries in abnormalities in genes that regulate the alternate pathway of complement. Many cases of aHUS may even have antecedent diarrhea. Compared with classic HUS, the prognosis for aHUS is worse. Fifty percent may progress to ESRD compared with 85% of cases of typical HUS who recover renal function. The use of eculizumab, a specific anti- C5 monoclonal antibody that blocks alternative complement pathway activation, has dramatically improved the outcome of aHUS patients with known or suspected mutations in complement regulatory genes.

Legendre CM, Licht C, Muus P, et al: Terminal complement inhibitor eculizumab in atypical hemolytic-uremic syndrome, *N Engl J Med* 368:2169–2181, 2013.
Kaplan BS, Ruebner RL, Copelovitch L: An evaluation of the results of eculizumab treatment of atypical hemolytic uremic syndrome, *Expert Opin Orphan Drugs* 2:167–176, 2013.

29. What are indications for dialysis in AKI?

A helpful pneumonic is **AEIOU:** **A**cidemia, **E**lectrolyte abnormalities, **I**ncreased blood pressure, **O**verload (volume), and **U**remia

- Severe metabolic acidemia that cannot be controlled with sodium bicarbonate
- Elevated blood urea nitrogen (BUN) and creatinine concentrations in the context of anuria or uncontrolled metabolic abnormalities. There are no established critical levels of BUN or creatinine above which dialysis needs to be instituted. However, when the creatinine reaches 10 mg/dL or the BUN is ≥100 mg/dL, the GFR is usually markedly reduced, and this results in one or more of the following abnormalities:
  - Hyperkalemia that is either rapidly rising or stable at a dangerously high level, especially with ECG changes, that is not controlled by infusions of insulin, bicarbonate, calcium, or Kayexalate-binding resin; other severe electrolyte disturbances, including symptomatic hyponatremia, hypocalcemia, hyperphosphatemia, and hyperuricemia
  - Volume-dependent hypertension or signs of CHF not responsive to diuretic treatment
  - Urgent need for a blood transfusion in the presence of fluid overload and/or hypertension
  - Acute signs or symptoms of encephalopathy

CHRONIC KIDNEY DISEASE

30. Based on GFR estimations and serum creatinine levels, how are AKI and chronic kidney disease (CKD) defined?

Criteria for AKI: GFR <60 mL/min per 1.73 m^2 for <3 months, OR decrease in GFR by >35% or increase in serum creatinine (SCr) by >50% for <3 months

Criteria for CKD: Presence of AKI criteria for >3 months

Kidney Disease: Improving Global Outcomes (KDIGO) CKD Work Group: KDIGO 2012 clinical practice guideline for the evaluation and management of chronic kidney disease, *Kidney Inter* 3S:1S–150S; 2013.

31. What are the stages of CKD?

There are 5 stages of CKD (Table 12-3). The stages are based on GFR.

Table 12-3. Stages of Chronic Kidney Disease

STAGE	GFR*	DESCRIPTION	TREATMENT
1	90+	Normal kidney function but urine or imaging abnormalities	Observation, control blood pressure
2	60-89	Mildly reduced function	Observation, control blood pressure control
3A 3B	45-59 30-44	Moderately reduced function	Observation, control blood pressure and risk factors
4	15-29	Severely reduced function	Plan for end stage renal failure
5	<15 or on dialysis	End-stage kidney disease	Discuss treatment choices

*GFR = Glomerular filtration rate (min/1.73 m^2).
Kidney Disease: Improving Global Outcomes (KDIGO) CKD Work Group: KDIGO 2012 Clinical Practice Guideline for the Evaluation and Management of Chronic Kidney Disease, *Kidney Int* 3S:1–150; 2013.

32. What are the main causes of CKD in children that result in renal transplantation?

- Obstructive uropathy
- Aplastic, hypoplastic, and dysplastic kidneys
- Focal segmental glomerulosclerosis

Whyte DA, Fine RN: Chronic kidney disease in children, *Pediatr Rev* 29:335–340, 2008.

33. Your nephrology attending likes to use the Socratic method of teaching. "What are four major endocrine and cardiac medications that have dramatically improved the lives and outcomes of children with CKD?" is a favorite question.
    - Use of *erythropoietin*, a hormone normally produced in the kidney, has largely eliminated the need for blood transfusions in children with CKD.
    - Use of *1,25-dihydroxycholecalciferol*, an active form of vitamin D normally produced in the kidney, has dramatically prevented or treated osteodystrophy.
    - Growth hormone (GH) is not produced by the kidney. However, *recombinant GH* administration results in growth acceleration in growth-retarded children with CKD.
    - Inhibition of the renin-angiotensin-aldosterone system with *ACE inhibitors* or *angiotensin receptor blockers (ARBs)* has helped control hypertension and also prevented progression of glomerular fibrosis.

34. What is the new term for renal osteodystrophy?
    Renal osteodystrophy has traditionally been the term used to describe the bone and mineral pathology caused by the endocrine and electrolyte derangements in CKD. The moniker **"chronic kidney disease–mineral and bone disorder (CKD–MBD)"** was recommended by an international consensus committee in 2009 to better describe the systemic changes that take place in CKD.

35. What hormonal elevation is key in the pathogenesis of CKD–MBD?
    Hyperparathyroidism is key. Decreased GFR results in retention of phosphate and hyperphosphatemia. Additionally, there is decreased renal 1,25-dihydroxyvitamin D production. These two factors lead to decreased absorption of calcium from the gastrointestinal tract and decreased responsiveness of bone to parathyroid hormone (PTH), which results in hypocalcemia. The hypocalcemia leads to an increased release of PTH, which then increases bone resorption. A long-term sequela of this secondary hyperparathyroidism from CKD can be bone marrow fibrosis.

36. Why is it important to recognize CKD–MBD at an early stage?
    Recognition of osteodystrophy, (which begins when the GFR is half of the normal rate) is important because early intervention with calcitriol, vitamin D, and phosphate binders can prevent and/or heal the bone disease (but not necessarily enhance growth). Furthermore, in states of chronic acidosis, the skeleton acts as a buffer for the net acid retained. This results in the release of calcium, which contributes to further osteopenia and bone disease.

37. Why is FGF23 an important evolving concept in CKD–MBD?
    Changes in calcium/phosphate metabolism in CKD are characterized by hyperphosphatemia, hypocalcemia, calcitriol deficiency, and hyperparathyroidism. A key regulator of this complex system is *FGF23*, a circulating peptide produced in the osteocyte that regulates renal phosphate excretion. PTH is still the most important biomarker, but novel biomarkers, such as FGF23, and noninvasive imaging techniques are emerging that can allow for individual classification and monitoring in progression of CKD-MBD.

Kemper MJ, van Husen M: Renal osteodystrophy in children: pathogenesis, diagnosis and treatment, *Curr Opin Pediatr* 26:180–186, 2014.

38. What are the ciliopathies?
    This is an important question because the answer opens up a whole new book in the understanding of many inherited renal conditions (Table 12-4). Diverse developmental and degenerative single-gene disorders such as polycystic kidney disease, nephronophthisis, retinitis pigmentosa, Bardet–Biedl syndrome, Joubert syndrome, and Meckel syndrome are categorized as ciliopathies, a recent concept that describes diseases characterized by dysfunction of a hairlike cellular organelle called the cilium. Most of the proteins that are altered in these single-gene disorders function at the level of the cilium–centrosome complex.

Hildebrandt F, Benzing T, Katsanis N: Ciliopathies, *N Engl J Med* 364:1533–1543; 2011.

Table 12-4. Prominent Single-Gene Ciliopathies

Dominant Disorders	Autosomal Dominant Polycystic Kidney Disease Von Hippel–Lindau Disease
Recessive Disorders	Autosomal Recessive Polycystic Kidney Disease Nephronophthisis
	Bardet–Biedl syndrome
	Retinal–Renal Syndromes
	Senior–Løken syndrome).
	Joubert Syndrome
	Meckel Syndrome

39. **Nephronophthisis is difficult to pronounce and spell, but what is it?**
   Nephronophthisis (one of the ciliopathies) is the most frequent genetic cause of ESRD in the first 3 decades of life (median age: 13 years) and is characterized by cysts restricted to the corticomedullary junction. Kidney size is normal or small. Mutations in more than 11 recessive genes (*NPHP1* to *NPHP11*) have been identified as causes of nephronophthisis. Mutations in *NPHP1* cause juvenile nephronophthisis type 1. Clinical features of juvenile nephronophthisis include anemia, polyuria, polydipsia, isosthenuria, growth failure, and progression to end stage kidney disease.

40. **Which is more common in children: autosomal dominant polycystic kidney disease (ADPKD) or autosomal recessive polycystic kidney disease (ARPKD)?**
   ADPKD is the more common, and it also is the most prevalent monogenic disorder in humans. Cysts are typically diagnosed incidentally (e.g., affected parent, imaging study for another reason). ADPKD may present with pain, hematuria, UTI, hypertension, and calculi and can even be diagnosed *in utero*. There is a large interfamilial and intrafamilial variation with genetic heterogeneity and modifier genes. Two polycystic kidney (PKD) genes have been identified: PKD1 (85% of cases) and PKD2 (15% of cases).

41. **What anatomic features characterize ADPKD?**
   Bilateral renal cysts are the predominant feature, but involvement of other organs can include cysts (liver, seminal vesicles, pancreas, arachnoid); intracranial aneurysms; mitral valve prolapse; diverticulosis; and rarely, aortic root dilatation and aortic aneurysms.

42. **How is ADPKD diagnosed and managed?**
   A **renal ultrasound** is usually adequate. Deoxyribonucleic acid (DNA) studies are rarely indicated. Presymptomatic diagnosis in children outweighs any benefits until effective treatments are available. It is important to counsel presymptomatic individuals before testing.
      Monitor blood pressure and urine in individuals with a family history of ADPKD. Avoid contact sports. Use of ACE inhibitors to control blood pressure has improved outcomes. Encourage water intake to suppress antidiuretic hormone (ADH) and retard cyst growth. The prognosis is excellent in children.

Torres VE, Harris PC, Pirson Y: Autosomal dominant polycystic kidney disease, *Lancet* 369:1287–1301, 2007.
Polycystic Kidney Foundation: www.PKDcure.org. Accessed on Mar. 20, 2015.
PKD Alliance: www.arpkdchf.org. Accessed on Mar. 20, 2015.

43. **Why was the term *infantile polycystic kidney disease* replaced with ARPKD?**
   This is because some patients have been diagnosed in adulthood with moderate renal insufficiency and ESRD. The characteristic dilatation of the renal collecting ducts begins during development and can present at any stage from infancy to adulthood. Renal insufficiency often occurs *in utero* and may lead to early abortion or oligohydramnios and lung hypoplasia. However, there are affected neonates who have no evidence of renal dysfunction. Up to 30% of patients die in the perinatal period, and those surviving the neonatal period can reach ESRD in infancy, early childhood, or adolescence. The clinical spectrum of ARPKD includes bilateral renal enlargement with microcysts, arterial hypertension, and intrahepatic biliary dysgenesis. Affected infants develop congenital hepatic

fibrosis and some have nonobstructive dilation of the intrahepatic bile ducts (Caroli disease). Cholangitis, variceal bleeding, and hypersplenism are serious complications. ARPKD is caused by mutations in the PKDHD1 gene on chromosome 6.

Büscher R, Büscher AK, Weber S, et al: Clinical manifestations of autosomal recessive polycystic kidney disease (ARPKD): kidney-related and non-kidney-related phenotypes, *Pediatr Nephrol* 29:1915–1925, 2014.

ENURESIS/DYSFUNCTIONAL VOIDING

44. How common is nocturnal enuresis in older children?

    At the age of 5 years, about 20% of children (boys more than girls) wet the bed at least once monthly. Nightly wetting is not as common (<5%). By the age of 7 years, the overall rate is down to 10%, and by the age of 10 years, it is down to 5%. As a general rule, after age 7 years, nocturnal enuresis resolves at a rate of 15% per year so that by age 15 years, about 1% to 2% of teenagers still have nocturnal enuresis.

45. Why does nighttime bed-wetting persist in some children?

    Ninety-seven percent or more of the causes are nonpathologic, and a number of explanations have been theorized: maturational delay of neurodevelopmental processes, small bladder capacity, genetic influences, difficulties with waking, and decreased nighttime secretion of ADH. No data support the belief that wetting occurs during "deep sleep." Genetic influences are quite strong. If both parents were enuretic, a child's likelihood is about 75%; if one parent was involved, the likelihood is about 50%. Psychological problems are unlikely to cause nocturnal enuresis, but they are more common if daytime symptoms are present.

Graham KM, Levy JB: Enuresis, *Pediatr Rev* 30:165–172, 2009.

46. What treatments are available for nocturnal enuresis?

    The therapeutic approach depends in large part on the age of the patient, the effect of the problem on the patient, and the parents' attitude. It is important to realize that 15% of patients per year will spontaneously improve.

    Dry bed training: Self-waking routines, cleanliness training, bladder training, and rewards for dry nights; generally not effective as a sole intervention

    Enuresis alarms: Portable alarms (auditory and/or vibratory) worn by the child at night and designed to awaken the child to the sensation of a full bladder; success rates as high as 70%; safe, but requires parental and child motivation

    Desmopressin: Synthetic analog of vasopressin that, at the renal level, increases distal tubular reabsorption of water, thus diminishing nighttime bladder volume; available in oral and nasal forms; up to 70% effective; high relapse rate after discontinuation (similar to placebo); possible adverse effects, including nasal irritation and hyponatremia; expensive

    Imipramine: Bladder effects include increasing capacity and decreasing detrusor excitability; high relapse rate; important central nervous system side effects in 10% (e.g., drowsiness, agitation, sleep disturbances)

47. A 7-year-old presents with problems of intermittent daytime urinary incontinence with a normal urinalysis and a negative urine culture. What evaluation is needed?

    The differential diagnosis is broad with considerable clinical overlap, including problems with bladder storage (overactive bladder or urge syndrome) and dysfunctional voiding, in which the child habitually contracts the external urinary sphincter during micturition. Keys to diagnosis are a good history of the pattern and circumstances of the incontinence, urinalysis/urine culture, a bladder diary, uroflowmetry (and assessment of postvoid residual), and baseline renal ultrasonography with efforts to exclude any neurogenic, infectious, or anatomic abnormalities. The prevalence in school-age children of daytime incontinence is remarkably high, almost 1 in 5, in some studies. The problem can have profound psychosocial effects, so attempts at a diagnosis are key. Urology referral is often required.

Deshpande AV, Craig JC, Smith GHH, et al: Management of daytime urinary incontinence and lower urinary tract symptoms in children, *J Paed Child Health* 48:e44–e52, 2012.

48. **What is the term for extraordinary daytime urinary frequency?**
    Pollakiuria is characterized by a very high daytime frequency of micturition (as high as 50 times per day). Symptoms are limited to the daytime. It is seen around 4 to 6 years in either gender and is associated with a history of recent death or life-threatening event in the family. It usually runs a benign, self-limiting course over 6 months. No specific treatment, apart from reassurance, is necessary. Children presenting with frequency, however, merit clinical investigation to exclude other pathologic causes.

49. **Why is giggle incontinence not a laughing matter?**
    This uncommon form of daytime incontinence usually occurs in school-age girls. There is moderate to large amounts of urinary leakage triggered by laughing. The accepted theory is that of a central inactivation (cataplexy) in association with laughter resulting in incontinence. It is a diagnosis of exclusion and is usually established on history and is supplemented by the absence of other voiding symptoms and normal investigations. Giggle incontinence has a significant adverse effect on social life, and this is often why medical assistance is sought.

50. **What is the normal bladder capacity in children?**
    Bladder capacity is a reflection of voided volumes and is an important factor in the evaluation of children with voiding dysfunction. It is estimated (in mL) by the formula: **[30 + (age in years × 30)].** The formula is useful up to age 12 years, after which age the estimated bladder capacity is 390 mL (an approximate adult value).

Nevéus T, von Gontard A, Hoebeke P, et al: The standardization of terminology of lower urinary tract function in children and adolescents: report from the Standardisation Committee of the International Children's Continence Society, *J Urol* 176: 314–324, 2006.

GLOMERULAR DISEASES

51. **What constellation of findings defines nephrotic syndrome?**
    The nephrotic syndrome is defined by **proteinuria, hypoalbuminemia, edema**, and **hypercholesterolemia**. There are, however, patients with nephrotic-range proteinuria and mild-to-moderate hypoalbuminemia or even normal albumin levels in whom there is no hyperlipidemia or peripheral edema. A proportion of such patients have focal segmental glomerulosclerosis (FSGS).

52. **What differentiates nephrotic syndrome from nephritis?**
    The suffix "-itis" implies evidence of glomerular inflammation. On biopsy, this is an increased number of the cells within the glomerulus and/or the presence of leukocytes. Glomerular inflammation disrupts glomerular basement membrane structure and function and leads to hematuria and proteinuria. The proteinuria may be minimal to massive, depending on the type and severity of the nephritis. The finding of RBC casts (Fig.12-1) in the urine is, with rare exceptions, diagnostic of glomerulonephritis.

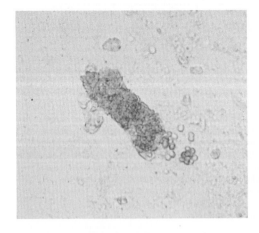

Figure 12-1. Red blood cell cast from a patient with streptococcal glomerulonephritis. These casts are almost always associated with glomerulonephritis or vasculitis and virtually exclude extrarenal disease. *(From Zitelli BJ, Davis HW: Atlas of Pediatric Physical Diagnosis, ed 4. St. Louis, 2002, Mosby, p 458.)*

Nephrosis is another term for the nephrotic syndrome. There are many causes of the nephrotic syndrome, and confusingly several different histopathological changes even with the same cause. Lupus nephritis is a classic example. Not only are there several causes of lupus (e.g., genetic, drugs such as hydralazine) but also at least five classes of renal pathologic changes. Most glomerulopathies present with a nephritic or a nephrotic syndrome. Many patients present with a mixed picture of nephritic/nephrotic syndrome.

53. **A 12-year-old girl complains of a sore throat and passes painless coke-colored urine for 2 days. When you see her a few days later she has amber colored urine, microscopic hematuria, 2+ proteinuria, RBC casts, and no other complaints or clinical findings. What is the most likely cause of this presentation?**
IgA nephropathy (IgAN) is by far the most likely cause. The simultaneous occurrence of upper respiratory symptoms and gross hematuria make poststreptococcal glomerulonephritis less likely. IgAN has a more benign clinical course in children than adults; pediatric patients are more likely to have minimal histologic lesions and less likely to have advanced chronic lesions. IgAN is the most common type of primary glomerular disease worldwide. The clinical and histological features of IgAN are variable and include microscopic hematuria, synpharyngitic hematuria (i.e., hematuria after upper respiratory infection [URI]), recurrent hematuria, proteinuria, nephrotic syndrome, nephritic syndrome, and acute renal failure. Glomerular deposits of IgA characterize IgAN (Fig. 12-2). There is no proven therapy, but ACE inhibitors may retard or prevent sclerosis.

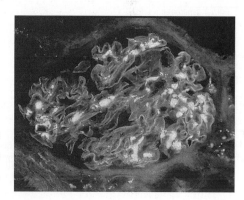

Figure 12-2. Diffuse mesangial IgA nephropathy is seen on indirect immunofluorescence with fluorescein isothiocyanate—anti-IgA. *(From Johnson RJ, Feehally J, Floege J:* Comprehensive Clinical Nephrology, *ed 5. Philadelphia, 2015, Saunders, pp 266–277.)*

54. **What is the long-term prognosis for patients with IgAN?**
IgAN is the most common form of glomerulonephritis that results in ESRD. Twenty percent to 25% of patients will progress to ESRD over 25 years. Risk factors for developing ESRD include elevated serum creatinine, proteinuria of ≥ 1 g/day, hypertension and the severity of interstitial fibrosis, tubular atrophy, and the extent of glomerular sclerosis.

Haas M: IgA nephropathy in children and adults: comparison of histologic features and clinical outcomes, *Nephrol Dial Transplant* 23:2537–2545, 2008

55. **During the evaluation of a patient with hematuria, what features suggest acute glomerulonephritis, chronic glomerulonephritis, or nephrotic syndrome?**
The three major presentations of glomerular involvement are
- *Acute glomerulonephritis:* Edema, proteinuria of 1+ or greater, hypertension, oliguria, dysmorphic RBCs, or RBC casts on urinalysis
- *Chronic glomerulonephritis:* Minimal acute symptoms; may have chronic fatigue, failure to thrive, normochromic normocytic anemia, hypertension, abnormal urinalysis, high BUN and creatinine concentrations (azotemia), metabolic acidosis, hypocalcemia, and hyperphosphatemia
- *Nephrotic syndrome:* Proteinuria of > 40 mg/m^2 per hour, edema, hypoalbuminemia, and hypercholesterolemia

56. If glomerulonephritis is suspected, what laboratory tests should be considered?

    First-line tests: dipstick urinalysis; urine microscopy; serum electrolytes; BUN and serum creatinine; serum C3 and C4; streptococcal serology (anti-streptolysin O titer or Streptozyme),throat culture; skin culture if impetigo is present; serum albumin

    Second-line tests: antinuclear antibody (ANA), anti-DNA antibodies (if lupus nephritis is suspected); hepatitis B and C serology (for patients in endemic areas, those previously transfused or individuals who engage in high-risk behavior); antineutrophil cytoplasmic antibody (ANCA) (if rapidly progressive glomerulonephritis or vasculitis is suspected)

57. Which glomerulonephritides have a genetic basis?

    See Table 12-5.

Table 12-5. Glomerular Diseases With Genetic Causes

	MUTATION	INHERITANCE
Congenital nephrotic syndrome	NPHS1	Recessive
Diffuse mesangial sclerosis	WT1	Recessive
Denys-Drash syndrome	WT1	Recessive
Frazier syndrome	KTS	Recessive
FSGS	NPHS2, TRPC6, ACTN4, INF2 and PLCE1	Recessive or dominant
Alport syndrome	COL4A5	X-linked Recessive, dominant
Nail-patella syndrome	LMX1B	Dominant
Steroid resistant NS with sensorineural deafness	COQ6	Dominant
C3 glomerulopathy	factor H, CFHR	Recessive

Hildebrandt F: Genetic kidney diseases, *Lancet* 375;1287-1295, 2010.
Carney EF: Glomerular disease: Frequency of podocyte-related gene mutations in FSGS, *Nat Rev Nephrol* 10:184, 2014.

58. Which types of glomerulonephritis are associated with hypocomplementemia?

    - Postinfectious glomerulonephritis, including poststreptococcal (ASPGN); staphylococcus in subacute bacterial endocarditis
    - Lupus nephritis
    - Membranoproliferative glomerulonephritis
    - C3 glomerulopathy
    - aHUS

59. Does the treatment of streptococcal skin or pharyngeal infections prevent ASPGN?

    No. Treatment of impetigo or pharyngitis does not prevent glomerulonephritis in the index case. However, treatment lessens the likelihood of contagious spread to children who may be susceptible.

60. What is the usual time course for ASPGN?

    Symptoms and signs begin about **7 to 14 days after pharyngitis** and **as long as 6 weeks after a pyoderma** with Lancefield group A β-hemolytic streptococci. Children typically have tea-colored urine and edema. The acute phase (hypertension, gross hematuria, oliguria) can last as long as 3 weeks. Serum C3 levels may remain depressed for up to 8 weeks, but persistence beyond this point suggests another diagnosis. Chronic microscopic hematuria can persist for up to 2 years. In pediatric patients, full recovery is expected, and progression to chronic renal insufficiency is rare.

61. What percentage of children with ASPGN have elevated levels of serum anti-streptolysin O titers?

About 80% to 85% of children with documented pharyngeal streptococcal infections develop elevated antistreptolysin (ASO) titers. Streptolysin O is bound to lipids in the skin, so that the percentage of individuals with streptococcal impetigo who develop positive ASO titers is much lower. For this reason, a normal ASO titer does not rule out recent streptococcal infection. Screening for other streptococcus-associated antigens, antihyaluronidase, and anti-DNAase B titers or the use of the Streptozyme test, which measures four of the streptococcal antigens, will be positive in more than 95% of children with documented streptococcal infection.

62. If pharyngitis and the brown urine occur on the same day or within 1 or 2 days, does this make ASPGN less likely?

Yes. The occurrence of upper respiratory symptoms and gross hematuria at the same time (synpharyngitic) is more characteristic of IgA nephropathy (IgAN). Serum C3 is normal in IgAN. These children may have recurrent episodes of synpharyngitic (i.e., at the time of or shortly after a URI) gross hematuria.

63. A 7-year-old girl has a typical presentation of poststreptococcal glomerulonephritis with positive ASO titers and low serum C3, but over the next 3 months she has recurrent episodes of gross hematuria and her C3 remains very low. What diagnosis should be considered?

Recurrent gross hematuria and persistently low C3 are extremely rare in ASPGN. **C3 glomerulopathy** is a recently characterized disease that includes dense deposit disease (DDD) and C3 glomerulonephritis (C3GN). Evaluation includes testing for alternative complement regulatory genes, presence of C3 nephritic factor (C3NeF), and a kidney biopsy. The histological feature is glomerular deposits of C3 or dense deposits in the glomerular basement membrane. Genetic abnormalities occur in the complement alternative pathway (AP). The serum C3 level is often low but C4 is normal. Acquired alternate pathway (AP) dysregulation in DDD and C3GN may be induced by C3 nephritic factor (C3NeF), which is found in 80% of patients with DDD and 45% with C3GN. C3GN may lead to ESRD within 10 years of the diagnosis in 36% to 50% of patients. Recurrences may occur after renal transplantation. Inhibition of complement C3 or C5 is a promising treatment option.

Prasto J, Kaplan BS, Russo P, et al: Streptococcal infection as possible trigger for dense deposit disease (C3 glomerulopathy), *Eur J Pediatr* 173:767–772, 2014.

Servais A, Noël LH, Frémeaux-Bacchi V, et al: C3 glomerulopathy, *Contrib Nephrol* 181:185–193, 2013.

64. You are on rounds and a know-it-all nephrology fellow asks you "what are the renal complications of HIV infection?"

The short answer is "any and every renal syndrome or condition." Human immunodeficiency virus (HIV) nephropathy can result from direct kidney infection with HIV or from the adverse effects of antiretroviral drugs. Patients with HIV disease are also at risk for developing prerenal azotemia due to volume depletion as a result of salt wasting, poor nutrition, nausea, or vomiting.

When faced with a known clinical problem with an unexpected complication, ask yourself three questions:

- Is the complication related to the disease itself?
- Is it related to the treatment of the disease?
- Is it unrelated to either?

This approach led to the observation that tenofovir was the cause of rickets and renal Fanconi syndrome in a boy with congenital HIV infection.

Wood SM, Shah SS, Steenhoff AP, et al: Tenofovir-associated nephrotoxicity in two HIV-infected adolescent males, *AIDS Patient Care STDS* 23:1–4, 2009.

HEMATURIA

65. **How common is hematuria in children?**

    Microscopic hematuria (>5 RBCs/high-power field [HPF]) is common (0.5% to 2% of school-age children) and often transient. In 70% to 80% of cases, no etiology is identified.

66. **What is the most identifiable cause of microscopic hematuria?**

    Hypercalciuria, defined as elevated urinary calcium excretion without concomitant hypercalcemia. In areas of the southeastern United States, often called "the stone belt," this is a common cause of isolated hematuria; nearly one-third of children with microscopic hematuria have hypercalciuria as the cause. It is less common in other parts of the United States. Overall, 3% to 6% of children have idiopathic hypercalciuria.

    Srivastava T, Schwaderer A: Diagnosis and management of hypercalciuria in children, *Curr Opin Pediatr* 21: 214–219, 2009.

67. **What distinguishes lower from upper tract bleeding?**

    As a general rule, brown, tea-colored, or cola-colored urine suggests *upper tract bleeding*, whereas bright red blood suggests *lower tract bleeding* (Table 12-6). The darker urine has had more time to become oxidized in the urinary tract. However, exceptions occur. Rapid upper tract bleeding may be red, and a dissolving clot within the bladder may produce brown urine. Establishing the source of microscopic hematuria can be difficult. *Glomerular bleeding* produces small and dysmorphic RBCs with blebs or burr cells as opposed to the normal-sized RBCs in lower tract bleeding. These changes are best observed with phase-contrast microscopy, which is not readily available in most clinical settings. The presence of significant proteinuria also suggests upper tract (kidney) disease.
    The presence of even a single RBC or hemoglobin cast indicates a glomerular (or, rarely, tubular) etiology.

Table 12-6. Glomerular and Nonglomerular Hematuria

	GLOMERULAR HEMATURIA	NONGLOMERULAR HEMATURIA
History		
Burning on micturition	No	Urethritis, cystitis
Systemic complaints	Edema, fever, pharyngitis, rash, arthralgia	Fever with urinary tract infections.
Pain	IgA nephropathy—flank pain	Calculi—costovertebral pain, radiating pain to groin
Trauma	No	Bright red urine
Family history	Deafness in Alport syndrome, renal failure	May be positive with calculi
Physical Examination		
Hypertension	Often present	Unlikely
Edema	May be present	No
Abdominal mass	No	Wilms tumor, polycystic kidneys
Rash, arthritis	Lupus erythematosus, Henoch-Schönlein	No
Urinalysis		
Color	Brown, tea, cola	Bright red
Proteinuria	Often present	No
Dysmorphic red blood cells	Yes	No
Red blood cell casts	Yes	No
Crystals	No	May be informative in patients with calculi

Kaplan BS, Pradhan M: Helping the pediatrician to interpret urinalysis, *Pediatr Ann* 42:45–51, 2013.

68. **Why does recurrent macroscopic hematuria "gross" us out?**
    Gross hematuria is problematic because we may not determine a cause and the uncertainty results in parental anxiety and second/third opinions. The most common diagnoses in children with glomerular gross hematuria are IgA nephropathy and Alport syndrome. No cause will be found in the majority of children with glomerular gross hematuria. The most common diagnoses in patients with nonglomerular gross hematuria are hypercalciuria, urethrorrhagia, and hemorrhagic cystitis. Recurrences of gross hematuria are uncommon. In nearly half of the patients with nonglomerular gross hematuria no diagnosis can be established, but their long-term prognosis appeared to be good.

Youn T1, Trachtman H, Gauthier B: Clinical spectrum of gross hematuria in pediatric patients, *Clin Pediatr* 45:135–141, 2006.

69. **If a healthy 10-year-old boy has bright red blood at the end of a previously clear urine stream, what is the likely diagnosis?**
    Urethrorrhagia. In a preadolescent or early adolescent male, terminal hematuria, which may present with bloodstained underpants, often reflects engorged vessels around the entry of the prostatic duct into the urethra at the veru montanum. Although the etiology is unclear, it is a benign condition associated with hormonal changes at adolescence. It resolves spontaneously in weeks to months and does not require cystoscopy or other investigations.

70. **A concerned mother of infant twins brings in a diaper from each with one having pink urine stains and the other blue urine stains. Which is more worrisome?**
    Blue diaper syndrome is more worrisome because it is a rare, autosomal recessive inborn error of amino acid metabolism caused primarily by defects in tryptophan intestinal absorption. Increased intestinal bacterial degradation of tryptophan results in increased production and absorption of indican (a protein breakdown product). Increased indicanuria occurs, which on exposure to air oxidizes to an indigo blue color. The condition can be associated with visual problems, hypercalcemia, and nephrocalcinosis.
    Pink diaper syndrome, on the other hand, is a benign condition often misinterpreted as hematuria. The red-brown spotting is caused by normal urate crystals, which turn pink on exposure to air and form a powder (unlike blood) that can be scraped from the diaper (unlike blood).

71. **What evaluations should be considered during the evaluation of isolated hematuria?**
    This is a subject of endless debate. There are two main approaches—one is an unfocused approach and the other is a tailored approach. The thoughtful approach considers hematuria as a symptom of a clinical problem. A careful history and examination must be done.
    If the urine is coffee or coke colored and proteinuria and RBC casts are present, consider a glomerulonephritis:
    1. Check BUN, serum creatinine, and electrolytes; serologic studies for evidence of a recent streptococcal infection (unless hematuria is recurrent or present for several months); and serum C3.
    2. Check antineutrophil cytoplasm antibodies (ANCA) if there is evidence of a vasculitis (fevers, arthralgias, rashes, lung disease).
    3. Check antinuclear antibody (ANA) and DNA-binding activity if there are clinical features of systemic lupus erythematosus (SLE). Isolated hematuria almost never occurs in lupus nephritis.
    4. Obtain a formal hearing test if there is a family history of Alport disease.
    If the urine is bright red and painless:
    1. Obtain a renal ultrasound to rule out a Wilms tumor or bladder cancer.
    2. Obtain a renal ultrasound to rule out renal calculi (they are not always painful).
    3. Obtain a renal ultrasound if there is a history of blunt abdominal trauma to rule out a large renal cyst, dominant polycystic kidney disease, or hydronephrosis.
    4. Obtain a hemoglobin electrophoresis if sickle cell trait or disease is suspected.
    If the urine is bright red with dysuria:
    1. Obtain a renal ultrasound to rule out renal calculi.
    2. Obtain a calcium-to-creatinine ratio to rule out hypercalciuria.
    3. Obtain a urine culture for a bacterial cause if there are symptoms of a urinary tract infection (UTI).

KEY POINTS: MICROSCOPIC HEMATURIA

1. This is a common finding. Asymptomatic microscopic hematuria is detected in 0.5% to 2% of schoolchildren by the dipstick test.
2. Asymptomatic microscopic hematuria is benign in the majority of individuals.
3. Further evaluation is costly and of no value in the absence of proteinuria, RBC casts, or a family history of renal disease or renal calculi.
4. Hypercalciuria (>4 mg/kg per day) is the most frequent identifiable cause.
5. Patients with significant proteinuria along with hematuria are much more likely to have underlying pathology.
6. If the dipstick assessment is positive for blood, but microscopic urinalysis is negative for RBCs, consider red dyes from beets or candy, hemolysis (hemoglobinuria) or rhabdomyolysis (myoglobinuria).
7. Take a careful family history of renal disease and of deafness to consider Alport syndrome.
   RBC, Red blood cell.

72. **What condition should be suspected in a 9-year-old with a history of hearing loss and visual deficits who presents with hematuria?**
    Alport syndrome, also known as **hereditary nephritis** should be considered. The cause is one of several genetic mutations that alter a type IV collagen protein essential for glomerular basement membrane function, for integrity of the inner ear organ of Corti, and for maintaining the shape of the lens. The inheritance pattern is mixed: 80% of cases are X-linked,15% are autosomal recessive, and 5% are autosomal dominant.

HYPERTENSION

73. How is hypertension defined in children?
    The diagnosis of hypertension is made on the basis of *comparison* with the normal blood pressures (BP) of healthy children of a similar age, sex, and height. Blood pressure tables are found in the 2004 Fourth Report cited below and on the International Pediatric Hypertension Association (IPHA) website: www.iphapediatrichypertension.org.
    Prehypertension: BP readings between the 90th and 95th percentile or >120/80 mm Hg in adolescents.
    Hypertension: systolic BP and/or diastolic BP ≥95th percentile for age, sex, and height (on 3 repeated measurements on different [nonconsecutive] days).

    Stage 1 hypertension: BP ≥ the 95th percentile and less than the 99th percentile + 5 mm Hg.
    Stage 2 hypertension: BP > 99th percentile + 5 mm Hg.

National High Blood Pressure Education Program Working Group on High Blood Pressure in Children and Adolescents. The fourth report on the diagnosis, evaluation, and treatment of high blood pressure in children and adolescents, *Pediatrics* 114:555–576, 2004.
International Pediatric Hypertension Association (IPHA): www.iphapediatrichypertension.org. Accessed on Nov. 25, 2014.

KEY POINTS: HYPERTENSION

1. Common causes of artifactual elevation: The blood pressure cuff is too small, the arm is below the level of the heart, the child is talking and feet are off the ground, or the child is given no time to relax.
2. Common causes of artifactual decrease: The arm is above the level of the heart.
3. Essential (no detectable cause): There is often a strong family history of hypertension.
4. Secondary (detectable lesion) hypertension: The higher the blood pressure and younger the child the more likely there is a secondary cause for the hypertension.
5. Most cases of secondary hypertension in children are caused by renal disease (renal anomalies, renal parenchymal disease) or renovascular disease.

74. **Why are repeat visits necessary to diagnose hypertension?**
Children and adolescents have very **labile BP** with prompt response to internal and external stimulae and will have substantial reductions in BP between the first and third visits to a new doctor, in part because of decreased anxiety. Among patients diagnosed as being hypertensive on a first visit to a new physician, there is a mean 15/7 mm Hg fall in the BP by the third visit, with some patients not reaching a stable value until the sixth visit. This does not apply to children or adolescents with repeat BP measurements at a *single* visit that indicate the presence of stage 2 hypertension. These children need immediate evaluation.

75. **How do you determine the optimum cuff size for obtaining a blood pressure?**
The length of the inflatable bladder inside the cuff (easily palpated) should almost completely encircle the arm and will overestimate the blood pressure if it is too short. Additionally, the height of the cuff should be the largest size that comfortably fits from the axilla to the elbow. A cuff that is too small can produce falsely elevated blood pressure readings.

76. **Which Korotkoff sound best represents diastolic blood pressure?**
The *Korotkoff* sounds are produced by the flow of blood as the constricting blood pressure cuff is gradually released. There are five phases of Korotkoff sounds. The first appearance of a clear, tapping sound is called phase I and represents the systolic pressure. As the cuff continues to be released, soft murmurs can be auscultated; this is phase II. These are followed by louder murmurs during phase III, as the volume of turbulent blood passing through the partially constricted brachial artery increases. The sounds become abruptly muffled in phase IV and disappear in phase V (usually within 10 mm Hg of phase IV). In studies that compare intravascular blood pressure determinations with auscultatory readings, true diastolic pressure is most closely related to **phase V** (the disappearance of sound). In some young children, muffled sounds can be heard to "zero" and don't clearly correlate with diastolic pressure. In these instances, it is best to record both the phase IV (the point at which sounds become muffled) and the phase V readings (e.g., 80/45/0).

77. **What is ambulatory blood pressure monitoring (ABPM)?**
ABPM is a noninvasive technique for measuring multiple BP readings over a 24-hour period during regular activities and during sleep. It has emerged as an increasingly important tool in the diagnosis and management of children with hypertension. ABPM is performed using an approved ABPM monitor. An appropriately sized BP cuff is placed on the nondominant arm and attached to a small monitor. For 24 hours, BP recordings are taken every 20 minutes while the patient is awake and every 30 minutes while asleep. ABPM is considered satisfactory if there is a minimum of 40 readings during the 24 hours with at least 6 "sleep" readings.

78. **What are the advantages and limitations of ABPM?**
Advantages: ABPM measurements are made outside of the health-care environment and second multiple parameters of BP can be assessed (mean 24-hour, daytime and nighttime readings, nocturnal dipping, and BP variability). In the general adult population, nocturnal nondipping, nocturnal hypertension, and increased BP variability are predictive of cardiovascular morbidity and mortality. ABPM also permits diagnosis of masked hypertension (normal office BP but ambulatory BP >95th percentile for sex and height).
    Limitations: There is uncertainty about normative BP measures, difficulty in defining ambulatory hypertension, technical limitations and costs.

Flynn JT, Daniels SR, Hayman LL, et al: Update: ambulatory blood pressure monitoring in children and adolescents. A scientific statement from the American Heart Association, *Hypertension* 63:1116–1135, 2014.

79. **In what settings is ABPM particularly useful?**
White-coat hypertension (WCH): WCH is defined as BP levels that are ≥95th percentile when measured in the office but are completely normal (average BP <90th percentile) outside of the clinical setting. Office measurements often fail to account for this transient, stress-induced elevation of BP. WCH is extremely common in children. Children and adolescents with WCH have increased body mass index (BMI) and a

tendency toward an elevated left ventricular mass index, thereby strengthening the suggestion for clinical ABPM follow-up of WCH.

Masked hypertension: This is the opposite. Patients are truly hypertensive, but the diagnosis is missed in office measurements. The incidence of this phenomenon can be particularly high in children with CKD.

Chaudhuri A: Pediatric ambulatory blood pressure monitoring: diagnosis of hypertension, *Pediatr Nephrol* 28:995–999, 2013.

KEY POINTS: WAYS TO AVOID MISDIAGNOSING HYPERTENSION

1. Properly sized cuff (age-dependent) with arm supported and kept at heart level
2. Quiet room, quiet patient, seated, feet on the floor or on a stool
3. Repeated measurements over time and the use of averaged values
4. Get rid of the white coat
5. Sit at the child's level when taking the measurement

80. **When should hypertension be treated in the neonate?**
    As a general rule, hypertension is defined as a blood pressure >90/60 mm Hg in term neonates and >80/45 mm Hg in preterm infants, but strict definitions are unavailable given limited data. A sustained systolic blood pressure of >100 mm Hg in the neonate should be investigated and treated. The most common cause is renovascular disease.

Batisky DL: Neonatal hypertension, *Clin Perinatol* 41:529–542, 2014.

81. **What are the indications for the pharmacologic treatment of hypertension in children and in adolescents?**
    - Symptomatic hypertension (e.g., headaches, visual disturbances, seizures)
    - Stage 2 hypertension
    - Stage 1 hypertension (without target-organ damage) not responding to 4 to 6 months of nonpharmacologic therapy (e.g., weight reduction, exercise, decreased salt intake)
    - Secondary hypertension
    - Hypertensive target-organ damage (left ventricular hypertrophy on ECG)
    - Diabetes (types 1 and 2)

National High Blood Pressure Education Program Working Group on High Blood Pressure in Children and Adolescents: the fourth report on the diagnosis, evaluation, and treatment of high blood pressure in children and adolescents, *Pediatrics* 114:555–576, 2004.

82. **During the evaluation of a child with elevated blood pressure, what risk factors should be considered for identification and/or reduction?**
    Important risk factors for hypertension in children:
    - Family history (If one parent has hypertension, the risk is about 25%; if both parents have hypertension, the risk is 45%.)
    - Genetic factors including ethnicity (Blacks have twice the incidence of hypertension compared with whites, beginning in adolescence.)
    - Obesity
    - History of renal disease
    - Dietary factors (mainly salt intake)
    - Low birth weight
    - Since hypertension is a critical risk factor for cardiovascular disease, additional important cardiovascular risk factors should also be assessed. These include diet, serum lipids, tobacco use, and lack of exercise.

83. What historical information suggests a secondary cause of hypertension?
    - Known UTI; recurrent abdominal or flank pain with frequency, urgency, dysuria; and secondary enuresis are suggestive of a secondary cause of hypertension.
    - Joint pains, rash, fever, edema suggest a vasculitis.
    - A complicated neonatal course requiring use of an umbilical artery catheter suggests renal artery stenosis.
    - Renal trauma suggests renal artery stenosis.
    - Hypertension suggested by drug use (sympathomimetics, anabolic or corticosteroids, NSAIDs, oral contraceptives, illicit drugs) may be responsible for drug-induced hypertension.
    - Aberrant course or timing of secondary sexual characteristics or virilization suggests an adrenal disorder.
    - Nervousness, personality changes, sweating, flushing suggest a pheochromocytoma or hyperthyroidism.

84. What is the most common cause of renal artery stenosis in children in the United States?

    Fibromuscular dysplasia, a nonatherosclerotic, noninflammatory arterial disease of unclear cause is the most common cause. In Asian children, it may be Takayasu arteritis (a vasculitis). This contrasts with adults for whom atherosclerosis is the most common cause. Gold standard for diagnosis is catheter angiography, but other less invasive tests, such as magnetic resonance angiography (MRA), are useful (Fig. 12-3). The vessel narrowing results in afferent arterioles of the kidney sensing a decreased systemic blood pressure due to reduced blood flow. The renin-angiotensin-aldosterone system is activated, which can contribute to hypertension.

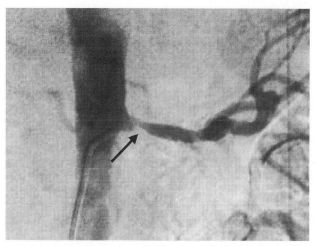

Figure 12-3. Renal arteriogram showing renal artery stenosis *(arrow)* secondary to fibromuscular dysplasia. *(From Kaplan BS, Meyers KEC: Pediatric Nephrology and Urology: The Requisites in Pediatrics. Philadelphia, 2004, Elsevier Mosby, p 119.)*

85. List the features on physical examination that suggest a secondary cause of hypertension

    See Table 12-7.

Table 12-7. Physical Findings That Suggest a Secondary Cause of Hypertension

PHYSICAL FINDING	POSSIBLE SECONDARY CAUSE
Blood pressure: >140/100 mmHg at any age	Multiple secondary causes
Leg < arm blood pressure, decreased or delayed leg pulses	Coarctation of the aorta
Adenotonsillar hypertrophy	Obstructive sleep apnea
Muscle weakness	Hyperaldosteronism
Joint swelling	Lupus nephritis, collagen vascular disease
Poor growth	Chronic renal disease
Turner syndrome	Coarctation of the aorta
>5 café-au-lait spots or neurofibromas	Renal artery stenosis, pheochromocytoma
Bruits over large vessels	Arteritis
Bruits over mid abdomen	Renal artery stenosis
Flank or upper quadrant mass	Renal malformation, renal or adrenal tumor
Excess sweating, increased resting heart rate	Pheochromocytoma, hyperthyroidism
Excessive virilization or secondary sex characteristics inappropriate for age	Adrenal disorder
Edema	Renal disease

86. What are the categories of antihypertensive medications used for outpatient management of hypertensive children?
    - ACE inhibitors
    - Angiotensin receptor blockers (ARB)
    - Calcium channel blockers (CCB)
    - α-Blockers and β-blockers
    - Central α-agonists
    - Vasodilators
    - Diuretics

Chaturvedi S, Lipszyc DH, Licht C, et al: Pharmacological interventions for hypertension in children. *Cochrane Database Syst Rev* 2:CD008117, 2014.

87. A 12-year-old girl is referred for evaluation of severe hypertension. She has hypernatremia, hypokalemia, and metabolic alkalosis, and plasma renin activity (PRA) on an ACE-inhibitor is not detectable. What is the most likely diagnosis?
    Low renin monogenic hypertension. Arterial hypertension in childhood may be due to single gene mutations inherited in an autosomal dominant or recessive fashion. Consider a genetic cause if there are abnormal potassium levels (low or high) in the presence of suppressed renin secretion and metabolic alkalosis or acidosis.

Simonetti GD, Mohaupt MG, Bianchetti MG: Monogenic forms of hypertension, *Eur J Pediatr* 171:1433–1439, 2012.

88. Why should patients with hypertension and/or those using diuretics avoid true licorice?

True licorice contains glycyrrhizic, which indirectly has mineralocorticoid properties (i.e., fluid and sodium retaining, potassium reducing). However, most American licorice contains only licorice flavoring without any such properties. Some chewing tobacco and chewing gum also contains licorice and has been associated with an excessive mineralocorticoid syndrome. Think of this if you are called to evaluate an edematous Boston Red Sox batboy.

de Klerk GJ, Nieuwenhuis MC, Beutler JJ: Hypokalaemia and hypertension associated with use of liquorice flavoured chewing gum, *BMJ* 314:731–732, 1997.

PROTEINURIA/NEPHROTIC SYNDROME

89. How does the dipstick test for urine protein compare with the sulfosalicylic method?

Dipstick assessment relies on the reaction of protein (primarily albumin) with tetrabromophenol blue in a citrate buffer impregnated on the dipstick patch. Mild false-positive reactions can occur (1+ to 2+) when the patient's urine is alkaline or when the dipstick is allowed to sit in the urine for too long and the buffer strength is overcome. The results are reported qualitatively as 1+ to 3+, which corresponds to a range of 30 to 500 mg/dL.

Sulfosalicylic acid test precipitates protein in the urine and allows for a comparison with a group of previously prepared aqueous standards; it is reported in the same way as those standards. In contrast with the dipstick assessment, all proteins—not just albumin—are precipitated, as are iodinated contrast material and some antibodies. Finding heavy proteinuria by sulfosalicylic acid testing with minimal proteinuria by dipstick testing suggests the presence of large amounts of non-albumin protein. This occurs in adults as the result of multiple myeloma and the excretion of Bence Jones proteins and in children in X-linked Dent disease (a renal tubulopathy).

90. What is microalbuminuria?

Microalbuminuria refers to the presence of small (micro) amounts of albumin in urine. It does not refer to small-sized albumin!

91. In what clinical setting is microalbuminuria a particularly important finding?

Type 1 diabetes mellitus. Long-term complications include blindness, kidney damage, cardiovascular disease, and neuropathy. Care for persons with diabetes is focused on early detection and prevention of nephropathy, which occurs in 10% to 20% of diabetics. The earliest evidence of nephropathy is microalbuminuria (MA), defined as the presence of small quantities of albumin in the urine (30 to 300 mg/24 hours). Prompt treatment of MA may delay or prevent complications. A first morning sample is recommended, but a random sample is acceptable. MA may be increased with exercise, illness, hypertension, marked hyperglycemia, and diurnal patterns. Therefore, it is advisable to obtain 3 samples over 3 months to avoid false-positive screening results.

Montgomery KA, Ratcliffe SJ, Baluarte HJ, et al: Implementation of a clinical practice guideline for identification of microalbuminuria in the pediatric patient with type 1 diabetes, *Nurs Clin North Am* 48: 343–352, 2013.

92. What is the best *spot* method for determining the amount of proteinuria?

Urine protein/creatinine excretion ratio (PCR). A 24-hour urine collection for protein is difficult to obtain in children and is imperfect in adults. Although both the dipstick and the sulfosalicylic methods estimate the concentration of protein in urine, small amounts of protein in very concentrated urine will register as more positive than the same amount of protein in dilute urine. The PCR approximates the total 24-hour urinary protein excretion. On a random sample, a PCR of <0.2 to 0.25 reflects normal daily protein excretion, whereas values of >2 suggest the presence of nephrotic-range proteinuria. This test is effective for the diagnosis of the nephrotic syndrome and for follow-up evaluations in children with prolonged and difficult-to-manage proteinuria. However, the test may overestimate protein excretion in individuals with low muscle mass and therefore lower creatinine excretion. Multiplying the ratio by 0.63 gives an approximation for the 24-hour protein excretion in g/24 hours.

93. **An asymptomatic 11-year-old boy is found to have 2+ protein on dipstick testing during a routine checkup. How should he be evaluated?**

Assuming that he is healthy and without subtle signs of renal disease (e.g., short stature, pallor, hypertension), and assuming that this is isolated proteinuria without hematuria, always determine whether the proteinuria is **orthostatic**, **intermittent**, or **persistent**.

- *Intermittent (transient) proteinuria* is entirely benign and does not require any evaluation.
- *Persistent proteinuria* may or may not be benign. The presence of persistent proteinuria can be determined by rechecking the urine at least 3 times over 2 to 3 weeks. One of these tests should be performed on a first-morning urine specimen (ask the child to void before going to bed the night before).
- *Orthostatic proteinuria* is determined in the same way. Orthostatic proteinuria is benign. Causes of transient or orthostatic proteinuria include fever, vigorous exercise, dehydration, stress, cold exposure, and seizures.

94. **How is the diagnosis of orthostatic proteinuria established?**

By definition, individuals with orthostatic proteinuria, who are usually adolescents, have normal rates of protein excretion when recumbent, but have increased excretion rates when upright/ambulant. Although all individuals excrete more protein when standing, some have an exaggerated response and may excrete as much as 1 g/day of protein. The adolescent is instructed to empty the bladder before going to bed and collect a first-morning urine specimen immediately on arising. Protein excretion is then assessed with a urine dipstick or in the laboratory as the PCR. In a concentrated first-morning urine specimen (urine specific gravity $\geq$1.018), a trace or negative value by dipstick assessment or sulfosalicylic acid precipitation rules out proteinuria. At any urine specific gravity, a urine PCR of <0.25 is normal. Remember, even individuals with renal disease may have increased protein excretion when standing and lower protein excretion rates when recumbent. The diagnosis of orthostatic proteinuria requires that protein excretion is truly normal when recumbent, elevated when ambulatory, and the individual is otherwise entirely healthy.

95. **What additional evaluation should be done for a patient with persistent proteinuria?**

If the proteinuria is persistent and not orthostatic, the amount of protein excretion must be determined. A timed 24-hour urine collection may be difficult to obtain in children because variable amounts of urine are often lost. The standard definition of proteinuria is the excretion of >4 mg/m^2 of protein per hour (or 100 mg every 24 hours for a 30-kg child). In practice, however, the urine PCR is used more frequently to assess proteinuria. The evaluation of a child with persistent proteinuria includes the same tests required to evaluate glomerulonephritis. Staged investigations include:

Stage 1: Assess BUN, serum creatinine, serum electrolytes, serum albumin, C3 and C4 levels.
Stage 2: Assess ANA, anti-DNA antibodies, and ANCA depending on clinical findings.
Stage 3: Renal imaging studies and renal biopsy may be necessary for diagnosis.

96. **What is the natural history of orthostatic proteinuria?**

The long-term outcome of children and adolescents is benign. Most agree that the prognosis is excellent, although the etiology remains unclear.

97. **What level constitutes significant proteinuria?**

Protein excretion of more than 4 mg/m^2 per hour on a timed urine collection is abnormal. Children with nephrotic syndrome excrete more than 40 mg/m^2 per hour. The upper limit of protein excretion in adults is 150 mg/day, but adolescents may excrete as much as 250 mg/day. A urine protein/creatinine ratio of >0.5 in children <2 years old and of >0.2 in older children is abnormal.

98. **In a child with hematuria, can proteinuria be attributed to the protein that is contained in whole blood?**

Only in a child with grossly bloody urine. If the urine is normal in color (yellow or clear), any amount of protein above trace is abnormal.

99. **Can proteinuria be caused by leukocytes or mucus in the urine?**

Probably not, although this untested statement is passed on from one generation of physicians to the next. Regardless of whether mucus or leukocytes can yield a positive dipstick test for albumin, it is important to do a spot protein/creatinine ratio if the test is >1 positive.

100. **At what serum albumin concentration does edema develop?**

Edema starts to manifest when the serum albumin decreases to <2.5 g/dL. Edema is almost always present at concentrations of <1.8 g/dL unless the child is receiving a diuretic or suffers from the rare condition of congenital analbuminemia (a very rare condition of low levels of albumin due to impaired synthesis but compensated by increased amounts of other circulating plasma proteins).

101. **What is the most common form of nephrotic syndrome in childhood?**
Minimal-change nephrotic syndrome (MCNS), previously known as *lipoid nephrosis* and *nil disease,* is the most common form. Most patients with MCNS have favorable therapeutic responses and prognoses. Unfortunately, many have frequent relapses, some are steroid dependent, and a minority is steroid resistant. The etiology of MCNS is unknown, but the pathogenesis is related to abnormal T-lymphocyte function.

102. **What is the most important historical factor to consider when assessing a patient for possible MCNS?**
The only definitive way to prove MCNS is with a renal biopsy, but this is rarely indicated. **Age at presentation** is the most important characteristic. Between 75% and 80% of children with nephrotic syndrome have MCNS, and about 80% of those present within the first 8 years of life. It is unusual to manifest before a year of age. Early onset in the first 6 months of life suggests a diagnosis of one of the types of congenital nephrotic syndrome or a secondary cause such as congenital syphilis.

103. **What are the typical clinical features and therapeutic responses seen in patients with MCNS?**
Edema is generally present, blood pressure is normal to slightly increased, and gross hematuria is absent, but up to one-third may have microscopic hematuria without RBC casts. In the absence of significant intravascular volume depletion, BUN, creatinine, and serum electrolytes are all within normal limits. Serum calcium is low because of hypoalbuminemia. Children who present with these findings should be started on daily prednisone. Up to 90% respond in 1½ to 4 weeks and have steroid-sensitive nephrotic syndrome (SSNS). A response is indicated by a diuresis and a negative or trace dipstick test for protein. If therapy is prolonged for an additional month, another 4% will respond. About 3% of children with biopsy-proven MCNS will be steroid resistant despite 2 months of therapy.

104. **What are the indications for furosemide and albumin infusions in patients with nephrotic syndrome?**
Indications are severe edema with **incapacitating anasarca, cellulitis, skin breakdown,** or **respiratory embarrassment from pleural effusions**. Albumin alone is helpful for a patient with a rising BUN caused by decreased renal perfusion, which is most often seen after vigorous diuretic therapy. Infusion of a 25% albumin solution in a dose of 0.5 to 1 g/kg of albumin over 1 to 2 hours, followed by furosemide (1 to 2 mg/kg), can be used to induce diuresis in a child with nephrotic syndrome who is unresponsive to furosemide alone. This measure is only temporary because the rise in albumin will lead to increased protein excretion, thereby returning the serum level to the previous steady-state value.

105. **Name two important complications of MCNS**
- **Hypercoagulable state**, which may result in sagittal sinus, cavernous sinuses, and renal veins thrombosis
- **Peritonitis** caused by *S. pneumoniae* or *E. coli*

106. **What are the prognostic factors in MCNS?**
The most important prognostic feature in MCNS is a **complete response to corticosteroid therapy**. However, even a partial response, with a decrease in protein excretion, appears to improve the prognosis. Persistent proteinuria beyond 4 to 6 weeks is a poor prognostic sign and is an indication for cyclophosphamide or tacrolimus treatment and may be an indication for a kidney biopsy.

107. **A 5-year-old child presents with puffy eyes and the laboratory features of the nephrotic syndrome, but fails to respond to corticosteroids within 6 weeks. What is the most likely diagnosis?**
Focal segmental glomerulosclerosis (FSGS). This important type of nephrotic syndrome (accounting for about 20% of cases in children) can progress to ESRD. FSGS is believed to represent a group of clinical-pathologic syndromes that share a common glomerular lesion, which is identified by renal biopsy (Fig. 12-4). A positive biopsy does not confer a disease diagnosis, but represents the beginning of an exploratory process that may lead to identification of a specific etiology and its appropriate treatment. No causes have been found in many cases but increasing numbers of genetic causes are being found, most with autosomal recessive (podocin mutations) and others with dominant modes of inheritance

(ACTN4 mutations). These mutations affect podocyte structure, actin cytoskeleton, calcium signaling, and lysosomal and mitochondrial function. HIV nephropathy and morbid obesity are important causes of secondary FSGS. Patients with a genetic cause of FSGS do not respond to prednisone treatment. Some patient's may benefit from ACE inhibitors.

Jefferson JA, Shankland SJ: The pathogenesis of focal segmental glomerulosclerosis, *Adv Chronic Kidney Dis* 21:408–416, 2014.
D'Agati VD, Kaskel FJ, Falk RJ: Focal segmental glomerulosclerosis, *N Engl J Med* 365:2398–2411, 2011.

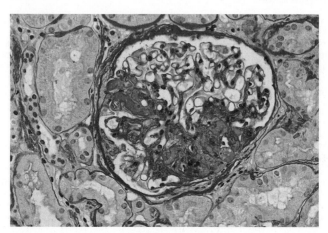

Figure 12-4. Focal segmental glomerulosclerosis with partial and segmented sclerosis and lesions of increased extracellular matrix and hyalinosis in light microscopic view with Periodic acid-Schiff staining. *(From Johnson RJ, Fehally J, Floege J, editors:* Comprehensive Clinical Nephrology, ed 5. *Philadelphia, Saunders, 2015, p 222.)*

RENAL FUNCTION ASSESSMENT AND URINALYSIS

108. **What is the simplest way to estimate the glomerular filtration rate (eGFR) in the absence of a timed urine collection?**
Devising a simple and reliable eGFR is one of the Holy Grails of nephrology. The previous most often used device, the Schwartz formula devised in the mid-1970s, was believed to overestimate GFR. A modified Schwartz formula is now felt to be a more accurate method of estimating GFR. It requires only a serum creatinine concentration and the height of the child in centimeters. No urine collection is necessary. The modified formula is [0.413 × (height in cm/serum creatinine in mg/dL)]. This formula may underestimate eGFR in muscular adolescents and is only validated for CKD stages III through V.

Schwartz GJ, Muñoz A, Schneider MF, et al: New equations to estimate GFR in children with CKD, *J Am Soc Nephrol* 20:629–637, 2009.

109. **How can you be confident that a 24-hour urine collection (for any determination) is complete?**
Creatinine is produced continuously and is eliminated only through the kidneys. Therefore, a given amount, determined largely by muscle mass, will be excreted daily, independent of the level of renal function. Thus, the determination of total urine creatinine in a timed sample can give a reasonable estimate of whether the collection approximates that of 24 hours. The guidelines for expected creatinine excretion applicable to children and adolescents are as follows: for males, 15 to 25 mg/kg per day; for females, 10 to 20 mg/kg per day.

110. **When should routine urinalyses (UA) be performed in the pediatric age group?**
There has been some controversy regarding the use of the UA as a routine screening tool. It is a simple, inexpensive, and noninvasive study that is quite sensitive and specific, but the likelihood of this test

uncovering significant, previously undiagnosed renal dysfunction is very low. Because of this, the likelihood of false-positive results is high, leading to unnecessary evaluations. The American Academy of Pediatrics (AAP) in 2007 made the recommendation to discontinue routine urine dipsticks in healthy children as a screen for CKD.

Sekhar DL, Wang L, Hoffenbeck CS, et al: A cost effectiveness analysis of screening urine dipsticks in well-child care, *Pediatrics* 125:660–663, 2010.

American Academy of Pediatrics: Committee on Practice and Ambulatory Medicine: Recommendations for preventive pediatric health care, *Pediatrics* 120:1376, 2007.

111. **What are the maximal and minimal renal dilutional and concentrating capabilities?**

    Maximally dilute urine has a specific gravity of 1.001 and an osmolality of 50. Maximally concentrated urine has a specific gravity of about 1.032 and an osmolality of about 1200. Urine that is neither concentrated nor dilute (isosthenuric) has a specific gravity of about 1.010 and a corresponding osmolality of 300. Infants born prematurely do not concentrate urine as effectively.

112. **What is the difference between urine specific gravity (SG) and urine osmolality?**

    Both tests measure the concentration or dilution of the urine, and the relationship between the two is linear and direct, although osmolality is more physiologically correct. *Specific gravity* is determined by the density (and thus the weight and size) of solute in solution. *Osmolality* depends on the number of particles (independent of their size) in solution and their effect on changing its freezing point. Therefore, when there are solutes with a relatively large molecular weight (albumin, glucose, contrast material) in the urine, specific gravity will disproportionately increase, and osmolality will be a better indicator of true urine concentration. A urine SG of 1.040 cannot be achieved by the human kidney. Consequently, levels that high in a child with nephrotic syndrome do not represent supernormal concentrating capacity but the effect of heavy proteinuria on the specific gravity.

113. **Which urinary crystals are always pathologic?**

    Cystine crystals. These flat, simple, hexagon-shaped crystals are evidence for the amino acid transport disorder cystinuria (Fig. 12-5). In classic cystinuria, the dibasic amino acids (cystine, ornithine, arginine, and lysine) are affected. The condition would be of little clinical significance except for the fact that cystine is very insoluble and results in nephrolithiasis.

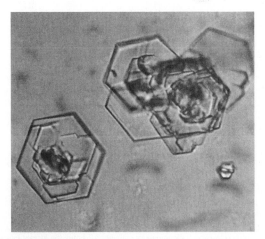

Figure 12-5. Cystine crystal with hexagonal structure. *(From Brown TA, Sonali SJ: USMLE Step 1 Secrets, ed 3. Philadelphia, 2013, Elsevier, pp 67–96.)*

SURGICAL ISSUES

114. **What is the most common cause of urinary tract obstruction in the newborn?**
Posterior urethral valves. These occur only in boys. The obstruction is frequently associated with high intravesicular pressures, which may damage the renal parenchyma resulting in renal dysplasia if not corrected. Thus, even with prompt recognition and treatment, renal insufficiency may progress.

115. **What is the most common renal abnormality detected on antenatal ultrasound?**
Hydronephrosis (also known as **renal pelvic dilatation**) with an incidence between 0.5% and 1% is most common. A renal pelvic diameter ≥ 5 mm is typically viewed as a cutoff point with grading (0 to IV) of hydronephrosis based on the degree of dilatation, number of calyces observed and evidence of any parenchymal atrophy. Likelihood of CAKUT increases with the severity of hydronephrosis. A repeat ultrasound is advised at 48 to 72 hours and at 4 to 6 weeks after birth. Based on those results, follow-up studies for vesicoureteral reflux and urology referral may be required. For patients with isolated antenatal hydronephrosis (without evidence of obstruction), routine prophylactic antibiotics are not indicated. Ninety-eight percent of patients with mild hydronephrosis (renal pelvic diameter <12 mm) resolve, stabilize, or improve at follow-up.

Becker AM: Postnatal evaluation of infants with abnormal antenatal renal sonogram, *Curr Opin Pediatr* 21:207–213, 2009.

116. **What are the possible causes of prenatal hydronephrosis?**
   - Ureteropelvic junction obstruction (most common)
   - Posterior urethral valves
   - Vesicoureteral reflux
   - Ectopic ureter or ureterocele
   - Megaureter (obstructive and nonobstructive)
   - Urethral atresia in the prune belly syndrome

117. **What is the most common cause of kidney disease of children worldwide?**
Congenital anomalies of the kidney and urinary tract (CAKUT), which includes obstructive uropathies, ureteropelvic junction obstruction, solitary kidney, renal hypoplasia, and vesicoureteral reflux, present as isolated findings or part of genetic syndromes. CAKUT accounts for up to 40% to 50% of cases of ESRD in children and 7% of ESRD in adults. The genetic mutations that cause CAKUT usually are sporadic and have been identified in a variety of signaling pathways regulating nephrogenesis. Currently, $<10\%$ of affected patients have identified mutations, and most affected patients may have unique genetic diagnoses. There are presently no benefits of offering genetic testing to patients and their relatives with CAKUT.

Copelovitch L, Furth SL: Genetics and urinary tract malformations, *Am J Kidney Dis* 63:183–185, 2014.

118. **Is unilateral renal agenesis (URA) a benign condition?**
Yes and no. We used to think so but now we are not so sure. A literature analysis was based on 2684 individuals of whom 63% were males. The incidence of URA was 1 in 2000. Associated CAKUT were identified in 32% of patients, of which VUR was identified in 24% of patients. Extrarenal anomalies were found in 31% of patients. Hypertension was identified in 16% of patients and 21% of patients had microalbuminuria. Ten percent of patients had a lower GFR (<60 mL/min/1.73 m^2).

Westland R, Schreuder MF, Ket JC, van Wijk JA: Unilateral renal agenesis: a systematic review on associated anomalies and renal injury, *Nephrol Dial Transplant* 28:1844–1855, 2013.

119. **Should a child with a single kidney be allowed to play football?**
This is a frequently asked question. Most pediatric nephrologists prohibit contact/collision sports participation by individuals with a single kidney, particularly football. The incidence of catastrophic sports-related kidney injury is 0.4 per 1 million children per year from all sports. Cycling was the most common cause of sports-related kidney injury causing >3 times the kidney injuries as football.

In addition, kidney injury from sports is much less common than catastrophic brain, spinal cord, or cardiac injury. Restricting participation of patients with a single, normal kidney from contact/collision sports is *unwarranted*. Therefore, let the family decide. Keep in mind that a large majority of physicians would ban participation, especially in American football.

Grinsell MM, Showalter S, Gordon KA, Norwood VF: Single kidney and sports participation: perception versus reality, *Pediatrics* 118:1019–1027, 2006.

TUBULAR DISORDERS

120. **In what settings should renal tubular acidosis (RTA) be considered?**
Primary RTA is characterized by *chronic hyperchloremic metabolic acidosis* with an inability to acidify the urine and a normal serum anion gap. Primary RTA is separated into three main types. Signs and symptoms that are common with all forms of RTA are growth failure, polyuria, polydipsia, recurrent dehydration, and vomiting. RTA can also occur secondarily to an acquired renal injury.

121. **What are defects in each type of primary RTA?**
Type 1 (distal) RTA: *Inability of the distal tubule to secrete hydrogen;* in the presence of significant acidosis, urine is not maximally acidified (pH <5.5)
Type 2 (proximal) RTA: *Decreased ability of the proximal tubule to reabsorb filtered HCO_3* at normal plasma HCO_3 concentrations
Type 4 RTA: Acquired or inherited *tubular insensitivity to aldosterone* or to an *absence of aldosterone*

122. **What are clinical and laboratory features of the primary RTAs?**
See Table 12-8.

Table 12-8. Clinical and Laboratory Manifestations of Various Renal Tubular Acidoses

	TYPE 1 (CLASSIC DISTAL)	TYPE 2 (PROXIMAL)	TYPE 4 (ALDOSTERONE DEFICIENCY)
Growth failure	+++	++	+++
Serum potassium	Normal or low	Normal or low	High
Nephrocalcinosis	Frequent	Rare	Rare
Low citrate excretion	+++	±	±
Fractional excretion of filtered HCO_3 at normal serum HCO_3 levels	<5%	5-10%	<10%
Daily alkali treatment (mEq/kg)	1-3	5-20	1-3
Daily potassium requirement	Decreases with correction	Increases with correction	
Urine pH	>5.5	<5.5	<5.5
Presence of other tubular defects	Rare	Common	Rare

123. **How is determining the urine anion gap helpful in the evaluation of metabolic acidosis?**
Investigation of any child with a persistent metabolic acidosis must consider some form of RTA in the differential diagnosis. The urinary anion gap is a convenient and accurate screening test for RTA. It is an indirect estimate of *urinary ammonium excretion* (and thus urinary acid excretion) and is calculated by the following formula after determining urinary electrolyte concentrations:

$$\text{Urinary anion gap} = Na^+ + K^- - Cl^-$$

If the anion gap is negative, it suggests a large chloride excretion and thus adequate ammonium excretion. The urinary anion gap is negative in hyperchloremic metabolic acidosis as a result of diarrhea, untreated proximal RTA, or prior administration of an acid load. If the anion gap is positive, it suggests an acidification defect, as is seen in patients with distal RTA. Results are not reliable if there are large amounts of unmeasured anions such as ketoacids, penicillin, or salicylates.

124. How is RTA diagnosed with utilizing a urine anion gap in a patient with a hyperchloremic metabolic acidosis and a normal serum anion gap? See Figure 12.6.

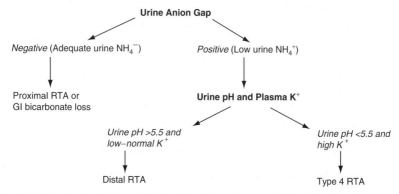

Figure 12-6. Diagnosis of renal tubular acidosis in patients with hyperchloremic metabolic acidosis and normal serum anion gap. *GI*, Gastrointestinal; *RTA*, renal tubular acidosis. *(Adapted from Lash JP, Arruda JA: Laboratory evaluation of renal tubular acidosis,* Clin Lab Med *13:117-129, 1993.)*

125. What is the recommended alkali therapy for the treatment of various forms of RTA?
The goals of RTA therapy are to improve growth, correct metabolic bone disease, prevent nephrolithiasis and nephrocalcinosis, and control underlying disease processes.
Alkali therapy (sodium citrate or sodium bicarbonate) is required for all forms of RTA, with the goal of normal plasma HCO_3 level. Patients with distal RTA generally require only 2 to 3 mEq of alkali/kg/day. However, infants may also experience some increased urinary bicarbonate wasting and require up to 10 mEq/kg/day. Patients with proximal RTA require large quantities of alkali (5 to 20 mEq/kg/day). For type 4 RTA, patients usually need low-dose alkali therapy (1 to 3 mEq/kg/day) plus a potassium-restricted diet and mineralocorticoid therapy if there is hypoaldosteronism.

126. What is most common cause of the *renal* Fanconi syndrome?
The *renal* Fanconi syndrome is the manifestation of multiple disorders of transport in the proximal tubule. It is characterized by the abnormal excretion of substances normally reabsorbed by the proximal tubule and for which there is no distal mechanism sufficient to recapture the unabsorbed molecules. Thus, there is abnormal excretion of glucose, phosphate, potassium, amino acids, and bicarbonate. The phosphaturia and hypophosphatemia result in metabolic bone disease. Bicarbonate loss causes metabolic acidosis. **Cystinosis,** a lysosomal storage disease with abnormal accumulation of the amino acid cystine, is the most common cause. Consider galactosemia, tyrosinemia, and fructose intolerance in any neonate or infant with severe jaundice, acidosis, and glucosuria, which could be a presentation of renal Fanconi syndrome.

127. A 2-year-old girl, generally healthy with height just below the 5th percentile, was noted to have blinking problems and glucose in her urine. Can you connect the two in a single diagnosis?
Patients with **cystinosis** can have photophobia and renal Fanconi syndrome. Cystine-depleting medical therapy and kidney transplantation has transformed this previously fatal disease into a treatable disorder with a life expectancy of >50 years. Early diagnosis and appropriate therapy are critically important.

Nesterova G1, Gahl WA: Cystinosis: the evolution of a treatable disease, *Pediatr Nephrol* 28:51–59, 2013.

128. **Glucosuria is detected on repeated urine dipstick testing in a 5-year-old boy, but the blood glucose is always normal. What is going on here?**

In the absence of clinical symptoms, hypokalemia, metabolic acidosis, or an elevated serum creatinine, the diagnosis is **renal glucosuria**. This is a benign condition. Because it is commonly familial, genetic abnormalities in renal glucose reabsorption are the likely culprit. Mild glucosuria is typical; heavy glucosuria is rare.

129. **What is the clinical presentation of acute interstitial nephritis (AIN)?**

AIN is caused by an immune-mediated inflammatory response that initially involves the renal interstitium and tubules, usually sparing the glomeruli and vasculature. AIN has a wide array of clinical presentations that range from isolated tubular disorders (e.g., Fanconi syndrome) to acute renal failure. Additional findings, fever, rash, and arthralgias, may suggest a hypersensitivity reaction.

130. **What medications are causes of AIN?**
- Antibiotics, especially penicillin analogs, cephalosporins, sulfonamides, and rifampin
- NSAIDs
- Diuretics, especially thiazides and furosemide

131. **What laboratory abnormalities are seen in patients with AIN?**

The urine sediment is often bland and may be normal aside from a low specific gravity.
- Urinary sediment: May contain RBCs, leukocytes (eosinophils), leukocyte casts
- Urinary protein excretion: Less than 1 g/day; with NSAID use, may be >1 g/day
- Fractional excretion of sodium: Usually >1%
- Proximal tubular defects: Glucosuria, bicarbonaturia, phosphaturia, aminoaciduria
- Distal tubular defects: Hyperkalemia, sodium wasting
- Medullary defects: Sodium wasting, urinary concentrating defects

Meyers CM: Acute interstitial nephritis. In: Greenberg A, editor: *Primer on Kidney Diseases. National Kidney Foundation.* San Diego, 1998, Academic Press, p 278.

URINARY TRACT INFECTIONS

132. **What two features on the dipstick test are used to evaluate possible UTIs?**

Nitrite: This test examines urine for the possible presence of nitrites, which can be produced by bacteria possessing the enzyme nitrate reductase, which reduces nitrates to nitrites. False negatives can occur. Not all urinary pathogens possess the enzyme (e.g., certain *Serratia* species). The test is more likely to be positive in the setting of a UTI if urine has been present in the bladder for several hours. The test is less effective in infants because of their increased micturition frequency.

Leukocyte esterase: This enzyme, present in white blood cells (WBCs), is typically present when urine is infected. However, since pyuria can be due to other nonbacterial causes and even NSAIDs, the test is less specific.

133. **How helpful are dipstick testing and microscopic analysis of urine as screening tests for UTIs?**

Sensitivity is the probability that test results will be positive among patients who have UTIs and specificity is the probability that test results will be negative among patients who do not have UTIs. The sensitivity and specificity of the components of the urinalysis individually and in combination as screening tools for the diagnosis of a UTI are summarized in Table 12-9. Dipstick testing, in particular, is much more effective as a diagnostic tool for UTIs in children >2 years than in younger children.

Mori R, Yonemoto N, Fitzgerald A: Diagnostic performance of urine dipstick testing in children with suspected UTI: a systematic review of relationship with age and comparison with microscopy, *Acta Paediatr* 99:581–584, 2010.

Table 12-9. Rapid Screening Tests for Urinary Tract Infection in Children: Sensitivity and Specificity

MICROSCOPY	SENSITIVITY (%) (RANGE)	SPECIFICITY (%) (RANGE)
≥5 WBC/HPF	67 (55, 88)	79 (77, 84)
Any bacteria/HPF	81 (16, 99)	83 (11, 100)
≥5 WBC or bacteria/HPF	99 (97, 100)	65 (67, 74)
Dipstick		
Any LE	83 (64, 89)	84 (71, 95)
Any nitrite only	50 (16, 72)	98 (95, 100)
Any nitrite or LE	88 (71, 100)	93 (76, 98)

LE = leukocyte esterase; HPF = high-power field; WBC = white blood cell.
Data from Christensen AM, Shaw K: Urinary tract infection in childhood. In: Kaplan BS, Meyers KEC, editors: Pediatric Nephrology and Urology: The Requisites in Pediatrics. *Philadelphia, 2004, Elsevier/Mosby, p 320.*

134. **Can the diagnosis of UTI be made on the basis of urinalysis alone?**
No. A urine culture is the only accurate means of diagnosing a UTI. Urinalysis is valuable for selecting individuals for the prompt initiation of treatment while awaiting results of the urine culture. In older children (in whom UTI symptoms are more reliable indicators of infection), a negative nitrite test, a negative leukocyte esterase test, and the absence of UTI symptoms are highly correlated with the absence of infection. However, babies require a culture to exclude UTI.

KEY POINTS: URINARY TRACT INFECTION

1. *Escherichia coli* bacteria cause 90% of cases.
2. Antibiotic sensitivity testing is important because of the increasing incidence of ampicillin-resistant *E. coli*.
3. Infections may be caused by bacteria ascending from the urethral area.
4. Clean bagged specimens are unreliable for diagnosis because of their high contamination rate.
5. Uncircumcised male infants have a 10-fold greater risk for infection than circumcised male infants.

135. **What bacterial counts constitute a positive urine culture?**
- **Suprapubic aspiration**: At least 100 colony-forming units (CFU)/mL
- **Catheterization**: At least 10,000 CFU/mL
- **Midstream clean catch**: At least 100,000 CFU/mL of a single organism; 10,000 to 100,000 CFU/mL is suspicious for a UTI and requires reculturing; less than 10,000 CFU/mL usually indicates contamination
- **Urine bag**: May be helpful if negative, but even when counts are ≥100,000 CFU/mL, there is a 40% to 85% false-positive result.

136. **A child has painful, frequent urination and a culture revealed a UTI, but the original urinalysis had a negative nitrite study. What is the most likely reason?**
Members of the gram-negative, rod-shaped *Enterobacteriaceae* family can reduce dietary nitrate to nitrite. However, the bacteria need hours for this conversion to occur. A first-morning void is more likely to be positive compared with the urinalysis of a child who has been urinating frequently with insufficient time to incubate in the bladder. A false-negative result is common with the nitrite test.

Patel HP: The abnormal urinalysis, *Pediatr Clin North Am* 53:325–337, 2006.

137. **What factors can cause a low colony count despite a definite urinary infection?**
- High urine volume
- Recent antimicrobial therapy
- Fastidious and slow-growing organisms (enterococci, *Staphylococcus saprophyticus*)

- Low urine pH(<5.0) and Specific gravity (<1.003)
- Bacteriostatic agents in the urine
- Complete obstruction of a ureter
- Chronic or indolent infection
- Use of inappropriate culture techniques

Bock GH: Urinary tract infections. In: Hoekelman RA, Adam HM, Nelson HM, et al: editors: *Primary Pediatric Care*, ed 4. St. Louis, 2001, Mosby, p 1896.

138. **Why should urine specimens be refrigerated if they cannot be immediately processed?**
Storage of urine specimens at room temperature is the most common causes of false-positive results. At room temperature, enteric organisms in specimens have a growth-doubling time of 12.5 minutes, and thus colony counts become an unreliable guide. If a urine specimen cannot be processed within 15 minutes, it should be refrigerated at less than 4°C to stop *in vitro* bacterial replication.

139. **What are the common presenting signs and symptoms of a UTI in an infant?**
The presenting findings are nonspecific and include fever, vomiting, diarrhea, irritability, hyperbilirubinemia, and poor feeding. These same findings are often seen in infants without UTIs, underscoring the importance of urine cultures in febrile infants.

140. **How common are UTIs in young febrile infants?**
In infants and toddlers between 2 and 24 months with unexplained fever ($>38.3°C$) the prevalence is about 7%, but it ranges between 2% and 9% depending on age and sex. The younger the child, the more likely the presence of a UTI. Girls have twice as many infections (or more) as circumcised boys. White female infants are twice as likely to have a UTI as black infants. In the first 3 months of life, uncircumcised males with fever have a 10-fold increased risk compared with circumcised boys. In infants younger than 2 months, 7.5% are likely to have UTIs, with boys having more than girls. Needless to say, the possibility of a UTI should always be considered in younger infants, particularly those without an identifiable source of infection, because UTIs now constitute the most likely source of an occult bacterial infection by a wide margin.

Greenhow TL, Hung YY, Herz AM, et al: The changing epidemiology of serious bacterial infections in young infants, *Pediatr Infect Dis J* 33:595–599, 2014.
Shaikh N, Morone ME, Bost JE, et al: Prevalence of urinary tract infection in childhood: a meta-analysis, *Pediatr Infect Dis J* 27:302–308, 2008.

141. **What pathogens are associated with UTIs in children?**
Between 80% and 90% of initial UTIs are caused by *E. coli*. Other organisms include *Proteus mirabilis*, *Klebsiella pneumoniae*, *Pseudomonas*, *Enterobacter*, and some *Staphylococcus* species.

142. **How is cystitis distinguished clinically from pyelonephritis?**
This can be difficult. Pyelonephritis tends to have more constitutional symptoms, such as fever, rigors, flank pain, and back pain, whereas cystitis has more bladder symptoms, such as enuresis, dysuria, frequency, and urgency. The presence of WBC casts or impaired urinary-concentrating ability is more indicative of pyelonephritis. Patients with pyelonephritis tend to have higher sedimentation rates, C-reactive protein levels, and serum procalcitonin levels, but these results can also be seen in some patients with cystitis. Renal dimercaptosuccinic acid (DMSA) scintigraphy may be useful for identifying acute pyelonephritis. However, for most children, the treatments for cystitis and of pyelonephritis are the same.

143. **What is the diagnostic approach for a possible UTI for a female infant 3 to 24 months of age with no known urinary tract abnormalities?**
One algorithmic approach uses risk factors and likelihood ratios (a number <1 is less likely, >1 more likely) and urinalysis results to categorize the probability of UTI (Fig. 12-7). Additional diagnostic algorithms are also available at the *JAMA* reference for febrile males ages 3 to 24 months and for verbal children >24 months with urinary or abdominal symptoms.

Shaikh N, Morone NE, Lopez J, et al: Does this child have a urinary tract infection? *JAMA* 298:2895–2904, 2007.

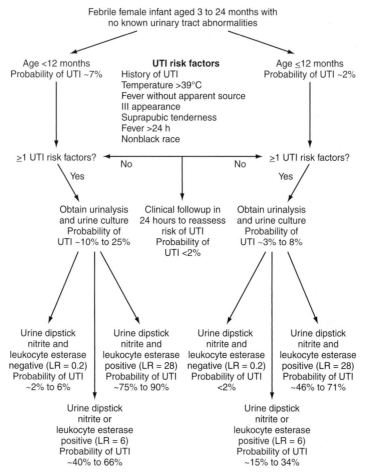

Figure 12-7. Diagnostic algorithm for febrile female infants 3 to 24 months of age suspected of having a urinary tract infection. *LR*, Likelihood ratio; *UTI*, urinary tract infection. *(From Shaikh N, Morone NE, Lopez J: Does this child have a urinary tract infection? JAMA 298:2902, 2007.)*

144. Which patients with UTIs require hospitalization and parenteral antibiotics?
   - Any patient who is toxic, dehydrated, or unable to tolerate oral antibiotics.
   - A patient with an underlying urinary tract abnormality in which pyelonephritis is suspected.
   - Many centers will hospitalize any infant <2 months because of a concern of an increased risk for urosepsis or other serious concomitant infections. However, recent studies indicate that low-risk infants (i.e., not clinically ill, no significant past medical history, normal WBC indices) may be at very low risk for bacteremia or clinical decompensation and might be managed with brief hospitalization or as outpatients. That debate is ongoing.

Schnadower D, Kuppermann N, Macias CG, et al: Outpatient management of young febrile infants with urinary tract infections, *Pediatr Emerg Care* 30:591–597, 2014.
Schnadower D, Kuppermann N, Macias CG, et al: Febrile infants with urinary tract infections at very low risk for adverse events and bacteremia, *Pediatrics* 126: 1074–1083, 2010.

145. **Should all pediatric patients with clinical pyelonephritis be hospitalized?**
The short- and long-term outcomes of patients (even as young as 2 months old) with uncomplicated pyelonephritis are the same whether they are treated initially with intravenous antibiotics or with oral, third-generation cephalosporins. A decision about outpatient therapy mandates the ability to tolerate oral antibiotics with no concerns regarding compliance and careful and reliable follow-up.

Strohmeier Y, Hodson EM, Willis NS, et al: Antibiotics for acute pyelonephritis in children, *Cochrane Database Syst Rev* 7:CD003772, 2014.

146. **What is the expected resolution of fever after a child is started on an antibiotic for a UTI?**
In one study of 128 infants younger than 60 days with UTI treated with parenteral antibiotics, 85% became afebrile within 24 hours. Only 4% were febrile after 48 hours. In another study of 364 patients 1 week to 18 years of age, 32% had fever beyond 48 hours. Older age is a risk factor for protracted fever.

Dayan RS, Hanson E, Bennett JE, et al: Clinical course of urinary tract infections in infants younger than 60 days of age, *Pediatr Emerg Care* 20:85–88, 2004.
Currie ML, Mitz L, Raasch CS, et al: Follow-up urine cultures and fever in children with urinary tract infection, *Arch Pediatr Adolesc Med* 157:1237–1240, 2003.

147. **What is the duration of antibiotic therapy for a UTI?**
Data to support a precise duration are insufficient. Standard duration of therapy for cystitis/lower UTIs varies from 7 to 14 days (oral or combined oral plus parenteral). Some experts lean toward 14 days of treatment for pyelonephritis. When IV antibiotics are given, a short IV course (2 to 4 days) followed by oral antibiotics is as effective as a longer course (7 to 10 days) of IV therapy. If the patient has not clinically improved within 2 to 3 days of starting therapy, the urine culture should be repeated and antibiotics adjusted, if indicated. Short-course (2- to 4-day) therapy compared with standard-duration (7- to 14-day) therapy for lower UTIs have shown clinical equivalency in some studies. Single-day or single-dose therapy is less effective and is not recommended.

Strohmeier Y, Hodson EM, Willis NS, et al: Antibiotics for acute pyelonephritis in children, *Cochrane Database Syst Rev* 7: CD003772, 2014.
Fitzgerald A, Mori R, Lakhanpaul M, et al: Antibiotics for treating lower urinary tract infection in children, *Cochrane Database Syst Rev* 8:CD006857, 2012.

148. **Are repeat cultures required at the end of therapy for a patient without symptoms?**
Although done commonly in the past as a "test of cure," follow-up urine cultures for a clinically improving patient >2 months of age are not indicated because the yield is extremely low (<.0.5%).

Oreskovic NM, Sembrano EU: Repeat urine cultures in children who are admitted with urinary tract infections, *Pediatrics* 119:e325–e329, 2007.

149. **In what patients are prophylactic antibiotics indicated for UTIs?**
This is controversial. Prophylaxis for recurrent UTI may actually increase the likelihood of infections. The recommendations are watchful waiting and rapid assessment when clinical concerns arise. It is also unclear whether preventing recurrent UTIs will prevent renal scarring. Consequently, prophylaxis for recurrent UTI in children *with normal urinary tract anatomy* is debatable, particularly for younger infants. Prophylaxis is generally indicated:
- In infants or children with their first UTI, who have finished their first course of antibiotic therapy and are awaiting the completion of studies (e.g., renal ultrasound).
- In patients with known urologic abnormalities that place them at high risk for recurrent UTIs (e.g., severe voiding disorders, high-grade VUR); however, the value of antibiotics in these situations is also questioned.

Dai B, Liu Y, Jia J, et al: Long-term antibiotics for the prevention of recurrent urinary tract infections in children: a systematic review and meta-analysis, *Arch Dis Child* 95:499–508, 2010.
Conway PH, Cnaan A, Zaoutis T, et al: Recurrent urinary tract infection in children: risk factors and association with prophylactic antimicrobials, *JAMA* 298:179, 2007.

150. **Is cranberry juice helpful in the management of recurrent UTIs in children?**
The use of cranberry juice as a urine-acidifying agent and treatment for UTI has been popular for adults since the 1920s and was used in the 1800s for disorders of the bladder. Studies of adults have shown it to be helpful for diminishing the frequency of bacteriuria, possibly because of its antiadhesive properties against *E. coli*. Results in pediatric studies are mixed, but more highly concentrated juice may have some limited value in recurrent UTI in children with no urologic abnormalities.

Afshar F, Stothers L, Scott H, et al: Cranberry juice for the prevention of pediatric urinary tract infection: a randomized controlled trial, *J Urol* 188:1584–1587, 2012.

151. **Do patients with an initial UTI require imaging studies?**
Approaches are controversial because of uncertainties regarding any causal relationship between UTIs, VUR, and renal scarring. In 1999, AAP guidelines recommended renal ultrasonography and voiding cystourethrogram (VCUG) in children < 2 years with a UTI to search for anomalies or the presence of vesicoureteral reflux. In 2011, these AAP guidelines were revised to recommend a follow-up ultrasound in all cases, but no VCUG routinely after the first UTI. A VCUG was recommended only if ultrasonography revealed hydronephrosis, scarring, or other findings that would suggest either high-grade VUR or obstructive uropathy. VCUG was also recommended in atypical or complex circumstances and for recurrent UTIs. The value of these studies, particularly their role in preventing long-term renal sequelae, continues under reexamination. Since the revised guidelines, clinical trends do indicate a more limited use of imaging studies with emphasis on higher-risk patients and a reduction in the use of the VCUG. Guidelines in the United Kingdom rely on ultrasound and radionuclide studies rather than the VCUG.

Coulthard MG, Lambert HJ, et al: Guidelines to identify abnormalities after childhood urinary tract infections: a prospective audit, *Arch Dis Child* 99:448–451, 2014.
Roberts KB, Subcommittee on Urinary Tract Infection, Steering Committee on Quality Improvement and Management: Urinary tract infection: clinical practice guideline for the diagnosis and management of the initial UTI in febrile infants and children 2 to 24 months, *Pediatrics* 128: 595–610, 2011.
Friedman AL: Acute UTI: What you need to know, *Contemp Pediatr* 25:68–76, 2008.
DeMuri GP, Wald ER: Imaging and antimicrobial prophylaxis following the diagnosis of urinary tract infection in children, *Pediatr Infect Dis J* 27:553–554, 2008.

152. **What imaging studies can be used for patients with UTIs who warrant evaluation?**
   - Renal ultrasound, to screen for urinary tract obstruction or other structural genitourinary abnormalities
   - VCUG or radionuclide cystogram, to evaluate for vesicoureteral reflux (the most common abnormality found in children with UTIs)
   - Renal cortical DMSA or MAG-3 (^{99m}Tc-mercaptoacetyltriglycine) scanning, recommended by some authorities to determine whether there is evidence of acute pyelonephritis or permanent renal scarring (Fig.12-8)

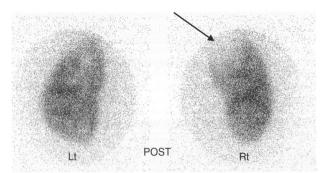

Figure 12-8. DMSA renal scan showing renal scarring *(arrow)* from pyelonephritis. *Lt*, left; *Rt*, right. *(From Kaplan BS, Meyers KEC: Pediatric Nephrology and Urology: The Requisites in Pediatrics. Philadelphia, 2004, Elsevier Mosby, p 119.)*

UROGENITAL ISSUES

153. What are risks associated with circumcision?

Rare complications are bleeding and infection. With poor technique, injury or amputation of the glans can occur. Meatal stenosis as a consequence of meatal ulceration is another potential complication.

154. Is circumcision now medically indicated?

We have watched the AAP's position statements on circumcision transform over the past 40 years. In the 1970s, circumcision was viewed as more of a negative. In 1999, the stance was modified to one of neutrality. In the 2012 policy statement, the positive benefits of circumcision were emphasized. Benefits have been found to exceed risks by at least 100 to 1 and that over the course of a lifetime, half of uncircumcised males will require treatment for a medical condition associated with retention of the foreskin. These benefits included protection against UTIs, sexually transmitted infections (particularly HIV infections), balanitis, and phimosis, and a lower incidence of penile cancer. No study has identified any adverse effect on sexual function or pleasure.

Although medical benefits can be emphasized, the decision at present still rests primarily on nonmedical family and cultural considerations.

As of 2013, CDC data indicate that the circumcision rate in the United States is about 80%. Clear racial differences were documented with rates of 91% among whites, 76% among blacks and 44% among Hispanics.

Morris BJ, Bailis SA, Wiswell TE: Circumcision rates in the United States: Rising or falling? What effect might the new affirmative pediatric policy statement have? *Mayo Clin Proc* 89:677–686, 2014.
American Academy of Pediatrics Task Force on Circumcision: Circumcision policy statement, *Pediatrics* 130: e756–e785, 2012.

155. What distinguishes phimosis and paraphimosis?

Phimosis is a narrowing of the distal foreskin, which prevents its retraction over the glans of the penis. In newborns, retraction is difficult because of normal adhesions that gradually self-resolve. Chronic inflammation or scarring can cause true phimosis with persistent narrowing and may require circumcision.

Paraphimosis is incarceration of a retracted foreskin behind the glans. It occurs when the retracted foreskin is not repositioned. Progressive edema results, which, if uncorrected, can lead to ischemic breakdown. Local anesthesia, ice, and manual reduction usually correct the problem, but if these are unsuccessful, surgical reduction is necessary.

Huang CJ: Problems of the foreskin and glans penis, *Clin Pediatr Emerg Med* 10:56–59, 2009.

156. What is hypospadias?

Hypospadias is a congenital defect in which the urethral opening is displaced to the underside of the penis. It results from the failure or delay of the midline fusion of the urethral folds. It is often associated with a ventral band of fibrous tissue (chordee) that causes ventral curvature of the penis, especially with an erection. Incidence is 1 to 2 per 1000 live births. When assessing hypospadias, it is useful to describe where the urethral meatus appears (i.e., glandular, distal shaft, proximal shaft, or perineal) and also the degree and location of chordee. The treatment of hypospadias is surgical repair, usually as a one-step procedure. With the advent of microsurgical techniques, the optimal time for repair appears to be 6 to 12 months of age.

157. How common are undescended testicles at birth?

The answer is very much dependent on gestational age. About 3% of term male infants are affected, but that increases to up to one-third of premature infants. The more premature the infant, the higher the likelihood of an undescended testicle.

158. When should undescended testicles be repaired?

The optimal time for surgery on an undescended testicle is **12 months of age or shortly thereafter**. Traditional teaching is that the majority of newborn cryptorchidism resolves without intervention with 75% percent of full-term infants and 90% of preterm cryptorchid newborns having full testicular descent by the age of 9 months. Some newer studies suggest the rate of spontaneous descent may be lower. Spontaneous descent after 9 months is unlikely. The AAP recommends surgery around 1 year of age to prevent testicular degeneration and to decrease the risk of testicular cancer. During the second year of life, ultrastructural changes in the seminiferous tubules of the undescended testes begin to appear, but these may be halted by orchiopexy.

Yiee JH, Saigal DS, Lai J, et al: Timing of orchiopexy in the United States: a quality-of-care indicator, *Urology* 80:1121–1126, 2012.

Wenzler DL, Bloom DA, Park JM: What is the rate of spontaneous testicular descent infants with cryptorchidism? *J Urol* 171:849–851, 2004.

159. How do you treat labial adhesions?
    Labial adhesions are a relatively common gynecologic finding in girls between 4 months 6 years of age. They may be complete or partial and are thought to result from local inflammation in a low-estrogen setting with resulting skin agglutination. Treatment consists of eliminating the underlying inflammation (if caused by an infection), sitz baths twice daily, maintenance of good perineal hygiene, and topical application of a 1% conjugated estrogen cream over the entire adhesion at bedtime for 3 weeks. The use of estrogen has an 80% to 90% cure rate and may be followed by the application of a petroleum jelly for 1 to 2 months nightly. It should be noted that the natural history of untreated asymptomatic labial adhesions is self-resolution: 50% resolve within 6 months, and nearly 100% resolve by 18 months. Surgical correction is almost never required.

Leung AKC, Robson WLM, Kao CP, et al: Treatment of labial fusion with topical estrogen therapy, *Clin Pediatr* 44:245–247, 2005.

UROLITHIASIS

160. Why are kidney stones increasing in frequency in children in the United States?
    There has been a 5-fold increase over the past 2 decades. A leading theory is that increased salt intake (consumption of salty snacks and processed foods) and insufficient fluid intake have led to increased urinary calcium and oxalate concentrations and stone formation. The increasing obesity is also paralleling increasing urolithiasis in children.

Copelovitch L: Urolithiasis in children, *Pediatr Clin North Am* 59: 881–896, 2012.

161. What are the clinical findings in pediatric urolithiasis?
    Patients present most commonly with flank pain, usually unilateral, with nausea and vomiting. Although hematuria (>2 RBCs/HPF) is common, up to 15% may have not have detectable hematuria. In about one-third of cases, there is a family history of urolithiasis. Fever, dysuria, and costovertebral angle tenderness lower the likelihood of stones and make infection more likely, although both may occur together.

Persaud AC, Stevenson MD, McMahon DR, Christopher NC: Pediatric urolithiasis: clinical predictors in the emergency department, *Pediatrics* 124:888–894, 2009.

162. What is the composition of kidney stones in children?
    Calcium (58%), struvite (25%), cysteine (6%), uric acid, urate (9%), others (2%)

163. What is the most common cause of pediatric urinary calculi?
    Idiopathic hypercalciuria is the most common cause of pediatric urinary calculi. Other causes include:
    • Hypercalcemia
    • Hypocitraturia
    • Hyperoxaluria
    • Cystinuria
    • Renal tubular dysfunction (usually Type 2 dRTA)
    • Endocrine (hypothyroidism, adrenocorticoid excess, hyperparathyroidism)
    • Bone metabolism disorders (immobilization, rickets, malignancies, juvenile rheumatoid arthritis)
    • Drugs (loop diuretics, excess vitamin D, corticosteroids)
    • UTI
    • Polycystic kidneys (dominant and recessive)
        A comprehensive metabolic evaluation is indicated in all children with calculi because of the high risk of recurrences in children with idiopathic hypercalciuria and hypocitraturia and

the importance of excluding rare but treatable conditions such as primary hyperoxaluria and cystinuria.

Copelovitch L: Urolithiasis in children, *Pediatr Clin North Am* 59: 881–896, 2012.
Spivacow FR, Negri AL, del Valle EE, et al: Metabolic risk factors in children with kidney stone disease, *Pediatr Nephrol* 23:1129–1133, 2008.

164. **How is hypercalciuria defined in pediatrics?**
    The strict definition of hypercalciuria in a child is >4 mg of urinary calcium/kg/24 hr on a normal, unrestricted diet for the child's age. Random urine collections are used to screen for hypercalciuria. The urine calcium-to-creatinine ratio varies with age. Morning nonfasting urine ratios that exceed the following criteria correlate with quantitative hypercalciuria:

Age (years)	Ratio
>7	>0.24
5-7	>0.30
3-5	>0.41
1-2	>0.56
<1	>0.81

165. **What are the appropriate laboratory studies for the initial evaluation of children with renal stones?**
    - Serum electrolytes, calcium, phosphorus, and creatinine
    - 24-hour urine collection for sodium, calcium, creatinine, urate, citrate, uric acid, oxalate, and cystine
    - Urine pH (by meter), urinalysis, and urine culture (if indicated)
    - Stone analysis on an available stone
    - Serum parathyroid hormone and vitamin D in patients with hypercalciuria, hypercalcemia, or hypophosphatemia

Nicoletta JA, Lande MB: Medical evaluation and treatment of urolithiasis, *Pediatr Clin North Am* 53:479–491, 2006.

166. **When is lithotripsy or surgery indicated for children with kidney stones?**
    Most stones up to 5 mm will pass spontaneously. Shock wave lithotripsy (SWL) is useful for children with pelvic or bladder stones that are radiopaque in whom fluoroscopy can be used to focus the shock waves. In general, SWL has a success rate of less than 50% with stones larger than 2 cm. Surgery (percutaneous nephrolithotomy) is reserved for stones causing urinary tract obstruction in children and for staghorn calculi in older patients. Cystine stones are difficult to fragment by SWL. Distal urethral stones are removed by ureteroscopy.

Mandeville JA, Nelson CP: Pediatric urolithiasis, *Curr Opin Urol* 119:419–423, 2009.

VESICOURETERAL REFLUX

167. **How is vesicoureteral reflux (VUR) graded?**
    VUR, the retrograde flow of urine from the bladder into the upper urinary tract, is typically divided into five grades, as shown in Fig. 12-9.

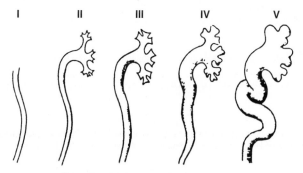

Figure 12-9. The five grades of vesicoureteral reflux.

168. **What is the natural history of VUR?**

The likelihood that reflux will resolve spontaneously is influenced by the severity of the reflux at the time of the initial diagnosis. About 80% to 90% of patients with grade I to II reflux, 70% (<age 2 years) and with grade III reflux, and 60%% with unilateral grade IV reflux will experience spontaneous resolution within 5 years. Spontaneous resolution of grade V reflux is uncommon. The chances for resolution are better in younger children and those with unilateral—rather than bilateral—reflux, especially for the higher grades of reflux.

Elder JS, Peters CA, Arant BS Jr, et al: Pediatric Vesicoureteral Reflux Guidelines Panel summary report on the management of primary vesicoureteral reflux in children, *J Urol* 157:1846–1851, 1997.

169. **How is VUR managed: medically or surgically?**

This is controversial. There are significant institutional differences given differing opinions on the role of VUR as a predisposing factor to acute pyelonephritis, renal scarring, and CKD, as well as the value of prophylactic antibiotics.

Grades I to II: These grades are usually managed medically, usually without prophylactic antibiotics, and given a higher likelihood of spontaneous resolution and a lower likelihood of significant sequelae.

Grades III to IV: If followed expectantly, these types of reflux will resolve slowly, at a rate of about 10% per year. Surgical intervention at the ureterovesicular junction will result in the elimination of this degree of reflux in the vast majority of patients, but randomized studies have not shown any significant difference in long-term renal outcome (e.g., renal scarring, hypertension, reduced function) when comparing medical versus surgical treatment. Prophylactic antibiotics are commonly used for these grades.

Grade V: Surgical intervention is typically indicated, particularly if the patient is older (>6 years) and significant renal scarring has been noted.

Martin AD, Iqbal MW, Sprague MD, et al: Most infants with dilating vesicoureteral reflux can be treated nonoperatively, *J Urol* 191(5 Suppl):1620–1626, 2014.

Peters CA, Skoog CJ, Arant BS Jr, et al: Summary of the American Urological Association guidelines on management of primary vesicoureteral reflux in children, *J Urol* 184:1134–1144, 2010.

170. **Are antibiotics effective to prevent recurrent UTIs in children with reflux?**

The effectiveness of antibiotics in the setting of significant reflux has been controversial and the results mixed. A 2014 well-designed Randomized Intervention for Children with Vesicoureteral Reflux (RIVUR) trial has found that treatment of children with VUR (grades I to IV) with a prophylactic antibiotic (trimethoprim-sulfamethoxazole), compared with placebo, was associated with a substantially reduced risk of recurrent UTIs but not of renal scarring for children treated following a first or second UTI. The authors questioned whether this decrease in recurrences in the setting of reflux might spur a reevaluation of the AAP's recommendation to not routinely do a reflux imaging study after a first UTI.

RIVUR Trial Investigators, Hoberman A, Greenfield SP, et al: Antimicrobial prophylaxis for children with vesicoureteral reflux, *N Engl J Med* 370:2367–2376, 2014.

171. **Should asymptomatic siblings of a patient with VUR have urologic imaging done as a screen for reflux?**

Some studies have demonstrated reflux in 33% to 45% of siblings of patients with reflux. Among identical twins, the rate is 80%. Typically, the reflux is milder (grades I to II) with only 2% of siblings in published studies having reflux of grades IV or V. Although the incidence of reflux is higher in siblings, data are still lacking that the screening and treatment of asymptomatic siblings decreases renal scarring.

Routh JC, Grant FD, Kokorowski P, et al: Costs and consequences of universal sibling screening for vesicoureteral reflux: a decision analysis, *Pediatrics* 126:865–871, 2010.

Acknowledgment

The editors gratefully acknowledge contributions by Drs. Michael Norman, Thomas Kennedy, James Prebis, and Stephen J. Wassner that were retained from the first three editions of *Pediatric Secrets*.

CHAPTER 13

NEUROLOGY

Tiffani L. McDonough, MD and James J. Riviello, Jr., MD

ANTIEPILEPTIC DRUGS

1. **Should treatment with antiepileptic drugs (AEDs) be started after the first afebrile seizure in a child?**
   Children with an isolated, uncomplicated seizure usually do not require AED therapy. Epidemiologic studies have shown that about one-third of children with an uncomplicated single seizure, a normal neurologic examination, and normal electroencephalogram (EEG) will experience a second. "Delaying" treatment until after the second seizure does not adversely affect the long-term chance of epilepsy remission. In fact, delaying treatment until 10 seizures may not affect remission, depending upon the underlying epilepsy syndrome.

   AEDs are not without risks and side effects, both dose related and idiosyncratic. Other factors, including EEG results, antecedent neurologic history, family history, and imaging (in selective cases), influence the risk for recurrence and should be considered. Risk for recurrent seizures is sharply increased if the seizure was nocturnal, the neurologic status is not normal, there is a positive family history, if no immediate precipitating cause can be identified, and the EEG reveals epileptiform discharges. Not even status epilepticus as the initial seizure increases the overall risk of seizure recurrence, but does increase the risk that the next seizure could be status epilepticus.

Haut SR, Shinnar S: Considerations in the treatment of a first unprovoked seizure, *Semin Neurol* 3:289–296, 2008.
Hirtz D, Berg A, Bettis D, et al, Quality Standards Subcommittee of the American Academy of Neurology; Practice Committee of the Child Neurology Society: Practice parameter: treatment of the child with a first unprovoked seizure. Report of the Quality Standards Subcommittee of the American Academy of Neurology and the Practice Committee of the Child Neurology Society, *Neurology* 60:166–172, 2003.

2. **What is the advantage of monotherapy chosen according to the epilepsy syndrome?**
   - Chronic toxicity is directly related to the number of drugs consumed.
   - As compared with monotherapy, intellectual and sensorium impairment is increased for any given AEDs (despite "normal" drug levels).
   - Drug interactions may paradoxically lead to loss of seizure control.
   - It is difficult to identify the cause of an adverse reaction.

Menkes JH, Sankar R: Paroxysmal disorders. In Menkes JH, Sarnat HB, Maria BL, editors: *Child Neurology*, ed 7, Philadelphia, 2006, Lippincott Williams & Wilkins, pp 891–893.

3. **Which AEDs are recommended for primary generalized tonic-clonic seizures in children over 1 month of age?**
   The "traditional" AEDs (phenobarbital, primidone, phenytoin) are no longer considered the drugs of choice for grand mal seizures for many age groups because of side effects. Studies have shown that most of the major anticonvulsants are comparable for reducing or eliminating seizure recurrences.

   Class I evidence demonstrates that topiramate, lamotrigine, levetiracetam, valproate, and zonisamide are effective for the treatment of primary generalized tonic-clonic seizures. Carbamazepine and oxcarbazepine may cause an increased frequency of primary generalized seizures, especially absence and myoclonic types, and are the drugs of choice for localization-related (focal) epilepsies.

Note that phenobarbital remains the first-line drug of choice for neonatal seizures.

Sankaraneni R, Lachhwani D: Antiepileptic drugs—a review, *Pediatr Ann* 44:e36–e42, 2015.

French JA, Kanner AM, Bautista J, et al: Therapeutics and Technology Assessment Subcommittee of the American Academy of Neurology; Quality Standards Subcommittee of the American Academy of Neurology; American Epilepsy Society: Efficacy and tolerability of the new antiepileptic drugs I: treatment of new onset epilepsy. Report of the Therapeutics and Technology Assessment Subcommittee and Quality Standards Subcommittee of the American Academy of Neurology and the American Epilepsy Society, *Neurology* 62:1252–1260, 2004.

Shankar R: Initial treatment of epilepsy with antiepileptic drugs: pediatric issues, *Neurology* 63:S30–S39, 2004.

4. What is the drug of choice for absence epilepsy?

Ethosuximide (Zarontin), **valproate** (divalproex sodium or Depakote), and **lamotrigine** (Lamictal) are all effective for eliminating or substantially reducing the number of absence attacks. Ethosuximide is traditionally the drug of choice, for several reasons:

- It works well for many patients. It not only stops the clinical attacks of absence, but it often normalizes the EEG by actually eliminating the 3/second spike-wave discharges.
- It is well tolerated by most patients. Although rare cases of serious bone marrow, liver, or dermatologic disorders have occurred, routine or frequent blood tests are not considered obligatory by most physicians.
- It has a relatively long serum half-life (40 hours). Thus, once- or twice-daily dosing is appropriate and represents a real convenience to the patient.
- It is relatively inexpensive.

A disadvantage is that ethosuximide protects only against absence seizures. Children with coexisting generalized convulsions should be treated with valproate or lamotrigine. Disadvantages of valproate include the risks for idiosyncratic liver toxicity, especially with an underlying metabolic disease, pancreatopathy, thrombocytopenia (dose and duration-related), low vitamin D levels, osteopenia, weight gain, and teratogenicity. Lamotrigine should also be considered, with the relative risk for rash (risk increases with valproic acid) and generally favorable cognitive profile taken into account.

Glauser TA, Cnaan A, Shinnar S, et al: Ethosuximide, valproic acid, and lamotrigine in childhood absence epilepsy, *N Engl J Med* 362:790–799, 2010.

5. Can AEDs paradoxically cause a worsening of seizures?

A paradoxic worsening of seizure control by various AEDs has been noted for decades. In fact, every AED may aggravate seizures. Mechanisms may include nonspecific effects of drug intoxication. In addition, specific medications may exacerbate specific seizure types. For example, carbamazepine may worsen the absence, myoclonic, and astatic seizures seen in generalized epilepsy syndromes; phenytoin and vigabatrin may also worsen generalized seizures; and gabapentin and lamotrigine may worsen myoclonic seizures. The clinical trap to avoid is assuming that increasing seizures are related to the underlying epilepsy and that increasing doses are needed. With a paradoxic worsening, seizures will continue to worsen or not improve.

Perucca E, Gram L, Avanzini G, Dulac O: Antiepileptic drugs as a cause of worsening seizures, *Epilepsia* 39:5–17, 1998.

6. When should blood levels be obtained if seizures are poorly controlled, compliance is questionable, or drug toxicity suspected?

Trough serum drug levels should be obtained to detect subtherapeutic or toxic concentrations. It is most helpful to check the serum level right before the dose, preferably in the morning before any medication is given. An inadequate serum concentration is the most common cause of persistent seizures, but drug toxicity, especially with phenytoin, may also manifest by deteriorating seizure control. There generally will be less variation in blood concentrations with tablets or capsules compared with liquid preparations; suspensions in particular result in notoriously inconsistent dosages. If drug toxicity is suspected, peak serum levels may be preferable to trough serum levels.

Stepanova D, Beran RG: The benefits of antiepileptic drug (AED) blood level monitoring to complement clinical management of people with epilepsy, *Epilepsy Behav* 42:7–9, 2015.

7. What are the suggested therapeutic ranges of AEDs?

See Table 13-1.

Table 13-1. Drug/Trade Name Target Plasma Drug Concentration Range*

DRUG (GENERIC)	BRAND NAME	TARGET DRUG LEVEL
Carbamazepine	Tegretol/Carbatrol	4-12 mcg/mL
Clobazam	Onfi	Not done
Ethosuximide	Zarontin	40-100 μg/mL
Felbamate	Felbatol	30-100 μg/mL
Gabapentin	Neurontin	4-20 μg/mL
Lacosamide	Vimpat	5-10 μg/mL
Lamotrigine	Lamictal	2-20 mcg/mL
Levetiracetam	Keppra	10-60 μg/mL
Oxcarbazepine	Trileptal	10-40 μg/mL
Phenobarbital	Luminal	10-45 μg/mL
Phenytoin	Dilantin, Fosphenytoin	10-20 mcg/mL
Primidone	Mysoline	5-10 mg/mL
Rufinamide	Banzel	3-30 μg/mL
Tiagabine	Gabitril	20-200 ng/mL
Topiramate	Topamax	2-25 μg/mL
Valproate	Depakene/Depakote	50-100 mcg/mL
Vigabatrin	Sabril	Not done
Zonisamide	Zonegran	10-40 μg/mL

*Therapeutic ranges are just guidelines for dosing. Seizures may respond to a low level, and toxicity may occur at a low level. Levels above "normal" may be needed to control seizures and can be used, if tolerated. It is important to treat the patient and not the "level."

8. **What are the typical dose-related side effects of AEDs?**
   Dose-related side effects occur somewhat predictably and can be anticipated, particularly as the medication dose is initiated and escalated. Common dose-related side effects include sedation, headache, gastrointestinal irritation, unsteadiness, and dysarthria. Management commonly consists of reducing the dose by 25% to 50% and waiting about 2 weeks for tolerance to develop. In addition, behavioral and cognitive side effects can occur in some patients; these can be subtler, and controversy exists regarding the relative effects of various AEDs.

   Dose-related side effects are referred to as "nuisance" side effects, which typically resolve either with dose-reduction or tolerance, compared with direct organ toxicity (liver, pancreas, bone marrow).

Guerrini R, Zaccara G, la Marca G, Rosati A: Safety and tolerability of antiepileptic drug treatment in children with epilepsy, *Drug Saf* 35: 519–533, 2012.

9. **What idiosyncratic drug reactions are associated with antiepileptic medications?**
   Idiosyncratic reactions occur unpredictably, are potentially fatal, and do not correlate with dose of medication.
   - **Carbamazepine:** leukopenia, aplastic anemia, thrombocytopenia, hepatic dysfunction, rashes
   - **Ethosuximide:** leukopenia, pancytopenia, rashes
   - **Phenobarbital:** rashes, Stevens-Johnson syndrome, hepatic dysfunction
   - **Phenytoin:** hepatic dysfunction, lymphadenopathy, movement disorder, Stevens-Johnson syndrome, fulminant hepatic failure
   - **Valproic acid:** fulminant hepatic failure (especially in at-risk patients, see question 10), hyperammonemia, pancreatitis, thrombocytopenia, rash, stupor
   - **Lamotrigine:** stevens-Johnson syndrome, toxic epidermal necrolysis, hepatic failure, DRESS syndrome (**D**rug **R**ash with **E**osinophilia and **S**ystemic **S**ymptoms), aseptic meningitis

10. **Which children are most susceptible to valproic acid–induced acute hepatic failure?**

The highest incidences occur in **children younger than 2 years who are receiving polytherapy** (1 in 540). In children younger than 2 years who are receiving valproic acid monotherapy, the rate is reduced to about 1 in 8000. The complication is unrelated to dosage and typically occurs during the first 3 months of therapy. Up to 40% of individuals who receive valproic acid will have dose-related elevations of liver enzymes that are transient or resolve with dosage adjustments. However, liver function test monitoring is not helpful for predicting acute hepatic failure. It has been hypothesized that valproic acid may cause carnitine deficiency, hyperammonemia, and hepatotoxicity. Despite a lack of data from clinical trials, some clinicians recommend prophylactic carnitine supplementation.

In addition, Alpers syndrome is a rare, autosomal recessive neurometabolic disease, often presenting with intractable seizures and psychomotor regression. The disease is caused by a mutation in POLG, which encodes for a mitochondrial DNA polymerase. Children with Alpers syndrome are at increased risk for fulminant hepatic failure with valproic acid administration, and this agent should be used with caution if this condition is suspected.

Saneto RP, Lee IC, Koenig MK, et al: POLG DNA testing as an emerging standard of care before instituting valproic acid therapy for pediatric seizure disorders, *Seizure* 19:140–146, 2010.

Bryant AE, Dreifuss FE: Valproic acid hepatic fatalities, *Neurology* 48:465–469, 1996.

11. **What are the warning signs and symptoms of hypersensitivity syndromes to AEDs?**

Symptoms often occur early, within the first months of treatment. Families need to be educated about the potential for drug reactions. Concerning symptoms include:

- body temperature higher than 40 °C
- protracted vomiting
- lethargy
- exfoliation of the skin (palm or sole) or mucosal lesions
- facial edema or swelling of the tongue
- confluent erythema, palpable purpura
- protracted bleeding from minor cuts
- lymph node enlargement
- wheezing (indicating anaphylaxis)

Multiple studies have shown that families fail to appreciate evolving symptoms of idiosyncratic reactions and continue to administer the offending agent. Laboratory abnormalities may include eosinophilia, atypical lymphocytosis, and abnormal liver function enzymes. Routine surveillance of blood chemistries and complete blood counts (every 3 to 6 months) is standard practice, but they are unlikely to identify potentially life-threatening conditions.

Ye YM, Thong BY, Park HS: Hypersensitivity to antiepileptic drugs, *Immunol Allergy Clin North Am* 34:633–643, 2014.

12. **What is Diastat?**

Diazepam rectal gel (Diastat) has been approved for the treatment of status epilepticus and severe recurrent convulsive seizures in children. It is prescribed for home use by parents as an emergency medication. Dosages (as they are for most medications in pediatric patients) are based on weight, and the medication is available in various premixed concentrations with syringe applicators. Parents are generally counseled to administer the medication for a seizure lasting greater than 5 minutes and to call 911 with administration because respiratory depression can occur with administration of benzodiazepines.

13. **Are there other options for outpatient treatment of severe recurrent and prolonged seizures in children?**

As of 2014, rectal diazepam is the only formulation approved in the United States by the FDA for out-of-hospital treatment. However, clinical trials are in progress for alternatives such as intranasal midazolam, diazepam and lorazepam, buccal midazolam (approved in the European Union), sublingual lorazepam, and intramuscular diazepam by autoinjection.

McKee HR, Abou-Khalil B: Outpatient pharmacotherapy and modes of administration for acute repetitive and prolonged seizures, *CNS Drugs* 29:55–70, 2015.

14. **After what period can AEDs be safely discontinued?**
The withdrawal of AEDs should be considered when the child is free of seizures for 2 years because well-controlled investigations have shown that the risk for relapse in children whose seizures have been in remission for 2 years is low. A 4-year period of seizure freedom was the previous standard. Although there is no uniform agreement about factors that are predictive of outcome, the highest remission rate appears to occur in those who are otherwise neurologically normal and in whom the EEG at the time of discontinuation lacks specific epileptiform features and displays a normal background. The prognosis is the worst for children with symptomatic epilepsies, persistently abnormal EEGs, and abnormal neurologic examinations. Remission also depends upon the underlying epilepsy syndrome.

Camfield P, Camfield C: When is it safe to discontinue AED treatment? *Epilepsia* 49S:25–28, 2008.
Smith R, Ball R: Discontinuing anticonvulsant medication in children, *Arch Dis Child* 87:259–260, 2002.

15. **When the decision is made to discontinue AEDs, should the tapering period be long or short?**
In practice, all AEDs should be tapered gradually rather than abruptly discontinued, although there is no actual withdrawal state produced by a "cold turkey" reduction of most AEDs (e.g., phenytoin, carbamazepine, valproate, ethosuximide). By contrast, a withdrawal syndrome of agitation, signs of autonomic overactivity, and seizures follows the sudden elimination of habitually consumed benzodiazepines (diazepam, clonazepam, clobazam, lorazepam) or short-acting barbiturates (e.g., secobarbital). The long elimination half-life of phenobarbital lessens the risk for withdrawal symptoms after abrupt discontinuation.

In a study of more than 100 children who had been seizure free for either 2 or 4 years, the risk for seizure recurrence during tapering and after discontinuation of the AED was no different if the period of taper was 6 weeks or 9 months. Rapid tapering appears to be an acceptable means of discontinuation.

Tennison M, Greenwood R, Lewis D, Thorn M: Discontinuing antiepileptic drugs in children with epilepsy: a comparison of a six-week and a nine-month taper period, *N Engl J Med* 330:1407–1410, 1994.

CEREBRAL PALSY

16. **What is cerebral palsy?**
Cerebral palsy (CP) describes a *heterogeneous* group of nonprogressive (static) motor and posture disorders of cerebral or cerebellar origin that typically manifest early in life. The primary impairment involves *significant deficits in motor planning and control*. Nonprogressive, clinical manifestations often change over time as the functional expression of the underlying brain is modified by brain development and maturation. However, motor function that is affected results from the part of the brain that is injured. Causes include cerebral malformations, metabolic and genetic causes, infection (both intrauterine and extrauterine), stroke, hypoxia-ischemia, and trauma.

American Academy for Cerebral Palsy and Developmental Medicine: www.aacpdm.org. Accessed on March 5, 2015.
United Cerebral Palsy Association: www.ucp.org. Accessed on March 5, 2015.

17. **What are the most common brain lesions seen on magnetic resonance imaging (MRI) in children with cerebral palsy?**
Periventricular white matter lesions are the most common and can be seen in 19% to 45% of children with CP (particularly formerly premature infants). Other common lesions include gray matter injuries of the basal ganglia and thalamus (21%), developmental cortical malformations (11%), and focal cortical infarcts (10%). Up to 15% of cases of CP do not have an identifiable lesion on MRI. The varied MRI findings are believed to be emblematic of the neurodevelopmental heterogeneity of CP.

Hadders-Algra M: Early diagnosis and early intervention in cerebral palsy, *Front Neurol* 5:185, 2014.

18. **What are the Levine (POSTER) criteria for the diagnosis of CP?**
    - **P**osturing/abnormal movements
    - **O**ropharyngeal problems (e.g., tongue thrusts, swallowing abnormalities)

- Strabismus
- Tone (hypertonia or hypotonia)
- Evolutional maldevelopment (primitive reflexes persist or protective/equilibrium reflexes fail to develop [e.g., lateral prop, parachute reflex])
- Reflexes (increased deep tendon reflexes/persistent Babinski reflex)
  Abnormalities in four of these six categories strongly point to the diagnosis of CP.

Feldman HM: Developmental-behavioral pediatrics. In Zitelli BJ, Davis HW, editors: *Atlas of Pediatric Diagnosis,* ed 5, St. Louis, 2007, Mosby, p 82.

19. What are the types of cerebral palsy?
    Clinical classification is based on the nature of the movement disorder and muscle tone and anatomic distribution. A single patient may have more than one type. Spastic cerebral palsy is the most common, accounting for about two-thirds of cases.
    Spastic (or pyramidal) CP: Characterized by neurologic signs of upper motor neuron damage with increased "clasp knife" muscle tone, increased deep tendon reflexes, pathologic reflexes, and spastic weakness. Spastic CP is subclassified based on distribution:
    - *Hemiplegia*: Primarily unilateral involvement, arm usually more than leg
    - *Quadriplegia*: All limbs involved, with legs often more involved than arms
    - *Diplegia*: Legs much more involved than arms, which may show no or only minimal impairment (more common in the premature infant)
    Dyskinetic (nonspastic or extrapyramidal) CP: Characterized by prominent involuntary movements or fluctuating muscle tone, with choreoathetosis the most common subtype. Distribution is usually symmetric among the four limbs.
    Ataxic CP: Primarily cerebellar signs (including ataxia, dysmetria, past pointing, nystagmus)
    Mixed types: Features of multiple types of cerebral palsy

Richards CL, Malouin F: Cerebral palsy: definition, assessment and rehabilitation, *Handb Clin Neurol* 111: 183–195, 2013.
Murphy N, Such-Neibar T: Cerebral palsy diagnosis and management: the state of the art, *Curr Probl Pediatr Adolesc Health Care* 33:146–169, 2003.

20. What proportion of CP is related to birth asphyxia?
    In contrast with popular perception, large clinical epidemiologic and longitudinal studies indicate that perinatal asphyxia is an important—but relatively minor—cause. Estimates range from a low of 3% to a high of 21%. In most cases, the events leading to CP occur in the fetus before the onset of labor or in the newborn after delivery.

McIntyre S, Blair E, Badawi N, et al: Antecedents of cerebral palsy and perinatal death in term and late preterm singletons, *Obstet Gynecol* 122:869–877, 2013.
Nelson KB: Can we prevent cerebral palsy? *N Engl J Med* 349:1765–1769, 2003.

21. How well do Apgar scores correlate with the development of CP?
    Large studies have mixed results. A 1981 study of 49,000 infants found that a low Apgar score correlated poorly with the development of CP. Of term infants with scores of 0 to 3 at 1 or 5 minutes, 95% did not develop CP. Conversely, nearly 75% of patients with CP had 5-minute Apgar scores of 7 to 10. More recent studies have found a stronger association between low Apgar scores and cerebral palsy in term infants, but there is no clear association for low birth weight or premature infants. A 2010 population study of over 500,000 Norwegian infants found an association between an Apgar score <4 at 5 minutes and cerebral palsy, which was strongest for infants with normal birth weight and for patients later diagnosed with quadriplegia.

Lie KK, Groholt E-K, Eskild A: Association of cerebral palsy with Apgar score in low and normal birthweight infants: population based cohort study, *BMJ* 341:c4990, 2010.
Nelson KB, Ellenberg JH: Apgar scores as predictors of chronic neurologic disability, *Pediatrics* 68:36–44, 1981.

22. **Why is CP difficult to diagnose clinically during the first year of life?**
Unlike adults with acute neurologic deficits, which may be focal, young children may manifest generalized and nonspecific neurologic dysfunction following an acute neurologic insult:
- Hypotonia is more common than hypertonia in the first year following an acute insult and spasticity typically develops later, both of which makes the prediction of CP difficult. Hypertonia, especially in the antigravity muscles, develops to compensate for weakness. Initial hypertonia may be seen with a basal ganglia insult.
- The early abundance of primitive reflexes (with variable persistence) may confuse the clinical picture.
- An infant has a limited variety of volitional movements for evaluation.
- Substantial myelination takes months to evolve and may delay the clinical picture of abnormal tone and increased deep tendon reflexes.
- Most infants who develop CP do not have identifiable risk factors; most cases are not related to labor and delivery events (intrapartum).
Most cases of cerebral palsy can be diagnosed by 18 to 24 months of life.

Hadders-Algra M: Early diagnosis and early intervention in cerebral palsy, *Front Neurol* 5:185, 2014.
Shapiro BK, Capute AJ: Cerebral palsy. In McMillan JA, DeAngelis CD, Feigin RD, Warshaw JB, editors: *Oski's Pediatrics, Principles and Practice*, ed 3, Philadelphia, 1999, Lippincott Williams & Wilkins, pp 1910–1917.

KEY POINTS: CEREBRAL PALSY

1. Apgar scores correlate relatively poorly with the ultimate diagnosis of cerebral palsy.
2. During the first year of life, hypotonia is more common than hypertonia in patients who are ultimately diagnosed with the disease.
3. Keep an eye on the eyes: As many as 75% of children with cerebral palsy have ophthalmologic problems (e.g., strabismus, refractive errors).
4. Spastic hemiplegia is the most common type of cerebral palsy that is associated with seizures.
5. Monitor regularly for hip subluxation, especially in patients with spastic diparesis, because earlier identification assists therapy.

23. **What behavioral symptoms during the first year should arouse suspicion about the possibility of CP?**
- Excessive irritability, constant crying, and sleeping difficulties (severe colic is noted in up to 30% of babies who are eventually diagnosed with CP)
- Early feeding difficulties with difficulties in coordinating suck and swallow, frequent spitting up, and poor weight gain
- "Jittery" or "jumpy" behavior, especially at times other than when hungry
- Easily startled behavior
- Stiffness when handled, especially during dressing, diapering, and handwashing
- Paradoxically "precocious" development, such as early rolling (actually a sudden, reflexive roll rather than a volitional one) or apparent early strength, such as the stiff-legged "standing" with support of an infant with spastic diplegia

Bennett FC: Diagnosing cerebral palsy—the earlier the better, *Contemp Pediatr* 16:65–76, 1999.

24. **What gross motor delays are diagnostically important in the infant with possible CP?**
- Inability to bring the hands together in midline while in a supine position by the age of 4 months
- Head lag persisting beyond 6 months
- No volitional rolling by 6 months
- Inability to independently sit straight by 8 months
- No hands-and-knees crawling by 12 months

Bennett FC: Diagnosing cerebral palsy—the earlier the better, *Contemp Pediatr* 16:65–76, 1999.

25. What problems are commonly associated with CP?
    - **Mental retardation:** Two-thirds of total patients; most commonly observed in children with spastic quadriplegia
    - **Failure to thrive, growth retardation**
    - **Feeding problems** (including dysphagia, sialorrhea [excessive salivation])
    - **Gastrointestinal problems** (gastroesophageal reflux, constipation)
    - **Learning disabilities**
    - **Ophthalmologic abnormalities** (strabismus, amblyopia, nystagmus, refractive errors)
    - **Hearing deficits**
    - **Communication disorders**
    - **Epilepsy:** One-half of total patients; most commonly observed in children with spastic hemiplegia and related to the degree of neuroimaging abnormality.
    - **Behavioral and emotional problems** (especially attention-deficit hyperactivity disorder, depression, sleep problems)
    - **Urinary problems** (incontinence, voiding dysfunction, urinary tract infections)
    - **Spinal column changes** (kyphosis, scoliosis)
    - **Respiratory problems** (upper airway obstruction, chronic aspiration)

Sewell MD, Eastwood DM, Wimalasundera N: Managing common symptoms of cerebral palsy in children, *BMJ* 349: g4596, 2014.

Dodge NN: Cerebral palsy: medical aspects, *Pediatr Clin North Am* 55:1189–1207, 2008.

26. What features in an infant suggest a progressive central nervous system (CNS) disorder rather than CP as the cause of a motor deficit?
    Abnormally increasing head circumference: Possible hydrocephalus, tumor, or neurodegenerative disorder
    Eye anomalies: Cataracts, retinal pigmentary degeneration, optic atrophy (possible neurodegenerative disease), coloboma, chorioretinal lacuna, optic nerve hypoplasia (possible Aicardi syndrome or septo-optic dysplasia)
    Skin abnormalities: Vitiligo, café-au-lait spots, nevus flammeus, port-wine stain (possible Sturge-Weber syndrome or neurofibromatosis)
    Hepatomegaly and/or splenomegaly (possible metabolic or lysosomal storage disease)
    Decreased or absent deep tendon reflexes
    Sensory abnormalities: Diminished sense of pain, position, vibration, or light touch
    Developmental regression or failure to progress: Rett syndrome or Leigh disease

Taft LT: Cerebral palsy, *Pediatr Rev* 16:411–418, 1995.

27. What therapies are used to treat the spasticity and dystonia of cerebral palsy?
    Casting: Serial "inhibitive" casting can reduce tone and allow improved gait and weight-bearing activities
    Nerve blocks, motor point blocks, botulinum toxin: Injected to target spasticity in particular muscle groups
    Oral and intrathecal medications: Including baclofen, dantrolene, carbidopa-levodopa, clonazepam
    Tendon-lengthening surgeries: At ankle, knee, wrist, or elbow to prevent or delay joint contractures
    Selective dorsal rhizotomy: A neurosurgical procedure that interrupts the afferent component of the deep tendon (stretch) reflex

Ailon T, Beauchamp R, Miller S, et al: Long-term outcome after selective dorsal rhizotomy in children with spastic cerebral palsy, *Childs Nerv Syst* 31: 415-423, 2015.

Copeland L, Edwards P, Thorley M, et al: Botulinum toxin A for nonambulatory children with cerebral palsy: a double-blind randomized controlled trial, *J Pediatr* 165:140–146, 2014.

CEREBROSPINAL FLUID

28. What is normal cerebrospinal fluid (CSF) pressure?
    CSF pressure as measured during a lumbar puncture varies with age, positional technique, and combativeness of the patient. For truly accurate pressures, the child should be relaxed with legs extended.

CSF can be seen in the manometer varying with respirations when the needle has been properly placed. As a general guide, the normal ranges of CSF opening pressures are:
- *Neonate:* 80 to 100 mm H_2O /CSF
- *1 month to 4 years:* 10 to 100 mm H_2O
- *8 years to adolescent-adult:* 100 to 200 mm H_2O
- *Adolescent to adult:* 100 to 250 mm H_2O (may reach 280 in obese or sedated patients). Any opening pressure >250 mm H_2O should be considered suspicious for intracranial hypertension. Some evidence exists that in the obese or sedated patient, a cutoff of 280 mm H_2O may be considered the upper limit of normal. Both elevated body mass index (BMI) and deep sedation may increase the opening pressure.

Avery RA: Interpretation of lumbar puncture opening pressure measurements in children, *J Neuroophthalmol* 34: 284–287, 2014.
Ellis R 3rd: Lumbar cerebrospinal fluid opening pressure measured in flexed lateral decubitus position in children, *Pediatrics* 93:622–623, 2003.

29. **What are the normal CSF volumes in an infant, child, and adolescent?**
Estimates for the volume of the ventricular system are:
- 40 to 50 mL in a term newborn
- 65 to 100 mL in an older child
- 90 to 150 mL in a teenager or adult
The choroid plexus actively secretes a distillate of CSF at a rate of 0.3 to 0.4 mL/minute in children and adults, which equals about 20 mL/hour or 500 mL/day. This equates to an hourly CSF volume turnover rate of about 15%.

30. **What are the common causes of an elevated CSF protein?**
Elevated CSF protein (>30 mg/dL) is a nonspecific finding that is encountered in various neurologic disorders. Several common etiologies should be considered:
Infection: Tuberculous meningitis, acute bacterial meningitis (pneumococcal, meningococcal, *Haemophilus influenzae*), syphilitic or viral meningitis, encephalitis
Inflammation: Guillain-Barré syndrome (GBS), multiple sclerosis, peripheral neuropathy, postinfectious encephalopathy
Tumor of the cerebral hemispheres or spinal cord; A CSF block may cause a very elevated CSF protein.
Vascular accidents, such as cerebral hemorrhage (including subarachnoid hemorrhage, subdural hemorrhage, intracerebral hemorrhages) or stroke as a result of cranial arteritis, diabetes mellitus, or hypertension
Degenerative disorders involving white-matter disease (e.g., Krabbe disease)
Metabolic disorders (e.g., uremia)
Toxins (e.g., lead)
Prematurity, related to immaturity of the blood-brain barrier

31. **What CSF findings suggest metabolic disease as a cause of neurologic signs and symptoms?**
- **Elevated CSF protein concentration** is characteristic of metachromatic leukodystrophy and globoid cell encephalopathy.
- **Low CSF glucose concentration** is consistent with hypoglycemia caused by a defect of gluconeogenesis or a defect in the transport of glucose across the blood-brain barrier (GLUT-1 deficiency syndrome).
- **Low CSF folate concentration** suggests a defect involving folate metabolism.
- **Presence in the CSF of amino acids, specifically glycine, glutamate, and γ-aminobutyric acid (GABA),** may be diagnostic of nonketotic hyperglycinemia, pyridoxine-dependent epilepsy, or another defect in GABA metabolism.
- **Lactate** and **pyruvate** values are elevated in CSF disorders of cerebral energy metabolism, including pyruvate dehydrogenase deficiency, pyruvate carboxylase deficiency, numerous disturbances of the respiratory chain, and Menkes syndrome.
- **Low CSF lactate** value may be seen in the GLUT-1 deficiency syndrome.
- **Abnormal CSF biogenic amines** suggest several disorders that are associated with disturbed neurotransmission.

32. **Why is a stylet used during a lumbar puncture?**

A stylet is typically used during a lumbar puncture to prevent epidermis (which might lodge in an open-ended needle) from being introduced into the subarachnoid space, where an epidermal tumor might form. There is debate about whether the stylet should be kept in place after the needle passes the subcutaneous space or removed at that point to allow a better assessment of CSF flow when the needle enters the subarachnoid space. After fluid has been collected, some experts advocate reinserting the stylet to minimize the potential to prevent attached arachnoid strands from causing prolonged CSF leakage through the dura, which may cause prolonged headaches. In newborns, it has been more common to not use a stylet, although this practice should be avoided.

Ellenby MS, Tegtmeyer K, Lai S, Braner DAV: Videos in clinical medicine. Lumbar puncture, *N Engl J Med* 355:e12:2006.
Baxter AL, Fisher RG, Burke BL, et al: Local anesthetic in stylet styles: factors associated with resident lumbar puncture success, *Pediatrics* 117:876–881, 2006.
Strupp M, Brandt T, Muller A: Incidence of post-lumbar puncture syndrome reduced by reinserting the stylet: a randomized prospective study of 600 patients, *J Neurol* 245:589–592, 1998.

33. **As tests of meningeal irritation, what constitutes a positive Kernig or Brudzinski sign?**

- *Kernig sign,* or the straight-leg-raising sign, consists of flexing the hip to 90 degrees and attempting to extend the knee. The limitation of knee extension as a result of painful resistance is a positive sign.
- *Brudzinski sign* is a positive sign, and it is present if a reflex flexion of the thighs occurs when a patient's neck is passively flexed.

It should be noted that these signs may not be present in the infant or young child (<18 to 24 months).

34. **How do the manifestations of increased intracranial pressure (ICP) differ in an infant compared with an older child?**

- *Infant:* Increasing head circumference, delayed closure of the fontanel, suture separation, bulging fontanel, failure to thrive, macrocephaly, paresis of upward gaze (known as setting-sun sign) shrill cry
- *Older child:* Headache (especially in the early morning, awakening the child from sleep, or association with vomiting), nausea, persistent vomiting, personality and mood changes, lethargy, anorexia, fatigue, somnolence, diplopia as a result of sixth-nerve palsy or third-nerve palsy with uncal herniation, papilledema (Fig. 13-1)

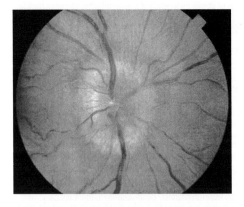

Figure 13-1. Papilledema. Signs include swelling of the optic disc with blurring of normally sharp margins, venous engorgement, and curvature of blood vessels due to elevation of the disc. *(From Douglas G, Nicol F, Robertson C, editors:* MacLeod's Clinical Examination, *ed 13. London, 2013, Elsevier, Ltd., p 285.)*

35. **What comprises the Cushing triad?**

The *Cushing triad* consists of the development of **slow or irregular respirations, decreased heart rate,** and **elevated blood pressure** (particularly an increased systolic pressure with a widening pulse pressure) resulting from an increase in ICP. The Cushing triad may be observed in children with increased ICP or compression of the posterior fossa, which houses the medullary circulatory control center. It is a very late finding of increased ICP.

36. How is hydrocephalus classified?

Communicating hydrocephalus is caused by an inability to normally reabsorb CSF by the arachnoid granulations, which can occur from meningeal scarring as a result of bacterial meningitis, intraventricular hemorrhage, or intrathecal chemotherapy. It can be diagnosed if a tracer dye injected into one lateral ventricle appears in the lumbar CSF.

Noncommunicating hydrocephalus refers to conditions causing intraventricular obstruction and alteration of the flow of dye into the lumbar CSF. Congenital malformations (especially aqueductal stenosis and Dandy-Walker syndrome with cystic dilation of the fourth ventricle) and mass lesions (e.g., tumors, arteriovenous malformations) can cause noncommunicating hydrocephalus.

Hydrocephalus *ex vacuo* describes increases in CSF volume without increased CSF pressure, which is seen in conditions of reduced cerebral tissue (e.g., malformation, atrophy).

37. What is the normal growth rate of head circumference during the first year of life?

Head circumference at birth is about 34 to 35 cm for the term infant. The head circumference normally grows by 2 cm/month for the first 3 months of life, 1 cm/month for months 4 to 6, and 0.5 cm/month up to 1 year of life. The measurement of head circumference should be part of the examination of any child and should be plotted at every visit. The head circumference represents brain growth, but it is also influenced by hydrocephalus and subdural or epidural fluid collections.

38. What are the complications of ventricular shunts?

Ventricular shunts drain CSF from the ventricles in patients whose normal outflow or absorption has been blocked. The fluid may be drained to a variety of different locations, including the peritoneum, kidney, or cardiac atrium. Shunts draining CSF have remarkably improved the outcome of children with hydrocephalus, but they are subject to obstruction, infection, or mechanical malfunction. Shunt malfunctions present with signs of increased ICP. Children with shunt infections may have a low-grade fever, as well as signs of increased ICP. Because it is impossible to know the compliance properties of the ventricular system, children with shunt malfunction or infection are at risk for sudden, catastrophic decompensation. Children suspected of having shunt malfunctions or infection require urgent attention, and they should be closely observed until the shunt has been fully evaluated.

Rogers EA, Kimia A, Madsen JR, et al: Predictors of ventricular shunt infection among children presenting to a pediatric emergency department, *Pediatr Emerg Care* 28:405–409, 2012.
Piatt JH Jr, Garton HJL: Clinical diagnosis of ventriculoperitoneal shunt failure among children with hydrocephalus, *Pediatr Emerg Care* 24:210–210, 2008.

39. What are the characteristic features of idiopathic intracranial hypertension?

Idiopathic intracranial hypertension consists of increased ICP in the absence of a demonstrable mass lesion and with a normal CSF formula. The condition was formerly called *pseudotumor cerebri* or *benign intracranial hypertension*. The term *"benign"* has been de-emphasized because the problem has the potential to cause significant visual loss and to disrupt normal activities of daily living. Characteristic features include the following:

- Headache, fatigue, vomiting, anorexia, stiff neck, and diplopia from increased ICP
- Normal neurologic examination except for papilledema or a third- or sixth-nerve palsy
- Visual field constriction (usually nasal field) and enlargement of the blind spot on confrontational testing
- Normal computed tomography scan, except sometimes for small ventricles
- Normal CSF profile with the exception of an elevated opening pressure >250 mm H_2O

Glatstein MM, Oren A, Amarilyio G, et al: Clinical characterization of idiopathic intracranial hypertension in children presenting to the emergency department: the experience of a large tertiary care pediatric hospital, *Pediatr Emerg Care* 31:6–9, 2015.
Krishnakumar D, Pickard JD, Czosnyka Z, et al: Idiopathic intracranial hypertension in childhood: pitfalls in diagnosis, *Dev Med Child Neurol* 56:749–755, 2014.

40. What causes idiopathic intracranial hypertension?

Although there are multiple possible causes, more than 90% of cases are idiopathic. Among the reported causes are the following:

- **Drugs:** Tetracycline, nalidixic acid, nitrofurantoin, corticosteroids, excess vitamin A (polar bear liver)

- **Endocrine disorders:** Obesity, hyperthyroidism, Cushing syndrome, hypoparathyroidism
- **Thrombosis** of the dural venous sinuses as a result of head trauma, otitis media, mastoiditis, or obstruction of jugular veins in the superior vena cava syndrome

41. What treatment is recommended for severe cases of idiopathic intracranial hypertension?

Patients with sustained visual field loss or severe refractory headache are candidates for treatment. Specific treatment depends on the presence of an identifiable precipitant, which should be removed when possible. For example, the cessation of the offending medication (e.g., tetracycline) or weight reduction in obese patients is recommended. Nonspecific treatment includes the administration of acetazolamide, furosemide, or hydrochlorothiazide and, sometimes, corticosteroids. In severe cases, surgical intervention is available through installation of a lumboperitoneal shunt or optic nerve sheath decompression.

Rogers DL: A review of pediatric idiopathic intracranial hypertension, *Pediatr Clin North Am* 61:579–590, 2014.

CLINICAL ISSUES

42. What are the key questions in a neurologic evaluation?
    - **Localization** of the lesion (Where is the lesion?)
    - **Identification** of the lesion (What is the lesion?)
    - **Time course** of the disorder (Is it paroxysmal, acute, subacute, or chronic?)
    - Presence of any **regression** (Is there a worsening of previously learned skills?)
    - **Development** of the nervous system (Is it age appropriate?)

43. What are general rules that govern localization of a potential neurologic problem?

Localization starts with the neurologic examination. The questions that need to be addressed are (1) is the examination normal or abnormal, and if abnormal, (2) is the abnormality focal, multifocal, or diffuse?

A problem can occur anywhere along the neuron axis: cerebrum, cerebellum, brainstem, spinal cord, nerve, neuromuscular junction, and muscle.

- **Cerebrum:** May present with seizures, mental status changes, headaches, unilateral signs (such as hemiparesis)
- **Cerebellum:** May involve ataxia, disturbances of speech, disorders of limb movement, nystagmus
- **Brainstem:** Combination of cranial nerve abnormalities and long-tract signs (symmetric weakness with or without sensory changes)
- **Spinal cord:** Defined level of impairment with motor and/or sensory changes below involved area and normal examination above
- **Neuropathy:** Distal more than proximal weakness with or without sensory changes
- **Muscle disease:** Proximal more than distal weakness with decreased deep tendon reflexes and normal sensation

Goldstein JL: Pediatric neurology in the emergency department: localization followed by differential diagnosis, *Clin Pediatr Emerg Med* 9:87, 2008.

44. What distinguishes the pediatric neurologic examination?

Observation. The most useful information is often acquired by *watching the child move and play*. The level of interaction, creativity, and degree of sustained attention can be observed and are all important components of the mental status examination. By observing eye movements, response to sounds, the child's reaction to visual stimuli introduced into the peripheral visual field, and the symmetry of facial movements, most of the cranial nerves can be tested. Persistent asymmetries of spontaneous motor activity (e.g., consistently reaching across midline for an object) are reliable signs of weakness. Inspection of the seated posture and gait of the child provides an assessment of the cerebellum and cerebellar outflow pathways.

45. What are the advantages and disadvantages of various imaging procedures used in pediatric neurologic evaluation?
    - **Skull films** are useful for detection of fractures, lytic lesions, and widened sutures. They have poor sensitivity and specificity for intracranial pathology in the setting of trauma.

- **CT scan without contrast** is the best imaging technique for neurologic emergencies to screen a patient with significant head trauma for skull fractures, signs of herniation, or acute intracranial hemorrhage. It can also be used to screen for acute strokes and subarachnoid hemorrhages. Midline or ventricular shifts due to masses and cerebral edema or increased ICP can be noted. CT identifies bone clearly. This rapid study allows routine monitoring and is less expensive than MRI. There is a small but defined risk associated with radiation from CT scans.

- **CT scan with contrast** uses radiodense contrast material to allow better identification of disruptions in the blood-brain barrier or of highly vascular structures, significantly improving detection of tumors, edema, focal inflammation, hemangiomas, and arteriovenous malformations.

- **MRI without contrast** is the preferred modality for most nonurgent examinations. It defines structures of brain more precisely than CT, especially within spinal cord, posterior fossa, and cisterns. It is more effective for subtle hemorrhages (especially subacute and chronic) and for tumors or masses. Different tissue-specific relaxation constants, called T1 and T2, and proton density allow for better definition of white and gray matter. It also provides an image in three dimensions. Its longer testing time may require sedation. Also, monitoring patients is more difficult in closed units. There are no known biologic hazards from MRI, which measures the emission of radio waves released when protons return to a lower energy state after excitation within characteristic tissue environments. MRI is contraindicated in patients with metallic implants that are ferromagnetic; this may heat and damage tissue.

- **MRI with contrast** is helpful in defining brain metastases and distinguishing postoperative scarring from other pathology.

- **Magnetic resonance angiography (MRA)** is a special type of MRI that displays larger arteries and veins without the use of contrast. It is less invasive than traditional arteriograms, and it is useful in defining arterial stenosis and identifying intracranial hemangiomas, arteriovenous malformations, and vascular aneurysms.

- **MR spectroscopy (MRS)** allows for *in vivo* examination of some chemical constituents of the brain including N-acetylaspartate (NAA), a neuronal marker; choline; creatine; and lactate (a marker of energy metabolism).

- **Functional MRI (fMRI)** allows for *in vivo* anatomic localization of the motor and sensory cortex, the visual cortex, and components of expressive and receptive language.

- **Positron emission tomography (PET)** detects localized functional abnormalities using short half-life isotopes of carbon, nitrogen, oxygen, and fluorine. Labeled glucose ligands are useful in the evaluation of epileptic foci before surgery. These are areas of reduced cerebral glucose metabolism during interictal periods. Evaluation of specific isotopes, such as the uptake value of alpha-[11C] methyl-L-tryptophan (AMT) for the epileptic tuber in tuberous sclerosis, may be beneficial in certain disorders.

- **Single-photon emission computed tomography (SPECT)** uses gamma-ray emission of lipophilic isotopes in the measurement of cerebral blood flow and is also used in the study of refractory epilepsies.

- **Magnetoencephalography (MEG)** provides real-time measures of neuronal electrical activity (localization of epileptic focus).

Menkes JH, Moser FG, Maria BL: Neurologic examination of the child and infant. In Menkes JH, Sarnat HB, Maria BL, editors: *Child Neurology*, ed 7, Philadelphia, 2006, Lippincott Williams & Wilkins, pp 18–27.

46. A child presents with progressive left leg weakness and diplopia, especially when looking toward the left. Where is the lesion?

The described history, in combination with an examination showing upper motor neuron nerve dysfunction, long tract signs, brisk reflexes, upgoing toe (Babinski sign), and a contralateral third-nerve palsy (down and out), localizes the lesion to the **right pyramidal tract before the decussation** (crossing over) and involves a lesion of the **right third-nerve nucleus**. The progressive course suggests a slow-growing lesion, such as a pontine glioma.

47. A dilated and unreactive pupil indicates the compression of what structure?

The third cranial nerve. This may be the result of compression anywhere along the course of the nerve. Uncal herniation is a medial displacement of the uncus of the temporal lobe and may cause this sign.

48. Pinpoint pupils and respiratory changes indicate the compression of what structure?
Progressive central herniation of the brain downward through the foramen magnum causes compression of the **pons** and can produce this finding.

49. How does the presentation of stroke differ between infants and older children?
Infants usually have a seizure, whereas older children have acute hemiplegia. Neonates almost always present with focal seizures.

Calder K, Kokorowski P, Tran T, Henderson S: Emergency department presentation of stroke, *Pediatr Emerg Care* 19:320–328, 2003.
Children's Hemiplegia and Stroke Association: www.chasa.org. Accessed on March 5, 2015.
Pediatric Stroke Network: www.pediatricstrokenetwork.com. Accessed on March 11, 2015.

50. What is the differential diagnosis of stroke in children?
Cerebrovascular disease, or *stroke*, can be the result of primary vascular disease, bleeding disorder (hemorrhagic stroke), or a variety of secondary problems that lead to thrombotic or embolic occlusions (most commonly of the middle cerebral artery). Diagnostic possibilities include the following:
- **Cardioembolic:** Cyanotic congenital heart disease, atrial myxoma, endocarditis, rheumatic or other valvular heart disease
- **Hematologic:** Hemoglobinopathies (especially sickle cell disease), hypercoagulable states (antithrombin III deficiency, protein C or S deficiency), hyperviscosity (leukemia, hyperproteinemia, thrombocytosis), coagulation disorders (lupus-associated antibodies, hemophilia, thrombocytopenia, factor V abnormalities, hyperhomocysteinemia)
- **Circulatory:** Vasculitis (infectious or inflammatory), occlusive (homocystinuria, arteriosclerosis, fibromuscular dysplasia of the internal carotid artery, posttraumatic carotid scarring), carotid or vertebral artery dissection, moyamoya disease, atrioventricular malformation with steal syndrome, anomalous circulation, posttraumatic air embolism, arterial aneurysm, hemiplegic migraine
- **Metabolic:** Mitochondrial disease

Gumer LB, Del Vecchio M, Aronoff S: Strokes in children: a systematic review, *Pediatr Emerg Care* 30:660–664, 2014.
Freundlich CL, Cervantes-Arsianian AM, Dorfman DH: Pediatric stroke, *Emerg Med Clin North Am* 30:805–828, 2012.

51. What is the derivation of "moyamoya" in moyamoya disease?
Moyamoya, which is Japanese for "puff of smoke," refers to the cerebral angiographic appearance of patients with this primary, vascular disease that results in stenosis of the arteries of the circle of Willis and carotid arteries, resulting in prominent arterial collateral circulation. It occurs in a wide variety of conditions, such as neurofibromatosis type 1, sickle cell disease, Down syndrome, and tuberous sclerosis, in addition to the idiopathic, likely genetic, vasculopathy that is endemic in Japan. Because it is a chronic condition, fine vascular collaterals can develop, and it is these collaterals that create the "puff of smoke" appearance on angiography (Fig. 13-2).

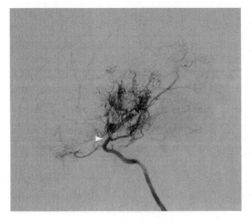

Figure 13-2. Injection of the internal carotid artery (ICA) demonstrates findings consistent with moyamoya disease: stenosis of the distal ICA *(arrowhead)*, diminished filling of the middle and anterior cerebral artery branches, and the proliferation of collateral vessels, the "puff of smoke" finding. *(From Winn HR, editor:* Youmans Neurological Surgery, *ed 6. Philadelphia, 2011, Saunders Elsevier, p 2145.)*

Patients with moyamoya present with transient ischemic attacks, ischemic strokes, and seizures, although in children, the predominant manifestation is ischemia.

Kleinloog R, Regli L, Rinkel GJ, Klijn CJ: Regional differences in incidence and patient characteristics of moyamoya disease, a systematic review, *J Neurol Neurosurg Psychiatry* 83:531–536, 2012.
Scott RM, Smith ER: Moyamoya disease and moyamoya syndrome, *N Engl J Med* 360:1226–1237, 2009.

52. A child who develops weakness, incontinence, and ataxia 10 days after a bout of influenza likely has what diagnosis?

Acute disseminated encephalomyelitis (ADEM) is thought to be a postinfectious or parainfectious process that is targeted against central myelin. Any portion of the white matter may be affected. Multiple lesions with a perivenular lymphocytic and mononuclear cell infiltration and demyelination are seen on pathologic examination. ADEM has been associated with mumps, measles, rubella, varicella-zoster, influenza, parainfluenza, mononucleosis, and some immunizations. An associated transverse myelitis may be acute (developing over hours) or subacute (developing over 1 to 2 weeks), with both motor and sensory tract involvement. Bladder and bowel dysfunction are often early and severe. CSF examination shows a mild increase of pressure and up to 250 cells/mm^3, with a predominance of lymphocytes. The MRI shows an increased T2 signal intensity. Prognosis, particularly with the use of intravenous corticosteroids, is generally good.

53. In patients with acute injury to the brain, what two types of edema may occur?

- **Vasogenic edema** results from increased permeability of the capillary endothelium with resulting exudation. It is more marked in cerebral white matter and occurs as a result of inflammation (meningitis and abscess), focal processes (hemorrhage, infarct, or tumor), vessel pathology, or lead or hypertensive encephalopathy. On cranial CT scan, vasogenic edema shows up best with the administration of contrast.

- **Cytotoxic edema** results from the rapid swelling of cells, especially astrocytes, and also from neurons and endothelial cells as a result of dysfunction of the membranes and ionic pumps from energy failure, which may lead to cellular death. Hypoxia caused by cardiac arrest, hypoxic-ischemic encephalopathy (HIE), various toxins, severe infections, status epilepticus, infarct, or increased ICP is also a possible cause.

54. What are the treatments for increased ICP?

- **Hyperventilation:** The usual goal is to lower the Pco$_2$ to 25 to 30 mm. This causes vasoconstriction, which decreases the intracranial vascular volume.

- **Fluid restriction, osmotic diuretics,** and **hypertonic mannitol solution** all work to shrink brain water content, provided there is an intact blood-brain barrier (none of these are evidence-based for newborn infants).

- **Head elevation** in a midline position to 30 degrees maximizes venous return. Head elevation may worsen ICP in the presence of hypovolemia.

- **External ventricular drain** (EVD) is sometimes placed, both to monitor pressure and to allow for a minimal amount of CSF withdrawal. An EVD may typically be used with intraventricular hemorrhage.

- **Normalization of physiologic parameters:** It is important to avoid significant hypotension, hypoxia, hypoglycemia, and hyperthermia.

55. How is brain death defined?

Brain death is defined by an irreversible absence of cortical and midbrain activity. Determination of brain death in term newborns, infants, and children is a clinical diagnosis based on the absence of neurologic function with a known irreversible cause of coma. Spinal cord, peripheral nerve, or reflex muscular activity may persist despite brain death. Decorticate or decerebrate posturing, however, is inconsistent with brain death. The examination must remain unchanged over time. Other countries have defined brain death as the absence of brainstem function alone, but in the United States, the absence of cortical function also must be demonstrated. The clinical hallmark of brain death is deep, unremitting, unresponsive coma.

De Georgia MA: History of brain death as death: 1968 to the present, *J Crit Care* 29:673–678, 2014.
Banasiak KJ, Lister G: Brain death in children, *Curr Opin Pediatr* 15:288–293, 2003.

56. How is the diagnosis of brain death in children made?

Patients with suspected brain death should be observed and tested on two separate occasions (including neurologic exam and apnea testing) over 12 to 24 hours for the following:

- Unresponsive coma and the absence of eye opening, extraocular movements, vocalizations, or other cerebral-generated activity
- The complete absence of brainstem function, including nonresponsive, midposition, or fully dilated pupils; no spontaneous or reflexive eye movements on oculovestibular testing ("doll's eyes" and calorics); no bulbar muscle function (i.e., corneal, gag, cough, sucking, and rooting reflexes); and no respirations on apnea testing
- Apnea testing with a rise of arterial P_{CO_2} at least 20 mm Hg above baseline and ≥ 60 mm Hg overall with no respiratory effort
- Ancillary testing (EEG and radionuclide cerebral blood flow) is not required and should not be used as a substitute, but may be used to supplement the neurologic examination and apnea testing.

Nakagawa TA, Ashwal S, Mathur M, et al: Clinical report—Guidelines for the determination of brain death in infants and children: an update of the 1987 Task Force recommendations, *Pediatrics* 128:e720–e740, 2011.

57. Compare the persistent vegetative state with the minimally conscious state.

- The **persistent vegetative state** is "a form of eyes-open permanent unconsciousness in which the patient has periods of wakefulness and physiologic sleep/wake cycles, but at no time is the patient aware of himself or herself or the environment." If this state persists for more than 3 months in children, the long-term outlook is grim.
- The **minimally conscious state** occurs on emergence from the persistent vegetative state, and a patient must demonstrate a reproducible action in one or more of four types of behavior: (1) simple command following; (2) gestural or verbal "yes/no" responses; (3) intelligible verbalization; or (4) purposeful behaviors.

Hirschberg R, Giacino JT: The vegetative and minimally conscious states: diagnosis, prognosis and treatment, *Neurol Clin* 29:773–786, 2011.

58. What is the differential diagnosis of an intracranial bruit?

An *intracranial bruit* can be found in normal children and may be augmented by contralateral carotid compression. Disorders that may be associated with an intracranial bruit include vascular malformations and conditions characterized by increased cerebral blood flow:

- Fever
- Cerebral angioma
- Intracerebral tumors
- Thyrotoxicosis
- Cerebral aneurysm
- Any cause of increased ICP
- Anemia
- Cerebral arteriovenous malformations
- Meningitis
- Cardiac murmurs

Mace JW, Peters ER, Mathies AW Jr: Cranial bruits in purulent meningitis in childhood, *N Engl J Med* 278: 1420–1422, 1968.

59. In a previously normal child who develops acute ataxia, what are the two most common diagnoses?

- **Drug ingestion,** especially of AEDs, heavy metals, alcohol, and antihistamines, is a common diagnosis.
- **Acute postinfectious cerebellitis,** most commonly after varicella, is a diagnosis of exclusion if drug screening, CT or MRI, CSF evaluation, and other tests are negative.

Prasad M, Ong MT, Setty G, et al: 15 minute consult: The child with acute ataxia, *Arch Dis Child Educ Pract Ed* 98: 212–216, 2013.

60. **What are the causes of toe walking?**
    - CP (spastic diplegia)
    - Hereditary spastic paraplegia (HSP)
    - Muscular dystrophy
    - Spinal dysraphism
    - Hereditary or acquired polyneuropathies
    - Intraspinal and filum terminale tumor
    - Equinovarus deformity
    - Isolated congenital shortening of the Achilles tendon
    - Variation of normal in early stages of walking
    - Normal development pattern in some toddlers

Oetgen ME, Peden S: Idiopathic toe walking, *J Am Acad Orthop Surg* 20:292–300, 2012.

61. **What is the significance of a positive Babinski response?**
    Stimulation of the lateral aspect of the sole of the foot to the distal metatarsals may elicit an extensor plantar response (i.e., dorsiflexion of the big toe), known as a positive Babinski response or sign. Its presence can be normal up to 12 months of age. When it persists after this age, it can be a sign of disturbed pyramidal tract function. The stimulus elicits a number of sensory pathways with competing functions (including grip and withdrawal) and is somewhat dependent on the state of the infant and the examiner's technique. Its value as a localizing sign in the neonate is more controversial, but a consistent asymmetry is abnormal.

62. **A 7-year-old child with progressive ataxia, kyphoscoliosis, nystagmus, pes cavus (high arch), and an abnormal electrocardiogram (ECG) likely has what diagnosis?**
    Friedreich ataxia. This heredodegenerative disease is an autosomal recessive disorder with childhood onset of gait ataxia, absent tendon reflexes, and extensor plantar responses. The spinal cord shows degeneration and sclerosis of the spinocerebellar tracts, the posterior column, and the corticospinal tracts. The condition is rare. The gene for Friedreich ataxia has been mapped to chromosome 9q13, contains a trinucleotide repeating sequence (GAA), and encodes for a protein called frataxin. A deficiency of frataxin leads to the accumulation of iron in the mitochondria and to oxidative stress, which leads to cell death.

Anheim M, Tranchant C, Koenig M: The autosomal recessive cerebellar ataxias, *N Engl J Med* 366:636–646, 2012.
Alper G, Narayanan V: Friedreich's ataxia, *Pediatr Neurol* 28:335–341, 2003.

63. **What clinical features help distinguish peripheral from central vertigo?**
    Peripheral vertigo implies dysfunction of the labyrinth or vestibular nerve, whereas *central vertigo* is associated with abnormalities of the brainstem or temporal lobe.
    Peripheral
    - Hearing loss, tinnitus, and otalgia may be associated.
    - Past pointing and falling in the direction of unilateral disease occur.
    - In bilateral disease, ataxia occurs with the eyes closed.
    - Vestibular and positional nystagmuses are present.
    Central
    - Cerebellar and cranial nerve dysfunction are frequently associated.
    - No hearing loss is present.
    - An alteration of consciousness may be associated.
    - Vertigo is a common symptom with migraine.

Fenichel GM: *Clinical Pediatric Neurology: A Signs and Symptoms Approach*, ed 6. Philadelphia, 2009, Elsevier, p 365.

64. **In what settings is hyperacusis noted?**
    Hyperacusis, or increased sensitivity to sound, is found in patients with injury to the facial nerve (CN VII), which innervates the stapedius muscle, or in those with injury to the trigeminal nerve (CN V), which innervates the tensor tympani muscle. Exaggerated startle response to sound or vibration occurs in patients with lysosomal storage diseases (e.g., sphingolipidoses such as Tay-Sachs disease, GM_1

gangliosidosis, and Sandhoff disease), Williams syndrome, hyperkalemia, tetanus, and strychnine poisoning.

65. What is the most common cause of neonatal asymmetric crying facies?

In this entity with an incidence of approximately 1 per 160 live births, one side of the lower lip depresses during crying (on the normal side), and the other does not (Fig. 13-3). Often misdiagnosed as a facial nerve palsy resulting from forceps delivery, the most common cause is **congenital absence or hypoplasia of the depressor anguli oris muscle** of the lower lip. Although it is usually an isolated finding in most cases, the condition can be associated with 22q11.2 deletion syndrome and other congenital malformations, especially of the cardiovascular system.

Pasick C, McDonald-McGinn DM, Simbolon C, et al: Asymmetric crying facies in the 22q11.2 deletion syndrome: implications for future screening, *Clin Pediatr* 52:1144–1148, 2013.

Sapin SO, Miller AA, Bass HN: Neonatal asymmetric crying facies: a new look at an old problem, *Clin Pediatr* 44:109–119, 2005.

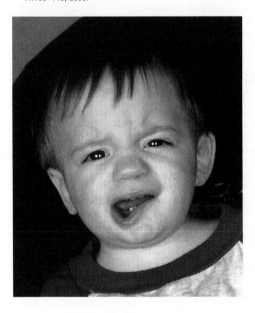

Figure 13-3. Asymmetric crying facies. *(From Terzis JK, Anesti K: Developmental facial paralysis: a review, J Plast Reconst Aesthet Surg 64:1318–1333, 2011, p 1324.)*

66. What are the common causes of peripheral seventh-nerve palsy?

Facial weakness caused by a lesion of the facial nerve (cranial nerve VII) is common. The facial weakness involves both the upper and lower face and affects both emotional and volitional facial movements. Any part of the nerve can be disturbed: the nucleus itself, the axon as it passes through the pons, or the peripheral portion of the nerve. A seventh-nerve palsy is either central or peripheral in location. Etiologies include the following:

- Trauma
- Developmental hypoplasia or aplasia, including the Möbius anomaly
- Bell palsy (usually idiopathic, but may follow nonspecific viral infections)
- Infections, including Ramsay Hunt syndrome (herpes zoster invasion of the geniculate ganglion producing herpetic vesicles behind the ear and painful paralysis of the facial nerve); Lyme disease; local invasion from suppurative mastoiditis or otitis media; mumps, varicella, Epstein-Barr virus, cytomegalovirus, rubella, human immunodeficiency virus, or enterovirus neuritis; sequelae of bacterial meningitis; and parotid gland infection, inflammation, or tumor
- Guillain-Barré syndrome
- Tumor of the brainstem or cerebellar pontine angle tumors
- Inflammatory disorders such as sarcoidosis

67. **How is *peripheral* seventh-nerve palsy distinguished from *central* seventh-nerve palsy?**

    The patient with a suspected palsy is asked to wrinkle the forehead, raise the eyebrows, and close the eyes tightly. In *peripheral* seventh-nerve palsy, no forehead furrows are noted, and the affected eye does not open as wide as the unaffected eye. In *central* seventh-nerve palsy, forehead furrowing and relatively good eye opening occur because the cells of the facial nucleus that innervate the upper face receive bilateral innervation from fibers from both cerebral hemispheres. Lower facial muscles are innervated from only the single contralateral cerebral hemisphere.

    Gilden DH: Bell's palsy, *N Engl J Med* 351:1323–1331, 2004.

68. **During recovery from Bell palsy, why do the eyes water at mealtime?**

    These are **crocodile tears**. The facial nerve supplies autonomic motor function to the lacrimal and salivary glands. Because of aberrant reinnervation during the course of healing from a facial nerve palsy, tasting a meal can trigger tearing rather than salivation. Folklore has it that crocodiles feel compassion for their victims and weep while munching. This is called synkinesis, which may also involve the other muscles of the facial nerve or may be congenital.

69. **When are "doll's eyes" movements considered normal or abnormal?**

    The *oculovestibular reflex* (also called *oculocephalic, proprioceptive head-turning reflex*, or *doll's eyes reflex*) is used most commonly as a test of brainstem function. The patient's eyelids are held open while the head is briskly rotated from side to side. A positive response is contraversive conjugate eye deviation (i.e., as the head rotates to the right, both eyes deviate to the left). Doll's eyes movements are interpreted as follows:

    - In healthy awake newborn infants (who cannot inhibit or override the reflex with willful eye movements), the reflex is easy to elicit and is a normal finding. It can be used to test the range of the extraocular movements of infants during the first weeks of life.
    - In healthy, awake, mature individuals, normal vision overrides the reflex, which is thus normally absent, and so the eyes follow the head turning.
    - In a patient in a coma with preserved brainstem function, the depressed cortex does not override the reflex, and doll's eyes movements occur in rapid head rotation. Indeed, the purpose of eliciting this reflex in the comatose patient is to demonstrate that the brainstem still functions normally.
    - In a patient in a coma with brainstem damage, the neural circuits that carry out the reflex are impaired, and the reflex is abolished.

70. **How are cold calorics done?**

    As a test of brainstem function in an obtunded or comatose individual, 5 mL of ice-cold water is placed in the external ear canal (after ensuring the integrity of the tympanic membrane), with the head elevated at 30 degrees. A normal response occurs with deviation of the eyes to the side in which the water was placed. No response indicates severe dysfunction of the brainstem and the medial longitudinal fasciculus. If done in the waking state, ipsilateral deviation occurs with nystagmus in the opposite direction.

71. **What causes pinpoint pupils?**

    Pupillary size represents a dynamic balance between the constricting influence of the third nerve (representing the parasympathetic autonomic nervous system) and the dilating influence of the ciliary nerve (which conducts fibers of the sympathetic nervous system). Pinpoint pupils indicate that the constricting influence of the third cranial nerve is not balanced by opposing sympathetic dilation. Possible etiologies include the following:

    - **Structural lesion in the pons** through which the sympathetic pathways descend (most commonly, hemorrhage)
    - **Opiates,** such as heroin or morphine
    - **Other agents,** including propoxyphene, organophosphates, carbamate insecticides, barbiturates, clonidine, meprobamate, pilocarpine eyedrops, and mushroom or nutmeg poisoning

72. **What is the differential diagnosis of ptosis?**

    Ptosis is the downward displacement of the upper eyelid as a result of dysfunction of the muscles that elevate the eyelid. A drooping eyelid may represent pseudoptosis caused by swelling of the eyelid as a result of local edema or active blepharospasm. True ptosis results from weakness of the eyelid muscles or interruption of its nerve supply. Etiologies include the following:

- **Muscular:** Congenital ptosis, which may occur alone or in the setting of Turner or Smith-Lemli-Opitz syndrome, myasthenia gravis (associated with marked daytime fluctuation), botulism, or some muscular dystrophies
- **Neurologic:** Horner syndrome, which results from the interruption of the sympathetic supply to Müller smooth eyelid muscle, and third-nerve palsy, which innervates the levator palpebral muscle; brainstem or orbital tumor (concerning if blurred vision also present)

73. **What does the Marcus Gunn pupil detect?**

    An **afferent pupillary defect (APD)**. The pupils are normally equal in size (except for patients with physiologic anisocoria) as a result of the consensual light reflex: light entering either eye produces the same-strength "signal" for the constriction of both the stimulated and nonstimulated pupil. Some diseases of the maculae or optic nerves affect one side more than the other, such as multiple sclerosis or optic neuritis. For example, a meningioma may develop on one optic nerve sheath. As a result of unilateral or asymmetric optic nerve dysfunction, a Marcus Gunn pupil may result.

74. **How is the swinging flashlight test done to detect a Marcus Gunn pupil?**

    - The patient is examined in a dim room, and fixation is directed to a distant target. This permits maximal pupillary dilation because of a lack of direct light and accommodation reflexes.
    - Light presented to the "good" eye produces the equal constriction of both pupils. A flashlight is swung briskly over the bridge of the nose to the eye with the "defective" optic nerve. The abnormal pupil remains momentarily constricted from the lingering effects of the consensual light response. However, the impaired eye with its reduced pupillomotor signal soon escapes the consensual reflex and actually dilates, despite being directly stimulated with light. The pupil that paradoxically dilates to direct light stimulation displays the afferent defect.

EPILEPSY

75. **What is epilepsy?**

    Epilepsy describes a syndrome of recurrent, unprovoked seizures, typically two or more, not the result of fever or a systemic medical condition. It is derived from the Greek verb *epilepsia* meaning "to seize upon" or "to take hold of." The early Greeks referred to it as the sacred disease, but Hippocrates debunked this notion and argued from clinical evidence that it arose from the brain. Epilepsy is not an entity or even a syndrome but rather a symptom complex arising from disordered brain function that itself may be the result of a variety of pathologic processes.

Chang BS, Lowenstein DH: Epilepsy, *N Engl J Med* 349:1257–1266, 2003.
American Epilepsy Society: www.aesnet.org. Accessed on March 14, 2015.
Epilepsy Foundation: www.epilepsy.com. Accessed on March 5, 2015.

76. **What is the long-term outcome for children with epilepsy?**

    There are many different causes of epilepsy, and, in large part, the outcome relates to the underlying etiology. Children with idiopathic or genetically determined epilepsy have the best prognosis, whereas children with antecedent neurologic abnormalities fare less well. Nearly 75% of children will enter into a sustained remission 3 to 5 years after the onset of their epilepsy. There is no evidence that antiepileptic medications as they are currently used in clinical practice are neuroprotective or that they alter the long-term outcome of patients. Although there is a favorable prognosis for the remission of seizures, children with epilepsy are at an increased risk for having other long-term comorbidities, including difficulties achieving social, educational, and vocational goals. Treatment with antiepileptic medications is one important part of the management of the child, but other critical aspects of the physician–patient interaction, including educating, counseling, and advocacy, are equally important.

77. **How often are EEGs abnormal in healthy children?**

    About 10% of "normal" children have mild, nonspecific abnormalities in background activity. About 2% to 3% of healthy children have unexpected incidental epileptiform (i.e., spikes or sharp wave) patterns. Some may have heritable, familial EEG abnormalities without a clinical seizure disorder (e.g., centrotemporal spikes seen in benign seizure-susceptibility syndromes such as rolandic epilepsy). In patients with migraines, the EEG may frequently have epileptiform features.

78. **Should an EEG be done on all children who have a first afebrile seizure?**
This is a major controversial issue. Of new-onset seizures in children, about one-third do not involve fever. The American Academy of Neurology has recommended that all children with a first seizure without fever undergo an EEG in an effort to better classify the epilepsy syndrome. Others argue that the quantity of expected information from obtaining EEGs for all cases is too low to affect treatment recommendations in most patients. They suggest that a selective approach to EEG use should be pursued, particularly for children with a seizure of focal onset, for children younger than 1 year, and for any child with unexplained cognitive or motor dysfunction or abnormalities on neurologic examination.

Khan A, Baheerathan A: Electroencephalogram after first unprovoked seizure in children: Routine, unnecessary or case specific, *J Pediatr Neurosci* 8:1–4, 2013.
Hirtz D, Ashwal S, Berg A, et al: Practice parameter: evaluating a first nonfebrile seizure in children. Report of the Quality Standards Subcommittee of the American Academy of Neurology, the Child Neurology Society, and the American Epilepsy Society, *Neurology* 55:616–623, 2000.

79. **In a patient with a suspected seizure disorder, but a normal EEG, how can the sensitivity of the EEG be increased?**
    - Repeat the EEG.
    - Obtain following sleep deprivation.
    - Use hyperventilation and photic stimulation (e.g., strobe lights).
    - Obtain a continuous video EEG (>24 hours).

80. **Which types of epilepsy are characterized by specific EEG findings?**
    - **Rolandic epilepsy:** Bicentral spikes (only during sleep in 30%); "midtemporal spikes" is a misnomer, related to the positioning of the EEG electrodes in the temporal regions.
    - **Benign epilepsy with occipital focus:** Continuous unilateral or bilateral occipital high-voltage spike waves
    - **Panayiotopoulos syndrome:** Also known as early-onset occipital epilepsy; abnormal spikes in one or both occipital lobes.
    - **Absence epilepsy:** Characteristic 3-Hz spike-wave pattern
    - **Juvenile absence epilepsy:** Characteristic fast spike-wave pattern (>3 Hz)
    - **Juvenile myoclonic epilepsy:** Fast spikes and polyspike-wave patterns
    - **Infantile spasms:** Hypsarrhythmia, a markedly disorganized pattern
    - **Lennox-Gastaut syndrome:** Slow spike-wave forms at <3-Hz frequency
    - **Landau-Kleffner syndrome:** Sleep activated spike-wave discharges, may be in pattern of electrical status epilepticus of sleep (ESES)

81. **Should all children with a new-onset afebrile, unprovoked generalized seizure have a CT or MRI evaluation?**
Although most adults with new-onset seizures should have a head imaging study (preferably MRI), the relatively high frequency of idiopathic seizure disorders in children often obviates a scan in those with generalized seizures, nonfocal EEGs, and normal neurologic examinations. Consider obtaining a cranial imaging study in the following situations:
    - Any seizure with focal components (other than mere eye deviation)
    - Newborns and young infants with seizures
    - Status epilepticus at any age
    - Focal slowing or focal paroxysmal activity on EEG

Weeke LC, Groenendaal F, Toet MC, et al: The aetiology of neonatal seizures and the diagnostic contribution of cerebral magnetic resonance imaging, *Dev Med Child Neurol* 57:248–256, 2015.
Hirtz D, Berg A, Bettis D, et al: Quality Standards Subcommittee of the American Academy of Neurology; Practice Committee of the Child Neurology Society: Practice parameter: treatment of the child with a first unprovoked seizure. Report of the Quality Standards Subcommittee of the American Academy of Neurology and the Practice Committee of the Child Neurology Society, *Neurology* 60:166–175, 2003.

82. **Which disorders commonly mimic epilepsy?**
Many conditions are characterized by the sudden onset of transient abnormal consciousness, awareness, reactivity, behavior, posture, tone, sensation, or autonomic function. Syncope, breath-holding spells, migraine, hypoglycemia, narcolepsy, cataplexy, sleep apnea, gastroesophageal reflux, and parasomnias (night terrors, sleep walking, sleep talking, nocturnal enuresis) feature an abrupt or "paroxysmal" alteration of brain function and suggest the possibility of epilepsy.

83. What are ways to distinguish psychogenic nonepileptic seizures (PNES) from epileptic seizures?

PNES consist of changes in behavior (including motor manifestations) or consciousness that are not accompanied by electrophysiological changes. PNES were formerly called pseudoseizures or hysterical seizures, but these terms are now discouraged. Features that help identify PNES include:

History: Patient is more likely to have a history of psychiatric problems including depression, anxiety, posttraumatic stress disorder and somatoform disorder. Common precipitating factors: school-related difficulties and interpersonal conflict.

Clinical: PNES are usually longer than 2 minutes, eyes are forcefully closed (compared to eyes typically open in epileptic seizures), motor activity is waxing and waning, vocalizations are commonly present (uncommon in epileptic seizures), incontinence is less common, awakening and reorientation are more rapid than epileptic seizures, and recall of event is more common in PNES than with an epileptic seizure.

Studies: Video-EEG (most reliable to rule-out epileptic seizures); ambulatory EEG; prolactin levels (typically elevated 15-20 minutes after an epileptic seizure but not after PNES).

Reilly C, Menlove L, Fenton V, Das KB: Pyschogenic nonepileptic seizures in children: a review, *Epilepsia* 54:1715–1724, 2013.
Avbersek A, Sisodiya S: Does the primary literature provide support for clinical signs used to distinguish psychogenic nonepileptic seizures from epileptic seizures? *J Neurol Neurosurg Psychiatry* 81:719–725, 2010.
Korff CM, Nordlii DR Jr: Paroxysmal events in infants: persistent eye closure makes seizures unlikely, *Pediatrics* 116: e485–e486, 2005.

84. What are the categories of seizures in children?

The syndrome classification as codified in the International Classification of Epileptic Seizures by the International League Against Epilepsy (ILAE) distinguishes seizures on the basis of *type* rather than *etiology* (Table 13-2). The classification was revised in 2010 with an elimination of terms previously used for focal seizures such as "simple partial," "complex partial," and "partial seizures secondarily generalized" as being too imprecise. The current classification includes *generalized seizures*, which occur in and rapidly engage bilaterally distributed networks while *focal seizures* are more limited to one hemisphere, either discretely localized or more widely distributed in that hemisphere. While the classification for generalized seizures was straightforward, the ILAE believed that there was inadequate information to create a scientific classification for focal seizures, but that focal seizures should be described according to their manifestations (e.g., dyscognitive with impairment of consciousness/awareness, focal motor).

Table 13-2. International League Against Epilepsy Classification of Seizures

Generalized
Tonic-clonic (in any combination)
Absence
Typical
Atypical
Absence with special features
Myoclonic absence
Eyelid myoclonic
Myoclonic
Myoclonic
Myoclonic atonic
Myoclonic tonic
Clonic
Tonic
Atonic
Focal seizures
Unknown
Epileptic spasms (infantile spasms)

Adopted from Berg AT, Berkovic SF, Brodie MJ, et al: Revised terminology and concepts for organization of seizures and epilepsies: Report of the ILAE Commission on Classification and Terminology, 2005-2009, Epilepsia 51:678, 2010.

Additionally, previous terminology by the ILAE categorized the causes of seizures into *symptomatic* (due to a known disorder of the CNS), *cryptogenic* (due to a hidden or occult cause) or *idiopathic* (no known cause except a possible hereditary predisposition). This terminology was believed to be confusing and was eliminated. New etiologic categories involve three groups: *genetic, structural/metabolic,* and *unknown.*

Berg AT, Berkovic SF, Brodie MJ, et al: Revised terminology and concepts for organization of seizures and epilepsies: Report of the ILAE Commission on Classification and Terminology, 2005-2009, *Epilepsia* 51:676–685, 2010.

85. **What are structural and metabolic causes of seizures?**
See Table 13-3.

Table 13-3. Structural and Metabolic Causes of Seizures

Fever
- Simple febrile seizures
- Complicated febrile seizures

Trauma
- Impact seizures
- Early posttraumatic seizures
- Late posttraumatic seizures

Hypoxia
- Complicated breath-holding spells
- Hypoxic seizures

Metabolic
- Acquired metabolic disorders
- Neurologic effects of systemic disease
- Inborn errors of metabolism

Toxins
- Drugs
- Drug withdrawal
- Biologic toxins

Stroke
- Ischemic stroke
- Embolic stroke
- Hemorrhagic stroke

Intracranial Hemorrhage
- Subdural hemorrhage
- Subarachnoid hemorrhage
- Intracerebral hemorrhage

CNS Malformation
- Cerebral atrophy
- Cortical dysplasia
- Microcephaly

CNS = Central nervous system.
Adapted from Evans OB: Symptomatic seizures, Pediatr Ann *28:231–237, 1999.*

86. **If a previously normal child has an afebrile, generalized tonic-clonic seizure, what should parents be told about the risk for recurrence?**
Studies indicate that the recurrence rate is between 25% and 50%. The EEG is an important predictor of recurrence. A subsequent normal EEG reduces the 5-year recurrence risk to 25%. Occurrence of the seizure during sleep increases the risk to 50%. Half of recurrences will occur during the first 6 months after the first seizure; two thirds will occurs within 1 year, and 90% or more will have occurred within

2 years. The child's age at the time of the first seizure and the duration of the seizure do not affect the recurrence risk.

Shinnar S, Berg AT, Moshe SL, et al: The risk of seizure recurrence after a first unprovoked afebrile seizure in childhood: an extended follow-up, *Pediatrics* 98:216–225, 1996.

87. **What are the most common inherited seizure or epilepsy syndromes?**
    - Febrile convulsions
    - Rolandic epilepsy, childhood absence epilepsy
    - Juvenile myoclonic epilepsy (of Janz)

88. **What are the clinical features of rolandic epilepsy?**
    Rolandic epilepsy is an idiopathic localization-related epilepsy that represents 10% to 15% of all childhood seizure disorders.
    - It begins in school-age children (4 to 13 years old) who are otherwise healthy and neurologically normal.
    - Seizures are idiopathic or familial (autosomal dominant inheritance with age-dependent penetrance).
    - Seizures may be simple or complex and partial or generalized. Classically, there is a history of one-sided facial paresthesias and twitching and drooling that may be followed by hemiclonic movements or hemitonic posturing. Consciousness is typically preserved. The seizures are primarily nocturnal and may secondarily generalize.
    - Often referred to as *benign* because the individual is developmentally normal, seizures are usually rare and nocturnal, and they most often resolve after puberty.
    - Many children may have one or only several seizures, so AED treatment is not mandatory, especially when seizures are nocturnal.
    - Treatment is indicated when seizures occur in the daytime (diurnal) or if escalating in frequency.

89. **What distinguishes typical and atypical absence seizures?**
    Typical absence
    - *EEG*: 3-Hz spike wave; may be activated by hyperventilation or intermittent photic stimulation
    - *Observations*: Abrupt onset and ending (typically 5 to 10 seconds)
    - *Simple subtype*: Unresponsiveness with no other associated features except minor movements (e.g., lip smacking or eyelid twitching)
    - *Complex subtype*: Unresponsiveness with more prolonged (>5 to 10 seconds) mild atonic, myoclonic, or tonic features or automatisms
    Atypical absence (most common in Lennox-Gastaut syndrome)
    - *EEG*: 2-Hz (or slower) spike wave
    - *Observations*: Gradual onset and ending; frequency is more cyclic; unresponsive with more prolonged and pronounced atonic, tonic, myoclonic, or tonic activity

90. **In a child who is suspected of having absence seizures, how can a seizure be elicited during an examination?**
    Hyperventilation for at least 3 minutes is a useful provocative maneuver to precipitate an absence seizure. Young patients may be coaxed into overbreathing by making a game of it. Hold a tissue paper or pinwheel in front of the child's mouth, and then instruct the patient to keep breathing fast enough to keep the tissue aloft or the pinwheel spinning.

91. **What percentage of patients with absence seizures also have occasional grand mal seizures?**
    About 30% to 50%; these may occur years later.

92. **What is the prognosis for children with absence epilepsy?**
    The prognosis for patients with childhood absence epilepsy has been studied prospectively, and nearly 90% of patients who have normal intelligence, normal neurologic examination, normal EEG background activity, no family history of convulsive epilepsy, and no history of tonic-clonic convulsions will have seizures that remit. Conversely, the complete absence of favorable factors is associated with a poor

prognosis for the cessation of seizures. It may be that absence seizures are expressed on a spectrum from typical childhood absence epilepsy (with the typical absence seizure that is genetic in origin to the Lennox-Gastaut syndrome) to the atypical absence seizure, which is symptomatic of brain injury.

93. **A teenager, like his father, develops brief, bilateral, intermittent jerking of his arms. What seizure disorder is he likely to have?**

Juvenile myoclonic epilepsy, which is also called *myoclonic epilepsy of Janz,* is a familial form of primary idiopathic generalized epilepsy that typically involves "fast" 3- to 5-Hz spike-wave discharges on EEG ("impulsive petit mal") and autosomal dominant inheritance. The distinctive clinical features of this type of epilepsy include morning myoclonic jerks, generalized tonic-clonic seizures upon awakening, normal intelligence, a family history of similar seizures, and onset between the ages of 8 and 20 years.

94. **What are myoclonic seizures?**

These seizures are characterized by rapid, bilateral, symmetric muscle contractions of short duration— "quick jerks." They may be isolated, or they may occur repetitively. Myoclonic seizures may be the sole manifestation of epilepsy, or more commonly, they may be associated with absence seizures or tonic-clonic seizures. By definition, a myoclonic seizure lasts less than 100 μsec.

KEY POINTS: EPILEPSY

1. Definition: Repeated, unprovoked seizures
2. Classified as localization-related: focal or generalized
3. Main etiologic categories: genetic, structural/metabolic, and unknown
4. Compared with older children with new-onset seizures, infants are more likely to have results from electroencephalogram (EEG) and neuroimaging that affect diagnosis and prognosis.
5. Proper classification of epilepsy syndromes provides guidance for treatment options and prognoses.

95. **What distinguishes atonic and akinetic seizures?**

An atonic seizure involves the sudden and usually complete loss of tone in the limb, neck, and trunk muscles. Muscle control is lost without warning, and the child may be seriously injured. This situation is often aggravated by the occurrence of one or more myoclonic jerks immediately before muscle tone is lost so that the fall is associated with an element of propulsion. Atonic seizures are particularly common in children with static encephalopathies, and they may prove refractory to therapy. In an **akinetic seizure,** movement is arrested without a significant loss of muscle tone; this is rare.

96. **Which seizure types constitute the "epileptic encephalopathies"?**

Epileptic encephalopathies constitute a group of diverse disorders that occur early in life with generalized or focal seizures resistant to pharmacology, persistent severe EEG abnormalities, and cognitive dysfunction with deterioration. The prototypical genetic epilepsy in this category is Dravet syndrome, also known as severe myoclonic epilepsy of infancy (SMEI), which is characterized by mutations in the sodium channel SCN1A gene. Other ion channel and non–ion-channel genetic defects are being identified. Other epileptic encephalopathies include Ohtahara syndrome, Lennox-Gastaut syndrome, Landau-Kleffner syndrome, and epileptic (infantile) spasms.

Nieh SE, Sherr EH: Epileptic encephalopathies: new genes and new pathways, *Neurotherapeutics* 11:796–806, 2014.

Covanis A: Epileptic encephalopathies (including severe epilepsy syndromes), *Epilepsia* 53(Suppl 4): 114–126, 2012.

97. **What is the classic triad of epileptic (infantile) spasms?**

Spasms, hypsarrhythmia, and developmental regression. Epileptic (infantile) spasms are also known as West syndrome. The condition is named for the physician who first described the condition in his own son in 1841.

98. **What characterizes hypsarrhythmia?**

The term means "mountainous slowing," and it describes the classic interictal EEG of epileptic (infantile) spasms that is characterized by extremely high-voltage (>300 μV), slow, and disorganized brain waves with multifocal spike activity. Hypsarrhythmia may either precede or follow the onset of epileptic spasms. This EEG configuration may appear first or most obviously in non–rapid eye movement sleep and confirms the clinical diagnosis of epileptic spasms.

It should be noted that the presence of hypsarrhythmia is not a prerequisite for epileptic spasms.

99. How commonly is a cause identified in epileptic spasms?

A cause can be identified in **up to 90%** of children with epileptic spasms, particularly in those who are symptomatic at the time of the initial seizure. Of identifiable causes, three-fourths are prenatal or perinatal, and one-fourth are postnatal. All patients with epileptic spasms should have detailed neuroimaging and metabolic and genetic studies. Causes, including some possible specific examples, include the following:

- **Prenatal and perinatal:** Neurocutaneous disorders (tuberous sclerosis), brain injury (HIE), intrauterine infection (cytomegalovirus), brain malformations (lissencephaly, agenesis of the corpus callosum), inborn metabolic errors (nonketotic hyperglycinemia, phenylketonuria, maple syrup urine disease, pyridoxine dependency)
- **Postnatal:** Infectious (herpes encephalitis), HIE, head trauma

100. What is the prognosis for infants with epileptic spasms?

Prognosis in large part depends on the underlying etiology and the clinical state at the time of the first seizure. In the group with an unknown cause (10% to 15%), development, neurologic examination, and imaging studies are usually normal at the onset. With adrenocorticotropic hormone (ACTH) treatment, up to 40% will have a complete or near-complete recovery with normal cognitive development. In the group with a known structural/metabolic cause (85% to 90%), neurologic deficits, developmental delays, or cranial abnormalities are typically present before the first seizure. In this group, complete or near-complete recovery is achieved by only 5% to 15%. Twenty-five to 50% will develop Lennox-Gastaut syndrome.

Regression may be seen before the onset of epileptic spasms, especially in visual or motor function.

Widjaja E, Go C, McCoy B, Snead OC: Neurodevelopmental outcome of infantile spasms: a systematic review and meta-analysis, *Epilepsy Res* 109:155–162, 2015.
Kivity S, Lerman P, Ariel R, et al: Long-term cognitive outcomes of a cohort of children with cryptogenic infantile spasms treated with high-dose adrenocorticotropic hormone, *Epilepsia* 45:255–262, 2004.

101. What is the treatment of choice for epileptic spasms?

Currently in the United States, most children with epileptic spasms are treated with ACTH as the first treatment option with positive response rate of approximately three-fourths of patients. Vigabatrin has been shown to be superior to ACTH for children with tuberous sclerosis with a 95% spasm cessation rate. Vigabatrin may cause visual field defects, including visual field constriction and retinal toxicity, which may increase with duration of treatment and mandates periodic assessment with electroretinograms. Vigabatrin may also cause abnormal enhancement or restricted diffusion on MRI of the deep gray matter (thalamus, basal ganglia, and brainstem), which is reversible after cessation of treatment.

Hsieh DT, Jennesson MM, Thiele EA: Epileptic spasms in tuberous sclerosis complex, *Epilepsy Res* 106:200–210, 2013.
Go CY, Mackay MT, Weiss SK, et al: Evidence-based guideline update: medical treatment of infantile spasms. Report of the Guideline Development Subcommittee of the American Academy of Neurology and the Practice Committee of the Child Neurology Society, *Neurology* 78:1974–1980, 2012.

102. What is the most likely diagnosis in a child of Ashkenazi descent with stimulus-sensitive seizures, cognitive deterioration, and a cherry-red spot?

The classic lysosomal lipid storage disorder presenting symptoms of a progressive encephalopathy during infancy is **Tay-Sachs disease**. The infantile forms of GM_2 gangliosidosis includes Tay-Sachs disease, which is caused by a deficiency of hexosaminidase A, and Sandhoff disease, which is caused by a deficiency of hexosaminidase A and B. Tay-Sachs is an autosomal recessive disorder that is localized to chromosome 15, with an incidence of 1 in 3900 in the Ashkenazi Jewish population of Eastern or Central European descent. The enzymatic defect leads to intraneuronal accumulation of GM_2 ganglioside. Normal development is seen until 4 to 6 months of age, when hypotonia and a loss of motor skills occur, with the subsequent development of spasticity, blindness, and macrocephaly. The classic cherry-red spot is present in the ocular fundi of more than 90% of patients (Fig. 13-4).

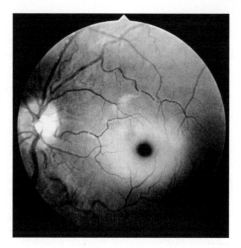

Figure 13-4. A cherry red spot in a patient with GM$_1$ gangliosidosis. Note the whitish ring of sphingolipid-laden ganglion cells surrounding the fovea. *(From Kleigman RM, Stanton BF, Schor NF, et al, editors: Nelson Textbook of Pediatrics, ed 19. Philadelphia, 2011, Elsevier Saunders, p 2072.)*

103. A patient with seizures, microcephaly, and a low CSF glucose but a normal serum glucose has what likely condition?

The **GLUT-1 deficiency syndrome,** previously referred to as the *glucose transporter protein deficiency syndrome*, was first described in 1991. The clinical phenotype is variable, but the child usually presents symptoms during the first years of life with seizures and delays of motor and mental development. Movement disorders, including dystonia, ataxia, myoclonus, and spasticity, are also seen. The head circumference decelerates during the first years of life. The diagnosis should be suspected if CSF reveals low glucose (and lactate) concentrations without evidence of inflammation, and serum blood sugars are normal. The ketogenic diet is the gold standard of treatment, although a modified Atkins diet has also been shown to be effective.

De Giorgis V, Vegglotti P: GLUT1 deficiency syndrome 2013: current state of the art, *Seizure* 10:803–811, 2013.
Pong AW, Geary BR, Engelstad KM, et al: Glucose transporter type 1 deficiency syndrome: epilepsy phenotypes and outcomes, *Epilepsia* 53: 1503–1510, 2012.

104. What is the clinical triad of the Lennox-Gastaut syndrome?

Lennox-Gastaut syndrome is characterized by **mental retardation, seizures** of various types, and disorganized **slow spike-wave activity** on an EEG. The seizures usually begin during the first 3 years of life and are characteristically severe and refractory to anticonvulsant drugs. Prognosis is poor, with more than 80% of children continuing to have seizures into adulthood.

Arzimanoglou A, French J, Blume WT, et al: Lennox-Gastaut syndrome: a consensus approach on diagnosis, assessment, management, and trial methodology, *Lancet Neurol* 8:82–93, 2009.

105. A 5-year-old with a history of normal language development who develops seizures and inattention to speech with severe regression of language skills has what likely condition?

Landau-Kleffner syndrome. First described in 1957, this is a condition of acquired epileptic aphasia with nocturnal EEG abnormalities, reduction in language function, and problems with attention. Despite the use of various AEDs and/or ACTH, recovery is often delayed, and communication problems persistent.

Caraballo RH, Cejas N, Chamorro N, et al: Landau-Kleffner syndrome: a study of 29 patients, *Seizure* 23:98–104, 2014.

106. How is status epilepticus defined?
- Because of uncertainty regarding at precisely what time morbidity ensues in the course of a prolonged seizure, there is a *variance* in definitional length regarding status epilepticus. In general, >30 minutes of continuous or sequential seizure activity has previously defined status epilepticus. The operational definition for status epilepticus, however, is 5 minutes, at which time a prolonged seizure is likely to become continuous, and thus treatment should be considered or started.
- Recurrent seizures without full recovery of consciousness between seizures.

107. Why is status epilepticus so dangerous?
With the onset of a seizure, catecholamine release and sympathetic discharge result in increased heart rate and blood pressure. Cerebral flow increases dramatically to compensate for the increased metabolic needs of the brain. With persistence of the seizure, compensatory mechanisms begin to fail. Respiratory acidosis and metabolic acidosis develop. Systemic blood pressure falls. ICP increases. The inability to meet the increased oxygen demands of the brain results in an intracranial switch to anaerobic metabolism with acidosis, increased CSF lactate, and cerebral edema. The prolonged electrical discharges by themselves may also cause neuronal damage, referred to as excitotoxicity.

Miskin C, Hasbani DM: Status epilepticus: immunologic and inflammatory mechanisms, *Semin Pediatr Neurol* 21: 221–225, 2014.

108. What should be done in the first 10 minutes for a child who presents with an ongoing seizure?
- **0 to 5 minutes:** Confirm the diagnosis. Maintain noninvasive airway protection by head positioning or oropharyngeal airway. Administer 100% nasal oxygen. Suction as needed. Obtain and frequently monitor vital signs using pulse oximetry and ECG. Establish an intravenous or intraosseous line. Obtain venous blood for laboratory determinations (e.g., glucose, serum chemistries, hematology studies, liver function studies, toxicology screen, culture, anticonvulsant levels if patient is a known epileptic). Administer antipyretics as indicated.
- **5 to 10 minutes:** If hypoglycemic (or if a rapid reagent strip for glucose testing is not available), administer 2 mL/kg of $D_{25}W$ or 5 mL/kg of $D_{10}W$. If IV/IO access is present, administer lorazepam, 0.1 mg/kg (max: 4 mg) IV/IO at 2 mg/min. If IV/IO access cannot be established, options include (1) diazepam: 2 to 5 years, 0.5 mg/kg; 6 to 11 years, 0.3 mg/kg; $\geq$ 12 years, 0.2 mg/kg (max: 20 mg); (2) midazolam: intranasal, 0.2 mg/kg (max: 10 mg); buccal, 0.5 mg/kg (max: 10 mg). Repeat lorazepam or one-half midazolam dose in 5 to 10 minutes if seizure persists.

Abend NS, Loddenkemper T: Pediatric status epilepticus management, *Curr Opin Pediatr* 26:668–674, 2014.

109. What is the most common cause of refractory seizures?
An **inadequate serum concentration of antiepileptic medication** is the most common cause of persistent seizures, but other causes should be considered:
- **Drug toxicity,** especially with phenytoin, may manifest by deteriorating seizure control.
- **Electrolyte disorders,** especially with an acute illness, may be causative.
- **Metabolic abnormalities,** particularly in patients with inborn errors of metabolism, such as a mitochondrial disorder, should be considered.
- **Medications** may have a paradoxic reaction and exacerbate certain types of seizures, particularly in children with mixed seizure disorders. For example, carbamazepine or phenytoin may control generalized tonic-clonic seizures in patients with juvenile myoclonic epilepsy, but may aggravate myoclonic and absence seizures.
- **Incorrect identification** of the epilepsy syndrome may be a cause. Partial seizures may masquerade as a generalized form of epilepsy in the very young child (bilateral symmetric tonic posturing may be seen in partial seizures). Conversely, generalized forms of epilepsy may first appear as partial seizures (severe infantile myoclonic epilepsy). Treatment based on an epilepsy syndrome rather than ictal semiology usually improves control in these circumstances.

110. What is the role of the ketogenic diet for the treatment of seizures?
The *ketogenic diet* is effective for the treatment of all seizure types, particularly in children with myoclonic forms of epilepsy. The diet involves supplying most calories through fats, with concurrent

limitation of carbohydrates and protein. The mechanism of seizure control is unclear, but it is perhaps related to a switch in the cerebral metabolism from the use of glucose to the use of β-hydroxybutyrate. After 24 hours of fasting, the child is placed on a high-fat diet in which the ratio of fats to carbohydrates and protein combined is 3:1 to 4:1. Anticonvulsant drugs may be reduced or eliminated entirely if the diet is effective. The regimen must be followed closely, and parents must understand the demands of close adherence to the diet. A skilled dietitian is instrumental for providing variety and palatability to the diet. It is important to recall that the diet may have adverse effects, including serious, potentially life-threatening complications such as hypoproteinemia, lipemia, and hemolytic anemia. Variants of the ketogenic diet include the modified Atkins diet and the low glycemic index. β-Hydroxybutyrate levels are used to assess the degree of acidosis (similar to a drug level).

Kossoff EH, Zupec-Kania BA, Rho JM: Ketogenic diets: an update for child neurologists, *J Child Neuro* 24:979–988, 2009.

111. **What is the role of the vagus nerve stimulator in seizure control?**
The *vagus nerve stimulator* (VNS) is a surgically implanted device that intermittently stimulates the left vagus nerve. Why this decreases seizure frequency is not well understood, although it causes alterations in epinephrine release and is thought to increase GABA levels in the brainstem. It is a palliative—not curative—procedure that has been performed in adults and children with intractable complex partial seizures or generalized tonic seizures that are not considered candidates for definitive surgical cure. The VNS has been placed in children as young as 2 to 3 years old.

Elijamel S: Mechanism of action and overview of vagus nerve stimulation technology, In Elijamel S, Slavin KV, editors: *Neurostimulation: Principles and Practice*, Oxford, 2013, Wiley Blackwell, pp 111–120.

112. **What should a teenager with epilepsy be told about the potential of obtaining a driver's license?**
State requirements vary regarding individuals with epilepsy and the right to drive. The most common requirement is a specified seizure-free period and submission of a physician's evaluation of the patient's ability to drive safely. Many states require the periodic submission of medical reports while the license is active. In addition, many states allow exceptions under which a license may be issued for a shorter seizure-free period (e.g., if a seizure occurred in isolation as a result of medication change or intercurrent illness), or they may issue licenses with restrictions (e.g., daytime driving only). A summary of requirements for each state is available from the Epilepsy Foundation.

Epilepsy Foundation: www.epilepsy.com. Accessed on March 5, 2015.

113. **What are some common seizure triggers about which families should be counseled?**
- Sleep deprivation, insufficient sleep, being overtired
- Fever and illnesses, particularly viral
- Low blood sugar, poor oral intake
- Flashing bright lights or patterns
- Association with menses
- Alcohol or drug use
- Stress
- Excess caffeine

Epilepsy Foundation: www.epilepsy.com/learn/triggers-seizures. Accessed on March 6, 2015.

114. **When should a child be referred for possible epilepsy surgery?**
Although many epilepsy syndromes in childhood have spontaneous remission, 20% of incident epilepsy is intractable, and 5% of patients with intractable epilepsy may benefit from epilepsy surgery. Indications for surgery include failure of two AEDs, intractable disabling seizures, and/or deteriorating development. In general, outcome is determined by the completeness of the evaluation and the congruence of the data, the completeness of the resection, and the etiology of the seizures.

Ryvlin R, Cross JH, Rheims S: Epilepsy surgery in children and adults, *Lancet Neurol* 13:1114–1126, 2014.

FEBRILE SEIZURES

115. How are febrile seizures defined?

Febrile seizures are defined as a convulsion caused by a fever (temperature $\geq$ 100.4 °F or 38 °C by any method) that is without evidence of CNS pathology or acute electrolyte imbalance that occurs in children between the ages of 6 months and 60 months with a peak at the end of the second year of life). Children with a history of epilepsy who have an exacerbation of seizures with fever are excluded. Febrile seizures occur in 2% to 5% of children. There is often a positive family history of febrile convulsions.

116. What is the likelihood of recurrence of a febrile seizure?

The likelihood of recurrence increases with a younger age of onset, with a recurrence rate about 1 in 2 if the patient is <1 year of age when the initial seizure occurs and 1 in 5 if the patient is >3 years of age at the time of the initial seizure. About half of recurrences are within 6 months of the first seizure; three-fourths occur within 1 year, and 90% occur within 2 years. Other risk factors for recurrence are a lower temperature (close to 38 °C) at the time of seizure, <1 hour's duration of fever before the seizure, and a family history of febrile seizures. Overall, the recurrence rate in the pediatric population is about 30%.

AAP Subcommittee on Febrile Seizures: Clinical practice guideline—febrile seizures: guideline for the neurodiagnostic evaluation of the child with a simple febrile seizure, *Pediatrics* 127:389–394, 2011.

117. What features make a febrile seizure complex rather than simple?

- **Simple febrile seizure:** Relatively brief (<15 minutes long) and occurs as a solitary event (one attack in 24 hours) in the setting of fever not caused by CNS infection
- **Complex (also called atypical or complicated) febrile seizure:** Focal features either at the onset or during the seizure, extended in duration (>15 minutes long), or occurring more than once in 1 day

118. Why are complex febrile seizures more worrisome than simple febrile seizures?

They suggest a more serious problem. For example, a focal seizure raises concern of a localized or lateralized functional disturbance of the CNS. An unusually long seizure (>15 minutes) also raises the suspicion of primary CNS infectious, structural, or metabolic disease. Repeated seizures within a 24-hour period likewise imply a potentially more serious disorder or impending status epilepticus.

119. When should a lumbar puncture (LP) be performed as part of the evaluation of a child <12 months of age with a simple febrile seizure?

This had traditionally been a difficult question when a well-appearing infant or young toddler was examined after a febrile seizure, but the widespread use of immunizations in the United States for two of the most common causes of bacterial meningitis, *H. influenzae* type b (Hib) and *S. pneumoniae*, has significantly lowered the incidence of bacterial meningitis. Current data no longer support a routine LP in a well-appearing, fully immunized child with a simple febrile seizure.

The American Academy of Pediatrics recommends a LP in any child who presents with a fever and seizure if the child has meningeal signs and symptoms (neck stiffness, Kernig and/or Brudzinski signs) or any history or exam suggestive of intracranial infection. An LP should be *considered*:

- **If the patient is between 6 to 12 months of age and has not received scheduled immunizations (especially Hib and pneumococcal vaccinations) or when the immunization status cannot be determined.** This child is at increased risk for bacterial meningitis. Patients >12 months should have recognizable symptoms of bacterial meningitis.
- **If a patient has been pretreated with antibiotics because antibiotic treatment can mask the signs and symptoms of meningitis**

AAP Subcommittee on Febrile Seizures: Clinical practice guideline—febrile seizures: guideline for the neurodiagnostic evaluation of the child with a simple febrile seizure, *Pediatrics* 127:389-394, 2011.

120. Are EEG or neuroimaging studies indicated for a child with a simple febrile seizure?

No. An EEG done shortly after or within a month after a seizure does not predict either the recurrence of febrile seizures or the development of afebrile seizures/epilepsy in the ensuing 2 years. CT or MRI studies are not indicated because children who are neurologically healthy before a simple febrile seizure have a low likelihood of a clinically important intracranial structural abnormality.

AAP Subcommittee on Febrile Seizures: Clinical practice guideline—febrile seizures: guideline for the neurodiagnostic evaluation of the child with a simple febrile seizure, *Pediatrics* 127:389–394, 2011.

121. **Do prolonged febrile seizures result in an increased peripheral white blood cell count?**

A common clinical question in children is whether a leukocytosis, if found, can be explained on the basis of a prolonged seizure as a stress reaction. In a study of 203 children with seizures and fever, 61% had a normal peripheral white blood cell count. No association was found between blood leukocytosis and febrile seizure duration in children.

van Stuijvenberg M, Moll HA, Steyerberg EW, et al: The duration of febrile seizures and peripheral leukocytosis, *J Pediatr* 133:557–558, 1998.

122. **What ancillary testing should be considered in a patient with a complex febrile seizure?**

Most children with their first complex febrile seizure should undergo a LP for a CSF examination to rule out intracranial infection. Children with focal motor seizures or postictal lateralized deficits (motor paresis, unilateral sensory or visual loss, sustained eye deviation, or aphasia) should be considered for emergent neuroimaging to exclude a structural abnormality before the LP. A LP could result in cerebral herniation if ICP is increased because of a mass effect. However, if the patient is neurologically normal, data suggest an emergent CT may not be necessary. The immediate performance of an EEG offers limited insight into the patient's disease. Prominent generalized postictal slowing is not unexpected. Definite focal slowing suggests a possible structural abnormality. For a simple febrile seizure, an EEG is not indicated because it is not predictive of either the risk for recurrence of febrile seizures or the development of epilepsy.

Teng D, Dayan P, Tyler S, et al: Risk of intracranial pathologic conditions requiring emergency intervention after a first complex febrile seizure episode among children, *Pediatrics* 117:304–308, 2006.
DiMario FJ: Children presenting with complex febrile seizures do not routinely need computed tomography scanning in the emergency department, *Pediatrics* 117:528–530, 2006.

123. **What is the risk for epilepsy after a simple febrile seizure?**

The risk depends on several variables. In otherwise normal children with a simple febrile seizure, the risk for later epilepsy is about 2%. The risk for epilepsy is higher if any of the following is present:
- There is a close family history of nonfebrile seizures.
- Prior neurologic or developmental abnormalities exist.
- The patient had an atypical or complex febrile seizure, defined as focal seizures, seizures lasting at least 15 minutes, and/or multiple attacks within 24 hours.

One risk factor increases the risk to 3%. If all three risk factors are present, the likelihood of later epilepsy increases to 5% to 10%.

Graves RC, Oehler K, Tingle LE: Febrile seizures: risks, evaluation, and prognosis, *Am Fam Physician* 85:149–153, 2012.
Waruiru C, Appleton R: Febrile seizures: an update, *Arch Dis Child* 89:751–756, 2004.

KEY POINTS: FEBRILE SEIZURES

1. Simple: Brief and lasting <15 minutes
2. Complex: Focal, >15 minutes long, or recurrence within 1 day
3. Risk for recurrent febrile seizure increases if positive family history or seizure occurs at <1 year of age and/or body temperature of <40°C
4. Risk for developing future nonfebrile seizures is low (only 2% by age 7 years)
5. Normal long-term intellect and behavior compared with controls
6. Increased risk for developing epilepsy if complex febrile seizure, prior neurologic abnormality, or family history of seizure disorder

124. **What is the long-term outcome for children with febrile seizures?**

In a previously normal child, the risk for death, neurologic damage, or persistent cognitive impairment from a single benign febrile seizure is near zero. These potential complications are more likely with complex febrile seizures, but the risk is still exceedingly low. Impaired cognition in the latter group is more likely if afebrile seizures subsequently develop. Febrile status epilepticus has a very low mortality with proper treatment. However, the potential development of hippocampal injury (mesial temporal sclerosis) is currently being evaluated in the United States in the FEBSTAT study.

Scott RC: Consequences of febrile seizures in childhood, *Curr Opin Pediatr* 26:662–667, 2014.
Verity CM, Greenwood R, Golding J: Long-term intellectual and behavioral outcomes of children with febrile convulsions, *N Engl J Med* 338:1723–1728, 1998.

125. **After a febrile seizure, should a child be treated with prophylactic AEDs?**
    For most children, a simple febrile seizure is an unwanted but transient disruption of their health, and treatment is not necessary. Treatment interventions, either continuous or intermittent (at the time of fever) have been evaluated for valproate, pyridoxine, phenobarbital, phenytoin, diazepam, and clonazepam. Adverse effects were noted in up to 30% in the phenobarbital group (lower comprehension scores) and up to 36% in the benzodiazepine treated group. Long-term prophylaxis does not improve the prognosis in terms of subsequent epilepsy or motor or cognitive ability. In general, the side effects of prophylaxis (especially the hepatotoxicity and pancreatopathy associated with valproic acid therapy) outweigh the relatively minor risks of recurrence. Exceptions could include the very young child if febrile seizures recur frequently, children with preexisting neurologic abnormalities or children with recurrent complex febrile seizures.

Offringa M, Newton R: Prophylactic drug management for febrile seizures in children, *Cochrane Database Syst Rev* 18: CD003031, 2012.

126. **Is the aggressive use of antipyretic therapy at the start of a febrile illness effective in reducing the likelihood of a febrile seizure?**
    Despite being recommended frequently by pediatricians, aggressive antipyretic use has not been shown to be effective in preventing recurrence of a febrile seizure.

Offringa M, Newton R: Prophylactic drug management for febrile seizures in children, *Cochrane Database Syst Rev* 18: CD003031, 2012.
Strengell T, Uhari M, Tarkka R, et al: Antipyretic agents for preventing recurrences of febrile seizures: randomized controlled trial, *Arch Pediatr Adolesc Med* 163:799–804, 2009.

HEADACHE

127. **What are the emergency priorities when evaluating a child with a severe headache?**
    As with all common presenting symptoms, the main priority is to rule out diagnostic possibilities that may be life-threatening:
    • Increased ICP (e.g., mass lesion, acute hydrocephalus)
    • Intracranial infections (e.g., meningitis, encephalitis)
    • Subarachnoid hemorrhage
    • Stroke
    • Malignant hypertension
    • Acute angle closure glaucoma (may appear as a headache, but rare in children)

128. **When should neuroimaging be considered in a child with headache?**
    • Abnormal neurologic signs (oculomotor abnormalities, gait ataxia, papilledema, focal weakness)
    • Headache increasing in frequency and severity
    • Headache occurring in early morning or awakening child from sleep
    • Headache made worse by straining or by sneezing or coughing (may be a sign of increased ICP)
    • Headache associated with severe vomiting without nausea
    • Headache worsened or helped significantly by a change in position
    • Macrocephaly
    • Fall off in linear growth rate
    • Recent school failure or significant behavioral changes
    • New-onset seizures, especially if seizure has a focal onset

- Migraine headache and seizure occurring in the same episode, with vascular symptoms preceding the seizure (20% to 50% risk for tumor or arteriovenous malformation)
- Cluster headaches in any child or teenager

Lewis DW, Ashwal S, Dahl G, et al, Quality Standards Subcommittee of the American Academy of Neurology; Practice Committee of the Child Neurology Society: Practice parameter: evaluation of children and adolescents with recurrent headaches. Report of the Quality Standards Subcommittee of the American Academy of Neurology and the Practice Committee of the Child Neurology Society, Neurology 59:490–498, 2002.

KEY POINTS: CLASSIC HEADACHE OF INCREASED INTRACRANIAL PRESSURE

1. Awakens patient from sleep at night
2. Pain present upon awakening in the morning
3. Vomiting without associated nausea
4. Made worse by straining, sneezing, or coughing
5. Intensity of pain changes with changes in body position
6. Pain lessens during the day

129. **What are the three primary headache disorders in children?**
These are recurrent headaches not attributable to underlying physical disease.
- **Migraine:** Most common type in children (4% in childhood, with a male predominance; after adolescence, more common in females)
- **Tension type:** Features different from migraine—bilateral, non-pulsating, not aggravated by activity; school problems with stress and absences and family dysfunction are frequently noted
- **Cluster:** Uncommon in childhood; consist of severe unilateral orbital or supraorbital pain with conjunctival injection and tearing

130. **What are the clinical features of migraine headaches in children?**
Migraine is a periodic disorder with symptom-free periods characterized by headaches with a throbbing nature, unilateral in older children and commonly bilateral in younger children, lasting 1 to 72 hours, pulsating with moderate or severe intensity, aggravated by routine physical activity and exercise, and associated with nausea and/or photophobia and phonophobia. There may be a history of recurrent vomiting, motion sickness, or vertigo. There is often a family history of migraine, and the genetics may be multifactorial.
- *Migraine with aura:* Previously called *classic migraine*, this is less common in children. The aura is a prodrome of variable focal neurologic features such as visual scotoma, sensory symptoms (numbness, tingling), sluggishness, and difficulty concentrating or motor features (weakness, dysphasia).
- *Migraine without aura:* Previously called common migraine, these are the more frequent type in childhood.
Other clinical syndromes that are considered migraine variants in childhood include cyclic vomiting syndrome; abdominal migraine; benign paroxysmal vertigo of childhood; and possibly, infantile colic.

Headache Classification Subcommittee of the International Headache Society: The international classification of headache disorders, *Cephalalgia* 24(Suppl 1):1–160, 2004.

---

131. **Which physical findings are important during the initial evaluation of possible migraine headache?**
- Height and weight should be normal for age. Pituitary tumor, craniopharyngioma, and partial ornithine transcarbamylase deficiency may all result in growth failure and mimic migraine headache. Head circumference should be normal, ruling out hydrocephalus.
- Skin should be checked for abnormalities. Throbbing headaches are common in neurofibromatosis and systemic lupus erythematosus, both of which have easily recognizable skin manifestations.
- Blood pressure should be normal.

- Check for sinus tenderness or pain with sinus percussion or head movement (implying cervical spine disease). The patient should be examined for carious teeth, misaligned bite, or disordered chewing and jaw opening (temporomandibular joint dysfunction).
- Auscultation should reveal no cranial bruits (if present, these suggest possible arteriovenous malformation or mass lesion).
- The neurologic examination should be normal.

132. **When do children begin to have migraine headaches?**
About 20% suffer their first headache before the age of 10 years.
   Infantile migraine does occur, and often manifests as vomiting, pallor, vertigo, and ataxia, with or without headache, which can occur in a periodic fashion and frequently improves with sleep.

Barlow CF: Migraine in the infant and toddler, *J Child Neurol* 9:92–94, 1994.

133. **Which foods have been associated with the development of migraine headaches?**
Tyramine-rich foods (cheese, red wine), foods with monosodium glutamate (Asian food, adobo seasoning), nitrate-rich foods (smoked and lunch meats, salami), alcoholic beverages, caffeinated beverages, chocolate, citrus fruits, and sulfites (food coloring) have been associated with the development of migraine headaches.

134. **What is familial hemiplegic migraine?**
Familial hemiplegic migraine is an autosomal dominant disorder that is clinically characterized by transient hemiparesis and aphasia followed by migraine headache. About 20% are affected by progressive cerebellar ataxia. Mutations in CACNA1A (which encodes a neuronal calcium channel) on chromosome 19 are found in half of affected families.

Wessman M, Kaunisto MA, Kallela M, et al: The molecular genetics of migraine, *Ann Med* 36:462–473, 2004.

135. **What is the likely diagnosis for a 10-year-old girl with a history of headaches and a family history of migraines who has had 10 minutes of a spinning sensation and double vision followed by an occipital headache and has a normal neurologic examination in the office?**
Basilar-type migraine, which occurs in 3% to 19% of childhood migraines, is a likely diagnosis. Symptoms related to balance, gait, and visual disturbance are followed by headache, which, unlike most migraines, is occipital. Patients with basilar artery migraine may have drop attacks with altered awareness. Syncope is also more common in patients with migraine compared with the general population.

Lewis DW: Pediatric migraine, *Pediatr Rev* 28:43–53, 2007.

136. **How do the triptans work to treat an acute migraine headache?**
Triptans are serotonin receptor subtype-selective drugs, which were thought initially to work primarily through their vasoconstrictive effects on arterial smooth muscle in cranial blood vessels. However, there are questions whether the primary mechanism is central or peripheral. Triptans act on peripheral nerve endings, preventing the release of proinflammatory and vasoactive peptides, including substance P and calcitonin gene–related peptide (GCRP). Also unclear is the apparent selectivity of triptans for migraine pain but not other kinds of somatic pain.

Pringsheim T, Becker WJ: Triptans for symptomatic treatment of migraine headache, *BMJ* 348:g2285, 2014.

137. **What nonpharmacologic therapies are available for the prevention of migraine?**
- Migraine elimination diet
- Vitamin therapy: riboflavin, coenzyme Q10, magnesium
- Normalization of sleep habits
- Discontinuance of possible triggering medications (e.g., analgesic overuse, bronchodilators, oral contraceptives)
- Biofeedback

- Relaxation therapy
- Family counseling (if family stress is a trigger)
- Self-hypnosis

Nicholson RA, Buse DC, Andrasik F, Lipton RB: Nonpharmacologic treatments for migraine and tension-type headache: how to choose and when to use, *Curr Treat Options Neurol* 13:28–40, 2011.

138. **What categories of medication are available for the prevention of migraine in children?**

As with many therapies used for children, most studies involve adults with extrapolation to children for whom the medications may not work as well. These medications are regularly used by clinicians but are not yet approved by the U.S. Food and Drug Administration for children. Keys to therapy are gradually increasing the dose until effectiveness is or is not established or adverse effects intervene.

- Antidepressants (e.g., tricyclics such as amitriptyline)
- Antihistamine (e.g., cyproheptadine, which has antiserotonergic effects)
- Antihypertensives (e.g., β-blockers such as propranolol and calcium channel blockers)
- Anticonvulsants (including divalproex sodium and topiramate)

Damen L, Bruijn JK, Verhagen AP, et al: Prophylactic treatment of migraine in children. Part 2. A systematic review of pharmacological trials, *Cephalalgia* 26:373–383, 2006.

139. **Who should be started on prophylactic medication for migraine headaches?**

There are no precise criteria, but generally prophylactic treatment should be considered if any of the following are present:

- Headaches with aura occur frequently.
- Headaches with aura are poorly responsive to abortive medication.
- School attendance is significantly affected.
- Headaches, although infrequent, last for several days.

140. **How long are the prophylactic medications continued?**

The optimal duration of therapy remains unclear, but many authorities suggest a treatment duration of 3 to 6 months followed by an attempt at weaning. Less than 50% will require the reinitiation of medication.

141. **What distinguishes tension-type headaches from migraines?**

Unlike migraines, these headaches are bilateral with a pressing and tightening quality (as opposed to the pulsatile quality of migraines) and usually of mild or moderate intensity. They are not associated with nausea or vomiting and typically not worsened by light or sound. Pericranial muscle tenderness is common.

Psychological stress is associated with and can aggravate tension-type headaches. Activation of hyperexcitable peripheral afferent neurons from head and neck muscles, as well as abnormalities in central pain processing and pain sensitivity, likely contributes to the problem.

Loder E, Rizzoli R: Tension-type headache, *BMJ* 336:88–92, 2008.

MOVEMENT DISORDERS

142. **What are the various types of pathologic hyperkinetic movements?**

- **Tremors:** Rhythmic oscillatory movements, both supination-pronation and flexion-extension, seen in resting state or with activity
- **Chorea:** Quick dancing movements of proximal and distal muscles with irregular unpredictable random jerks
- **Athetosis:** Irregular, slow, distal writhing movements
- **Stereotypy:** Repetitive, purposeless motions (e.g., body rocking, head rolling) that resemble voluntary movements often associated with akathisia (sensory and motor restlessness); often seen in autism spectrum disorders

- **Dystonia:** Slow, twisting, sustained movements; may result in abnormal postures and progress to contractures
- **Ballismus:** Abrupt, random, violent, flinging movements, often proximal and unilateral
- **Myoclonus:** Abrupt, brief, jerky contractions of one or more muscles, often stimulus sensitive
- **Tics:** Rapid, sudden, repetitive movements or vocalizations

143. **What techniques can be used to elicit abnormal movements (particularly chorea)?**
Methods of provocative testing include the maintenance of posture in extension against gravity, hyperpronation (or "spooning," especially above the head), tongue protrusion ("trombone tongue"), squeezing the finger of the examiner ("milk-maid's grip"), pouring liquid, and drawing a spiral.

144. **What disorders are commonly associated with the various hyperkinetic movements?**
- **Tremors, resting:** Primary juvenile Parkinson disease, secondary Parkinson disease
- **Tremors, kinetic:** Essential (familial) tremor, cerebellar disorders, brainstem tumors, hyperthyroidism, Wilson disease, electrolyte disturbance (e.g., glucose, calcium, magnesium), heavy-metal intoxication (e.g., lead, mercury), multiple sclerosis
- **Chorea:** Sydenham chorea (associated with rheumatic fever), Huntington disease, hyperthyroidism, infectious mononucleosis, pregnancy, anticonvulsants, neuroleptic drugs, closed head injury, systemic lupus erythematosus, carbon monoxide poisoning, Wilson disease, hypocalcemia, polycythemia, parainfectious and infectious encephalopathies (e.g., rubeola, syphilis)
- **Athetosis:** CP, other static encephalopathies, Lesch-Nyhan syndrome, kernicterus
- **Stereotypy:** Autism, Rett syndrome, neuroleptic drugs (i.e., tardive dyskinesia), schizophrenia
- **Dystonia:** Idiopathic primary dystonias (e.g., torsion dystonia), Sandifer syndrome, spasmus nutans, neuroleptic drugs, static encephalopathy, perinatal asphyxia, familial dystonia (sometimes dopa-responsive)
- **Ballismus:** Encephalitis, closed head injury
- **Myoclonus:** Sleep myoclonus, benign myoclonus of infancy, postanoxic encephalopathy, uremic encephalopathy, hyperthyroidism, urea cycle defects, side effects of tricyclic therapy, slow virus infections, Wilson disease, myoclonus-opsoclonus, neuroblastoma, epileptic encephalopathies, mitochondrial disease, prion disease, Tay-Sachs disease, startle disease, sialidosis

145. **What constitutes a tic?**
Tics are brief, sudden, repetitive, stereotyped, involuntary, and purposeless movements or vocalizations. They most commonly involve muscles of the head, neck, and respiratory tract. Their frequency can be increased by anxiety, stress, excitement, and fatigue. They are decreased during sleep and relaxation; during activities involving high concentration; and, at times, through voluntary action. In some cases, premonitory feelings (e.g., irritation, tickle, temperature change) can precipitate the motor or vocal response.

146. **What is the range of clinical tics?**
- **Motor (simple clonic):** Eye blinking, eye deviation, head twitching, shoulder shrugging
- **Motor (simple dystonic):** Bruxism, abdominal tensing, shoulder rotation
- **Motor (complex):** Grunting, barking, sniffing, snorting, throat clearing, spitting
- **Vocal (complex):** Coprolalia (obscene words), echolalia (repeating another's words), palilalia (rapidly repeating one's own words)

147. **What are the causes of a tic?**
Transient and chronic tic disorders usually do not have an identifiable cause. However, dyskinesias such as tics can be found in association with a number of other conditions:
- **Chromosomal abnormalities:** Down syndrome, fragile X syndrome
- **Developmental syndromes:** Autism, pervasive developmental disorder, Rett syndrome
- **Drugs:** Anticonvulsants, stimulants (e.g., amphetamines, cocaine, methylphenidate, pemoline)
- **Infections:** Encephalitis, post-rubella syndrome

148. **How should simple tics be treated?**
Simple motor tics are common and occur in more than 5% to 21% of school-age children. Simple tics generally do not require pharmacologic intervention and can be treated expectantly by developing relaxation techniques, minimizing stresses that exacerbate the problem, avoiding punishment for tics,

and decreasing fixation on the problem. Most simple tics self-resolve in 2 to 12 months. Moderate or severe tics, especially when significant patient distress is involved, may warrant pharmacologic treatment.

149. **What comorbidities occur in children with tics?**

The prevalence of tic disorder is higher in younger children and in males and is associated with school dysfunction, learning disabilities, obsessive-compulsive disorder, and attention-deficit/hyperactivity disorder. In addition, separation anxiety, overanxious disorder, simple phobia, social phobia, agoraphobia, mania, major depression, and oppositional defiant disorder were found to be significantly more common in children with tics.

150. **When do tics warrant pharmacologic intervention?**

Tics that have a significant disabling impact on a child's educational, social, or psychological well-being (particularly if they have been present for >1 year) may require intervention. When the complexity of tics increases or the diagnosis of Tourette syndrome is suspected, pharmacotherapy should also be considered. Most theories point to a hyper-dopaminergic state of the basal ganglia as the most likely etiology for unregulated movements. Pharmacologic management includes α_2-agonists (e.g., clonidine, guanfacine) or the administration of atypical neuroleptics (e.g., risperidone, haloperidol) and/or the cessation of any stimulant drugs that can cause dopamine release. Because of the high associated incidence of obsessive-compulsive disorder and attention-deficit/hyperactivity disorder, other medications may be needed, and consultation with a pediatric psychiatrist or neurologist is often warranted.

151. **What are the diagnostic criteria for Tourette syndrome?**

In 1885, Gilles de la Tourette described a syndrome of motor tics and vocal tics with behavioral disturbances and a chronic and variable course. *Diagnostic and Statistical Manual of Mental Disorders* (DSM-V) criteria for Tourette syndrome require the following:
- Two or more motor tics *and* at least one vocal tic
- Presence of tics for more than 1 year (usually on a daily basis, but can be intermittent)
- Onset before the age of 18 years
- Not caused by medications or any identifiable medical etiology

American Psychiatric Association: *Diagnosis and Statistical Manual of Mental Disorders,* ed 5, Washington, DC, 2013, American Psychiatric Association.

152. **What is coprolalia?**

Coprolalia is an irresistible urge to utter profanities, occurring as a phonic tic. Only 20% to 40% of patients with Tourette syndrome have this phenomenon, and it is not essential for the diagnosis.

153. **What behavioral problems are associated with Tourette syndrome?**
- Obsessive-compulsive disorder
- Attention-deficit/hyperactivity disorder
- Severe conduct disorders
- Learning disabilities (particularly math)
- Sleep abnormalities
- Depression, anxiety, and emotional lability

Tourette Syndrome Association: www.tsa-usa.org. Accessed on March 6, 2015.
Robertson MM: The Gilles De La Tourette syndrome: the current status, *Arch Dis Child* 97:166–175, 2012.

154. **Why is the diagnosis of Tourette syndrome commonly delayed?**
- Tendency to associate unusual symptoms with attention-getting or psychological problems
- Incorrect belief that all children with Tourette syndrome must have severe tics
- Attribution of vocal tics to upper respiratory infections, allergies, or sinus or bronchial problems
- Diagnosis of eye blinking or ocular tics as ophthalmologic problems
- Mistaken belief that coprolalia is an essential diagnostic feature

Singer HS: Tic disorders, *Pediatr Ann* 22:22–29, 1993.

155. **What is the cause of tardive dyskinesia?**
Tardive dyskinesia is a hyperkinetic disorder of abnormal movements, most commonly involving the face (e.g., lip smacking or pursing, chewing, grimacing, tongue protruding). Tardive dyskinesia occurs during treatment with neuroleptics (e.g., chlorpromazine, haloperidol, metoclopramide) or within 6 months of their discontinuance. This disorder is thought to be a result of dopaminergic dysfunction of the basal ganglia because these drugs act as dopamine-receptor blockers.

156. **For a patient taking neuroleptic medication, how long must therapy last before symptoms of tardive dyskinesia can develop?**
About 3 months of continuous or intermittent treatment with neuroleptics is needed before the risk for tardive dyskinesia increases.

157. **What is neuroleptic malignant syndrome?**
Neuroleptic malignant syndrome is a syndrome of movement (rigidity, tremor, chorea, and dystonia), autonomic dysfunction (fever, hypertension, tachycardia, diaphoresis, irregular respiratory pattern, urinary retention), alteration of consciousness, and rhabdomyolysis with an elevation of creatinine kinase. It occurs within weeks of starting neuroleptics, and there is a 20% associated mortality rate in adults.

158. **Which movement disorder in children presents with "dancing eyes and dancing feet"?**
Opsoclonus-myoclonus (infantile polymyoclonus syndrome or acute myoclonic encephalopathy of infants) is a rare but distinctive movement disorder in children that is seen during the first 1 to 3 years of life. Opsoclonus is characterized by wild, chaotic, fluttering, irregular, rapid, conjugate bursts of eye movements (saccadomania). Myoclonus is sudden, shocklike muscular twitches of the face, limbs, or trunk. The anatomic site of pathology is the cerebellar outflow tracts. The etiology may be direct viral invasion, postinfectious encephalopathy, or neuroblastoma. Immunomodulatory therapy with corticosteroids (ACTH, dexamethasone), intravenous immunoglobulin (IVIG), and rituximab may be useful.

NEONATAL SEIZURES

159. **How are neonatal seizures classified?**
Although there is no universally accepted standard classification system, one based on clinical criteria is commonly used. It divides neonatal seizures into four types:
- **Subtle** (ocular phenomena, oro-buccal-lingual movements, limb bicycling, autonomic phenomena, apneic seizures)
- **Tonic** (focal or generalized)
- **Clonic** (focal or multifocal)
- **Myoclonic** (focal, multifocal, or generalized)

All seizure types are recognized as paroxysmal alterations in behavioral, motor, or autonomic function. Not all clinically observed phenomena, however, are accompanied by associated epileptic surface-EEG activity, and this electroclinical disassociation is increased after AED treatment. Partial clonic, tonic, and myoclonic seizures have been shown to have the most consistent EEG ictal correlate.

160. **Why are generalized seizures uncommon in newborns?**
Generalized seizures are rarely seen in neonates because of **incomplete myelination**, which tends to prevent highly organized, synchronized ictal motor activity from occurring.

161. **What is the most common type of clinical seizure during the neonatal period?**
The so-called **subtle seizure** is the most common. Rather than arising as an abrupt dramatic "convulsion" with obvious forceful twitching or posturing of the muscles, the subtle seizure appears as unnatural, repetitive, stereotyped choreography, featuring oral-buccal-lingual movements, eye blinking, nystagmus, lip smacking, or complex integrated limb movements (swimming, pedaling, or rowing) and other fragments of activity drawn from the limited repertoire of normal infant activity. These neonates frequently have HIE and moderately to markedly abnormal EEGs, and they are at significantly greater risk for mental retardation, CP, and epilepsy.

162. **What are the causes of neonatal seizures?**
- Hypoxic-ischemic encephalopathy caused by birth asphyxia
- Infection
- Toxins (e.g., inadvertent fetal injection with local anesthetic; cocaine, including withdrawal)

- Metabolic abnormalities (e.g., hypoglycemia, hypocalcemia, hypomagnesemia, pyridoxine deficiency, inborn errors)
- CNS malformations
- Cerebrovascular lesions (e.g., intraventricular, periventricular hemorrhage, subarachnoid hemorrhage, infarction, arterial cerebral occlusion)
- Benign familial neonatal-infantile seizures (e.g., a sodium channelopathy)

Glass HC: Neonatal seizures: advances in mechanisms and management, *Clin Perinatol* 41:177–190, 2014.
Zupanc ML: Neonatal seizures, *Pediatr Clin North Am* 51:961–978, 2004.

163. **In premature and full-term infants, how do the causes of seizures vary with regard to relative frequency and time of onset?**
See Table 13-4.

Table 13-4. Variance in Relative Frequency and Time of Onset of Causes of Seizures

	Postnatal Time of Onset		Relative Frequency	
ETIOLOGY	0-3 DAYS	>3 DAYS	PREMATURE	FULL-TERM
Hypoxic-ischemic	+		+++	+++
Intracranial hemorrhage*	+	+	++	+
Hypoglycemia	+		+	+
Hypocalcemia	+	+	+	+
Intracranial infection[†]	+	+	++	+
Developmental defects	+	+	++	++
Drug withdrawal	+	+	+	+

*Hemorrhages are principally germinal matrix-intraventricular in the premature infant and subarachnoid or subdural in the term infant.
[†]Early seizures occur usually after intrauterine nonbacterial infections (e.g., toxoplasmosis, cytomegalovirus infection), and later seizures usually occur with herpes simplex encephalitis or bacterial meningitis.
Adapted from Volpe JJ, editor: Neurology of the Newborn, *ed 3. Philadelphia, 1995, WB Saunders, p 184.*

164. **What is an acceptable workup in a newborn with seizures?**
- A careful prenatal and natal history and a complete physical examination are needed.
- Laboratory studies should include blood for glucose, electrolytes, calcium, phosphorus, and magnesium.
- A lumbar puncture should be performed to rule out meningitis.
- Neuroimaging studies (cranial ultrasound, CT scan, or preferably, MRI) are mandatory.
- Additional studies may include blood levels for ammonia, lactate, and pyruvate; additional CSF studies (e.g., lactate, pyruvate, glucose, glycine, CSF neurotransmitters if metabolic disease is suspected); and urine studies for organic and amino acid analysis for possible inborn errors of metabolism.
- Serial use of EEG polygraphy can document persistent seizures, especially the persistence of electrographic seizures without clinical seizures after initial treatment.

165. **In what settings should an inborn error of metabolism be suspected as a cause of neonatal seizures?**
- The onset of seizures is beyond day 1 of life. (The exception is pyridoxine deficiency, which can occur on day of life 1; patients may have a history of seizures *in utero*.)
- The infant becomes symptomatic after the introduction of enteral or parenteral nutrition.
- The seizures are intractable and do not respond to conventional AEDs.
  Characteristic EEG patterns may be seen in maple syrup urine disease, propionic acidemia, and pyridoxine deficiency.

Scher MS: Neonatal seizures. In Polin RA, Yoder MC, editors: *Workbook in Practical Neonatology*, ed 4. Philadelphia, 2007, Saunders Elsevier, p 363.

166. How are seizures differentiated from tremors in the neonate?
     See Table 13-5.

Table 13-5. Tremors Versus Seizures

CLINICAL FEATURE	TREMORS	SEIZURES
Suppressibility	+	0
Abnormality of gaze or eye movement	0	+
Movements are exquisitely stimulus sensitive	+	0
Predominant movement	Tremor	Clonic jerking
Movements cease with passive flexion	+	0
Autonomic changes	0	+

167. What are the treatment options for neonatal seizures?
     Neonatal seizures may be treated with phenobarbital. Studies of the pharmacokinetics of phenobarbital in neonates have indicated that it is most appropriate to load with a full 20 mg/kg rather than smaller fractions. If seizures persist, additional increments of phenobarbital to total loading doses of 40 mg/kg can be given. Continued seizures may be treated with a loading dose of 20 mg/kg of phenytoin (or phenytoin equivalents in the case of fosphenytoin). The usual maintenance dose for phenobarbital is between 3 and 6 mg/kg per day and between 4 and 8 mg/kg per day for phenytoin. Efficacy from either of these two agents is low, with only one-third of patients showing an immediate complete response. Even after apparently successful intravenous treatment with phenobarbital and phenytoin with the resolution of clinical seizures, electrographic seizures may continue unabated. The significance of this finding is unclear, and the need to suppress electrographic seizures without clinical accompaniments is controversial.
     Other agents, such as levetiracetam and topiramate, have some evidence for efficacy, but are not at this time considered first-line agents for neonatal seizures. Lidocaine and midazolam have also been used in the treatment of neonatal status epilepticus.

Slaughter LA, Patel AD, Slaughter JL: Pharmacological treatment of neonatal seizures: a systematic review, *J Child Neurol* 28: 351–364, 2013.
Abend NS, Gutierrez-Colina AM, Monk HM, et al: Levetiracetam for treatment of neonatal seizures, *J Child Neurol* 26:465-470, 2011.
Glass HC, Poulin C, Shevell MI: Topiramate for the treatment of neonatal seizures, *Pediatr Neurol* 244:439–442, 2011.

168. What is the treatment for refractory seizures in the neonate?
     Frequent and recurrent seizures are not uncommon in newborns and are especially common in the setting of asphyxia. If seizures are refractory to full dosing of phenobarbital and phenytoin, the addition of drugs in the benzodiazepine family (e.g., diazepam, lorazepam, midazolam) is generally effective. It is important to ensure that no underlying biochemical disturbance is present before the serum levels of anticonvulsants are raised to maximal concentrations. Although pyridoxine-dependent seizures are rare, a trial dose of pyridoxine should be administered intravenously to infants with recurrent seizures of uncertain etiology. If possible, simultaneous EEG recordings should be performed to document the cessation of seizure activity and the normalization of the EEG within minutes of pyridoxine treatment. Infants with pyridoxine-dependent epilepsy may have profound autonomic dysfunction (apnea, bradycardia, and hypotension) in response to initial pyridoxine administration and should be monitored carefully. Folinic acid is allelic to pyridoxine deficiency and pyridoxal phosphate (P5P) is used in pyridoxine-resistant seizures.

169. Of what prognostic value is the interictal EEG in a neonate with seizures?
     This study can have significant prognostic value. Severe interictal EEG abnormalities (e.g., burst suppression, marked voltage suppression, flat or isoelectric) are highly predictive (90%) of a fatal outcome or severe neurologic sequelae. Conversely, a normal interictal EEG in a term infant with

seizures confers a very low (10%) likelihood of significant neurologic impairment. Moderate abnormalities (e.g., voltage asymmetries, immature patterns) have a mixed outcome.

Laroia N, Guillet R, Burchfiel J, McBride MC: EEG background as predictor of electrographic seizures in high risk neonates, *Epilepsia* 39:545–551, 1998.

170. **After an infant has recovered from a seizure, how long should medication be continued?**
There are no clear guidelines for duration of therapy after neonatal seizures. Maintenance therapy typically involves the use of phenobarbital because it is difficult to achieve therapeutic levels of phenytoin with oral administration in infancy, and others are less well studied. Although phenobarbital is generally well tolerated, it may have deleterious effects on behavior, attention span, and possibly brain development. It does not prevent the later development of epilepsy. Many authorities recommend discontinuing therapy if the neurologic examination has normalized. In addition, if the neurologic examination is abnormal but an EEG by the age of 3 months reveals no seizure activity, consideration can also be given to stopping phenobarbital.

171. **In patients with neonatal seizures, how does the cause affect the prognosis?**
See Table 13-6.

Table 13-6. Relationship Between Cause and Prognosis of Neonatal Seizure

ETIOLOGY	FAVORABLE OUTCOME*	MIXED OUTCOME	UNFAVORABLE OUTCOME*
Toxic-metabolic	Simple late-onset hypocalcemia Hypomagnesemia Hyponatremia Mepivacaine toxicity	Hypoglycemia Early-onset complicated hypocalcemia Pyridoxine dependency	Some aminoacidurias
Asphyxia	—	Mild hypoxic-ischemic encephalopathy	Severe hypoxic-ischemic encephalopathy
Hemorrhage	Uncomplicated subarachnoid hemorrhage	Subdural hematoma Intraventricular hemorrhage (grades I and II)	Intraventricular hemorrhage (grades III and IV)
Infection	—	Aseptic meningoencephalitis; some bacterial meningitides	Herpes simplex encephalitis; some bacterial meningitides
Structural	—	Simple traumatic contusion	Malformations of the central nervous system

*Favorable prognosis implies at least an 85% to 90% chance of survival and subsequent normal development. Unfavorable prognosis implies a high likelihood (85% to 90%) of death or serious handicap in survivors.
From Scher MS: Neonatal seizures. In Polin RA, Yoder MC, editors: Workbook in Practical Neonatology, ed 4. Philadelphia, 2007, Saunders Elsevier, p 370.

NEUROCUTANEOUS SYNDROMES

172. **What are the three most common neurocutaneous syndromes?**
Neurocutaneous syndromes (also called *phakomatoses*) are disorders characterized by the presence of tumors in various parts of the body (including the ocular and central nervous systems) and characteristic dermatologic findings of varying severity. The three most common are
- Neurofibromatosis
- Tuberous sclerosis complex
- Sturge-Weber syndrome

173. **What are the inheritance patterns of the various neurocutaneous syndromes?**
- **Neurofibromatosis:** Autosomal dominant
- **Tuberous sclerosis complex:** Autosomal dominant

- **von Hippel-Lindau syndrome:** Autosomal dominant
- **Incontinentia pigmenti:** X-linked dominant
- **Sturge-Weber syndrome:** Sporadic
- **Klippel-Trénaunay-Weber syndrome:** Sporadic

174. What are the diagnostic criteria for neurofibromatosis-1 (NF1)?

Two or more of the following:

- Café-au-lait spots (6 or more that are >0.5 cm in diameter before puberty; 6 or more that are >1.5 cm in diameter after puberty)
- Skinfold freckling (axillary or inguinal region)
- Neurofibromas (two or more) of any type, or at least one plexiform neurofibroma
- Iris hamartomas, also called *Lisch nodules* (two or more)
- Characteristic osseous lesion (i.e., sphenoid dysplasia, thinning of the cortex of the long bones with or without pseudoarthrosis)
- First-degree relative with NF1 diagnosed by the above criteria

Williams VC, Lucas J, Babcock MA, et al: Neurofibromatosis type 1 revisited, *Pediatrics* 123:124–133, 2009.

175. How does NF1 differ from NF2?

NF1, which is also known as *classic von Recklinghausen disease*, is much more common (1 in every 3000 to 4000 births) than NF2 and accounts for up to 90% of cases of neurofibromatosis. NF2 (1 in every 50,000 births) is characterized by bilateral acoustic neuromas, intracranial and intraspinal tumors, and affected first-degree relatives. NF1 has been linked to alterations on chromosome 17, whereas NF2 is linked to alterations on chromosome 22. Dermatologic findings and peripheral neuromas are rare in NF2. Other rarer subtypes of neurofibromatoses (e.g., segmental distribution) have been described.

Asthagiri AR, Parry DM, Butman JA, et al: Neurofibromatosis type 2, *Lancet* 373:1974–1986, 2009.

176. How common are café-au-lait spots at birth?

Up to 2% of black infants will have three café-au-lait spots at birth, whereas one café-au-lait spot occurs in only 0.3% of white infants. White infants with multiple café-au-lait spots at birth are more likely than black infants to develop neurofibromatosis. In older children, a single café-au-lait spot that is more than 5 mm in diameter can be found in 10% of white and 25% of black children.

Hurwitz S: Neurofibromatosis. In Hurwitz S, editor: *Clinical Pediatric Dermatology*, ed 2. Philadelphia, 1993, WB Saunders, pp 624–629.

177. If a 2-year-old child has seven café-au-lait spots that are larger than 5 mm in diameter, what is the likelihood that neurofibromatosis will develop, and how will it evolve?

Up to 75% of these children, if followed sequentially, will develop one of the varieties of neurofibromatosis, most commonly type 1. In a study of nearly 1900 patients, 46% with sporadic NF1 did not meet criteria by the age of 1 year. By the age of 8 years, however, 97% met the criteria, and by the age of 20 years, 100% did. The typical order of appearance of features is café-au-lait spots, axillary freckling, Lisch nodules, and neurofibromas. Yearly evaluation of patients with suspicious findings should include a careful skin examination, ophthalmologic evaluation, and blood pressure measurement.

DeBella K, Szudek J, Friedman JM: Use of the National Institutes of Health criteria for the diagnosis of neurofibromatosis 1 in children, *Pediatrics* 105:608–614, 2000.
Korf BR: Diagnostic outcome in children with multiple café-au-lait spots, *Pediatrics* 90:924–927, 1992.

178. What are Lisch nodules?

Pigmented iris hamartomas (Fig. 13-5). Although these are not usually present at birth in patients with NF1, up to 90% will develop multiple Lisch nodules by the age of 6 years. Hamartomas are focal malformations that are microscopically composed of multiple tissue types, and these can resemble neoplasms. However, unlike neoplasms, they grow at similar rates as normal components and are unlikely to pathologically compress adjacent tissue.

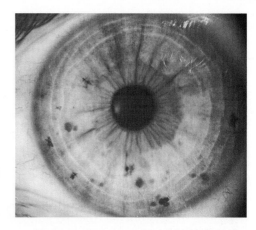

Figure 13-5. Pigmented iris hamartomas (Lisch nodules). *(From Habif TP, editor:* Clinical Dermatology: A Color Guide to Diagnosis and Therapy, *ed 5. Philadelphia, 2010, Elsevier, p 985.)*

179. **How common is a positive family history in cases of NF1?**
Because of the high spontaneous mutation rate for this autosomal dominant disease, only about 50% of newly diagnosed cases are associated with a positive family history.

180. **What are the primary diagnostic criteria for tuberous sclerosis complex (TSC)?**
TSC is characterized by hamartomatous growths that occur in multiple tissues. The National Institutes of Health Consensus Conference in 1998 revised the diagnostic criteria for TSC on the basis of major or minor features. Definite TSC consisted of two major features or one major and two minor features; probable and possible TSC had fewer features (Table 13-7). No single finding was considered pathognomonic for TSC. Two gene site abnormalities, TSC1 (chromosome 9) and TSC2 (chromosome 16), have been identified. Genetic testing is now available.

Crino PB, Nathanson KL, Henske EP: The tuberous sclerosis complex, *N Engl J Med* 355:1345–1356, 2006.

Table 13-7. Diagnostic Features for Tuberous Sclerosis Complex

MAJOR FEATURES	MINOR FEATURES
Facial angiofibromas	Dental enamel pits
Nontraumatic ungual or periungual fibroma	Bone cysts
Hypomelanotic macules (>3)	Hamartomatous rectal polyps
Shagreen patch	Gingival fibromas
Multiple retinal nodular hamartomas	Cerebral white matter migration tracts
Cortical tuber	
Subependymal nodule or giant cell astrocytoma	
Cardiac rhabdomyoma, single or multiple	

181. **What is the classic triad of TSC?**
- **Seizures**
- **Mental retardation**
- **Facial angiofibroma (adenoma sebaceum)**
  However, less than one-third of patients will develop these classic features.

Staley BA, Vail EA, Thiele EA: Tuberous sclerosis complex: diagnostic challenges, presenting symptoms, and commonly missed signs, *Pediatrics* 127:e117–e125, 2011.

182. **What is the most common presenting symptom of TSC?**
Seizures. About 85% of patients have seizures, and epileptic (previously called infantile) spasms are the most common. The first-line treatment of epileptic spasms in TSC is vigabatrin (as opposed to ACTH in other etiologies of epileptic spasm). Tonic and atonic seizures are also seen. Complex partial seizures are frequently seen in conjunction with other seizure types. Mental retardation is especially common with the onset of seizures before the age of 2 years. Autism and other behavioral disturbances are also frequently seen in children with TSC.

Staley BA, Vail EA, Thiele EA: Tuberous sclerosis complex: diagnostic challenges, presenting symptoms, and commonly missed signs, *Pediatrics* 127:e117–e125, 2011.
Curatolo P, Bombardieri R, Jozwiak S: Tuberous sclerosis, *Lancet* 372:657–668, 2008.

183. **What are skin findings in patients with tuberous sclerosis?**
See Table 13-8.

Table 13-8. Skin Findings in Tuberous Sclerosis

AGE AT ONSET	SKIN FINDINGS	INCIDENCE (%)
Birth or Later	Hypopigmented macules	80
2-5 yr	Angiofibromas	70
2-5 yr	Shagreen patches	35
Puberty	Periungual and gingival fibromas	20-50
Birth or Later	Café-au-lait spots	25

184. **Why is the term *adenoma sebaceum* a misnomer when used to describe patients with tuberous sclerosis?**
On biopsy, these papules are actually *angiofibromas*. They have no connection to sebaceous units or adenomas. This rash occurs in about 75% of patients with tuberous sclerosis, usually developing on the nose and central face between the ages of 5 and 13 years. It is red, papular, and monomorphous, and it is often mistaken for acne (Fig. 13-6). The diagnosis of tuberous sclerosis should be entertained in children who develop a rash that is suggestive of acne well before puberty.

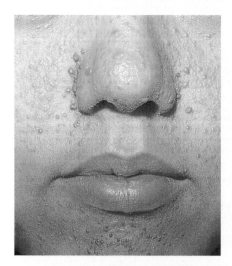

Figure 13-6. Adenoma sebaceum in patient with tuberous sclerosis. These angiofibromas first appear as flat, pink macules and later become papular. Lesions may bleed easily. *(From Habif TP: Clinical Dermatology: A Color Guide to Diagnosis and Therapy, ed 5. Philadelphia, 2010, Elsevier, p 988.)*

185. **What is the "tuber" of tuberous sclerosis?**
These 1- to 2-cm lesions consist of small stellate neurons and astroglial elements that are thought to be primitive cell lines resulting from abnormal differentiation. They may be located in various cortical regions. They are firm to the touch, like a small potato or tuber.

186. **What is the tissue type of a shagreen patch?**
A shagreen patch is an area of cutaneous thickening with a pebbled surface that, on biopsy, is a **connective tissue nevus**. The term *shagreen* derives from a type of leather that is embossed by knobs during the course of processing.

187. **Which types of facial port-wine stains are most strongly associated with ophthalmic or CNS complications?**
Port-wine stains can occur as isolated cutaneous birthmarks or, particularly in the areas underlying the birthmark, in association with structural abnormalities in the following areas: (1) the choroidal vessels of the eye, thereby leading to glaucoma; (2) the leptomeningeal vessels of the brain, thus leading to seizures (Sturge-Weber syndrome); and (3) hemangiomas in the spinal cord (Cobb syndrome). Glaucoma or seizures are most often associated with port-wine stains in children demonstrating the following:
- Involvement of the eyelids
- Bilateral distribution of the birthmark
- Unilateral involvement of all three branches (V_1, V_2, V_3) of the trigeminal nerve
- Ophthalmologic assessment and radiologic studies (CT or MRI) are indicated for children exhibiting these findings.

Sudarsanam A, Ardern-Holmes SL: Sturge-Weber syndrome: from the past to the present, *Eur J Paediatr Neurol* 18: 257–266, 2014.
Tallman B, Tan OT, Morelli JG, et al: Location of port-wine stains and the likelihood of ophthalmic and/or central nervous system complications, *Pediatrics* 87:323–327, 1991.

188. **What are the three stages of incontinentia pigmenti?**
Incontinentia pigmenti is an X-linked dominant disorder that is associated with seizures and mental retardation. Ectodermal tissues, such as eyes, nails, hair, and teeth, are also affected. The condition is presumed to be lethal to boys *in utero* because nearly 100% of cases are female. There are rare cases of XY patients with incontinentia pigmenti. It is caused by mutations in the NEMO (**N**F-kappaB **e**ssential **mo**dulator) gene, which is involved in cellular signal transduction.
- **Stage 1—Vesicular stage:** Lines of blisters are present on the trunk and extremities of the newborn that disappear in weeks or months. They may resemble herpetic vesicles. Microscopic examination of the vesicular fluid demonstrates eosinophils.
- **Stage 2—Verrucous stage:** Lesions develop in the patient at about 3 to 7 months of age that are brown and hyperkeratotic, resembling warts; these disappear over 1 to 2 years.
- **Stage 3—Pigmented stage:** Whorled, swirling, (marble cake–like), macular, hyperpigmented lines develop. These may fade over time, leaving only remnant hypopigmentation in late adolescence or adulthood (which is sometimes considered a fourth stage).

189. **What is the likely diagnosis for a 7-year-old who is noted to have recurrent nosebleeds, cutaneous telangiectasias on his lips, and an intracranial arteriovenous malformation on MRI?**
This child has **hereditary hemorrhagic telangiectasia,** which has also been known as *Osler-Weber-Rendu disease.* This condition may affect up to 1 in 5000 in the United States. The condition consists of nosebleeds; skin, lip, and oral mucosal lesions (Fig. 13-7); visceral manifestations due to arteriovenous malformations in the lung, liver, gastrointestinal tract, and CNS; and a positive family history. Genetic mutations involve transforming growth factor-β, which causes abnormalities in blood vessel formation.

Giordano P, Lenato GM, Lastella P, et al: Hereditary hemorrhagic telangiectasia: arteriovenous malformations in children, *J Pediatr* 163:179–183, 2013.

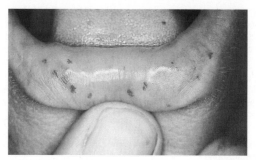

Figure 13-7. Hereditary hemorrhagic telangiectasia with lip telangiectasia. *(From Habif TP, editor:* Clinical Dermatology: A Color Guide to Diagnosis and Therapy, *ed 5. Philadelphia, 2011, Elsevier, p 911.)*

NEUROMUSCULAR DISORDERS

190. How can the anatomic site responsible for muscle weakness be determined clinically?
See Table 13-9.

Table 13-9. Clinical Determination of Anatomic Site Responsible for Muscle Weakness

	UPPER MOTOR NEURON	ANTERIOR HORN CELL	NEURO-MUSCULAR JUNCTION	PERIPHERAL NERVE	MUSCLE
Tone	Increased (may be decreased acutely)	Decreased	Normal, variable	Decreased	Decreased
Distribution	Pattern (e.g., hemiparesis, paraparesis) Distal > proximal	Variable, asymmetric	Fluctuating, cranial nerve involvement	Nerve distribution	Proximal > distal
Reflexes	Increased (may be decreased early	Decreased to absent	Normal (unless severely involved)	Decreased to absent	Decreased
Babinski	Extensor	Flexor	Flexor	Flexor	Flexor
Other	Cognitive dysfunction, atrophy only very late	Fasciculations, atrophy, no sensory involvement	Fluctuating course	Sensory nerve involvement, atrophy, rare fasciculations	No sensory deficits; may be tenderness and signs of inflammation

Adapted from Packer RJ, Berman PH: Neurologic emergencies. In Fleisher GR, Ludwig S, editors: Textbook of Pediatric Emergency Medicine, *ed 3. Baltimore, 1993, Williams & Wilkins, p 584.*

191. What are the causes of acute generalized weakness?
- **Infectious and postinfectious conditions:** Acute infectious myositis, GBS, enteroviral infection
- **Metabolic disorders:** Acute intermittent porphyria, hereditary tyrosinemia
- **Neuromuscular blockade:** Botulism, tick paralysis
- **Periodic paralysis:** Familial (hyperkalemic, hypokalemic, normokalemic)

Fenichel GM: *Clinical Pediatric Neurology: Signs and Symptoms Approach*, ed 5. Philadelphia, 2009, Elsevier, p 197.

192. **If a child presents with weakness, what aspects of the history and physical examination suggest a myopathic process?**

History
- Gradual rather than sudden onset
- Proximal weakness (e.g., climbing stairs, running) rather than distal weakness (more characteristic of neuropathy) predominates
- Absence of sensory abnormalities, such as "pins-and-needles" sensations
- No bowel and bladder abnormalities

Physical examination
- Proximal weakness is greater than distal weakness (except in myotonic dystrophy)
- Positive Gowers sign (see question 193)
- Neck flexion weaker than neck extension
- During the early stages, reflexes normal or only slightly decreased
- Normal sensory examination
- Muscle wasting but no fasciculations
- Muscle hypertrophy seen in some dystrophies

Weiner HL, Urion DK, Levitt LP: *Pediatric Neurology for the House Officer*, Baltimore, 1988, Williams & Wilkins, pp 136–138.

193. **What is the significance of a Gowers sign?**
Weakness of truncal and proximal lower extremity muscles. Most classically seen in Duchenne muscular dystrophy, the sign describes the manner in which children turn prone to rise and then rise from a sitting position by grasping and pushing on the knees and thighs ("climbing up the thighs") until they are standing (Fig. 13-8). The adaptation of a prone position before rising is an important early feature because only 6.5% of healthy children still roll prone before standing. After age 3 years, any child with a need to turn prone before rising should be followed closely for a possible underlying neuromuscular condition.

Wallace GB, Newton RW: Gower's sign revisited, *Arch Dis Child* 64:1317–1319, 1989.

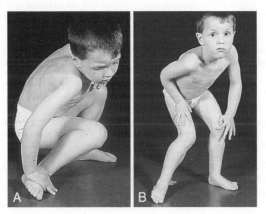

Figure 13-8. Gowers sign. **(a)** A child turns prone to rise and begins to use his hands to push his body upright, **(b)** finally pushing off his knees/thighs before standing *(From Lissauer T, Clayden G, Craft A: Illustrated Textbook of Paediatrics, ed 4. London, 2012, Elsevier Ltd, p 488.)*

194. **How does electromyography help differentiate between myopathic and neurogenic disorders?**
Electromyography measures the electrical activity of resting and voluntary muscle activity. Normally, the action potentials are of standardized duration and amplitude, with two to four distinguishable phases. In **myopathic** conditions, the durations and amplitudes are shorter than expected, called brief,

small-amplitude potentials (BSAPs); in **neuropathies,** they are longer. In both conditions, extra phases (i.e., polyphasic units) are usually noted.

195. How is pseudoparalysis distinguished from true neuromuscular disease?
     Pseudoparalysis (hysterical paralysis) or weakness may be seen in conversion reactions (i.e., emotional conflicts presenting as symptoms). In conversion reactions, sensation, deep tendon reflexes, and Babinski response are normal; movement may also be noted during sleep. *Hoover sign* is also helpful in cases of unilateral paralysis. With the patient lying supine on the table, the examiner places a hand under the heel of the affected limb and asks the patient to raise the unaffected limb. In pseudoparalysis, the examiner will feel pressure on the hand as the patient involuntarily extends the weak hip.

196. Why is it important to localize the cause of hypotonia?
     Localization of the level of the lesion is critical for determining the nature of the pathologic process. In the absence of an acute encephalopathy, the differential diagnosis of hypotonia is best approached by asking the question, "Does the patient have normal strength despite the hypotonia, or is the patient weak and hypotonic?" The combination of weakness and hypotonia usually points to an abnormality of the anterior horn cell or the peripheral neuromuscular apparatus, whereas hypotonia with normal strength is more characteristic of brain or spinal cord disturbances.

KEY POINTS: HYPOTONIA

1. Localization of lesion is critical for determining pathologic process.
2. Most important question: Is strength normal or abnormal?
3. Hypotonia *with weakness*: Think abnormality in anterior horn cell or peripheral neuromuscular apparatus.
4. Hypotonia *without weakness*: Think brain or spinal cord disturbance.

197. How can you detect myotonia clinically?
     Myotonia is a painless tonic spasm of muscle that follows voluntary contraction, involuntary failure of relaxation, or delayed muscle relaxation after a contraction. It can be elicited by grip (e.g., handshake), forced eyelid closure (or delayed eye opening in crying infants), lid lag after upward gaze, or percussion over various sites (e.g., thenar eminence, tongue).

198. How do the presentations of the two forms of myotonic dystrophy differ?
     The presentation of **congenital** myotonic dystrophy is during the immediate newborn period. Symptoms include hypotonia; facial diplegia with "tenting" of the upper lip; and, frequently, severe respiratory distress as a result of intercostal and diaphragmatic weakness, especially in the right hemidiaphragm. Feeding problems as a result of poor suck and gastrointestinal dysmotility are also present. The **juvenile** presentation of this condition is during the first decade of life. This form is characterized by progressive weakness and atrophy of the facial and sternocleidomastoid muscles and shoulder girdle, impaired hearing and speech, and excessive daytime sleepiness. Clinical myotonia is more likely, and there may be mental retardation.

199. In a newborn with weakness and hypotonia, what obstetric and delivery features suggest a diagnosis of congenital myotonic dystrophy?
     A history of **spontaneous abortions, polyhydramnios, decreased fetal movements, delays in second-stage labor, retained placenta,** and **postpartum hemorrhage** all raise the concern for *congenital myotonic dystrophy*. Because the mother is nearly always affected in congenital myotonic dystrophy (although previously diagnosed in only one-half of the cases), a careful clinical and electromyographic evaluation of the mother is essential. It is always important to shake the hand of the mother (barring religious exclusions) because affected women may not be able to release their hand after a handshake.

200. How is myotonic dystrophy an example of the phenomenon of "anticipation"?
     Genetic studies have shown that the defect in myotonic dystrophy is an expansion of a trinucleotide (CTG) in a gene on the long arm of chromosome 19 that codes for a protein kinase. The gene product was named myotonin-protein kinase, and it is thought to be involved in sodium- and chloride-channel

function. In successive generations, this repeating sequence has a tendency to increase, sometimes into the thousands (normal is <40 CTG repeats), and the extent of repetition correlates with the severity of the disease. Thus, each succeeding generation is likely to get more extensive manifestations and earlier presentations of the disease (i.e., the phenomenon of "anticipation"). This trinucleotide repeat phenomenon is also seen in Huntington disease and Fragile X syndrome.

201. **How does the pathophysiology of infant botulism differ from that of food-borne and wound botulism?**
   - *Infant botulism* results from the ingestion of *Clostridium botulinum* spores that germinate, multiply, and produce toxin in the infant's intestine. This is called a toxi-infection. The source of the spores is often unknown, but it has been linked to honey in some cases, and spores have been found in corn syrups. Therefore, these foods are not advised for infants younger than 1 year old.
   - *Food-borne botulism* involves cases in which preformed toxin is already present in the food. Improper canning and anaerobic storage permit spore germination, growth, and toxin formation, which result in symptoms if the toxin is not destroyed by proper heating.
   - *Wound botulism* occurs if spores enter a deep wound and germinate.

202. **What is the earliest indication for intubation in an infant with botulism?**
   Intubation is indicated if there is a **loss of protective airway reflexes**. This occurs before respiratory compromise or failure because diaphragmatic function is not impaired until 90% to 95% of the synaptic receptors are occupied. An infant with hypercarbia or hypoxia is at very high risk for imminent respiratory failure.

Schreiner MS, Field E, Ruddy R: Infant botulism: a review of 12 years' experience at the Children's Hospital of Philadelphia, *Pediatrics* 87:159–165, 1991.

203. **In an infant with severe weakness and suspected botulism, why is the use of aminoglycosides relatively contraindicated?**
   The botulism toxin acts by irreversibly blocking acetylcholine release from the presynaptic nerve terminals. Aminoglycosides, tetracyclines, clindamycin, and trimethoprim also interfere with acetylcholine release; therefore, they have the potential to act synergistically with the botulinum toxin to worsen or prolong neuromuscular paralysis.

204. **What are the two most common symptoms in children with juvenile myasthenia gravis?**
   Ptosis and **diplopia.** Myasthenia gravis is characterized by a highly variable clinical course of fluctuating weakness (characteristically with increasing contractions) that initially involves muscles that are innervated by the cranial nerves. It is caused by a defect in neuromuscular transmission that is caused by an autoimmune antibody-mediated attack on the acetylcholine receptors.

205. **What are the risks to a neonate who is born to a mother with myasthenia gravis?**
   Passively acquired neonatal myasthenia develops in about 10% of infants born to myasthenic mothers because of the transplacental transfer of antibody directed against acetylcholine receptors (AChR) in striated muscle. Signs and symptoms of weakness typically arise within the first hours or days of life. Pathologic muscle fatigability commonly causes feeding difficulty, generalized weakness, hypotonia, and respiratory depression. Ptosis and impaired eye movements occur in only 15% of cases. The weakness virtually always resolves as the body burden of anti-AChR immunoglobulins diminishes. Symptoms typically persist for about 2 weeks but may require several months to disappear completely. General supportive treatment is usually adequate, but oral or intramuscular neostigmine may help diminish symptoms.

206. **How does the pathophysiology of juvenile versus congenital myasthenia gravis differ?**
   Juvenile (and adult) myasthenia gravis is caused by circulating antibodies to the AChR of the postsynaptic neuromuscular junction. Occurrence is rare before the age of 2 years. *Congenital myasthenia gravis* is a nonimmunologic process. It is caused by morphologic or physiologic features affecting the presynaptic and postsynaptic junctions, including defects in ACh synthesis, end-plate acetylcholinesterase deficiency, and end plate AChR deficiency. *Neonatal myasthenia gravis* refers to the transient weakness that occurs in infants of mothers with myasthenia gravis.

207. How is the edrophonium (Tensilon) test done?

Edrophonium is a rapid-acting anticholinesterase drug of short duration that improves symptoms of myasthenia gravis by inhibiting the breakdown of ACh and increasing its concentration in the neuromuscular junction. A test dose of 0.015 mg/kg is given intravenously; if it is tolerated, the full dose of 0.15 mg/kg (up to 10 mg) is given. If measurable improvement in ocular muscle or extremity strength occurs, myasthenia gravis is likely. Because edrophonium may precipitate a cholinergic crisis (e.g., bradycardia, hypotension, vomiting, bronchospasm), atropine and resuscitation equipment should be available.

208. Does a negative antibody test exclude the diagnosis of juvenile myasthenia gravis?

No. Up to 90% of children with juvenile myasthenia have measurable anti-AChR antibodies, but, in the other 10%, continued clinical suspicion is necessary because their symptoms are usually milder (e.g., ocular muscle weakness, minimal generalized weakness). In these children, other tests (e.g., edrophonium, electrophysiological studies, single-fiber electromyography) may be needed to make the diagnosis.

Della Marina A, Trippe H, Lutz S, Schara U: Juvenile myasthenia gravis: recommendations for diagnostic approaches and treatment, *Neuropediatrics* 45:75–83, 2014.

209. What are the four characteristic features of damage to the anterior horn cells?

Weakness, fasciculations, atrophy, and **hyporeflexia.**

210. What processes can damage the anterior horn cells?
- **Degenerative** (spinal muscular atrophy): Werdnig-Hoffmann, Kugelberg-Welander
- **Metabolic:** Tay-Sachs disease (hexosaminidase deficiency), Pompe disease, Batten disease (ceroid-lipofuscinosis), hyperglycinemia, neonatal adrenoleukodystrophy
- **Infectious:** Poliovirus, Coxsackie virus, echoviruses

211. What is the primary genetic abnormality in infants and children with spinal muscular atrophy (SMA)?

Disruption of the **survival motor neuron 1 (SMN1) gene**. SMAs are a group of diseases that affect the motor neuron, resulting in widespread muscular denervation and atrophy. Incidence is estimated at 1 in 6000 to 10,000 newborns with a carrier frequency between 1 in 40 to 60. SMAs are the second most common hereditary neuromuscular disease after Duchenne muscular dystrophy. Extra copies of the SMN2 gene (a companion protein-coding gene) modify the clinical outcome. How changes in the SMN protein result in the disease process and phenotypic variability is unclear.

Nurputra DK, Lai PS, Harahap NI, et al: Spinal muscular atrophy: from gene discovery to clinical trials, *Am Hum Genet* 77:435–463, 2013.
Spinal Muscular Atrophy Association: www.smafoundation.org. Accessed March 6, 2015.

212. How are the inherited progressive spinal muscular atrophies distinguished?

See Table 13-10.

213. What are muscular dystrophies?

A *muscular dystrophy* is an inheritable myopathy that affects limbs or facial muscles and is progressive, with pathologic evidence of degeneration or regeneration without any abnormal storage material.

Muscular Dystrophy Association: www.mdausa.org. Accessed on March 6, 2015.

214. What is the clinical importance of dystrophin?

Dystrophin is a muscle protein that is presumed to be involved in anchoring the contractile apparatus of striated and cardiac muscle to the cell membrane. As a result of a gene mutation, this protein is completely missing in patients with Duchenne muscular dystrophy. On the other hand, muscle tissue from patients with Becker muscular dystrophy contains reduced amounts of dystrophin or, occasionally, a protein of abnormal size.

215. How are Duchenne and Becker muscular dystrophies distinguished?

See Table 13-11.

Table 13-10. Progressive Spinal Muscular Atrophies (SMAs)

DISORDER	INHERITANCE	AGE OF ONSET	CLINICAL FEATURES
Acute infantile SMA (Werdnig-Hoffmann disease, SMA type 1)	Autosomal recessive	*In utero* to 6 mo	Frog-leg posture; areflexia; tongue atrophy and fasciculations, progressive swallowing, and respiratory problems; survival <4 yr
Intermediate SMA (chronic Werdnig-Hoffmann disease, SMA type 2)	Autosomal recessive; rarely autosomal dominant	3 mo to 15 yr	Proximal weakness; most sit unsupported; decreased or absent reflexes; high incidence of scoliosis, contractures; survival may be up to 30 yr
Kugelberg-Welander disease (SMA type 3)	Autosomal recessive; rarely autosomal dominant	5-15 yr	May be part of the spectrum of SMA 2; hip girdle weakness; calf hypertrophy; decreased or absent reflexes; may be ambulatory until fourth decade
Adult-onset SMA (SMA type 4)	Autosomal recessive	After age 30 years	Mild to moderate muscle weakness, most commonly proximal; tremors, twitching; normal life

Adapted from Parke JT: Disorders of the anterior horn cell. In McMillan JA, DeAngelis CD, Feigin RD, Warshaw JB, editors: Oski's Pediatrics: Principles and Practice, ed 3. Philadelphia, 1999, JB Lippincott, p 1959.

Table 13-11. Duchenne Versus Becker Muscular Dystrophy

	GENETICS	DIAGNOSIS	MANIFESTATIONS
Duchenne	1 in 3500 male births X-linked Several different deletions, point mutations in dystrophin gene result in a completely nonfunctional protein New mutations occur Carrier females may have mild weakness or cardiomyopathy	Whole-blood DNA may reveal a deletion in about 65%; otherwise, electromyogram and muscle biopsy studies are definitive	Clinically evident at 3-5 years of age Regular, stereotyped course of progressive proximal weakness Calf hypertrophy Loss of ambulation by 9-12 years Worsening scoliosis and contractures Eventual dilated cardiomyopathy and/or respiratory failure Life expectancy of 16-19 years
Becker	1 in 20,000 male births X-linked Various mutations in dystrophin gene result in reduced amount of or partially functional protein	More benign clinical course Reduced dystrophin levels in muscle cells (by immunostaining) or abnormal dystrophin	Clinically evident during early second decade Milder, slower course as compared with Duchenne Calf pseudohypertrophy Pes cavus Cardiac and central nervous system involvement unusual Ambulatory until 18 years or beyond Life expectancy twice as long as compared with Duchenne

Adapted from Tsao VY, Mendell JR: The childhood muscular dystrophies: making order out of chaos. Semin Neurol 19:9–23, 1999.

216. **What causes the calf hypertrophy seen in Duchenne muscular dystrophy?**

Calf hypertrophy (Fig. 13-9) occurs primarily from replacement of muscle fibers with fat and fibrous tissue. When palpated, the calf has an unusually firm rubbery feel. Other muscles, including the tongue, can be enlarged with replacement tissues.

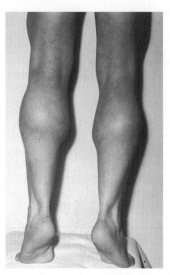

Figure 13-9. Calf enlargement in Duchenne muscular dystrophy. *(From Perkin GD, Miller DC, Lane R, et al, editors: Atlas of Clinical Neurology, ed 3. Philadelphia, 2011, Saunders Elsevier, p 58.)*

217. **Is corticosteroid therapy effective for the treatment of Duchenne muscular dystrophy?**

Several studies have documented an improvement in strength with an optimal dose of prednisone of 0.75 mg/kg per day. The strengthening effect lasts for up to 3 years while the steroid is continued. Despite mediation and supportive care, loss of ambulation, respiratory failure, and compromised cardiac function remain the inevitable outcomes. However, clinical trials are currently underway using gene therapy, which could eventually revolutionize the treatment of the disease.

Al-Zaidy S, Rodino-Klapac L, Mendell JR: Gene therapy for muscular dystrophy: moving the field forward, *Pediatr Neurol* 51:607–618, 2014.

218. **What is the most likely diagnosis in a child with progressive walking difficulties evolving over several days?**

Guillain-Barré syndrome (GBS) is an acute demyelinating neuropathy that is characterized by ascending, acute, progressive peripheral and cranial nerve dysfunction and paresthesias. In younger children (<6 years), it may be heralded by pain. It is frequently preceded by a viral respiratory or gastrointestinal illness. The disease is characterized by the presence of multifocal areas of the inflammatory demyelination of nerve roots and peripheral nerves. As a result of the loss of the healthy myelin covering, the conduction of nerve impulses (action potentials) may be blocked or dispersed. Axonal injury may also occur. The resulting clinical effects are predominantly motor (i.e., the evolution of flaccid, areflexic paralysis). There is a variable degree of motor weakness. Some individuals have mild brief weakness, whereas fulminant paralysis occurs in others. Autonomic signs (e.g., tachycardia, hypertension) and sensory symptoms (e.g., painful dysesthesias) are not uncommon, but they are overshadowed by the motor signs. More than half of these patients develop facial involvement, and mechanical ventilation may be required.

Yuki N, Hartung H-P: Guillain-Barré syndrome, *N Engl J Med* 366:2294–2304, 2012.

219. **What are subtypes of GBS?**

Subtypes are classified based on the clinical picture, laboratory results (including antiglycoside autoantibody patterns) and results of electromyography (EMG) and nerve conduction velocity (NCV) studies, which differentiate the relative effect of damage from either demyelination or axonal injury. One commonly used classification is:

- **AIDP: A**cute **I**nflammatory **D**emyelinating **P**olyneuropathy. This is the primary demyelinating form. EMG/NCV studies show evidence of demyelination of both motor and sensory nerves. In North America and Europe, 90% of cases of GBS involve this type.
- **AMSAN: A**cute **M**otor-**S**ensory **A**xonal **N**europathy. The axon of the nerve is considered to be the primary target, with secondary loss of myelin. Motor nerves alone are affected without sensory loss.
- **AMAN: A**cute **M**otor **A**xonal **N**europathy. Motor nerves alone are affected without sensory loss. EMG does not show demyelination. Axonal variants (AMSAN and AMAN) are much more frequent in Asia, accounting for 40% to 50% of cases.
- **Variants:** *Miller Fisher syndrome (MFS)* is characterized by gait ataxia, areflexia, and ophthalmoparesis. *Bickerstaff encephalitis* is brainstem encephalitis with encephalopathy in addition to the features seen in MFS. Both are associated with autoantibodies to glycoside GQ1b.

Arcila-Londono X, Lewis RA: Guillain-Barré syndrome, *Semin Neurol* 32:179–132, 2012.

220. **What CSF findings are characteristic of GBS?**

The classic CSF finding is the **albuminocytologic** dissociation. Most common infections or inflammatory processes generate an elevation of white blood cell count and protein. The CSF profile in GBS includes a normal cell count with elevated protein, usually in the range of 50 to 100 mg/dL; however, at the onset of disease, the CSF protein concentration may be normal.

221. **Outline the management of acute GBS.**

Early clinical monitoring is focused on the development of bulbar or respiratory insufficiency. Bulbar weakness manifests as unilateral or bilateral facial weakness, diplopia, hoarseness, drooling, depressed gag reflex, or dysphagia. Frank respiratory insufficiency may be preceded by air hunger, dyspnea, or a soft muffled voice (hypophonia). The autonomic nervous system is occasionally involved, and this is signified by the presence of cardiac arrhythmia, labile blood pressure and body temperature, and urinary retention. The management of GBS includes the following:

- Observation in an intensive care unit is critical, with frequent monitoring of vital signs.
- The early institution of IVIG or plasmapheresis shortens the clinical course and lessens long-term morbidity; corticosteroid therapy is thought to be ineffective.
- If bulbar signs are present, the patient should receive nothing orally, and the mouth is suctioned frequently. Hydration is maintained intravenously, and nutritional support is provided by nasogastric feedings.
- The vital capacity (VC) is measured frequently. In children, the normal VC may be calculated as $VC = 200\ mL \times$ age in years. If the VC falls below 25% of normal, endotracheal intubation is performed. Careful pulmonary toilet is conducted to minimize atelectasis, aspiration, and pneumonia.
- Meticulous nursing care includes careful patient positioning to prevent pressure sores, compression of peripheral nerves, and venous thrombosis.
- Physical therapy is conducted to prevent the development of contractures by passive range-of-movement exercises and splinting to maintain physiologic hand and limb postures until muscle strength returns.

Hughes RA, Swan AV, van Doorn PA: Intravenous immunoglobulin for Guillain-Barré syndrome, *Cochrane Database Syst Rev* 9:CD002063, 2014.

Agrawal S, Peake D, Whitehouse WP: Management of children with Guillain-Barré syndrome, *Arch Dis Child Educ Pract Ed* 92:161–168, 2007.

222. **What is the prognosis for children with GBS?**

Children appear to recover more quickly and more fully than adults. Most have good neurologic recovery, although approximately 20% to 40% may have some longer term residual symptoms (including paresthesias and fatigue). In children, the long-term outcome is not substantially different among the GBS subtypes. In rare cases, the neuropathy may recur as a chronic inflammatory demyelinating polyneuropathy (CIDP). There is debate whether CIDP is a long-term continuation of AIDP or a separate illness with a different pathogenesis.

Roodbol J, de Wit MC, Aarsen FK, et al: Long-term outcome of Guillain-Barré in children, *J Peripher Nerv Syst* 19:121–126, 2014.
Vajsar J, Fehlings D, Stephens D: Long-term outcome in children with Guillain-Barré syndrome, *J Pediatr* 142:305–309, 2003.
GGS/CIDP Foundation International: www.gbs-cidp.org. Accessed on March 6, 2015.

223. **Does multiple sclerosis (MS) present during childhood?**
     Uncommonly. It is estimated that about 3% to 5% of patients with multiple sclerosis experience their first attack <18 years of age and onset <10 years is quite uncommon (<1%). Studies of affected children demonstrate a variable predominance of boys during early childhood and females during adolescence. Ataxia, muscle weakness, and transient visual or sensory symptoms are relatively common presentations. CSF examination may demonstrate mild (<25 cells/mm^3) mononuclear pleocytosis with an increasing probability of oligoclonal bands with each recurrence. MRI is the single most useful diagnostic test: the presence of multiple, periventricular white matter plaques (bright areas on T2 images) confirms the diagnosis.

Bigi S, Banwell B: Pediatric multiple sclerosis, *J Child Neurol* 27:1378–1383, 2012.

SPINAL CORD DISORDERS

224. **Which sacral dimples and coccygeal pits in a newborn are concerning for an occult spinal dysraphism (OSD)?**
     These occur in up to 4% of newborns. Isolated simple sacral dimples are rarely associated with a significant spinal abnormality. However, certain features are more likely to be associated with an OSD (such as tethered cord syndrome) and warrant a screening ultrasound.
     - Location above the gluteal crease (typically >2.5 cm from the anus)
     - Deep dimples (if base cannot be visualized, do not probe because of risk for introducing an infection if a direct communication with the spinal canal is present)
     - Larger size (>0.5 cm)
     - Pits with cutaneous markers (lipoma, hypertrichosis, hemangioma)

Kucera JN, Coley I, O'Hara S, et al: The simple sacral dimple: diagnostic yield of ultrasound in neonates, *Pediatr Radiol* 45:211–216, 2015.
Williams H: Spinal sinuses, dimples, pits and patches: what lies beneath? *Arch Dis Child Educ Pract Ed* 91:75–80, 2006.

KEY POINTS: NEONATAL SACRAL FINDINGS SUGGESTIVE OF OCCULT SPINAL DYSRAPHISM

1. Location above the gluteal crease (typically >2.5 cm from the anus)
2. Deep dimples
3. Larger dimple size (>0.5 cm)
4. Sacral pits with cutaneous markers (lipoma, hypertrichosis, hemangioma)

225. **What are the two main features of the Chiari malformations?**
     Cerebellar elongation and **protrusion of the foramen magnum into the cervical spinal cord**. Anatomic anomalies of the hindbrain and skeletal structure result in different positioning of the various structures relative to the upper cervical canal and foramen magnum with different clinical features.

226. **What are the types of Chiari malformations?**
     Type I is the most common, but clinically the least severe and is generally asymptomatic during childhood. It is often diagnosed as an incidental finding on cervical MRI scans for neck pain and/or headache. The presentation of a Chiari I malformation may be insidious. There may be paroxysmal

vertigo, drop attacks, vague dizziness, and headache, which may be increased by the Valsalva maneuver. Occipital headache precipitated by exertion may progress to torticollis, down-gaze nystagmus, periodic nystagmus, and oscillopsia (objects in the visual field oscillate). MRI findings include malformations of the base of the skull and of the upper cervical spine, including hydromyelia and syringomyelia, which is a cyst (or syrinx) in the spinal cord that can expand and elongate over time. Surgical treatment is typically reserved only for symptomatic patients or those with a syrinx.

Type II is the so-called "classic" Chiari malformation (known historically as Arnold-Chiari malformation). Medulla and cerebellum, together with part or the entire fourth ventricle, are displaced into the spinal canal (Fig. 13-10). A variety of cerebellar, brainstem, and cortical defects can occur. This type is strongly associated with noncommunicating hydrocephalus and lumbosacral myelomeningocele.

Type III comprises any of the features of types I and II, but the entire cerebellum is herniated throughout the foramen magnum, with a cervical spina bifida cystica. Hydrocephalus is a common feature.

Baisden J: Controversies in Chiari I malformations, *Surg Neurol Int* 3(Suppl 3):S232–237, 2012.

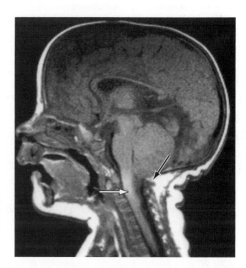

Figure 13-10. A midsagittal T1-weighted MRI of patient with type II Chiari malformation. The cerebellar tonsils *(white arrow)* have descended below the foramen magnum *(black arrow)*. Note the small, slitlike fourth ventricle, which has been pulled into a vertical position. *(From Kleigman RM, Stanton BF, Schor NF, et al, editors:* Nelson Textbook of Pediatrics, *ed 19. Philadelphia, 2011, Elsevier Saunders, p 2009).*

KEY POINTS: EARLY CLUES TO SPINAL CORD COMPRESSION

1. Scoliosis producing sustained poor posture
2. Back or abdominal pain beginning abruptly during sleep
3. Increased sensitivity of spinal column to local pressure or percussion
4. Bowel or bladder dysfunction
5. Diminished sensation in the anogenital region and lower limbs

227. What are types of spina bifida?

Spina bifida refers to malformations that result from failure of closure at the caudal end of the neural tube, as well as the overlying vertebral arches during embryogenesis. This can range from an asymptomatic defect such as spina bifida occulta in which the two halves of the vertebral arch fail to close to increasing displacement of the spinal cord (myelomeningocele) to the most severe form, myeloschisis, with exposed nervous tissue surrounded by no membrane (Fig. 13-11).

DIFFERENT TYPES OF SPINA BIFIDA

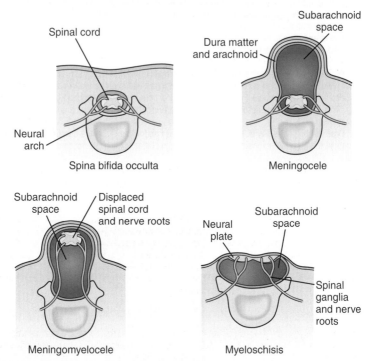

Figure 13-11. The different types of spinal bifida. *(From Perkin GD, Miller DC, Lane R, et al, editors: Atlas of Clinical Neurology, ed 3. Philadelphia, 2011, Saunders Elsevier, p 267.)*

228. **How common are asymptomatic spinal anomalies in normal children?**
Up to 5% of children have *spina bifida occulta*, an incomplete fusion of the posterior vertebral arches, which is usually noted as an incidental radiographic finding. The defect most commonly involves the lower lumbar lamina of L5 and S1.

229. **What is the full anatomic expression of myelomeningocele?**
- The presence of unfused or excessively separated vertebral arches of the bony spine (spina bifida)
- Cystic dilation of the meninges that surround the spinal cord (meningocele)
- Cystic dilation of the spinal cord itself (myelocele)
- Hydrocephalus and the spectrum of congenital cerebral abnormalities

230. **What is the likelihood that a patient with myelomeningocele will have hydrocephalus?**
Hydrocephalus is seen in 95% of children with thoracic or high lumbar myelomeningocele. The incidence decreases progressively with more caudal spinal defects to a minimum of 60% if the myelomeningocele is located in the sacrum.

231. **What is the usual cause of stridor in a child with myelomeningocele?**
The stridor is usually caused by **dysfunction of the vagus nerve,** which innervates the muscles of the vocal cords. In their resting position, the edges of the cords meet in the midline; during speech, they move apart. Hence, in bilateral palsies of the vagus nerve, the free edges of the vocal cords are closely opposed and obstruct air flow, thereby resulting in stridor. In symptomatic patients, the motor nucleus of the vagus nerve may be congenitally hypoplastic or aplastic. More commonly, the vagal dysfunction is believed to arise from a mechanical traction injury caused by hydrocephalus, which produces

progressive herniation and inferior displacement of the abnormal hindbrain. Shunting the hydrocephalus may alleviate the traction and improve the stridor. Sometimes the later recurrence of stridor indicates the reaccumulation of hydrocephalus as a result of ventriculoperitoneal shunt failure.

232. **What are the principal options for managing urinary incontinence in patients with myelomeningocele?**

About 80% of patients have a neurogenic bladder, which most commonly manifests as a small, poorly compliant bladder and an open and fixed sphincter. Options include the following:
- Clean intermittent catheterization, which results in more complete emptying than simple Credé maneuvers
- Artificial urinary sphincter to increase outlet resistance
- Surgical urinary diversion (e.g., suprapubic vesicostomy), which is uncommonly used
- Augmentation cystoplasty to increase bladder capacity in combination with the use of oxybutynin (a smooth muscle antispasmodic)

Mourtzinos A, Stoffel JT: Management goals for the spina bifida neurogenic bladder: a review from infancy to adulthood, *Urol Clin North Am* 37:527–535, 2010.

233. **How frequently is myelomeningocele associated with intellectual disability?**

Only 15% to 20% of patients have associated intellectual disability (mental retardation). Hydrocephalus *per se* does not cause the mental retardation that is associated with this syndrome. Children with appropriately treated congenital hydrocephalus caused by simple aqueductal stenosis usually have normal psychomotor development. Only severe hydrocephalus with a very thick cortical mantle predicts lower intelligence. Intellectual disability is usually attributed to acquired secondary CNS infection or subtle microscopic anomalies of neuronal migration and differentiation, which may coexist with the macroscopically visible malformation of the hindbrain.

234. **In an infant born with myelomeningocele, how does the initial evaluation predict long-term ambulation potential?**

The level of motor function—and not the level of the defect—is most predictive of ambulation.
- **Thoracic:** No hip flexion is noted. Almost no younger children will ambulate, and only about one-third of adolescents will ambulate with the aid of extensive braces and crutches.
- **High lumbar (L1, L2):** The patient is able to flex the hips, but there is no knee extension. About one-third of children and adolescents will ambulate, but only with extensive assistive devices.
- **Mid-lumbar (L3):** The patient is able to flex the hips and extend the knee. The percentage of those able to ambulate is midway between those with high and low lumbar lesions.
- **Low lumbar (L4, L5):** The patient is able to flex the knee and dorsiflex the ankle. Nearly half of younger children and nearly all adolescents will ambulate, with varying degrees of braces or crutches.
- **Sacral (S1-S4):** The patient is able to plantar flex the ankles and move the toes. Nearly all children and adolescents will ambulate, with minimal or no assistive devices.

Acknowledgment

The editors and the author gratefully acknowledge contributions by Drs. Kent R. Kelly, Douglas R. Nordli, Jr., Peter Bingham, and Robert R. Clancy that were retained from the first five editions of *Pediatric Secrets*.

CHAPTER 14

ONCOLOGY

Kerice Pinkney, MBBS and Alice Lee, MD

CHEMOTHERAPY AND RADIATION THERAPY

1. **What was the first cytotoxic chemotherapeutic agent used for the treatment of children with leukemia?**
   In 1948, Sidney Farber reported success using aminopterin (4-aminopteroyl-glutamic acid) in 16 children with acute leukemia. Aminopterin was a precursor to the antifolate drug, methotrexate, which is commonly used today.

   Farber S, Diamond LK, Mercer RD, et al: Temporary remissions in acute leukemia in children produced by folic acid antagonist, 4-amino-pteroylglutamic acid (aminopterin), *N Engl J Med* 238:787–793, 1948.

2. **Name the common cytotoxic chemotherapeutic drug classes.**
   Chemotherapeutic drugs are usually classified by their primary site and mechanism of action or source. The most common are the **alkylators, antimetabolites, antitumor antibiotics,** and **plant toxins**.

3. **We can thank the guinea pig for a major (albeit serendipitous) breakthrough in the treatment of childhood acute lymphoblastic leukemia (ALL). What role did our rodent friend the *Cavy* play?**
   In 1953, investigators discovered that whole guinea pig serum could bring about regression of certain transplanted lymphosarcomas in inbred mice. By 1961, it was determined that the fraction of guinea pig serum responsible for its antileukemic effect contained significant asparaginase activity. Most leukemic lymphoblasts were then found to be asparagine autotrophs, requiring exogenous asparagine for survival. A bacterial source (*Escherichia coli*) of asparaginase was identified, and pharmaceutical production of L-asparaginase began, increasing the complete remission rate for children with ALL from about 80% to more than 95%.

4. **Which chemotherapeutic agents are cell cycle dependent? In which phase are they most active?**
   See Figure 14-1.

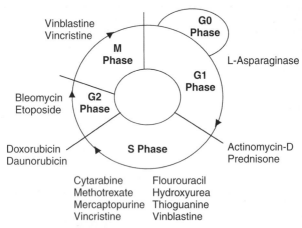

Figure 14-1. Phases in which cell cycle–dependent chemotherapy agents are most active. *G0*, resting phase (nonproliferation); *G1*, gap1 (pre-DNA synthesis with diploid RNA and protein synthesis); *S*, DNA synthesis; *G2*, gap2 (post-DNA synthesis); *M*, mitosis. *(From Weiner MA, Cairo MS: Pediatric Hematology/Oncology Secrets. Philadelphia, 2000, Hanley & Belfus, p 96.)*

5. **What is the difference between adjuvant and neoadjuvant chemotherapy?**
   Adjuvant chemotherapy is administered *after* the primary treatment of a tumor (surgical resection or radiation therapy), when there is no remaining gross tumor that can be assessed for response to the chemotherapy.

   Neoadjuvant chemotherapy is administered *before* the delivery of definitive local treatment and then continues afterward in the adjuvant setting. For children with solid tumors, several cycles of neoadjuvant chemotherapy are often administered to improve the chances of achieving complete surgical resection and improved local control of a primary tumor.

6. **Why are most chemotherapeutic drug dosages based on body surface area (BSA)?**
   In theory, *BSA* correlates better than body weight with cardiac output and hence hepatic and renal perfusion. Because most drug clearance occurs by hepatic and renal mechanisms, anticancer drugs that have a very narrow therapeutic index are usually dosed in a manner that is normalized to BSA. The exception is made for infants, who have a very high BSA-to-body weight ratio; infants receive chemotherapy based on body weight. BSA can be estimated using height and weight. One estimate can be obtained with the following formula:

$$BSA\ (m^2) = \sqrt{[(weight \times height)/3600]}$$

7. **What is the difference between pharmacokinetics and pharmacodynamics?**
   Pharmacokinetics refers to the effect of the body on the drug. It is the study of how drugs are absorbed, distributed, metabolized, and eliminated from the body. Common parameters include elimination half-life, peak concentration, clearance, and area under the concentration-time curve.

   Pharmacodynamics refers to the effect of the drug on the body. A pharmacodynamic effect can be a toxicity measurement (decrease in blood counts) or an anticancer measurement (decrease in the size of a tumor) after chemotherapy.

8. **What are the phases of clinical trials?**
   - **Phase I:** *The dose determination phase.* This phase is designed primarily to recommend a dose for further testing in children, usually the maximal tolerated dose. Pharmacokinetic studies are performed during phase I trials to help learn whether children handle a drug differently than adults. Phase 1 trials typically enroll 18 to 30 children.
   - **Phase II:** *The efficacy phase.* Usually a group of children with the same diagnosis are studied, and the percentage of patients in whom the drug causes a tumor to decrease in size is determined. Phase II trials enroll 30 to 150 children, depending on how many different tumor types are being studied.
   - **Phase III:** *The comparative phase.* This phase studies whether a new drug (or a new combination of drugs) that was found to be efficacious in a phase II trial can improve therapy relative to the best current therapy. Phase III trials are randomized and can enroll hundreds to thousands of children.

Balis FM, Fox E, Widemann BC, Adamson PC: Clinical drug development for childhood cancers, *Clin Pharmacol Ther* 85:127–129, 2009.

9. **What is the major dose-limiting toxicity for the alkylating agents?**
   Myelosuppression. Alkylating agents are chemically reactive compounds that covalently add an alkyl group; this is most important with regard to macromolecules involved in DNA synthesis, damaging templates, and inhibiting synthesis. Agents include the nitrogen mustards, oxazaphosphorines (including cyclophosphamide and ifosfamide), busulfan, and cisplatin.

10. **If one had to choose a single laboratory test to obtain before administering high-dose methotrexate, which one should it be?**
    Determination of serum creatinine is essential before administering high-dose methotrexate. The kidneys eliminate more than 90% of methotrexate. In the presence of abnormal renal function, high-dose methotrexate carries a high risk for severe or fatal toxicity.

Widemann BC, Adamson PC: Understanding and managing methotrexate nephrotoxicity, *Oncologist* 11:694–703, 2006.

11. **What factors are associated with an increased risk for developing anthracycline-induced cardiotoxicity?**

    Total cumulative dose, mediastinal radiotherapy, young age, and **female gender** are associated with an increased risk for developing anthracycline (doxorubicin, daunorubicin)-induced cardiotoxicity. Cumulative anthracycline dose has long been associated with an increased risk, with the incidence of clinically apparent congestive heart failure rising significantly with doxorubicin doses exceeding 450 mg/m^2. Late cardiotoxicity appears to be more common in children than in adults because the heart is unable to grow in proportion to the child, resulting in a small, poorly compliant left ventricle. Thus, younger children, particularly children younger than 5 years, are at higher risk. There is also some evidence that girls have a higher incidence of abnormal cardiac findings at any given cumulative dose than boys. Trisomy 21 and black patients may also be at increased risk. Dexrazoxane, a cardioprotective agent, has been used in adults receiving anthracyclines, but the FDA has limited pediatric use because of possible higher rates of second malignancies and acute myelogenous leukemia (AML) in patients treated for different cancers.

Lipshultz SE, Sambatakos P, Maguire M, et al: Cardiotoxicity and cardioprotection in childhood cancer, *Acta Haematol* 132:391–399, 2014.

Barry E, Alvarez JA, Scully RE, et al: Anthracycline-induced cardiotoxicity: course, pathophysiology, prevention and management, *Expert Opin Pharmacother* 8:1039–1058, 2007.

12. **How did a periwinkle plant contribute to some longstanding chemotherapeutic agents?**

    Extractions from the pink Madagascar periwinkle plant have been used for centuries as natural remedies. When used (unsuccessfully) as a treatment for diabetes mellitus, myelosuppression was noted. In the 1950s, the active components were noted to be vinca alkaloids. This property led to studies in oncology with vincristine (one of the alkaloids) licensed by the Food and Drug Administration (FDA) in 1963.

Moudi M, Go R, Yien CY, et al: Vinca alkaloids, *Int J Prev Med* 11:1231–1235, 2013.

13. **What is the mechanism of action of vincristine?**

    Vincristine binds to tubulin, which disrupts microtubules and arrests mitosis in metaphase. Thus, it is most effective in rapidly dividing cell types. It is used in all phases of ALL therapy including induction, consolidation, and maintenance. It has also played a role in the treatment of a variety of other pediatric oncologic diseases, including non-Hodgkin lymphoma, Hodgkin lymphoma, Wilms tumor, and neuroblastoma.

Liesveld J, Asselin B: It's ALL in the liposomes: vincristine gets a new package, *J Clin Oncol* 20:657–659, 2013.

14. **What agent can limit the complication of hemorrhagic cystitis that occurs in some chemotherapeutic regimens?**

    Mesna is the acronym for 2-mercaptoethane sodium sulfonate, a sulfhydryl compound. The oxazaphosphorines (cyclophosphamide, ifosfamide) are widely used in clinical practice for their antitumor activities. However, urinary excretion of their urotoxic metabolite, acrolein, can lead to hematuria and hemorrhagic cystitis. Mesna acts as a detoxifying agent. It is given as an adjuvant therapy and binds to acrolein in the urine, which creates an inert thioether that is excreted.

Andriole GL, Sandlund JT, Miser JS, et al: The efficacy of mesna (2-mercaptoethane sodium sulfonate) as a uroprotectant in patients with hemorrhagic cystitis receiving further oxazaphosphorine chemotherapy, *J Clin Oncol* 5:799–803, 1987.

15. **What is a vesicant?**

    A *vesicant* is an agent that produces a vesicle; in oncology, it is a chemotherapeutic drug that can cause a severe burn if the drug infiltrates around the intravenous catheter. The anthracyclines (doxorubicin, daunorubicin), dactinomycin, and the vinca alkaloids (vincristine, vinblastine) are all vesicants. These drugs must be administered either through a central venous catheter or through a newly placed, free-flowing intravenous catheter that does not cross over a joint space.

16. **Which classes of chemotherapeutic agents have most commonly been implicated in causing secondary leukemias?**

    The **alkylating agents** (e.g., cyclophosphamide) and **topoisomerase II inhibitors** (etoposide) increase the risk for developing secondary leukemia. Etoposide-induced leukemias tend to occur earlier, usually within 2 to 3 years of exposure.

17. **Why is intrathecal chemotherapy dose based on patient age, whereas systemic (oral, intravenous) dosing is based on weight or BSA?**

    The brains of children grow disproportionately more quickly than their bodies (hence the tendency of infants who have recently learned to sit to readily tip over). The cerebrospinal fluid (CSF) increases in parallel with central nervous system (CNS) growth, such that by the age of 3 years, CSF volume is 80% that of adult CSF volume. Scaling intrathecal doses to body size would undertreat younger children, whereas scaling doses in adolescent patients, whose CNS size has plateaued relative to body size, would unnecessarily expose them to potentially more toxic drug concentrations.

18. **What antiemetic agents are most effective in the management of chemotherapy-induced nausea and vomiting?**

    The **serotonin receptor antagonists** (ondansetron and granisetron) act as the foundation of prophylactic therapy for chemotherapy with significant emetogenic potential. The **neurokinin (NK1) receptor antagonists** (e.g., aprepitant), are the newest class of effective antiemetic agents and have shown extremely promising results. Aprepitant blocks the NK-1 receptors in the vomiting centers in the CNS, which are activated by substance P, released as an unwanted consequence of chemotherapy. Corticosteroids are useful for chemotherapeutic agents with low emetic potential; however, they are most effective when used in combination with other agents. Less effective agents include metoclopramide, phenothiazines, cannabinoids, and olanzapine, all of which have a greater potential for adverse side effects.

Hargreaves R, Ferreira JC, Hughes D, et al: Development of aprepitant, the first neurokinin-1 receptor antagonist for the prevention of chemotherapy-induced nausea and vomiting, *Ann NY Acad Sci* 1222:40–48, 2011.

Hesketh PJ: Chemotherapy-induced nausea and vomiting, *N Engl J Med* 2008; 358:2482–2494, 2008.

19. **Who develops the "somnolence syndrome"?**

    Transient symptoms attributed to temporary demyelination have been observed 6 to 8 weeks after **completion of CNS radiation**, most commonly for CNS prophylaxis for ALL. Children who develop the somnolence syndrome have lethargy, headache, and anorexia that last for about 2 weeks. Computed tomography (CT) and CSF studies show no consistent abnormality, but an electroencephalogram often reveals a slow-wave activity consistent with diffuse cerebral disturbance. The use of steroids during irradiation appears to minimize the occurrence of the syndrome.

20. **What is radiation recall?**

    Radiation recall is a delayed effect that results from the interaction of certain chemotherapeutic agents (doxorubicin, daunorubicin, or actinomycin-D) with radiation. After radiation therapy, an erythematous rash in the previous radiation field develops. The rash is geographic, usually precisely following the outline of the radiation field. Many of these occur months after the radiation treatment.

21. **What is a "fraction" of radiation?**

    Radiation therapy is coordinated so that a patient receives a maximally tolerated total amount of radiation dose. However, exposure to large amounts of radiation in one instance does not necessarily result in optimal cellular destruction, and it may have significant side effects. As a result, radiation is "fractionated" into smaller doses. Patients may receive up to dozens of individual fractions to achieve total radiation doses. For solid tumors, radiation is delivered over 2 to 6 weeks.

22. **A 10-year-old girl is being treated for AML with a combination of high-dose cytarabine and daunorubicin. Five days after the initiation of therapy, she develops the onset of nystagmus, ataxia, and dysmetria, and a brain CT reveals no focal abnormalities. What is the most likely cause of her symptoms?**

    High-dose cytarabine can result in an **acute cerebellar syndrome** leading to nystagmus, ataxia, dysmetria, and dysdiadochokinesia. Imaging at the onset of symptoms is typically normal. In most cases, neurologic symptoms resolve within a week, but as many as 30% of patients do not regain full cerebellar function. The risk for developing cerebellar syndrome is related to the dose and schedule of cytarabine, with the highest risk being observed with administration of high doses over 6 or more days.

23. **What are the long-term sequelae of chemotherapy?**
Today, approximately 80% of children with cancer are cured. However there are significant long-term effects from chemotherapy that have come to the forefront with a growing population of survivors. The effects are based on the type of treatment received and the age at which the patient was treated. The major sequelae include **cognitive defects**, **cardiac defects** (particularly with anthracyclines), **endocrinopathies** (especially thyroid dysfunction and hypopituitarism), **infertility**, and unfortunately **secondary malignancies**. There is a significant component of **psychosocial morbidity**, including depression and anxiety, which has been reported.

Skinner R: Long-term effects of cancer therapy in children—functional effects, late mortality and long-term follow-up, *Paediatr Child Health* 22(6):248–252, 2012.
Skinner R: Long-term effects of cancer therapy in children—organs, systems and tissues, *Paediatr Child Health* 22:201–206, 2012.

24. **Radiation therapy: what are its long-term effects?**
Radiation therapy is an important component of treatment for many pediatric cancers. However, it is associated with the development of **secondary neoplasms** (solid tumors), **obesity** following cranial radiation, **thyroid dysfunction,** and **pulmonary** and **cardiac** complications. The majority of these complications arise within the field of exposure. Limiting the dose and the extent of radiation exposure is key in reducing the long-term effects.

Armstrong GT, Stovall M, Robison LL: Long-term effects of radiation exposure among adult survivors of childhood cancer: results from the Childhood Cancer Survivor Study, *Radiation Res* 174:840–850, 2010.

CLINICAL ISSUES

25. **A patient has a central venous catheter and develops a fever. What should be done?**
The risk for bacteremia is increased in patients with central venous catheters. As such, any patient with an indwelling central venous catheter and a fever (temperature usually $\geq$38.5 °C) should have paired blood cultures drawn from the catheter (one or more catheter lumens) and from a peripheral vein before any antibiotic administration. Intravenous antibiotics are typically administered until evidence of a negative blood culture is provided. Removal of the catheter should be considered if the patient has signs of sepsis, significant worsening erythema, or purulence. Removal of the catheter is generally advised if blood cultures are positive with a suspected pathologic organism. If the catheter is left in place, it should be removed if bloodstream infection continues despite >72 hours of antimicrobial therapy to which the infecting microbes are susceptible. If catheter removal is required, the catheter tip should be cultured.

Mermel LA, Allon M, Bouza, et al: Clinical practice guidelines for diagnosis and management of intravascular catheter-related infection, 2009 update by the Infectious Diseases Society of America, *Clin Infect Dis* 49:1-45, 2009.
Rackoff WR, Ge J, Sather HN, et al: Central venous catheter use and the risk of infection with acute lymphoblastic leukemia: a report from the Children's Cancer Group, *J Pediatr Hematol Oncol* 21:260–267, 1999.

26. **Describe three different types of infection that are associated with central venous catheters, and how the treatment approaches to these infections differ.**
For external catheters (e.g., Hickman, Broviac), an **exit site infection,** manifested as inflammation and occasionally exudate limited to where the catheter emerges through the skin, can usually be managed with a combination of local care and systemic antibiotics. Patients with indwelling catheters are at increased risk for **bloodstream infections.** Many bacterial blood infections associated with central lines can be cleared with intravenous antibiotics administered through the central catheter, rotating lumens for multiline catheters. The potentially most serious bacterial infection is a **tunnel infection,** manifested by inflammation and tenderness along the entire subcutaneous tract of the catheter. These infections mandate prompt removal of the catheter and administration of intravenous antibiotics.

27. **A patient undergoing chemotherapy is neutropenic and has a fever. What should be done?**
Because neutropenic patients are at risk for invasive bacterial infections, patients who are neutropenic (absolute neutrophil count <500/mm^3 or <1000/mm^3 and falling) should have blood

cultures obtained and receive broad-spectrum antibiotics. Antibiotic coverage should include both gram-negative and gram-positive organisms, including antibiotics that are active against *Pseudomonas aeruginosa*. Broad-spectrum antibiotics are continued until blood cultures have been negative for 48 hours, a patient has been afebrile for at least 24 hours, and there is marrow evidence (with increasing neutrophil counts) that indicates signs of recovery.

Lehmbecher T, Phillips R, Alexander S, et al: Guideline for the management of fever and neutropenia in children with cancer and/or undergoing hematopoietic stem-cell transplantation, *J Clin Oncol* 30:4427–4438, 2012.

28. **A patient remains febrile and neutropenic despite appropriate antibiotics for several days. Is there cause for concern?**
    Although it is not uncommon for a neutropenic patient to remain febrile for many days despite administration of broad-spectrum antibacterial agents, persistent fever is associated with an **increased likelihood of invasive fungal infection**. Pediatric patients at particular risk for invasive fungal disease are those with AML or relapsed acute leukemia, those receiving highly myelosuppressive chemotherapy for other malignancies, and those undergoing stem-cell transplantation with fever $\geq$96 hours despite broad-spectrum antibiotic therapy and with neutropenia expected to continue >10 days. Because the ability to recover fungi in routine blood cultures is limited, the approach to such patients is to empirically add antifungal coverage after a period of persistent fever. Choices of empirical antifungal therapy have expanded over recent years and now include liposomal formulations of amphotericin B, azoles (e.g., voriconazole), and echinocandins (e.g., caspofungin).

Lehmbecher T, Phillips R, Alexander S, et al: Guideline for the management of fever and neutropenia in children with cancer and/or undergoing hematopoietic stem-cell transplantation, *J Clin Oncol* 30:4427–4438, 2012.

29. **How should a patient who has oral candidiasis or esophageal candidiasis be treated?**
    Candida species of yeast are a common cause of oral or esophageal infections in immunocompromised hosts. Topical antifungals (e.g., nystatin) may be tried in cases of simple oral candidiasis, and these can be added to regimens to treat esophageal candidiasis. However, systemic therapy is usually indicated in cases of esophageal candidiasis. Fluconazole is the first-line agent that can be used against candidal mucosal infections.

30. **After receiving broad-spectrum antibiotic therapy for 4 days for fever and neutropenia, a patient develops a new fever that is associated with abdominal cramps and bloody diarrhea. What is the most likely diagnosis?**
    The patient most likely has ***Clostridium difficile* colitis** brought on by treatment with broad-spectrum antibiotics. The diagnosis should be confirmed by detection of the *C. difficile* toxins in the stool, and either metronidazole (preferred) or oral vancomycin should be initiated promptly.

31. **A 10-year-old in her second year of treatment for ALL has had all medications voluntarily stopped by her parents for 8 weeks. What is the likely diagnosis when she presents to the emergency department (ED) with cough, tachypnea, hypoxia, and a chest x-ray that reveals widespread pulmonary infiltrates?**
    ***Pneumocystis jiroveci* pneumonia (PJP).** Formerly called *pneumocystis carinii*, *pneumocystis jiroveci* are yeast-like fungi that can result in opportunistic infections in individuals with compromised immune systems. Although classified as a fungus, PJP is nonresponsive to antifungal treatment. Children with cancer are immunosuppressed both because of their underlying diagnosis and the chemotherapy they receive. As a result, they require PJP prophylaxis (typically trimethoprim-sulfamethoxazole), which is given as 2 to 3 consecutive days of dosing per week. In this case, a compliance failure likely resulted in pneumonia. Clinical signs of *pneumocystis* pneumonia can be highly variable, but a classic feature is an arterial oxygen level (PaO$_2$) that is distinctly lower than expected given the clinical findings.

32. **What paraneoplastic syndromes can occur in childhood?**
    Paraneoplastic signs or symptoms are those that are unrelated to a malignancy but that can herald cancer. They occur more commonly in adults than children. However, unexplained high calcium, watery diarrhea, polymyositis, dermatomyositis, unexplained high hemoglobins, hypertension, precocious puberty, encephalitis, and opsoclonus or myoclonus can be associated with childhood malignancies.

Wells EM, Dalmau J: Paraneoplastic neurologic disorders in children, *Curr Neurol Neurosci Rep* 11:187–194, 2011.

33. **What are the metabolic abnormalities in the tumor lysis syndrome?**
Tumor lysis syndrome is an oncologic emergency that occurs when there is spontaneous or chemotherapy-induced massive breakdown of tumor cells. The subsequent release of the cells' contents into the circulation leads to **hyperkalemia, hyperuricemia, hyperphosphatemia,** and **secondary hypocalcemia.** Hyperkalemia is the most dangerous aspect of tumor lysis syndrome because of the high risk of sudden death. As such, patients at risk for tumor lysis syndrome should have no potassium placed in their IV fluids, have frequent electrolyte checks, and may need to be placed on a cardiac monitor.

Howard SC, Jones DP, Pui CH: The tumor lysis syndrome, *N Engl J Med* 364:1844–1845, 2011.

34. **In what settings is tumor lysis syndrome more likely to occur?**
Tumor lysis syndrome has been most frequently observed in patients with non-Hodgkin lymphoma and other hematologic malignancies (such as ALL) after the initiation of cytotoxic chemotherapy. It may also occur in other tumor types with a high proliferative rate or high sensitivity to cytotoxic therapy, as well as in the presence of a large tumor burden. In addition, the presence of preexisting renal impairment is widely regarded as a contributory factor.

Cairo MS, Coiffier B, Reiter A, et al: Recommendations for the evaluation of risk and prophylaxis of tumour lysis syndrome (TLS) in adults and children with malignant diseases: an expert TLS panel consensus, *Br J Haematol* 149(4):576-586, 2010.

35. **What are the current recommendations regarding management of tumor lysis syndrome?**
Prevention is the key in the management of tumor lysis syndrome and is done through aggressive intravenous (IV) hydration. The goal of IV hydration is to quickly improve renal perfusion and glomerular filtration, which results in high urine output that minimizes the likelihood of uric acid or calcium phosphate precipitation in the tubules. There is no current consensus regarding the role of urinary alkalinization by using sodium bicarbonate in these patients. Reducing the level of uric acid through pharmacologic measures is also recommended.

36. **What two pharmacologic agents can be used to prevent or treat hyperuricemia caused by tumor lysis syndrome?**
Allopurinol inhibits the enzyme xanthine oxidase, a key enzyme required for the formation of uric acid. Its administration blocks further uric acid *production.* **Rasburicase** is a recombinant enzyme that catalyzes the conversion of uric acid to allantoin, which is more soluble than uric acid, and more readily *excreted* by the kidney.

37. **A child with newly diagnosed leukemia experiences a rapid decline in hemoglobin soon after administration of rasburicase. What is the basis for this drug-related adverse event?**
Rasburicase is contraindicated in patients with glucose-6-phosphate dehydrogenase (G6PD) deficiency because of the risk for hemolysis and development of methemoglobinemia.

38. **A child undergoing induction chemotherapy for leukemia develops right lower quadrant pain and tenderness. What diagnosis should be considered?**
Typhlitis. Although patients with cancer or those receiving chemotherapy may develop appendicitis, typhlitis is a severe necrotizing infection of the ileocolonic junction that occurs in neutropenic patients.

39. **What is the difference between a Broviac and a Port-A-Cath?**
Children who require repeated blood draws or intravenous medications often have a semipermanent central venous catheter placed.
- A **Broviac catheter** is tunneled through the subcutaneous tissues of the chest and emerges as a thin plastic tube, usually at the level of the second or third rib.
- A **Port-A-Cath** contains a subcutaneous reservoir and is implanted under the skin of the chest. It is not visible, but it must be accessed by inserting a small needle through the skin and into the reservoir.

Gallieni M, Pittiruti M, Biffi R: Vascular access in oncology patients, *CA Cancer J Clin* 58:323–346, 2008.

40. **What is the differential diagnosis of an anterior mediastinal mass?**
    The five "T's" can be used to remember the differential diagnosis of an anterior mediastinal mass: **t**eratoma (germ-cell tumor), **t**hymoma, **t**hyroid tumor, **T**-cell leukemia, and **t**errible lymphoma (Fig. 14-2).

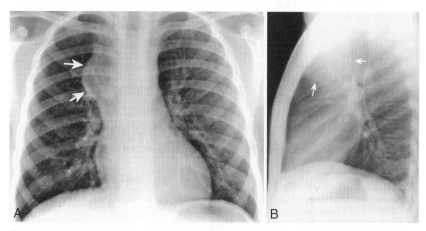

Figure 14-2. (A) Frontal radiograph in a child with "leukemia/lymphoma" syndrome, demonstrating an anterior mediastinal mass *(arrows)*. **(B)** Lateral film illustrates the anterior nature of the mass *(arrows)* with posterior displacement of the trachea. *(From Blickman JG, Parker BR, Barnes PD: Pediatric Radiology: The Requisites, ed 3. Philadelphia, 2009, Mosby, p 42.)*

41. **What is superior mediastinal syndrome? How is it managed?**
    Superior mediastinal syndrome, also called superior vena cava syndrome, results from the presence of an anterior mediastinal mass that compresses the trachea and the superior vena cava. Patients have a cough and dyspnea, particularly when supine, and they have swelling of the head and upper extremities as a result of venous compression. Patients with a large mediastinal mass must not be anesthetized because of the risk for complete airway obstruction and vascular collapse. The optimal management of a mediastinal mass is prompt diagnosis and the initiation of appropriate treatment. Irradiation of the mass may provide emergent relief while the diagnosis is being made.

42. **Which tumor is the most common cause of superior mediastinal syndrome in children?**
    Non-Hodgkin lymphoma. Less frequent causes are Hodgkin disease, neuroblastoma, and sarcomas. Nonmalignant infectious causes are unusual but can include histoplasmosis or tuberculosis. The most frequent nonmalignant cause in children, however, is *iatrogenic,* resulting from vascular thrombosis after surgeries for congenital heart disease, shunting procedures for hydrocephalus, or central catheterization for venous access.

43. **Why is a generous mediastinal shadow on a radiograph much more worrisome in a teenager than in an infant?**
    Among infants, the incidence of Hodgkin disease is extremely low. The thymus normally has a distinctive shape with flaring at the base and indentations from the ribcage ("sail sign"), which can usually be delineated on plain film. In teenagers, thymic enlargement has a higher likelihood of malignancy, particularly Hodgkin disease, which is usually accompanied by lymphadenopathy in other areas of the mediastinum, particularly the paratracheal, tracheobronchial, and hilar regions.

44. **Which neoplasms are associated with hemihyperplasia?**
    Wilms tumor, hepatoblastoma, adrenal cortical carcinoma, and **leiomyosarcomas** are associated with hemihyperplasia (formerly called hemihypertrophy) either as part of a syndrome (such as Beckwith-Wiedemann syndrome) or in isolation. Hemihyperplasia results in one side or portion of the body being larger than the other. The difference can be subtle (noted only when a patient lies on a flat surface) or more obvious when posture or gait is observed. Between 1% and 3% of Wilms tumor patients have hemihyperplasia.

45. **Which cancers are often associated with splenomegaly?**
Acute leukemia, chronic myeloid leukemia, chronic myelomonocytic leukemia, Hodgkin disease, and non-Hodgkin lymphoma are often associated with splenomegaly. Solid tumors rarely metastasize to the spleen to the point of causing splenomegaly.

46. **What are the predictors of malignancy in the pediatric patient with peripheral lymphadenopathy?**
A common clinical problem is determining which patients with enlarged lymph nodes require biopsy for diagnosis. Risk for malignancy is increased with increasing size (>1 cm in the neonatal period, >2 cm and increasing in older children despite antibiotic therapy), increasing number of adenopathy sites, and concurrent systemic symptoms (i.e., prolonged fever, night sweats, weight loss). Supraclavicular location, abnormal chest radiograph, abnormal complete blood count (CBC), and fixed nodes are also significantly predictive of malignancy.

King D, Ramachandra J, Yeomanson D: Lymphadenopathy in children: refer or reassurance? *Arch Dis Child Educ Pract Ed* 99:101–110, 2014.
Soldes OS, Younger JG, Hirschl RB: Predictors of malignancy in childhood peripheral lymphadenopathy, *J Pediatr Surg* 34:1447–1452, 1999.

47. **What is the function of the Langerhans cells?**
These are antigen-presenting immune cells, dendritic in appearance, that are found in all layers of the skin and mucosal surfaces and in lymph nodes. The ultrastructural hallmark of the cell is the Birbeck granule, a cytoplasmic organelle that is shaped like a tennis racquet.

48. **What are the features of Langerhans cell histiocytosis (LCH)?**
LCH is a multifaceted disorder and replaces the diseases grouped under the term *histiocytosis X.*
The presenting symptoms of LCH may be isolated bone lesions (eosinophilic granuloma), bone lesions with exophthalmos and diabetes insipidus (Hand-Schüller-Christian disease), or bone lesions with disseminated disease (Letterer-Siwe disease). Other features include skin rashes that resemble seborrheic dermatitis, chronic otitis externa, lymphadenopathy, hepatosplenomegaly, pancytopenia, neurologic deficits, and pulmonary disease. Mild forms of the disease tend to wax and wane even without treatment, whereas disseminated disease is often resistant to therapy.

49. **What is an eosinophilic granuloma?**
Eosinophilic granuloma is a lytic tumor of bone that is accompanied by pain and sometimes swelling. Its histology is identical to that of LCH, with which it is now classified. Biopsy of an isolated eosinophilic granuloma is often curative, although lesions may also regress spontaneously.

50. **What are the common indications for transfusion support for children with cancer?**
Although there are no absolute criteria, in most centers, packed red blood cells are given when a patient has a hemoglobin level in the range of 6 to 8 g/dL, even if asymptomatic, or at higher levels if a patient has symptoms or if ongoing marrow suppression is anticipated. Platelets are empirically administered for a platelet count of less than 10,000 to 20,000/mm^3 in an otherwise well patient; a higher threshold may be used if there is active bleeding, disseminated intravascular coagulation (DIC), or a planned procedure. Granulocyte transfusions may be effective in neutropenic patients with a refractory infection caused by a gram-negative organism. Transfusions with plasma may be used for the treatment of coagulopathies.

Roseff SD, Luban NL, Manno CS: Guidelines for assessing appropriateness of pediatric transfusion, *Transfusion* 42:1398–1413, 2002.

51. **What are the most common symptoms experienced by oncology patients receiving end-of-life care?**
Fatigue, pain, and **dyspnea.** Parents report that these symptoms are managed effectively in less than one-third of children. As compared with adults, twice as many children die in hospitals (usually an ICU) during the final stages of disease, half on ventilators, and only 10% to 20% of dying children receive hospice care. This is despite the fact that 70% of families would choose for their child to die at home if

support were adequate. Insufficient attention to palliative care has been a large problem, although an appreciation of its importance is growing.

Epelman CL: End-of-life management in pediatric cancer, *Curr Oncol Rep* 14:191–196, 2012.
Wolfe J, Grier HE, Klar N, et al: Symptoms and suffering at the end of life in children with cancer, *N Engl J Med* 342:326–333, 2000.
National Hospice and Palliative Care Organization: www.nhpco.org/pediatrics. Accessed on Jan. 9, 2015.

EPIDEMIOLOGY

52. Although in psychic lore a "seer" can look into the future, SEER has a different connotation for cancer researchers. What is it?
SEER stands for the **S**urveillance, **E**pidemiology, and **E**nd-**R**esults database. SEER collects cancer incidence, prevalence, and survival data in specific geographic areas in the United States. These areas represent about 26% of the U.S. population. SEER data are freely available to qualified investigators and can be used to study epidemiologic trends in cancer incidence, prevalence, and survival.

National Cancer Institute: www.seer.cancer.gov. Accessed on Jan. 9, 2015.

53. How do the types of cancers differ between adults and children?
As a general rule, in *adults*, most cancers are carcinomas (of epithelial origin). In *children*, the origin of most cancers are reticuloendothelial (e.g., leukemia, lymphoma), embryonal (e.g., blastomas) or mesenchymal (e.g., sarcomas).

54. What is the most frequently occurring childhood cancer?
Leukemia is the most frequently occurring with ALL being the most frequent single cancer diagnosis.

55. How do the types and frequency of childhood cancers vary by age?

Children *(Ages: 0 to 14 years)*	Adolescents *(Ages: 15 to 19 years)*
• Acute lymphoblastic leukemia: 26%	• Hodgkin lymphoma: 15%
• Brain and CNS tumors: 21%	• Thyroid carcinoma: 11%
• Neuroblastoma: 7%	• Brain and CNS tumors: 10%
• Non-Hodgkin lymphoma: 6%	• Testicular germ cell tumors: 8%
• Wilms tumor: 5%	• Non-Hodgkin lymphoma: 8%
• Acute myeloid leukemia: 5%	• Acute lymphoblastic leukemia: 8%
• Hodgkin lymphoma: 4%	• Bone tumors: 7%
• Rhabdomyosarcoma: 3%	• Melanoma: 6%
• Retinoblastoma: 3%	• Acute myeloid leukemia: 4%
	• Ovarian germ cell tumors: 2%

Ward E, DeSantis C, Robbins A, et al: Childhood and adolescent cancer statistics, 2014, *Ca Cancer J Clin* 64:83–103, 2014.

56. Where does cancer rank as a cause of death in younger children?
While cancer is the leading cause of *disease-related* mortality in children 5 to 14 years of age, it is overall the second leading cause of death in this age group in the United States. It accounts for ≈12% of deaths in children younger than 14 years. Unintentional injuries, primarily motor vehicle accidents, are the most frequent cause of death in children ages 5 to 14 years.

Murphy SL, Xu J, Rochanek KD: Deaths: Final report for 2010. National Vital Statistics Report, Volume 62, No. 6, Hyattsville, MD, 2013, National Center for Health Statistics.

57. Is cancer the leading cause of death in teenagers and young adults?
No. Unintentional injuries are the leading cause of death for adolescents and young adults, accounting for more than 40% of deaths. Homicides and suicides are responsible for almost 30% of deaths in this age group, with cancer being a distant third at 6.4%.

Murphy SL, Xu J, Rochanek KD: Deaths: Final report for 2010. National Vital Statistics Report, Volume 62, No. 6, Hyattsville, MD, 2013, National Center for Health Statistics.

58. What are the relative risks for children to develop leukemia?
See Table 14-1.

Table 14-1. Relative Risk for Children to Develop Leukemia

POPULATION AT RISK	ESTIMATED RISK
U.S. white children	1 in 2800
Siblings of a child with leukemia	1 in 700
Identical twin of a child with leukemia	1 in 5
Children with:	
Down syndrome	1 in 75
Fanconi syndrome	1 in 12
Bloom syndrome	1 in 8
Ataxia-telangiectasia	1 in 8
Exposures:	
Atom bomb within 100 m	1 in 60
Ionizing radiation	?
Benzene	1 in 960
Alkylating agents	1 in 2000?

Data from Mahoney DH Jr: Neoplastic diseases. In McMillan JA, DeAngelis CD, Felgin RD, Warshaw JB, editors: Oski's Pediatrics, Principles and Practice, ed 3. Philadelphia, 1999, JB Lippincott, p 1494.

59. Does cell phone usage increase the risk of cancers, specifically brain tumors?
Any connection between cell phones and cancer is controversial. Studies have been conflicting. A number suggested a relationship between long-term use (>10 years) of mobile and cordless phones and the development of certain CNS tumors, primarily gliomas and acoustic neuromas. However, the largest study to date, the INTERPHONE study involving 13 countries, found no increased risk. Cell phones emit radiofrequency electromagnetic fields (RF-EMFs) and obviously the brain is proximate during typical usage. In 2011, the International Agency for Research on Cancer (IARC) classified RF-EMFs as "possible" human carcinogens. Data are currently epidemiologic. Theories on the role of RF-EMF as potential initiators and promoters of stages of carcinogenesis at present remain speculative, but certainly do raise concern given the high degree of cell phone usage and exposure in younger children and teenagers.

INTERPHONE Study Group: Brain tumour risk in relation to mobile telephone use: results of the INTERPHONE international case-control study, *Int J Epidemiol* 39:675–694, 2010.

60. Which cancers have a significant racial predilection?
Wilms tumor has a higher incidence among black female infants. **Ewing tumor** is about 30 times more common in whites than in blacks. **Hodgkin disease** is rare in those of East Asian descent.

61. What cancers are most commonly associated with a second neoplasm?
See Table 14-2.

Table 14-2. Cancers Most Commonly Associated With a Second Neoplasm

PRIMARY TUMORS	SECONDARY TUMORS
Retinoblastoma	Osteosarcoma
	Pineoblastoma
Hodgkin disease	Acute nonlymphoblastic leukemia
	Non-Hodgkin lymphoma

Table 14-2. Cancers Most Commonly Associated With a Second Neoplasm (*Continued*)

PRIMARY TUMORS	SECONDARY TUMORS
	Sarcoma (in radiation field)
	Thyroid carcinoma
	Breast carcinoma (in radiation field)
Acute lymphoblastic leukemia	Brain tumors
	Non-Hodgkin lymphoma
Sarcomas	Sarcomas

62. Are there any known transplacental carcinogens?

Diethylstilbestrol, which was used to prevent spontaneous abortion, has been associated with an increased risk for vaginal cancer in the female offspring. It has also been reported that there is a 10-fold increased risk for monoblastic leukemia in the infants of mothers who smoke **marijuana**. It has been suggested that sedatives and a number of nonhormonal drugs are transplacental carcinogens, but this has not been proven. It also has not been proven if cigarette smoke and the use of oral contraceptives are transplacental carcinogens.

63. Is prenatal ultrasound associated with a risk for leukemia later in childhood?

No. In vitro, ultrasound has been shown to cause cell membrane changes, and thus concern has been expressed regarding potential effects on embryogenesis and prenatal and postnatal development. However, the available evidence on both fetal development and neonatal outcomes following ultrasound exposure is strongly reassuring, including no increased risk of childhood cancer. Of note, the only known association of prenatal ultrasound with alterations in development has been a slight preference among males for non–right handedness (i.e., use of both hands equally or left handedness). One concern is that most of the longer-term outcome studies were begun before 1990, when ultrasound was not performed as frequently and when the allowable output potential of the ultrasound equipment was relatively reduced.

Houston LE, Odibo AO, Macones GA: The safety of obstetrical ultrasound: a review, *Prenat Diagn* 13:1204–1212, 2009.
Salvesen KA, Elk-Nes SH: Ultrasound during pregnancy and subsequent child non-right handedness: a meta-analysis, *Ultrasound Obstet Gynecol* 13:241–246, 1999.

64. Do children living near electrical power lines have an increased risk for developing cancer?

Although a few small studies have suggested an association between power lines and an increased risk for ALL, evidence has been inconsistent, but largely negative.

Bunch KJ, Keegan TJ, Swanson J, et al: Residential distance at birth from overhead high-voltage power lines: childhood cancer risk in Britain, 1962-2008, *Br J Cancer* 110:1402–1408, 2014.
Linet MS, Hatch EE, Kleinerman RA, et al: Residential exposure to magnetic fields and acute lymphoblastic leukemia in children, *N Engl J Med* 337:1–7, 1997.

LEUKEMIA

65. What are the most common clinical findings in the initial presentation of ALL?

- **Hepatosplenomegaly:** 70% (10% to 15% of children have marked enlargement of the liver or spleen to a level below the umbilicus)
- **Fever:** 40% to 60%
- **Lymphadenopathy:** 25% to 50% with moderate or marked enlargement
- **Bleeding:** 25% to 50% with petechiae or purpura
- **Bone and joint pain:** 25% to 40%
- **Fatigue:** 30%
- **Anorexia:** 20% to 35%

KEY POINTS: ACUTE LYMPHOBLASTIC LEUKEMIA

1. Most common childhood malignancy
2. Increased risk: Patients with Down syndrome, congenital immunodeficiency syndrome, exposure to ionizing radiation; sibling of patient with acute lymphoblastic leukemia
3. Chemotherapy phases: Induction (to achieve remission), delayed intensification, maintenance
4. Survival (if in standard risk group) >80% at 5 years after completion of therapy
5. Most common sites of relapse: Bone marrow, central nervous system, testis

66. **What are the typical hematologic findings noted during the presentation of ALL?**
    Leukocyte count (mm^3)
    - <10,000: 45% to 55%
    - 10,000 to 50,000: 30% to 35%
    - >50,000: 20%

    Hemoglobin (g/dL)
    - <7.5: 45%
    - 7.5 to 10.0: 30%
    - >10: 25%

    Platelet count (mm^3)
    - <20,000: 25%
    - 20,000 to 99,000: 50%
    - >100,000: 25%

67. **What studies of tumor cells are useful for determining a patient's prognosis?**
    Cytogenetics and ploidy (number of chromosomes): Cytogenetics and DNA index (ratio of DNA content in abnormal cells compared with normal reference cells) are determinants of the number and structure of chromosomes and chromosomal material in tumor cells. More than 50 chromosomes or a DNA index of >1.16 is favorable, whereas <46 is a poor prognostic indicator. Certain chromosomal translocations are unfavorable.

    Immunophenotyping is also useful and involves the determination of B- or T-cell lineage, with maturity or immaturity of cells. Mature B-cell and precursor T-cell types have poorer prognosis.

Harrison CJ: Cytogenetics of paediatric and adolescent acute lymphoblastic leukaemia, *Br J Haematol* 144:147–156, 2009.
Pui C-H, Relling MV, Downing JR: Acute lymphoblastic leukemia, *N Engl J Med* 350:1535–1548, 2004.

68. **Which patients with ALL have a poorer prognosis: younger or older children?**
    The prognosis for children diagnosed with **ALL ≤12 months** has remained poor. Infant ALL appears to be a biologically distinct entity in comparison with ALL in older children, with infants generally having a conglomeration of adverse factors including *MLL* gene rearrangement (observed in up to 80% of infants with ALL, see question 69), high presenting leukocyte counts, hepatosplenomegaly, CNS disease, and slow early response to therapy.

Silverman LB: Acute lymphoblastic leukemia in infancy, *Pediatr Blood Cancer* 49(7 Suppl):1070–1073, 2007.

69. **What is the significance of translocations of the *MLL* gene?**
    The term *MLL* gene refers directly to the mixed lineage leukemia gene, present at chromosome 11, band q23. This region is frequently involved in a variety of chromosomal translocations and rearrangements in pediatric leukemia. Translocations involving the *MLL* gene are found primarily in infant ALL, where they confer a poor prognosis. They are also found in infant AML and confer an intermediate risk. The presence of *MLL* translocations results in increased intensification of chemotherapy.

Chowdhury T, Brady HJ: Insights from clinical studies into the role of the MLL gene in infant and childhood leukemia, *Blood Cells Mol Dis* 40:192–199, 2008

70. Although many prognostic factors have come and gone for childhood ALL, which two have remained significant for the past 40 years?

The two most consistent prognostic factors are **age** and **elevation of presenting white blood cell count**. Children <1 year or >10 years have a worse prognosis, as do those with a presenting white blood cell count of 50,000/mm^3 or greater. Prognostic factors are important because, although 95% of ALL patients achieve remission (<5% lymphoblasts in bone marrow), 25% relapse. Identifying patients at higher risk is important so that more aggressive or novel therapy can be considered.

71. Why do boys with ALL fare more poorly than girls?

In boys, after a full course of chemotherapy with remission, testicular involvement is a common site of relapse, occurring in up to 10% of cases. In older boys and teenage boys, there is a higher incidence of T-cell disease than in girls. T-cell disease is associated with adverse prognostic factors (high white blood cell count, hepatosplenomegaly, and mediastinal masses) and alone carries a poorer prognosis. In girls, ovarian relapse is very rare.

72. Are race and ethnicity related to treatment outcome in patients with acute leukemia?

Race and ethnicity appear to be related to outcome in ALL. Black, Hispanic, and American Indian/Alaskan Native children have a somewhat poorer outcome than white children. Asian/Pacific Islander children fare slightly better than white children. Although the reasons are not known, these differences may be the result of either host or leukemia characteristics.

Kadan-Lottick NS, Ness KK, Bhatia S, et al: Survival variability by race and ethnicity in childhood acute lymphoblastic leukemia, *JAMA* 290:2008–2014, 2003.

KEY POINTS: HIGHER-RISK GROUPS WITH POORER PROGNOSIS OF PATIENTS WITH ACUTE LYMPHOBLASTIC LEUKEMIA

1. Age: <1 year and >10 years
2. White blood cell count: >50,000/mm^3
3. Chromosomal translocation abnormalities, specifically t(8;14), t(9;22), and t(4;11)
4. Hypoploidy (<45 chromosomes)
5. Malignant cells, with mature B-cell or T-cell immunophenotyping
6. Central nervous system involvement
7. Black and Hispanic patients
8. Males

73. In the United States, what are the four most common types of pediatric leukemia, and about how many children are diagnosed each year with each type?

ALL, with about 2500 new diagnoses yearly; **AML,** with about 500 new diagnoses yearly; **chronic myelogenous leukemia** (CML), with about 100 new diagnoses yearly; and **juvenile myelomonocytic leukemia** (JMML), with about 50 new diagnoses yearly.

74. What is MRD and how is it used?

MRD stands for *minimal residual disease*, which is typically detected by flow cytometry at several time points during therapy. In ALL, MRD detects patients who have a normal appearing bone marrow by light microscopy, but in fact have an increased risk for relapse owing to low-level, persistent disease. MRD use in AML is not as well defined as in ALL.

75. Is there a relationship between MRD and prognosis in children with ALL?

Yes. A 2008 study indicated that MRD after induction therapy is the *most important prognostic factor* for outcome in children with ALL.

Borowitz MJ, Devidas M, Hunger SP, et al: Clinical significance of minimal residual disease in childhood acute lymphoblastic leukemia and its relationship to other prognostic factors: a Children's Oncology Group study, *Blood* 111:5477–5485, 2008.

76. **What is the acute risk for a very elevated blast count noted at the time of the initial diagnosis of leukemia?**

An elevated blast count at diagnosis may cause **CNS leukostasis and stroke.** The risk is higher in patients with AML because myeloblasts are larger and may have procoagulant activity that increases the risk for stroke or hemorrhage. Leukocytapheresis is sometimes used to reduce the blast count before initiating therapy, but its impact on improving outcome remains unproved.

77. **What are the most common sites of extramedullary relapse of ALL?**

The most common is the **meninges,** and this is followed by **testicular relapse.** Testicular disease is accompanied by painless testicular swelling (usually unilateral). The diagnosis must be confirmed by biopsy. Patients with testicular disease require irradiation in addition to intensive retreatment with chemotherapy.

78. **What are known risk factors for acute myeloid leukemia?**

See Table 14-3.

Table 14-3. Risk Factors for AML

GENERALLY ACCEPTED RISK FACTORS	SUGGESTIVE OF INCREASED RISK	SUGGESTIVE OF DECREASED RISK	LIMITED EVIDENCE
• Down Syndrome • Fanconi anemia • Familial monosomy 7 • Ataxia telangiectasia • Shwachman-Diamond syndrome • Bloom syndrome • Ionizing radiation in utero	• Older maternal age • Increasing birth order • Prior fetal loss • Maternal alcohol use • Maternal exposure to pesticides • High birth weight • Low birth weight	• Long term breast-feeding	• Paternal exposure to benzene • Parental smoking • Maternal exposure to benzene • Maternal use of antibiotics • Maternal dietary consumption of DNA topoisomerase II inhibitors

AML = Acute myelogenous leukemia; DNA = deoxyribonucleic acid.
From Puumala SE, Ross JA, Aplenc R, Spector LG: Epidemiology of childhood acute myeloid leukemia Pediatr Blood Cancer 60:728–733, 2013.

79. **What is a chloroma?**

A *chloroma* is a tumor that is formed by a coalescence of AML blasts. It may appear in bones, skin, soft tissue, or other sites. Its name is derived from its green appearance on its cut surface.

80. **What are the two major classes of lymphomas?**

Lymphomas can be divided into **Hodgkin** and **non-Hodgkin lymphomas (NHL)**. Lymphomas as a group are the third most common pediatric malignancy with NHL accounting for approximately 7% of pediatric cancers. Whereas lymphomas in adults generally are defined as low grade or intermediate, almost all lymphomas in pediatrics are high grade. Higher grade lymphomas are faster growing and more aggressive.

81. **What is the malignant cell of Hodgkin disease?**

The **Reed-Sternberg cell.** Its normal cell of origin remains unclear, with the predominance of evidence indicating a B or T lymphocyte. However, the cells alone are not pathognomonic of Hodgkin disease and may be seen in infectious mononucleosis, non-Hodgkin lymphoma, carcinomas, and sarcomas.

82. **How is Hodgkin disease staged?**

The Ann Arbor staging system with Cotswolds modifications is the current staging system for Hodgkin lymphoma. Individuals are defined as being in one of four different numeric stages (stages I to IV).

- **Stage I**: Involvement of a single lymph node region
- **Stage II**: Involvement of two or more lymph node regions on the same side of the diaphragm
- **Stage III**: Involvement of lymph node regions on both sides of the diaphragm
- **Stage IV**: Diffuse or disseminated disease

Patients are then further subclassified based on the absence (A) or presence (B) of one or more of the following "B" symptoms: fever, night sweats, or unexplained weight loss.

83. **What is the difference between clinical and pathologic staging as it relates to Hodgkin disease?**
Clinical staging refers to staging based on history, physical examination, and imaging (preferably PET-CT) following a single diagnostic biopsy. *Pathologic staging* was based on staging laparotomy with splenectomy, liver biopsy, multiple lymph node biopsies, and bone marrow biopsy. Pathologic staging is no longer performed.

84. **What is the histologic classification of Hodgkin disease?**
See Table 14-4.

Table 14-4. The Rye, New York, Histologic Classification*

TYPE	LYMPHOCYTES	REED-STERNBERG CELLS	OTHER	INCIDENCE (%)
Lymphocyte predominant	Many	Few	Histiocytes	10-15
Nodular sclerosing	Many	Few or many	Bands of refractile fibrosis	40-70
Mixed cellularity	Many	Few or many	Eosinophils, histiocytes	20-30
Lymphocyte depletion	Few	Many	No refractile fibrosis	<5

*Based on the relative number of lymphocytes and Reed-Sternberg cells.

85. **What is the prognosis for the various stages of Hodgkin disease?**
The prognosis for children with Hodgkin disease is excellent in that most are cured. For stages I and IIA, the 5-year relapse-free survival rate is higher than 80% for patients treated with radiation only, and it may be higher than 90% for patients treated with radiation and chemotherapy. For stage IIB, prognosis is not as good, especially if there is a massive mediastinal tumor, but 5-year survival is still higher than 80%. The same survival figures pertain to stage IIIA disease, but treatment generally is more extensive than that for a limited stage II disease. For stage IV disease, the 5-year relapse-free survival rate is 70% to 90%.

86. **From what cells do non-Hodgkin lymphoma (NHL) derive?**
NHL constitutes a variety of lymphoid malignancies with different cell types including B and T cell progenitors; mature B and T cells; and rarely, natural killer (NK) cells.

87. **How is childhood NHL classified?**
The 2008 World Health Organization (WHO) system for classification is the one most commonly used. It relies on (1) cell immunophenotype (i.e., B lineage, T lineage, or NK lineage) and (2) differentiation (i.e., precursor versus mature cell). Although a large number of subtypes are categorized on the basis of histology and genetic studies, NHL of childhood and adolescence falls into three main categories, which are based in large measure on the clinical features and the therapeutic response to treatment.
- **Mature B-cell NHL** (Burkitt and Burkitt-like lymphoma/leukemia and diffuse large B-cell lymphoma): These account for about 40% to 50% of U.S. NHL pediatric cases.
- **Lymphoblastic lymphoma** (primarily precursor T-cell lymphoma and, less frequently, precursor B-cell lymphoma): These account for about 20% of U.S. cases.
- **Anaplastic large cell lymphoma** (mature T-cell or null-cell lymphoma, which lacks characteristic markers of both T and B cells): These account for about 10% of U.S. cases.

Jaffe ES, Harris NL, Stein H, et al: Introduction and overview of the classification of the lymphoid neoplasms. In: Swerdlow SH, Campo E, Harris NL, et al, editors: *WHO Classification of Tumors of Haematopoietic and Lymphoid Tissues*, ed 4. Lyon, France, 2008, International Agency for Research on Cancer, pp 157–166.

88. Are there specific chromosomal abnormalities in Burkitt lymphoma?
    Yes. Burkitt lymphoma is associated with three chromosomal translocations resulting in the inappropriate expression of the c-Myc oncogene. The translocations are t(8;14) (most frequent) and t(8;22) or t(2;8) (relatively rare), each of which juxtaposes the c-Myc gene located on chromosome 8 (specifically, 8q24) with an immunoglobulin heavy chain locus regulatory element. C-Myc is a proto-oncogene, which is involved in cellular proliferation.

89. What is the role of geography in the classification of Burkitt lymphoma?
    The rapid onset of Burkitt lymphoma and its uneven geographic distribution has suggested a possible infectious etiology by a vectored pathogen as key to the disease. This peculiar epidemiology led the WHO to classify Burkitt lymphoma into three clinical entities: *endemic* (found primarily in countries where malaria is endemic, such as Africa and Papua New Guinea), *sporadic* (the predominant type found in the United States and in nonmalarial areas), and *immunodeficiency-related* (seen most often in individuals with HIV). Each entity has different clinical presentations and genetic features. The endemic variant most commonly presents as a jaw or facial bone tumor, while the sporadic form has an abdominal presentation with ascites. Epstein-Barr virus is found to be associated with almost all cases of the endemic variant, less frequently so with the immunodeficiency variant and rarely in the sporadic variant.

Molyneux EM, Rochford R, Griffin B, et al: Burkitt's lymphoma, *Lancet* 379:1234–1244, 2012.

90. Who was Burkitt?
    Denis Burkitt was an Irish surgeon who, while living in Uganda, noted a series of children with swellings at the angles of the jaw and began to investigate the tumors. He published his case series in 1958, concluding that these represented a new previously unrecognized tumor complex. He later became a prominent proponent of increased dietary fiber, having noted that many Western diseases were rare in Africa. He was one of the first to suggest a fiber-depleted etiology for colorectal cancer, although subsequent epidemiologic studies did not support that hypothesis. He died in 1993 at the age of 82.

Smith O: Denis Parsons Burkitt (1911-93), Irish by birth, Trinity by the grace of God, *Brit J Haematol* 156:770–776, 2012.

91. What differentiates B- and T-cell precursor leukemia from lymphoma?
    The **bone marrow blast percentage** is used to differentiate B- and T-cell precursor leukemia from lymphoma. If the bone marrow blast percentage is greater than or equal to 25%, the diagnosis of leukemia is given. If the blast percentage is less than 25% and the patient has other sites of malignant disease, the diagnosis of lymphoma is given.

NERVOUS SYSTEM TUMORS

92. How are CNS tumors classified?
    Most are typically classified on the basis of histology:
    - **Glioma:** Arises from supportive tissue (astrocytes)
    - **Ependymoma:** Arises from the ependymal cells that line the ventricles
    - **Germ cell tumor:** Arises from totipotent germ cells
    - **Rhabdoid:** Arises from an unknown cell type
    - **Craniopharyngioma:** Arises from embryonic precursors to anterior pituitary gland

KEY POINTS: CENTRAL NERVOUS SYSTEM TUMORS

1. Second most common neoplasm of childhood, after leukemia
2. Older children (>1 year): Most tumors are infratentorial (cerebellar or brainstem)
3. Younger children (<1 year): Most tumors are supratentorial
4. Gold standard for diagnosis: MRI with and without gadolinium enhancement
5. Back pain, extremity weakness, and/or bowel and bladder dysfunction suggestive of spinal cord lesions or metastases

93. Where is the most common area for each tumor to occur?
    - **Glioma:** Cerebellum and optic pathway (more commonly benign and low grade); cerebrum or brainstem (more commonly malignant and higher grade)

- **Ependymoma:** Fourth ventricle; less commonly the spinal cord
- **Germ cell tumor:** Pineal or supracellar region
- **Primitive neuroectodermal tumor (PNET) medulloblastoma:** Midline of the cerebellum
- **Rhabdoid:** Posterior fossa
- **Craniopharyngioma:** Choroid plexus
  See Figure 14-3.

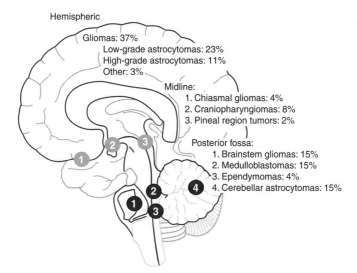

Hemispheric

Gliomas: 37%
Low-grade astrocytomas: 23%
High-grade astrocytomas: 11%
Other: 3%

Midline:
1. Chiasmal gliomas: 4%
2. Craniopharyngiomas: 8%
3. Pineal region tumors: 2%

Posterior fossa:
1. Brainstem gliomas: 15%
2. Medulloblastomas: 15%
3. Ependymomas: 4%
4. Cerebellar astrocytomas: 15%

Figure 14-3. Relative frequency of brain tumor histologic types and anatomic distribution. *(From Kleigman RM, Stanton BF, Schor NF, et al: Nelson Textbook of Pediatrics, ed 19, Philadelphia, 2011, Elsevier Saunders, p 1748.)*

94. What are the most common supratentorial brain tumors? What are their symptoms?
    Supratentorial tumors include tumors of the cerebrum, basal ganglia, thalamus, and hypothalamus. They can be gliomas, ependymomas, PNETs, germ cell tumors, choroid plexus tumors, or craniopharyngiomas. These tumors can show signs of increased intracranial pressure, such as headache and vomiting. In addition, these tumors may be accompanied by focal deficits, such as memory loss, weakness, and visual changes.

Hawley DP, Walker DA: A symptomatic journey to the centre of the brain, *Arch Dis Child Educ Pract Ed* 95:59–64, 2010.

95. What are the most common infratentorial tumors? What are their symptoms?
    Infratentorial tumors include tumors of the cerebellum and brainstem. They can be astrocytomas, medulloblastoma, ependymomas, or gliomas. If infratentorial tumors block CSF outflow, headache and vomiting may be the presenting signs; they can also become apparent with localizing signs such as cranial nerve palsies or ataxia.

96. Which common parameters should be closely monitored in a child after resection of a brain tumor?
    It is important to closely monitor **urine output** and **serum sodium** in children undergoing CNS surgery. Resection of a hypothalamic glioma, germ cell tumor, or craniopharyngioma can directly disrupt the function of the pituitary gland and lead to diabetes insipidus. Alternatively, some patients may develop a cerebral salt-wasting syndrome after resection.

97. Which cranial nerve abnormality is most common in children showing signs of increased intracranial pressure as the result of a posterior fossa tumor?
    Inability to abduct one or both eyes **(cranial nerve VI palsy)** may result from an elevation in intracranial pressure and can be a false localizing sign for the primary brain tumor.

98. What are the three "E's" of the diencephalic syndrome?

Diencephalic syndrome is the constellation of symptoms that result from the presence of a hypothalamic tumor: **euphoria, emaciation,** and **emesis.**

99. What is Parinaud syndrome?

Parinaud syndrome is the result of increased intracranial pressure at the dorsal midbrain, causing downgaze, papillary dilation, and nystagmus.

100. In addition to imaging studies, what should be included in the evaluation of a possible CNS germ cell tumor?

Both serum and cerebrospinal **tumor α-fetoprotein** and **human chorionic gonadotropin** should be obtained. Significant elevation of these markers is diagnostic of CNS germ cell tumor in a patient with an intracranial mass.

101. What are the key evaluations for a child with a newly-diagnosed medulloblastoma?

Medulloblastomas may spread contiguously to the cerebellar peduncle, to the floor of the fourth ventricle, into the cervical spine, or above the tentorium. In addition, medulloblastomas may disseminate through the CSF. Every patient should thus be evaluated with diagnostic imaging (magnetic resonance imaging [MRI]) of the spinal cord and of the whole brain. Examination of CSF should be performed after resection of the primary tumor.

Bartlett F, Kortmann R, Saran F: Medulloblastoma, *Clin Oncol (R Coll Radiol)* 25:36–45, 2013.

102. What is a "dropped met"?

Most brain tumors do not metastasize; they are fatal because of local invasion. A **dropped metastasis** occurs when a primary brain tumor spreads through CSF pathways, thereby resulting in meningeal deposits along the spinal cord. These metastases have "dropped" from their original site down to the spinal cord or cauda equina.

103. What are the differences among a glioma, an astrocytoma, and glioblastoma multiforme?

- A **glioma** (from the Greek word *glia* for glue and the suffix *-oma* for tumor) is a neoplasm that is derived from one of the various types of cells that form the supporting interstitial tissue of the CNS, such as astrocytes, oligodendria, and ependymal cells. Of the gliomas, astrocytomas of variable malignancy are the most prevalent.
- **Astrocytomas** are subdivided into categories (grades) on the basis of the degree of tumor anaplasia and the presence or absence of necrosis. The juvenile pilocytic and subependymal astrocytoma are low-grade gliomas. Anaplastic astrocytomas (grade 3) grow more rapidly than the more differentiated astrocytomas.
- **Glioblastoma multiforme** is the highest grade astrocytoma (grade 4).

Ullrich NJ, Pomeroy SL: Pediatric brain tumors, *Neurol Clin* 21:897–913, 2003.

104. What is the most common benign brain tumor found in children?

Juvenile pilocytic astrocytoma (JPA). This is a type of low grade astrocytoma (glioma), most commonly found in the cerebellum. JPAs are associated with the genetic diagnosis of neurofibromatosis type I and involvement of the optic nerve is a classic finding. Fifteen percent of neurofibromatosis type I patients develop JPAs. The tumor is very slow growing.

105. Is resection curative for patients with juvenile pilocytic astrocytoma?

If complete resection is possible, no additional treatment is required. However, for many patients a full resection is not possible because of the tumor's location and size. In this situation, the surgical resection could have debilitating and neurologically devastating consequences. A number of chemotherapy and radiation regimens may be used to treat residual or recurrent tumors, but they are frequently noncurative.

Karajanis M, Allen J, Newcomb E: Treatment of pediatric brain tumors, *J Cell Physiol* 217:584-589, 2008.

106. **Why is the prognosis for children with brainstem gliomas so poor?**
Location. A basic tenet of CNS tumors is that a gross total resection is necessary to achieve the greatest chance of long-term cure. Brainstem tumors most commonly are fully intrinsic to the pons and unresectable. Although radiation can improve symptoms, there currently is no known curative therapy for most children with brainstem gliomas.

107. **What is leukocoria?**
White pupillary reflex. It can be obvious or it can be a subtle asymmetry on pupillary red reflex evaluation. Although other diagnoses can accompany leukocoria, the most significant one is retinoblastoma.

108. **What is the heredity of retinoblastoma?**
Although most cases are sporadic, retinoblastoma can be inherited as an autosomal dominant trait with nearly complete penetrance. Of all cases, 60% are nonhereditary and unilateral, 15% are hereditary and unilateral, and 25% are hereditary and bilateral. Families of patients with retinoblastoma should have genetic counseling.

109. **What is the "two-hit" hypothesis of cancer, particularly retinoblastoma?**
Alfred Knudson's "two-hit" hypothesis is a basic tenet of malignant transformation. In 1971, Knudson calculated the genetic probabilities of developing retinoblastoma and hypothesized that patients with bilateral disease first inherited a germline mutation and then underwent a second somatic mutation to develop the disease. Patients with unilateral or sporadic disease developed two somatic mutations during early childhood. The identification of the genes associated with the first of the "two hits" correctly predicted the presence of tumor suppressor genes.

Knudson A: Two genetic hits (more or less) to cancer, *Nat Rev Cancer* 1:157–162, 2001.

110. **In what age group does retinoblastoma usually occur?**
Retinoblastoma most often occurs in younger children, with 80% of cases diagnosed before the age of 5 years. Retinoblastoma is usually confined to the eye, with more than 80% of children being cured with current therapy.

Shields CL, Shields JA: Basic understanding of current classification and management of retinoblastoma, *Curr Opin Ophthalmol* 17:228–234, 2006.

111. **Patients with retinoblastoma are at increased risk for other tumors. How significant a risk is this?**
Patients with the hereditary type of retinoblastoma have a markedly increased frequency of second malignant neoplasms. The cumulative incidence is about $26\% \pm 10\%$ in nonirradiated patients and $58\% \pm 10\%$ in irradiated patients by 50 years after diagnosis of retinoblastoma. Most of the second malignant neoplasms are osteosarcomas, soft tissue sarcomas, and melanomas.

112. **What is the cell of origin of neuroblastoma?**
Neuroblastoma is an embryonal tumor of the autonomic nervous system. The tumors originate in tissues of the sympathetic nervous system, most frequently in the adrenal medulla or paraspinal ganglia. Hence neuroblastomas may present as mass lesions in the abdomen, pelvis, neck or chest.

113. **What is the most common cancer in younger children?**
While leukemias may constitute the most common group of pediatric cancer diagnoses overall, **neuroblastomas** are the most commonly occurring cancer in children <1 year of age.

Maris JM: Recent advances in neuroblastoma, *N Engl J Med*, 362:2202–2211, 2010.

KEY POINTS: NEUROBLASTOMA

1. Most common pediatric extracranial solid tumor
2. Most common malignant tumor among infants
3. Majority of children <4 years old
4. Poorer prognosis: >1 year old, metastatic disease, Myc-N amplification
5. Most metastatic at diagnosis

6. Paraneoplastic syndromes: VIP syndrome (diarrhea as a result of increased vasoactive intestinal peptide), opsoclonus-myoclonus ("dancing eyes, dancing feet"), and catecholamine excess (with flushing, sweating, headache, and hypertension)

114. **What are the most common presentations of neuroblastoma?**
Children with disseminated neuroblastoma are irritable and ill, and they often have exquisite bone pain, proptosis, and periorbital ecchymoses. Seventy percent of neuroblastomas arise in the abdomen; half of these arise in the adrenal gland, and the other half arise in the parasympathetic ganglia and are distributed throughout the retroperitoneum and the paravertebral area in the chest and neck. The tumor produces and excretes catecholamines, which can on occasion cause systemic symptoms such as sweating, hypertension, diarrhea, and irritability. Children with localized neuroblastoma may have symptoms referable to a mass.

Maris JM: Recent advances in neuroblastoma, *N Engl J Med* 362:2202–2211, 2010.

115. **What is Horner syndrome?**
Ptosis, miosis (with unequal pupils), and **anhidrosis** (Fig. 14-4). The syndrome results from unilateral disruption of sympathetic neural pathways. The condition can occur from congenital

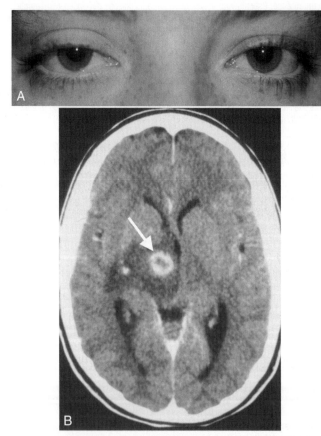

Figure 14-4. (A) Right Horner syndrome due to a T-cell lymphoma involving the right thalamus and hypothalamus. **(B)** Ring-enhancement *(arrow)* and edema are seen on the axial CT scan. *(From Liu GT, Volpe NJ, Galetta SL, editors: Neuro-Ophthalmology: Diagnosis and Management, ed 2. Philadelphia, 2010, Elsevier, p 431.)*

brachial plexus injury, but acquired Horner syndrome requires evaluation for intrathoracic (preganglionic); cervical (postganglionic); or intracranial (central) pathology, particularly neuroblastoma.

116. **Where does neuroblastoma tend to metastasize?**
Neuroblastoma spreads to the **liver; the bone;** the **bone marrow;** and less commonly, the skin.

117. **What is meant by "dancing eyes, dancing feet"?**
"Dancing eyes, dancing feet" is a descriptive term for *opsoclonus-myoclonus*, a condition in which children with neuroblastoma develop horizontal nystagmus and involuntary lower extremity muscle spasm. These symptoms are thought to arise from a nonspecific antibody reaction to neuroblastoma that cross-reacts with the motor end plate. These symptoms do not always improve, despite appropriate neuroblastoma therapy.

118. **What urinary test aids in the diagnosis of neuroblastoma?**
Urinary concentrations of catecholamines and metabolites, including dopamine, homovanillic acid, and vanillylmandelic acid, are often increased (>3 standard deviations above the mean per milligram creatinine for age) in children with neuroblastoma.

119. **Which molecular abnormality is associated with a more aggressive form of neuroblastoma?**
Myc-N amplification is often seen in patients with stage 4 neuroblastoma. The presence of myc-N amplification renders a patient at higher risk for recurrence regardless of staging.

120. **What does the S stand for in stage 4S neuroblastoma?**
Stage 4S is a "special" type of neuroblastoma that is found only in children <1 year of age. Along with a primary tumor, these infants also may have bone marrow, liver, and skin disease. Even without therapy, these cancers spontaneously regress and disappear over time. Treatment is only indicated if the patient is symptomatic from the underlying disease (e.g., large abdominal mass, liver disease).

121. **How can the site of spinal cord compression be clinically localized?**
Spinal tenderness on percussion correlates with localization in up to 80% of patients. In addition, **neurologic evaluation** of strength, sensory level changes, reflexes, and anal tone can help pinpoint the location in the spinal cord, the conus medullaris (the terminal neural portion of the spinal cord), or the cauda equina. Progression is rapid with spinal cord compression but may be rapid or variable with compression of the conus medullaris or the cauda equina. Spinal cord compression most commonly occurs in the thoracic area (70%) compared with the lumbar (20%) and cervical (10%) regions.

SOLID NON-NERVOUS SYSTEM TUMORS

122. **What are the peak ages of incidence of the most common solid tumors of childhood?**
Neuroblastoma and Wilms tumor are tumors of early childhood. Ewing sarcoma and osteosarcoma are more prevalent during adolescence. Rhabdomyosarcoma occurs throughout childhood and the teenage years.

123. **What are "blastemal" tumors?**
Many pediatric solid tumors are thought to arise from a primitive blastemal cell. A *blastema* is a mass of embryonic cells from which an organ or a body part develops. Thus, these cells are undifferentiated and, if mutated, may develop into tumors such as neuroblastoma, pleuropulmonary blastoma, hepatoblastoma, or Wilms tumor, to name a few.

124. **What is the average age of diagnosis for Wilms tumor?**
Wilms tumor is a primary malignant renal tumor of large histologic diversity. Average age of diagnosis is **3 to 4 years**. The tumor becomes less common as children grow older and is an uncommon occurrence after 6 years of age.

125. What are the three histologic components of a Wilms tumor?

Wilms tumors are considered triphasic, consisting of a **blastemal** (immature) component, an **epithelial** (tubular) component, and a **stromal** (muscular) component.

126. How is Wilms tumor distinguished radiographically from neuroblastoma?
- **Wilms tumor:** CT images will show intrinsic distortion of the kidney parenchyma and the collecting system. Only 10% of children with Wilms tumor have calcifications.
- **Neuroblastoma:** This is almost always extrarenal and causes displacement—not distortion—of the renal parenchyma and collecting system. Calcifications are seen in more than 50% of children with abdominal neuroblastoma.

127. Where does Wilms tumor tend to metastasize?

Locally, Wilms tumor can grow through the renal capsule, invade the renal veins, extend into the vena cava, and even progress into the chambers of the heart. The lungs, regional lymph nodes, and liver are the most common sites of metastasis.

128. What is a stage V Wilms tumor?

Bilateral Wilms tumor is known as a stage V tumor. Each tumor is staged independently; prognosis with bilateral disease is not necessarily poor.

129. What factors influence the prognosis of a patient with Wilms tumor?

Overall, Wilms tumor carries a good prognosis. Factors that influence the prognosis include tumor stage and histology, as well as chromosomal abnormalities such as loss of heterozygosity (LOH). LOH for markers on the distal arm of chromosome 16 has been found in about 20% of Wilms tumors, whereas loss of the short arm of chromosome 1 has been found in about 10% of cases. LOH of either locus portends an adverse prognosis, independent of tumor stage and histology.

130. "Small, round, blue cell tumor" is often used in the description of which childhood tumors?

Neuroblastoma, rhabdomyosarcoma, Ewing sarcoma, lymphoblastic leukemia, and **lymphoma**. All appear as small, round, blue cells on low-power microscopic examination. High-power microscopic examination, usually in combination with a panel of immunohistochemical stains and molecular diagnostics, is required for definitive diagnosis.

131. Where are the most common locations of Ewing sarcoma?

The **pelvis, leg, upper arm**, and **rib.** These tumors arise in extraskeletal (soft tissue) locations and can locally invade the bone.

132. What molecular abnormality is commonly seen in Ewing sarcoma?

The **t(11:22) translocation** is pathognomonic of Ewing sarcoma. This translocation results in the fusion gene *EWS-FLI1*, which is thought to disrupt transcriptional regulatory pathways. About 85% of Ewing sarcomas carry this translocation.

133. What are the two most common sites of metastases for patients with Ewing sarcoma?

Ewing sarcoma often metastasizes to the **lungs** and somewhat less frequently to other **bones.** In general, lymph nodes are not involved, which suggests that dissemination of this tumor is primarily hematogenous.

134. What type of tumor is an osteosarcoma?

An osteosarcoma is a **malignant spindle cell tumor** in which the cells produce neoplastic osteoid. It is the most common primary malignancy of bone in children.

135. Osteosarcoma generally arises in which part of the bone?

The **metaphyses of long bones** of the extremities. Between 60% and 80% of tumors are located in the metaphyses of the knee (i.e., the proximal tibia or the distal femur) (Fig. 14-5).

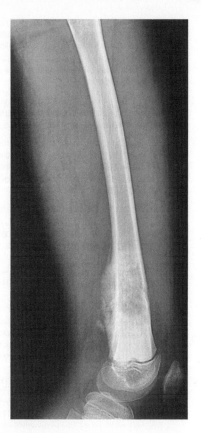

Figure 14-5. Radiograph of an osteosarcoma of the distal femur with typical "starburst" appearance of bone formation. *(From Kleigman RM, Stanton BF, Schor NF, et al: Nelson Textbook of Pediatrics, ed 19, Philadelphia, 2011, Elsevier Saunders, p 1764.)*

136. **Do all patients with osteosarcoma require surgical resection of the primary tumor?**
Surgical resection of the primary tumor is a requirement for curative treatment of osteosarcoma. In contrast to Ewing sarcoma, osteosarcoma is a relatively radiation-resistant tumor, and thus surgical resection after neoadjuvant chemotherapy is a mainstay of treatment.

137. **For patients with localized osteosarcoma, what factor is most predictive of a favorable outcome?**
Patients with **more than 95% necrosis** of the primary tumor (as determined by pathologic examination) **after neoadjuvant chemotherapy** have a better prognosis than those with lesser amounts of necrosis.

138. **What do Ewing sarcoma and osteosarcoma have in common?**
Both are treated with neoadjuvant chemotherapy, which is an initial 2- to 3-month period of chemotherapy, followed by local control with surgery. For select cases of Ewing sarcoma, radiation therapy is also used. Both tumors can develop distant metastases in the lungs and in other bones, and both tumors are cancers of adolescence. Although both Ewing sarcoma and osteosarcoma appear to be soft tissue tumors arising in bone, only osteosarcoma is truly a tumor of bone, whereas Ewing sarcoma is a primitive neuroectodermal tumor.

139. **In what solid tumor has the surgical resection of pulmonary metastases been shown to result in long-term cure?**
Although many pediatric sarcomas metastasize to the lungs, only surgical resection of pulmonary metastases from **osteosarcoma** has been definitively shown to contribute to cure, and only, in general, when the metastases are few in number. The role of the surgical resection of pulmonary metastases arising from other sarcomas (e.g., rhabdomyosarcoma, Ewing sarcoma) is less clear and is only undertaken in select circumstances.

140. What is a limb salvage procedure?

In an attempt to save as much natural tissue as possible, patients with soft tissue sarcomas often undergo a "limb salvage" surgery, in which cancerous tumor is removed from the bone without amputation. Because of the proximity of osteosarcomas to the knee joint, this often results in the removal of the joint as well. Patients who undergo a limb salvage procedure will require a prosthesis or crutches to ambulate.

141. What type of tumor is a rhabdomyosarcoma?

A rhabdomyosarcoma is a **soft tissue tumor** that arises from cells that give rise to striated skeletal muscle. It is the most common soft tissue tumor of childhood.

142. Where do rhabdomyosarcomas usually arise?

The four most common areas are as follows: (1) **head and neck**; (2) **genitourinary region**; (3) **extremities**; and (4) **orbit**. The survival rate for those with tumors in other areas is dependent on the amount, if any, of tumor left after resection and the presence or absence of metastatic disease.

143. What sites of disease are associated with the best outcomes for children with rhabdomyosarcoma?

Favorable locations include the orbit, the head and neck (except for parameningeal tumors), the vagina, and the biliary tract. Unfavorable locations include the extremities, retroperitoneum, and trunk.

Mazzoleni S, Bisogno G, Garaventa A, et al: Outcomes and prognostic factors after recurrence in children and adolescents with nonmetastatic rhabdomyosarcoma, *Cancer* 104:183–190, 2005.

144. What are the two major histologic subtypes of rhabdomyosarcoma?

Alveolar rhabdomyosarcoma, a name derived from its superficial appearance histologically to lung tissue, tends to occur in older children and adolescents. Most of these tumors carry the t(2;13) translocation, and they carry a higher risk for recurrence. **Embryonal rhabdomyosarcomas** tend to occur in younger children, and they are the predominant histology associated with favorable site tumors.

145. Which germ cell tumor is usually seen in young children?

Most germ cell tumors that appear in young children are **benign teratomas** occurring in the sacrococcygeal region. In general, patients with mature teratomas are managed by surgical resection, with care taken for sacrococcygeal tumors to be sure that the entire coccyx is removed.

146. Why are tumor markers assessed before surgery for teratomas and other germ cell tumors?

Tumor markers (e.g., α-fetoprotein, β-HCG) are assessed in anticipation of postoperative monitoring for possible recurrence and malignant transformation. If elevated at diagnosis, these levels should be obtained monthly for the first 6 months because this is the highest risk period. If no elevation is noted, intermittent monitoring should be continued for a total of 3 years after resection.

147. Virilization may be associated with which childhood cancer?

Tumors that cause virilism are most commonly those that produce large quantities of dehydroepiandrosterone, a 17-ketosteroid. Tumors that produce testosterone may also cause virilization. Most commonly, these are **benign tumors of the adrenal gland**; rarely are they malignant. However, the distinction between carcinoma and benign adenoma is frequently difficult. Occasionally, males with primary hepatic neoplasms may become virilized because of the production of androgens by the tumor.

148. How great is the risk for malignant transformation in undescended testes?

The risk for malignancy may be **5 to 10 times higher** in the undescended testis than in a normal testis. The risk in the contralateral testis may also be increased. Orchidopexy decreases, but does not eliminate, the risk for subsequent malignant transformation.

149. What are the most common primary liver tumors of childhood?

Hepatoblastoma and **hepatocellular carcinoma**. Hepatoblastomas usually develop in infants and young children, whereas hepatocellular carcinomas develop throughout childhood. Infection with hepatitis B and C virus is the greatest risk factor for the occurrence of hepatocellular carcinoma.

150. Which tumor marker is most likely to be elevated in children with hepatic tumors?

Most patients with either hepatoblastoma or hepatocellular carcinoma have an elevated concentration of **α-fetoprotein** that parallels disease activity. Lack of a significant decrease of α-fetoprotein with treatment may signify a poor response to therapy. Occasionally, hepatoblastomas produce β-human chorionic gonadotropin and can result in isosexual precocity.

151. Lance Armstrong's treatment for metastatic testicular germ cell tumor had an important modification from standard therapy. What was it and why did this seven-time winner (albeit later discredited) of the *Tour de France* find this important?

Lance Armstrong had a testicular germ cell tumor with metastases to the brain. The therapy for germ cell tumors is typically a combination of cisplatin, etoposide, and bleomycin. Bleomycin is a glycopeptide antibiotic that can result in pulmonary fibrosis and impaired lung function. Fortunately, a number of other agents have excellent activity in the treatment of germ cell tumors, including ifosfamide and etoposide, and thus Mr. Armstrong was effectively treated *without* administration of bleomycin. Pulmonary toxicity from bleomycin could certainly have affected bicycle climbs through the Pyrenees. In general, gonadal germ cell tumors, even when metastatic, have a good prognosis.

STEM CELL TRANSPLANTATION

152. What are the two main types of hematopoietic stem cell (HSC) transplant?
- **Allogeneic**: The recipient receives stem cells from an HLA identical, haploidentical, or mismatched donor.
- **Autologous**: The recipient and the donor are the same person.

153. What is the importance of HLA matching in HSC transplant recipients?

The genes for HLA, the major histocompatibility complex, are closely linked on chromosome 6. Matching donor and recipient for human leukocyte antigen (HLA) class I (A, B, and C) and class II (DRB1 and DQB1) haplotypes is vital to successful allogeneic HSC transplant. There is a progressive decrease in posttransplant survival with each HLA allele mismatch.

Fürst D, Müller C, Vucinic V, et al: High-resolution HLA matching in hematopoietic stem cell transplantation: a retrospective collaborative analysis, *Blood* 122:3220–3229, 2013.

154. What is the chance of siblings having the same human leukocyte antigen (HLA) type?

The HLAs, which are located on chromosome 6, approximate simple Mendelian inheritance, with two siblings having a 1 in 4 chance of having the same typing. A 1% crossover of material may also occur during meiosis. The larger the family, the more likely a match becomes, as shown by the formula $[1 - (0.75)^n]$, with n being the number of siblings. Thus, a child with five brothers and sisters has a 76% chance of having a sibling with an HLA match.

155. What is the chance of finding an HLA-matched unrelated donor?

Although in theory the number of possibilities would equal or even exceed the world's population, thereby making a match astonishingly unlikely, HLA types cluster in individuals of similar genetic and racial backgrounds. In one estimate of persons of European ancestry, about 200,000 individuals would need to be screened to reach a 50% chance of finding a match.

Gahrton G: Bone marrow transplantation with unrelated volunteer donors, *Eur J Cancer* 27:1537–1539, 1991.

156. What are the different sources of stem cells for transplantation?

Stem cells may be obtained either from the **peripheral blood**, the **bone marrow** itself, or the **umbilical cord blood** of a newborn. Peripheral blood stem cells are collected by leukocytapheresis, whereas bone marrow stem cells are collected by multiple bone marrow aspirates. Cord blood is harvested from the placenta at the time of delivery. Stored placental or cord blood is a useful source for patients without a related histocompatible donor because of less graft-versus-host disease (GVHD).

Copelan EA: Hematopoietic stem-cell transplantation, *N Engl J Med* 354:1813–1826, 2006.

157. **What are the advantages and disadvantages of umbilical cord blood as the source for a stem cell transplantation?**
Advantages
- No risk to mother or infant
- Available on demand after cryopreservation
- Can target minority families
- Donors not lost as a result of age, illness, or relocation

Disadvantages
- Limited number of stem cells in collection
- Possible lack of availability of additional donor cells if graft failure or relapse occurs
- Undiagnosed medical condition may be present in newborns

158. **How are stem cells collected?**
Bone marrow is collected by repeated bone marrow aspirates while the donor is under general or local anesthesia. Marrow is generally obtained from the posterior iliac crests. Peripheral blood contains low levels of circulating stem cells. However, the administration of hematopoietic growth factor (e.g., granulocyte-macrophage colony-stimulating factor [GM-CSF]), greatly increases this circulating number. Peripheral blood stem cells are generally obtained after the donor has been given G-CSF and with collection by apheresis. Umbilical cord blood contains high numbers of hematopoietic stem cells at the time of delivery. Cord blood is harvested from the placenta at the time of delivery and these cells can be processed and cryopreserved in cord blood banks.

159. **What is the rationale behind an autologous transplant?**
Autologous transplants are used in situations where high dose chemotherapy will increase the response rate in chemosensitive tumors, but toxicity from the intense chemotherapy is a limiting factor. This limitation can be overcome by harvesting HSCs from the patient, cryopreserving and then subsequently reinfusing the HSCs once they have received the chemotherapy and/or radiotherapy.

160. **Are there nonmalignant indications for an HSC transplant?**
The list of nonmalignant indications is growing, both for hereditary disorders that trace their origin to the hematopoietic stem cell (e.g., sickle cell disease, thalassemia major) and more recently for nonhematopoetic hereditary disorders in which engraftment of stem cells might ameliorate damage in target organs. These latter diseases have included epidermolysis bullosa and Fanconi anemia.

Tolar J, Mehta PA, Walters MC: Hematopoietic cell transplantation for nonmalignant disorders, *Biol Blood Marrow Transplant* 18(1 Suppl):S166–S171, 2012.

161. **In transplant medicine, to what does the term "conditioning" refer?**
Conditioning refers to the preparative regimen necessary to achieve bone marrow ablation and immune suppression for successful donor engraftment to occur. This conditioning regimen is also important in eradicating the underlying disease for which the individual is receiving the transplant.

162. **What are the three most common categories of conditioning regimens?**
- **Myeloablative:** These are comprised of single or combination agents that completely destroy the HSCs in a patient's bone marrow. The result is severe pancytopenia that is often irreversible and may be fatal without the infusion of a stem cell rescue. Current myeloablative regimens may include total body irradiation or high dose busulfan.
- **Nonmyeloablative:** This causes minimal cytopenia (but severe lymphopenia) and does not require stem cell support.
- **Reduced intensity:** An intermediate category of regimens, which may lead to prolonged cytopenias (although not frequently irreversible) and may require stem cell infusion for support.

Bacigalupo A, Ballen K, Rizzo D, et al: Defining the intensity of conditioning regimens: working definitions, *Biol Blood Marrow Transplant* 15:1628–1633, 2009.

163. **What are the major side effects from total-body irradiation used in conditioning?**
In the short term, total-body irradiation may cause **interstitial pneumonitis** and **nephritis**. Over the long term, total-body irradiation may lead to cataracts, growth retardation, hypothyroidism, other endocrine dysfunction, infertility, and secondary malignancies. The long-term effects of total-body irradiation on pulmonary, cardiac, and neuropsychiatric function continue to be studied.

164. Which prophylactic measures should be taken after stem cell transplantation?
Patients may receive antibiotics for gut decontamination. An oral antifungal agent such as fluconazole is also frequently administered. Patients should receive *P. jiroveci* prophylaxis and replacement of immunoglobulins with intravenous immunoglobulin. Acyclovir may also be administered.

165. What is the most common early complication seen in patients after HSC transplant?
Mucositis is the most common early complication seen in patients after autologous or allogeneic hematopoietic stem cell transplant. It frequently occurs in the setting of myeloablative preparative regimens and the use of methotrexate for GVHD prophylaxis. If the mucositis is severe enough, the patient may be unable to tolerate oral intake and may require total parenteral nutrition to maintain their daily caloric needs.

166. What are the major features of graft-versus-host disease (GVHD)?
Acute GVHD typically begins with a fever that is followed by a salmon-colored rash on the palms and soles. The rash may be pruritic and may desquamate. Hepatitis (with jaundice and transaminase elevation) and gastroenteritis (with diarrhea, weight loss, and abdominal pain) may also occur.

167. How is GVHD managed?
Doses of methotrexate, cyclosporine, or tacrolimus during the immediate posttransplantation period may be given in an attempt to prevent the development of acute GVHD. T-cell depletion of the bone marrow graft also decreases the incidence of GVHD. For the treatment of acute GVHD, steroids, cyclosporine, or tacrolimus may be used alone or in combination, depending on the extent of donor-recipient mismatch and the severity of GVHD.

Carpenter PA, MacMillan ML: Management of acute graft-versus-host disease in children, *Pediatr Clin North Am* 57:273–295, 2010.

168. What are the risk factors for GVHD?
There are multiple risk factors for GVHD. First and foremost is the relatedness of the donor to the recipient. An unrelated donor transplant will have a higher risk for GVHD than a matched related donor transplant. Second, the number of T cells received is a risk factor with higher T-cell numbers associated with a higher risk of GVHD. Donor age and parity status are also risk factors, with older donors and multiparous donors having higher risks of GVHD.

169. What is the most likely diagnosis for a patient who experiences weight gain, right upper quadrant pain, and hepatomegaly 10 days after stem cell infusion?
The patient most likely has **venoocclusive disease (VOD),** also known as **sinusoidal obstruction syndrome (SOS).** VOD/SOS is due to damage to the hepatic endothelial cells that then leads to activation of the clotting cascade within the hepatic sinusoids and subsequent reversal of blood flow through the liver. Severe VOD/SOS may be characterized by more than 10% weight gain, respiratory failure, hepatorenal syndrome, and mental status changes. The treatment of VOD centers on maintaining adequate intravascular volume without compromising respiratory function and administration of defibrotide.

Acknowledgments

The editors gratefully acknowledge contributions by Drs. Richard Aplenc, Emily Lipsitz and Peter Adamson, as well as from all of the previous authors, that were retained from prior editions of *Pediatric Secrets*.

CHAPTER 15

ORTHOPEDICS

Benjamin D. Roye, MD, MPH

CLINICAL ISSUES

1. **What is torticollis?**
   Torticollis, also called a "cock-robin" deformity, is a combined head tilt in one direction with rotation in the opposite direction. This deformity may be fixed or flexible.

2. **What is the differential diagnosis for torticollis?**
   Torticollis is a *symptom* that has a variety of underlying etiologies:

   Osseous: Atlanto-occipital anomalies, unilateral absence of C1, Klippel-Feil syndrome (fusion of cervical vertebrae), atlantoaxial rotatory displacement, basilar impression
   Nonosseous: Congenital muscular torticollis, Sandifer syndrome (severe gastroesophageal reflux), ocular dysfunction (strabismus, oculogyric crisis), infections (cervical adenitis, retropharyngeal abscess), central nervous system tumors, syringomyelia, Arnold-Chiari malformation, abnormal skin webs (pterygium colli)

3. **An x-ray of a 10-year-old boy taken to rule out an ankle fracture reveals a 4-mm, well-circumscribed lytic lesion in the cortex of the tibia, which is away from where he is having symptoms. What is the most likely diagnosis?**
   There are a variety of incidental findings on x-ray that carry little clinical significance, sometimes called "incidentalomas." The lesion described here could easily be a fibrous cortical defect also called a **nonossifying fibroma**. This is the *most common benign tumor* in childhood and typically resolves spontaneously. Very large lesions can rarely weaken the bone enough to pose a fracture risk, and a small percentage of these lesions present with a pathologic fracture.

4. **What are two other common types of benign bone tumors in children?**
   Unicameral bone cysts (UBC) and **aneurysmal bone cysts (ABC).** These lesions tend to occur in the metaphyses of long bones and typically have a "bubbly" lytic appearance on x-ray although they typically have well-defined borders because they are slow growing. Both are usually treated with surgery with curettage of the cyst and placement of bone graft to facilitate healing.

5. **How and why is it important to differentiate between an ABC and a UBC?**
   Although the x-ray appearance of ABCs and UBCs can be very similar, fluid-fluid levels seen on magnetic resonance imaging (MRI) are pathognomonic for ABCs and will not be seen in UBCs (which are sometimes called "simple cysts" for this reason). The fluid-fluid levels seen in ABCs represent the two fluids in the cyst, the cyst fluid and blood. It is very important to differentiate between these two lesions before surgery! Although both lesions are benign, **ABCs can be locally aggressive and have a much higher recurrence rate. ABCs are often associated with other tumors** including giant cell tumor, chondroblastoma, and fibrous dysplasia. As such, typically a more aggressive open surgery will be performed for an ABC while less aggressive percutaneous procedures are often attempted for UBCs.

6. **What is rickets?**
   Rickets is the failure of osteoid to calcify in a growing child, most commonly caused by a lack of vitamin D. The adult equivalent is osteomalacia.

7. **What are the physical signs that are suggestive of rickets?**
   The anatomic abnormalities of rickets result primarily from the inability to normally mineralize osteoid; the bones become weak and subsequently distorted. Signs of rickets include the following:
   - Femoral and tibial bowing
   - Delayed suture and fontanel closure
   - Pectus carinatum or "pigeon breast" (anterior protrusion of the sternum)
   - Frontal thickening and bossing of the forehead

- Defective tooth enamel
- Harrison groove (a rim of rib indentation at the insertion of the diaphragm)
- Widened physes at wrists and ankles
- "Rachitic rosary" (enlarged costochondral junctions)

8. **Which bones are known to develop aseptic (also called avascular) necrosis?**
   The **osteochondroses** are a group of disorders in which aseptic necrosis of epiphyses occurs with subsequent fragmentation and repair (Table 15-1). The exact cause is unknown in most cases. However, systemic steroid use has been associated with the development of aseptic necrosis. The patient usually presents with pain at the affected site.

Table 15-1. Typical Age of Onset of Osteochondroses

LOCATION	EPONYM	TYPICAL AGE OF ONSET (YR)
Tarsal navicular bone	Köhler disease	6
Capitellum of distal humerus	Panner disease	9-11
Carpal lunate	Kienböck disease	16-20
Distal lunar epiphysis	Burns disease	13-20
Head of femur	Legg-Calvé-Perthes disease	3-5

9. **What are the inheritance patterns and clinical features of osteogenesis imperfecta?**
   Of the several types of *osteogenesis imperfecta*, the most common is type IV, which occurs in 1 in 30,000 live births. The clinical features vary and depend on the severity of the condition (Table 15-2).

Table 15-2. Types of Osteogenesis Imperfecta

TYPE	INHERITANCE	CLINICAL FEATURES
I	Autosomal dominant	Bone fragility, blue sclerae, onset of fractures after birth (most at preschool age)
Type A		*Without* dentinogenesis imperfecta
Type B		*With* dentinogenesis imperfecta
II	Autosomal recessive	Lethal in perinatal period, dark blue sclerae, concertina femurs, beaded ribs
III	Autosomal recessive	Fractures at birth, progressive deformity, normal sclerae and hearing

10. **McCune-Albright syndrome is associated with what skeletal abnormalities?**
    Polyostotic fibrous dysplasia (i.e., fibrous tissue replacing bones). The fibrous dysplasia occurs most commonly in the long bones and the pelvis and may result in deformity and/or increased thickness of bone. Fibrous dysplasia associated with precocious puberty and café-au-lait spots is known as *McCune-Albright syndrome.*

11. **What are the causes of in-toeing gait (pigeon-toeing)?**
    In-toeing can be due to problems in the foot, tibia or hip:
    Foot:
    - Metatarsus adductus
    - Talipes equinovarus (clubfoot)

Leg:
- Tibial torsion (internal)

Hip:
- Femoral anteversion (medial femoral torsion)
- Paralysis (polio, myelomeningocele)
- Spasticity (cerebral palsy)
- Maldirected acetabulum

Tunnessen WW Jr: *Signs and Symptoms in Pediatrics*, ed 3. Philadelphia, 1999, Lippincott Williams & Wilkins, pp 693–695.

12. **Is in-toeing a problem?**
   The majority of cases of in-toeing are not pathologic problems. There is a normal range of foot placement during gait that can range from slightly internally rotated to slightly externally rotated. Many children will improve their walking as they get older: most children do not have a mature gait pattern until around age 7. Many elite runners turn their feet in when running because they are faster this way. Most parents love this piece of information.

13. **When, if ever, does in-toeing need to be treated?**
   In-toeing rarely requires treatment other than reassurance to the family that their child's walking will improve with time. Femoral anteversion and tibial torsion almost never require treatment in the neurologically normal child. Traditional treatments such as the infamous boots and bars and orthopedic shoes do nothing to change the natural history of these problems. Metatarsus adductus frequently resolves in the first 2 years of life, but feet that are rigid (i.e., the foot cannot easily be manipulated into a normal position) or severe cases may require casting; straight-laced shoes; or in extreme cases, surgery. Children with extreme rotational problems or very asymmetric rotation occasionally benefit from surgery to derotate the affected bone (femur or tibia).

14. **A 15-year-old with tibial pain (worse at night and relieved by nonsteroidal anti-inflammatory drugs) has a small lytic area surrounded by reactive bone formation on x-ray. What is the likely diagnosis?**
   Osteoid osteoma, a benign bone-forming tumor, is typically seen in older children and adolescents and exhibits a male predominance (male-to-female ratio, 2:1). Most children complain of localized pain, usually in the femur and tibia; however, arms and vertebrae may also be involved. Radiographs may demonstrate an osteolytic area surrounded by densely sclerotic reactive bone, and bone scans reveal "hot spots." Computed tomography (CT) scans will show a "nidus" in the middle of the lesion, which is pathognomonic for this diagnosis. The site is usually <1 cm in diameter and arises at the junction of old and new cortex. Pathologically, the lesion is highly vascularized fibrous tissue with an osteoid matrix and poorly calcified bone spicules surrounded by a dense zone of sclerotic bone. Treatment is surgical excision.

15. **What is the clinical significance of limb-length discrepancy?**
   A significant portion of the population has mild limb-length discrepancy. Limb-length discrepancies of <2 cm in a skeletally mature individual usually require no treatment. However, larger discrepancies can lead to problems including limp and low back pain. Over time other problems may be seen including Achilles contractures in the short leg and late hip arthritis.

16. **What are the possible causes of a limb-length discrepancy?**
   - **Congenital anomalies**: Congenital short femur, proximal femoral focal deficiency, congenital absence of fibula, posteromedial bowing of tibia, tibial hypoplasia, congenital hemihypertrophy
   - **Tumors**: Neurofibromatosis, fibrous dysplasia, enchondromatosis, hereditary multiple exostosis, Klippel-Trénaunay-Weber syndrome
   - **Trauma**: Physeal injuries, fracture
   - **Infection**: Septic arthritis, osteomyelitis (the infection can damage the growth plates)
   - **Inflammatory**: Juvenile idiopathic arthritis

17. **What are the general management principles for a limb-length discrepancy?**
   - *0 to 2 cm:* No treatment
   - *2 to 6 cm:* Shoe lift, epiphysiodesis

- *6 to 20 cm:* Limb lengthening
- *>20 cm:* Prosthetic fitting

There is flexibility in these guidelines to account for factors such as environment, motivation, intelligence, compliance, emotional stability, patient and parent wishes, predicted final height, and associated pathology in the limbs.

Friend L, Widmann RF: Advances in the management of limb length discrepancy and lower limb deformity, *Curr Opin Pediatr* 20:46–51, 2008. Guidera KJ, Helal AA, Zuern KA: Management of pediatric limb length inequality, *Adv Pediatr* 42:501–543, 1995.

18. What is a nursemaid elbow?

Also known as a "pulled elbow," a *nursemaid elbow* is a subluxation of the radial head under the orbicular (or annular) ligament resulting from axial traction applied to the extended arm of a young child (Fig. 15-1). Given the pathology, some experts also prefer either the term "annular ligament entrapment" or "annular ligament displacement." Clinically, the child is unwilling to move the affected limb (pseudoparalysis) and there is tenderness directly over their radial head. Attempts to supinate the forearm cause significant pain. The diagnosis is typically made by history and physical examination. Radiographs are normal and not indicated if the mechanism of injury is consistent with this diagnosis. If there is direct trauma or twisting trauma or if a child has significant localized tenderness or swelling on exam, a radiograph should be considered to evaluate for fracture.

Rudloe TF, Schutzman S, Lee LK, et al: No longer a "nursemaid's" elbow: mechanisms, caregivers and prevention, *Pediatr Emerg Care* 28:771–774, 2012.

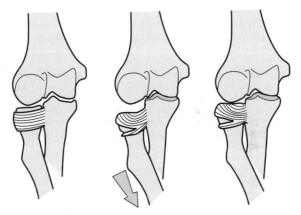

Figure 15-1. Pathology of nursemaid elbow. When the arm is pulled, the radial head moves distally. When traction is discontinued, the ligament is carried into the joint. *(From Kleigman RM, Stanton BF, Schor NF, et al, editors:* Nelson Textbook of Pediatrics, *ed 19. Philadelphia, 2011, Elsevier Saunders, p 2384.)*

19. How is a nursemaid elbow reduced?

Two methods can be utilized. In one, the subluxed radial head is reduced by supinating the extended forearm followed by fully flexing the elbow. In the other, the forearm is hyperpronated. When there is a successful reduction, an audible and palpable click is often present. The child will begin to use his or her arm spontaneously (usually after a few minutes of crying). Limited studies have found that the pronation method may be more effective and less painful than the supination method as a technique for reduction.

Gunaydin YK, Katirci Y, Duymaz, et al: Comparison of success and pain levels of supination-flexion and hyperpronation maneuvers in childhood nursemaid's elbow cases, *Am J Emerg Med* 31:1078–1081, 2013.

20. **What signs and symptoms suggest a serious cause of back pain in a child that warrants further evaluation?**

    Symptoms: age <4 years; pain interfering with daily activities in school, play, or athletics; pain lasting longer than 4 weeks; night pain (often associated with tumor); pain radiating down the leg; fever or other systemic symptoms; limp or altered gait; bowel or bladder changes

    Signs: postural changes; clawing of the toes, gait changes, bowel and bladder habit changes, other neurologic abnormalities; reproducible point tenderness; pain with hyperextension of the back; bruising

Davis PJC, Williams HJ: The investigation and management of back pain in children, *Arch Dis Child Educ Pract Ed* 93:73–83, 2008.

21. **What is the differential diagnosis of back pain in children?**
    - **Infectious**: Discitis, vertebral osteomyelitis, vertebral tuberculosis
    - **Developmental**: spondylolysis, spondylolisthesis, Scheuermann kyphosis, scoliosis
    - **Traumatic**: Herniated disc, muscle strain, fractures, vertebral apophyseal fracture
    - **Inflammatory**: Juvenile idiopathic arthritis, ankylosing spondylitis
    - **Neoplastic**: Eosinophilic granuloma, osteoid osteoma or osteoblastoma, aneurysmal bone cyst, leukemia, lymphoma, Ewing sarcoma, osteosarcoma
    - **Visceral**: Urinary tract infection, hydronephrosis, ovarian cysts, inflammatory bowel disease

Thompson GH: Back pain in children, *J Bone Joint Surg Am* 75:928–937, 1993.

22. **Do school backpacks contribute to back pain?**

    Probably, but this is controversial. Some experts suggest that the limits of maximum loads lifted by children should be 5% to 20% of body weight. In some studies, more than a third of students carried more than 30% of their body weight at least once during the school week. With an apparent increasing incidence of back pain in children and adolescents (particularly those with open physes), the bulging backpack may be one contributing cause.

Dockrell S, Simms C, Blake C: Schoolbag weight limit: can it be defined? *J Sch Health* 83:368–377, 2013.

23. **What constitutes an orthopedic emergency?**

    There are few true emergencies in orthopedics that require immediate attention, but conditions that fall into this category include: open fractures, impending compartment syndrome, femoral neck fractures (including unstable slips of the proximal femoral physis or SCFE), dislocation of major joints (i.e., knee, hip, spine), septic arthritis, cauda equina syndrome.

KEY POINTS: PEDIATRIC ORTHOPEDIC EMERGENCIES—NO DELAY!

1. Open fracture
2. Impending compartment syndrome
3. Dislocation of major joints
4. Septic arthritis
5. Arterial injury

FOOT DISORDERS

24. **Do infants and children need shoes?**

    Barefoot is the natural state of the foot. Humans evolved without shoes and individuals who spend most of their lives unshod have stronger feet and fewer foot deformities than those who wear shoes. Before they begin walking, infants do not need foot coverings other than to keep their feet warm. Once the child begins to walk, shoes will offer protection from the cold and from sharp objects. The AAP recommends soft, light, flexible shoes for new walkers—not bulky, heavy supportive shoes.

25. **What is the most common congenital foot abnormality?**
Metatarsus adductus, also known as metatarsus varus, is the most common abnormality. In patients with this condition, the forefoot is turned toward the midline as a result of adduction of the metatarsal bones at the tarsometatarsal joints. The hindfoot (heel) is normal (Fig. 15-2). Most cases are mild and flexible, with the foot easily straightened by passive stretching. A simple test to determine if the kidney-shaped curvature is within normal limits is to draw a line that bisects the heel. When extended, this line normally falls between the second and third toe space. If it falls more laterally, metatarsus adductus is present. In many cases, *in utero* positioning is the suspected cause of the condition. It is seen more frequently in firstborn children, presumably because primigravida mothers have stronger muscle tone in their uterine and abdominal walls.

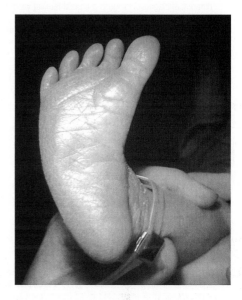

Figure 15-2. Metatarsus adductus. *(From Clark DA: Atlas of Neonatology. Philadelphia, 2000, WB Saunders, p 224.)*

26. **How is metatarsus adductus treated?**
If the foot can be passively abducted beyond neutral, the prognosis is excellent for a spontaneous correction without any therapeutic intervention. In those feet that are stiffer, a program of passive stretching is in order. The parents are taught to hold the heel in a neutral position and manually abduct the forefoot using their thumb placed over the cuboid as a fulcrum. This exaggerated position should be held for a few seconds and the stretching repeated 10 times each session. These sessions should occur with bathing and diaper changing. If this fails to improve the foot, bracing and/or casting can be of help.

27. **How is clubfoot distinguished from severe metatarsus adductus?**
Clubfoot, or *talipes equinovarus,* is distinguished pathologically by a combination of forefoot and hindfoot abnormalities, which result in a fixed (rigid) equinus and varus deformity of the hindfoot. Metatarsus adductus is often a component of clubfeet, but in isolated metatarsus adductus the hindfoot (heel) is *normal.* If the ankle can be dorsiflexed to neutral or beyond, metatarsus is the most likely diagnosis.

28. **How are clubfeet treated?**
Most clubfeet respond well to serial casting using the Ponseti method. The casts should be applied soon after birth, and they are changed weekly. Over the course of 3 to 8 casts significant improvement in the shape of the foot can be expected. About 80% of the feet that are corrected with casting will require an Achilles tenotomy to correct the equinus deformity. Those feet that are not adequately corrected with casting require a more extensive surgical release.

Smith PA, Kuo KN, Graf AN, et al: Long-term results of comprehensive clubfoot release versus the Ponseti method: which is better? *Clin Orthop Relat Res* 472:1281–1290, 2014.

29. **What is a calcaneovalgus foot?**
This common deformity, a sort of anti-clubfoot, is the result of an *in utero* "packaging defect" and is considered a normal variant. The deformity is the exact opposite of the clubfoot: the foot lies in an acutely dorsiflexed position, with the top of the foot in contact with the anterolateral surface of the leg. The heel is in severe valgus, and the forefoot is markedly abducted. Overall the foot is flexible, and both the heel and the forefoot can be corrected into a neutral position. Spontaneous correction is the norm. However, having parents passively stretch the foot is often beneficial (and makes the parents feel better and proactive).

30. **What should be suspected when pes cavus is noted on examination?**
Pes cavus, or high-arched feet (often associated with claw toes), can result from contractures or disturbed muscle balance (Fig. 15-3). A neurologic etiology should always be considered and looked for. The differential diagnosis includes a normal familial variant, Charcot-Marie-Tooth disease, spina bifida or other spinal cord anomaly, peroneal muscle atrophy, Friedreich ataxia, Hurler syndrome, and polio. Neurology consult and/or MRI of the spine is often indicated.

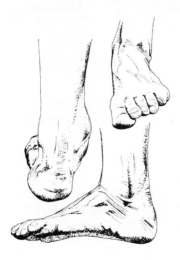

Figure 15-3. Pes cavus. *(From Mellion MB, Walsh WM, Shelton GL: The Team Physician's Handbook, ed 2. Philadelphia, 1997, Hanley & Belfus, p 603.)*

31. **Should children with flexible flat feet be given corrective shoes?**
Only very rarely. Flexible flat feet (*pes planovalgus*) is a common finding in infants and children and approximately 15% of adults. During weight-bearing activity, the ligaments supporting the medial longitudinal arch stretch, and the arch becomes flattened. The heel may also go into an increased valgus (outward) position. There are no radiographic parameters that define a flexible flat foot; it is felt to be a normal variant that results from ligamentous laxity. Children typically do not complain of pain, and an arch can be created easily by removing weight from the feet, having the child stand on his/her toes or by dorsiflexing the great toe. This condition is distinguished from pathologic flat feet in which lack of weight bearing does not lessen the flatness, and rigidity is present on physical examination. Prospective studies have shown that corrective shoes or orthotic insets are not necessary in young children with asymptomatic flexible flat feet because the arch can spontaneously develop during the first 8 years of life and even when it does not, arches do not change the natural history.

Dare DM, Dodwell ER: Pediatric flatfoot: cause, epidemiology, assessment and treatment, *Curr Opin Pediatr* 26:93–100, 2014.

32. **When should I worry about a child with flat feet?**
Flat feet become concerning if they are rigid (as opposed to flexible), painful, or if they cause a disability (such as decreased walking or running endurance). If any of these conditions occurs, the child should be evaluated by a specialist for possible treatment including physical therapy (to stretch the Achilles tendon and strengthen the foot and ankle muscles); orthotics; or in rare cases, surgery.

33. How does the cause of foot pain vary by age?
    - **0 to 6 years:** Ill-fitting shoes, foreign body, occult fracture, osteomyelitis, juvenile idiopathic arthritis (if other joints are involved), rheumatic fever (hypermobile flat foot)
    - **6 to 12 years:** Ill-fitting shoes, foreign body, accessory navicular bone, occult fracture, tarsal coalition (peroneal spastic flat foot), ingrown toenail, hypermobile flat foot
    - **12 to 19 years:** Ill-fitting shoes, foreign body, ingrown toenail, pes cavus, hypermobile flat foot with tight Achilles tendon, ankle sprains, stress fracture

---

Gross RH: Foot pain in children, *Pediatr Clin North Am* 33:1395–1409, 1986.

34. A 10-year-old boy with recurrent ankle sprains and painful flat feet should be evaluated for what possible diagnosis?
    Tarsal coalition. Fusion of various tarsal bones via fibrous or bony bridges can result in a stiff foot that inverts with difficulty. When inversion of the foot is done during an examination, tenderness occurs on the lateral aspect of the foot, and peroneal tendons become very prominent. Thus, this condition is also referred to as "*peroneal spastic flat foot.*" Unless the condition is very severe and warrants surgery, corrective shoes are usually adequate treatment. Other possible causes of a rigid flat foot include rheumatoid arthritis, septic arthritis, posttraumatic arthritis, neuromuscular conditions, and congenital vertical talus.

FRACTURES

35. What are the fractures patterns unique to children?
    Children can suffer from **physeal (growth plate) fractures, buckle fractures, greenstick fractures,** and **plastic deformation** injuries. Most fractures in children incorporate one or more of these patterns.

36. What is a buckle fracture?
    Children's bones are softer and more plastic than adult bones. Their bones can bend without actually breaking. A *buckle (or torus) fracture* occurs when a bone is bent (usually as a result of a fall), and compressive forces cause the cortex to actually buckle out, causing a bump in the bone. This is analogous to what happens to the sheet metal in a car involved in a collision. While this is a fracture, the bone is still in one piece and stable, which is why these fractures are often diagnosed a week or two after injury, much to the surprise and chagrin of the parents who had been ignoring their child's complaints.

37. What is a greenstick fracture?
    A *greenstick* is an incomplete fracture of a long bone. It is called thus because the fracture pattern is similar to what happens when you try to snap a still living branch (or green stick) in half: the branch will break on one side but not all the way through. Similarly, in a greenstick fracture only one cortex fractures while the other cortex remains intact, although usually bent.

38. What does plastic deformation mean?
    The softness, or plasticity, of a child's bones allows them to bend without breaking. When you take a metal rod and bend it just a little, it tends to spring back to its original position. However, if you bend it more, it may spring back, but not all the way, leaving you with a bent rod. The same thing happens in children's bones. Depending on how much force and energy is imparted into the bone as a result of an injury, the bone will first bend, then buckle, then break. So a little bit of force will bend the bone, leaving the child with a bent forearm (far and away the most common location for this pattern of injury). A little more force may cause the cortex to buckle, and even more force will cause a fracture line to extend across the bone. It's important to realize that plastically deformed bones *do not remodel* because there is no healing response as there is when the bone is actually cracked. Therefore, patients with plastically deformed bones usually require them to be straightened (in the operating room or under sedation). This maneuver often results in a complete fracture occurring, which may require internal fixation with rods, wires or plates.

39. Where are the most frequent sites of fractures among children?
    - Clavicle
    - Distal radius
    - Distal ulna

40. What is an open fracture?
    In an *open fracture*, the fracture site communicates with the external environment, usually as a result of the bone piercing the skin. Often times the bone pokes out than falls back beneath the skin, so any laceration of a

fracture site must be presumed to be an open fracture until proven otherwise. Open fractures have higher incidence of infection and a higher degree of soft-tissue damage when compared with closed fractures.

41. **What is a toddler fracture?**

A *toddler fracture* is a fracture of the tibia in a child 9 months to 3 years old as a result of low-energy rotational forces. Typically, these fractures have a spiral appearance and are not displaced. The fibula is rarely fractured. The child will limp, or more commonly, refuse to bear weight. If the child is comfortable at rest, no immobilization is required, but some children (and families) will be more comfortable in a cast or splint for around 2 to 3 weeks.

42. **How are growth-plate fractures classified?**

The Salter-Harris classification of growth-plate (physis) injuries (Fig. 15-4) was devised in 1963. Physeal fractures can result in growth disturbances, and the probability of those happening increases as the classification goes from I to V:

- **Type I:** Epiphysis and metaphysis separate; usually no displacement occurs as a result of the strong periosteum; radiograph may be normal; tenderness over the physis may be the only sign; normal growth after 2 to 3 weeks of cast immobilization
- **Type II:** Fragment of metaphysis splits with epiphysis; usually closed reduction; casting is for 3 to 6 weeks (longer for lower extremity than upper extremity); growth usually not affected, except distal femur and tibia
- **Type III:** Partial plate fracture involving a physeal and epiphyseal fracture to the joint surface; occurs when growth plate is partially fused; closed reduction more difficult to achieve
- **Type IV:** Extensive fracture involving epiphysis, physis, metaphysis, and joint surface; high risk for growth disruption unless proper reduction (usually done operatively) is obtained
- **Type V:** Crush injury to the physis; high risk for growth disruption

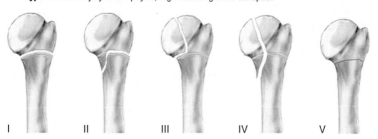

| I | II | III | IV | V |

Figure 15-4. Salter-Harris classification. *(From Katz DS, Math KR, Groskin SA, editors:* Radiology Secrets. *Philadelphia, 1998, Hanley & Belfus, p 403.)*

43. **In a patient with suspected fracture, what are the key points on physical examination?**

Assess "the five P's" in the affected extremity:

- **P**ain and point tenderness
- **P**ulse (distal to the fracture)—to evaluate vascular integrity
- **P**allor—to evaluate vascular integrity
- **P**aresthesia (distal to the fracture)—to assess for sensory nerve injury
- **P**aralysis (distal to the fracture)—to assess for motor nerve injury

    Examine for pain above and below the suspected injury site because multiple fractures can occur in the same limb. The involved extremity should also be carefully examined for deformity, swelling, crepitus, discoloration, and open wounds. A primary concern in any evaluation is a distal neurovascular compromise, which may require immediate surgical intervention. Although the neurologic examination can be challenging in the setting of pain, especially in the younger child who is not cooperative, it is very important to do as thorough an exam as possible.

44. **What are the signs of compartment syndrome?**

The five P's noted in the preceding question are seen in impending or established *compartment syndrome*, a condition in which circulation and function in tissues in a closed space (e.g., thigh, lower leg) is compromised by increased pressure due to swelling, which results in distal ischemia. However, the most important symptom is **pain**, especially pain that does not respond to pain medication and pain with passive range of motion of the digits (fingers or toes) distal to the fracture. If one waits for numbness and paralysis to make the diagnosis of compartment syndrome, it is too late—permanent damage has likely been done. Compartment syndrome is often unrecognized in unconscious patients so a high index of suspicion must be maintained in patients with severe injuries and an altered mental status. In addition, a frightened young child or infant may be very difficult to examine. If there is any concern about compartment syndrome, the compartment pressures must be measured.

45. **What is the treatment of compartment syndrome?**

Compartment syndrome is a true orthopedic emergency. Increased pressure in a compartment is relieved by incising the skin and fascia encompassing the involved compartment. The wound is left open and covered with sterile dressing until swelling decreases. Dressing changes, debridements, and partial wound closure are usually done in the operating room every day or two until the skin can be closed. In some cases, skin grafts are necessary.

46. **How do you treat clavicle fractures?**

These fractures are best managed with a sling and activity restriction. Union occurs in 2 to 4 weeks, but the sling may be removed once the child is comfortable. The residual bump (fracture callus) may take up to 2 years to smooth out (remodel), but there always may be some bump left, especially in older children. Although some studies in adults have suggested improved outcomes with operative management, nonoperative outcomes are good even in older adolescents.

47. **Is surgery ever indicated in clavicle fractures?**

Surgical treatment of clavicular fractures is a very rare event. Traditionally, surgery has been considered necessary in children in only a few extreme scenarios: open fractures, neurovascular injury, or skin compromise. In the adult, there has been growing enthusiasm supporting surgical fixation of clavicular fractures with significant shortening of the bone (>2 to 3 cm) because these can cause problems with weakness and deformity in the affected shoulder. However, there is no similar literature to support surgery in a pediatric population. All studies in children show close to a 100% healing rate for these fractures without surgery. Of note, studies looking at outcomes with surgery show that these cases represent approximately only 1% of all the clavicle fractures.

Randsborg P-H, Fuglesang HFS, et al: Long-term patient-reported outcome after fractures of the clavicle in patients aged 10 to 18 years, *J Pediatr Orthop* 34:393–399, 2014.

Kubiak R, Slongo T: Operative treatment of clavicle fractures in children: a review of 21 years, *J Pediatr Orthop* 2002;22:736–739.

48. **A teenager who punches a wall in anger typically incurs what fracture?**

Boxer fracture. This is a fracture of the distal fifth metacarpal, usually with apical dorsal angulation (Fig. 15-5). Up to 35 degrees of angulation can be accepted without compromise of function. Reduction may be held with a cast, although at times it may require pin fixation.

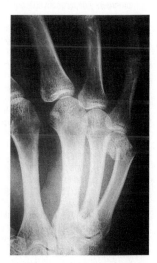

Figure 15-5. Boxer fracture with fracture of fifth (and fourth) metacarpal with volar displacement of the distal fragments after a punching injury. *(From Katz DS, Math KR, Groskin SA, editors:* Radiology Secrets. *Philadelphia, 1998, Hanley & Belfus, p 440.)*

49. Children who fall on outstretched arms often suffer what type of fractures?
Colles fractures. This is a group of complete fractures of the distal radius with varying displacement of the distal fragment. The fall, with the hand outstretched, wrist dorsiflexed, and forearm pronated, often results in a classic "dinner-fork" deformity of the wrist on examination.

50. What does the presence of the posterior fat pad on an elbow x-ray suggest?
Of the two fat pads that overlie the elbow joint, only the anterior one typically is visible on a lateral x-ray. If fluid accumulates in the joint space, as it does in cases involving bleeding, inflammation, or fracture, the fat pads are displaced upward and outward. The position of the anterior pad changes, and the posterior pad becomes visible. In the setting of acute trauma, the presence of a posterior fat pad is associated with a nearly 75% chance of occult fracture and the elbow should be immobilized in a cast or splint with close follow-up scheduled. The most common injuries would be a radial head fracture and a nondisplaced supracondylar humerus fracture.

51. For a teenager with wrist trauma, why is palpation of the anatomic "snuff box" a critical part of the physical exam?
The *anatomic snuff box* (the inpouching formed by the tendons of the abductor pollicis longus and extensor pollicis longus when the thumb is abducted [in hitchhiker fashion]) sits just above the scaphoid (carpal navicular) bone. The scaphoid is the carpal bone most commonly fractured, and it is at high risk for nonunion or avascular necrosis. Snuff box tenderness, pain on supination with resistance, and pain on longitudinal compression of the thumb should increase suspicion for fracture of the scaphoid bone. Even when an x-ray is negative, if there is significant snuff box tenderness, a fracture should be suspected and the wrist and thumb immobilized. A repeat x-ray in 2 to 3 weeks may better reveal a fracture. The use of computed tomography (CT) or MRI can be used to more reliably identify a scaphoid fracture when the plain film is negative and the clinical suspicion is high.

Evenski AJ, Adamczyk MJ, Steiner RP, et al: Clinically suspected scaphoid fractures in children, *J Pediatr Orthop* 29:352–355, 2009.

52. Name the eight carpal bones of the wrist.
Disdaining some of the classic (mostly obscene) mnemonics, remember what will happen if a wrist fracture is missed: **S**inister **L**awyers **T**ake **P**hysicians **T**o **T**he **C**ourt **H**ouse, which helps identify the bones in order of proximal to distal, lateral to medial: **s**caphoid, **l**unate, **t**riquetrum, **p**isiform, **t**rapezium, **t**rapezoid, **c**apitate, and **h**amate.

53. What is the difference between open and closed reductions?
A fracture reduction means realignment of the bone to its original shape. A *closed reduction* occurs by simply pushing on the bone and holding it in place with a splint or a cast. This may be done in the emergency department (ED) or the operating room; some form of anesthesia is usually required. An *open reduction* implies that an incision is required to expose the fracture site, help realign the bone, and use an internal implant (if needed) to stabilize the bone. This often occurs when the fracture is already exposed (an open fracture), when there is soft tissue interposed between the fragments blocking reduction, or when a joint surface is involved. Joints do not remodel and perfect alignment is critical to prevent post-traumatic arthritis. Other indications for open reduction include children with polytrauma (multiple fractures and/or head injuries to facilitate their mobilization) and those with Salter-Harris III and IV fractures where a good reduction can reduce the risk of physeal arrest.

54. In pediatric fractures, what amount of angulation is acceptable before reduction is recommended?
Acceptable angulation or displacement varies with the location of the fracture and the child's age. Younger children have remarkable healing potential to remodel with minimal to no residual deformity or limitation of rotation. As a rule, wrist fractures in children up to 8 years old, as much as 30 degrees of angulation *in the plane of motion* will heal satisfactorily without reduction. This means that a fracture that is flexed or extended in the wrist (in the direction the wrist typically moves) can be expected to model well. Less angulation is accepted in the midshaft of the forearm; typically 15 to 20 degrees will be allowed. However, displacement with angulation towards the radius or ulna will not remodel so reliably and rotational malalignment will not remodel at all. The degree of remodeling diminishes with age and growth remaining. In general, fractures closer to the growth plate will remodel more readily than midshaft fractures.

Boutis K: Common pediatric fractures treated with minimal intervention, *Pediatr Emerg Care* 26:152–162, 2010.

55. **In which fractures will remodeling of bone *not* occur?**
Remodeling, or reshaping of the bone to its original configuration, is a common phenomenon in pediatric fractures, which lessens the need for surgery for many fracture patterns. Remodeling occurs most readily when the fracture is close to the growth plate, and the deformity is in the plane of motion (e.g., a distal femur fracture is bent in flexion as opposed to being in varus or valgus). Interestingly, **extension-type supracondylar humerus fractures**, the most common surgically treated elbow fracture in children, do not remodel very well even though they are close to the physis, and the deformity is in the plane of motion (extension usually). The following fractures also have a low chance of remodeling and may require closed or open reduction: **intra-articular fractures** (these must always be reduced anatomically to preserve joint function); **plastic deformation** (see above), and **fractures with excessive shortening or rotation**. Angulation and translation deformities may remodel, but if the severity is too great, they may not remodel completely with the sequelae of residual deformity and possible dysfunction.

56. **How long should fractures be immobilized?**
Children's fractures generally heal more quickly than their counterparts in adults. The exact length of immobilization depends on several variables, including the child's age, the location of the fracture, and the type of treatment. As a rule of thumb, physeal, epiphyseal, and metaphyseal fractures heal more rapidly than diaphyseal fractures because they have a better blood supply. On average, epiphyseal, physeal, and metaphyseal fractures heal in children within 3–5 weeks, whereas diaphyseal fractures may heal within 4–6 weeks. The big exception is the tibial shaft fractures, which can take up to 12 weeks to heal even in healthy children.

Castroom: The Casters and Bracers Home: www.castroom.net. Accessed on Mar. 27, 2015.

57. **How long do fractured clavicles and femurs take to heal?**
   - **Newborn:** *Clavicle*, 10 to 14 days; *femur*, 3 weeks
   - **16-year-old child:** *Clavicle*, 6 weeks; *femur*, 6 to 10 weeks

HIP DISORDERS

58. **Why has DDH replaced CHD?**
The term *developmental dysplasia of the hip* (DDH) has replaced congenital hip dislocation (CHD) to reflect the evolutionary nature of hip problems in infants during the first months of life. About 2.5 to 6.5 infants per 1000 live births develop problems, and a significant percentage of these are not present on neonatal screening examinations. Therefore, the overt pathologic process may not be present at birth, and the term *congenital* does not apply to all cases of hip dysplasia and has been dropped. As such, periodic examination of the infant's hip is recommended at each routine well-baby examination until the age of 1 year.

DDH also refers to the *entire spectrum* of abnormalities involving the growing hip, ranging from dysplasia to subluxation to dislocation of the hip joint. Unlike CHD, DDH refers to alterations in the hip growth and stability *in utero*, during the newborn period, and during infancy. If other diseases are involved (e.g., cerebral palsy), "hip dysplasia" alone is a sufficient term. Hip dislocation as a result of neurologic disease or joint contracture syndromes (e.g., spina bifida, arthrogryposis) is more correctly labeled "teratologic dislocation."

Nemeth BA, Narotam V: Developmental dysplasia of the hip, *Pediatr Rev* 33:553–561, 2012.

59. **What are the Ortolani and Barlow maneuvers?**
The most reliable clinical methods of detection remain the Ortolani reduction and the Barlow provocative maneuvers. The infant should be lying quietly supine. Both examinations begin with the hips flexed to 90 degrees. To perform the *Ortolani maneuver*, the hip is abducted, as the examiner's index finger gently pushes up on the greater trochanter. This is a reduction maneuver that allows a dislocated femoral head to "clunk" back into the acetabulum (Fig. 15-6, *A*). The *Barlow maneuver* is performed by adducting the flexed hip and gently pushing the thigh posteriorly in an effort to dislocate the femoral head (Fig. 15-6, *B*). After 3 to 6 months of age, these tests are no longer useful because the hip becomes fixed in its dislocated position over time.

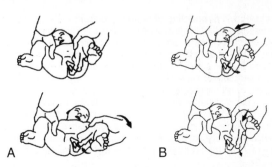

Figure 15-6. A, Ortolani maneuver. **B,** Barlow maneuver. *(From Staheli LT, editor:* Pediatric Orthopaedic Secrets. *Philadelphia, 1998, Hanley & Belfus, p 166.)*

KEY POINTS: THE FOUR F'S OF INCREASED RISK FOR DEVELOPMENTAL DISLOCATION OF THE HIP

1. First born
2. Female
3. Funny presentation (breech)
4. Family history (positive for developmental dysplasia of the hip)

---

60. What is a positive Galeazzi sign?

    The *Galeazzi test* is performed by flexing both hips and knees together while evaluating the relative height of the knees. A positive Galeazzi sign is present if one knee is significantly higher than the other. This can mean one of two things: the hip on the low side is dislocated or the femur on the low side is short. As opposed to the Ortolani and Barlow signs, the Galeazzi sign remains positive, and in fact usually becomes more obvious, as the child gets older.

61. What is the significance of a "hip click" in a newborn?

    A *hip click* is the high-pitched sensation felt at the very end of abduction when testing for development dysplasia of the hip with the Barlow and Ortolani maneuvers; it occurs in ≤10% of newborns. Classically, it is differentiated from a hip "clunk," which is heard and felt as the hip goes in and out of joint. Although a debatable point, the hip click is felt to be benign. Its cause is unclear and may be the result of movement of the ligamentum teres between the femoral head and the acetabulum or the hip adductors as they slide over the cartilaginous greater trochanter. Worrisome features that might warrant evaluation (e.g., hip ultrasound, hip x-ray) include late onset of the click, associated orthopedic abnormalities, and other clinical features suggestive of developmental dysplasia (e.g., asymmetric skin folds/creases, unequal leg length).

Witt C: Detecting developmental dysplasia of the hip, *Adv Neonatal Care* 3:65–75, 2003.

---

62. What is the most reliable physical finding for a dislocated hip in the older child?

    Limited hip abduction. This is the result of shortening of the adductor muscles.

63. What other diagnostic signs are suggestive of a dislocated hip?

    - **Asymmetry of the thigh and gluteal folds:** However, these may be present in many normal infants and it is an unreliable sign if all other tests are normal.
    - **Waddling gait, hyperlordosis of lumbar spine:** This is seen in older patients with bilateral dislocations.
    - **Unilateral toe walking** is consistent with a significant leg length discrepancy as can be seen in a unilateral hip dislocation

64. **What radiographic studies are most valuable for diagnosing DDH during the newborn period?**

In infants <6 months old, the acetabulum and the proximal femur are predominantly cartilaginous and thus not visible on plain x-ray. In this age group, these structures are best visualized with **ultrasound**. In addition to morphologic information, ultrasound provides dynamic information about the stability of the hip joint.

Omeroğlu H: Use of ultrasonography in developmental dysplasia of the hip, *J Child Ortho* 8:105–113, 2014.

65. **Should all infants be routinely screened by ultrasound for DDH?**

The answer is not clear. Because physical examination is not completely reliable and the incidence of late-diagnosed DDH has not declined, some investigators have recommended routine ultrasonographic screening. However, others argue that ultrasonography can lead to overdiagnosis and treatment. At present, the issue remains controversial. Universal screening is more commonly done in Europe, whereas in the United States, selective screening on the basis of risk factors and physical examination findings is more the norm.

Shorter D, Hong T, Osborn DA: Screening programmes for developmental dysplasia of the hip in newborn infants, *Cochrane Database Syst Rev* 9:CD004595, 2011.

66. **Who is at a higher risk for DDH?**

Dislocated, dislocatable, and subluxable hip problems occur in about 1% to 5% of infants; 70% of dislocated hips occur in girls, and 20% occur in infants born in breech position. Other risk associations include the following:

- Congenital torticollis
- Skull or facial abnormalities
- First pregnancy
- Positive family history of dislocation
- Metatarsus adductus
- Calcaneovalgus foot deformities in infants <2500 g
- Amniotic fluid abnormalities (especially oligohydramnios)
- Prolonged rupture of membranes
- Large birth weight

MacEwen GD: Congenital dislocation of the hip, *Pediatr Rev* 11:249–252, 1990.

67. **What is the recommended timing for ultrasound evaluation when screening is indicated?**

The AAP recommends both static and dynamic assessments 3 weeks after birth. The American College of Radiology endorses ultrasound 2 or more weeks after birth. Earlier use of ultrasound can result in a high rate of false-positive studies due to physiologic ligamentous laxity, which resolves spontaneously.

Nemeth BA, Narotam V: Developmental dysplasia of the hip, *Pediatr Rev* 33:553–561, 2012.

68. **How is DDH treated?**

If the hip is dislocated, the first goal is to obtain a reduction and maintain that reduction to provide an optimal environment for femoral head and acetabular development. This is accomplished by keeping the legs abducted and the hips and knees flexed. The most commonly used device is a Pavlik harness for infants younger than age 6 months. Frequent follow-up is necessary for harness adjustments. Early initiation of harness therapy (at <2 months of age) results in stable hips in >95% of cases of DDH.

Double and triple diapers have *no role* in the treatment of DDH; they provide the parents with a false sense of security and do not provide reliable stabilization or positioning. If the hip is merely shallow or loose and not frankly dislocated, the treatment is the same, but the harness or splint can come off once a day for an hour for bathing or play time.

Cooper AP, Doddabasappa SN, Mulpuri K: Evidence-based management of developmental dysplasia of the hip, *Orthop Clin North Am* 45:341–354, 2014.

69. **What is the natural history of untreated DDH?**
A child with a unilateral hip dislocation may have a leg-length discrepancy and painless (Trendelenburg) limp throughout childhood and young adulthood. If the hip is subluxed, osteoarthritis of the hip joint may develop at some point during the third through fifth decades of life. Hip fusion and total hip arthroplasty are surgical treatment options for the symptomatic hip in young adults. Children with bilateral DDH often have no leg-length inequality and no appreciable limp. They tend to walk with hyperextension of the lumbar spine (hyperlordosis) and have a waddling gait. As with patients with unilateral dislocations, these patients tend to develop early osteoarthritis. Total hip arthroplasty is the treatment of choice for adults with symptomatic bilateral DDH.

70. **What is the significance of a Trendelenburg gait?**
A *Trendelenburg gait* results from functionally weakened hip abductor muscles. It is commonly seen in children with a dislocated hip and Legg-Calvé-Perthes disease. With a dislocated hip, the abductor muscles are at a mechanical disadvantage and are effectively weakened, which makes it difficult for them to support the child's body weight. As a result, the pelvis tilts away from the affected hip. In an effort to minimize this imbalance during the stance phase of gait, children lean over the affected hip. This constitutes a positive Trendelenburg sign (Fig. 15-7).

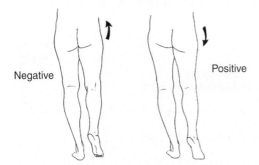

Negative

Positive

Figure 15-7. Trendelenburg sign. The pelvis tilts toward the normal hip when weight is borne on the affected side. *(From Goldstein B, Chavez F: Applied anatomy of the lower extremities, Phys Med Rehabil State Art Rev 10:601–603, 1996.)*

71. **What is the most common cause of a painful hip in a child <10 years old?**
Transient synovitis is a self-limited inflammatory condition that occurs before adolescence, has no known cause, and generally has a benign clinical outcome. Some theorize that it is an immune response to a viral illness, and many patients give a history of having a recent viral illness; however, viral illnesses are very common in childhood. This disorder, although benign, can cause considerable anxiety among physicians and family members during its clinical course because it can mimic other, more sinister, conditions such as septic arthritis, osteomyelitis, Legg-Calvé-Perthes disorder, juvenile idiopathic arthritis, slipped capital femoral epiphysis, and tumor. It may occur anytime from the toddler age group to the late juvenile years, but the peak age of onset is between 3 and 6 years, and it is more common among boys. Acute transient synovitis remains a diagnosis of exclusion. Treatment consists of rest and calming of the synovitis with anti-inflammatory agents. Most patients experience complete resolution of their symptoms within 2 weeks of onset; the remainder may have symptoms of lesser severity for several weeks.

Nouri A, Walmsley D, Pruszczynski B, et al: Transient synovitis of the hip: a comprehensive review, *J Pediatr Orthop B* 23:32–36, 2014.

72. **How can transient synovitis be differentiated from septic arthritis?**
See Table 15-3.

Table 15-3. Transient Synovitis versus Septic Arthritis

	TRANSIENT SYNOVITIS	**SEPTIC ARTHRITIS**
History	Preceding upper respiratory infection ± low-grade fever Hip or referred knee pain Limp	Fever Usually large joint involvement (hip, ankle, knee, shoulder, elbow)
Physical	Refusal to bear weight Can delicately elicit range of motion in affected hip joint	Exquisite pain, swelling, warmth Marked resistance to mobility
Laboratory	ESR normal or mildly elevated Mild peripheral leukocytosis Negative blood culture Joint fluid cloudy Negative Gram stain	ESR markedly elevated Leukocytosis with left shift Often positive blood culture Joint fluid purulent Often positive Gram stain

ESR, Erythrocyte sedimentation rate.

73. What is LCP disease?

LCP disease (also called Perthes, Legg-Perthes or Legg-Calvé-Perthes after the three physicians who independently described it) is a disorder of the femoral head of unknown etiology that is characterized by ischemic necrosis, collapse, and subsequent repair (Fig. 15-8). Children typically present with a limp that is often painless. Over time they often develop pain that localizes to the groin or is referred to the thigh or knee.

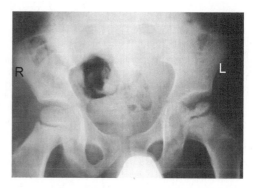

Figure 15-8. Anteroposterior view of the pelvis demonstrates fragmentation and irregularity of the left femoral head in a patient with Legg-Calvé-Perthes disease. The right hip is normal. *(From Katz DS, Math KR, Groskin SA, editors:* Radiology Secrets. *Philadelphia, 1998, Hanley & Belfus, p 405.)*

74. What are the pathologic stages of LCP disease?

LCP is a condition of aseptic necrosis of the femoral head involving children primarily between the ages of 4 and 10 years.

- **Incipient or synovitis stage**: Lasting 1 to 3 weeks, this first stage is characterized by an increase in hip-joint fluid and a swollen synovium associated with reduced hip range of motion.
- **Avascular necrosis**: Lasting 6 months to 1 year, the blood supply to part (or all) of the head of the femur is lost. That portion of the bone involved dies, but the contour of the femoral head remains unchanged.
- **Fragmentation or regeneration and revascularization**: In the last and longest pathologic stage of LCP, which lasts 1 to 3 years, the blood supply returns and causes both the resorption of necrotic bone and the laying down of new immature bone. As the dead bone is removed, the integrity of the head is weakened and it collapses. Permanent hip deformity can occur during this last stage.

It is important to note that plain radiographs may lag behind the progression of the disorder by as much as 3 to 6 months. Radionuclide bone scans and MRI are much better tests because ischemia and avascular necrosis can be detected much earlier.

75. **What is the prognosis for children with LCP disease?**
The two main prognostic factors for LCP disease include the **age of the child at diagnosis** and the **amount of epiphyseal involvement**. Children <6 years of age tend to have a more favorable prognosis, and those with less epiphyseal involvement also tend to have a better prognosis. Epiphyseal involvement has been classified by Salter into type A (those with <50% epiphyseal involvement) and type B (those with >50% head involvement).

76. **What condition does the child in Figure 15-9 have?**
This is **femoral anteversion** (or medial femoral torsion), which is a common cause of in-toeing in younger children. The child is demonstrating the reverse tailor, or "W" position, which is a sign of the internally rotated hip.

Staheli LT: Torsional deformity, *Pediatr Clin North Am* 33:1382, 1986.

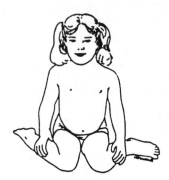

Figure 15-9. Reverse tailor position or "W" position.

77. **How is the extent of femoral anteversion measured?**
With the child lying prone and knees flexed at 90 degrees, the hip normally cannot be rotated internally (i.e., feet pushed outward) more than 60 degrees (angle A in Fig. 15-10, *A*). In addition, external rotation (angle B in Fig. 15-10, *B*) should exceed 20 degrees. A normal child averages approximately 35 degrees. Motion outside these ranges indicates that the cause of in-toeing is likely the result of physiologic femoral anteversion (or, less commonly, hip capsular contractions as are seen in patients with cerebral palsy).

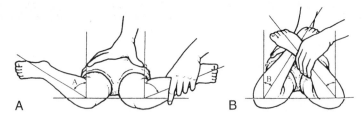

A   B

Figure 15-10. Measurement of femoral anteversion. *(From Dormans JP: orthopaedic management of children with cerebral palsy, Pediatr Clin North Am 40:650, 1993.)*

78. **Is sitting in the "W" position harmful?**
In a word, **no**. While there is great confusion about this amongst many physicians and patients alike, there is absolutely no evidence that sitting in the "W" position has a harmful effect on the development of the hip and knee. Similarly use of special orthopedic shoes or the infamous boots and bars that hold the feet turned in has no effect on the bony alignment of the proximal femur.

79. **Is there ever an indication to treat femoral anteversion?**
The neurologically normal child almost never requires treatment for anteversion. While they may walk with their feet turned in, especially early in life, this tends to improve as they age and improve in strength, coordination, and balance. An exception is the child with so-called *miserable malalignment syndrome* who has severe femoral anteversion along with external tibial torsion. This child walks with their feet straight ahead (the tendency to in-toe is counterbalanced by the external rotation of the foot through the tibia), but the knees are pointed in and this places severe stress across the patellofemoral joint. Significant knee pain and disability follow. The treatment is quite significant, involving osteotomies of the femurs and tibias, but most patients respond well with improved knee mechanics and decreased pain.

80. **What symptoms do children with slipped capital femoral epiphysis (SCFE) have?**
SCFE involves progressive displacement of the hip with external rotation of the femur on the epiphyseal growth plate. The patient has intermittent or constant hip, thigh, or knee pain that has often been present for weeks or months. A limp, a lack of internal rotation, and an inability to flex the hip without also abducting may be noted. It is important to realize that any patient with knee pain may have underlying hip pathology.

81. **What systemic conditions are associated with SCFE?**
Children with SCFE tend to have delayed skeletal maturation and obesity and usually present between the ages of 8 to 14 years. It is more common in boys and in black children. Systemic conditions associated with SCFE include **hypothyroidism, panhypopituitarism, hypogonadism, rickets,** and **irradiation**.

82. **What does FAI stand for?**
Femoral acetabular impingement syndrome. This is a relatively recently recognized entity thought to be a significant cause of hip pain and disability in adolescents and young adults. Similar to the way the rotator cuff of the shoulder can be damaged when impinged between the humeral head and acromion, the labrum of the hip (a structure analogous to the meniscus in the knee) can be torn when pinched between the acetabulum and femoral head or neck.

Philippon MJ, Patterson DC, Briggs KK: Hip arthroscopy and femoroacetabular impingement in the pediatric patient, *J Pediatr Orthop* 33S: S126–S130, 2013.

83. **What new treatments are available for the treatment of hip pathology including DDH, FAI, and SCFE?**
Over the last decade, hip arthroscopy has come into much more frequent use to diagnose and treat hip pain due to labral tears and to recontour the bony aspects of the hip joint when some types of dysplasia exist. Even more recently, some hip centers around the country have been describing their experience with repairing hip pathology through surgical dislocation of the hip. This technique has been eschewed in the past because of concerns of osteonecrosis of the femoral head as a complication. However, newer techniques have shown extremely low rates of this complication and this procedure allows more direct and effective treatment of many hip problems including unstable SCFE and FAI.

Jayakumar P, Ramachandran M, Youm T, et al: Arthroscopy of the hip for paediatric and adolescent disorders: current concepts, *J Bone Joint Surg Br* 94:290–296, 2012.

INFECTIOUS DISEASES

KEY POINTS: OSTEOMYELITIS

1. The most common causative organisms in healthy children are *Staphylococcus aureus* and beta-hemolytic streptococci.
2. In children (unlike adults), spread of bacteria to bone is hematogenous rather than by local trauma.
3. In children with a puncture wound through a sneaker and osteomyelitis, think of *Pseudomonas aeruginosa*; however, the most common organism is still *S. aureus*.

4. Because of intravascular sludging and infarction, patients with sickle cell disease are at increased risk, especially for *Salmonella* infections.
5. Bone changes on x-ray may not occur for 10 to 15 days.

84. **What percentage of septic arthritis is "culture negative"?**
Several studies have established that 30% to 60% of patients with clinically apparent septic arthritis have negative cultures of joint fluid. Reasons (both postulated and confirmed) for this observation include the fastidious nature of some causes of infectious arthritis (e.g., *Kingella kingae*), the loss of viability of some organisms on transport to the laboratory (e.g., *Neisseria* species), and perhaps a substance or cell population in the aspirate fluid that is bacteriostatic during *in vitro* culture conditions. Prompt processing of specimens and the use of several culture techniques (e.g., solid media plus liquid-culture systems such as those used for blood cultures) can increase the yield of joint fluid cultures.

85. **Where does acute hematogenous osteomyelitis most commonly localize in children?**
Approximately two-thirds of all cases involve the **femur**, **tibia** or **humerus**.

86. **What is the most common cause of acute hematogenous osteomyelitis?**
Staphylococcus aureus, particularly methicillin-resistant *S. aureus* (MRSA), is responsible for 70% to 90% of cases for which a bacterial pathogen is identified. Most cases of MRSA infection have additional virulence factors, such as Panton-Valentine leukocidin, which causes tissue necrosis. A variety of other organisms may be involved but rates of *Haemophilus influenzae* type b and *S. pneumonia* have declined since universal vaccination against these pathogens began. *Kingella kingae* (an anaerobic, β-hemolytic, gram-negative organism) is the second most common cause (beyond gram-positive cocci) of osteoarticular infections, particularly septic arthritis, in children younger than age 4 years in the United States. For children with sickle cell disease, *Salmonella* is an important cause of infection. Neonatal causes are more varied compared with older children, with *S. agalactiae*, coagulase-negative staphylococci, and gram-negative bacilli as additional possible causes. Fungal causes are rare.

Yagupsky P, Porsch MA, St. Geme III JW: *Kingella kingae:* an emerging pathogen in young children, *Pediatrics* 127:557–565, 2011.
Harik NS, Smeltzer MS: Management of acute hematogenous osteomyelitis in children, *Expert Rev Anti Infect Ther* 8:175–181, 2010.

87. **How often are blood cultures positive in patients with osteomyelitis?**
Blood cultures are positive 50% of the time or less. Because this rate is relatively low, direct bone aspiration should be strongly considered, especially in the setting of an abscess. Aspiration raises the yield to 70% to 80% and can facilitate antibiotic therapy.

88. **As osteomyelitis progresses, how soon do x-ray changes occur?**
- **3 to 4 days:** Deep muscle plane shifted away from periosteal surface
- **4 to 10 days:** Blurring of deep tissue muscle planes
- **10 to 15 days:** Changes in bone occur (e.g., osseous lucencies, punched-out lytic lesions, periosteal elevation)
- **>30 days:** Bone sclerosis may be evident

89. **What is the best way to confirm the diagnosis of osteomyelitis?**
Bone infections in children are typically accompanied by fever, local pain, and decreased use of the affected body part (e.g., limp or failure to bear weight). Although point tenderness is often elicited, plain radiographs may appear normal during the first 10 to 14 days of infection, until a sufficient portion of cortex is damaged and the periosteal reaction becomes apparent. Early during the course of infection, other imaging studies (triphasic radioisotope scanning with [99m]technetium, CT or MRI) and/or direct aspiration with Gram stain and culture can be of use for confirming the diagnosis. MRI is especially valuable in the assessment because it can simultaneously assess the osseous, articular, and muscular structures without ionizing radiation exposure (Fig. 15-11).

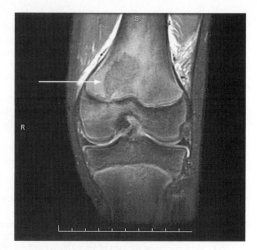

Figure 15-11. MRI image of the distal femur showing metaphyseal lesion *(arrow)* and overlying inflammatory edema of muscles, consistent with osteomyelitis. *(From Bergelson JM, Shah SS, Zaoutis TE: Pediatric Infectious Diseases: The Requisites in Pediatrics. Philadelphia, 2008, Elsevier Mosby, p 239.)*

90. **How long should antibiotics be continued in patients with osteomyelitis and septic arthritis?**
   The precise answer is unclear. Traditionally, a minimum of 4 to 6 weeks was believed to be necessary for the treatment of *S. aureus* infections. Newer studies have indicated that a combination of intravenous and oral therapy for 3 to 4 weeks is associated with therapeutic success in uncomplicated cases. Longer durations may be required if there is delayed or incomplete surgical evacuation or distant foci of infection (e.g., endocarditis).

Peltola H, Pääkhönen M: Acute osteomyelitis in children, *N Engl J Med* 370:352–360, 2014.

91. **Which marker, C-reactive protein (CRP) or erythrocyte sedimentation rate (ESR), is more sensitive to assess inflammation both diagnostically and therapeutically?**
   C-reactive protein. CRP has a serum circulation life of approximately 1 day. The ESR is most influenced by the fibrinogen level, which has a circulatory life of approximately 4 days. Thus, the ESR may be normal or only mildly elevated during the first days of evolving osteomyelitis and later declines more slowly. CRP rises more quickly in the setting of infection and then declines more quickly with appropriate therapy.

Conrad DA: Acute hematogenous osteomyelitis, *Pediatr Rev* 31:464–470, 2010.

92. **When is open surgical drainage indicated in cases of osteomyelitis?**
   - Abscess formation in the bone, subperiosteum, or adjacent soft tissue
   - Bacteremia persisting more than 49 to 72 hours after the initiation of antibiotic treatment
   - Continued clinical symptoms (e.g., fever, pain, swelling) after 72 hours of therapy
   - Development of a sinus tract
   - Presence of a sequestrum (i.e., detached piece of necrotic bone)

Darville T, Jacobs RF: Management of acute hematogenous osteomyelitis in children, *Pediatr Infect Dis J* 23:255–257, 2004.

93. **Why are treatment failures more common in osteomyelitis than in septic arthritis?**
   - Antibiotic concentrations are much greater in joint fluid than in inflamed bone. Concentrations in joint fluid may actually exceed peak serum concentrations, whereas those in bone may be significantly less than serum concentrations.
   - Devitalized bone may serve as an ongoing nidus for infection, and it has no blood flow to bring in antibiotics.
   - Diagnosis of osteomyelitis is more likely to be delayed than that of septic arthritis.

94. How is the diagnosis of discitis established?

Discitis, which is the infection and/or inflammation of the intervertebral disc, most commonly occurs in children between the ages of 4 and 10 years. The etiology is often unclear, but a bacterial cause (particularly *S. aureus*) is identified by blood cultures in about 50% of cases. The diagnosis can be difficult because the symptoms can be vague and vary greatly. Symptoms include generalized back pain with or without localized tenderness, limp, refusal to stand or walk, back stiffness with loss of lumbar lordosis, abdominal pain, and unexplained low-grade fever.

As with osteomyelitis, a helpful laboratory test is an elevated CRP or ESR. White blood cells may often be normal, and early x-rays (<2 to 4 weeks of symptoms) may not show changes. Technetium-99 bone scans will demonstrate abnormalities early during the course of illness. MRI studies can help distinguish between discitis and vertebral osteomyelitis.

Treatment consists of 3 to 6 weeks of antistaphylococcal antibiotics, with variable amounts of immobilization and bracing to control symptoms. Persistent or atypical cases may require biopsy to identify the etiology, but this is unusual.

Early SD, Kay RM, Tolo VT: Childhood diskitis, *J Am Acad Orthop Surg* 11:413–420, 2003.

95. What is the most important variable that influences mortality in necrotizing fasciitis?

Time to surgical debridement. *Necrotizing fasciitis* is a relatively uncommon deep soft-tissue infection that can rapidly cause necrosis of fascial planes and surrounding tissue. The infection most commonly follows trauma, but even minor insults (e.g., scrape, insect bite) can be implicated. High clinical suspicion is key to early diagnosis. Pain out of proportion to clinical findings is an important clue to the diagnosis. Aggressive and early surgical debridement, coupled with antibiotic therapy, constitute the primary treatment for this disease, which has been called "flesh-eating bacteria syndrome" in the popular media.

Bellaplanta JM, Ljungquist K, Tobin E, et al: Necrotizing fasciitis, *J Am Acad Orthop Surg* 17:174–182, 2009.

96. What is the role of bone scintigraphy in children with obscure skeletal pain?

In the child with vague symptoms who is not clearly localizing to a specific anatomic location, a bone scan can help localize an abnormality in the bones, joints, or soft tissues. Once localized, the region can be further evaluated with three-dimensional imaging, if indicated, such as MRI or CT scan. Bone scans are very sensitive but not very specific. So, a negative bone scan makes the likelihood of a serious problem such as infection or tumor unlikely, which can be comforting to the physician and family. A bone scan should be considered only after a careful history and physical examination have been performed and plain x-rays of the abnormal area are obtained. The scan is most useful for ruling out an occult infection or bone tumor.

97. What are the phases of a bone scan?

There are three phases in a bone scan defined by the time elapsed since injection of the radionuclide dye.
- **Phase I**—Angiographic phase: During the first few seconds, the dye passes through the large blood vessels and provides early assessment of regional vascularity and perfusion.
- **Phase II**—Blood pool phase: Usually obtained during the first minutes after an injection, this phase highlights the movement of the dye into the extracellular spaces of soft tissue and bone.
- **Phase III**—Delayed phase: By 1.5 to 3 hours after injection, the dye localizes in the bone with minimal soft-tissue imaging.

The three-phase process is used to differentiate soft tissue from bony abnormalities. At times, a Phase IV study may be done by rescanning for the same dye at 24 hours, which further minimizes soft-tissue background activity.

KNEE, TIBIA, AND ANKLE DISORDERS

98. What is the difference between valgus and varus deformities?

Some things seem to be destined to be learned, forgotten, and relearned many times as a rite of passage: the Krebs cycle is one; this is another. The terms refer to angular deformities of the musculoskeletal system. If the distal part of the deformity points toward the midline, the term is *varus*. If the distal part points away from the midline, it is *valgus*. For example, in patients with knock knees, the lower portion of the deformity points away, so the term is genu valgum.

Another method is to consider the body in the supine (anatomic) position. Draw a circle around the body. All angles conforming to the curve of the circle are *varus*; all angles going against the circle are *valgus*. Bowleggedness conforms to the circle around the body and is, therefore, genu varum.

99. **Are children normally knock-kneed or bowlegged?**
The answer is *yes*. Both can be normal depending on the age of the child. Most children at birth are bowlegged (genu varum) up to 20 degrees, but this tendency progressively diminishes until about 24 months, when the trend toward knock knees (genu valgum) begins. Knock knees are most noticeable at around the age of 3 years (up to 15 degrees) and then begin to diminish. By 8 years of age, most children are—and will remain—in neutral alignment, meaning that with their knees extended their knees and ankles both touch (Fig. 15-12).

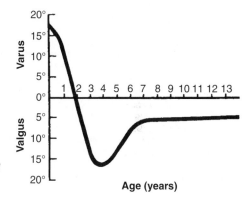

Figure 15-12. Development of the tibiofemoral angle during growth. *(From Bruce RW, Jr: Torsional and angular deformities,* Pediatr Clin North Am *43:875, 1996.)*

100. **Which bowlegged infants or toddlers require evaluation?**
Radiographs should be considered if bowleggedness demonstrates any of the following features:
- Present after 24 months (the age when most children start to develop physiologic genu valgum)
- Progressive varus develops after age 1 as the infant begins to bear weight and walk
- Unilateral deformity
- Visually >20 degrees of varus angulation across the knee

It's important to remember that clinical or radiographic evaluation of alignment in the legs requires the knees to be pointed straight ahead. If the knees are pointed in or out, flexion at the knee can be easily mistaken for bowing of the legs.

101. **What are the causes of pathologic genu varum (bowleggedness) or genu valgus (knock knees)?**
Genu varum
- Physiologic bow legs
- Infantile tibia vara
- Hypophosphatemic rickets
- Metaphyseal chondrodysplasia
- Focal fibrocartilaginous dysplasia

Genu valgum
- Hypophosphatemic rickets
- Previous metaphyseal fracture of the proximal tibia (Cozen fracture)
- Multiple epiphyseal dysplasia
- Pseudoachondroplasia

Sass P, Hassan G: Lower extremity abnormalities in children, *Am Fam Physician* 68:461–468, 2003.

102. **Which children are more likely to develop Blount disease?**
Tibia vara, or Blount disease, is a medial angulation of the tibia in the proximal metaphyseal region as a result of a growth disturbance in the medial aspect of the proximal tibial epiphysis. In the

infantile type, the child is usually an obese early walker, and he or she develops pronounced bowlegs during the first year of life. Black females are particularly at risk for severe deformity. In the adolescent variety, the onset occurs during late childhood or early adolescence, and the deformity is usually unilateral and milder. While bracing may be effective in some infantile cases diagnosed in the first 2 years of life, correction of severe deformity usually requires surgical intervention.

103. **How does tibial torsion change with age?**
Tibial torsion, the most common cause of in-toeing in children between the ages of 1 and 3 years, gradually rotates externally with age. For excessive internal rotation, bracing was used extensively in the past, but its efficacy is questionable because the natural history of the condition is self-resolution. Measurement is done by measuring the angle made by the long axis of the foot and the thigh when the knee is flexed 90 degrees.

104. **How effective is the Denis Browne splint for the treatment of tibial torsion?**
Not at all. The splint consists of a metal bar connected to shoes and holds the feet in varying degrees of external rotation. The splint was used frequently in the past for children with internal tibial torsion. However, there is absolutely no scientific evidence that this device alters the natural history of tibial torsion, and the use of this device for treatment of tibial torsion by pediatric orthopedics has essentially disappeared.

105. **Why are ligamentous injuries less common in children?**
In children, ligaments tend to be stronger than the cartilaginous growth plates, and thus the growth plate will often fail (i.e., fracture) before the ligament tears.

106. **How are ankle sprains graded?**
Between 80% and 90% of ankle sprains are the result of excessive inversion and/or plantar-flexion resulting in injury to the lateral ligaments (anterior talofibular and calcaneofibular). A **grade 1 ankle sprain** is a mild, partial tear of the ankle ligament and results in no instability. A **grade 2 sprain** is a high grade partial tear. Clinically differentiating between a grade 1 and 2 can be challenging. A **grade 3 sprain** is a complete tear of the ligament. This will result in some instability of the ankle, which can be detected with the ankle drawer test. This test is performed by immobilizing the lower tibia with one hand as the other hand grasps the heel and pulls the foot forward. There is always some motion (test the unaffected side to get an idea of what is normal for that patient) but with a complete tear, there is marked laxity with a poor endpoint.

107. **Which ankle sprains should be evaluated with an x-ray?**
More than 5,000,000 radiographs are estimated to be taken annually in children and adults for ankle injuries. Various guidelines have been proposed including the Low Risk Ankle Rules (LRAR) and the Ottawa Ankle Rules. The LRAR advises that x-rays are not necessary if a child has swelling and tenderness that is isolated to the distal fibula and/or adjacent lateral ligaments distal to the tibial anterior joint line. The Ottawa Rules advise obtaining an x-ray if there is malleolar pain and one or both of the following conditions is present: (1) the inability to bear weight for four steps immediately after the injury and during office or ED evaluation; and/or (2) bone tenderness at the posterior edge or tip of either malleolus. Use of these simple criteria can reduce unnecessary x-rays by 25% to 50% or more with low likelihood of missing a fracture.

Boutis K, Grootendorst P, Willan A, et al: Effect of the Low Risk Ankle Rule on the frequency of radiography in children with ankle injuries, *CMAJ* 185:E731–738, 2013.

108. **Should ankle sprains be casted?**
No. If inversion ankle sprains are not complicated by a fracture or peroneal tendon dislocation, casting is not warranted. Randomized trials have shown that casts have no benefit over early immobilization with functional removable braces, and in fact, complete immobilization may actually delay rehabilitation.

109. **What is the most significant mistake made during the evaluation of knee pain?**
Failure to evaluate the hip as a source of the pain. Hip pathology frequently masquerades as knee or distal thigh pain (e.g., Perthes' disease, slipped capital femoral epiphysis). More than one knee has undergone a diagnostic arthroscopy for hip pathology.

110. **In acute injury, what injuries typically cause bleeding into the knee joint?**
Acute hemarthrosis will occur when there is an injury to an *intra-articular* structure. Injuries outside the knee joint capsule cannot cause bleeding into the joint. Injuries commonly associated with a hemarthrosis include:
- Rupture of the anterior or posterior cruciate ligaments
- Peripheral meniscal tears
- Intra-articular fractures (such as avulsion of the tibial spine)
- Major disruption or tear in the joint capsule

111. **A 5-year-old boy with a painless swelling in the back of his knee has what likely condition?**
Popliteal cyst. Also called Baker cysts, these occur more frequently in boys, are usually found on the medial side of the popliteal fossa, and are painless. In children, the cysts are rarely associated with intra-articular pathology. The mass should transilluminate on physical exam, confirming the fluid-filled nature of the lesion. The natural history is for the cyst to disappear spontaneously after 6 to 24 months. Surgery is not required except in extraordinary circumstances such as unremitting pain. Atypical findings (e.g., tenderness, firmness, history of rapid enlargement, pain) are justification for further diagnostic evaluation.

Herman AM, Marzo JM: Popliteal cysts: a review, *orthopaedics* 37:e678–e684, 2014.

112. **How does patellofemoral stress syndrome occur?**
This major cause of chronic knee pain in teenagers results from **malalignment of the extensor mechanism of the knee**. It is most commonly seen as an "overuse" entity in sports that involve running and full-knee flexion (e.g., track, soccer). It has been inappropriately called *chondromalacia patella*, which is a specific pathologic diagnosis of an abnormal articular surface that occurs in a minority of these patients. The patella serves as the fulcrum on which the quadriceps extends the knee. The multiple muscle bellies of the quadriceps may act asymmetrically causing greater stress on the lateral aspect of the patella. This is particularly a problem for individuals with problems placing them at risk for patellar symptoms including: femoral anteversion, external tibial torsion, high (alta) patella, abnormally developed quadriceps, excessive flattening of the trochlear groove, or an increased Q angle. Treatment consists of ice, rest, nonsteroidal anti-inflammatory drugs, quadriceps strengthening, hamstring stretching, and possibly patellar-stabilizing braces.

113. **What is the Q angle?**
This angle describes the lines of force acting on the patella. The angle is formed by the intersection of a line drawn from the anterior-superior iliac spine to the patella, and a line from the patella to the tibial tubercle. For teenage males, the average Q angle is 14 degrees, and, for females, it is 17 degrees. Angles of >20 degrees create a bowstringing effect, which places a lateral stress on the patella and predisposes individuals (particularly runners) to chronic knee pain.

SPINAL DISORDERS

KEY POINTS: SCOLIOSIS

1. Scoliosis of >10 degrees is relatively common (1% to 2%), but progression to ≥25 degrees and the need for treatment is rare.
2. Bracing does not permanently correct scoliosis, but it can prevent progression.
3. Establishing the maturity level of the skeleton is important because the risk of progression is increased with immaturity.
4. In adolescents, progressive curves are seven times more likely to appear in girls than in boys.
5. All scoliosis is not idiopathic: assess for limb-length discrepancy, congenital anomalies, and neurologic abnormalities, especially reflexes.

114. **What are the different forms scoliosis?**
Scoliosis is a lateral curvature of the spine (i.e., coronal plane deformity) that has several general causes. The most common form is **idiopathic scoliosis** that arises in otherwise

normal children for reasons that are not fully understood, but there is an underlying genetic cause. Idiopathic scoliosis is subdivided according to age at which the disease is diagnosed. Previously, three age groups were considered, but most now split idiopathic scoliosis into two groups: early-onset ($<$9 years) and adolescent ($\geq$10 years). **Congenital scoliosis** occurs when there is a problem with the way the vertebrae form during embryogenesis. This form of scoliosis may be associated with anomalies of the cardiac and renal systems, which are developing at the same time. **Neurogenic scoliosis** is associated with a variety of spastic and paralytic neuromuscular diseases such as cerebral palsy, muscular dystrophy, and myelomeningocele. Finally there are **miscellaneous**, typically syndromic, causes of scoliosis that can be associated with connective tissue disorders like Marfan and Ehlers-Danlos syndromes. Scoliosis is also seen in increased rates in children who underwent major abdominal or thoracic surgery in infancy (such as open heart surgery or congenital diaphragmatic hernia repair). Scoliosis has been reported after ligation of a patent ductus arteriosus.

Konieczny MR, Senyurt H, Krauspe R: Epidemiology of adolescent idiopathic scoliosis, *J Child Orthop* 7:3–9, 2013.
National Scoliosis Foundation: www.scoliosis.org. Accessed on Nov. 24, 2014.

115. **Is scoliosis more common in boys or girls?**
    It depends on the age and the cause of the scoliosis. For idiopathic scoliosis seen in infancy, males outnumber females by a 3:2 margin. As age increases, females catch up and by adolescence, females are five to seven times more likely than males to have scoliosis.

Weinstein SL, Dolan LA, Wright JG, et al: Effects of bracing in adolescents with idiopathic scoliosis, *N Engl J Med* 369:1512–1521, 2013.

116. **How likely is the progression of scoliosis?**
    Idiopathic scoliosis, characterized by a lateral curvature of the spine with a Cobb angle (see question 120) of 10 degrees or more is believed to occur in about 3% of children younger than 16 years of age. Only 0.3% to 0.5% will have progression of curves that will require treatment.

117. **What are the risk factors for progression of idiopathic scoliosis?**
    Idiopathic scoliosis is a growth phenomenon, and the rate of progression of the curve is proportional to the rate of growth. This is why many curves become clinically apparent in adolescence just after the growth spurt. Therefore, the risk of progression is greater in younger children (who have more growth remaining) and the larger the curve, the more likely it is to progress. Most other risk factors for progression are a surrogate for growth remaining such as skeletal age and menarchal status.

Hresko MT: Idiopathic scoliosis in adolescents, *N Engl J Med* 368:834–841, 2013.

118. **How is screening for spinal deformity performed?**
    The child should be undressed or dressed only in underwear with a gown open at the back. The child is asked to bend forward while standing and the contour of the back is examined from behind and the side. This exam is then repeated with the child sitting. The following signs can suggest scoliosis:
    • Shoulder or scapular asymmetry
    • Asymmetry of paraspinal muscles or rib cage (the so-called rib hump) in the thoracic spine noted on forward bending ($>$0.5 cm in lumbar region and $>$1.0 cm in thoracic region; a scoliometer may be used for this determination)
    • Sagittal plane deformity such as increased kyphosis when viewed from the side
    • Waist-crease asymmetry that does not disappear when sitting (many waist-crease asymmetries are the result of leg-length discrepancies). This finding is very helpful in obese patients whose paraspinal prominence may be obscured by their subcutaneous adipose tissue.

119. **What constitutes an abnormal scoliometer measurement?**
    The *scoliometer* (also called an inclinometer) is a type of protractor used to measure the vertebral rotation and rib prominence that is seen in scoliosis with the forward-bending test (Fig. 15-13). An angle of $\leq$5 degrees is usually insignificant while an angle of $\geq$7 degrees warrants

orthopedic referral and consideration of standing posteroanterior and lateral radiographs for more precise assessment of curvature. This is different from the measurement of the scoliosis made on radiographs, which is known as the Cobb angle. Although it can vary dramatically, the Cobb angle is often about three times as large as the scoliometer measure. Usually orthopedists discuss the Cobb angle when describing scoliosis, and it is the Cobb angle that typically dictates treatment.

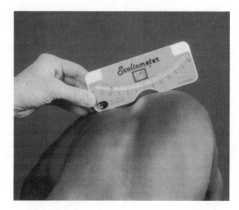

Figure 15-13. Use of scoliometer demonstrating 20 degrees of trunk rotation. *(From Dormans JP:* Pediatric Orthopaedics and Sports Medicine: The Requisites in Pediatrics. *Philadelphia, 2004, Elsevier Mosby, p 150.)*

120. **How is scoliosis measured by the Cobb method?**
 This is the standard technique used to quantify scoliosis in posteroanterior radiographs. One line is drawn along the vertebra tilted the most at the top of the curve, and another is drawn at the bottom of the curve. The curvature is represented by angle "a," which can be measured in two ways, as illustrated in Figure 15-14.

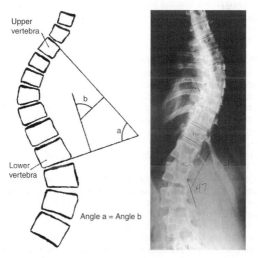

Figure 15-14. Measurement of the Cobb angle. *(From Kaz DS, Math KR, Groskin SA, editors:* Radiology Secrets. *Philadelphia, 1998, Hanley & Belfus, p 321.)*

121. **How valuable are school-based screening programs for scoliosis?**
    This is controversial. Many states in the United States mandate school scoliosis screening. Experts in favor of these programs contend that reliable screening procedures exist and that early identification will lead to earlier nonoperative care and the prevention of progression and of the need for surgical intervention. Opponents argue that the low incidence of children requiring treatment, the low positive-predictive value of screening programs, and high numbers of children unnecessarily referred do not justify the programs.

Burton MS: Diagnosis and treatment of adolescent idiopathic scoliosis, *Pediatr Ann* 42: 224–228, 2013.
Richards BS, Vitale MG: Screening for idiopathic scoliosis in adolescents, *J Bone Joint Surg Am,* 90:195–198, 2008.

122. **What is the natural history of untreated severe idiopathic scoliosis?**
    Untreated idiopathic scoliosis that is greater than 50 degrees at skeletal maturity is likely to continue to progress throughout life. The rate of progression tends to be slow, on the order of 1 degree per year, but over the expected lifetime of the patient that could be 60 or more degrees of progression. However, even with this progression, adolescent idiopathic scoliosis (AIS) is generally not a fatal disease and there is little excess mortality seen in the few long-term natural history studies. Only when curves are greater than 90 to 100 degrees is there a clinically important effect on cardiopulmonary function. Some studies have shown psychosocial problems related to the patient's dissatisfaction with their appearance, but not all studies have reproduced this finding. Back pain may be increased in this population compared with age-matched norms, but there is no indication that surgery improves upon this.

Weinstein SL, Dolan LA, Spratt KF, et al: Health and function of patients with untreated idiopathic scoliosis: a 50-year natural history study, *JAMA* 289: 559–67, 2003.

123. **When should surgery be considered for idiopathic scoliosis?**
    As seen in the natural history, idiopathic scoliosis continues to progress throughout life once **larger than 50 degrees**, so this is usually the criterion for surgery in AIS.

124. **What type of surgery is typically performed for scoliosis correction?**
    The surgery is usually a **fusion procedure** in which the vertebrae involved in the curve are instrumented with metal implants and connected to a rod to correct the curve, to balance the spine and to stabilize the bones to allow them to fuse together. Clearly, this eliminates motion and prevents growth in the operated segment of the spine. Most children with AIS are undergoing surgery in adolescence and as such do not have a lot of growth remaining. The height gained by straightening the spine typically offsets any potential loss of growth from fusing those vertebrae.

125. **Are the spines of young children fused as well?**
    Not anymore. Scoliosis in toddlers and young children is one of the most difficult problems seen in pediatric orthopedics. Originally, these curves were corrected and fused with the theory being that a short straight spine is better than a longer crooked one. However, long-term follow-up found that fusing spines before the age of 8 or 9 resulted in small thoraxes and limited lung development. The result was that many patients were dying from respiratory insufficiency in early adulthood because their lungs were unable to keep up with the needs of their adult bodies.

126. **So how are large curves in young children treated?**
    This is a challenging question with no good answer. Currently there are several options available—casting, bracing, or growing implants. We know that fusing small spines is a bad idea, so implants that stabilize the spine while still allowing it to grow (sort of an internal brace) have been used with some success for a couple of decades. Current generation "growing rods" attach to the ribs, spine, and/or pelvis. These rods need to be lengthened periodically to compensate for the growth that is occurring in the spine and to maintain the correction of the scoliosis. In the United States, these rods until very recently have required multiple surgeries to be lengthened with high complication rates. However, some patients are candidates for a rod that can be lengthened in the office using a magnetically controlled gearing mechanism. This device, available

in Europe for several years but only since 2014 in the US, is not indicated for all patients, but has the promise to greatly reduce the number of surgeries for many patients.

Hickey BA, Towriss C, Baxter G, et al: Early experience of MAGEC magnetic growing rods in the treatment of early onset scoliosis, *Eur Spine J* 23S:S61–S65, 2014.
Akbarnia BA, Blakemore LC, Campbell RM Jr, et al: Approaches for the very young child with spinal deformity: what's new and what works, *Instr Course Lect*, 59:407–424, 2010.

127. Are casts still used to treat scoliosis?

The first fusion procedure for scoliosis was performed about 100 years ago, and for decades casts were used to stabilize the spine for months until the fusion could take hold. The advent of metal implants obviated the need for casts, but casting has become popular again as a treatment for scoliosis *in the very young*. A derotational casting technique has proven quite effective for many patients and can even be curative in some cases. While no open surgery is involved, the casts do require traction under anesthesia, and thus they are performed in the operating room.

Sanders JO, D'Astous J, Fitzgerald M, et al: Derotational casting for progressive infantile scoliosis, *J Pediatr Orthop* 29:581–587, 2009.

128. Is bracing an effective treatment for scoliosis?

There has long been a history of bracing in the orthopedic literature, and the results of studies have been somewhat mixed. Furthermore, the quality of many of these studies has been low and many orthopedists were unsure if bracing was an effective treatment. However, a 2013 multi-center study funded by the NIH found dramatic improvements in children who were braced compared with unbraced controls. Patients in the study were 10 to 15 years of age, required Cobb angles between 20 and 40 degrees, and wore the brace for at least 18 hours daily with reassessment by x-rays every 6 months. This BrAIST (Bracing in Adolescent Idiopathic Scoliosis Trial) study is the first to prove the effectiveness of bracing in premenarchal adolescent girls.

Weinstein SL, Dolan LA, Wright JG, et al: Effects of bracing in adolescents with idiopathic scoliosis, *N Engl J Med* 369:1512–1521, 2013.

129. What diagnosis should you consider in a teenage male with very poor posture that is not flexible?

Scheuermann kyphosis. This is a wedge-shaped deformity of the vertebral bodies of unclear etiology that causes juvenile kyphosis (abnormally large dorsal thoracic or lumber curves). Common in teenagers, it is distinguished from simple poor posture ("postural round-back deformity") by its sharp angulation and inability to correct by having the patient stand up straight or lie on top of a bolster. X-ray studies reveal anterior vertebral body wedging and irregular erosions of the vertebral endplate. Treatment consists of exercise; bracing; and rarely, surgical correction (for severe, painful deformities).

130. What is the difference between spondylolysis and spondylolisthesis?

Spondylolysis is a condition in which there is a defect in the pars interarticularis (vertebral arch) of a vertebra that is most common at L5. This can be a congenital problem but is commonly seen as a stress fracture in athletes who do a lot of hyperextension of the lower back (classically gymnasts and football offensive linemen). *Spondylolisthesis* is a condition (often resulting from spondylolysis) that is characterized by forward slippage of one vertebra on the lower vertebrae. Pain is the most common presenting symptom for both conditions. The etiology is unclear, but various theories relate it to hereditary factors, congenital predisposition, trauma, posture, growth, and biomechanical factors. Treatment includes watchful waiting, limitation of activity, exercise therapy, bracing, casting, and surgery, depending on the patient's age, the magnitude of the slippage, the extent of pain, and the predicted likelihood of progression of the deformity.

Foreman P, Griessenauer CJ, Watanabe K, et al: L5 spondylolysis/spondylolisthesis: a comprehensive review with an anatomic focus, *Childs Nerv Syst* 29:209–216, 2013.

SPORTS MEDICINE

131. A 12-year-old baseball player presents complaining of elbow pain. What diagnosis do you need to consider?

    Little league elbow, an apophysitis of the medial epicondyle of the elbow, is a tension injury to the growth plate seen in pitchers' (and other throwers') elbows. Treatment includes rest and avoiding all throwing activities for a minimum of 4 to 6 weeks, followed by gradual resumption of throwing under the close guidance of a therapist and/or coach.

132. Which is worse for a baseball pitcher's elbow: throwing curveballs or fastballs?

    Conventional wisdom has held that curveballs are more stressful on the thrower's elbow than fastballs. There are recommendations that curveballs not be thrown until an athlete is approaching skeletal maturity, which is around 14 years of age. However, recent research has found that the amount of mechanical stress on an elbow is not different when throwing a curveball or fastball. There may be other reasons to limit or delay throwing curveballs in younger athletes, but increased stress at the elbow does not seem to be one of them.

Nissen CW, Westwell M, Ounpuu S, et al: A biomechanical comparison of the fastball and curveball in adolescent baseball pitchers, *Am J Sports Med* 37:1492–1498, 2009.

133. How can elbow and shoulder injuries be prevented in pitchers?

    The use of **pitch counts** to protect the arms of throwers at all levels of baseball from little league to the majors has come into the spotlight in recent years. There is evidence showing that pitch count is more important than the type of pitch thrown in protecting the elbow. Little league baseball has standardized the number of pitches allowed and the amount of rest mandated between pitching days.

Tjoumakaris FP, Pepe MD, Bernstein J: Eminence-based medicine versus evidence-based medicine: it's okay for 12-year-old pitchers to throw curveballs; it's the pitch count that matters, *Phys Sportsmed* 40:83–86, 2012.

134. Do meniscal tears occur in younger children?

    Meniscal tears rarely occur before the age of 12 years. An exception is a patient with a discoid meniscus, which is a congenitally abnormal meniscus shaped like a hockey puck instead of the normal "C" appearance. Because there is meniscus in the weight-bearing portion of the knee (and the meniscus is not designed for this), all eventually tear and become symptomatic. Meniscal tears in children not associated with a discoid meniscus are typically associated with significant injuries. Be sure to look for an associated injury to the anterior cruciate ligament.

135. If a ninth-grade soccer player with knee swelling "felt a pop" while scoring a goal, what are three possible diagnoses?

    A pop or snap sensation in the setting of acute knee injury is usually associated with the following:
    - **Anterior cruciate ligament injury**
    - **Meniscal injury**
    - **Patellar subluxation**

136. How is meniscal integrity assessed on examination?

    Apley compression and **McMurray test**. The Apley test involves compression with pain in the knee suggesting injury. The McMurray test assesses lateral and medial tears by applying valgus stress/internal rotation and varus stress/external rotation, respectively, while feeling for pops/clicks and tenderness over the joint line, which, if present, could indicate injury (Fig. 15-15).

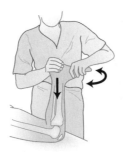

Apley compression test

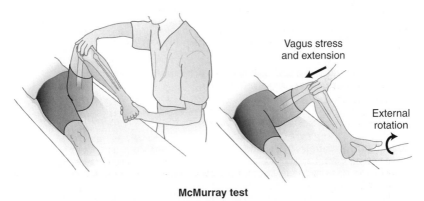

Vagus stress
and extension

External
rotation

McMurray test

Figure 15-15. *Apley compression test* is performed with the patient prone and the examiner's knee over the patient's posterior thigh. The tibia is externally rotated while a downward compressive force is applied over the tibia. The *McMurray test* is performed with the patient supine and the examiner standing on the side of the affected knee. *(From Kleigman RM, Stanton BF, Schor NF, et al:* Nelson Textbook of Pediatrics, *ed 19. Philadelphia, 2011, Elsevier Saunders, p 2415.)*

137. **What is the typical mechanism for an anterior cruciate ligament (ACL) tear?**
The ACL sits in the knee joint and prevents the tibia from subluxing anteriorly out from under the femur. This ligament is under stress when weight is applied to a slightly flexed knee. When rotation and a valgus stress (a force pushing the knee toward the midline) are applied to the knee at the same time, the ligament is most susceptible to tearing. This combination of forces typically occurs when an athlete lands on the leg and tries to change direction.

138. **How is ACL stability tested on examination?**
Anterior drawer test and **Lachman test**. Both assess any possible abnormal forward movement of the tibia with the thigh/femur and foot stabilized. Excessive movement, compared with the opposite knee, suggests ACL injury (Fig. 15-16).

139. **Why are girls and young women more susceptible to ACL tears than their male counterparts?**
Rates of ACL tears in females are 3 to 8 times higher than in males. Suspected reasons include: (1) **anatomic factors**, such as a narrower intercondylar notch in the knee and a wider pelvis than males; (2) **biochemical factors**, such as increased estrogen, which makes ligaments more elastic; and (3) **neuromuscular factors** in the way women activate muscles during jumping and landing. Researchers from Oregon have described additional risk factors that include chronic fatigue (three

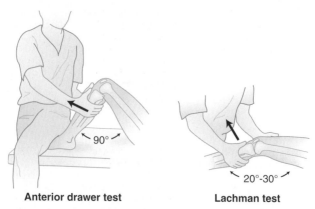

Anterior drawer test   **Lachman test**

Figure 15-16. *Anterior drawer test* is performed with the patient supine and the knee in 90 degrees of flexion. The *Lachman test* is conducted with the patient supine and the knee flexed 20 to 30 degrees. *(From Kleigman RM, Stanton BF, Schor NF, et al: Nelson Textbook of Pediatrics, ed 19. Philadelphia, 2011, Elsevier Saunders, p 2415.)*

times more likely in high school girls than boys) and dietary problems that range from poor nutritional intake to frank eating disorders.

Elliot DL, Goldberg L, Kuehl KS, et al: Young women's anterior cruciate ligament injuries: an expanded model and prevention paradigm, *Sports Med* 40:367–376, 2010.

140. Are ACL tears treated differently in children, adolescents, and adults?
A resounding **yes**. Traditional ACL reconstruction procedures involve drilling a large tunnel across where the physis would be in the proximal tibia and distal femur. In children with open physes, the concern for growth arrest is great. Current recommendations are generally for using a *physeal-sparing* technique in prepubescent children, which is not as stable as traditional techniques and technically more difficult to perform. For younger adolescents, a *transphyseal* reconstruction is permitted, but the graft is entirely soft tissue and the sutures or screws used to stabilize the graft are placed far from the growth plate. In older adolescents, a standard trans-physeal technique is used, although no bone is placed across the growth plate (a technique sometimes used in adults).

Vavken P, Murray MM: Treating anterior cruciate ligament tears in skeletally immature patients, *Arthroscopy* 27:704–716, 2011.
Finlayson CJ, Nasreddine A, Kocher MS: Current concepts of diagnosis and management of ACL injuries in skeletally immature athletes, *Phys Sportsmed* 38:90–101, 2010.

141. Are there ways to prevent ACL tears?
Most ACL tears are a result of noncontact plays (e.g., landing a jump or making a cut on the field, rather than being tackled or hit). The number of prevention programs has exploded across the country in recent years, typically involving neuromuscular exercises to retrain athletes regarding the best way to jump, land, and cut. These studies have often been very successful. A recent meta-analysis showed that on average these programs reduced ACL tears 50% in women and up to 80% in men.

Sadoghi P, von Keudell A, Vavken P: Effectiveness of anterior cruciate ligament injury prevention training programs, *J Bone Joint Surg Am* 94:769–776, 2012.

142. A teenager has chronic knee pain, swelling, and occasional "locking" of the knee joint, and his x-ray reveals increased density and fragmentation at the weight-bearing surface of the medial femoral condyle. What condition does he likely have?
Osteochondritis dissecans. In this disease, there is focal necrosis of a region of subchondral bone, typically in the lateral half of the medial femoral condyle. The cause is unknown, but

antecedent trauma is common and children (usually boys) with this condition are typically very active. These cases present with activity-related pain; locking, buckling, and stiffness may be seen as well. A plain radiograph can reveal the diagnosis, but an MRI is more sensitive when the clinical suspicion is high and radiographic findings are equivocal. Extended immobilization and activity restriction is the primary treatment in skeletally immature patients who have a favorable natural history. The lesions typically heal without surgery. For older adolescents and skeletally mature individuals, surgery is frequently required to stabilize the lesion and encourage healing. If the fragment does not heal, it may detach and become a loose body. This is a major problem because the lost articular cartilage cannot be replaced and the risk for arthritis is high.

143. **What is the most likely diagnosis if a 12-year-old basketball player has painful swelling below both knees?**
Osgood-Schlatter disease. This is a traction apophysitis and results from repetitive stress (pull of the patellar tendon) on the tibial tubercle, which is connected to the tibial shaft through a cartilaginous plate. The cartilage is unable to handle the tensile forces created by the quadriceps muscle, and it hypertrophies and becomes inflamed. This process often occurs around the time of the adolescent growth spurt and is related to the level of physical activity. Physical examination reveals tenderness to palpation and a very prominent tibial tubercle. The pain is exacerbated with resisted knee extension.

Appropriate clinical management includes the judicious use of anti-inflammatory medications, restricted activities, quadriceps stretching and strengthening, and cross training. The condition is usually self-limited and resolves with skeletal maturity, although the bump remains. Immobilization, which may lead to diffuse atrophy, is rarely necessary.

144. **What is the likely diagnosis in a fifth-grade football player with heel pain and a positive "squeeze test"?**
Sever disease, or apophysitis of the calcaneus. Caused by traction on the calcaneus at the insertion sites of the gastrocnemius-soleus muscles, microavulsions occur where bone meets cartilage. Pain is reproduced with compression of the medial and lateral aspects of the heel (the "squeeze test"). Treatment involves Achilles stretching, viscoelastic heel cups, and nonsteroidal anti-inflammatory drugs. Failure to improve suggests a possible calcaneal stress fracture, and immobilization may be required.

Soprano JV, Fuchs SM: Common overuse injuries in the pediatric and adolescent athlete, *Clin Pediatr Emerg Med* 8, 8–11, 2007.

145. **Which sports injuries are the most common in school-age children and adolescents?**
Some 75% of injuries in school-age children involve the lower extremities, and a majority of injuries to the knee and ankle are reinjuries as a result of incomplete healing from a previous problem. Contusions and sprains are the most common types of injury, with fractures and dislocations accounting for an additional 10% to 20%. Cranial injuries are the most common cause of sports fatality.

Adolescent boys who participate in contact team sports, particularly football and wrestling, are at the highest risk for injuries. Among girls, softball and gymnastics have the highest injury rate.

Only 10% of sports injuries are caused by an opponent; most injuries are caused by stumbling, falling, or misstepping. The latter finding suggests that improving intrinsic factors (e.g., raising the level of physical fitness, avoiding overuse, and strengthening joint stability) may be more important for the prevention of injuries than external factors (e.g., rule changes, equipment).

146. **What are the definitions of concussion and postconcussion syndrome?**
In 2004, the Second International Conference on Concussion in Sports defined a sports **concussion** as a complex physiological process following head trauma resulting in rapid onset of short-lived functional impairment, though in some cases associated with prolonged post-concussive symptoms, and typically associated with a normal CT scan. **Postconcussion syndrome** has been defined as the persistence beyond 7 to 10 days of the injury of any one of the following symptoms not present before injury: headaches, easy fatigability, sleep disturbances, dizziness, irritability, aggressiveness,

anxiety, depression, missed work, relationship troubles, personality change, trouble with simple math, and trouble with short-term memory.

Eisenberg MA, Meehan WP III, Mannix R: Duration and course of post-concussive symptoms, *Pediatrics* 133:999–1006, 2014.
ME, Walter KD, and the Council on Sports Medicine and Fitness: Clinical report—sport-related concussion in children and adolescents, *Pediatrics* 126:597–615, 2010.

147. **What is the value of "brain rest" in the treatment of concussion?**
Cognitive rest was proposed in 2004 based on the theory that activities that require concentration and attention may exacerbate the symptoms of concussion and thus delay recovery. Reduction of activities such as reading, text messaging, video game playing, computer use, and performing schoolwork has been urged by some as vital in concussion management. The underlying theory is that concussion results in a cerebral metabolic disruption with a decreased supply of adenosine triphosphate (ATP). Instituting cognitive rest conserves ATP supplies for injury recovery. Although the cognitive rest concept has been subject to debate, an increasing number of studies support its role as a tool in the management of concussions.

Brown NJ, Mannix RC, O'Brien MJ, et al: Effect of cognitive activity level on duration of post-concussion symptoms, *Pediatrics* 133:e299–e304, 2014.
Halstead ME, McAvoy K, Devore CD, et al: Returning to learning following a concussion, *Pediatrics* 132: 948–957, 2013.

148. **When should an athlete who has suffered a concussion be allowed to return to play?**
No athlete should be allowed to return to the playing field on the day of the concussion nor thereafter if they are symptomatic at rest or with exertion. Although most overt symptoms will resolve within 1 week, younger athletes may require a longer recovery period for full cognitive function. Thus, a more conservative approach is used for pediatric and adolescent patients compared with adults. *Graded return-to-play protocols* with escalating exercises are recommended with a system in place to monitor symptoms and cognitive function. Postinjury neuropsychological testing (such as ImPACT testing) is often used as a guide to return, especially if preinjury testing is available for comparison.

Heads Up to Clinicians: Concussion Training: www.cdc.gov/concussion/headsup/return_to_play.html. Accessed on Nov. 24, 2014.

Acknowledgments

The editors gratefully acknowledge contributions by Drs. Francis Y. Lee, John P. Dormans, Richard S. Davidson, Mark Magnusson, David P. Roye, and Joshua E. Hyman that were retained from the first four editions of Pediatric Secrets.

PULMONOLOGY

Robert W. Wilmott, MD and Bradley A. Becker, MD

CHAPTER 16

ALLERGIC RHINITIS

1. How common is allergic rhinitis?
   Very common. Up to 40% of children experience rhinitis, which is the most common manifestation of allergic disease and one of the most common chronic diseases of childhood.

2. In addition to chronic or recurrent nasal congestion, what features on history and physical examination suggest allergic rhinitis?
   - "Allergic facies": Open mouth, midface hypoplasia
   - "Allergic nasal crease": Nasal crease on bridge of nose as a result of chronic upward rubbing with the palm of the hand (the allergic salute)
   - Diminished sense of taste and smell
   - Dental malocclusion
   - Allergic "shiners" (dark circles under the eyes)
   - Multiple infraorbital folds
   - Cobblestoning of the posterior oropharynx (Fig. 16-1)
   - Pale, boggy appearance of the nasal mucosa

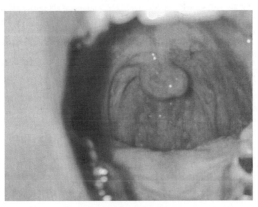

Figure 16-1. Cobblestone appearance of the posterior pharynx from postnasal drip. (From Terasaski G, Paauw DS: Evaluation and treatment of chronic cough, *Med Clin North Am* 98:391–403, 2014.)

3. What are three early-life risk factors for allergic rhinitis?
   1. Male gender (Females have a higher incidence of rhinitis in adulthood.)
   2. Not having early contact with siblings at home or children in daycare
   3. Not having early contact with pets or not living on a farm

Matheson MC, Dharmage SC, Abramson MJ, et al: Early-life risk factors and incidence of rhinitis: results from the European Community Respiratory Health Study—an international population-based cohort study, *J Allergy Clin Immunol* 128:816–823, 2011.

4. **How does the time of year help identify the potential cause of allergic rhinitis?**
Tree pollen is usually associated with the onset of the growing season. After local tree pollination, grass pollens appear; this may occur earlier in locales where there are short winters. Weed pollen other than ragweed, is associated with the late-summer pollen peak. In the autumn, ragweed is the major pollen allergen. It pollinates from mid-August until the first freeze in most of the U.S. Counts are especially high in eastern and central North America. Fungal aeroallergens span the growing season. Relative concentrations of household animal allergens, dust mites, and indoor fungi generally increase when doors and windows are closed. However, dust mites and molds proliferate in areas of high humidity and may cause perennial symptoms.

Naclerio R, Solomon W: Rhinitis and inhalant allergens, *JAMA* 278: 1842–1848, 1997.

5. **When are allergy blood tests used?**
   - A patient is taking a medication that blocks allergy skin testing, such as an antihistamine that cannot be stopped for at least 3 days.
   - A patient has a skin condition such as eczema or psoriasis without sufficient unaffected areas to do skin testing
   - Blood testing would be better tolerated, such as in an infant or young child.

American College of Allergy, Asthma and Immunology: www.acaai.org. Accessed on Jan. 13, 2015.

6. **What is an antigen-specific IgE ImmunoCAP?**
An IgE ImmunoCAP (Thermo-Fisher Scientific Inc., Uppsala, Sweden) is an *in vitro* automated laboratory method used to quantify the amount of allergen-specific IgE in a patient's serum. The test allergen is bound to a solid phase matrix and then incubated with the serum. If it contains the allergen-specific IgE, the patient's IgE will bind to the ImmunoCAP antigen. Nonspecific IgE is removed by washing. Fluorescent-labeled anti-IgE is then added and binds to the IgE-antigen complex. Fluorescence is measured and compared to a standard curve.

Johansson SG: ImmunoCAP specific IgE test: an objective tool for research and routine allergy diagnosis, *Expert Rev Mol Diagn* 4:273–279, 2004.

7. **Summarize the pros and cons of skin testing versus *in vitro* testing (e.g., IgE ImmunoCAP) for allergies**
   ***In vitro* tests**
   - No risk for anaphylaxis
   - Results not influenced by medications (e.g., antihistamines), dermatographism, or extensive dermatologic disease
   - More costly
   - Better predictive value for some common food allergens

   Skin testing
   - Less costly
   - More sensitive than *in vitro* tests
   - Results immediately available

8. **What are the recommended treatments for children with allergic rhinitis?**
   - **Environmental control** measures for allergen avoidance are the mainstay of treatment. Relevant allergens are recommended for exposure reduction on positive skin or serum-specific IgE testing correlated with the presence of symptoms on allergen exposure.
   - **Pharmacotherapy**, including nasal corticosteroid sprays, antihistamines (given orally or by nasal spray), oral antileukotrienes, or combinations of these medications are effective treatments.
   - **Immunotherapy** is reserved for those with persistent symptoms despite the above treatment and for those who want control of symptoms with less medications.

American Academy of Allergy, Asthma and Immunology: www.aaaai.org. Accessed on Jan. 13, 2015.

KEY POINTS: ALLERGIC RHINITIS

1. History (symptoms, family history, and worsening with environmental exposure) is the key to diagnosis.
2. With two atopic parents, the risk to the child is 50% to 70%.
3. Sensitivity of testing ranks as follows: intradermal (may yield false-positive results) > skin prick > IgE ImmunoCAP.
4. IgE ImmunoCAP testing is indicated in patients with severe skin disorders or those unable to temporarily discontinue H_1-blocking antihistamines.
5. Allergic features include Shiners (dark circles under eyes), increased infraorbital folds, transverse nasal bridge crease, boggy pale-blue nasal mucosa, and cobblestoning of conjunctiva and posterior oropharynx.
6. Immunotherapy should be considered when allergen avoidance and pharmacotherapy have produced suboptimal results.

9. **What are the major indoor (year-round) allergens?**
House dust mites, animal danders, cockroach, and **molds.**

10. **How can you decrease cat allergen in the home?**
   - Consider a "felinectomy."
   - Remove upholstered furniture, carpet, and other sources harboring the allergen.
   - Use high-efficiency particulate air (HEPA) air filters and vacuum cleaners.
   - Wash the cat weekly if feasible.

11. **Is there truly a dog breed that is "hypoallergenic"?**
Alas, the hypoallergenic dog appears to be a **myth**. Although certain dogs (e.g., poodles; Spanish waterdogs; Airedale terriers; and the newer hybrid, the Labradoodle) are commonly marketed as "hypoallergenic," comparison of the quantity of the dog allergen (Can f 1) in hair and coat samples and in the surrounding surface environment found no differences compared with control breeds. In the United States, about 78 million dogs occupy homes, so this is not good news to the 20% of the general population who may be allergic to dogs.

Vredegoor DW, Willemse T, Chapman MD, et al: Can f 1 levels in hair and homes of different dog breeds: lack of evidence to describe any dog breed as hypoallergenic, *J Allergy Clin Immunol* 130:904.e7–909.e7, 2012.

12. **Which children should be considered for immunotherapy?**
Allergen immunotherapy is an effective treatment for allergic rhinitis, asthma, and the prevention of venom anaphylaxis. It also may be of benefit in atopic dermatitis. For allergic rhinitis and allergic asthma, immunotherapy should be considered in patients who are not well-controlled despite attempts at allergen exposure reduction and pharmacotherapy or in patients who wish to take less medication. Subcutaneous or sublingual routes (for certain inhalant allergens) are approved in the United States. In children, immunotherapy has been shown to prevent the progression of allergic rhinitis to asthma and may prevent sensitization to new allergens in monosensitized individuals.

Jones SM, Burks W, Dupont C: State of the art on food allergen immunotherapy: oral, sublingual, and epicutaneous, *J Allerg Clin Immunol* 133:318–323, 2014.
Burks AW, Calderon MA, Casale T, et al: Update on allergy immunotherapy: American Academy of Allergy, Asthma & Immunology/European Academy of Allergy and Clinical Immunology/PRACTALL consensus report, *J Allergy Clin Immunol* 131:1288–1296, 2013.

13. **How common is exercise-induced bronchospasm in children with allergic rhinitis?**
Exercise is a trigger of bronchospasm in 40% to 50% of children with allergic rhinitis, compared with 90% of those diagnosed with asthma and 10% of those not known to have asthma or

respiratory allergies. *Exercised-induced bronchospasm* is defined as a 10% drop in FEV_1 or peak expiratory flow rate from the value before exercise.

Randolph C: Exercise-induced bronchospasm in children, *Clinic Rev Allerg Immunol* 34:205–216, 2008.

ASTHMA

14. **If both parents are asthmatic, what is the risk that their child will have asthma?**
    The risk is **60%**. For a child with only one parent with asthma, the risk is estimated to be about 20%. If neither parent has asthma, the risk is 6% to 7%.

15. **When does asthma usually have its onset of symptoms?**
    About 50% of childhood asthma develops before the age of 3 years, and nearly all has developed by the age of 7 years. The signs and symptoms of asthma, including chronic cough, may be evident much earlier than the actual diagnosis but may be erroneously attributed to recurrent pneumonia.

American Lung Association: www.lungusa.org. Accessed on Jan. 13, 2015.

16. **Which children with wheezing at an early age are likely to develop chronic asthma?**
    Although about one-third of children will have an episode of wheezing before they are 1 year old, most (80%) do not develop persistent wheezing after age 3 years. Risks factors for persistence include the following:
    - Positive family history of asthma (especially maternal)
    - Increased IgE levels
    - Atopic dermatitis
    - Rhinitis not associated with colds
    - Secondhand smoke exposure

Taussig LM, Wright AL, Holberg CJ, et al: Tuscon Children's Respiratory Study: 1980 to present, *J Allergy Clin Immunol* 111:661–675, 2003.

17. **What historical points are suggestive of an allergic basis for asthma?**
    - Seasonal nature with concurrent rhinitis (suggesting pollen)
    - Symptoms worsen when visiting a family with pets (suggesting animal dander)
    - Wheezing occurs when carpets are vacuumed or bed is made (suggesting mites)
    - Symptoms develop in damp basements or barns (suggesting molds)

18. **What are other potential triggers for asthma?**
    - Cold air
    - Emotional extremes (stress, fear, crying, laughing)
    - Environmental (pollutants, cigarette smoke)
    - Exercise
    - Foods, food additives
    - Gastroesophageal reflux disease
    - Hormonal (menstrual, premenstrual)
    - Irritants (strong odors, paint fumes, chlorine)
    - Medications (nonsteroidal anti-inflammatory drugs, aspirin, β-blockers)
    - Substance abuse
    - Upper airway infections (rhinitis, sinusitis)
    - Weather changes

American Academy of Allergy, Asthma and Immunology: www.aaaai.org. Accessed on Jan. 13, 2015.

19. **What distinguishes EIA from EIB?**
    Exercise-induced asthma (EIA) is a common component of those who have been diagnosed with asthma. Significant symptoms (e.g., cough, chest tightness, wheezing, dyspnea) are noted after

exercise in up to 90% of asthmatic children, although abnormal pulmonary function tests can be found in nearly 100% of these patients. *Exercise-induced bronchospasm (EIB)* now more commonly refers to those with airway narrowing in response to exercise who have not been diagnosed with asthma. Up to 12% of adolescent athletes and 40% of college varsity athletes may manifest EIB. Among atopic children, the incidence of EIB has been estimated to be as high as 40%.

Parsons JP, Kaeding C, Phillips G, et al: Prevalence of exercise-induced bronchospasm in a cohort of varsity college athletes, *Med Sci Sports Exerc* 39:1487, 2007.

20. **What is the time course of EIB?**
Symptoms, most commonly cough, peak 5 to 10 minutes after the conclusion of exercise and usually resolve within 30 to 60 minutes.

21. **How is EIB diagnosed?**
    - **Exercise challenge:** EIB is likely if the peak flow rate or FEV_1 drops by 15% after 6 minutes of vigorous exercise, either in a laboratory or field setting. This exercise can include jogging on a motor-driven treadmill (15% grade at 3 to 4 mph), riding a stationary bicycle, or running up and down a hallway or around a track in field testing. The greatest reduction in EIB is usually seen 5 to 10 minutes after exercise. As further verification of the diagnosis, if the patient has developed a decreased peak flow (and possibly wheezing), two puffs of a β_2-agonist should be administered to attempt to reverse the bronchospasm.
    - **Eucapnic voluntary hyperventilation (EVH)** involves breathing a dry gas at an increased respiratory rate in an effort to induce bronchospasm and a decrease of FEV_1 of $>10\%$.
    - **Osmotic challenge** is the inhalation of hypertonic saline or dry powder mannitol to induce bronchospasm.
    - **Pharmacologic challenge** is a direct measurement using agents that act on smooth muscle (e.g., histamine, methacholine). The threshold concentration required to induce bronchospasm is determined and compared with that required in healthy controls.

Cuff S, Loud K: Exercise-induced bronchospasm, *Contemp Pediatr* 25:88–95, 2008.

22. **A 15-year-old with repeated shortness of breath after track practice has suspected exercise-induced bronchospasm, but pulmonary function tests are normal, bronchoprovocation testing is negative, and he has no response to treatment with asthma medications. What is a likely alternative?**
Exercise-induced laryngeal obstruction (EILO). This group of diagnoses includes *vocal cord dysfunction* and *exercise-induced laryngomalacia.* In the former, during exercise, the vocal cords adduct during inspiration to cause shortness of breath, chest tightness, cough, or stridor. In the latter, there is inspiratory prolapse of supraglottic structures, which causes dyspnea and/or stridor. In both cases, there is paradoxic laryngeal motion—narrowing occurs when a bigger breath is taken. The precise reasons are unclear but may be related to smaller airway dimensions, inhibition of laryngeal reflexes, or impaired innervation and/or power of the laryngeal muscles. The gold standard test for diagnosis is flexible nasoendoscopy with continuous video recording of the larynx throughout exercise.

Tilles SA, Ayars AG, Picciano JF, et al: Exercise-induced vocal cord dysfunction and exercise-induced laryngomalacia in children and adolescents: the same clinical syndrome? *Ann Allergy Asthma Immunol* 111:342–346, 2013.
Nielsen EW, Hull JH, Backer V: High prevalence of exercise-induced laryngeal obstruction in athletes, *Med Sci Sports Exerc* 45:2030–2035, 2013.

23. **What mechanisms lead to airway obstruction during an acute asthma attack?**
The main causes of airflow obstruction in acute asthma are airway inflammation, including edema, bronchospasm, and increased mucous production. Chronic inflammation eventually results in airway remodeling, which may not be clinically apparent.

24. **All that wheezes is not asthma. What are other noninfectious causes?**
    - **Aspiration pneumonitis:** Especially in a neurologically impaired infant or an infant with gastroesophageal reflux, and especially if there is coughing, choking, or gagging with feedings. If there is a clear association with feedings, consider the possibility of tracheoesophageal fistula.

- **Bronchiolitis obliterans:** Chronic wheezing often after adenoviral infection
- **Bronchopulmonary dysplasia:** Especially if there has been prolonged oxygen therapy or a ventilatory requirement during the neonatal period
- **Ciliary dyskinesia:** Especially if recurrent otitis media, sinusitis, or situs inversus is present
- **Congenital malformations:** Including tracheobronchial anomalies, tracheomalacia, lung cysts, and mediastinal lesions
- **Cystic fibrosis:** If wheezing is recurrent, and associated with failure to thrive, chronic diarrhea, or recurrent respiratory infections
- **Congenital cardiac anomalies:** Especially lesions with large left-to-right shunts
- **Foreign-body aspiration:** If associated with an acute choking episode in an infant >6 months
- **Vascular rings, slings, or airway compression**

25. How is the severity of an acute asthma attack estimated?
   See Table 16-1.

Table 16-1. Classifying Severity of Asthma Exacerbations in the Urgent or Emergency Care Setting

	SYMPTOMS AND SIGNS	INITIAL PEF (OR FEV_1)	CLINICAL COURSE
Mild	Dyspnea only with activity (assess tachypnea in young children)	PEF ≥70% predicted or personal best	• Usually cared for at home • Prompt relief with inhaled SABA • Possible short course of oral systemic corticosteroids
Moderate	Dyspnea interferes with or limits usual activity	PEF 40-69% predicted or personal best	• Usually requires office or ED visit • Relief from frequent inhaled SABA • Oral systemic corticosteroids; some symptoms last for 1-2 days after treatment is begun
Severe	Dyspnea at rest; interferes with conversation	PEF <40% predicted or personal best	• Usually requires ED visit and likely hospitalization • Partial relief from frequent inhaled SABA • Oral systemic corticosteroids; some symptoms last for >3 days after treatment is begun • Adjunctive therapies are helpful
Subset: Life threatening	Too dyspneic to speak; perspiring	PEF <25% predicted or personal best	• Requires ED/hospitalization; possible ICU • Minimal or no relief from frequent inhaled SABA • Intravenous corticosteroids • Adjunctive therapies are helpful

ED = emergency department; FEV_1 = forced expiratory volume in 1 second; ICU = intensive care unit; PEF = peak expiratory flow; SABA = short-acting beta$_2$-agonist.
Adapted from the National Asthma Education and Prevention Program Expert Panel Report 3, 2007.

26. Is a chest radiograph necessary for all children who wheeze for the first time?
   A chest radiograph should be considered for a first-time wheezing patient in the following situations:
   - Findings on physical examination that may suggest other diagnoses
   - Marked asymmetry of breath sounds (suggesting a foreign-body aspiration)
   - Suspected pneumonia
   - History suggestive of foreign-body aspiration
   - Hypoxemia or marked respiratory distress
   - Older child with no family history of asthma or atopy
   - Suspected congestive heart failure
   - History of trauma that may have caused injury to the airway (e.g., burns, scalds, blunt or penetrating injury)

27. **What are the usual findings on arterial blood gas sampling during acute asthma attacks?**

The most common finding is **hypocapnia** (i.e., low $Paco_2$) because of hyperventilation and hypoxemia may also be present unless the child is being treated with oxygen. Hypercapnia is a serious sign that suggests that the child is tiring or becoming severely obstructed. This finding should prompt reevaluation and consideration of admission to a high-acuity unit.

28. **What are the indications for hospital admission in children with asthma?**

After therapy in the emergency department, admission is advisable if a child has any of the following:

- Depressed level of consciousness
- Incomplete response with moderate retractions, wheezing, peak flow of <60% predicted, pulsus paradoxus of >15 mm Hg, Sao_2 of 90% or less, Pco_2 of 42 mm Hg or more
- Breath sounds diminished significantly
- Evidence of dehydration
- Pneumothorax
- Residual symptoms and history of severe attacks involving prolonged hospitalization (especially if intubation was required)
- Parental unreliability

An equally difficult (and very unpredictable) challenge relates in predicting which patients will relapse after responding to therapy and subsequently require hospitalization. This is a major problem because rates of relapse in asthma can approach 20% to 30%.

29. **List the possible acute side effects of albuterol and other β-agonists**

- **General:** Hypoxemia, tachyphylaxis
- **Renal:** Hypokalemia
- **Cardiovascular:** Tachycardia, palpitations, premature ventricular contractions, atrial fibrillation
- **Neurologic:** Headache, irritability, insomnia, tremor, weakness
- **Gastrointestinal:** Nausea, heartburn, vomiting

Fortunately, these side effects are uncommon.

30. **What is the role of magnesium sulfate in acute asthma attacks?**

Magnesium sulfate is a known smooth muscle relaxant most commonly used in the treatment of preeclampsia. In asthmatic patients, when used in conjunction with standard bronchodilators and corticosteroids, intravenous magnesium sulfate can provide additional bronchodilation with a reduced likelihood of hospital admission. It is most commonly used when severely ill patients have failed to respond to conventional therapy. Inhaled magnesium sulfate as an adjuvant therapy in children is currently under study. Adult studies have demonstrated significant improvements in respiratory function and lower hospital admission rates.

Shan Z, Rong Y, Yang W, et al: Intravenous and nebulized magnesium sulfate for treating acute asthma in adults and children: a systematic review and meta-analysis, *Resp Med* 107:321–330, 2013.

31. **How is chronic asthma severity classified among children 5 to 11 years of age?**

The National Heart, Lung, and Blood Institute and National Asthma Prevention Program (NAEPP) define severity in terms of impairment and risk. Four categories are listed: **intermittent, mild persistent, moderate persistent,** and **severe persistent.** Categorization which is also separately done for 0 to 4 years and ≥12 years, helps guide therapy (Table 16-2).

National Asthma Education and Prevention Program Expert Panel Report 3: *Guidelines for the Diagnosis and Management of Asthma. Full Report 2007*, Bethesda, MD, August 2007, National Heart, Lung, and Blood Institute. NHLBI publication 08-4051. Available at http://www.nhlbi.nih.gov/guidelines/asthma/asthgdln.htm. Accessed on Jan. 13, 2015.

32. **What is the treatment of choice for patients with *persistent* asthma?**

Inhaled corticosteroids. Daily administration significantly improves symptoms, reduces exacerbations, and allows healing of the chronic inflammatory changes that have taken place in

Table 16-2. Classifying Asthma Severity and Initiating Therapy in Children

CLASSIFYING ASTHMA SEVERITY AND INITIATING THERAPY IN CHILDREN

COMPONENTS OF SEVERITY		Intermittent Ages 0-4	Intermittent Ages 5-11	Persistent Mild Ages 5-11	Persistent Mild Ages 0-4	Persistent Moderate Ages 5-11	Persistent Moderate Ages 0-4	Persistent Severe Ages 0-4	Persistent Severe Ages 5-11
Impairment	Symptoms	≤2 days/week	≤2 days/week	>2 days/week but not daily	>2 days/week but not daily	Daily	Daily	Throughout the day	Throughout the day
	Nighttime awakenings	0	≤2 ×/month	3-4 ×/month	1-2 ×/month	>1 ×/week but not nightly	3-4 ×/month	>1 ×/week	Often 7x/week
	Short-acting beta2-agonist use for symptom control	≤2 days/week	≤2 days/week	>2 days/week but not daily	>2 days/week but not daily	Daily	Daily	Several times per day	Several times per day
	Interference with normal activity	None	None	Minor limitation	Minor limitation	Some limitation	Some limitation	Extremely limited	Extremely limited
	Lung function • FEV_1 (predicted) or peak flow (personal best) • FEV_1/FVC	N/A	Normal FEV_1 between exacerbations >80% >85%	>80% >80%	N/A	60–80% 75–80%	N/A	N/A	<60% <75%
Risk	Exacerbations requiring oral systemic corticosteroids (consider severity and interval since last exacerbation)	0-1/year	≥2 ×/year (see notes) Relative annual risk may be related to FEV_1		≥2 exacerbations in 6 months requiring oral synthetic corticosteroids or ≥4 wheezing episodes/1 year lasting >1 day and risk factors for persistent asthma.				

FEV_1 = Forced expiratory volume in 1 second; FVC = forced expiratory capacity; ICS = inhaled corticosteroids; ICU = intensive care unit; N/A = not applicable.
Adapted from the National Asthma Education and Prevention Program Expert Panel Report 3, 2007.

the airways over time. Dosing and the use of adjunctive medications (e.g., long-acting inhaled β_2-agonists, leukotriene-receptor antagonists) depend on the severity of the persistence.

Bel EH: Mild asthma, *N Engl J Med* 369:549–557, 2013.
Rachelefsky G: Inhaled corticosteroids and asthma control in children: assessing impairment and risk, *Pediatrics* 123:353–366, 2009.

33. Do inhaled steroids affect growth in children?

Results are conflicting but tend to indicate that mild growth suppression occurs among children receiving moderate to high doses, particularly in children with more severe asthma and primarily during the first year of therapy (about 1 cm). The reduction in growth is generally not progressive. Asthma *per se* can also inhibit growth, and inhaled steroid therapy does not appear to affect eventual adult height. It is important that children who require the extended use of inhaled steroids are monitored for height and height velocity and also for cataracts.

Zhang L, Prietsch SO, Ducharme FM: Inhaled corticosteroids in children with persistent asthma: effects on growth, *Cochrane Database Sys Rev* 7:CD009471, 2014.
Kelly HW, Sternberg AL, Lescher R, et al: Effect of inhaled glucocorticoids in childhood on adult height, *N Engl J Med* 367:904–912, 2012.

34. What is anti-IgE treatment for asthma?

Omalizumab is a humanized monoclonal anti-IgE antibody approved for adjunctive therapy of severe persistent asthma in patients aged 12 years and older with an elevated total IgE and sensitivity to perennial allergens. It prevents free serum IgE from binding to its high-affinity receptors on mast cells and basophils. Omalizumab has been shown to reduce asthma exacerbations. It should be considered as an add-on for children >6 years of age who have inadequately controlled severe persistent allergic IgE-mediated asthma who require continuous or frequent oral corticosteroids. Rarely, symptoms of anaphylaxis may develop up to 24 hours after administration, so the clinician administering the drug should be prepared to treat anaphylaxis, and the patient should carry self-injectable epinephrine for 1 day after administration.

Normansell R, Walker S, Milan SJ, et al: Omalizumab for asthma in adults and children, *Cochrane Database Syst Rev* 1: CD003559, 2014.

35. Is there a role for complementary and alternative medicines in the treatment of asthma?

There are no clear directions or guidelines for the use of complementary and alternative medicines for children with asthma, although these therapies are often independently used by families. Hypnosis, yoga, relaxation techniques, acupuncture, and massage have shown benefit in some studies, but a review of studies involving mind-body techniques, relaxation, manual therapies, and diet has found a tendency to little or no significant difference between sham (placebo) and active therapy.

Snyder J, Brown P: Complementary and alternative medicine in children: an analysis of the recent literature, *Curr Opin Pediatr* 24:539–546, 2012.
Markham AW, Wilkinson JM: Complementary and alternative medicines (CAM) in the management of asthma: an examination of the evidence, *J Asthma* 41:131–139, 2004.

36. How useful are pulmonary function tests when evaluating and following children with asthma?

Spirometry is used for both the diagnosis and monitoring of asthma in children 5 years of age and older. The diagnosis of asthma requires airflow obstruction with at least a 12% improvement, or reversibility, in FEV_1 from baseline with the inhalation of a short-acting β-agonist. Patient history and physical examination do not adequately predict the degree of a patient's airflow obstruction. Spirometry is also used to monitor asthma after diagnosis and treatment. The goals of asthma therapy include normal or near-normal lung function with treatment. Spirometry should be performed on the patient after treatment has been initiated or changed, based on abnormal lung function, to assess improvement. It should also be performed during periods of prolonged loss of asthma control. Otherwise, in symptomatically controlled patients, it should be repeated at least yearly to monitor the patient long term. *Hand-held peak flow* measurements are useful for monitoring patients, but not for initial diagnosis.

National Asthma Education and Prevention Program Expert Panel Report 3: *Guidelines for the Diagnosis and Management of Asthma. Full Report 2007*, Bethesda, MD, August 2007, National Heart, Lung, and Blood Institute. NHLBI publication 08-4051. Available at http://www.nhlbi.nih.gov/guidelines/asthma/asthgdln.htm. Accessed on Jan. 13, 2015.

KEY POINTS: ASTHMA

1. Asthma is characterized by recurrent reversible airway obstruction and inflammation, often with identifiable triggers.
2. Typical abnormalities on spirometry include the following: decreased FEV_1 and FEV_1/FVC ratio; increase in FEV_1 ($>12\%$) with bronchodilator.
3. Classification is based on frequency of symptoms and exacerbations; nighttime awakenings; limitation of normal activities; use of oral steroids; and lung function—intermittent, mild persistent, moderate persistent, and severe persistent.
4. $Paco_2$ measurements that are normal (40 mm Hg) or rising in an asthmatic patient with tachypnea, or significant respiratory distress, are worrisome for evolving respiratory failure.
5. Signs of impending respiratory failure include severe retractions, accessory muscle use (especially sternocleidomastoids), decreased muscle tone, and altered mental status.

37. **What proportion of asthmatic children "outgrow" their symptoms?**
Popular pediatric teaching has been that most children with asthma outgrow their symptoms. However, studies suggest that this is erroneous and that only 30% to 50% become free of symptoms, primarily those with milder disease. Many children who appear to outgrow symptoms have recurrences during adulthood. Studies also indicate that many infants who wheeze with viral infections and are asymptomatic between illnesses tend to outgrow their asthma. Children with (1) early-onset asthma (age <3 years) with a positive parental history for asthma, (2) atopic dermatitis, or (3) sensitization to aeroallergens are more likely to have persistent or recurrent bronchospasm. Although the overall trend is for asthma to become milder, a large percentage of adults have persistent obstructive disease, both recognized and unrecognized.

Link HW: Pediatric asthma in a nutshell, *Pediatr Rev* 35:287–297, 2014.
Sears MR, Greene JM, Willan AR, et al: A longitudinal, population-based, cohort study of childhood asthma followed to adulthood, *N Engl J Med* 349:1414–1422, 2003.

38. **What diagnosis should be considered in a patient with poorly controlled asthma with recurrent infiltrates who has central bronchiectasis on a chest computed tomography (CT) scan and peripheral blood eosinophilia?**
Allergic bronchopulmonary aspergillosis. This is a T-cell mediated hypersensitivity response to *Aspergillus fumigatus* (a ubiquitous fungus) that can cause migrating pulmonary infiltrates and central bronchiectasis. The condition occurs as a complication primarily in patients with asthma and cystic fibrosis. Diagnosis relies on an abnormal chest radiograph and CT scan, skin prick reactivity to *A. fumigatus*, elevated total serum IgE >417 IU/L, and positive serum antibodies to *A. fumigatus* (IgE and/or IgG).

Greenberger PA: Chapter 18: Allergic bronchopulmonary aspergillosis, *Allergy Asthma Proc* 33S: S61–S63, 2012.

BRONCHIOLITIS

39. **What is the most important cause of lower respiratory tract disease among infants and young children?**
Respiratory syncytial virus (RSV). Up to 100,000 children are hospitalized annually in the United States as a result of this pneumovirus, which is different from—but closely related to—the

paramyxoviruses. Disease most commonly occurs during outbreaks in winter or spring in the United States and during the winter months of July and August in the southern hemisphere. In the first 2 years of life, 90% of children will become infected with RSV, and up to 40% will develop some lower respiratory disease.

Hall CB, Weinberg GA, Iwane MK, et al: The burden of respiratory syncytial virus infection in young children, *N Engl J Med* 360:588–598, 2009.

40. What other agents cause bronchiolitis?

RSV is estimated to cause 50% to 80% of cases. Other agents responsible for bronchiolitis include human metapneumovirus (second most common cause), parainfluenza virus, influenza virus types A and B, and adenovirus. Of these, adenovirus is most likely to result in rare serious sequelae, such as obliterative bronchiolitis.

Teshome G, Gattu R, Brown R: Acute bronchiolitis, *Pediatr Clin North Am* 60:1019–1034, 2013.

41. What are the best predictors of the severity of bronchiolitis?

The single best predictor at an initial assessment appears to be **oxygen saturation,** which can be determined by pulse oximetry. An Sao_2 of $<95\%$ correlates with more severe disease; a low Sao_2 is often not clinically apparent, and objective measurements are necessary. An arterial blood gas with a Pao_2 of 65 or less or a $Paco_2$ of >40 mm Hg is particularly worrisome. Other predictors of increased severity include the following:

- An ill or "toxic" appearance
- History of prematurity (gestational age <34 weeks)
- Atelectasis on chest radiograph
- Respiratory rate of >60 breaths/minute
- Infant <3 months old

42. What are the typical findings on a chest radiograph in a child with bronchiolitis?

The picture is varied. Most commonly, there is hyperinflation of the lungs. About 25% of hospitalized infants have atelectasis or infiltrates. Bilateral interstitial abnormalities with peribronchial thickening are common, or patients may have lobar, segmental, or subsegmental consolidation that can mimic bacterial pneumonia. Bacteremia or secondary bacterial pneumonia, however, is unusual in patients with bronchiolitis. With the possible exception of atelectasis, the chest radiograph findings do not correlate well with the severity of the disease.

43. Which patients with bronchiolitis are at risk for apnea?

Apnea in patients hospitalized with bronchiolitis has ranged from 3% to 7% in studies. Concerns of apnea are often used as rationale for hospitalization. In one study, higher-risk patients were those born at term and <1 month, preterm infants (<37 weeks of gestation) and <48 weeks postconception, and those with an observed apneic episode before evaluation. If none of these clinical criteria were present, the risk of apnea was $<1\%$. In another study, independent predictors of apnea were age <2 weeks, birth weight <2.3 kg, reported apneic event during current illness, and preadmission oxygen saturation $<90\%$.

Schroeder AR, Mansbach JM, Stevenson M, et al: Apnea in children hospitalized with bronchiolitis, *Pediatrics* 132: e1194-e1201, 2013.
Willwerth BM, Harper MB, Greenes DS: Identifying hospitalized infants who have bronchiolitis and are at high risk for apnea, *Ann Emerg Med* 48:4441–4447, 2006.

44. Is the use of steroids justified for bronchiolitis?

Although corticosteroids have been used by clinicians for many years for the treatment of bronchiolitis, the preponderance of multiple controlled studies has shown no immediate or long-term advantage with their use, either by the systemic or inhaled route.

Schroeder AR, Mansbach JM: Recent evidence on the management of bronchiolitis, *Curr Opin Pediatr* 26: 328–333, 2014.

45. **Is inhalation therapy effective for bronchiolitis?**

    Bronchodilators: The use of bronchodilator therapy for bronchiolitis is controversial, but in general, evidence has not supported significant efficacy. A 2010 meta-analysis found that outpatient use did not reduce the rate of hospitalization and that inpatient use did not shorten length of stay. Lack of benefit in bronchiolitis compared with asthma may be explained by the fact that bronchiolitis is characterized by bronchial wall edema and epithelial sloughing and not bronchospasm. Despite little support in the literature of its value, bronchodilator therapy continues to be widely practiced.

    Epinephrine: Some centers tout epinephrine, a therapy with α-agonistic vasoconstrictive properties, but recent evidence indicates no benefits compared with inhaled saline.

    Hypertonic saline: In theory, hypertonic saline might be efficacious through the absorption of mucosal water in the bronchioles and enhancement of mucociliary clearance. Results of early clinical trials indicated some possible reduction in hospital length of stay, but multiple recent studies have demonstrated no benefit.

Schroeder AR, Mansbach JM: Recent evidence on the management of bronchiolitis, *Curr Opin Pediatr* 26:328–333, 2014.

Jacobs JD, Foster M, Wan J, et al: 7% Hypertonic saline in acute bronchiolitis: a randomized controlled trial, *Pediatrics* 133: e8–e13, 2014.

46. **Is there a vaccine to prevent RSV infection?**

    No, there is not yet a safe and effective vaccine against RSV, although vaccines are in development. Palivizumab (Synagis), a monoclonal antibody directed against RSV, is effective for prophylaxis of RSV infection in high-risk infants. It is given intramuscularly and must be given once per month during the RSV season. This drug is not indicated for the treatment of RSV infection.

KEY POINTS: BRONCHIOLITIS

1. The most common causes are respiratory syncytial virus and metapneumovirus.
2. The illness severity is greatest between 2 and 6 months of age.
3. Atelectatic changes on chest radiograph are common.
4. In most cases, supportive care is all that is needed.
5. In more severe cases, the value of bronchodilators and corticosteroids is controversial.

47. **Does infection with RSV confer lifelong protection?**

    No. In fact, reinfection is very common. In day care centers, up to 70% of infants who acquire RSV infections during the first year of life are reinfected during the subsequent 2 years. Primary infections tend to be the most severe episodes, with subsequent illnesses being milder. In older children and adults, RSV infections present with the same symptoms as "colds," and reinfection is also common.

48. **If a 5-month-old child is hospitalized as a result of RSV bronchiolitis, what should the parents be told about the likelihood of future episodes of wheezing?**

    In follow-up studies, 40% to 50% of these infants have subsequent recurrent episodes of wheezing, usually during the first year after illness. Subclinical pulmonary abnormalities may also persist. The question of whether the pulmonary sequelae are the result of the bronchiolitis or of a genetic predisposition to wheezing or asthma remains unclear. Factors such as pulmonary abnormalities before the illness, passive cigarette smoke exposure, atopic diathesis, and immunologic responses of virus-specific IgE determine the risk for recurrence.

CLINICAL ISSUES

49. **How is hemoptysis differentiated from hematemesis?**

    See Table 16-3.

Rosenstein BJ: Hemoptysis. In Hilman BC, editor: *Pediatric Respiratory Disease*, Philadelphia, 1993, WB Saunders, p 533.

Table 16-3. Hemoptysis Versus Hematemesis

	HEMOPTYSIS	HEMATEMESIS
Color	Bright red and frothy	Dark red or brown
pH	Alkaline	Acid
Consistency	May be mixed with sputum	May contain food particles
Symptoms	Preceded by gurgling Accompanied by coughing	Preceded by nausea Accompanied by retching

50. **What are the indications for surgical repair of pectus excavatum?**
    This is still an area of considerable controversy. Nearly 1 in 400 children have this congenital chest wall anomaly. Children with pectus excavatum (Fig. 16-2) tend to have reduced total lung capacity, reduced vital capacity, increased residual volume, and reduced cardiac stroke volume during maximal exercise. However, most patients are still in the normal range for these values. The most common complaints relate to poor self-image and decreased exercise tolerance. Counseling is often sufficient for the cosmetic aspects, but many older patients report an improvement in exercise tolerance following repair, despite what appear to be minor changes in cardiac function. Whether the reason is cosmetic or to improve maximal exercise, operative repair should be delayed until the child is >16 years of age to decrease the risk for recurrence during the pubertal growth spurt.

Obermeyer RJ, Goretsky MJ: Chest wall deformities in pediatric surgery, *Surg Clin North Am* 92:669–684, 2012.

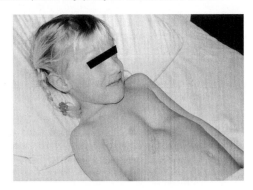

Figure 16-2. Pectus excavatum. *(From James EC, Corry RJ, Perry JF:* Principles of Basic Surgical Practice. *Philadelphia, 1987, Hanley & Belfus, p 173.)*

51. **What are the most common causes of chronic cough?**
    Postnasal drip and **asthma**. The differential diagnosis of chronic cough is very long and includes congenital anomalies, infectious or postinfectious cough, gastroesophageal reflux, aspiration, physical and chemical irritation, and psychogenic cough. After a thorough history and physical examination, evaluation with a chest radiograph and spirometry can also help establish the diagnosis.

Acosta R, Bahna SL: Chronic cough in children, *Pediatr Ann* 43:e176–e183, 2014.
Asilsoy S, Bayram E, Agin H, et al: Evaluation of chronic cough in children, *Chest* 134:1122–1128, 2008.

52. **When should the diagnosis of psychogenic cough be considered?**
    A *psychogenic cough* should be considered in children with a persistent dry, honking, explosive daytime cough that disappears with sleep or at the weekend. It often starts after an upper respiratory infection (URI). The patient complains of a tickle or "something in the throat." Physical examination and laboratory work are normal, and conventional therapies are ineffective. A behavioral approach with training in how to reduce the cough is the preferred treatment, although, in some cases, psychological intervention is required; hypnosis has also been employed successfully.

53. **What medications are most effective for cold symptoms in children?**

Multiple studies have failed to show benefit over placebo of any particular medication, including dextromethorphan, diphenhydramine, codeine, and echinacea. In addition, because the use of over-the-counter cold and cough products with antihistamines and decongestants have been implicated with many adverse events, a U.S. Food and Drug Administration advisory committee has recommended against their use in children <6 years of age. Many manufacturers have voluntarily removed such products intended for children <2 years of age. Supportive care with patience and self-resolution of symptoms (tincture of time) remain the mainstay of treatment.

Isbister GK, Prior F, Kilham HA: Restricting cough and cold medicines in children, *J Paediatr Child Health* 48:91–98, 2012.

54. **Which is the more effective for cough in children: antihistamines, antitussives, mucolytics, decongestants, or honey?**

Honey. Numerous studies have demonstrated that honey is a safe and effective treatment for cough associated with URI in children >1 year of age. Honey should not be given to children <1 year of age because of the risk of botulism. Since 2007, a number of advisory agencies, including the FDA, have cautioned against the use of over-the-counter cough and cold medications in children younger than 2 to 6 years of age because of a lack of proven efficacy and reported cases of misuse and overdose with severe adverse clinical effects and deaths.

Mazer-Amirshahi M, Reid N, van de Anker J, Litovitz T: Effect of cough and cold medication restriction and label changes on pediatric ingestions reported to United States Poison Centers, *J Pediatr* 163:1372–1376, 2013
Cohen A, Rozen J, Kristal H, et al: Effect of honey on nocturnal cough and sleep quality: a double-blind, randomized, placebo-controlled study, *Pediatrics* 130:465–471, 2012

55. **What constitutes passive cigarette smoke?**

Passive cigarette smoke consists of both the smoker's exhalation (mainstream smoke, about 15% of total) and the more noxious sidestream (the unfiltered burning end of the cigarette, about 85% of total).

56. **What are the possible risks of passive cigarette smoke exposure?**

- Decreased fetal growth and persistent adverse effects on lung function across childhood from smoking in pregnancy
- Increased incidence of sudden infant death syndrome
- Increased incidence of acute and chronic middle ear effusions
- Increased frequency of upper and lower respiratory tract infections
- Appearance of wheeze illness at an earlier age with more frequent exacerbations
- Impaired lung function during childhood from second-hand smoke after birth
  Longer-term issues of increased cancer rates and cardiovascular disease remain under study.

In addition, if a parent smokes, a child is twice as likely to become a smoker.

U.S. Department of Health and Human Services: *The Health Consequences of Involuntary Exposure to Tobacco Smoke: A Report of the Surgeon General.* Available at www.surgeongeneral.gov/library/reports/secondhandsmoke/fullreport.pdf. Accessed on Jan. 13, 2015.

57. **How is clubbing diagnosed?**

Digital clubbing is the presence of increased amounts of connective tissue under the base of the fingernail. This may be determined by the following:

- **Rock the nail** on its bed between the examiner's finger and thumb. In patients with clubbing, the nail seems to be floating.
- **Visual inspection** reveals that the distal phalangeal depth (DPD), which is the distance from the top of the base of the nail to the finger pad, exceeds the interphalangeal depth (IPD), which is the distance from the top of the distal phalangeal joint to the underside of the joint. Normally, the DPD/IPD ratio is <1, but in patients with clubbing, it is >1.
- **The diamond (or Schamroth) sign:** Normally, if the nails of both index fingers or any other two identical fingers are opposed, there is a diamond-shaped window present between the nail bases (Fig. 16-3); this window disappears in patients with clubbing.

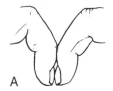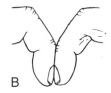

Figure 16-3. A, Normal child with a diamond-shaped window between the nail bases when the fingers are opposed. **B,** In digital clubbing, the diamond-shaped window is obliterated by the increased amount of soft tissue under the base of the nail.

58. **What are the causes of digital clubbing?**
    - **Pulmonary:** Bronchiectasis (as in cystic fibrosis, bronchiolitis obliterans, ciliary dyskinesia), pulmonary abscess, empyema, interstitial fibrosis, malignancy (bronchial carcinoma), pulmonary atrioventricular fistula
    - **Cardiac:** Cyanotic congenital heart disease, chronic congestive heart failure, subacute bacterial endocarditis
    - **Hepatic:** Biliary cirrhosis, biliary atresia, α_1-antitrypsin deficiency
    - **Gastrointestinal:** Crohn disease, ulcerative colitis, chronic amebic and bacillary diarrhea, polyposis coli, small bowel lymphoma
    - **Endocrine:** Thyrotoxicosis, thyroid deficiency
    - **Hematologic:** Thalassemia, congenital methemoglobinemia (rare)
    - **Idiopathic:** May be a variation of normal and not indicative of underlying disease
    - **Hereditary:** May be a variation of normal and not indicative of underlying disease

Modified from Hilman BC: Clinical assessment of pulmonary disease in infants and children. In Hilman BC, editor: *Pediatric Respiratory Disease.* Philadelphia, 1993, WB Saunders, p 61.

59. **What is the pathophysiology of clubbing?**
    The answer is unclear. The increased connective tissue under the nail beds that causes digital clubbing may be caused by the presence of vasoactive substances that are increased because of hypoxia, increased production in chronic inflammatory disease, or decreased lung clearance. Possible mediators include platelet-derived growth factor and prostaglandin E_2.

60. **Nasal polyps are associated with which conditions?**
    Children: Nasal polyps are rare in children except as a manifestation of cystic fibrosis (Fig. 16-4). About 3% of children with cystic fibrosis have nasal polyps, which are often a recurrent problem that becomes more frequent with increasing age
    - **Adolescents:** There is a wider range of possible diagnoses, including cystic fibrosis, allergic rhinitis, chronic sinusitis, malignancy, "triad asthma" (asthma, nasal polyps, aspirin sensitivity), and ciliary dyskinesia syndrome (e.g., Kartagener syndrome).

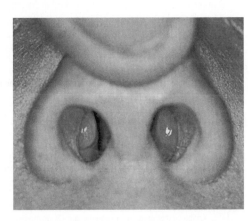

Figure 16-4. Nasal polyps in a patient with cystic fibrosis. *(From Zitelli BJ, Davis HW:* Atlas of Pediatric Physical Diagnosis, *ed 4. St. Louis, 2002, Mosby, p 550.)*

61. A patient with chronic sinusitis and recurrent pulmonary infections has a chest radiograph that demonstrates a right-sided cardiac silhouette. What diagnostic test should be considered next?

Bronchial or nasal turbinate mucosal biopsy for electron microscopic evaluation of cilia should be performed. **Kartagener syndrome** is one of the ciliary dyskinesia (or immotile cilia) syndromes. The presenting symptoms are a constellation of recurrent pulmonary infections, chronic sinusitis, recurrent otitis media, situs inversus, and infertility (in males). Structural ciliary abnormalities (most common are absent dynein arms) result in abnormal ciliary function and decreased clearance of respiratory secretions, thereby predisposing the patient to infection. In addition, because spermatozoa have tails with the same ultrastructural abnormalities as respiratory cilia, they move less well, causing infertility.

The cause of the situs inversus (Fig. 16-5) is not fully understood, but it occurs in about 50% of individuals with primary ciliary dyskinesia. It has been suggested that cilia are important for proper organ orientation during embryonic development and that dysfunctional cilia make organ orientation a random event, leading to situs inversus 50% of the time.

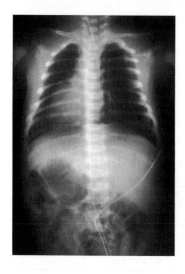

Figure 16-5. Dextrocardia with situs inversus. *(From Clark DA: Atlas of Neonatology. Philadelphia, 2000, WB Saunders, p 115.)*

62. What percentage of children snore?

Between 5% and 10% of preadolescent children are reported by their parents to snore at night.

63. In which children who snore should obstructive sleep apnea (OSA) be suspected?

At night, the child with OSA may have persistent snoring interrupted by periods of silence during which respiratory efforts are made, but there is no air movement. Increased work of breathing, with retractions; prominent mouth breathing; unusual sleep postures; frequent nighttime awakenings; enuresis; and night sweats are symptoms of OSA. During the day, there may be excessive daytime sleepiness, learning problems, morning headaches, or personality changes. It's estimated that 2% to 3% of the general pediatric population suffer from OSA; much higher rates are found in obese adolescents.

Reiter J, Rosen D: The diagnosis and management of common sleep disorders in adolescents, *Curr Opin Pediatr* 26:407–412, 2014.

64. What evaluations should be performed on a child with suspected OSA?

- **Physical examination** is used to assess for mouth breathing while awake, midface or mandibular hypoplasia, tonsillar hypertrophy, cleft palate, palatal deformity caused by adenoidal hypertrophy, failure to thrive (FTT), or obesity.
- **Lateral airway radiograph** is one of the easiest and most direct means of assessing upper airway caliber. Less commonly required are CT or magnetic resonance imaging (MRI).

- **Flexible nasopharyngoscopy** is useful for dynamic assessment of the nasal cavities, upper airway, and larynx.
- **Detailed nocturnal polysomnography** (overnight sleep study or polysomnogram [PSG]) is the gold standard for the definitive diagnosis of OSA until consistent clinical correlates can be found.
- **Cardiologic assessment** (chest radiograph, electrocardiogram, and echocardiography) is used for children with documented OSA and severe or sustained oxygen desaturation.

Wetmore RF: Sleep-disordered breathing. In Wetmore RF, editor: *Pediatric Otolaryngology: The Requisites*, Philadelphia, 2007, Mosby Elsevier, pp 190–201.

65. What are the potential long-term consequences of OSA?
The most severe complications of OSA in children are right ventricular hypertrophy, hypertension, polycythemia, respiratory acidosis with compensatory metabolic alkalosis, life-threatening cor pulmonale, and respiratory failure. Later in life, OSA is associated with an increased risk for cardiovascular morbidity and mortality. It is strongly implicated in the development of hypertension, ischemic heart disease, arrhythmias, and sudden death (in individuals with coexisting ischemic heart disease); it also contributes to the risk for stroke.

Capdevila OS, Kheirandish-Gozal L, Dayyat E, et al: Pediatric obstructive sleep apnea: complications, management, and long-term outcomes, *Proc Am Thorac Soc* 5:274–282, 2008.

66. What is the most common cause of infantile stridor?
Congenital laryngomalacia occurs as a result of prolapse of the poorly supported supraglottic structures—the arytenoids, the aryepiglottic folds, and the epiglottis—on inspiration (Fig. 16-6). Stridor is loudest after crying or exertion, but it typically does not interfere with feeding, sleep, or growth. Symptoms usually resolve by the time the infant is 18 months old.

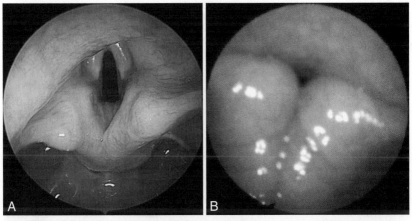

Figure 16-6. Laryngomalacia. **(A)** Normal position of supraglottic structures during expiration. **(B)** Collapse of arytenoids during inspiration. *(From Powitzky R, Stoner J, Fisher T, Digoy GP: Changes in sleep apnea after supraglottoplasty in infants with laryngomalacia,* Int J Pediatr Otolaryngol *75:1234–1239, 2011.)*

67. How can you clinically distinguish bilateral from unilateral vocal cord paralysis in an infant?
Normally, the vocal cords are tonically abducted, with voluntary adduction resulting in speech. With unilateral paralysis, one cord is ineffective for speech, and hoarseness results. The infant's cry may be weak or absent. Stridor is usually minimal but may be positional (e.g., sleeping on the side with the paralyzed cord up may allow it to fall to midline and produce obstructive sounds). With bilateral paralysis, hoarseness is less apparent, and the cry remains weak, but stridor (both inspiratory and expiratory) is usually quite prominent; in addition, the infant is more likely to have frank symptoms of pulmonary aspiration.

68. **What is the most common cause of chronic hoarseness in children?**
    Screamer's nodes. These are vocal cord nodules caused by vocal abuse, such as repetitive screaming, yelling, and coughing. They are the cause of a hoarse voice in >50% of children when hoarseness persists for >2 weeks.

69. **What are the most common symptoms and signs in children with suspected foreign body aspiration?**
    Coughing and **choking** (witnessed or by history) occur in up to 80% to 90%, which highlights the importance of questioning about choking in a child who is evaluated for cough. The classic triad of *cough, wheeze,* and *unilaterally decreased breath sounds* is found in only about one third to one-half of patients.

Tan HKKK, Brown K, McGill T: Airway foreign bodies: a 10-year review, *Int J Pediatr Otolaryngol* 56:91–99, 2000.

70. **Which other clinical features are suggestive of foreign-body aspiration?**
    Symptoms and history
    - Child <4 years old
    - Boys twice as common as girls
    - Hemoptysis
    - Respiratory infection not resolving with treatment
    - Difficulty breathing
    Signs
    - Wheezing in a child who has no history of asthma
    - Mediastinal shift
    - One nipple higher than the other as a result of unilateral hyperinflation
    - Stridor

71. **Are chest radiographs useful for evaluating a foreign-body aspiration?**
    Unfortunately, only about 10% to 20% of aspirated foreign bodies are radiopaque. Thus, inspiratory films are often normal. Features suggesting a foreign-body aspiration are as follows:
    - Expiratory chest radiograph showing asymmetry in lung aeration as a result of obstructive emphysema (The foreign body often acts as a ball-valve mechanism, allowing air in but not out.) (Fig. 16-7)

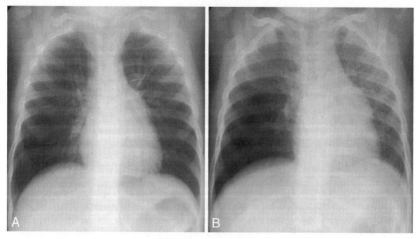

Figure 16-7. Right-sided foreign body aspiration. Compared to inspiratory film **(A)**, expiratory film **(B)** shows continued expansion on the right side due to air trapping caused by the foreign body. *(From Pinzoni F, Boniotti C, Molinaro SM: Inhaled foreign bodies in pediatric patients: review of personal experience,* Int J Pediatr Otolaryngol *71:1897–1903, 2007.)*

- Right and left lateral decubitus films that show the same asymmetry (These views are often used in uncooperative children who cannot or will not exhale on command.)
- Local hyperinflation
- Obstructive atelectasis

72. **On which side of the chest are foreign-body aspirations and aspiration pneumonias more common?**
Right side, particularly in older children and adolescents. This occurs because of anatomic considerations. The right main stem bronchus, compared with the left, is wider, has a larger airflow, and has a less acute angle with the trachea. This allows for easier passage of both small foreign bodies or aspirated liquids to enter the right side and its secondary airways. This angulation difference is less pronounced in infancy and increases as children age through puberty. Thus, the younger the child, the less likely is a right-sided predominance.

73. **What are the possible mechanisms for the development of lung abscesses in children?**
- **After pneumonia:** Particularly *Staphylococcus aureus, Haemophilus influenzae, Streptococcus pneumoniae,* and *Klebsiella pneumoniae*
- **Hematogenous spread:** Especially if an indwelling central catheter or right-sided endocarditis is present
- **Penetrating trauma**
- **Aspiration:** Especially in neurologically compromised patients
- **Secondary to infection of an underlying pulmonary anomaly:** Such as a bronchogenic cyst

Campbell PW: Lung abscess. In Hilman BC, editor: *Pediatric Respiratory Disease*, Philadelphia, 1993, WB Saunders, pp 257–262.

74. **What are the typical clinical findings in patients with bronchiectasis?**
Bronchiectasis is the progressive dilation of bronchi, most likely from acute and/or recurrent obstruction and infection. It may result from a variety of infections (e.g., adenoviral, rubeola, pertussis, tuberculosis), and it is often associated with underlying pulmonary susceptibility (e.g., cystic fibrosis, ciliary dyskinesia syndromes, immunodeficiencies). Clinical findings can be variable but usually include bad breath, persistent cough, chronic production of purulent sputum, recurrent fevers, and digital clubbing. Inspiratory crackles are often heard over the affected area. Hemoptysis and wheezing can occur but are uncommon.

75. **A novice teenage mountain-climber develops headache, marked cough, and orthopnea at the end of a rapid 2-day climb. What is the likely diagnosis?**
Acute mountain sickness with high-altitude pulmonary edema. This condition results from insufficient time to adapt to altitude changes above 2500 to 3000 meters, with alveolar and tissue hypoxia occurring as a result of pulmonary hypertension and pulmonary edema. In severe cases, cerebral edema can result. Treatment consists of returning the patient to a lower altitude and administering oxygen. If descent and supplemental oxygen are not available, portable hyperbaric chambers and nifedipine or phosphodiesterase-5 inhibitors should be used until descent is possible. If cerebral edema is suspected, dexamethasone is indicated.

Bärtsch P, Swenson ER: Acute high-altitude illnesses, *N Engl J Med* 368:2294–2302, 2013.

76. **What is the likely diagnosis of a child with diffuse lung disease, microcytic anemia, and sputum that contains hemosiderin-laden macrophages?**
Pulmonary hemosiderosis. This condition, the presenting symptoms of which can include chronic respiratory problems or acute hemoptysis, is characterized by alveolar hemorrhage and microcytic hypochromic anemia with a low serum iron level. Hemosiderin ingested by alveolar macrophages can often be detected in sputum or gastric aspirates after staining with Prussian blue. Most commonly, the condition is idiopathic and isolated, but it can be associated with cow milk hypersensitivity (Heiner syndrome), glomerulonephritis with anti–basement membrane antibodies (Goodpasture syndrome), and collagen vascular disease.

77. **How should a child with a spontaneous pneumothorax be managed?**

If the pneumothorax is small and the child is asymptomatic, observation alone is appropriate. Administration of 100% oxygen may speed resorption of the free air, but this technique is less effective in children in older age groups. If the pneumothorax is larger than 20% (as measured by the [diameter of pneumothorax]^3/[diameter of hemithorax]^3) and/or the patient has evolving respiratory symptoms, insertion of a thoracostomy tube and application of negative pressure should be considered. Signs of tension pneumothorax (e.g., marked dyspnea, tachypnea and tachycardia, unilateral thoracic hyperresonance with reduced breath sounds, tracheal shift) necessitate emergent aspiration and tube placement. Adolescents with spontaneous pneumothoraces have a high recurrence rate because of the common association with congenital subpleural blebs. As a follow-up measure, many authorities recommend chest CT with contrast because significant blebs can be treated thoracoscopically.

78. **Describe the clinical and radiographic features of a tension pneumothorax**
    - **Clinical:** Increasing respiratory distress, hypoxemia, hypercarbia, hypotension
    - **Radiographic:** Hyperlucency of the hemithorax, shifting of the mediastinum, flattening of the diaphragm, widening of the intercostal spaces (Fig. 16-8)

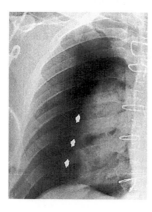

Figure 16-8. Tension pneumothorax. *(From Katz DS, Math KR, Groskin SA, editors:* Radiology Secrets. *Philadelphia, 1998, Hanley & Belfus, p 61.)*

79. **What physical examination features suggest a pleural effusion?**
    - Dullness to percussion ("stony dullness")
    - Diminished or absent breath sounds on the side of the effusion
    - Diminution in tactile fremitus
    - Presence of a friction rub on auscultation
    - Egophony ("e" to "a" changes)

80. **In children with pleural effusions, how are exudates distinguished from transudates?**

Exudative pleural effusions meet at least one of the following criteria:
    - Pleural fluid protein–to–serum protein ratio of 0.5 or greater
    - Pleural fluid lactate dehydrogenase (LDH)–to–serum LDH ratio of > 0.6
    - Pleural fluid LDH concentration is $>66\%$ of the upper limit of normal for serum

    If none of these criteria are met, the patient has a transudative pleural effusion. The criteria are extremely sensitive for the identification of exudates, but specificity is much lower. Twenty percent of transudates from congestive heart failure may be incorrectly identified as exudates, particularly in the setting of diuretic use, which increases protein and LDH concentration in pleural fluid.

Muzumdar H: Pleural effusion, *Pediatr Rev* 33:44-46, 2012.

81. **What pediatric diseases are associated with exudative and transudative pleural effusions?**

Exudates result from conditions of increased capillary permeability, whereas transudates occur with increased capillary hydrostatic pressure.

Exudative
- Pneumonia
- Tuberculosis
- Malignancy
- Chylothorax

Transudative
- Congestive heart failure
- Cirrhosis
- Nephrotic syndrome
- Upper airway obstruction

In children, the most common cause for a pleural effusion is pneumonia ("parapneumonic"), whereas, in adults, the most common etiology is congestive heart failure.

Beers SL, Abramo TJ: Pleural effusions, *Pediatr Emerg Care* 23:330–334, 2007.

82. **What are possible treatments for infected parapneumonic effusions?**

Although uncomplicated pleural effusions can usually be managed conservatively without the need for surgery, about 5% of patients with pleural effusions progress to empyema (Fig. 16-9). The precise approach to therapy is controversial and often varies by institution, but options include medical management alone or in combination with thoracentesis, chest tube drainage, video-assisted thorascopic surgery (VATS) with chest tube drainage, intrapleural fibrinolytic therapy, and thoracotomy. In general, a simple diagnostic and therapeutic thoracentesis is done with insertion of a chest tube in the early exudative phase of an empyema when fluid is accumulating. VATS therapy is more commonly the treatment of choice in early organizing empyemas (a fibrinopurulent phase), whereas thoracotomy, often combined with pleural stripping, is used in later, more advanced empyemas when scar formation can result in lung entrapment.

Shah SS, Hall M, Newland JG, et al: Comparative effectiveness of pleural drainage procedures for the treatment of complicated pneumonia in childhood, *J Hosp Med* 6:256–263, 2011.

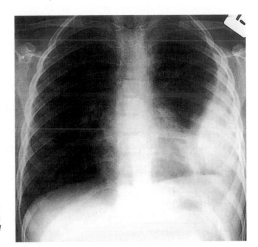

Figure 16-9. Large left empyema with passive atelectasis of the adjacent lung. *(From Chernick V, Boat TF, Wilmott RW, Bush A, editors:* Kendig's Disorders of the Respiratory Tract in Children, *ed 7. Philadelphia, 2006, WB Saunders, p 374.)*

83. **What is the value of chest physiotherapy (CPT) in patients with pediatric pulmonary disease?**

The main function of chest physiotherapy is to assist with the removal of tracheobronchial secretions to lessen obstruction, reduce airway resistance, enhance gas exchange, and reduce the work of breathing. A variety of techniques are used: chest wall percussion, vibration, and postural drainage. CPT has been advocated in patients with chronic sputum production (e.g., cystic fibrosis), primary pneumonia, and atelectasis; for intubated neonates; and for postextubation and postoperative patients. However, clinical benefits in each category—with the exception of diseases of chronic sputum production—remain highly anecdotal and understudied. Limited evidence does not support a role in bronchiolitis and asthma.

Chaves GS, Fregonezi GA, Dias FA, et al: Chest physiotherapy for pneumonia in children, *Cochrane Database Syst Rev* 9: CD010277, 2013.

Roque I, Figuis M, Giné-Garriga M, et al: Chest physiotherapy for acute bronchiolitis in paediatric patients between 0 and 24 months, *Cochrane Database Sys Rev* 2:CD004873, 2012.

American Association for Respiratory Care: www.aarc.org. Accessed on Jan. 13, 2015.

84. **Who was Ondine, and what was her curse?**

Ondine was a legendary water nymph who fell in love with Hans, a mortal. She put a curse on him with the stipulation that, should he ever betray her, he would suffocate by not breathing when he fell asleep. Unfortunately, Hans fell for the charms of Bertha, and he eventually succumbed to the curse while dozing. The term *Ondine curse* has been used to describe the syndrome of sleep apnea as a result of reduced respiratory drive, although the term *central hypoventilation syndrome* (CHS) is used more correctly. This rare condition is often associated with other abnormalities of brainstem function. CHS can be idiopathic, or it can be a complication of an earlier insult to the developing brain. In some families, it is genetic. Children with CHS are initially treated by tracheostomy and mechanical ventilation during sleep. Results with phrenic nerve pacing have been good in older infants and children. Familial recurrence of CHS has suggested a genetic etiology and mutations in the *PHOX2B* gene have been reported in studies from France and the United States.

Marion TL, Bradshaw WT: Congenital central hypoventilation syndrome and the *PHOX2B* gene mutation, *Neonatal Netw* 30:397–401, 2011.

CYSTIC FIBROSIS

85. **What is the basic defect in patients with cystic fibrosis (CF)?**

Patients with CF have a defect in the **CF transmembrane conductance regulator (CFTR) protein.** This is a key ion channel that regulates chloride and sodium transfer across the apical membrane of epithelial cells and other cells. In patients with CF, chloride is poorly secreted into the lumen, and there is increased absorption of sodium from the luminal surface of the airway or duct, thereby resulting in respiratory and pancreatic secretions that are relatively dehydrated and viscid. These hyperviscous secretions obstruct pancreatic ducts, resulting in steatorrhea from exocrine pancreatic insufficiency, and they interfere with pulmonary mucociliary clearance, thereby causing chronic respiratory disease. In the sweat gland, CFTR is involved in the reabsorption of chloride, and abnormal CFTR function in patients with CF leads to the production of sweat with increased sodium and chloride concentrations. More than 1900 mutations of the gene that codes for this protein have been identified.

O'Sullivan BP, Freedman SD: Cystic fibrosis, *Lancet* 373:1891–1904, 2009.

86. **What is the incidence of CF in various ethnic groups?**
- Whites: 1 in 3300 live births
- Hispanics: 1 in 8000 to 9500 live births
- Native Americans (in the United States): 1 in 11,200 live births
- Blacks: 1 in 15,300 live births
- Asians: 1 in 32,100 live births

Cystic Fibrosis Foundation: www.cff.org. Accessed on Jan. 13, 2015.

87. **What are the presenting signs and symptoms of CF?**
    These can be remembered with the acronym **CF PANCREAS**:
    - **C**hronic cough and wheezing
    - **F**ailure to thrive
    - **P**ancreatic insufficiency (signs of malabsorption, including bulky, foul stools)
    - **A**lkalosis and hyponatremic dehydration
    - **N**eonatal intestinal obstruction (meconium ileus) and **N**asal polyps
    - **C**lubbing of the fingers and **C**hest radiographs with changes
    - **R**ectal prolapse
    - **E**lectrolyte elevation in sweat (salty skin)
    - **A**bsence or congenital atresia of the vas deferens
    - **S**putum with *Staphylococcus* or *Pseudomonas* (mucoid)

Schidlow DV: Cystic fibrosis. In Schidlow DV, Smith DS, editors: *A Practical Guide to Pediatric Respiratory Diseases*, Philadelphia, 1994, Hanley & Belfus, p 76.

88. **How is the diagnosis of CF made?**
    The presence of one or more typical symptoms of CF, or a history of CF in a sibling, or an abnormal newborn screen plus laboratory evidence of CFTR dysfunction.
    Laboratory evidence of CFTR dysfunction can be in the form of a positive sweat test, demonstration of 2 known disease-causing mutations or abnormal nasal potential difference measurements.

89. **What constitutes an abnormal sweat test?**
    Sweat gland secretions should be obtained by pilocarpine iontophoresis. A level of sweat chloride of >60 mEq/L is abnormal; 40 to 60 mEq/L is borderline; and <40 mEq/L is normal. Note that sweat chloride values <40 mEq/L have occasionally been demonstrated in genetically proven cases of CF. In infancy, values greater than 30 mEq/L should be considered abnormal and lead to further evaluation.

90. **How are newborns screened for CF?**
    Newborns with CF have elevated levels of immunoreactive trypsinogen (IRT), a pancreatic enzyme precursor. If the initial screen for this compound is elevated (and sometimes a repeat IRT test to confirm elevation), mutational analysis of DNA or sweat testing is used to confirm the diagnosis. As of 2010, all states offer CF screening as part of their expanded newborn screening programs, and the sensitivity of the testing varies depending on the methodology and the reference ranges selected. In general, the testing is no more than 95% sensitive, so symptoms suggestive of CF in a child whose newborn screen was normal are an indication for sweat testing or mutational analysis.

Wagener JS, Zemanick ET, Sontag MK: Newborn screening for cystic fibrosis, *Curr Opin Pediatr* 24:329–325, 2012.

91. **When and why should children with cystic fibrosis be screened for possible CF-related diabetes mellitus?**
    Children with CF should be screened for possible CF-related diabetes mellitus **after 9 years of age.** Thick viscous secretions in CF patients cause obstructive damage to the exocrine pancreas, which ultimately can lead to islet cell destruction and diminishment of insulin production. Annual glucose tolerance testing is recommended after 9 years of age. The hemoglobin A_1C test is not sufficient as a screen because it underestimates glycemic control.

Paranjape SM, Mogayzel PJ Jr: Cystic fibrosis. *Pediatr Rev* 35:194–204, 2014.

92. **What are the mainstays of pulmonary therapy for children with CF?**
    - Airway clearance techniques (e.g., chest physiotherapy, mechanical vests, flutter valve)
    - Mucolytic agents (e.g., recombinant human DNAse, hypertonic saline aerosols)
    - Anti-inflammatory agents (e.g., ibuprofen, oral azithromycin)
    - Bronchodilators (e.g., inhaled β_2-agonists)
    - Antibiotics (oral, inhaled, and intravenous)

O'Sullivan BP, Freedman SD: Cystic fibrosis, *Lancet* 373:1891–1904, 2009.

93. What is the role of Ivacaftor in the treatment of CF patients?

Ivacaftor is an oral agent, classified as a CFTR potentiator that activates a defective CFTR at the cell surface in patients with a certain class III mutation (G551D). This mutation affects 4% to 5% of CF patients. Clinical trials involving patients with other mutations are underway. The resultant improvement in cellular channel function in airways increases chloride secretion, reduces excessive sodium and water absorption, and decreases secretion tenacity. However, it is one of the most expensive drugs ever marketed with a yearly cost in 2013 of over $300,000, which has prompted much criticism.

O'Sullivan B, Orenstein DM, Milla CE: Viewpoint: pricing for orphan drugs, will the market bear what society cannot? *JAMA* 310:1343–1344, 2013.
Ramsey BW, Davies J, McElvaney NG, et al: VX09-770-102 Study Group. A CFTR potentiator in persons with cystic fibrosis and the G551D mutation. *N Engl J Med* 365:1663–1672, 2011.

KEY POINTS: CYSTIC FIBROSIS

1. Cystic fibrosis (CF) is the most common lethal inherited disease in whites.
2. There are more than 1900 known mutations of the CF gene; ΔF508 is the most common in North America (75%).
3. The key to diagnosis is a sweat test (sweat chloride >60 mEq/L is abnormal).
4. CF is a chronic obstructive pulmonary disease.
5. Gastrointestinal manifestations can include pancreatic insufficiency, bowel obstruction, rectal prolapse, intussusception, gastroesophageal reflux, and cholelithiasis.
6. Pulmonary colonization with *Pseudomonas aeruginosa,* methicillin-resistant *S. aureus* (MRSA) or *Burkholderia cepacia* is a poor prognostic sign.

94. Which features of CF have prognostic significance?
   - **Gender:** Males have better survival rates than females, although the gap is narrowing.
   - **Colonization with virulent bacteria:** *Pseudomonas aeruginosa*, methicillin-resistant *S. aureus* (MRSA), and *Burkholderia cepacia* are more serious pathogens, which are often resistant to multiple drugs and difficult to clear after the patient becomes persistently infected. *Stenotrophomonas maltophilia* is an emerging problem; patients who are chronically colonized with these organisms have significantly poorer survival rates than other patients with CF.
   - **Diabetes mellitus** is a negative prognostic factor that is associated with increased rates of decline in pulmonary function.
   - **Malnutrition** is also associated with increased rates of decline in pulmonary function.
   - **Cor pulmonale** is one of the late complications of CF because progressive obstructive airway disease leads to the development of pulmonary hypertension and respiratory failure. The patient's prognosis is poor after the development of cor pulmonale.
   - **Pneumothorax** is associated with moderate to advanced lung disease in patients with CF. Therefore, air leak has traditionally been regarded as a poor prognostic sign. The prognosis has been improving now that pneumothoraces are being managed aggressively.
   - **Worsening pulmonary function tests:** Patients with an FEV$_1$ level that is <30% of predicted have an increased 2-year mortality rate.

Montgomery GS, Howenstine M: Cystic fibrosis, *Pediatr Rev* 30:302–309, 2009.
Kulich M, Rosenfeld M, Goss CH, Wilmott R: Improved survival among young patients with cystic fibrosis, *J Pediatr* 142:631–636, 2003.

PNEUMONIA

95. What agents cause pneumonia in children?
   See Table 16-4.

Table 16-4. Agents That Cause Pneumonia

AGE	VIRAL	BACTERIAL	ATYPICAL
Birth to 3 wk	Cytomegalovirus Herpes simplex virus	Group B streptococcus Gram-negative enteric bacilli (e.g., *Escherichia coli*) *Listeria monocytogenes*	*Ureaplasma* *urealyticum*
3 wk to 3 mo	Respiratory syncytial virus Parainfluenza viruses Human metapneumovirus Influenza A and B Adenovirus Bocavirus Rhinovirus	*Streptococcus* *pneumoniae* *Bordetella pertussis* *Staphylococcus aureus*	*Chlamydia* *trachomatis*
3 mo-5 yr	Respiratory syncytial virus Parainfluenza viruses Influenza A and B Human metapneumovirus Adenovirus Bocavirus Rhinovirus	*Streptococcus pneumoniae* *Haemophilus influenzae* (nontypeable) *Staphylococcus aureus*	*Mycoplasma* *pneumoniae* *Chlamydophila* *pneumoniae*
5 yr to adolescence	Influenza A and B	*Streptococcus pneumoniae* *Staphylococcus aureus*	*Mycoplasma* *pneumoniae* *Chlamydophila* *pneumoniae*

96. What are important trends in the etiology of pneumonia in the United States?
    - **Bacterial:** The introduction of the pneumococcal conjugate vaccines has substantially reduced hospitalizations for pneumonia.
    - **Viral:** Viral pneumonia is more common in younger age groups, and most frequently is RSV. Human metapneumovirus, described initially in 2001, can mimic the clinical picture of RSV.
    - **Atypical pneumonia:** Caused by *Mycoplasma pneumoniae* and *Chlamydophila* (formerly *Chlamydia*) *pneumoniae*, these infections were previously thought to be uncommon in preschool-age children. In this age group, the incidence is thought to be increasing. Both organisms become more prevalent in school-age children and are the most common etiology for pneumonia in older children.

Grijalva CG, Griffin MR, Nuorti JP, et al: Pneumonia hospitalizations among children before and after introduction of the pneumococcal conjugate vaccine—United States, 1997–2006. *MMWR* 58:1, 2009.

97. Are throat or nasopharyngeal cultures helpful for the diagnosis of pneumonia?
    As a rule, the correlation between throat and nasopharyngeal bacterial cultures and lower respiratory tract pathogens is poor and of limited value. Healthy children may be colonized with a wide variety of potentially pathologic bacteria (e.g., *S. aureus*, nontypeable *Haemophilus influenzae*), which can be considered part of the normal flora; *Bordetella* pertussis is an exception. Polymerase chain reaction studies to identify respiratory viruses, *C. pneumoniae*, or *M. pneumoniae* are more useful because these organisms are much less commonly carried asymptomatically.

98. How often are blood cultures positive in children with suspected bacterial pneumonia?
    Blood cultures are positive 10% of the time or less in hospitalized patients. In outpatients with community-acquired pneumonia, the likelihood is significantly lower (<3%). Thus, the sicker the patient, the greater the potential yield. The incidence of bacteremia is unclear because the true denominator in the equation (the number of true bacterial pneumonias) is difficult to ascertain because of the

imprecision with making a definitive diagnosis. The low rate of positive blood cultures does suggest that most bacterial pneumonias are not acquired by hematogenous spread.

Myers AL, Hall M, Williams DJ, et al: Prevalence of bacteremia in hospitalized pediatric patients with community-acquired pneumonia, *Pediatr Infect Dis J* 32:736–740, 2013.

99. **How often are pleural fluid cultures positive in children with suspected bacterial pneumonia?**
Between 60% and 85% are positive if antibiotics have not already been initiated. This high yield emphasizes the importance of recognizing a pleural effusion in patients with pneumonia and the value of early thoracentesis before starting antibiotic therapy.

100. **Can a chest radiograph reliably distinguish between viral and bacterial pneumonia?**
No. Viral infections more commonly have multifocal interstitial, perihilar, or peribronchial infiltrates; hyperinflation; segmental atelectasis; and hilar adenopathy. Effusions are uncommon. However, there can be considerable overlap in features with bacterial (and chlamydophilal and mycoplasmal) pneumonia. Bacterial pneumonia more commonly results in lobar and alveolar infiltrates, but the sensitivity and specificity of this finding are not very high.

Kronman MP, Shah SS: Pediatric community-acquired pneumonia, *Contemp Pediatr* 26:44–50, 2009.

101. **What are indications for hospital admission in children with pneumonia?**
- All who are toxic, dyspneic, or hypoxic
- Suspected staphylococcal pneumonia (e.g., pneumatocele on chest radiograph) (Fig. 16-10)
- Significant pleural effusion
- Suspected aspiration pneumonia (because of the higher likelihood of progression)
- Children who cannot tolerate oral medications or who are at significant risk for dehydration
- Suspected bacterial pneumonia in very young infants, especially with multilobar involvement
- Poor response to outpatient therapy after 48 hours
- Those whose family situation and chances for reliable follow-up are suboptimal

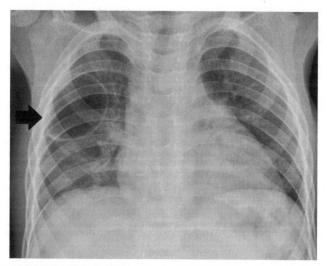

Figure 16-10. Pneumatocele after severe staphylococcal pneumonia (a thin-walled cyst in the right upper zone *(arrow)*). *(From Adam A, Dixon AK, Gillard JH, et al:* Grainger & Allison's Diagnostic Radiology, *ed 6. Philadelphia, 2015, Elsevier, p 1789.)*

102. **What clinical clues suggest atypical pneumonia?**

Atypical pneumonia refers to one caused by certain bacteria, including *Mycoplasma pneumoniae, Chlamydophila pneumoniae,* and *Legionella pneumophila.* Characteristically, these infections start gradually, have minimal or a nonproductive cough, and have frequent constitutional signs (e.g., headache, rash, and pharyngitis). Chest radiographs tend to show patchy, peribronchial infiltrates with only occasional lobar consolidation.

103. **What are the causes of "afebrile infant pneumonia" syndrome?**

The syndrome is usually the result of *Chlamydia trachomatis*, cytomegalovirus, *Ureaplasma urealyticum,* or *Mycoplasma hominis.* Affected infants develop progressive respiratory distress over several days to a few weeks, along with poor weight gain. A maternal history of a sexually transmitted infection is common. Chest radiographs reveal bilateral diffuse infiltrates with hyperinflation. There may be eosinophilia and elevated quantitative immunoglobulins (IgG, IgA, IgM). The etiologic causes overlap in the clinical picture, although a history of conjunctivitis suggests chlamydia.

104. **What are the clinical characteristics of chlamydial pneumonia in infants?**
- Illness occurs between 2 and 19 weeks after birth. Most infants show symptoms by 8 weeks of age.
- Onset is gradual, with upper respiratory prodromal symptoms lasting longer than 1 week.
- Nearly 100% of patients are afebrile.
- Less than half have inclusion conjunctivitis.
- Respiratory signs and symptoms include the following: staccato cough, tachypnea, diffuse crackles, and occasional wheezing.
- Chest radiograph reveals bilateral hyperexpansion and symmetric interstitial infiltrates.
- Seventy percent have an elevated absolute eosinophil count ($>400/mm^3$).
- More than 90% have increased quantitative immunoglobulins.

105. **How helpful are cold agglutinins in the diagnosis of *M. pneumoniae* infections?**

Cold agglutinins are IgM autoantibodies that are directed against the I antigen of erythrocytes, which agglutinate red blood cells at 4°C. Up to 75% of patients with mycoplasma infections will develop them, usually toward the end of the first week of illness, with a peak at 4 weeks. A titer of 1:64 supports the diagnosis. Other infectious agents, including adenovirus, cytomegalovirus, Epstein-Barr virus, influenza, rubella, *Chlamydia,* and *Listeria,* can also give a positive result. A single cold agglutinin titer of 1:64 is therefore suggestive but not conclusive evidence of infection with *M. pneumoniae.* More definitive testing requires IgG and IgM serology (especially acute and convalescent titers), quantitative polymerase chain reaction (FQ-PCR) and culture.

Qu J, Wu J, Dong J, et al: Accuracy of IgM antibody testing, FQ-PCR and culture in laboratory diagnosis of acute infection by *Mycoplasma pneumoniae* in adults and adolescents with community-acquired pneumonia, *BMC Infect Dis* 13:172, 2013.

106. **When do the radiologic findings of pneumonia resolve?**

Although there is a wide range, as a rule, most infiltrates that result from *S. pneumoniae* resolve in 6 to 8 weeks, and those that are caused by RSV resolve in 2 to 3 weeks. However, with some viral infections (e.g., adenovirus), it may take up to 1 year for radiographs to normalize. If significant radiologic abnormalities persist for >6 weeks, there should be a high index of suspicion for a possible underlying problem (e.g., unusual infection, anatomic abnormality, immunologic deficiency).

Regelmann WE: Diagnosing the cause of recurrent and persistent pneumonia in children, *Pediatr Ann* 22:561–568, 1993.

107. **Do children with pneumonia need follow-up radiographs to verify resolution?**

Generally, no. Exceptions would include children with pleural effusions, those with persistent or recurrent signs and symptoms, and those with significant comorbid conditions (e.g., immunodeficiency).

Mahmood D, Vartzelis G, McQueen P, Perkin MR: Radiological follow-up of pediatric pneumonia: principle and practice, *Clin Pediatr* 46:160–162, 2007.

108. What are the causes of recurrent pneumonia?
    - **Aspiration susceptibility:** Oropharyngeal incoordination, vocal cord paralysis, gastroesophageal reflux, tracheoesophageal fistula
    - **Immunodeficiency:** Congenital, acquired
    - **Congenital cardiac defects:** Atrial septal defect, ventricular septal defect, patent ductus arteriosus
    - **Abnormal secretions or reduced clearance of secretions:** Asthma, cystic fibrosis, ciliary dyskinesia
    - **Pulmonary anomalies:** Sequestration, cystic adenomatoid malformation
    - **Airway compression or obstruction:** Foreign body, vascular ring, enlarged lymph node, malignancy
    - **Miscellaneous:** For example, sickle cell disease, sarcoidosis

Brand PL, Hoving MF, de Groot EP: Evaluating the child with recurrent lower respiratory tract infections, *Paediatr Respir Rev* 13:135–138, 2012.
Kaplan KA, Beierle EA, Faro A, et al: Recurrent pneumonia in children: a case report and approach to diagnosis, *Clin Pediatr* 45:15–22, 2006.

KEY POINTS: PNEUMONIA

1. Effusion or pneumatocele suggests a bacterial cause.
2. Radiographic findings in patients with mycoplasmal infections are highly variable.
3. In half of patients with chlamydial pneumonia, conjunctivitis precedes pneumonia.
4. Hilar adenopathy suggests tuberculosis.
5. Yield of blood cultures for community-acquired pneumonia is very low.

109. How does the pH of a substance affect the severity of disease in aspiration pneumonia?
    A **low pH is more harmful** than a slightly alkaline or neutral pH, and it is more likely to be associated with bronchospasm and pneumonia. The most severe form of pneumonia is seen when gastric contents are aspirated; symptoms may develop in a matter of seconds. If the volume of aspirate is sufficiently large and the pH is <2.5, the mortality rate may exceed 70%. The radiographic picture may be that of an infiltrate or pulmonary edema. Unilateral pulmonary edema may occur if the child is lying on one side.

110. How should children with aspiration pneumonia be managed?
    Acute aspiration can often be treated supportively without antibiotics because the initial process is a chemical pneumonitis. If secondary signs of infection occur, antibiotics should be started after appropriate cultures; either penicillin or clindamycin is a reasonable choice to cover the oropharyngeal anaerobes that predominate. If the aspiration is nosocomial, antibiotic coverage should be extended to include gram-negative organisms.

PULMONARY PRINCIPLES

111. In addition to underlying immunologic immaturity, why are infants more susceptible to an increased severity of respiratory disease?
    - Very compliant chest wall (allows passage through birth canal but limits inspiratory effort as it distorts with increased respiratory loading)
    - Respiratory muscles more easily fatigued as a result of decreased muscle mass and fewer type I muscle fibers (slow twitch, high oxidative fibers)
    - Chest wall elastic recoil is low in infancy (airway closure occurs at a higher relative lung volume)
    - High airway compliance facilitates airway collapse and air trapping
    - Collateral ventilation poorly developed, thus increasing likelihood of atelectasis during illness
    - Higher airway mucous gland concentration in infants than in adults

112. At what age do alveoli stop increasing in number?
    Although extra-acinar airway development is complete by 16 weeks of gestation, alveolar multiplication continues after birth. Early studies suggested that postnatal alveolar multiplication

ends at 8 years of age. However, more recent studies have shown that it is terminated by 2 years of age and possibly between 1 and 2 years of age. After the end of alveolar multiplication, the alveoli continue to increase in size until thoracic growth is completed.

113. **What is the normal respiratory rate in otherwise healthy children?**
Rates in children who are awake can be widely variable, depending on their psychological state and activity. Rates while sleeping are much more reliable and are a good indicator of pulmonary health. As a general rule in an afebrile, otherwise healthy and calm, resting infant or child, the expected maximal respiratory rate declines with increasing age. In the absence of other signs and symptoms, term newborns breathe up to a mean of 50 breaths/minute, decreasing to 40 breaths/minute by 6 months and to 30 breaths/minute at 1 year. Beyond 1 year of age, the rate declines gradually, reaching the typical adult rate of 14 to 20 breaths/minute by the middle teenage years. Counting respiratory rates over 1 minute gives a more accurate measurement than extrapolating rates over shorter periods to 1 minute.

114. **What is the significance of grunting respirations?**
Grunting respirations are crying-like noises heard during expiration and are thought to be a physiologic attempt to maintain alveolar patency (PEEP). In patients seen in hospital settings, grunting is associated with a higher likelihood of serious infections, including pneumonia, pyelonephritis, and peritonitis.

Bilavsky E, Shouval DS, Yarden-Bilavsky H, et al: Are grunting respirations a sign of serious bacterial infection in children? *Acta Paediatr* 97:1086–1089, 2008.

115. **What is normal oxygen saturation in healthy infants who are <6 months?**
In a longitudinal study using pulse oximetry, baseline saturation was higher than 95% (normal was 98%, with the lower 10th percentile at 95%). However, acute desaturations are common; almost all are associated with brief episodes of apnea while sleeping.

Hunt CE, Corwin MJ, Lister G, et al: Longitudinal assessment of hemoglobin saturation in healthy infants during the first six months of life, *J Pediatr* 134:580–586, 1999.

116. **What is the difference among Kussmaul, Cheyne-Stokes, and Biot types of breathing patterns?**
   - **Kussmaul:** Deep, slow, regular respirations with prolonged exhalation; seen in diabetic ketoacidosis and salicylate ingestion
   - **Cheyne-Stokes:** Crescendo-decrescendo respirations alternating with periods of apnea (no breathing); causes include heart failure, uremia, central nervous system trauma, increased intracranial pressure, and coma
   - **Biot** (also known as ataxic breathing): Characterized by unpredictable irregularity; breaths may be shallow or deep and stop for short periods; causes include respiratory depression, meningitis, encephalitis, and central nervous system lesions involving the respiratory centers

117. **Why a sigh?**
A sigh is just a sigh in Casablanca, but it is also a very effective anti-atelectatic maneuver. By definition, it is a breath that is more than three times the normal tidal volume.

118. **Is there a respiratory basis for yawning?**
Although a respiratory function for yawning is frequently suggested, scientific support for this belief is minimal. Increasing the concentration of CO_2 in inspired air increases the respiratory rate but does not change the rate of yawning. Relief of hypoxia and opening areas of microatelectasis are other theories that are not supported by scientific studies. Some authors hypothesize that yawning may be an arousal reflex.

119. **At what concentration is inspired oxygen toxic?**
In addition to atelectasis, high oxygen concentration can cause alveolar injury with edema, inflammation, fibrin deposition, and hyalinization. The precise level of hyperoxia that results in injury is unclear and varies by age and underlying lung pathology, but a reasonable rule is to assume that a concentration

of more than 80% for longer than 36 hours is likely to result in significant ongoing damage; 60% to 80% is likely to be associated with more slowly progressive injury. An inspired oxygen concentration of 50%, even when administered for extended periods of time, is unlikely to cause pulmonary toxicity.

Jenkinson SG: Oxygen toxicity, *J Intensive Care Med* 3:137–152, 1988.

120. **Why is a child who is receiving 100% oxygen more likely to develop atelectasis than one who is breathing room air?**
Nitrogen is more slowly absorbed than oxygen by alveoli. In room air (with its 78% nitrogen), alveolar collapse is minimized by the continued presence and pressure of nitrogen gas (the "nitrogen stint"). With 100% oxygen breathing, however, the high solubility of oxygen in blood can lead to absorption atelectasis in areas of poor ventilation and intrapulmonary shunting.

121. **At what Pao_2 does cyanosis develop?**
Cyanosis develops when the concentration of desaturated (i.e., reduced) hemoglobin is at least 3 gm/dL centrally or 4 to 6 g/dL peripherally. However, multiple factors affect the likelihood that a given Pao_2 will result in clinically apparent cyanosis: anemia (less likely), polycythemia (more likely), reduced systemic perfusion or cardiac output (more likely), and hypothermia (more likely). Cyanosis is generally a sign of significant hypoxia. In a patient with adequate perfusion and a normal hemoglobin, central cyanosis is commonly noted when the Pao_2 is about 50 mm Hg.

122. **What are the causes of a reduced Pao_2 associated with an increased $A\text{-}aDo_2$ (alveolar-arterial oxygen tension difference or A-a gradient)?**
   - **Right-to-left shunting:** Intracardiac, abnormal arteriovenous connections; intrapulmonary shunts that result from perfusion of airless alveoli (e.g., pneumonia, atelectasis), often referred to as ventilation-perfusion mismatching
   - **Maldistribution of ventilation:** Asthma, bronchiolitis, atelectasis, and so forth
   - **Impaired diffusion:** An uncommon mechanism because many of the conditions previously thought to have a "diffusion block" (e.g., respiratory distress syndrome) also have a major component of shunting; may be seen when interstitial edema affects the septal walls (e.g., in early pulmonary edema and interstitial pneumonia)
   - **Decreased central venous oxygen content:** As a result of a sluggish circulation (e.g., shock) or increased tissue oxygen demands (e.g., sepsis)

123. **How does the pulse oximeter work?**
The key principle behind pulse oximetry is that oxygenated hemoglobin allows for more transmission of certain wavelengths of red light than does reduced hemoglobin. By contrast, transmission of infrared light is unaffected by the amount of oxyhemoglobin present. A light source of red and infrared wavelengths is applied to an area of the body thin enough that the light can traverse a pulsating capillary bed and be detected by a light detector on the other side. Each pulsation increases the distance the light has to travel, which increases the amount of light absorption. A microprocessor derives the arterial oxygen saturation by comparing absorbencies at baseline and during the peak of a transmitted pulse.

Sinha I, Magell SJ, Halfhide C: Pulse oximetry in children, *Arch Dis Child Educ Pract Ed* 99:117–118, 2014.

124. **What are the disadvantages or limitations of pulse oximetry?**
   - Patient movement disturbs measurements.
   - Poor perfusion states affect accuracy.
   - Fluorescent or high-intensity light can interfere with results.
   - It is unreliable if abnormal hemoglobin is present (e.g., methemoglobin).
   - It is unable to detect hypoxia until the Pao_2 decreases below 80 mm Hg.
   - Accuracy diminishes with arterial saturations below 70% to 80%.

125. **In infants with unilateral lung disease, should the good lung be up or down?**
The good lung should be **up**. This is another example of why children are not simply small adults. It is well established that adults with unilateral lung disease treated in a decubitus position will have an

increase in oxygen saturation when the good lung is placed down; this occurs because of an increase in ventilation to the dependent lung. Studies have shown that the opposite occurs in infants and children because ventilation is preferentially distributed toward the uppermost lung. This positional redistribution of ventilation appears to change to an adult pattern during the late teenage years.

Davies H, Helms P, Gordon I: Effect of posture on regional ventilation in children, *Pediatr Pulmonol* 12:227–232, 1992.

Acknowledgment

The editors gratefully acknowledge contributions by Drs. Ellen R. Kaplan, Carlos R. Perez, William D. Hardie, Barbara A. Chini, and Cori L. Daines that were retained from the first three editions of *Pediatric Secrets*.

CHAPTER 17

RHEUMATOLOGY

Carlos D. Rosé, MD, CIP, Elizabeth Candell Chalom, MD and Andrew H. Eichenfield, MD

CLINICAL ISSUES

1. What is an ANA?

   Antinuclear antibody (ANA) is made up of circulating γ-globulins directed against several known and unknown nuclear proteins. Unfortunately, the classic immunofluorescence technique is being replaced by a still nonvalidated enzyme-linked immunosorbent assay (ELISA) technique in order to save costs. When it is measured by an immunofluorescent technique, it is also called *fluorescent antinuclear antibody* (FANA). It is expressed as a titer, usually with a cutoff of 1:40. It is positive in 97% of patients with systemic lupus erythematosus (SLE), usually at a titer at or above 1:320, and in 60% to 80% of patients with juvenile idiopathic arthritis (JIA), usually at a lower titer. It is also positive in 10% to 30% of normal children, and because of that should not be used as a screening test when the child does not present objective physical findings of arthritis.

2. What is an ANA profile?

   Out of the many nuclear antigens that can make the FANA test positive, there are some with clinical value in pediatrics. They are grouped under the so-called ANA profile. These are individual antibodies measured by ELISA (commercial laboratories) or Western blot (specialized laboratories).

3. Should I order a profile instead of an ANA because it has more specificity?

   No. This test has value only in the right clinical context (see later) and when there is a documented positive ANA by immunofluorescence.

4. What is the significance of the various antibodies included in the ANA profile?

   - *Anti–double-stranded DNA:* Associated with SLE. This test has to be ordered separately; it is not usually part of the profile.
   - *Antihistone:* Associated with drug-induced lupus
   - *Anti-Ro* (also called anti-SS A): Associated with Sjögren syndrome and neonatal lupus
   - *Anti-La* (also called anti-SS B): Associated with Sjögren syndrome and neonatal lupus

5. A 6-year-old girl with a 2-month history of joint pain (onset after a viral illness) has a normal physical examination, complete blood cell count, and erythrocyte sedimentation rate (ESR), but a positive ANA titer of 1:160. What are some of the possible explanations for this positive ANA?

   - Laboratory variation
   - Nonspecific response to viral illness
   - Preclinical state of SLE (least likely)
   - Normal population frequency (about 8% at that titer)
   - Other autoimmune or paraneoplastic conditions

   Tan EM, Feltkamp TE, Smolen JS, et al: Range of antinuclear antibodies in "healthy" individuals, *Arthritis Rheum* 40:1601–1611, 1997.

6. Is Raynaud phenomenon a disease?

   In 1874, Maurice Raynaud, while still a medical student, described a triad of episodic pallor, cyanosis, and erythema after exposure to cold stress; the term *Raynaud phenomenon* describes this clinical triad. When this phenomenon is associated with a disease such as scleroderma or lupus, it is called *Raynaud syndrome*; when the phenomenon is seen as an isolated condition without any other rheumatic disorder, it is called *Raynaud disease*, although some patients on long-term follow-up may develop an associated disease (e.g., CREST syndrome [a limited form of systemic sclerosis]). Rheumatologists are commonly consulted for adolescents with blue dusky hands and feet. If there is no pallor, it is probably acrocyanosis (Crocq disease), a benign variant of no clinical relevance. It may occur in association with weight loss in athletes or children treated with amphetamine derivatives for attention-deficit/hyperactivity disorder.

Nigrovic PA, Fuhlbrigge RC, Sundel RP: Raynaud's phenomenon in children: a retrospective review of 123 patients, *Pediatrics* 111:715–721, 2003.

7. When is a child considered to have hypermobile joints?

The presence of three of the following features suggests true hypermobility:

- Apposition of the thumb to the flexor aspect of the forearm (Fig. 17-1)
- Hyperextension of the fingers so that they lie parallel to the dorsum of the forearm
- Hyperextension at the elbow of >10 degrees
- Knee hyperextension of >10 degrees
- Ability to touch the floor with the heel and also with the palms of the hands from a standing position without flexing the knee

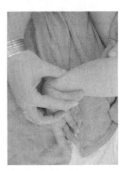

Figure 17-1. Abnormal contact between the thumb and forearm in a young girl with benign hypermobility joint syndrome.

8. Which children can demonstrate a Gorlin sign?

Gorlin sign is the ability to touch the tip of the nose with the tongue. It is seen in conditions associated with hypermobility syndromes, such as Ehlers-Danlos syndrome.

9. In what settings can reactive arthritis occur?

Reactive arthritis in its broadest sense refers to a pattern of arthritis associated with a nonarticular (remote) infection. By definition, it is an inflammatory arthritis, but a live organism cannot be isolated by culture of synovial fluid or synovial biopsy. A restricted definition of the syndrome includes arthritis after enteric (e.g., *Salmonella, Shigella, Yersinia, Campylobacter, Giardia*) or genitourinary infections (e.g., *Chlamydia*).

Morris D, Inman RD: Reactive arthritis: developments and challenges in diagnosis and treatment, *Curr Rheumatol Rep* 14:390–394, 2012.

10. What conditions are associated with gastrointestinal symptoms and arthritis?

Noninfectious

- Ulcerative colitis
- Crohn disease
- Behçet disease
- Henoch-Schönlein purpura
- Celiac disease

Infectious

- Salmonella
- Shigella
- Yersinia
- Campylobacter
- Tuberculosis
- Giardiasis

11. **One week after mild trauma, an 8-year-old girl has pain and tenderness in the right foot and leg, both of which are cold, exquisitely tender to the touch, with mottled discoloration. What is the likely diagnosis?**

    Complex regional pain syndrome, type 1. More commonly called *reflex sympathetic dystrophy*, or reflex neurovascular dystrophy, this poorly understood entity is often confused with arthritis because of localized severe pain in one of the extremities. However, several features separate it from arthritis. The pain is not confined to a single joint; it is regional in nature, involving portions of an extremity; and it often follows minor trauma (+/− immobilization or walking aid use). The pain is very severe, and even light touch causes pain (i.e., hyperesthesia). Several dysautonomic changes (e.g., mottling, color changes, sweating) may occur but not always. Laboratory findings are normal. Imaging techniques or nerve conduction studies are not needed unless the diagnosis is in question. Regional osteopenia as a result of disuse may develop in very severe cases.

    Because the role of the sympathetic nervous system is unclear and dystrophy may not occur in all cases, the terminology change has been revised by the International Association for the Study of Pain. In type 1, all of the features of the complex are present without definable nerve injury. In type 2, a definable nerve injury is present.

Rajapakse D, Liossi C, Howard RF: Presentation and management of chronic pain, *Arch Dis Child* 5:474–480, 2014.
Merskey H, Bogduk N, editors: *Classification of Chronic Pain*. IASP Press, 2002, Seattle, pp 41–43.

12. **How is complex regional pain syndrome managed?**

    Although many children are casted because of suspected hairline fractures, immobilization is contraindicated. Treatment is aimed at providing pain relief using analgesics and other nonmedical modalities. It is important that families be given a good explanation of the mechanism of pain and assurance that this condition is controllable. A physical therapy program should be started immediately, with emphasis on passive and active range of motion exercises and the maintenance of function and pain desensitization. Aquatic therapy is particularly useful in these children to initiate therapy. Desensitization of the painful area using one of several modalities (e.g., biofeedback, transcutaneous electrical nerve stimulation, visualization, acupuncture) can be part of the program. A positive attitude on the part of physicians and therapists is essential.

Katholi BR, Daghstani SS, Banez GA, et al: Noninvasive treatments for pediatric complex regional pain syndrome: a focused review, *PM&R* 6(10): 926–933, 2014.
Lee BH, Scharff L, Sethna NF, et al: Physical therapy and cognitive-behavioral treatment for complex regional pain syndromes, *J Pediatr* 141:135–140, 2002.

13. **Do children develop fibromyalgia?**

    Children as young as 9 years of age have been diagnosed with this syndrome. *Fibromyalgia* is a condition that is characterized by musculoskeletal aches and pains, fatigue, variable disturbed sleep patterns, and tenderness over various parts of the body. These tender points are useful for the diagnosis (Fig. 17-2). There should be tenderness over at least 4 of these 11 points for proper classification of individuals. In addition, there should be no tenderness over nonspecific sites such as the forehead or the pretibial region.

    Aches and pains are extremely common in children and may be the result of serious medical diseases (e.g., leukemia), mental illness (e.g., depression), and psychosocial stress. Differentiation of chronic musculoskeletal pain of nonorganic origin may be difficult in children and adolescents.

Criteria for diagnosis of fibromyalgia (American College of Rheumatology)

1. History of widespread pain
Pain is considered widespread when it occurs on both sides of the body above and below the waist. Axial skeletal pain must be present.

2. Pain in 11 of 18 bilateral tender point sites on digital palpation (using about 4 kg of pressure).

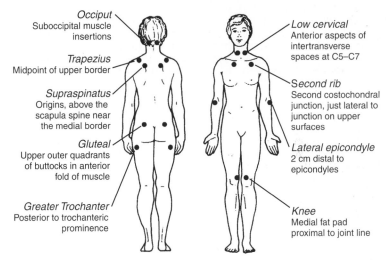

Occiput
Suboccipital muscle insertions

Trapezius
Midpoint of upper border

Supraspinatus
Origins, above the scapula spine near the medial border

Gluteal
Upper outer quadrants of buttocks in anterior fold of muscle

Greater Trochanter
Posterior to trochanteric prominence

Low cervical
Anterior aspects of intertransverse spaces at C5–C7

Second rib
Second costochondral junction, just lateral to junction on upper surfaces

Lateral epicondyle
2 cm distal to epicondyles

Knee
Medial fat pad proximal to joint line

Figure 17-2. American College of Rheumatology criteria for the diagnosis of fibromyalgia. *(From Ballinger S, Bowyer S: Fibromyalgia: the latest "great" imitator, Contemp Pediatr 14:147, 1997.)*

DERMATOMYOSITIS AND POLYMYOSITIS

14. **What are the criteria used for the diagnosis of juvenile dermatomyositis and polymyositis?**
    - Symmetric proximal muscle weakness (e.g., Gowers sign)
    - Elevated serum enzymes in muscle (creatine kinase [CK], lactic dehydrogenase [LDH], aspartate transaminase [AST], and/or aldolase)
    - Abnormal electromyogram (increased insertional activity, myopathic pattern, polymorphic potentials)
    - Inflammation and/or necrosis on muscle biopsy
    - Characteristic skin eruption
    The presence of rash distinguishes dermatomyositis from polymyositis. Three out of four criteria plus a pathognomonic rash establish the diagnosis of dermatomyositis, and a confirmatory biopsy is not necessary. If fewer criteria are met, a biopsy may be needed for diagnosis.

Huber A, Feldman BM: An update on inflammatory myositis in children, *Curr Opin Rheumatol* 25:630–635, 2013.

15. **What skin changes are pathognomonic for dermatomyositis?**
    Gottron patches (Fig. 17-3). These begin as inflammatory papules over the dorsal aspect of interphalangeal joints and the extensor aspect of the elbows and knee joints. The papules become violaceous and flat topped and may coalesce to become patches. Eventually, the lesions show atrophic changes and become hypopigmented.

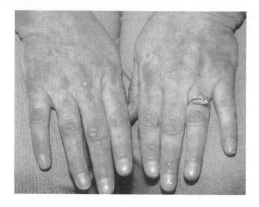

Figure 17-3. Gottron papules. *(From Fitzpatrick JE, Aeling JL: Dermatology Secrets, ed 2. Philadelphia, 2001, Hanley & Belfus, p 257.)*

16. **What are the other classic cutaneous findings of dermatomyositis among children?**
    - Periorbital edema and erythema with violaceous color of the upper eyelid (heliotrope rash)
    - Rash over the upper chest in the shawl distribution
    - Photosensitivity
    - Cutaneous vasculitis with ulceration
    - Nail-fold capillary abnormalities

17. **Which infectious agents are known to cause myositis?**
    - **Viral:** Notably Coxsackie (named after Coxsackie, NY) and influenza A and B
    - **Bacterial:** *Staphylococcus* and *Yersinia* (causing pyomyositis)
    - **Protozoal:** *Toxoplasma* and trichinosis
    - **Spirochetal:** *Borrelia*

    The most common cause of acute muscle disease associated with pain, difficulty walking, and a high level of creatine kinase is *viral myositis.*

JUVENILE IDIOPATHIC ARTHRITIS

18. **Why is JRA becoming juvenile idiopathic arthritis (JIA)?**
    The Europeans and Canadians have never liked the term "rheumatoid" embedded in J**R**A, which has been used in the United States since 1977, because it suggests homology with the adult disease (rheumatoid arthritis). In the same year of 1977 in the city of Basel, European investigators coined the term JCA, which included pretty much all forms of primary childhood arthritis. The International League of Associations of Rheumatology (ILAR) ended the transatlantic dispute and has come up with the new name— JIA (juvenile **idiopathic** arthritis). At least there is some consistency because the "J" and the "A" remain unchanged. "J" stands for *juvenile* (before the seventeenth birthday for disease onset), and "A" for *arthritis*, meaning joint inflammation. The new classification went through multiple revisions and is still a work in progress. The potential advantages are (1) an end to the confusion and (2) the hopeful beginning of a solution by at least recognizing that we do not know what causes the disease (it may pay to be humble).

19. **What is synovitis, and at what point is it considered chronic?**
    Synovial inflammation (synovitis) is the primary pathologic lesion in JIA. It is chronic at 6 weeks in the United States and at 3 months in Europe.

20. **What is the most common chronic arthritis seen in children?**
    JIA, with a point prevalence of about 1:1000.

21. **What are the diagnostic criteria for the classification of JIA?**
    JIA is a *diagnosis of exclusion.* Features include the following:
    - Onset at ≤16 years of age
    - Clinical arthritis with joint swelling or effusion, increased heat, and limitation of range of motion with tenderness
    - Duration of disease of ≥6 weeks

22. What are the characteristics of the seven main subsets of JIA?

The seven major subgroups are distinguished by the number of joints, presence of rheumatoid factor, and different combination of extra-articular manifestations (Table 17-1).

Table 17-1. Subsets of Juvenile Idiopathic Arthritis

SUBSET	NO. OF JOINTS	AGE	UVEITIS	RF	ANA	HLA-B27	RE-MISSION	OTHER SYMPTOMS
Systemic	Any	0-16 mo	—	—	—	—	50%	Fever, visceromegaly, serositis, rash
Oligopersistent	1–4	2 yr	++++	—	++++	—	60%	None
Oligoextended*	>5	2 yr	++++	—	++++	—	20%	None
Polyarticular RF(−)	>5	3 yr	+++	—	+++	—	15%	Subcutaneous nodules (small)
Polyarticular RF(+)	>5	12–17 yr	None	+	++	—	0%	Subcutaneous nodules (large)
Enthesitis-related arthritis	Any number	8–16	Acute	—	—	+	Unknown	Tendinous involvement Enthesitis†
Psoriatic arthritis	Any number	Any	+	—	+/−		Low	Dactylitis, psoriasis of nails and skin, tendinous involvement
Other arthritis‡		N/A	N/A	N/A	N/A	N/A	N/A	N/A

ANA = Antinuclear antibody; HLA = human leukocyte antigen; RF = rheumatoid factor.
*After a typical oligoarticular onset with an oligoarticular course for 6 months, the new joints become recruited.
†Inflammation at the insertion point of tendons, capsule, and ligaments.
‡Any form of chronic arthritis that fails to meet criteria for any of the other subsets.

23. What percent of pediatric JIA presents as systemic JIA?

Five percent to 15% of JIA presents as systemic in North America and Europe. In Asia, however, systemic JIA appears to account for a greater percentage of JIA cases with 25% in India and 50% in Japan.

24. What is the pattern of fever and characteristic rash of the systemic-onset subset of JIA?

Systemic-onset JIA (Still disease) accounts for about 15% of cases of children with JIA. Affected individuals typically have fever of unknown origin with once- or twice-daily (i.e., quotidian) temperature spikes, often higher than 40 °C. Shaking chills often precede the fever. The temperature characteristically returns to 37 °C or lower; continuous fever should suggest other diagnoses.

A blotchy, light pink, evanescent rash that blanches on compression and that may show perimacular pallor accompanies the fever in more than 90% of cases (Fig. 17-4). The rash of systemic JIA is diagnostic

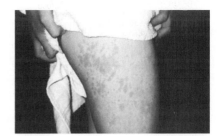

Figure 17-4. Typical rash of systemic-onset juvenile rheumatoid arthritis. *(From West S:* Rheumatology Secrets, *ed 2. Philadelphia, 2002, Hanley & Belfus, p 493.)*

only after the diagnosis is made (by exclusion). Arthritis may not be present during the first several weeks of illness. Serositis, hepatosplenomegaly, and lymphadenopathy are other significant findings in patients with this form of the disease.

Prakken B, Albani S, Martini A: Juvenile idiopathic arthritis, *Lancet* 377:2138–2149, 2011.

25. **In addition to different clinical features, how is systemic JIA distinguished from other subgroups of JIA?**
    - Equal sex distribution (other subgroups more commonly occur in females)
    - Rarely familial
    - Lack of autoantibodies (e.g., rheumatoid factor, ANA) and autoreactive T-cells
    - Lack of HLA associations
    - Greater responsiveness to interleukin-1 and interleukin-6 inhibition
    - Autoinflammatory, rather than autoimmune, disease (See question 101.)

Prakken B, Albani S, Martini A: Juvenile idiopathic arthritis, *Lancet* 377:2138–2149, 2011.

26. **Why is it sometimes difficult to distinguish systemic JIA (sJIA) from leukemia?**
    Up to 20% of patients with acute lymphoblastic leukemia (ALL) have some degree of musculoskeletal symptoms, including joint pain and occasional swelling that can mimic sJIA. In both diseases, there is anemia, fever, and weight loss. Both can involve hepatosplenomegaly and lymphadenopathy. In ALL, however, the fever is not usually spiking, and platelets and white blood cell counts tend to be low to low normal. In ALL, compared with sJIA, pain occurs more commonly at nighttime. A good examination of a peripheral smear is crucial. A high lactic dehydrogenase level is very suggestive of leukemia, and the technetium-99 bone scan shows a different pattern of uptake. More than one bone marrow biopsy may be necessary.

Marwaha RK, Kulkarni KP, Bansal D, Trehan A: Acute lymphoblastic leukemia masquerading as juvenile rheumatoid arthritis: diagnostic pitfall and association with survival, *Ann Hematol* 89:249–254, 2010.
Jones OY, Spencer CH, Bowyer SL, et al: A multicenter case-control study on predictive factors distinguishing childhood leukemia from juvenile rheumatoid arthritis, *Pediatrics* 117:e840–e844, 2006.

27. **In a patient with suspected rheumatic disease, what clinical features are more suggestive of malignancy?**
    Particularly concerning are **nonarticular bone pain**, **back pain** as the principal symptomatic feature, **bone tenderness**, and **severe constitutional symptoms**. Children with rheumatic joint problems are typically stiff, and they may complain about pain. The pain of malignancy is out of proportion to the amount of swelling around the joint, and it tends to be worse at night. It is vital to think about the possibility of malignancy in children with rheumatic complaints.

Cabral DA, Tucker LB: Malignancies in children who initially present with rheumatic complaints, *J Pediatr* 134: 53–57, 1999.

28. **What is the value of measuring ANA and rheumatoid factor (RF) in patients with JIA?**
    After JIA has been diagnosed on clinical grounds, results of these tests help assign the patient to the appropriate category (e.g., oligoarticular or RF-positive polyarticular). These tests are also useful as prognostic indicators. Because ANA can be present in 10% to 30% of normal children, this test should not be used as a screening test to diagnose JIA in children who experience noninflammatory pain. The presence of ANA increases the risk for uveitis, thereby making ophthalmologic surveillance more important. RF is valuable as a marker of poor functional prognosis in adolescents with polyarticular arthritis.

29. **Are radiographs helpful for diagnosing JIA?**
    No. There are no characteristic radiographic changes at onset. The value of radiology is to rule out other skeletal conditions and to provide a documented baseline status.

30. **A patient with JIA who becomes ill with thrombocytopenia, profound anemia, and markedly elevated transaminases probably has what complication?**
   Macrophage activation syndrome (MAS). This new conceptualization of an old problem is seen in children with systemic-onset JIA both at onset (even at presentation) and late during the course of disease. It is characterized by a massive upregulation of T-cell and macrophage function, with vast release of proinflammatory cytokines leading to *hemophagocytosis* (the hallmark). It is believed that, in most cases, MAS is triggered by a viral infection. MAS is the single most important contributor of mortality, together with gastrointestinal bleeding and infection among patients with systemic JIA. The name and nosologic classification of this entity are currently being debated by experts in the field.

Bennett TD, Fluchel M, Hersh AO, et al: Macrophage activation syndrome in children with systemic lupus erythematosus and children with juvenile idiopathic arthritis, *Arthritis Rheum* 64:4135–4142, 2012.

31. **What are the main features of the macrophage activation syndrome?**
   - Worsening of fever and rash
   - Anemia, frequently severe (due in part to hemophagocytosis), leukopenia, and thrombocytopenia
   - Disseminated intravascular coagulation with hypofibrinogenemia and pseudonormalization of ESR
   - Liver dysfunction
   - Hypertriglyceridemia
   - Hyponatremia (pseudo)
   - Massive increase in ferritin levels
   - Occasional central nervous system involvement
   - Generalized musculoskeletal pain

Ramanan AV, Schneider R: Macrophage activation syndrome—what's in a name! *J Rheum* 30:2513–2516, 2003.

KEY POINTS: JUVENILE IDIOPATHIC ARTHRITIS

1. Sine qua non: Persistence for ≥ 6 weeks
2. Seven subtypes differentiated by number of involved joints, presence of rheumatoid factor, and extra-articular involvement
3. Characteristic finding: Morning stiffness or soreness that improves during the day
4. No laboratory tests are diagnostic.
5. Patients <7 years old with antinuclear antibody–positive oligoarticular juvenile idiopathic arthritis at highest risk for uveitis

32. **What is the traditional first-line approach to JIA medical management?**
   The so-called first-line therapy consists of **nonsteroidal anti-inflammatory drugs (NSAIDs).** Given at the correct dose, they exert pain relief and suppress inflammation (decrease in morning stiffness), with a peak action at 4 to 6 weeks. The classic members of this group are aspirin, ibuprofen, naproxen, tolmetin, and indomethacin. Choice among them is made on the basis of availability in liquid form, half-life, side-effect profile, individual doctor preferences, and results of an individual trial. Most of their action is through inhibition of cyclooxygenase. About one-third of patients have their symptoms controlled through the use of NSAIDs; two-thirds require more aggressive drug therapy. For patients with oligoarticular disease, intra-articular injection of corticosteroids is also considered first-line therapy.

33. **What second-line agents have been used in the treatment of JIA?**
   - Gold salts
   - Penicillamine
   - Hydroxychloroquine
   - Sulfasalazine
   - Methotrexate

Of these, only methotrexate has been proved beneficial in a randomized, double-blind, placebo-controlled trial.

Giannini EH, Brewer EJ, Kuzmina N, et al.: Methotrexate in resistant juvenile rheumatoid arthritis: results of the USA-USSR double blind placebo controlled trial, *N Engl J Med* 326:1043–10499, 1992.

34. When are corticosteroids indicated for children with JIA?
    - Life-threatening disease (e.g., pericarditis, myocarditis)
    - Unremitting fever not responsive to NSAIDs
    - Unrelenting polyarthritis with severe limitations requiring intensive physical therapy to achieve ambulatory status
    - Topical therapy for uveitis (systemic steroids are rarely needed for children with aggressive uveitis unresponsive to topical therapy)
    - As intra-articular injections to treat unresponsive joints or single joint disease in the context of intolerance to or lack of efficacy of NSAIDs. Triamcinolone hexacetonide is the drug of choice.

35. What are the most common side effects of prolonged corticosteroid therapy?
    Effects can be minimized by alternate-day therapy, but sometimes the treatment is worse than the disease. Commonly encountered problems associated with high-dose corticosteroid use in children can be remembered using the mnemonic **CUSHINGOID MAP**:
    - **C**ataracts
    - **U**lcers
    - **S**triae
    - **H**ypertension
    - **I**nfectious complications
    - **N**ecrosis of bone (avascular)
    - **G**rowth retardation
    - **O**steoporosis
    - **I**ncreased intracranial pressure (pseudotumor cerebri)
    - **D**iabetes mellitus
    - **M**yopathy
    - **A**dipose tissue hypertrophy (obesity, "buffalo hump")
    - **P**ancreatitis

36. What are biologic agents?
    These are genetically engineered products that act by blocking specific immune pathways, such as cytokine signaling, to lessen inflammation. Etanercept, the first biologic agent used in the treatment of JIA, blocks the actions of tumor necrosis factor-α, a proinflammatory cytokine. A growing variety of other agents are used, including adalimumab, another antibody to tumor necrosis factor, and abatacept, which is a costimulation blocker that acts by blocking receptors on antigen-presenting cells. Newer biologics have been developed to control up-regulated IL-1 (anakinra, rilonacept and canakinumab) and IL-6 (tocilizumab). Canakinumab is approved for the treatment of systemic-onset JIA and tocilizumab for both systemic and polyarticular JIA. Biologic agents have become important therapeutic options for patients with JIA resistant to or intolerant of conventional treatments.

Sen ES, Ramanan AV: New age of biological therapies in paediatric rheumatology, *Arch Dis Child* 99:679–685, 2014.

37. Which children with JIA require the most frequent monitoring for uveitis?
    Uveitis (also called *iridocyclitis*) is inflammation of the iris and the ciliary body. It occurs on average in 20% of patients with **pauciarticular JRA** and in 5% of patients with **polyarticular disease**. Table 17-2 summarizes the American Academy of Pediatrics guidelines for frequency of slit-lamp examination developed by the sections of ophthalmology and rheumatology. Patients at high risk require quarterly examinations; those at moderate risk need biannual examinations; and those at low risk can be examined annually.

Qian Y, Acharya NR: Juvenile arthritis-associated uveitis, *Curr Opin Ophthalmol* 21:468–472, 2010.

Table 17-2. Frequency of Ophthalmologic Examination in Patients with JIA

TYPE	ANTINUCLEAR ANTIBODIES	AGE AT ONSET	DURATION OF DISEASE (YEARS)	RISK CATEGORY	EYE EXAMINATION FREQUENCY (MONTHS)
Oligo- or polyarthritis	+	≤6	≤4	High	3
	+	≤6	>4	Moderate	6
	+	≤6	>7	Low	12
	+	>6	≤4	Moderate	6
	+	>6	>4	Low	12
	−	≤6	≤4	Moderate	6
	−	≤6	>4	Low	12
	−	>6	N/A	Low	12
Systemic disease (fever, rash)	N/A	N/A	N/A	Low	12

JIA = juvenile idiopathic arthritis.
Frequency of Ophthalmologic Examination in Patients with JIA.
(Data from Cassidy J, Kivlin J, Lindsley C, Nocton J: Ophthalmologic examinations in children with juvenile rheumatoid arthritis. Pediatrics 117:1843-1845, 2006.)

38. **What is the earliest sign of uveitis among patients with JIA?**
When the anterior chamber of the eye is examined with a slit lamp, a "**flare**" is the earliest sign. This is a hazy appearance as a result of an increased concentration of protein and inflammatory cells. Later signs can include a speckled appearance of the posterior cornea (as a result of keratic precipitates), an irregular or poorly reactive pupil (as a result of synechiae between the iris and lens), band keratopathy, and cataracts (Fig. 17-5).

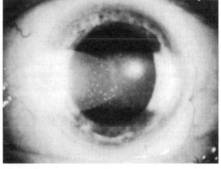

Figure 17-5. Uveitis. A slit-lamp examination shows "flare" in the fluid of the anterior chamber (caused by increased protein content) and keratic precipitates on the posterior surface of the cornea, representing small collections of inflammatory cells. *(From Cassidy JT, Laxer RM, Petty RE, Lindsley CB, editors: Textbook of Pediatric Rheumatology, ed 6. Philadelphia, 2011, Saunders, pp 305–314.)*

39. **What are the juvenile spondyloarthropathies under the revised classification system?**
The spondyloarthropathies are now considered one of the subsets of JIA and are recognized under the heading enthesitis-related arthritis (ERA).

40. **What are the characteristic clinical features of the juvenile spondyloarthropathies?**
    - Affect males >8 years of age
    - Enthesitis (inflammation of tendon, capsule, and ligament insertion sites) is characteristic
    - Prodromal oligoarthritis involving large joints of the lower extremities including the hip
    - Involvement of the sacroiliac joints and the back, which is manifested as pain, stiffness, and reduced range of motion (Fig. 17-6)
    - Associated with human leukocyte antigen (HLA-B27) (≤90% in children with ankylosing spondylitis and 60% of those with other spondyloarthropathies)
    - Seronegativity: ANA and rheumatoid factors typically negative

Ramanathan A, Srinivasalu H, Colbert RA: Update on juvenile spondyloarthritis, *Rheum Dis Clin North Am* 39:767–788, 2013.

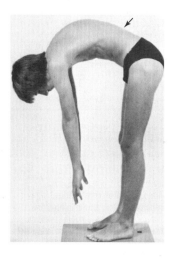

Figure 17-6. Fifteen-year-old boy shown in the position of maximal forward flexion. Note the flattened back *(arrow)*. Radiographs demonstrated bilateral sacroiliac arthritis but no abnormality of the lumbosacral spine. *(From Casssidy JT, Laxer RM, Petty RE, Lindsley CB, editors:* Textbook of Pediatric Rheumatology, *ed 6. Philadelphia, 2011, Saunders, pp 272–286.)*

41. **How is enthesitis diagnosed clinically?**
    The *enthesis* is the site of attachment of ligaments, tendons, capsule, and fascia to bone. Enthesopathy is unique to the spondyloarthropathies and appears as painful localized tenderness at the tibial tubercle (which may be mistaken for Osgood-Schlatter disease), the peripheral patella, and the calcaneal insertion of the Achilles tendon and plantar fascia (which may be mistaken for Sever disease). Thickening of the Achilles tendon and tenderness of the metatarsophalangeal joints are associated findings. Magnetic resonance imaging (MRI) can be extremely helpful. The T2-weighted image may show bone marrow edema adjacent to the enthesis.

42. **Why is the diagnosis of ankylosing spondylitis difficult to make in children?**
    A child may have undifferentiated spondyloarthritis (an enthesitis-related arthritis) that is characterized by enthesitis and recurrent episodes of lower-extremity oligoarthritis for several years before he or she develops back symptoms. To fulfill the criteria for ankylosing spondylitis, clinical features of lumbar spine pain, limitation of lumbar motion, and radiographic signs of sacroiliitis must be present. The average time from onset of symptoms to diagnosis in an adult with ankylosing spondylitis is 5 years; many adolescents are adults before they fulfill the criteria (Fig. 17-7). MRI (STIR [short T1 inversion recovery] or T2W [T2-weighted]) is very helpful to document early sacroiliitis. For sacroiliitis, no gadolinium is necessary.

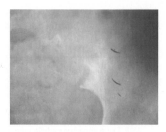

Figure 17-7. Periarticular sclerosis in a boy with chronic sacroiliitis and a diagnosis of spondyloarthropathy.

43. **Where are the dimples of Venus?**
The dimples of Venus are used to define a baseline for the Schober test. The dimples are prominent paravertebral indentations in the lower back of some individuals. A line drawn between the dimples marks the lumbosacral junction and this is the point from which one measures 10 cm above for an upper limit and 5 cm below for the lower limit to assess anterior flexion of the lumbosacral spine. After the patient bends over without flexing the knees one takes a second measurement of the distance. The change in length between the upper and the lower point should be now >5 cm from the baseline measurement.

LYME DISEASE

44. **What criteria are used to diagnose Lyme disease?**
Classification criteria (i.e., case definition) as determined by the Centers for Disease Control and Prevention include the following:
- Erythema migrans: enlarging circular erythematous lesion (minimum size, 5 cm), *or*
- At least one clinical manifestation (arthritis, cranial neuropathy, atrioventricular block, aseptic meningitis, radiculoneuritis) and isolation or serologic evidence of *Borrelia burgdorferi* infection

45. **What is the typical rash seen in Lyme disease?**
The classic rash of **erythema migrans (EM)**, believed to be pathognomonic for Lyme disease, is an expanding erythematous skin lesion (round or oval; ≥5 cm) that begins as a small macule or papule at the bite site. As the lesion expands over days to weeks, central or paracentral clearing gives the lesion an annular or targetlike appearance (Fig. 17-8). However, EM is not always classic. About 60% of cases have homogenous erythema, 30% with central erythema, 9% with central clearing, 7% with central vesicles or ulcerations, and 2% with central purpura.

Dandache P, Nadelman RB: Erythema migrans, *Infect Dis Clin North Am* 22:235–260, 2008.

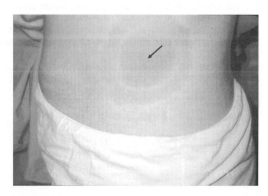

Figure 17-8. Erythema migrans (EM) with punctum *(arrow). (From Dandache P, Nadelman RB: Erythema migrans,* Infect Dis Clin North Am *22:237, 2008.)*

46. How long after a tick bite does the rash of Lyme disease appear?
Median time is **7 to 10 days**, but the rash can appear with a range of 1 to 36 days.

47. How is Lyme disease confirmed in the laboratory?
Although attempts to demonstrate borrelial DNA in infected tissues by polymerase chain reaction has met with some success and cultures occasionally render positive results, the main diagnostic tool continues to be serology. Immunoglobulin M (IgM) peaks about 4 weeks after infection, and IgG peaks at 6 weeks. This is the main reason why antibodies may not be detected during the early dermatologic and neurologic stages.

There are two detection techniques: ELISA and Western blot. Both are available for IgG and IgM. ELISA measures whole components of *Borrelia*. It is a very sensitive test, but with many false-positive results. A negative ELISA requires no further investigation at a given time. All positive ELISAs—particularly those with borderline positivity—should be confirmed by Western blot. This is the so-called two-tier system. The C6 peptide ELISA measures IgG to a relatively invariant lipoprotein on the spirochete, and as a single test, has been shown to be as sensitive and almost as specific as the two-tier system.

Steere AC, McHugh G, Damle N, et al: Prospective study of serologic tests for Lyme disease, *Clin Infect Dis* 47:188–195, 2008.

48. If infection ensues after a tick bite, how does Lyme disease progress?
- **Early localized disease:** 2 to 30 days. Sixty percent to 80% of children will develop EM. Some may have a flulike illness with fever, myalgia, headache, fatigue, arthralgia and malaise.
- **Early disseminated disease:** 3 to 12 weeks. Clinical manifestations reflect hematogenous spread to other sites; these include secondary EM (multiple lesions), cranial nerve palsies (primarily facial nerve), and aseptic meningitis. Much more rarely seen in children (compared with adults) are radiculoneuritis and carditis (with varying degrees of heart block).
- **Late disease:** 2 to 12 months. In children, the most common manifestation is arthritis. Rarely, encephalomyelitis can develop. There is controversy regarding chronic Lyme disease.

Shapiro ED: Lyme disease, *N Engl J Med* 370:1724–1731, 2014.
Feder HM Jr, Johnson BJB, O'Connell S, et al: A critical appraisal of "chronic Lyme disease." *N Engl J Med* 357:1422–1430, 2007.

49. How is the diagnosis of Lyme meningitis established?
The diagnosis is often inexact and is commonly made on the basis of the finding of cerebrospinal fluid pleocytosis and the presence of EM and/or positive serology. Both ELISA and Western blot testing may be negative or indeterminate early during the course of infection, when dissemination to the central nervous system has occurred. Testing of the cerebrospinal fluid for intrathecal production of specific antibody and demonstration of *B. burgdorferi* DNA by polymerase chain reaction testing is not readily available, and the latter is relatively insensitive.

50. How are Lyme disease and viral meningitis clinically differentiated?
Both are predominantly summertime illnesses, but the distinction is critical because Lyme meningitis requires weeks of intravenous antibiotics. In addition to the possible presence of EM, other areas of clinical distinction in patients with signs and symptoms of meningitis include the following:
- Cranial neuropathy, especially peripheral seventh-nerve palsy, is strongly suggestive of Lyme meningitis.
- Papilledema is more commonly seen in patients with Lyme meningitis.
- Longer duration (7 to 12 days versus 1 to 2 days) of symptoms, including headache before lumbar puncture, is more typical of Lyme meningitis.
- Rash of EM
- Cerebrospinal fluid pleocytosis should not have more than 10% neutrophils in Lyme meningitis
  Either the rash of EM, papilledema, or a cranial nerve palsy is seen in more than 90% of patients with Lyme meningitis but in almost none with viral meningitis.

Avery RA, Frank G, Glutting, Eppes SC: Prediction of Lyme meningitis in children from a Lyme disease-endemic region: a logistic-regression model using history, physical, and laboratory findings, *Pediatrics* 117:e1–e7, 2006.
Shah SS, Zaoutis TE, Turnquist JL, et al: Early differentiation of Lyme from enteroviral meningitis, *Pediatr Infect Dis J* 24:542–545, 2005.

51. Should lumbar punctures be done for patients with facial palsy and suspected Lyme disease?

This remains debated because studies in the late 1990s revealed "occult meningitis" (i.e., cerebrospinal fluid [CSF] pleocytosis) in patients without meningeal signs but with Lyme facial palsy. However, the clinical significance of an abnormal CSF is unclear, and there has been no apparent increase in late-stage Lyme disease in those treated with oral antibiotics alone. Consequently, most experts advise no lumbar puncture for suspected or confirmed Lyme facial palsy, unless there is severe or prolonged headache, nuchal rigidity, or other meningeal signs.

52. How is Lyme arthritis differentiated from septic arthritis?

The inflammation generated by Lyme arthritis is significantly less intense than septic arthritis. Lyme arthritis typically involves a single large joint (knee $\geq$90%), range of motion is less limited than septic arthritis, and weight bearing is sometimes possible. On joint aspiration, septic arthritis more typically shows >100,000 cells/mL^3. Septic arthritis is more commonly associated with an elevated peripheral white blood cell count and elevated sedimentation rate.

Deanehan JK, Kimia AA, Tan Tanny SP, et al: Distinguishing Lyme from septic knee monoarthritis in Lyme disease-endemic areas, *Pediatrics* 131:e695–e701, 2013.

53. What is the prognosis for children diagnosed with Lyme arthritis?

Multiple studies have shown that the long-term prognosis for treated patients is excellent, with little morbidity. Clinicians should be aware that persistent synovitis after the completion of a single course of 4 weeks of antibiotics is not rare and not the result of antibiotic failure. In fact, up to two-thirds of patients with Lyme arthritis require 3 months to achieve resolution, and 15% have symptoms of their arthritis for more than 12 months.

Smith BG, Cruz AI Jr, Milewski MD, Shapiro ED: Lyme disease and the orthopaedic implications of Lyme arthritis, *J Am Acad Orthop Surg* 19:91–100, 2011.
Gerber MA, Zemel LS, Shapiro ED: Lyme arthritis in children: clinical epidemiology and long-term outcome, *Pediatrics* 102:905–908, 1998.

54. What should be suspected if a patient with Lyme disease develops fever and chills after starting antibiotic treatment?

The **Jarisch-Herxheimer reaction.** This reaction consists of fever, chills, arthralgia, myalgia, and vasodilation, and it follows the initiation of antibiotic therapy in certain illnesses (most typically syphilis). It is thought to be mediated by endotoxin release as the organism is destroyed. A similar reaction occurs in 40% or less of patients treated for Lyme disease, and it may be mistaken for an allergic reaction to the antibiotic.

55. Should we follow Lyme disease course and response to therapy with titers?

No! As a result of the continued secretion of antibodies by memory cells, serology (particularly with ultrasensitive commercial kits) may remain positive for up to 10 years after microbial eradication. The misinterpretation of positive serology as a proxy for active infection is responsible for many unnecessary antibiotic courses in endemic areas.

Kalish RA, McHugh G, Granquist J, et al: Persistence of immunoglobulin M or immunoglobulin G antibody responses after active Lyme disease, *Clin Infect Dis* 33:780–785, 2001.

56. Is antibiotic prophylaxis indicated for all tick bites?

No. In most regions, the rate of tick infestation is low, and thus the likelihood of transmission is also low. Even in endemic areas, the risk for Lyme disease to a placebo group after tick bites was only 1.2%. The tick has to be attached for at least 24 to 48 hours before the transmission of infection occurs. Treating all tick bites with antibiotics is impractical (some children would be on oral antibiotics throughout the summer). One study did show that a single 200-mg dose was effective for preventing Lyme disease if it was given within 72 hours of the tick bite. Consequently, antibiotic prophylaxis is not routinely recommended, but, in unique circumstances (e.g., endemic areas, prolonged attachment, pregnancy), prophylaxis could be considered.

Nadelman RB, Nowakowski J, Fish D, et al, Tick Bite Study Group: Prophylaxis with single-dose doxycycline for the prevention of Lyme disease after an *Ixodes scapularis* tick bite, *N Engl J Med* 345:79–84, 2001.
Shapiro ED, Gerber MA, Holabird NB, et al: A controlled trial of antimicrobial prophylaxis for Lyme disease after deer-tick bites, *N Engl J Med* 327:1769–1773, 1992.

57. **What are other means of preventing Lyme disease?**
    - Avoidance of tick-infested areas
    - Use of light-colored, long-sleeved clothing, with pants tucked into sneakers
    - Insect repellents (N,N-diethyl-meta-toluamide [DEET]; permethrin)
    - "Tick checks" after potential exposures
    - Proper tick removal: Pulling straight out, with tweezers close to skin

---

Hayes EB, Piesman J: How can we prevent Lyme disease? *N Engl J Med* 348:2424–2430, 2003.

KEY POINTS: LYME DISEASE

1. Spirochete *Borrelia burgdorferi* is the culprit.
2. Only one-third of patients recall the tick bite.
3. The erythema migrans rash is virtually diagnostic.
4. Enzyme-linked immunosorbent assay testing has a high false-positive rate; confirm with Western blot analysis.
5. Potential complications include arthritis, aseptic meningitis, and cranial nerve palsies, and atrioventricular block.
6. Lyme meningitis (compared with viral meningitis): Cranial neuropathy and papilledema are more common, with longer duration of symptoms before diagnosis.

RHEUMATIC FEVER

58. **What is acute rheumatic fever?**
    Rheumatic fever is a postinfectious, immune-mediated, inflammatory reaction that affects the connective tissue of multiple organ systems (heart, joints, central nervous system, blood vessels, subcutaneous tissue) and that follows infection with certain strains of group A β-hemolytic streptococci (GABHS). The major manifestations are carditis, polyarthritis, chorea, erythema marginatum, and subcutaneous nodules. In the developing world, acute rheumatic fever and rheumatic heart diseases are the leading causes of cardiovascular death during the first 5 decades of life.

59. **What are the major Jones criteria for rheumatic fever?**
    The mnemonic **J ♥ NES** may be useful:
    - **J**oints: Migratory arthritis
    - **♥**: Heart disease
    - **N**odules: Subcutaneous nodules
    - **E**rythema: Erythema marginatum
    - **S**ydenham: Sydenham chorea

60. **What is acceptable proof of antecedent streptococcal pharyngitis when diagnosing acute rheumatic fever?**
    - **Throat culture:** This is the gold standard for diagnosis of GABHS. Positive cultures, however, do not distinguish GABHS pharyngitis from a carrier state.
    - **Streptococcal antigen tests:** Rapid diagnostic tests for the detection of GABHS antigens in pharyngeal secretions are acceptable evidence of infection because they are highly specific. Again, positive tests do not distinguish true infection from a carrier state.
    - **Antistreptococcal antibodies:** At the time of clinical presentation with rheumatic fever, throat cultures are usually negative. It is reasonable to assess the levels of antistreptococcal antibodies in all cases of suspected rheumatic fever because the antibodies should be elevated at the time of presentation.

Gerber MA, Baltimore RS, Eaton CB, et al: Prevention of rheumatic fever and diagnosis of acute streptococcal pharyngitis, *Circulation* 119:1541–1551, 2009.

---

61. **Which antistreptococcal antibodies are most commonly measured?**
    The most commonly employed test measures antibodies to **anti-streptolysin O**. The cutoff for a positive test in a school-age child is 320 Todd units (240 in an adult); levels peak 3 to 6 weeks

after infection. If the test is negative—as may be the case in 20% or less of patients with acute rheumatic fever (ARF) and in 40% of those with isolated chorea—other antistreptococcal antibodies may be detected. The most practically available of these identifies antibodies to **deoxyribonuclease B** (positive cutoff, 240 units in children, 120 in adults). Alternatively, subsequent convalescent samples run simultaneously with the acute sample may detect rising titers of either antistreptolysin O or antideoxyribonuclease B.

62. **What are the common manifestations of carditis in patients with ARF?**
In his *Etudes Médicales du Rhumatisme*, Lasègue remarked that "rheumatic fever licks the joints . . . and bites the heart," meaning that the severity of the two manifestations tends to be inversely related. In more recent outbreaks of ARF, 80% or less of patients have had evidence of carditis. ARF causes a pancarditis, which potentially affects all layers (from the pericardium through the endocardium) and may include the following:
- **Valvulitis:** This is heralded by a new or changing murmur. The most common manifestation is isolated mitral regurgitation, and this is followed in frequency by a mid-diastolic rumble of unclear pathophysiology (Carey-Coombs murmur), and then by aortic insufficiency in the presence of mitral regurgitation. Isolated aortic insufficiency is uncommon, and so are stenotic lesions.
- **Dysrhythmias:** Electrocardiogram abnormalities typically involve some degree of heart block.
- **Myocarditis:** When mild, this may manifest as resting tachycardia out of proportion to fever. However, when it is clinically more severe and in combination with valvular damage, myocarditis may lead to congestive heart failure.
- **Pericarditis:** Patients may have chest pain or friction rub. Pericarditis and myocarditis virtually never occur in isolation.

Messeloff CR: Historical aspects of rheumatism, *Med Life* 37:3–56, 1930.

63. **How quickly can valvular lesions occur in children with ARF?**
New murmurs appear within the first 2 weeks in 80% of patients, and they rarely occur after the second month of illness. Hence, during an episode, one normal echocardiogram in the first 2 weeks should be sufficient to eliminate carditis.

64. **What are the typical characteristics of arthritis in patients with ARF?**
Migratory polyarthritis is usually the earliest symptom of the disease, and it typically affects the large joints, the knees, the ankles, the elbows, and the wrists (hips are not commonly involved). The joints are extraordinarily painful; weight bearing may not be possible. Physical examination discloses warmth, erythema, and exquisite tenderness such that the weight of even bedclothes and sheets may not be tolerable. This tenderness is typically out of proportion with the degree of swelling.

65. **What is the effect of aspirin therapy on the arthritis of rheumatic fever?**
This type of arthritis is exquisitely sensitive to even modest doses of salicylates, which effectively arrest the process within 12 to 24 hours. If aspirin or other NSAIDs are employed early during the course of the condition, the arthritis will not migrate, and a delay in diagnosis may result. Such medications should be withheld until the clinical course of the illness has become clear. Conversely, if there is not a dramatic response to aspirin, a diagnosis other than rheumatic fever should be considered.

66. **What is the rash of rheumatic fever?**
Erythema marginatum. This rash occurs in less than 5% of cases of ARF. If you see it and call a colleague to the bedside to confirm it, it is likely to have disappeared in the meantime. It is an evanescent, pink to slightly red, non-pruritic eruption with pale centers and serpiginous borders; it may be induced by the application of heat, and it always blanches when palpated. The outer edges of the lesion are sharp, whereas the inner borders are diffuse (Fig. 17-9). It is most often found on the trunk and proximal extremities (but not the face). Erythema marginatum is seen almost solely in patients with carditis.

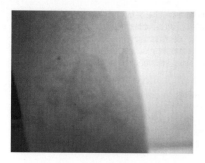

Figure 17-9. Classic rash of erythema marginatum on the arm of a child with acute rheumatic fever.

67. **What is Sydenham chorea?**

Purposeless, involuntary, irregular movements of the extremities that are associated with muscle weakness and labile emotional behavior. These symptoms are believed to result from inflammation of the cerebellum and of the basal ganglia.

Wei F, Wang J: Sydenham's chorea or St. Vitus's dance, *N Engl J Med* 369:e25, 2013.

68. **Who was Saint Vitus?**

Saint Vitus was a Sicilian youth who was martyred in the year 303 at the age of 14. In the Middle Ages, individuals with chorea would worship at shrines dedicated to this saint. Accordingly, Sydenham chorea is also known as "Saint Vitus dance." Saint Vitus is the patron saint of dancers and comedians. And chorea, by the way, means dance in Greek! St. Vitus was one of the 14 Holy Helpers. He was invoked to help people with epilepsy, nervous disorders, and Sydenham's chorea although at the time of Vitus, there was no Sydenham. Thomas Sydenham (the "British Hippocrates") was born in 1624.

69. **Are corticosteroids of benefit for the treatment of ARF?**

Controlled studies in the 1950s failed to show any definite benefit of corticosteroids for the treatment of rheumatic carditis. Nonetheless, it is generally recommended that patients with severe carditis (e.g., congestive heart failure, cardiomegaly, third-degree heart block) receive prednisone (2 mg/kg/day) in addition to conventional therapy for their heart failure. The unusual patient with well-documented rheumatic arthritis that does not respond to salicylates or NSAIDs will benefit symptomatically from prednisone.

70. **Can antibiotic prophylaxis for rheumatic fever ever be discontinued?**

The optimal duration of antistreptococcal prophylaxis after documented ARF is the subject of some debate. It is clear that the risk for recurrence decreases after 5 years have elapsed from the most recent attack. Most clinicians therefore recommend discontinuing prophylaxis in patients who have not had carditis after 5 years or on the twenty-first birthday (whichever comes later). Those at high risk for contracting streptococcal pharyngitis (e.g., school teachers, health care professionals, military recruits, others living in crowded conditions) and anyone with a history of carditis should receive antibiotic prophylaxis for longer periods. Recommendations vary, ranging from 10 years to the fortieth birthday (whichever is longer) to lifelong prophylaxis, depending on the extent of residual heart disease.

71. **Where do PANDAS live in the world of pediatric rheumatology?**

In 1989, Swedo and colleagues characterized the psychiatric abnormalities found in children with Sydenham chorea, noting a high prevalence of obsessive-compulsive disorder (OCD) behaviors. They also described a syndrome, which they dubbed **PANDAS** (**p**ediatric **a**utoimmune **n**europsychiatric **d**isorders **a**ssociated with **s**treptococcal infection), in which OCD and Tourette syndrome in some children appeared to be triggered or exacerbated by streptococcal infections in the absence of classic chorea or other manifestations of rheumatic fever. PANDAS has been expanded into **PANS** (pediatric acute-onset neuropsychiatric syndrome), which theorizes a wider possibility of antecedent triggers for acute OCD symptoms.

    The existence of PANDAS (and PANS) remains controversial. There has been no prospective study of group A streptococcal infection to confirm the association of streptococcal pharyngitis with these behavioral abnormalities. The symptoms of tic disorders and OCD tend to fluctuate spontaneously and may be nonspecifically exacerbated by illness. In some cases, the only link to streptococcal infection has been a single throat culture or serologic test, thereby bringing the specificity of the condition into question. PANDAS (the syndrome) currently remains an unproven hypothesis, PANDA the mammal (*Ailuropoda melanoleuca*) can be found both in central China and in zoos around the world.

Murphy TK, Gerardi DM, Leckman JF: Pediatric acute-onset neuropsychiatric syndrome, *Psychiatr Clin North Am* 37:353–374, 2014.
Swedo SE, Rapaport JL, Cheslow DL, et al: High prevalence of obsessive-compulsive symptoms in patients with Sydenham chorea, *Am J Psychiatry* 146:246–249, 1989.

SYSTEMIC LUPUS ERYTHEMATOSUS

72. What is systemic lupus erythematosus (SLE)?

SLE is a multisystem autoimmune disorder characterized by the production of autoantibodies and a wide variety of clinical and laboratory manifestations.

Lupus Foundation of America: www.lupus.org. Accessed Jan. 13, 2015.

73. What laboratory tests should be ordered in a child who is suspected of having SLE?

A useful study for SLE is the **ANA** test. Up to 97% of patients with SLE have positive ANAs at some point during their illness. In a patient with characteristic signs and symptoms, a positive ANA may help confirm suspicions of SLE. Unfortunately, however, around 10% of the normal childhood population may also have a positive ANA. Therefore, a positive ANA in the absence of any objective findings of SLE means very little. Other autoantibodies are much more specific, but they are less sensitive for SLE. These include antibodies to double-stranded DNA and the extractable nuclear antigen Sm. Complement levels are often depressed in patients with active SLE, and sedimentation rates are often elevated. The combination of a positive anti–double-stranded DNA antibody level and a low C_3 level is nearly 100% specific for SLE. Anemia, leukopenia, lymphopenia, and/or thrombocytopenia may also be seen.

Levy DM, Kamphuis S: Systemic lupus erythematosus in children and adolescents, *Pediatr Clin North Am* 59:345–364, 2012.
Tsokos GC: Systemic lupus erythematosus, *N Engl J Med* 365:2110–2121, 2011.

KEY POINTS: SYSTEMIC LUPUS ERYTHEMATOSUS

1. The hallmark of systemic lupus erythematosus (SLE) is the presence of autoantibodies at intermediate to high titers.
2. About 15% to 20% of SLE patients have the onset of disease during childhood.
3. Clinical presentations vary, but the most common presenting symptoms are arthritis, rash, and renal disease.
4. Neonatal SLE is caused by maternal autoantibodies; this leads to complete congenital heart block.
5. The presence of antiphospholipid antibodies predisposes the patient to venous thrombosis.

74. What are the most common manifestations of SLE in children?

- Arthritis: 80% to 90%
- Rash or fever: 70%
- Renal disease, such as proteinuria or casts (every patient with SLE is likely to have some abnormality demonstrated on renal biopsy): 70%
- Serositis: 50%
- Hypertension: 50%

- Central nervous system disease (psychosis/seizures): 20% to 40%
- Anemia, leukopenia, thrombocytopenia: 30% each

Iqbal S, Sher MR, Good RA, Cawkwell GD: Diversity in presenting manifestations of systemic lupus erythematosus in children, *J Pediatr* 135:500–505, 1999.

75. **What are the neurologic manifestations of SLE?**
    Lupus cerebritis is a term that implies an inflammatory etiology of central nervous system disease. Microscopically, however, widely scattered areas of microinfarction and noninflammatory vasculopathy are seen in brain tissue; actual central nervous system vasculitis is rarely observed. A lumbar puncture may reveal cerebrospinal fluid pleocytosis or an increased protein concentration, but it can be normal as well. Neuropsychiatric manifestations (e.g., psychoses, behavioral changes, depression, emotional lability) or seizures are most commonly observed. An organic brain syndrome with progressive disorientation and intellectual deterioration can be seen. Cranial or peripheral motor or sensory neuropathies, chorea, transverse myelitis, and cerebellar ataxia are less common manifestations of central nervous system lupus. Severe headaches and cerebral ischemic events have also been seen.

Steinlein MI, Blaser SI, Gilday DI, et al: Neurological manifestations of pediatric systemic lupus erythematosus, *Pediatr Neurol* 13:191–197, 1995.

76. **Which diseases should be considered in the differential diagnosis of children with a butterfly rash?**
    A malar rash is present in 50% of children with SLE. The typical butterfly rash involves the malar areas and crosses the nasal bridge, but it spares the nasolabial folds; occasionally, it is difficult to distinguish from the rash of dermatomyositis. See Fig. 17-10. (Erythematous papules on the extensor surfaces of the metacarpophalangeal and proximal interphalangeal joints are common in dermatomyositis, but these are not generally seen in patients with SLE.) Seborrheic dermatitis or a contact dermatitis may be similar to the rash of SLE. Vesiculation should suggest another disease, such as pemphigus erythematosus. A malar flush is clinically distinct and may be seen in children with mitral stenosis or hypothyroidism.

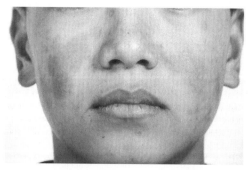

Figure 17-10. Malar rash of a 14-year-old patient with SLE. The distribution of this typical "butterfly" or malar rash includes the cheeks and crosses the nasal bridge but spares the nasolabial folds. *(From Firestein GS, editor:* Kelley's Textbook of Rheumatology, *ed 9. Philadelphia, 2013, Saunders, pp 1771–1800.)*

77. **Should children with SLE undergo a renal biopsy?**
    This is an area of controversy because nearly all children with SLE will have some evidence of renal involvement. Usually, clinical disease (e.g., abnormal urine sediment, proteinuria, renal function changes) correlates with the severity of renal disease on biopsy, but this is not always the case. Extensive glomerular abnormalities can be found on biopsy with minimal concurrent clinical manifestations.

For this reason, many authorities are aggressive with early biopsy. Three circumstances in particular warrant biopsy:

- A child with SLE and nephrotic syndrome—to distinguish membranous glomerulonephritis from diffuse proliferative glomerulonephritis (which would warrant more aggressive therapy)
- Failure of high-dose corticosteroids to reverse deteriorating renal function—to determine the likelihood of benefit from cytotoxic therapy
- A prerequisite to entry into clinical therapeutic trials

Silverman E, Eddy A: Systemic lupus erythematosus. In Cassidy JT, Petty RE, Laxer R, Lindsley C, editors: *Textbook of Pediatric Rheumatology*, ed 6, Philadelphia, 2011, WB Saunders, pp 315–343.

78. **How can the result of renal biopsy affect treatment of SLE?**
    Biopsy can reveal a spectrum of renal pathology, ranging from a normal kidney (rare) to mesangial nephritis or glomerulonephritis (focal or diffuse, proliferative or membranous). Histologic transformation from one group to another over time is not unusual. Treatment of lupus nephritis is based on the severity of the lesion. Mesangial disease may require little or no intervention. Patients with membranous nephropathy commonly have nephrotic syndrome and usually respond to prednisone. Focal proliferative glomerulonephritis is often controlled with corticosteroids alone, but diffuse proliferative glomerulonephritis often requires corticosteroids, intravenous pulse cyclophosphamide, and possibly other immunosuppressives. Among the latter group is mycophenolate mofetil and rituximab (a monoclonal antibody that depletes B cells). Because of the detrimental effects on fertility observed with cyclophosphamide, many investigators feel that mycophenolate should be used instead of cyclophosphamide (including children with diffuse proliferative glomerulonephritis).

79. **When should high-dose corticosteroid therapy be considered for SLE management?**
    High-dose corticosteroids usually consist of either intravenous pulse methylprednisolone (30 mg/kg per dose with a maximal dose of 1 g given daily or on alternate days given as an intravenous bolus for up to 3 doses) or oral prednisone (1 to 2 mg/kg/day). Often, intravenous pulses are then followed by high-dose oral steroids. The main indications for high-dose steroids in cases of SLE are as follows:
    - Lupus crisis (widespread acute multisystem vasculitic involvement)
    - Worsening central nervous system disease (as long as steroid psychosis is not thought to be the etiology)
    - Severe lupus nephritis
    - Acute hemolytic anemia
    - Acute pleuropulmonary disease

80. **What is the association of antiphospholipid antibodies and lupus?**
    Antiphospholipid antibodies can cause recurrent arterial and/or venous thromboses (e.g., stroke, phlebitis, renal vein thrombosis, placental thrombosis leading to fetal demise). Antiphospholipid antibodies are usually detected as anticardiolipin antibodies or lupus anticoagulant. These antibodies are often seen in patients with SLE, but their prevalence among patients with pediatric lupus varies widely (30% to 87% for anticardiolipin antibodies and 6% to 65% for lupus anticoagulant), depending on the study cited. The pathogenesis of thrombosis in patients with antiphospholipid antibodies remains unclear.

Von Scheven E, Athreya BH, Rosé CD, et al: Clinical characteristics of antiphospholipid antibody syndrome in children, *J Pediatr* 129:339–345, 1996.

81. **Which laboratory tests are useful for monitoring the effectiveness of therapy in patients with SLE?**
    Serologic studies can provide useful information about the activity of SLE. The ANA titer does not correlate with disease activity. However, anti–double-stranded DNA titers (if present) often drop, and complement levels may increase and return to normal with effective therapy. Sedimentation rates usually decrease, and complete blood cell counts may return to normal (or at least improve) with effective therapy and decreased disease activity.

82. **What are the most common manifestations of neonatal lupus erythematosus?**

The syndrome of *neonatal lupus erythematosus* (NLE) was first described in babies born to mothers with SLE or Sjögren syndrome; however, it has now been found that 70% to 80% of mothers with these conditions are asymptomatic. NLE is most likely caused by the transmission of maternal IgG autoantibodies. The main manifestations are as follows:

- **Cutaneous:** Skin lesions are found in about 50% of babies with NLE. Although the rash may be present at birth, it usually develops within the first 2 to 3 months of life. The lesions include macules, papules, and annular plaques, and they may be precipitated by exposure to sunlight. The lesions are usually transient and nonscarring.
- **Cardiac:** Complete congenital heart block (CCHB) is the classic cardiac lesion of NLE; 90% of all CCHB is due to neonatal lupus. Most cases of CCHB appear after the neonatal period, and 40% to 100% of these patients eventually require a pacemaker, usually before they are 18 years old.
- **Hepatic:** Hepatic involvement is seen in at least 15% of babies with NLE. Hepatomegaly with or without splenomegaly is usually seen. Hepatic transaminases are either mild or moderately elevated, or they may be normal. Clinically and histologically, the appearance is often one of idiopathic neonatal giant cell hepatitis.
- **Hematologic:** Thrombocytopenia, hemolytic anemia, and/or neutropenia may be seen.

Izmirly PM, Rivera TL, Buyon JP: Neonatal lupus syndromes, *Rheum Dis Clin North Am* 33:267–285, 2007.

83. **What is the pathophysiology of the CCHB of NLE?**

CCHB is caused by **maternal autoantibodies** that cross the placenta and deposit themselves in the conducting system—usually the atrioventricular node—of the fetal heart. This leads to a localized inflammatory lesion, which may then be followed by scarring with fibrosis and calcification. The autoantibodies found are usually anti-Ro antibodies, but anti-La antibodies can also be the etiologic agents.

84. **What are the common features of drug-induced lupus?**

Fever, arthralgias and arthritis, and serositis can be seen in patients with drug-induced lupus. ANA and antihistone antibodies are often positive, but antibodies to double-stranded DNA are usually negative, and complement levels remain normal. Renal involvement, central nervous system disease, malar rash, alopecia, and oral ulcers are not usually seen in patients with drug-induced lupus, and their presence should raise suspicion for SLE.

85. **What are the most common causes of drug-induced lupus in children?**

Antiepileptic medications (especially ethosuximide, phenytoin, and primidone) are the most common causes, and at least 20% of children taking antiepileptic drugs will develop a positive ANA. Minocycline, hydralazine, isoniazid, α-methyldopa, and chlorpromazine are also associated with drug-induced lupus, as are a variety of antithyroid medications and β-blockers. Actually, all the tetracyclines have been associated with a peculiar lupuslike syndrome that includes the following:

- Acute symmetric polyarthritis
- Positive ANA
- Mild liver dysfunction

Perhaps the most common agent associated with lupus currently is chronic use of minocycline (and other tetracyclines) in association with the treatment of acne. Drug-induced lupus usually resolves within 2 weeks of discontinuation of the medication, but it may last longer (months). It is characterized by arthritis, lupus rash, and hepatitis (persistent "transaminitis"). Other autoantibodies in addition to ANA can be seen as well.

El-Hallak M, Giani T, Yeniay BS, et al: Chronic minocycline-induced autoimmunity in children, *J Pediatr* 153:314-319, 2008.

VASCULITIS

86. **What clinical features suggest a vasculitic syndrome?**
A multisystem disease with **fever, weight loss,** and **rash** is often the presenting picture of a vasculitic disorder, which is characterized by the presence of inflammation in a blood vessel wall. Many different types of rashes may be seen, the more common of which are palpable purpura, urticarial vasculitis, and dermal necrosis. Central nervous system involvement, arthritis, myositis, and/or serositis may be seen.

Blanco R, Martinez-Taboada VM, Rodriguez-Valverde V, Garcia-Fuentes M: Cutaneous vasculitis in children and adults: associated diseases and etiologic factors in 303 patients, *Medicine* 77:403–418, 1998.

87. **How are the primary systemic vasculitides classified?**
One scheme proposed by an international consensus (EULAR/PRES: European League against Rheumatism/Paediatric Rheumatology European Society) has classified vasculitides on the basis of the size of the vessels that are predominantly affected as well as "other vasculitides," which do not fit well into a vessel size category. In the list below, conditions *in italics* are common pediatric diseases. Conditions marked with an asterisk (*) are not uncommon in pediatric rheumatology centers.
Predominantly large vessel vasculitis
- Takayasu arteritis*
Predominantly medium-sized vessel vasculitis
- Kawasaki disease
- Polyarteritis nodosa and its limb-limited variant*
Predominantly small vessel vasculitis
- Microscopic polyangiitis*
- Granulomatosis with polyangiitis (formerly Wegener granulomatosis)*
- Eosinophilic granulomatosis with polyangiitis (formerly Churg-Strauss syndrome)*
- Leukocytoclastic vasculitides
- Immune complex mediated: *Henoch-Schönlein purpura, lupus vasculitis, serum-sickness vasculitis, drug-induced immune-complex vasculitis, infection-induced immune-complex vasculitis,* Sjögren syndrome vasculitis,* hypocomplementemic urticarial vasculitis*
Other vasculitides
- Behçet disease*
- Paraneoplastic small vessel vasculitis (mostly with acute myelocytic leukemia, acute lymphoblastic leukemia, or asparaginase treatment)*
- Inflammatory bowel disease vasculitis, particularly ulcerative colitis–associated stroke and polyarteritis nodosa–like syndrome associated with Crohn disease*

Ozen S, Ruberto N, Dillon MJ, et al: EULAR/PReS endorsed consensus criteria for the classification of childhood vasculitides, *Ann Rheum Dis* 65:936–941, 2006.

88. **What are the two most common pediatric vasculitides?**
Henoch-Schönlein purpura and **Kawasaki disease** are the two most common pediatric vasculitides.

89. **Which infectious agents are associated with vasculitis?**
- **Viral:** Human immunodeficiency virus, hepatitis B and C viruses, cytomegalovirus, Epstein-Barr virus, varicella virus, rubella virus, and parvovirus B19
- **Rickettsial:** Rocky Mountain spotted fever, typhus, rickettsialpox
- **Bacterial:** Meningococcus, disseminated sepsis as a result of any organism, subacute bacterial endocarditis
- **Spirochete:** Syphilis
- **Mycobacterial:** Tuberculosis

90. **What are the conditions that are grouped under the term** *pulmonary-renal syndromes*?
These are medical syndromes with alveolar hemorrhage plus glomerulonephritis, which can occur spontaneously or weeks to months apart, and are usually manifestations of autoimmune conditions. Serum autoantibody patterns are helpful in distinguishing the causes (e.g., Goodpasture syndrome is

typically positive for antiglomerular basement membrane antibodies). Symptoms can include dyspnea, fever, and hemoptysis in combination with signs of glomerulonephritis (e.g., edema, hematuria).
- Goodpasture syndrome
- Granulomatosis with polyangiitis (GPA, formerly Wegener granulomatosis)
- Eosinophilic granulomatosis with polyangiitis (EGP, formerly Churg-Strauss syndrome)
- SLE

91. **What is the clinical triad of Behçet disease?**
Aphthous stomatitis, genital ulcerations, and **uveitis.** Behçet disease is a vasculitis of unclear etiology. In two-thirds of cases in children, polyarthritis and inflammatory gastrointestinal lesions occur, which can confuse the diagnosis with inflammatory bowel disease, particularly if the patient is younger than 5 years. Aseptic meningitis, sinus vein thrombosis, and other forms of deep vein thrombosis are characteristic of this disease.

92. **Should it be "Henoch-Schönlein purpura" or "Schönlein-Henoch purpura"?**
In 1837, Johann Schönlein described the association of purpura and arthralgia. Edward Henoch later added the other clinical features including gastrointestinal in 1874 and renal in 1899. Thus, purists would say that, more properly, the term should be "Schönlein-Henoch purpura." However, in 1801, William Heberden described a 5-year-old boy with joint and abdominal pains, petechiae, hematochezia, and gross hematuria in his *Commentaries on the History and Cure of Disease*, so the true purists might say that, most properly, the condition should be "Heberden syndrome."

93. **What are the characteristic laboratory findings of patients with Henoch-Schönlein purpura (HSP)?**
Acute-phase reactants, including the ESR and C-reactive protein, are commonly elevated, and there is frequently a mild leukocytosis. Thrombocytopenia is never seen. Microscopic hematuria and proteinuria are indicators of renal involvement. HSP purpura appears to be an IgA-mediated illness; elevated serum IgA has been noted and has been demonstrated by immunofluorescence in skin and renal biopsies. (The renal histology is indistinguishable from Berger disease.) Circulating immune complexes and cryoglobulins containing IgA are also commonly seen.

94. **What kinds of skin lesions are noted in patients with HSP?**
HSP is one of the *hypersensitivity vasculitides* and, as such, is characterized by leukocytoclastic inflammation of arterioles, capillaries, and venules. Initially, **urticarial** lesions predominate, and they may itch or burn; these develop into pink **maculopapules** (Fig. 17-11). With damage to the

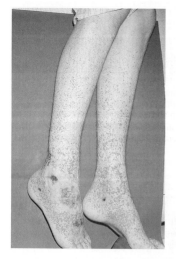

Figure 17-11. Numerous purpuric macules and papules on the legs and feet of a child with Henoch-Schönlein purpura. *(From Gawkrodger DJ: Dermatology: An Illustrated Colour Text, ed 3. Edinburgh, 2002, Churchill Livingstone, p 78.)*

vessel walls, there is bleeding into the skin, which results in nonthrombocytopenic **petechiae** and **palpable purpura**. A migrating soft tissue edema is also commonly seen in younger children.

95. **In addition to the skin, what other organ systems are typically involved in HSP?**
    Classically, HSP involves the musculoskeletal system, the gastrointestinal tract, and/or the kidneys.
    - The most common abdominal finding is gastrointestinal colic (70%). This is frequently associated with nausea, vomiting, and gastrointestinal bleeding. These findings may precede the skin rash in 30% of cases or less. Intussusception occurs in 5% of cases or less.
    - Renal involvement occurs in about 50% of reported cases, and it is usually apparent early during the course of the illness. It ranges in severity from microscopic hematuria to nephrotic syndrome.
    - Joint involvement is very common (80%) and can be quite painful. Periarticular swelling of the knees, ankles, wrists, and elbows—rather than a true arthritis—is usually seen.
    - Up to 15% of males can have scrotal involvement with epididymitis, orchitis, testicular torsion, and scrotal bleeding.
    - Pulmonary hemorrhage is a rare complication of HSP that is mainly seen among adolescents and adults. It is associated with significant mortality.

Trnka P: Henoch-Schönlein purpura in children, *J Paediatr Child Health* 49:995–1003, 2013.
Tizard EJ, Hamilton-Ayres MJJ: Henoch-Schönlein purpura, *Arch Dis Child Educ Pract Ed* 93:1–8, 2008.

96. **How often does chronic renal disease develop in children with HSP?**
    The long-term prognosis of patients with HSP depends mainly on the initial renal involvement. Overall, <5% of patients with HSP develop end-stage renal disease. However, up to two-thirds of children who have severe crescentic glomerulonephritis documented on biopsy will develop terminal renal failure within 1 year. Of those with nephritis or nephrotic syndrome at the onset of illness, almost half may have long-term problems with hypertension or impaired renal function as adults. Microscopic hematuria as the sole manifestation of HSP is common and is associated with a good long-term outcome.

Bogdanović R: Henoch-Schönlein purpura nephritis in children: risk factors, prevention and treatment, *Acta Paediatr* 12:1882–1889, 2009.
Coppo R, Andrulli S, Amore A, et al: Predictors of outcome in Henoch-Schönlein purpura in children and adults, *Am J Kidney Dis* 47:993–1003, 2006.

KEY POINTS: HENOCH-SCHÖNLEIN PURPURA

1. A small vessel vasculitis
2. The classic clinical triad is as follows: purpura, arthritis, and abdominal pain.
3. Half of patients have abnormal urinalyses (hematuria, proteinuria; usually mild).
4. Steroid therapy is debated, but it should be considered for painful arthritis, abdominal pain, nephritis, edema, and scrotal swelling.
5. A few patients have long-term renal complications.

97. **Why is the diagnosis of intussusception often difficult in patients with HSP?**
    - Intussusception can occur suddenly, without preceding abdominal symptoms.
    - Nearly half of cases of HSP intussusception are ileoileal (compared with non-HSP intussusceptions, of which 75% are ileocolic). This increases the likelihood of a false-negative barium enema.
    - The variety of possible gastrointestinal complications in patients with HSP (e.g., pancreatitis, cholecystitis, gastritis) can confuse the clinical picture.
    - The common occurrence (50% to 75%) of melena, guaiac-positive stools, and abdominal pain in HSP without intussusception may lead to a lowered index of suspicion.

98. **When are corticosteroids indicated for the treatment of HSP?**
    The precise indication for corticosteroids in patients with HSP remains controversial. Prednisone, 1 to 2 mg/kg/day (maximum: 80 mg/kg/day) for 5 to 7 days, is often used for severe intestinal symptoms and

may decrease the likelihood of intussusception. Corticosteroids may be helpful in the settings of significant pulmonary, scrotal, or central nervous system manifestations to minimize vasculitic inflammation; they are sometimes used if severe joint pain is present and NSAIDs are contraindicated. Steroids do not prevent the recurrence of symptoms, and symptoms may flare when steroids are discontinued. Controversy has arisen regarding the use of corticosteroids in all patients with HSP. Some epidemiologic studies have shown that the use of corticosteroids may shorten hospital course and prevent surgical complications. There is no controversy in the fact that corticosteroids make children with HSP feel a lot better rather quickly. However, the issue is whether to use a toxic medication for a disease that is benign most of the time. There is a great deal of controversy as well with regards to the early use of corticosteroids (oral or intravenous pulses) in patients with renal disease and their ability to improve long-term outcomes; no benefit has yet been demonstrated in randomized controlled trials.

Jauhola O, Ronkainen J, Koskimies O, et al: Outcome of Henoch-Schönlein purpura 8 years after treatment with a placebo or prednisone at disease onset, *Pediatr Nephrol* 27:933–939, 2012.
Weiss PF, Feinstein JA, Luan X, et al: Effects of corticosteroid on Henoch-Schönlein purpura: a systematic review, *Pediatrics* 120:1079–1087, 2007.

99. What is acute hemorrhagic edema of infancy (AHEI)?

A simplistic answer is that AHEI is an infantile version of HSP, appearing during the first year of life. Erythematous, palpable, large purpuric lesions develop and when confluent are quite dramatic in appearance. (The French call it the "rosette" and the English call it the "knot of ribbons.") Skin lesions are seen in the upper and lower extremities and on the face, particularly in the ears. IgA deposition is common around the vasculitic lesions. Renal and gastrointestinal involvements are rare, and recovery is the rule in 2 to 3 weeks. It is also known as *Finkelstein syndrome*.

McDougall CM, Ismail SK, Ormerod A: Acute haemorrhagic oedema of infancy, *Arch Dis Child* 90:316, 2005.

100. In which rheumatic diseases can "cauliflower ears" be seen?

In babies with AHEI and in older children with relapsing polychondritis—a potentially serious disease primarily affecting cartilage of the ears, airways, sclera, and aortic valve ring.

101. What is the difference between autoinflammatory and autoimmune diseases?

Autoinflammatory diseases are a group of conditions that involve deregulation of the inflammatory cascade in the absence of autoantibodies (such as ANA, RF, and ANCA). The autoinflammatory problem is believed to involve dysregulation of *innate immunity*. This is the branch of the immune system characterized by nonspecific immune defenses (e.g., neutrophils and monocytes). *Autoimmune diseases* result from problems with *adaptive (or acquired) immunity*, which refers to the more complex antigen-specific immune response (e.g., lymphocytes). Both conditions result in the immune system attacking the body's own tissues.

Autoinflammatory diseases are incompletely understood, but many are characterized by genetic mutations, which result in increased and frequent activation of inflammatory pathways. Inflammatory cytokines, such as interleukin-1β (IL-1β), interleukin-6 (IL-6), and tumor necrosis factor-α (TNF-α), are overproduced. Unlike autoimmune diseases, autoantibodies are not driving the inflammation. Autoinflammatory diseases are characterized by chronic and recurrent episodes of systemic and organ-specific inflammation with fever, particularly recurrent, as a prime symptom.

Hausmann JS, Dedeoglu F: Autoinflammatory diseases in children, *Dermatol Clin* 31:481–494, 2013.

102. Are all autoinflammatory diseases characterized by periodic fever and genetic mutations?

No, and this can make the diagnostic process difficult. More than 20 monogenetic auto-inflammatory diseases have been identified. These include familial Mediterranean fever, TNF-associated periodic fever syndrome (TRAPS), and hyperimmunoglobulin D syndrome (HIDS). However, PFAPA (periodic fever, aphthous stomatitis, pharyngitis, adenitis) syndrome, also known as Marshall syndrome, has no known genetic basis although it has many of the features of an auto-inflammatory disorder. In addition, Behçet syndrome (discussed previously) and systemic-onset JIA, both without a specific single gene mutation, are suspected to be autoinflammatory diseases.

Russo RAG, Brogan RA: Monogenic autoinflammatory diseases, *Rheumatology* 53:1927–1939, 2014.

INDEX

Note: Page numbers followed by *b* indicate boxes, *f* indicate figures and *t* indicate tables.